LECTURES

ON

HOMOEOPATHIC
MATERIA MEDICA

**TOGETHER WITH KENT'S *'NEW REMEDIES'*
INCORPORATED AND ARRANGED IN
ALPHABETICAL ORDER**

BY

JAMES TYLER KENT, A.M., M.D.

Late Professor of Materia Medica in Hering Medical College, Chicago.
Author of "Repertory of the Homoeopathic Materia Medica"
and "Lectures on Homoeopathic Philosophy"

INTRODUCTION BY

DR. JUGAL KISHORE, B.Sc., D.M.S. (Cal.)

Hony. Physician to the President of India. Author, 'Kishore Card
Repertory', and former Director, Nehru Homoeopathic
Medical College, New Delhi.

B. JAIN PUBLISHERS (P) LTD.

USA—Europe—India

LECTURES ON HOMOEOPATHIC MATERIA MEDICA

Second Rearranged Edition: 2009
43ith Impression: 2016

Note from the Publishers
Any information given in this book is not intended to be taken as a replacement for medical advice. Any person with a condition requiring medical attention should consult a qualified practitioner or therapist.

Published by Kuldeep Jain for
B. JAIN PUBLISHERS (P) LTD.
D-157, Sector-63, NOIDA-201307, U.P. (INDIA)
Tel.: +91-120-4933333 • Email: info@bjain.com
Website: www.bjain.com
Registered office: 1921/10, Chuna Mandi, Pahargani,
New Delhi-110 055 (India)

Printed at B. B. Press, Noida

ISBN: 978-81-319-0259-2

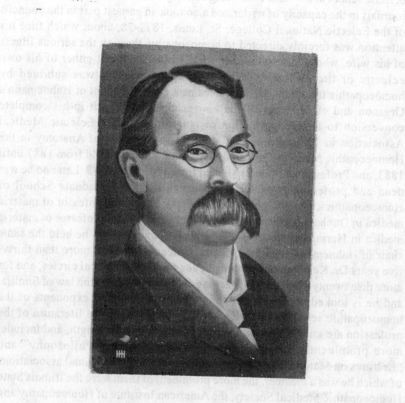

LIFE SKETCH OF DR. JAMES TYLER KENT

James Tyler Kent, A.M., Chicago, Illinois, Professor of Materia Medica in Hahnemann Medical College, Chicago physician and author of several valuable medical works, is a native of the town of Woodhull, Steuben county, New York, born in 1849, son of Stephen Kent and Caroline Tyler, his wife. His elementary and secondary education was acquired in Franklin Academy, Prattsburg, and his higher education in Madison (now Colgate) University, Hamilton, New York, where he came to his degree, Ph.D., in 1868; A. M., 1870. He was educated in medicine in the Eclectic Medical Institute, Cincinnati, Ohio, graduating there in 1871, and the Homoeopathic Medical College of Missouri, St. Louis, where he was awarded the diploma of that institution in 1889. Dr. Kent began his professional career in St. Louis as a physician of the eclectic school at the same time being actively connected with several eclectic journals in the capacity of writer and also took an earnest part in the councils of the Eclectic National College, St. Louis, 1877-78, about which time his attention was forcibly directed to homoeopathy, through the serious illness of his wife, whose case refused to yield to the treatment either of his own eclectic or the allopathic school practitioners, but was subdued by homoeopathic treatment. He then became a careful student of Hahnemann's Organon and other works of the new school, with result in his complete conversion to homoeopathy, his resignation from the Eclectic Medical Association in 1879 and his appointment to the chair of Anatomy in the Homoeopathic Medical College of Missouri, which he held from 1881 until 1883, and Professor of Materia Medica from 1883 until 1888. Later on he was dean and professor of Materia Medica in the Post-Graduate School of Homoeopathics, Philadelphia, Pennsylvania; dean and professor of materia medica in Dunham Medical College, Chicago; dean and professor of materia medica in Hering Medical College, Chicago; and in 1905 he held the same chair in Hahnemann Medical College, Chicago. Thus for more than thirty-five years Dr. Kent had been a conspicuous figure in medical circles, and for more than twenty-five years in teaching and practice under the law of Similia; and he is looked upon as one of the ablest teachers and exponents of the homoeopathic school in America. His contributions to the literature of the profession are known by their strength rather than their length, and include, more prominently, his "Repertory", "Homoeoapthic Philosophy" and "Lectures on Materia Medica". Among the various professional associations of which he was a member, the more prominent of them were the Illinois State Homoeopathic Medical Society, the American Institute of Homoeopathy and the International Hahnemannian Association, besides which he held a honorary corresponding membership in the British Homoeopathic Medical Society.

Kent died, on June 6, 1916 at Stevensville, Montana.

INTRODUCTION

I have been asked to write an introduction to this great monumental work on the Homoeopathic Materia Medica. A work like this which has stood the test of time and has been valued as a priceless treasure by the numerous students of homoeopathy all over the world needs no introduction.

The Homoeopathic Materia Medica is a very fascinating and yet an exasperating subject. Its simplicity, its vastness and its apparent similarity of symptoms in different drugs throw a tremendous challenge to the beginners. Kent said that there is no royal road to a perfect understanding of Materia Medica. It is at its worst a tedious drudgery. One can realise its vast extent by reading 138 printed pages on Sulphur in the Encyclopedia or 90 pages on Lachesis of Hering's Guiding Symptoms. It requires tremendous study, experience and insight to see some order in the maze of such a collection of symptoms.

Our Materia Medica is a record of actual occurrences, of events that really took place, of the results that were unquestionably produced upon healthy subjects.

Right from Hahnemann onwards, the records of provings prepared in schematic form were presented as Materia Medica. Before Kent, the best writers and teachers of materia medica were Hering, Dunham and Farrington. The materia medica was presented as a list of symptoms arranged according to Hahnemann's schema. It was obvious that it was not possible to memorise the symptoms. Kent held that materia medica can be learnt and not memorised. Of course it required a careful and diligent study. His emphasis was on the understanding of each remedy in its entirety and not on the memorising of unrelated symptoms.

In this direction Dr. Allen made an effort and tried to present remedies as distinctive individual entities so that a student could be saved from being lost in the maze of symptoms. It must be understood that the list of symptoms of a particular drug can never be exhausted. Human memory has a limited scope and even if one does remember all the symptoms, it is difficult to apply this knowledge for the relief of patient unless he knows the individual characteristics of a particular drug. All the same, the listing of symptoms has to be done as that is the ultimate charter of our applied materia medica.

Because of the complexity and uniqueness of Materia Medica, a large number of books were written on it. No other system of therapeutics possesses such a large number of books on materia medica. Each author tried to present the drugs as he understood them, according to his own experiences and his own genius. It was bound to happen. The facts are the same to the eye of every reader. But where one mind may see only confusion and a maze of unconnected words, another may discern order and light and the outline of a definite and consecutive chain of pathological processes, and consequently a clear indication for the use of drugs in treatment of the sick.

"The significance of a fact is measured by the capacity of the observer". Every teacher or student of Materia Medica sees the same facts in the drugs but in his evaluation and experience he emphasises certain aspects which may be completely ignored by another person. This is why the richness of our materia medica is increased by contributions from different authors.

Kent, like Hahnemann, was endowed with a keen analytical intellect coupled with a highly artistic temperament. His genius could see unity in diversity; an order and light in an apparent confusion of jumbled up symptoms. He was a strange mixture of an artist and a scientist. It is with a stroke of his rich imagination that he conceived a novel idea of presenting the drugs of our materia medica as individual pictures. In his lectures he was able to present well-defined but colourful pictures of each drug. This was a very bold and a great step forward in the development of our materia medica. Kent gave his lectures in a colloquial, semi-clinical form with the result that anybody who listened to his lectures was spell-bound and carried an indelible impression of the drug. He was able to create a continuity of a symptom-picture from all the disjointed symptoms listed in the other standard books.

So far the efforts at curing patients depended on one's ability in hunting through the mass of symptoms—the similar symptoms present in a particular case of sickness. The idea of evaluation of symptoms was still nebulous. Hahnemann had pointed out, as a guidance, the importance of rare, strange and peculiar symptoms. Kent was the first to see clearly how to present our materia medica to the beginners; how to lay down precise guidelines regarding the hierarchy of evaluations of different kinds of symptoms. One can see in his efforts at studying and teaching the materia medica a gradual progress and evaluation from one stage to a higher one. I am sure that thinking along these lines later on helped him in the making of his greatest work i.e. his Repertory. His comprehension of evaluation later on helped him to plan his Repertory. We can see in all his works a gradual progress and maturity. I can say that his Repertory came into being because of his being a serious and unusual student and teacher of Homoeopathic Materia Medica.

Many people have asked why it is that a number of symptoms present in his materia medica are not listed in his repertory. That is a very relevant question. Here one must understand the man, as Kent was. While making his repertory, he tabulated the rubrics and included the remedies as a true scientist— a person uninfluenced by his won prejudices or intuitive impressions. He rejected what was not known or proved definitely. Here he followed the great Hering. In his materia medica he could afford to give a little flight to his imagination and intuition. Here he could guide his students in placing together disjointed symptoms in one string by analogy based on his experiences. Here he was closer to Boenninghausen.

Every good teacher of Homoeopathic Materia Medica followed the great guide or source-material, the Hering's Guiding Symptoms. Kent was no exception. Farrington and Allen had done the same. The latter's characteristics are taken out of this great book and I say, very often haphazardly. Kent was able to see things deeper. Hence what he expressed and how he expressed had his own peculiar imprint enriched by experiences at the bed-side. Anybody who has gone through

Kent's lectures on Fluoric acid and Iodine and a few others will notice that in no other materia medica one can find such a beautiful picture. The symptoms that have been given there in that manner could not have been collected by anybody else. He was the one who could see a running red strand through all the symptoms and give us a living picture as if in flesh and blood.

Like me there are many people who could not have cured many difficult and chronic cases unless guided and inspired by his lectures. In the early days of my practice I cured a difficult case of Fluoric acid and I confirmed every word that Kent had written. No other book could guide me to this remedy. It appears, therefore, that Kent was endowed with an exceptional intuition and he could see what others did not. He could apply the existing knowledge of the drugs with uncanny foresight with the result that he gave more than he took, and our materia medica is richer by his experiences.

I can cite one small example of his special contribution. While studying Bromium I could hardly find any author mentioning it aggravated by being over-heated. Hering's Guiding Symptoms had mentioned this against a number of symptoms, and hence emphasised it in his materia medica. No one had done the same (neither Farrington nor Allen had mentioned it). This particular modality of Bromium was seen to be running through the entire picture. This symptom was incorporated in the repertory also giving it a second grade in evaluation. Yet, there are symptoms in the materia medica which could not find a place in the repertory as they did not stand the rigorous standards set out by Kent himself. That is why he refused to include Boger's additions in his repertory.

The publishers (Messrs B. Jain Publishers) of the present edition of Kent's Lectures have done a yeoman's service in publishing books on homoeopathy. In publishing the lectures they have included remedies from Kent's New Remedies. This is indeed a great advantage to the students as they find the remedies at one place and at much lesser cost. The greatest advantage however is that while many remedies in the New Remedies have been neglected as fewer people had access to them, now many more people will study them and apply them more effectively than has been the case in the past. Keeping the New Remedies in a hotch-potch of lesser writings, these

have been neglected and people have not paid proper attention
to them. However, I must sound a warning to all the serious
students. Many of the "New Remedies" are not proved at all.
Dr. Sherwood in the Preface to the New Remedies has
mentioned that Kent had published the provings in various
journals and the book is the result of his experiences. Let us
be honest to Kent's memory and admit that he never published
this book in his life-time. His friends and followers published
it. Very few of the remedies were thoroughly proved or
confirmed, whereas others were merely made up according to
a certain pattern. I stumbled upon this pattern while I was
making my additions to Kent's repertory for the preparation of
my Card Repertory. For example, the symptoms of remedies
like Aurum sulph., Barium sulph., Kali silicatum, Natrum
silicatum have been synthesised from Kent's repertory. If we
examine Aurum and Sulph in various rubrics in the Kent's
repertory and wherever these exist together in a particular
rubric, has been ascribed to the chemical compound Aur.
sulph. So the symptoms of the remedies like this are
compounded from their chemical components. Moreover, the
description of these symptoms as given is entirely different
from the description of drugs given by Kent elsewhere. (I think
Kent must have written down the symptoms from his repertory
as a sort of rough guiding indications for clinical
experimentation in the absence of proper provings or
pathogenetic symptoms of these apparently deep-acting
constitutional remedies. The publishers of Kent's New
Remedies might have considered them as proved remedies
and hence included them with other remedies. I hope the
readers will follow only what Kent himself intended to do and
not more than that). On the other hand there are some new
remedies like Cenchris which have been wonderfully well proved
by Kent and his associates and the symptom-picture given is
most dependable. Same is the case with Vespa vulgaris and
Wyethia. These remedies should be prescribed often enough.
The publishers are to be congratulated that they have
undertaken to bring all these remedies under one cover and
hence conferred a boon to the young students and scholars
alike.

One can only imagine the plight of homoeopathic students,
before books like Kent's Materia Medica appeared. The subject
which should have been most entertaining and out of sheer

necessity the most useful, remained a jumble of symptoms. Such an array of symptoms was more frightening than inspiring, with the result that they could scarcely make an effort to comprehend or unravel the beautiful mysteries of this branch of homoeopathic medicine. All the succeeding generations of homoeopaths cannot realise the immensity of the benefit conferred by the genius of Kent.

His method of narrating drugs is popularly known as 'Picture method'. His able and faithful student from Britain, Dr. Tyler, was another writer who gave us 'Drug Pictures' of homoeopathic medicines. It is no wonder that this book too has carved an important niche in our literature. Dr. Kent's lectures appeared first in his journal known as Journal of Homoeopathics as early as 1899. Later on they were collected together in a book form. Kent at that time was Professor of Materia Medica and Homoeopathics in the Philadelphia Post-Graduate School of Homoeopathics. The Journal of Homoeopathics was edited by Kent himself. It must be mentioned that before Kent embraced the homoeopathic system of medicine, he was an active worker, writer and speaker for the Eclectic National Medical Association. His earlier training stood him in good stead for giving his best talents to the homoeopathic literature. If we scan through early American literature, we find that Kent did not develop his method of teaching and writing materia medica all of a sudden. In his case too his methods developed slowly and gradually. For example, his description of drugs published earlier in the journals like Medical Advance is entirely different; the arrangement of the symptoms is more similar to other writers, although one gets glimpses of his future approach to the subject. He was a prolific contributor to the contemporary journals on the subject of materia medica and homoeopathic philosophy. One does wonder at the wide range of his genius. At one time he was a professor of anatomy. To jump from a subject like this to homoeopathic philosophy means a great elasticity and versatilitiy of his genius.

Although Kent's novel method of presenting materia medica was found to be very effective, he himself advised the students not to depend entirely on the drug pictures. They must go back to the larger textbooks giving the symptoms of the drugs.

More than that they must go to the repertories also for constant reference and comparative study. The materia medica and repertory go hand in hand and nobody can master either of the subjects without referring to the other. It has been found that great repertorians were also the masters of materia medica. Of course no repertory can be made or improved without constant study of our materia medicas. It is a hard and laborious study but the rewards are none the less as sweet.

The student can at least make an effort at emulating this great teacher. He was a thorough student. Whatever he undertook, he undertook with zeal and with all his heart and soul, with the result that whatever he produced, whatever he wrote, had the imprint of a genius.

Like Hering and some of the great men of homoeopathy, Kent was converted to homoeopathy in spite of himself. His first wife was seriously ill. No amount of eclectic and allopathic treatment helped her. She entreated her husband to seek medical advice and help from a known homoeopath in their neighbourhood. To satisfy her whim he called Dr. Phelan, the homoeopath. He watched him, with possibly contemptuous amusement, taking the case-history and later his giving her some globules to be dissolved in water and taken according to his directions until she fell asleep. Mrs. Kent had been suffering from sleeplessness for days and nothing had helped her the least in giving her some sleep. Kent chuckled within himself when Dr. Phelan mentioned about her getting sleep from the medicated water. He, however, fulfilled his part of the contract by giving her the first dose. The second dose to be given to her was delayed because Dr. Kent became absorbed in his books. When he remembered about the dose, he found her into such a natural and sound sleep. This incident transformed his thinking. Under the care of Dr. Phelan, Mrs. Kent made a steady progress from the next day onwards. This was enough for Kent to throw his heart and soul into the study of the homoeopathic science.

Later on Kent's first wife died and, like Hahnemann, he married another lady, a doctor who had come to see him as a patient. She was converted to homoeopathy and during his later years helped him in his great books : Homoeopathic Materia Medica, Homoeopathic Philosophy and Repertory. As in the case of Hahnemann, Kent's last few years were the most fruitful from every point of view.

Kent's Repertory is considered to be his greatest contribution. That was the result of years of most painstaking search and research and has not been surpassed so far. Materia Medica, Philosophy and Repertory are so closely interwoven into one another that no homoeopathic doctor can aspire to do anything worthwhile without the constant study of each of these disciplines and without constant reference to them.

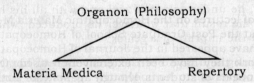

Organon (Philosophy)

Materia Medica   Repertory

Kent made original contributions to all the three. It is most befitting to his memory that we continue further from where he ended because that is what he would have wished the future generations to do.

DR. JUGAL KISHORE
B.Sc., D.M.S. (Cal.)

86, Golf Links
New Delhi
February 25, 1971.

PREFACE TO FIRST EDITION

The course of lectures on the Homoeopathic Materia Medica was delivered at the Post-Graduate School of Homoeopathics. Some of them have appeared in the Journal of Homoeopathics, but for this work they have been extensively revised. Owing to the strong appeals of students, though against the author's inclination, the colloquial style has been permitted to stand. The lectures are presented in the simple form to explain the author's plan of studying each remedy. The speech of laymen presents all sickness to the physician's mind, hence the Materia Medica must be reduced from technicalities to simple speech. No two remedies are studied exactly alike. Each has its own requirement in order to bring before the mind what is characteristic. Not all of the Materia Medica has been brought out, but the leading and fully proved remedies such as have strong characteristics have been presented for the purpose of showing how the Materia Medica must be evolved and used. There are other methods of studying a remedy, but this seems to the author the most natural way of giving to the student lasting idea of the nature of each remedy. It may be that it seems so because it is the only way the author could ever do it. The numerous repetitions of characteristic symptoms may subject the work to criticism, but experience has shown that it is the only way of giving the beginner a lasting grasp of the remedy.

Hahnemann's Materia Medica Pura, Hering's Guiding Symptoms, and the Encyclopedia of Pure Materia Medica have been the works that have given the most help in these studies.

They are not offered as being complete digests of the various remedies, but simply as the examinations of some of the most salient points. A complete digest would be endless. If some of the younger practitioners and students of the Materia Medica shall meet the assistance in this work they have been looking

11

for, it is all that can be expected. There is no royal road to a perfect understanding of the Materia Medica. It is tedious and drudgery at best, but no more so than any great science. Because of its greatness many will fail to undertake it even when it is for the saving of life and lessening of suffering, yet many will not decline to offer their services to the people knowing full well and confessing ignorance openly that the methods they offer are inadequate, useless, and often destructive. Some profess not to believe in this careful way of analyzing the symptomatology, but if some easy method is offered for a pretended mastery of it they wildly embrace it only to return to their primitive repulsive mental aversion crying out "sour grapes."

The Materia Medica can be learned by careful study and by using it. It can be understood but not memorized. All who would memorize the Materia Medica must ignominiously fail. To be constantly at hand, it must be constantly and correctly used. The continuous study of the Materia Medica by the aid of a full repertory for comparison is the only means of continuing in a good working knowledge. To learn the Materia Medica, one must master Hahnemann's Organon, after which the symptomatology and the Organon go "hand in hand". The Organon, the symptomatology and a full repertory must be the constant reference books, if careful homoeopathic prescribing is to be attained and maintained.

All who wish to make a more extensive examination of the reason for the methods used in the work are referred to the chapter on VALUE OF SYMPTOMS in the Lectures on HOMOEOPATHIC PHILOSOPHY.

October 29, 1904
108, N. State St., Chicago

JAMES TYLER KENT

CONTENTS

NEW ADDITIONS FROM
KENT'S NEW REMEDIES

HOMŒOPATHIC
MATERIA MEDICA

ABROTANUM

This very valuable remedy should be more frequently used. It is indicated in such conditions as are cured by *Bryonia* and *Rhus tox.,* but its symptoms mark out its own individual cases. Rheumatic conditions with heart irritation; epistaxis; bloody urine; anxiety and trembling, when there has been a history of diarrhœa. A suddenly checked diarrhœa will be followed by the above symptoms in a case requiring Abrot. A suddenly suppressed rheumatism of any joint followed by violent cardiac symptoms; it is much like *Ledum, Aurum* and *Kalmia.*

In marasmus of children it is a very useful remedy and not unfrequently indicated. The emaciation begins *in the lower limbs and gradually spreads upward,* so that the face is the last affected; that is the opposite of *Lycopodium, Natrum mur.* and *Psorinum.*

It has cured pleurisy after *Bryonia,* which seemed indicated, had failed. A woman lying in bed with dyspnœa, anxiety, cold sweat and pain in the heart was surrounded by friends to see her die. It was learned that she had suffered for many months with a rheumatism in one knee, that she had used crutches to get about the house, and that she had recently been speedily cured (?) by a strong liniment only a few days before this attack. Abrot. restored her to health promptly.

It has caused and cured burning ulcerative pains in the stomach with suspicious vomiting.

Metastasis is a marked feature in Abrot. The changing of one so-called disease into another always calls attention to Abrotanum. Inflammation of the parotid (mumps) changing to testes or mammx is generally cured by *Carbo v.* or *Pulsatilla,* but Abrot. has cured when these remedies have failed.

A suddenly checked diarrhœa followed by piles and acute rheumatism, with bleedings, as mentioned above, is further argument in favor of this idea.

The Abrot. patient is sensitive to cold air and cold damp weather. He suffers much from backaches, and his symptoms are worse during the night,

In boys it cures hydrocele. In infants it cures bleeding from the navel.

There is either diarrhœa or constipation; with the latter he is rheumatic, with the former he is at his best, as when the diarrhœa slacks up he is full of suffering. The diarrhœa is his great relief, like *Natrum sulph.* and *Zincum.*

Sharp pains here and there, but especially in ovaries ana joints.

ACETIC ACID

This remedy is useful in complaints of pale, sickly people. Patients who have been weak fox many years, who have inherited phthisis. Emaciation, weakness, anaemia, loss of appetite, burning thirst and copious pale urine are a combination calling for Acetic acid. Sensation of heat with pulsation coming and going, like orgasms; chlorosis in young girls; dropsical conditions in general; bad effects from stings and bites, have been cured by this remedy. Vinegar is an old remedy for bad effects from chloroform. It is useful in the hæmorrhagic constipation. Bleeding from various mucous membranes, nose, stomach, rectum, lungs and from ulcers. Sensitive to cold.

Confusion of mind; does not know her own children; forgets what has recently happened; attacks of anguish; constantly borrows trouble; thinks something is going to happen; peevishness, complaining.

Fainting spells in weak, anæmic subjects; headaches; face pale and waxy; epistaxis; one cheek pale and the other red; diphtheria in throat or larynx, unquenchable thirst; sensitive stomach; vomiting blood, and all food taken; ulceration of stomach; hot, sour eructations; frothy vomiting; gnawing pain; distension of stomach, with a constant commotion; burning in stomach and abdomen, ameliorated by lying on the stomach.

In the abdomen there is great pain, distension, flatulence or dropsy, sore to touch; diarrhœa, thin, bloody or pure blood; profuse bleeding from piles; chronic diarrhœa.

Copious watery urine. It has cured diabetes, with sugar in the urine or without, where there is great thirst, weakness and pallor and loss of flesh.

Weakness with seminal losses; relaxed genitals and swollen feet.

Uterine hæmorrhage; copious menses, or watery menstrual flow; scanty menses with chlorosis.

Weakness of larynx; croup; diphtheria. It has cured many cases of laryngeal diphtheria; hoarseness, with pale mucous membranes; chronic dry, hacking cough in sickly, pale persons, such as have inherited phthisis, with crdema of extremities, diarrhœa and dyspnœa, or night sweats; hæmorrhage from the lungs; burning in chest and stomach; rattling in chest; chronic bronchitis.

Weakness and lameness in extremities, with swelling, rheumatic or œdematous; dropsy of limbs, with diarrhœa.

It is a deep-acting, constitutional remedy, and when well studied will be very useful. *All substances abused as food become great remedies,* such as vinegar, coffee, common salt, etc. We should look to them oftener than we do for the stubborn chronic cases.

ACONITUM NAPELLUS

Aconite is a short-acting remedy. Its symptoms do not last long. It is a violent poison in large doses, either destroying life or passing away in its effects quite soon, so that if the patient recovers, the recovery is not delayed. There are no chronic diseases following it. Like a great storm, it comes and sweeps over and passes away. By a little meditation we will discover what kind of sickness all this is like, and what kind of a patient is most likely to have that short, sudden sickness. If we think a moment from experience and homœopathic observation, we will remember that vigorous, plethoric individuals, when they take cold, come down violently, whereas feeble people, sickly people, come down and recover slowly from acute diseases, and do not become so violently and so suddenly sick. From this, and from examining the sudden effects of Aconite, it will be easy to see that persons who come down with Aconite sicknesses are plethoric individuals. Strong, robust people, rugged children and infants become sick, not a very slight cold, or from slight exposure, but from more violent exposure. From being exposed with deficient clothing; from sudden, violent changes; from prolonged exposure to the cold, north, dry wind. A vigorous person caught out with thin clothing, or remaining out in the cold, dry air of mid-winter, with its sudden, violent changes, comes down even before night with violent symptoms. This is the class of patients, the plethoric and vigorous, who have a strong heart, active brain, vigorous circulation, and come down suddenly from violent exposure, that need Aconite.

Aconite has in its nature none of the results usually following inflammation. The storm is over so quickly that it seems mostly to conform to the earlier condition. In these vigorous patients sudden congestions are likely to be thrown off by good reaction. The patient seems to be threatened with a sudden and violent death, but recovery is quick. So, as was observed by Dunham, it is a great storm and soon over. Dunham's discussion of this remedy in his Materia Medica is very poetical and well worth reading.

Attacks come on suddenly from exposure to a dry, cold wind. In plethoric children we have an illustration of that in the sudden congestion of the brain with intense fever, or with convulsions. We get illustrations of its suddenness and violence in any organ of the body, the brain, the lungs, the liver, the blood, the kidneys. It is suited to the complaints that come on *suddenly from the very cold weather* of winter, or from the *intensely hot weather* of summer. It has the lung and brain complaints of winter, and the bowel inflammations and stomach disorders of summer. We know how these plethoric individuals become suddenly overheated and become violently sick. Their sudden attacks are frightful to look upon, All these inflammatory conditions are attended with great excitement of the circulation, violent action of the heart, a tremendous turmoil of the brain, a violent shock with intense fear.

The mind symptoms that are nearly always associated with Aconite conditions stand out in bold relief. The patient feels the violence of his sickness, for he is under great nervous irritation and excitement. Fear is depicted upon his countenance, and the heart's action is so overwhelming the first thing he thinks of is that he must die; this must mean death, which he fears. It stands out upon his countenance. He says: "Doctor, there is no use; I am going to die." Many times he actually predicts the moment or *the hour of his death.* If a clock is in the room, he may say that when the hour hand reaches a certain point he will be a corpse. *When we see this intense fear, this awful anxiety, great restlessness, the violence and the suddenness of these attacks,* we have a case, perhaps, that is dying from the poison of Aconite, or one who needs Aconite. One who has a sickness resembling the poison of Aconite needs the smallest possible dose of Aconite. It is a very short-acting medicine, and that must be remembered.

It hardly matters what part of the body we are considering we will find inflammatory conditions. But regardless of the region or the locality of the inflammation, that which I have described is the appearance of the patient. Such are the symptoms that will stand out, that you will observe first—the appearance of the fact, the mind symptoms, the restlessness, the intensity. Now, there are many little mental symptoms that are of much less importance than this fear, this anxiety, symptoms that will be masked by these marked symptoms that indicate the patient. He has lost all affection for his friends. He does not care what becomes of them, he has not the slightest interest in them. It sometimes may be a state of indifference.

What I have brought out will enable one to readily see that this picture does not belong to all the remedies in the Materia Medica. In fact, it belongs only to Aconite. No matter what remedy you compare this with, you would find it only under Aconite. You will find *some* of the features in the text under other remedies, but those which I have mentioned col-lectively will be found only under Aconite. Take the mental symptoms, intensity marks every one of them. If it is a delirium, it is an intense deli-rium, *with excitement, with fear, with anxiety.* Patients in delirium, with excitement and fear, will weep, as in great torment. *Great excitement, fear,*

fear of death. You wonder what she is weeping about. There are all sorts of moods intermingled also with the fear of Aconite. There is moaning and irritability, anger, throwing things away, all attended with *the violence and anxiety.* These features that I described as uppermost are intermingled with all the other symptoms.

"Screams with pain." The pains are like knives, they are stinging, cutting, stabbing. The intensity of the Aconite suffering is wonderful, so that if the nerves take on neuralgic pains *the pains are intense.* It is the feeling that some awful thing must be upon him or he could not have such dreadful suffering. It says in the text, "predicts the day of his death." This to a great extent is the result of the awfulness that seems to be overwhelming him. And this mental picture is always present, in pneumonia, in inflammatory conditions of any part of the body, in inflammation of the kidneys, of the liver, of the bowels, etc.

Dizziness prevails throughout all this symptom picture. "Vertigo, turning and whirling." A woman out shopping runs up suddenly against a dog and becomes violently dizzy, she cannot even get to her carriage. "Vertigo that comes on from fear, from sudden fear, and the fear of the fright remains." There is a remnant of that fear left, but it will lead you on more strongly towards *Opium.* "Complaints from fear. inflammation of the brain from fear, dizziness from fear." *Even congestion of parts as a result of fear.* A turmoil in the whole sensorium. Things go round and round.

The *headaches* can hardly be described, they come with such violence. Tearing burning in the brain, in the scalp, attended *with fear, with fever, with anguish;* headache from taking cold, from suppressing catarrh in the nose. Catarrh stops suddenly in plethoric people, from exposure, from riding in the dry, cold wind such as we have in this northern climate in winter. "Violent headache over the eyes. Congestion of the brain, with congestive headache, *with anxiety, with hot face."*

The symptoms that would lead you to give Aconite for affections of the eye are numerous. Eyes take on sudden inflammation. Congestion of the eye. Blood red appearance of the eye. Sudden inflammation of all the tissues; conjunctivitis, etc., from *taking cold, from exposure to dry, cold winds.*

There is a teaching that has long prevailed: give Aconite for the first stage of an inflammation. It is not good teaching, although it is recommended in all of our books. It does not say for what kind of a constitution, or how it comes about. Do not practice that way. Get all the elements for an Aconite case, if possible, or give a better remedy. Another practice has prevailed, viz., giving Aconite for fever. Aconite was the fever remedy of many of our early routinists, but it is a bad practice.

Aconite has an inflammation of the eyes that comes on so suddenly that

one wonders how that inflammation came in so short a time. The eyes take on
great swelling without any discharge, or only very watery mucus. The sudden
inflammations that come on with thick discharges would never be Aconite.
Aconite has no results of inflammation. Those conditions that are about to
take on the results of inflammation will always indicate some other remedy.
You are not to think of Aconite in fever unless the Aconite patient is present.
With the Aconite fever there will be sensitiveness to light. "Great restlessness
with fever." Eyes staring, with pupils contracted, "violent aching and
inflammation of the deep structures of the ball." Give Aconite only when the
symptoms agree. An inflammation that is about to run a prolonged course, to
take on suppuration, or if it is mucous membrane to take on discharge of pus,
will never show you the symptoms of Aconite. Never give Aconite in blood
poisoning, such as we find in scarlet fever, in typhoid fever, etc. We find
nothing of the violent symptoms of Aconite in such conditions. The nervous
irritation is never present, but the opposite, the stupor, the laziness, the purple
skin—whereas Aconite is bright red. Never give Aconite for any form of
zymosis, for it has no zymotic history. There should be no thought of Aconite
in the slow coming, continued fever. Aconite has no symptoms like the slow
types of continued fevers. The Aconite fever is generally one short, sharp
attack of fever. It is in no way related to an intermittent fever, as it has no such
symptoms. You might find something that would deceive you in one attack of
intermittent fever, but the very fact that there was a second one would shut
out Aconite. Some remedies have periodicity or waves, Aconite has no such
condition. The most violent attack of fever will subside in a night if Aconite
is the remedy. If it is not it is a pity that you made a mistake in giving it, for it
will sometimes do mischief. All things that exist in a sickness must be taken
into account, not only what the remedy does cover, but what it does not
cover.

Aconite has inflammation of the eyes, with burning and sudden swelling;
the lids swell so rapidly that they cannot be opened except with great difficulty,
and when they are forced open by seizing the margins of the lids with a pair
of forceps drops of hot water will fall out, but no pus. This comes on rapidly
from taking cold. Whenever there are inflammations or the mucous surfaces
bloody water is apt to flow. Suddenly the blood vessels become engorged
and ooze, the blood vessels rupture and the capillaries ooze.

Inflammation of the *ear* comes on just as suddenly. "Throbbing, intense,
cutting pains in the ear." The child comes home after being out in the cold
north wind, and is not sufficiently clad, and now it screams and puts its hand
to the ear. The attack comes on early in the evening, after being out in the
daytime. Fever and anxiety; child must be carried. The suffering is intense.
Noise intolerable. Music goes through every limb, so intense is the sense of

hearing. Everywhere in the body will we find that same intense condition of the nerves. Wherever there are complaints they are intense, violent, and the patient is always in a state of anxiety and irritability. "Stinging, burning, rending, tearing, cutting pains in the ear."

Coryza if attended with violent headache, coming on in the night after exposure and taking cold during the day, suddenly, this short-acting, very quick-acting remedy will be indicated. The coryza that comes on from *Carbo veg.* comes on several days after the exposure. The coryza that comes on from *Sulphur* also develops several days after the exposure. The *Carbo veg.* patient becomes overheated and takes cold by keeping on his overcoat when he comes into your office. In Aconite he goes out in cold air with his light clothing, and comes down, if he is a plethoric individual, before midnight.

But especially is it often indicated in the coryza of the rosy, chubby, plethoric baby. Not in the sickly or pale ones. These sickly ones will come down later; their vital activities are so reduced that their complaints do not come on sometimes for two or three days. So that if you take a sickly one and a vigorous one in the same family and expose them both one will have croup tonight and need Aconite, and the other will have it the next morning and need *Hepar.*

The symptoms likely to occur with coryza are nosebleed, headache, anxiety and fear. The anxious expression is one of the first things observed in the Aconite sufferer. The Aconite pneumonia will often show itself on the face. Look at the face; there is great anxiety. It shows much of the proving of Aconite. You know there is much in the expression of the face that will enable one to read all that is going on in the body; it tells the story. The pleasures and sadness, and the distress of the human family, much of which you can generalize, and see at a glance that some great thing has happened. You have only to guess once or twice before you hit it. Here you have the anxiety.

"One cheek red and the other pale" is in a good many remedies, but the anxious expression, and the fear, and the heat, and the restlessness, and the suddenness with which it comes on in a plethoric individual—yesterday it was very dry and windy—and you will at once place this one symptom with Aconite. But it might be one of several other remedies, were other conditions present. "Neuralgic pains in the face, like hot wires running along either side of the face." The individual rides in the cold, raw wind, and his face was exposed to the cold wind. He becomes numb, then pain sets in, intense pain. He cries out and shrieks with the knife-like cutting pains. Aconite will relieve. "Crawling, creeping like ants"; Aconite has that sensation along the course of the nerves. It has a sensation like ice water poured along the course of the nerves. Sciatica when the sensation is felt down the nerve like ice water. "Creeping, tingling and crawling in the face, with or without pain." There is intense heat, intense fever in the face. The side of the face laid on will often break into a sweat, and if the patient turns over, that side will at once become dry, and the other side will at once break out in a sweat.

Oh, what a comforting remedy it is for *toothache*. It has been so useful in toothache that nearly every old lady nowadays knows enough to put a drop of Aconite on a bit of cotton and put it in the old hollow tooth. It will quite often palliate. A dose of Aconite will act much better. But the violence of the toothache; again the same old story, from the dry, cold winds, plethoric individuals, with hollow teeth, pain intense, cutting, shooting pains in the teeth. Sometimes these pains are in sound teeth and affect the whole row of teeth. Violent pains from exposure, such as riding in the wind. The pains are relieved and go away speedily after a dose of Aconite.

Disturbances of taste, disordered stomach. *Everything tastes bitter,* except water; and, oh, how the Aconite patient longs for water. It seems almost impossible for him to get water enough and it agrees well.

Burning is a symptom that runs all through the remedy, you will find it descriptive of all the pains. Burning in the head, burning along the course of nerves, burning in the spine, burning in fever sometimes burning as if covered with pepper.

Aconite is a very useful medicine in inflammation of the *throat,* when there is burning, smarting, dryness, great redness of the tonsils, or the fauces, the whole throat. Sometimes the soft palate is greatly swollen. A high grade of inflammation, acute inflammation of all that can be seen and called throat. But that alone would not indicate Aconite. It cures that kind of case, it cures inflammation of the throat, but every homœopathic physician knows that forty or fifty remedies could be selected just as well as Aconite from all that I have said. I have only mentioned a nondescript case. No homœopathic physician could prescribe upon that kind of evidence. But you note the kind of throat every physician must ask himself the question: "What would make that kind of a throat an Aconite case?" And then the question would come up, could he not prescribe for it as well if he had not seen the throat? The throat does not do much towards representing, to an *intelligent physician,* the patient. If it was necessary to represent to the mind of the physician the inflamed part itself, how would he treat the liver? He cannot see it. How would he prescribe for the stomach? He cannot see it. We are then compelled to fall back upon that which represents to the intelligent physician the very nature of the patient himself, and then at once we will see the reason for some of these things. If you present the Aconite patient well before the mind you can prescribe. It would be well to see anything that is visible. If you could see the liver, I would say look at it. If you could see the heart, I would say examine it.

What is it in this throat that really represents the patient? Of course, any soreness of the throat makes it difficult to swallow. I mean to infer that there is nothing in the soreness to represent to the physician the Aconite patient. If that individual were a plethoric individual, if he had been riding in a cold, raw wind a good part of the day, and he had wakened in the night with a violent burning, tearing sore throat, and he could not swallow, and the fever came on high, and he had thirst for cold water and he could not get enough of it, he was in *an anxious, feverish state,* you have then a *patient* to prescribe for. Many times will patients become intelligent enough under your observation to write just what some member of the family acts like. You know just what the patient looks like. The black man will sometimes give the best kind of a description, better than the Vassar girl, who writes us: "Doctor, will you please send the medicine; I have looked into the throat and it is red."

With the stomach symptoms what an anxious patient we have! The pains are dreadful. Burning pains, tearing pains, with anxiety, with restlessness, with fever, coming on from taking cold—not from overeating, but from taking cold, which has settled in the stomach, from exposure to an ice bath, or in a very hot summer from intense heat, associated with an irritable brain in vigorous children. Vomiting and retching, tearing, as it were, the very inside out by the awful retching. The vomiting of blood, bright red blood. This is descriptive of the general stomach trouble. During this febrile state he craves bitter things, wine and beer, and brandy, but they will come up as soon as they reach the stomach. He craves pungent things, nothing tastes hitter enough. "If he could only get something bitter." And yet his food tastes bitter, everything he eats tastes bitter, everything except water.

The word in the text is a clinical word; it says "gastric catarrhs". It is a very sharp, acute inflammation of the stomach. Retching, vomiting, of bile, vomiting of blood. Ineffectual urging to vomit; when there is nothing in the stomach. With it there will be *anxiety, restlessness, fear of death.* The fear depicted upon the countenance makes an awful expression.

Aconite is a useful medicine in inflammation of the liver, when it comes suddenly. It is not very useful in repeated attacks, but in the first attack. Violent inflammation of the liver, with violent tearing pains and much burning. Then comes the restlessness, the awful *tortures of anxiety, moving constantly, fear of death, red face, glassy eyes, great thirst.* "Anxious restlessness" covers nearly all of these things.

In the abdomen there are shooting pains, burning, stinging pains, after exposure to cold, becoming chilled. We will soon come to think that it does not make much difference where the disorder occurs, we must have the Aconite patient. We also have inflammatory troubles of all the viscera of the abdomen. It may be a violent catarrhal inflammation. It may be a catarrhal condition of the lower portion of the colon, or a catarrhal condition of the rectum, when we will have a dysentery. In dysentery, that which is found in the commode is almost pure blood, blood and a little slime. It seems impossible for him to leave the commode. Vomiting a little blood and passing bloody mucus from the rectum. Always they will predict they will die tonight, or in a few hours. They look as if they realized the sensation of death. The whole body is in a state of anguish, but the tenesmus and cramp, the urging to stool are simply terrible. It has a watery diarrhœa, but that is not a very important symptom, although it is doubly marked in Hering. But when pure blood is passed, and mucus, with tenes-mus, or when a little green mucus is passed by infants with summer troubles, pure blood or grass-green discharges with fever coming on suddenly, in bright, rosy little ones, think of Aconite. Most of the bowel troubles come on from intense heat, in the children. The infant takes on inflammation of the liver from the heat, and the stool becomes white like milk, of putty consistency. The child becomes yellow and screams with pain.

It is useful in urinary troubles, bladder and kidney troubles. Inflammatory conditions, and with bloody urine. Scanty urine, suppressed urine, or retained urine. Retention from shock. This retention from shock makes it one of our best remedies for retention in the new-born. The infant just born into the world has undergone a shock. At your next visit the nurse says, "The child has not passed urine." The functions of that little one are not yet established, because of the great shock the little one has gone through.

Inflammation of the bladder, with cutting, tearing pains. Burning pains with burning urine. Urine is hot, dark, colored red; red and clear, or bloody. Retention from cold, especially in children, with crying and restlessness. With inflammatory conditions of the bladder, either in adults or in infants, there will be all the mental states representing the Aconite patient.

Aconite cures most violent cases of orchitis, which come on suddenly. Orchitis from cold, from being chilled, in plethoric men. But in the common orchitis from suppressed gonorrhoeal discharges Aconite is useless.

The woman is a natural Aconite patient, with her sympathetic natural sensitiveness. She usually takes on complaints from nervous shock, from fear, and she naturally takes on complaints from causes other than those from which men take on sickness. It is very seldom that fear will give a man inflammation, but fear is a common cause of inflammation of the uterus, and of the ovaries, in plethoric, vigorous, excitable women. Fear will often cause abortion, but when Aconite is given early enough it will check the abortion that comes from fear. We will have the stitching, burning, tearing pains of Aconite sometimes following fear or sudden emotion. Sometimes a pregnant woman will say, "Doctor, there is no use your planning for my confinement. I know I am going to die in that confinement." If there is any one thing that is a really strong symptom to prescribe on it is that. A dose of Aconite, and then change the subject, she goes away, and in a few days you ask her about that fear and she says, "Oh, never mind that." Many little things like that can be singled out. But that state of fear is a very peculiar thing, and really represents the whole nature and being of the woman. She predicts the day of her death. The reason that Aconite is so often the infant's remedy is because the infant is so often made sick from fright.

"Inflammation of the genitals in plethoric women." Aconite is more frequently indicated in women and children than in men. Sensitive, vigorous, excitable women. It is indicated in men in inflammatory conditions from becoming chilled in dry, cold air, and it is wonderful how you can convince a patient who needs Aconite what wonderful things there are in Homœopathy by showing him how rapidly, with Aconite, you can put him in a sweat and break up a sharp fever when that is a recent and single attack.

"After tedious and difficult parturition. Violent after-pains. Shooting, tearing after-pains, with febrile conditions." Uterine hæmorrhage with bright red blood and fear of death. It is wonderful what Aconite will do in some cases arising from taking cold in the puerperal state, but do not mix that up with puerperal fever. The first is a simple form, non-septic; perhaps the breast is involved, with soreness in the breast, suppression of the milk and febrile conditions; but if there is suppression of the lochia do not give Aconite.

New-born children, with difficulty of breathing, after the use of forceps, or from a tedious labor; the child is breathless, there is difficulty with the heart, and in a few hours fever comes on. Aconite is a very simple remedy. The retention of urine in the infant is so commonly an Aconite condition that you will hardly ever need to use any other medicine. The little one cannot yet talk, it cannot manifest very much, and, to a certain extent, the practitioner is compelled to be somewhat routine in these affairs, and the routine practitioners have been more or less successful with Aconite for the retention of the urine. Again, it is true that in many cases of retention of the urine in the mother, it will disappear after a dose of *Causticum*.

Aconite is a great routine croup remedy, one that is misused; but it is indicated in all those cases of croup which come on suddenly in plethoric children, from exposure to dry, cold wind, having been out in the cold wind with the mother during the day. The child is put to bed and rouses up from the first sleep, perhaps at 9 or 10 or 11 o'clock, grasps the throat, coughs violently, a croupy, choking cough, with hoarse bark. Hardly any other remedy can correspond to that rapidity of action, taking cold in the daytime and developing itself so suddenly. Croup that comes on from exposure today, and does not develop until tomorrow morning or tomorrow evening, may correspond to quite a number of other remedies, but especially *Hepar*, which is slower in its pace. And it is more suitable in children somewhat run down and subject to frequent attacks of croup. *Spongia* is also similar, but it lacks many of the elements more likely to occur in run-down children, those always taking cold. It would be a difficult matter to distinguish between the appearance of the Aconite and the *Spongia* croup so far as the croup is concerned, because both have all the anxious appearance found in croup. The Aconite croup is a violent croup, inflammation of the larynx, and, at the same time, spasms of the larynx coming on with great rapidity. The *Spongia* croup is less inflammatory, the inflammation grows with the spasms; but while *Spongia* may rouse up at 11 o'clock at night, suffocating and choking, it has not the intense febrile excitement that belongs to Aconite, nor the anguish, although it has all the dryness that is found in Aconite. Aconite conditions are dry as a usual thing, or there is only a little watery discharge. *Spongia* is entirely dry; if there is an inflamed mucous membrane, it is dry. We have in the croup symptoms in Aconite: Larynx sensitive to touch. "Croup, waking in first sleep, after exposure to dry, cold winds."

Aconite is full of disturbances of respiration, dyspnœa from contraction of the smaller bronchial tubes, which we find resembles asthma. It is indicated in that dyspnœa that belongs to capillary bronchitis, in that dyspnœa that belongs to cardiac excitement in plethoric persons, from taking cold, becoming exposed or from shock. Dyspnœa from fear, such as occurs in nervous women, excitable, easily affected, nervous, plethoric women. Breathing short, labored, anxious, quick. It is an asthmatic dyspnœa and there is usually dryness of the mucous membranes of the small bronchial tubes.

"Sits up straight and can hardly breathe." Aconite has such a sudden violent cardiac irritation, pulse fluttering, weak, full and bounding; sits up in bed, grasps the throat, wants everything thrown off; before midnight, a hot skin, great thirst, great fear—everything is associated together.

"Anguish with dyspnœa. Sudden attacks of pain in the heart, with dyspnœa." All go together. "Great suffocation." From this fear and from anxiety he breaks out in profuse sweat; he is drenched with sweat—and yet his skin is hot. When this anxiety passes off he becomes hot. So there is heat and sweat with this awful anxiety. Pulse like a thread.

"Better during expiration." The spasm of the larynx often comes on during inspiration. "Worse during inspiration. Constant short, dry cough. Difficult breathing. Breathes only with the diaphragm. Chest troubles, such as pneumonia." Aconite produces a very rapid inflammation of the viscera of the chest, of the pleura, of the lungs, of the mucous membrane lining the air passages. In pneumonia we have this dyspnœa, the suddenness with which it comes on. If it spreads rapidly it may go into pneumonia. Inflammation runs so high that the mucous membrane oozes blood, cherry red, or the mucus that comes up is white and heavily streaked with bright red blood. You go to the bedside of broncho-pneumonia and you will find in the pan mucus streaked with bright red blood. Now, take the violence with which that comes on, the restlessness and anxiety of the individual—he predicts the hour of his death— that would be the case with the Aconite patient. In the case of pneumonia where the lung is involved, it is likely to be the upper half of the left lung when Aconite is indicated. Sometimes the whole mucous membrane, the visible throat, the larynx, trachea, the bronchial tubes, will all ooze blood, sometimes a mouthful of blood, so violent is the inflammation. In these chest troubles there is much pain. Shooting, burning, tearing pains, and the patient is compelled to lie in a somewhat elevated position, on the back. Cannot lie upon either side, but upon the back. Lying on the side increases the pain. The dry cold winds. Sudden shocks, in persons of good, strong, vigorous circulation. The hæmoptysis that is. spoken of is not such as occurs in phthisis, but is involuntary; the blood comes up with a slight cough. Some one might be deceived to give it in such cases in broken down constitutions in sickly patients; but it is not to be administered in such cases, we have much better remedies. The patient does not always become a pneumonia patient, but inflammation of the small air passages may be all that is present.

"Dry cough, vomiting and retching, intense fever, spitting of blood." No expectoration except a little watery mucus and blood. It occurs a good deal in this way. Dry cough, sensation of dryness of the whole chest, sensation of dryness in the larynx and throat. Pours down great quantities of cold water, and once in a while after a violent coughing spell he gets up a little blood. But the expectoration is generally mucus.

Pneumonia is generally attended with an expectoration looking like iron rust, as if iron rust had been mixed in with it. Such medicines as *Bryonia* and *Rhus tox.* and a few others have that expectoration as a common feature, as natural to the remedies themselves, but Aconite *is the cherry red, bright red* expectoration. Its hæmorrhages *are bright red, and sometimes copious.*

All these coughs in pneumonia, in croup, and chest troubles come on suddenly, and if he goes to sleep he will have spasm of the larynx, with dryness of the larynx. He goes to sleep and the larynx becomes dry, and he wakes up and grasps his larynx; he thinks he is going to choke. All these come on from cold winds. Vigorous persons get into a draft and get a chill that will bring on Aconite symptoms.

Aconite has in all inflamed parts a sensation as if hot steam were rushing into the parts, as if warm blood were rushing into the parts, or "flushes of heat in the parts." Along nerves, a sensation of heat, or sensation of cold.

The pulse in the highest form of the fever is full and bounding; strong, vigorous pulse. When the attack is first coming on and the awful anxiety and nerve tension are present the pulse is very small, but after the heart's action is well established, then the pulse becomes stronger.

"Tearing pains down the spine. Painful, stiff neck. Crawling in the spine like insects." That is a peculiar feature, this crawling sensation; it comes from cold, from being suddenly chilled.

"Trembling of the hands" associated with these sudden acute attacks. "Creeping pains in the fingers" associated with these sudden acute inflammatory attacks. "Cold as ice. Feet cold as ice. Hot palms." Hot hands and cold feet are sometimes present. Rheumatic conditions of the joints. Those that come on as a first attack. Not old rheumatic and gouty attacks, but those that come on as acute rheumatism, those that come on from sudden exposure to cold, from long rides in a dry, cold wind. They also are attended with fever, with anxious restlessness, with a critical State of mind so often described.

"Trembling, tingling, convulsions of the muscles." But the *nerves* are full of Aconite symptoms and Aconite sufferings. Aconite is a wonderful remedy for neuritis in plethoric persons. Numbness along the course of the nerves, from cold, from exposure. Numbness and tingling, along the course of the nerves, especially those that run close to the surface. "Inflammation of the nerve sheaths. Nervous excitability. Excessive restlessness."

Sulphur has a strong relation to Aconite. It has many Aconite symptoms. In many of the old chronic cases where *Sulphur* would be used in strong, vigorous constitutions Aconite will be suitable for a sudden attack, and *Sulphur* for the chronic. In sudden attacks that Aconite conforms to, that is the whole attack, there may be left in that constitution a tendency to return of a similar attack. Aconite has no power over that tendency, but *Sulphur* has. Of course, most of the symptoms must agree, but it will seem to you frequently where Aconite has been suitable in the acute disease that Sulphur symptoms will follow, and many times a very violent attack leaves a weakness in the constitution which Aconite has no power to contend with. It has no power to keep off recurrent attacks. It does all that it is capable of doing, and that is the end of it. But it is not so with *Sulphur.*

After Aconite follow well *Arnica* and *Belladonna.* Sometimes it is true it will appear to you that Aconite is capable of coping with all there is in the disease. But there seems to be a lingering something that holds on, and such medicines as *Arn.* and *Bell.,* and *Ip.* and *Bry.,* do have to come in to finish up the attack—or sometimes *Sulphur.* Very commonly *Silica* So we have to study the relations of medicines.

If you have administered Aconite in too many doses, or given it too strong, and your patient is slow in recovering from the attack, or your patient has taken Aconite himself unwisely, then *Coffea* or *Nux* will often put the patient into a better condition.

ACTÆA RACEMOSA (BLACK COHOSH)

This remedy has been only meagerly proved, yet there are a few useful points in it. From its proving we can perceive that it is similar to diseased states in the human family, and especially in women, namely, hysterical and rheumatic conditions. The patient is always chilly, easily affected by cold, sensitive to cold and damp weather, which rouses the rheumatic state and develops a state of rheumatism not only in the muscles and joints all over the body, but also along the course of nerves. In the general nervous disturbance there is a lack of will balance, or great disturbance in the voluntary system, which is the underlying feature of hysteria, the symptoms are intermingled with rheumatism. With the pains we have soreness all over the body. Trembling, numbness, jerking of muscles. Inability to exercise the will over the muscles of the body, turmoil in the voluntary system, with stiffness.

Tendency to take cold and thereby she takes on sensitiveness in the glands and larger organs, such as the liver and uterus. Complaints in these organs come on from cold damp weather (*Dulcamara*) and from being chilled. The patient is sensitive to cold in all parts except the head, and is aggravated from becoming cold both in parts of the body and in general. The headaches, however, are better in the open air and from cold, which is an exception and a particular, for the *general* feature is aggravation from cold.

There is a terrible mental state that alternates with physical states. It is an overwhelming sadness or gloominess, she is bowed down with sorrow. Sits and mopes in great sadness, like *Psorinum* and *Pulsatilla.* This may pass off instantly, or be brought on and aggravated from motion, from fear, from excitement, from taking cold. Very commonly there is *muscular soreness, a bruised feeling all over,* with drawing and jerking. This will let up very suddenly and leave a nervous, hysterical girl in a state of sadness, and she will sit and say nothing. When questioned perhaps she will break into tears or express in various ways the overwhelming sadness. With the headache there is marked sadness. Changeable moods. The physical and the mental are all the time changing. Other symptoms alternate and change. The jerking has made physicians see the resemblance to chorea in these hysterio-rheumatic constitutions. The rheumatisms will change in a day into chorea, and again the choreic movements will keep on with the soreness throughout the muscles of the body. The jerking and soreness and numbness often keep on together.

There are certain features about the chorea that should be noted. Jerking of the muscles when in a state of emotion or from becoming chilled. If any part of the body is pressed upon jerking of the muscles of that part will take place. One of these nervous, rheumatic, hysterical subjects may not have chorea constantly, but as soon as she retires at night the *whole of the side lain on will commence to jerk and prevent her from going to sleep*. If she turns on the back the muscles of the back and shoulders will jerk and prevent sleep. She turns over on the other side, but after a little while the muscles pressed on commence to jerk. All this time she has become so restless and nervous that she is driven to distraction. The mind is full of all sorts of imaginations, and the body is full of all sorts of uneasiness, because she can find no place to rest upon. Sometimes the muscles are so sore that they cannot be lain upon for any length of time; sometimes it is a numbness, sometimes a jerking. These things are queer, but they belong to the patient, affecting not one part, but the whole economy.

Full of fear, anguish and restlessness. Fear of death, excitement, suspicious. "Will not even take the medicine because there is something wrong about it." It has a mania such as occurs in nervous, hysterical women, and it has cured puerperal mania. Puerperal mania from taking cold during or soon after confinement. The remedy belongs especially to women, because its symptoms are so commonly associated with the affections of women. Mental states following the disappearance of rheumatism is a strong feature. The rheumatism gets better, but the mental state becomes worse. Sometimes the rheumatism disappears in short order and the mind is not disturbed, but then it is because a diarrhœa has come on, with great soreness and aching in the bowels, or because a flow from the uterus has given relief. There must be some relief or a disturbance will take place like Abrotanum. Some flow must be established, and hence the menstrual flow or diarrhœa gives relief; otherwise the mind takes on trouble, the patient becomes gloomy, or has a low form of mental excitement. One of the symptoms is quite descriptive of this sadness I have referred to: "Sensation as if a black cloud had settled all over her," while at the same time it weighed like "lead upon the head." This is entirely figurative. It can all be expressed in the word "sadness." We will find "melancholy," "gloominess," "low spirited," etc., running all through our text, but the word "sadness" is just as broad as any of them.

The headaches are rheumatic. "Sore, bruised feeling all over the head. Bruised sensation in the occiput. Sore, bruised feeling in the top of the head, as if the top of the head would fly off." "As if cold air was blowing upon the brain." Yet most of these headaches are better by being in the cold air. "Headache brought on from catching cold, from the weather changes, cold, damp weather." There are many headaches. Pressing headache. Many of the headaches are intense, and described as if a bolt were extending down into the back of the neck. Soreness in the back of the neck. Pain in the back of the neck. Hysterical girls; *they have much pain in the back of the neck.* With the headache the eyeballs are very sore, "painful to turn in any direction." "Pain in the eyes, bruised pain in the head."

"Soreness in the abdomen; sore and bruised. Alternate diarrhœa and constipation. Alternation of diarrhœa and physical complaints."

We pass now to the female genitalia, which form a center for a great deal of trouble in the remedy. A routine saying about Actæa is that it makes confinement easy. That is not a legitimate saying concerning any remedy, and such expressions encourage routine practice. It is true that when this remedy has been given to pregnant women in accordance with its symptoms it has proved capable of making confinement easy. But the way it has been given has been the routine practice of giving it in the tincture or in the 2nd or 3rd, until the patient was under its influence even when it was not indicated, as it was not similar to the case. But the homœopathic physician never practices in this way. A remedy fits a general condition when the symptoms of that general condition are found in the remedy. Remember that it does so because *all the symptoms agree.*

"Pain in the uterine region, darting from side to side. Bearing down and pressing out." These bearing down sensations, taken with all the other states that relate to the patient in general, show that it is a very useful remedy in *prolapsus of the uterus.* It has the relaxation of the parts. Do not suppose that our remedies are not sufficient to cure these conditions, *when these symptoms agree.* It is true that remedies will cure prolapsus when the symptoms agree, and at *no other time.* If it fits the patient in general, these bearing down sensations will go away, the patient will be made comfortable, and an examination will finally show that the parts are in normal condition. You cannot prescribe for the prolapsus; you must prescribe for the woman. You cannot prescribe for one symptom, because there are probably fifty remedies that have that symptom.

There are menstrual disorders in these hysterical rheumatic constitutions. Irregularity of the menstrual flow. It may he copious, suppressed or scanty. Severe pain all through the flow. *The more the flow the greater the pain.* That is very peculiar. Generally the flow will relieve pain, but with this remedy the *pain is during the flow.* Generally the most severe and most painful attack is at the beginning of the flow, and with some women again just after the flow has ceased. Each woman is a law unto herself. In this remedy the sufferings are *during the menstrual flow as a rule.* The most severe mental symptoms, the most severe rheumatic symptoms, the most extreme jerking and cramping of the limbs and sleeplessness are during the menstrual flow.

During menses, epileptic spasms. All sorts of sufferings in the nerves. Soreness along the course of the nerves, soreness in the muscles or joints during the flow. Increase of mental symptoms. Cold and chilly, must be wrapped up. "Rheumatism. Dysmenorrhœa." "Soreness in the uterus and ovarian region. Lame, bruised feeling all over; painful menstruation," and some one has named that rheumatic dysmenorrhœa, not a bad name.

Many symptoms during pregnancy. It cures all sorts of conditions in this kind of constitution, these nervous, rheumatic, fidgety women with jerking in the muscles. So markedly do her troubles alternate with each other that alternation is in the nature of her case. You will commonly find that all the rest of her troubles have passed away, and that now nausea has come on. In all the years past she has had a hysterical constitution, but now. when she is pregnant she has nausea all the time. You will find when one set of symptoms becomes extremely severe others have temporarily subsided, and so they change about like *Pulsatilla.* But the symptoms have to be taken collectively to get at the image of the patient. A woman will come to you with one group of symptoms today and may come back to you with an entirely different group in a couple of weeks. These are very troublesome cases to prescribe for, and you have sometimes to take the symptoms a dozen times and put them all together as if she had left them all in one day, and so make your prescription. A hysterical patient is difficult to manage because of this changing of symptoms, and also because she has a tendency to deceive the doctor.

"Shivering in the first stage of labor. Hysterical manifestations through labor." Pains have all ceased or are irregular, so that they do no good. No dilatation has taken place. But when the regular pains come on we have some important symptoms. A pain comes on and it seems to be about to finish satisfactorily; it has been regular and prolonged until about two-thirds through, and all at once she screams out and grasps her hip—the pain has left the uterus and gone to the hip, causing a cramp in the hip, and she has to be rubbed and turned over. This medicine will regulate the pains, and when the next pain comes it will hold on to the end. So impressionable is this woman during confinement that if she is subjected to any emotion—such as having an emotional story told in the room—or if anything excitable occurs, the pain will stop. If she has passed through the labor and the lochia has been established, from such a cause the lochia will stop, as if she had taken cold, and she will have cramps and troublesome after-pains, the milk will be suppressed, she will feel sore and bruised all over, and have fever. This remedy should be compared with *Caulophyllum,* which has the following symptoms; Weakness in the reproductive system of the woman.

From weakness she is sterile, or she aborts in the early months of gestation. During parturition the contractions of the uterus are too feeble to expel the contents, and they are only tormenting. Labor-like pains during menstruation with drawing pains in the thighs and legs, and even the feet and toes. Uterine hæmorrhage from inertia of the uterus. Relaxation of muscles and ligaments. Heaviness, and even prolapsus. Subinvolution. Excoriating leucorrhœa. Menses too soon or too late. She is sensitive to cold and wants warm clothing—quite unlike *Pulsatilla*. She is hysterical, like *Ignatia*. She is fretful and apprehensive. She is rheumatic, like Actæa, only the small joints are most likely to be affected. Later she suffers from after-pains, and they are felt in the inguinal region. Rheumatic stiffness of the back and very sensitive spine. She is sleepless, restless and withal very excitable. This remedy has cured chorea at puberty when menstruation was late.

You need not be surprised that such an emotional subject has a fluttering, quick pulse, and irregular action of the heart, but many of the most marked hysterical features are present without any disturbances whatever in the action of the heart. "A feeling in the region of the heart as if the heart were sore, and as if it were enlarged."

"Back of head and neck sore." *The head is drawn back from contraction of the muscles at the nape. Violent aching down the back.* Rheumatism in the back. Impossible to lie upon the back because of the contraction of the muscles of the back. Impossible to lie upon the side of the body because of the contraction and jerking of the muscles. "Numbness of the limbs. Trembling. Soreness."

The symptoms of the nerves are simply a reiteration of what I have said. "Hysterical spasms. Convulsions. Trembling of the legs; hardly able to walk." The numbness is such as is associated with paralysis. Paralytic weakness.

The best effects have resulted from the 30th, 200th, 1000th and still higher potencies, and from the use of medicine in single doses.

It is similar in some of its conditions to the Blue Cohosh. Compare it with *Puls., Sepia, Natr. mur., Lit. t., Caulophyllum* and *Ign.*

ÆSCULUS HIPPOCASTANUM

A peculiar kind of *plethora* is found running through this remedy, a vascular fulness which affects the extremities and the whole body, and there are symptoms showing that the brain is similarly affected.

The conditions of Æsculus are *worse during sleep,* hence symptoms are observed on waking. He wakes up with confusion of mind, looks all around the room in confusion, bewildered, does not know the people, wonders where he is and what is the meaning of the things he sees. It is especially useful in children that rouse up in sleep frightened and in confusion, like *Lycopodium*. The remedy produces great *sadness, irritability,* loss of memory and aversion to work. There are times when there is a sense of bodily congestion, *fulness of the veins,* and then these symptoms are most marked. It is a *general venous stasis,* and is sometimes worse in sleep, worse from lying, better from bodily exertion. The symptoms pass away after considerable exertion; moving about, doing something, keeping busy relieves. You will find it useful in persons who suffer from palpitation when the pulsation extends to the extremities and the throbbing of the heart in sleep can be heard; an audible palpitation.

Now, as the mental symptoms are the most important in a proving, so are the mental symptoms in sickness the most important. Hahnemann directs us to pay most attention to the symptoms of the mind, because the symptoms of the mind constitute the man himself. The highest and innermost symptoms are the most important, and these are the mind symptoms. Æsculus has not been brought out in the finest detail, but we have the key to it. Extreme irritability is the very general state from which ramify a great many mental symptoms. Irritability and mental depression run through a great many remedies, and form the centre around which revolve all the mental symptoms in some cases. The reason that these are more interior than some other symptoms of the mind is that these relate to the affections themselves. The mental symptoms can be classified in a remedy. The things that relate to the memory are not so important as the things that relate to the intelligence and the things that relate to the intelligence are not so important as the things that relate to the affections or desires and aversions. We see in a state of irritability that the patient is not irritable while doing the things that he desires to do; if he wants to be talked to, for instance, you do not discover his irritability while talking to him. You never discover he is irritable if you do the things he wants you to do. But just as soon as you do something he does not want, this irritability or disturbance of the will is brought on, and this is the very innermost of the man's state. That which he wishes belongs to that which he wills, and the things that relate to what he wills are the most important things in every proving. You may say that an individual is sad, but he is sad because he lacks something that he wants; he desires something which he has not and becomes sad for it; sadness may go on to such an extent that the mind is in confusion.

Confusion of mind and vertigo. Make this distinction, vertigo is not a confusion of the intelligence. You have only to meditate upon it a moment and you will see that it is not. Confusion of the mind is a disturbance of the intellect, not a disturbance of the sensorium; you will make a distinction between staggering when walking and a period of disturbance of the mind, with inability to think clearly. Vertigo is a sensation of rolling, and belongs to the sensorium. A great mistake has been made in some of our repertories, in that confusions of mind are placed with vertigo under sensorium. These things must be thought out carefully, so that we are clear in our own minds as to what symptoms mean when they are given to us by patients. A patient may state that when walking in the street he is dizzy, or that it appears as though everything interiorly were turning around, yet he may be perfectly able to add up a column of figures; his mind may be clear. If we ourselves are perfectly clear as to the meaning of these expressions, we will commonly glean the meaning of the patient. It is important to record the language of the patient, yet often a patient will say something which you can see he does not mean at all, and it then becomes necessary to put in a parenthesis what he really means. For instance, a patient says: "I have such a pain in my chest," with the hand on the abdomen, or a woman when menstruating will say the pain is in the stomach when you know it is in the uterus. Patients must be questioned oftentimes as to their statements, or requested to place the hand upon the painful part. In the same way, therefore, patients talk about dizziness when they are not dizzy at all, but feel a confusion of mind, or they speak of confusion of mind when they mean that they stagger in the street.

It is in the nature of this remedy to have *flying pains* all over the body, like *Pulsatilla* and *Kali carb.* flitting, sharp, shooting, tearing pains, flying from one part to another; they seem at times to be scarcely more than skin deep. Sometimes they fly along the course of the nerves.

This remedy is full of *headache.* It has also dull aching pain, when it seems that the brain would be pressed out. But especially are these pains felt in the *back of the head, as if the head would be crushed;* hard aching pains, violent aching pains, fulness of the brain. "Dull frontal headache, from right to left, with constrictive feeling of skin of forehead." Fulness of the head, with dull, heavy pains, aching in the forehead; pain over the right eye. "Neuralgic pains in the right supraorbital region." "Shooting in left parietal bone, later in right." Formication of the scalp. If you examine the skin you will find formication, tickling and shooting and itching all over the body, so what there is in the scalp is only what belongs to the remedy in all parts.

Æsculus is a wonderful *eye* remedy, especially when the eyes have "hæmorrhoids." Does that convey any idea to you? By that I mean particularly enlarged blood vessels. *Great redness of the eyes, with lachrymation, burning eyeballs and vascular appearance.* This increased determination of blood is more or less painful; the eyeballs feel sore and ache; sharp, shooting pains in eyes. In almost every rubric of Æsculus we shall find stitching and shooting; little twinges; wandering pains with fulness; almost every kind of disturbance will intensify the fulness. Fulness of the hands and feet, not the fulness that pits upon pressure, that we call œdema, but a tenseness. Medicines having much trouble with the veins are often disturbed by hot bathing, weakness after a hot bath, weakness in warm weather, aversion to heat and desire for cold. It is the state of *Pulsatilla*. The *Pulsatilla* veins contract in cold weather, and the shrivelling up makes the patient feel better, but the veins fill and become engorged in the warm air and after a hot bath. A tepid bath sometimes makes a *Pulsatilla* patient feel better, but a Turkish bath is generally distressing. Many of the complaints of Æsculus are of this sort; Æsculus often feels better in cold air. The symptoms of Æsculus are often brought out by temperature, especially the little stinging pains. It is characteristic of these superficial pains that they are nearly always ameliorated by heat, while the deeper affections are oftentimes ameliorated from cold. Now, in *Pulsatilla,* the stinging pains of the scalp and those over the body, here and there, are often ameliorated by the local application of heat, while the patient himself wants to be in the cold; in the same way Æsculus stinging pains are better from heat, while the patient is often better from cold, although at times he is aggravated from cold, damp weather in rheumatic and venous conditions. Again, in *Secale,* we see that the little sharp pains that follow the course of the nerves are better from heat, but the patient himself wants to be in the cold air, or to be uncovered, except the spot of pain, which he wants kept warm. We notice the same thing running through *Camphor;* during the twinges of pain he wants the windows closed and wants hot applications; but as soon as the pain is over he wants the windows up and desires to be uncovered so that he can breathe. These are general things, things that are to be observed in Analyzing symptoms.

Æsculus then is a venous remedy, engorged and full, sometimes to bursting. Now, there is another feature I want to bring out. You will notice where congestion takes place that it is *purple* or blue in color. This remedy produces inflammation of the throat, the characteristic being that it is very dark. It has the tendency to produce varicose veins and ulceration, and round about these we have marked duskiness. Æsculus cures varicose leg ulcers *with a purplish areola.* When we study the hæmorrhoidal state we see *the tumor is purple,* looking almost as if it would slough. The remedy is not active in its inflammatory state, *it is sluggish and passive.* Certain remedies produce a slight inflammation with a high degree of redness, everything is violent and rapid, but in this medicine things are slow; the activities are reduced, the heart is laboring and the veins are congested.

"Eructations: sour, greasy, bitter." "Desire to vomit." *"Heart-burn and gulping up of food after eating."* It has a great *disturbance of digestion,* and we can see by these symptoms that we must class it with *Phosphorus* and *Ferrum.* As soon as the patient has swallowed the food, or a little while after, it becomes sour and he eructates it, until after a while he has emptied the stomach of its contents. Such is the state of *Phosphorus, Ferrum, Arsenicum,*

Æsculus and a few other medicines. Æsculus has also a state of congestion and ulceration of the stomach. "Constant distress and burning in the stomach. inclination to vomit." Such a state as this might be present in ulceration of the stomach.

The *abdomen* is full of trouble. If we read the symptoms of the right hypochondrium, of the abdomen and of the rectum, we shall see from the study of these that there must he a marked portal stasis. Digestion is slow, the bowels are constipated and there is protrusion of the rectum when at stool. It has most troublesome *hæmorrhoids* with *fulness of the right hypochondrium*. The liver is full of suffering. After eating there is distress in the bowels and rectum. Sticking, jagging, burning pains, as if the rectum were *full of sticks*. Great suffering with blind hæmorrhoids. The hæmorrhoidal veins are all distended and ulcerate. The stool becomes jammed into the rectum, against these distended veins, and then ulceration takes place with bleeding and great suffering. This remedy is often supposed to be suitable to hæmorrhoids that do not bleed, but it cures bleeding piles also. We find in the text over two pages devoted to the symptoms of the rectum. Great soreness; much pain; urging to stool; dark stool followed by white one, showing the liver engorgement. Chronic constipation.

The *back* is the seat of much trouble, especially low down in the back, through the sacrum and hips; although there is also aching all along the back and pain in the back of the neck. It is a very common thing for patients suffering from hæmorrhoids to have pain in the back of the neck and base of the brain, basilar headaches, and when these. hæmorrhoidal patients undertake to walk they have pain and aching across the sacrum into the hips. *This pain through the sacrum and into the hips, when walking, is a striking feature of* Æsculus, so striking that you may expect it to be present even when there are no hæmorrhoids.

Constant dull backache; walking is almost impossible; scareely able to rise or walk after sitting. You will see one suffering from the Æsculus backache, on attempting to rise from sitting, make many painful efforts before he finally succeeds. This is found in *Sulphur, Petroleum* and is also cured by *Agaricus.*

Æsculus is indicated oftentimes in the *troubles of women,* with great dragging pain in the pelvis. Many a time has Æsculus cured the dragging-down pain of the pelvis with copious leucorrhœa and *pressing pain in the hips when walking.* The woman feels that the uterus is engorged. She says that the lower part of the abdomen feels full, both before and during menstruation. There is much suffering at this time with pains in the hips. "Uterine soreness, with throbbing in the hypogastrium." "Old cases of leucorrhœa, discharge of a dark yellow color, thick and sticky." "Leucor-rhœa, *with lameness in the back across sacroiliac articulations. "* During pregnancy there are many complaints, with soreness and fulness and uneasy consciousness of the uterus and pain across the back when walking.

Æsculus is full of *gouty sufferings;* gout in all the joints, gouty rheumatic affections, neuralgic affections. Especially is this rheumatic tendency found from the elbows to the hands, in the forearm and hands. Rending, tearing pains, flying hither and thither without any particular order, relieved by heat. Varicose veins of the thighs and legs have been cured by Æsculus (*Fluoric acid*). This varicose tendency in the body we have already seen is a striking feature of Æsculus. After the sore throat has passed away, engorged veins are left, which Æsculus sometimes cures. After eye troubles have been cured, varicose veins remain in the eye. With rheumatic complaints there are varicose veins. It is one of the most frequently indicated remedies in the haemorrhoidal constitution, as it used to be called.

ÆTHUSA CYNAPIUM

Before Æthusa was known a certain class of cases of cholera infantum, and vomiting and diarrhœa in children, all resulted fatally, because there was no remedy that looked like such serious cases. Death is stamped on the face from the beginning, and if there are any remedies in the book that save life this is one of them. It applies to the cases that come on very suddenly in hot weather in infancy, with extreme prostration. The mother does not suspect the child is sick until she takes it from the crib; only a few hours before it was well; but when cholera infantum is prevalent in hot weather, this little one fills its stomach with milk and almost before it has had time to coagulate or form into curds the milk comes up partly in curds and partly liquid, and accompanying the vomiting there is a thin, yellow greenish, slimy stool. The child has the appearance as if it were dying, pale hippocratic face, there is a whitish-blue pallor around the lips, the eyes are sunken and there is a sunken condition around the nose. The mother is astonished and sends for the doctor hurriedly. The child sinks into an exhausted sleep. It wakes up and again fills the stomach with milk which comes up again in a few minutes, partly in curd and partly liquid, and again there is the awful exhaustion, deathly appearance and prolonged sleep. Without Æthusa, in two or three days the undertaker gets that child. That is pretty nearly the whole story of Æthusa.

It has delirium, it has excitement, it has mental disturbances of various kinds, but they are acute and accompany the brain troubles. A certain class of infants come down sick in the hot weather, in the hot nights, and they get brain trouble, and from that time the stomach quits business, the bowels become relaxed, and everything put into the stomach either comes up or goes right through. This occurs especially in those infants that have been fed as the ordinary everyday mother feeds her baby, and how is that? Every time it cries she puts it to the breast or feeds it. Well, now; let us think a bit. Every doctor ought to think a little, once in a while. Now meditate a trifle as to whether that is a wise or foolish thing to do. It takes about two hours or two hours and a half for the ordinary baby's stomach to transact good wholesome business in digesting the milk taken, and it ought to have a rest of half an hour or so, and when we get up to three hours and the baby cries then it is probably hungry and will be glad to take some more and digest it. Any shorter interval of feeding than that is bad practice. It would be just the same thing if the child should take half a teacupful of milk and let it partly digest, and in a little while take a little more, and then later add a little more. It commences to spit up its food and it is sour, and the very first spell of hot weather that comes brings on head trouble. Only the toughest children will stand this bad method. I have watched these children and seen them stand it until the summer. The doctor must put his foot down, and put it down violently, and make them see he means it. The old woman comes in and says: "That doctor does not know anything" and the baby must be fed. Now Æthusa suits improperly fed babies. It is at the head of the list of medicines for that condition; that is, when digestion has absolutely ceased from brain trouble. So far as busy doctors have discovered the call for this remedy, it has been mostly among babies, but adults sometimes take on an Æthusa state, when digestion has absolutely ceased from brain trouble and from excitement. It has cured dyspepsia from constant feeding, in those nibblers, those hungry fellows who are always eating, always nibbling, always taking crackers in their pockets until there comes a time when the stomach ceases to act. It also suits cases of indigestion from head troubles, with hot head, vomiting, exhaustion, sweat and long sleep.

Æthusa has convulsions in children. Sometimes the brain trouble does not affect the stomach, but the child goes into convulsions, with clammy hands, deathly countenance, and the sweat, exhaustion and sleep. "Convulsions, great weakness and prostration, with sleepiness. Dosing of the child after vomiting and after stool, with convulsions."

In the Æthusa patient there is much in the face and aspect to indicate a remedy; so much can be seen and comes within the observation, and so little questioning is necessary, that a sort of snap-shot prescribing can be done, but it is not to be recommended. A busy physician, one who really and truly studies his Materia Medica, and has learned the principles, will in time do a great deal of what seems to he snap-shot prescribing, but he really does not so, because he puts together many things that outsiders would not think of. Æthusa then shows itself upon the surface, whereas in many remedies there is nothing seen upon the surface, because they manifest themselves in inner or deeper sensations. Let me lay a case before you to illustrate this. For instance, take a robust looking fellow, who declares himself fairly well, out to lunch with you. You have noticed for some time that his nose is all the time peeling off; at once there is a star. He never talks about his health. Pretty soon, while lunching, the door slams and he jumps. That is the second point. Then he tells you how much he eats, how well it affects him, how good he feels after eating, and you have noticed yourself that he eats a good deal. You have not said one word about his health to him. You have not asked him to tell you any symptoms. Finally you shove the pitcher of milk over to him, and he says, "Oh, I can't drink milk; if I take milk it gives me diarrhœa; I never think of taking it." Who could not prescribe for that fellow without taking him into the office? Who would think of anything but *Natrum carb.* for such a case? Sometimes you can find out the whole story by getting a stubborn patient to go and dine with you.

AGARICUS MUSCARIUS

The most striking things running through this medicine are twitchings and tremblings. Jerkings of the muscles and trembling of the limbs; quivering and tremors, everywhere these two features are present in all parts of the body and limbs. The twitching of the muscles becomes so extensive that it is a well-developed case of chorea It has in its nature all that is found in chorea and has cured many cases. This is a general belonging to all parts, to all muscles. Throughout the body there is a sensation of creeping and crawling. It is hardly confined to the skin, it is felt as if in the flesh, a sensation as if of ants. Itching of the skin all over which changes place from scratching. No place is exempt from this. There are strange sensations here and there upon the skin or in parts, cold sensations, sensations of cold needles and of hot needles; stinging and burning where the circulation is feeble, about the ears, nose, back of hands and fingers and toes, red spots with itching and burning as if frostbitten. It is a great remedy for chilblains. The patient is extremely nervous and sensitive to cold. Itching, pricking, tingling, etc., come on from mental exertion and are relieved from physical exertion. All the symptoms of Agaricus are also aggravated after sexual intercourse. especially in the symptoms of the spinal cord. It is useful for the symptoms which come on after coition in young, nervous married women, hysterical fainting after coition.

The *mental* symptoms are such as you would expect. Great changeability, irritability, mental depression and complaints which come on from overexertion of the mind and prolonged study. The brain seems to be developed tardily.

Children are late in learning to talk and walk, thus combining the features of two remedies, *Natrum muriaticum,* which has the symptom "late learning to talk," and *Calcarea carb.,* which has the symptom "late learning to walk." It will be noticed in *Calcarea* that this is due to a defect in bone weakness. In Agaricus it is a mental defect, a slowly developing mind. Children with twitching and early fainting, nervous girls prior to puberty who have convulsions from being scolded, from excitement and shock; late in mental development. Children who cannot remember, make mistakes and are slow in learning. Nervous patients who on going over their manuscripts find out their mistakes in writing and spelling. The condition of the mind is one in which they are slow to grasp ideas; wrong words float in kaleidoscopically. When, we read in the book "the whole psychological sphere as if paralyzed," we must read between the lines. The whole mind and sensorium seem paralyzed; the patient is sluggish, stupid, at times seems to be delirious; there is confusion of the mind so nearly like delirium that it is not unlike intoxication. A delirium such as is produced by alcohol. He also becomes silly, says foolish and silly things, sings and whistles at an inopportune time, makes verses and prophesies; or he lapses into an opposite state, becomes indifferent to his surroundings. One who is mild and placid becomes self-willed, obstinate and conceited.

Difficulty in co-ordinating the movements of the muscles of the body. Incoordination of brain and spinal cord. Clumsy motion of the fingers and hands. In handling things she drops them. Fingers fly open spasmodically while holding things. You will sometimes cure Bridget in the kitchen with Agaricus or *Apis,* when the trouble is that she is continually breaking the dishes by letting them fall. These two remedies are opposites, Agaricus must stay near the fire, while *Apis* she wants to get out of the kitchen. The awkardness, clumsiness, etc., are both mental and bodily. Every sort of change is rung on the patient and the doctor. At times the patient is stupid, awkward and clumsy, at other times quick and poetical, can run off poetry without effort, *especially at night.* In the morning he is tired and sluggish and this may last till noon. The mental symptoms are worse in the morning and are relieved towards evening. All jerkings and twitchings subside during sleep. There is vertigo when walking in the open air. He is always chilly. On undertaking to do something he does the opposite. Vertigo and confusion of mind are mixed up.

It is a common feature for the headaches of this remedy to be associated with the spinal symptoms, the quivering and jerking. Headaches in spinal patients. Pain as though sharp ice touched the head, or as if from cold needles. That is general; we find it in other parts. Pain in the head as if from a nail. There is some bleeding in the morning, and the blood is thick, black and will hardly drop. Coldness in the head. In the scalp there are all sorts of queer sensations; icy coldness after itching or scratching. That runs all through the body. There is itching, although no eruption is visible; can't let it alone, and after scratching there is a sensation of icy coldness in the part or as if the wind was blowing on it. The head is in constant motion as in chorea. Itching of the scalp, especially in the morning on rising. There again we have the general aggravation in the morning. There are marked eruptions on the scalp. Eczema with crusts.

Twitching and jerking of the eyes. You will observe this about the Agaricus eyes; as the patient looks at you there is a pendulum-like action of the eyes, they go back and forth all the time; they oscillate, though he tries his best to fix his look on you. This stops only during sleep; all the motions subside during sleep. A few other medicines have cured this eye symptom, *Cicuta, Arsenicurn, Sulphur, Pulsatilla,* but Agaricus also produces and cures it. There is every conceivable kind of deception in colors and in vision. Flickering before the eyes; he reads with difficulty. Objects seem to be where they are not. Black flies before the eyes; black motes; sees double; floating flies before the eyes. Muscular weakness of the eyes. Irregularity of the motions of the eyes; pupils dilated; pupils contracted. Sensation as of a mist or cobweb before the eyes. Spasmodic twitching and jerking. The jerkings and twitchings are the most marked symptoms, as also the choreic movements about the eyes, and the deceptions in colors and figures before the eyes.

Redness, burning and itching of the ears as if they had been frostbitten. The sensation as of chilblains, the same sensation as found throughout; the same itching and tingling as of the remedy in general. Dulness of hearing. Deafness. Hearing acute. In the morning he is dumb, sluggish, stupid, tired, but when evening comes he brightens up, becomes warmed up, becomes excited, poetical and prophetical, wants to sit up late at night, is brilliant, wants to play games.

Nosebleed; profuse, fœtid discharge from the nose. Agaricus will cure the most inveterate chronic catarrhs with dryness and crusts, in tubercular constitutions, so deep-seated is it. It has cured many cases of incipient phthisis. It cures old coughs and catarrhs. Red nose, as if frostbitten. It is as good as *Ledum* and *Lachesis* for the red-tipped nose in old drunkards.

From what we have already seen we expect twitching of the muscles of the face, and itching and redness and burning as if frostbitten, paralytic weakness, etc., because these are general features, and just as we expect we see these things in the text. Choreic spasms. Expression as of idiocy. Now notice this: Some patients when going on with their own usual vocation are pretty smart, but if you put some new idea before them, something not in the routine of their work, they are perfectly idiotic. This is especially noticeable in the morning. He can't take in, anything new in the morning, but he is able to take in new ideas and is bright in the evening, like the effect produced by tea and coffee and alcoholic beverages. This remedy is a great antidote to alcoholic beverages. In this remedy and in *Zincum* the spine is affected and both of these have aggravation from stimulants.

Agaricus has cured many cases of epileptiform convulsions, more commonly the hysterio-epileptic type with frothing of the mouth, opisthotonos, drawing of the muscles of the face. The Agaricus patient has spells in which a little muscle of the face or a few fibres of a muscle will quiver for a few minutes and stop, and then in another part of the face the same thing, an eyelid will quiver, and then another set of fibres, sometimes so bad as to nearly drive him crazy. Such is an Agaricus state as well as *Nux vomica.*

The teeth feel too long and are sensitive to touch. The tongue quivers, twitches, jerks and causes disorderly speech; articulates violently. Tongue dry, tremulous. Learns to speak with difficulty. Spasms of the tongue, inarticulate speech. Phagedenic ulcer on the frænum of the tongue; eats it away. Soreness of the tongue. Mercurial aphthæ in roof of mouth. Little white blisters like nursing sore mouth. Chronic sore throat. Induration of tonsils. Burning thirst, ravenous appetite. Gnawing in stomach as if from hunger, without desire for food.

Flatus; distressing belching; great tympanites; rumbling; turmoil in abdomen; offensive flatus; rumbling and gurgling in belly. Everything ferments; rumbling and loud rolling; pinching colic. Horribly fœtid discharge. Tympanitic condition marked in typhoid; low type of typhoid; trembling and jerking of muscles; paralytic weakness; emaciation; mental symptoms.

Morning diarrhœa, great deal of hot flatus (*Alöe*), with burning in the rectum; soft stool; great tenesmus; urging to stool violent; involuntary straining before, during and after stool. Sensation as if rectum would burst, even after stool (*Merc.* and *Sul.*). Violent, sudden pains; can't wait; distressing, bursting sensation. *Before* stool, cutting and pinching in abdomen; urgent tenesmus; painful straining in rectum. *During* stool, colic and passing of flatus; burning, soreness, smarting and cutting in anus; sweat; pain in loins to legs, continuing after stool. *After* stool, headache relieved; biting in anus; *straining in rectum;* cutting pain in anus; griping in hypogastrium; distension in abdomen; heaviness in abdomen and around navel; pain in chest. Emphasize the *tenesmus after stool.*

May have constipation and paralytic feelings of the rectum; stool hard; straining at stool as if life depended on it and yet no stool. Beginning paralysis of the lower limbs, with twitching of the muscles and burning spine. In one case, after straining had been given up as unsuccessful would pass a stool involuntarily. This symptom only was known in *Arg. n.* (stool and urine). Desire to urinate as urgent as the desire for stool. Dribbling of urine. A peculiar feature of this remedy is that the urine feels cold on passing; while the urine dribbles, can count the cold drops along the urethra. "Urine passes slowly in a stream or in drops, has to press to promote the flow." "Urine watery, clear, lemon-colored, bright yellow; dark yellow and hot; red, flocculent, a powdery sediment; watery in the forenoon, in the afternoon milky, like whey, with a red or white sediment (phosphate of magnesia); iridizing on surface." Phosphates; milky urine. Oily surface, iridescent surface, greasy-like pellicle on urine, like petroleum. Scanty urine in rheumatic, gouty, hysterical subjects. Persons cold, feeble, pale, going into phthisis. Urine becomes scanty and a headache comes on. Goes many days and is constipated, and headache relieved by stool. In *Fluoric acid,* if he does not attend to the desire to urinate, a headache comes on.

Transformation takes place. The milk ceases in one day, but congestion of the brain or spine comes on. Metastasis, especially if milk ceases and complaints come on.

Genital organs cold and shrunken. The comparative examination of the symptoms of male and female sexual organs shows that the proving has not been extensively made on the female, but in the male there are many symptoms which have an analogous condition in the female. In the male, symptoms are worse after coition, but just as marked in the female. Complaints after sexual excitement, debauch, etc., in the woman, fainting; in the man, weakness. The trembling and twitching, or any of the Agaricus symptoms, may be worse after coition, because the sexual functions are related to the cord. Those suffering from spinal affections have distress after this act.

In the *male,* during coition, burning in the urethra comes from excoriation or a mice of hotness of the seminal fluid while being ejected, and hence can only be a symptom of the male. Burning in the prostate during ejaculation. Violent sexual excitement before and during, but at the time of ejaculation the orgasm is wanting, it is a passive and pleasureless ejaculation. This occurs in men with spinal weakness, nervous men who have tingling and crawling all over. It comes in the cure of old catarrhal discharge from the urethra, chronic gonorrhœa, gleet, after all sorts of local treatment have been used. The penis is cold and shrunken; excessively painful retraction in testes. In old gleety discharge where there is a continued itching tingling in the urethra and the last drop will remain, discharging for a long rime. There are two remedies better for this than many others, *Petroleum* and Agaricus.

The routine prescriber always thinks of *Puls., Sep., etc.,* for bearingdown pains in the female, but in a woman with spinal irritation, etc., with the dragging-down sensation as if the parts would drop into the world, this remedy is the best. Those slender, nervous, restless women with tingling and creeping, must have Agaricus. During menses, headache, toothache, etc. All the general symptoms are worse during the menstrual period, not to any great extent before or after. Aggravation of the heart symptoms and prolapsus just at the close of the menses.

Leucorrhœa very profuse, dark, bloody, acrid, excoriating in parts. This remedy has been mentioned in relation to *Fluoric acid.* There are many points of relation. They are like each other in the leucorrhœa especially; copious and *acrid,* so acrid that it keeps the parts raw and irritated around the genitals and the patient can't walk. In *Fluoric acid* there is, with the nervous symptoms, headache ameliorated by passing the urine, or headache if urination is not immediately attended to, with copious, acrid, excoriating leucorrhœa.

Agaricus is a great remedy in *chest* troubles, though seldom thought of. It has cured what seemed to he consumption. Catarrhal condition of the chest, with night sweats and history of the nervous symptoms. Violent cough in isolated attacks ending in sneezing. Convulsive cough, with sweat towards evening, with frequent pulse, expectoration of pus-like mucus, worse in the mornings and when lying on the back. Add to this the symptoms of Agaricus as described, and Agaricus will take hold of that case. Cases of incipient phthisis. It closely relates to the tubercular diathesis. I remember starting out to prove *Tuberculinum* on an individual I suspected would be sensitive to it from his history and symptoms. The first dose almost killed him, and, considering the use that that substance is put to in diagnosing the disease in cattle, it seemed to stir him up. He became emaciated and looked as if he would die. I let it alone and watched and waited patiently and the symptoms of Agaricus came up and established the relationship between these two remedies, and confirmed Hering's observation of the relationship of Agaricus to the tubercular diathesis. Agaricus cured him and fattened him up.

The remedy is full of nervous palpitation; worse in the evening. It cures shocks and thrills in the heart; spasms of the heart; internal manifestations of its jerking symptoms. These shocks come from sudden noise; from eructations; on coughing; when lying on the left side or back; worse at night; during fever; they often extend to other parts, as to abdomen or back or limbs. On the outer chest there is tingling and creeping as in general.

The *back* has many peculiar and general guiding symptoms. Stiffness of the whole spine. Feeling as if it would break when he attempts to bend. Feels as if something is so right that it will break when he stoops. Tightness in the muscles of the back. Tingling deep in the spine. Violent, shooting, burning pains. Pain along the spine, worse by stooping. Pains of all sorts in the spine. Pains go up the back and down the back. Sensitiveness of the spine to touch, especially in the back of the neck and dorsal region between the scapulæ? Sensitive to a hot sponge in the lumbar region in spinal irritation. Sensation as if cold air were spreading along the back like an aura epileptica.

Sensation of ice touching the body. Cold spots. Chilliness over the back, crawling, creeping and formication. Numbness of skin over the back. The most of the pains are in the back of the neck and the lumbo-sacral region. Pains in this region in connection with coition. Pain in the lumbar region and sacral region, especially during exertion, sitting, etc. Pain in the sacrum as if beaten, as if it would break. Pains below the waist in women.

In the limbs in general there are twitchings; they are numb, choreic; burning here and there; cold feelings in spots, paralyzed. Trembling of limbs, hands, awkwardness of all the movements. Rheumatism and gout of joints. Paralysis of the lower limbs. Trembling and weakness of the lower limbs.

Burning itching of the hands as if frozen. In the smaller joints, where the circulation is feeble, there are frostbite symptoms. Toes and fingers stiff.

Bones feel as if they would break during rest, especially in the lower limbs. Feeling as if the tibia would break. Aching in the tibia. Growing pains in children and they must sit at the fire or the extremities will get cold. Pains in the bones. Weight in the legs. Pains in the lower limbs; aching; stitching; tearing; better from warmth and from motion.

Paralytic weakness in the lower limbs soon after becoming pregnant. This comes with every pregnancy and she must go to bed. The symptoms may lead to Agaricus. Weight in the legs. Legs feel heavy. Trembling and jerking motion in the lower limbs.

AGNUS CASTUS

This wonderful remedy is often overlooked. It should come to mind for old sufferers who are broken from sexual excesses and secret vice. The pale sickly and sad mortals who lament over their misspent life. It is good for both sexes. Sexual weakness; relaxation of parts. Perversion of all the functions.

A woman who indulged extensively in secret vice, found after marriage that she had no sexual thrill, was cured by this remedy. Later she was confined and no milk came in her mammæ, again Agnus started the belated milk at the end of three weeks.

When the milk ceases after it has started, or becomes scanty when the above history is known, and the woman is sad, this remedy will, if not opposed, most likely cure.

It cures uterine hæmorrhage, and restores suppressed menses in young women with a history. The vagina is much relaxed, there is often prolapsus, and there is a copious white-of-egg-like. leucorrhœa.

But the pitiful, woebegone young man, heart-broken over his early life, now finds himself newly married, and impotent. He has had gonorrhœa; he has lived in excesses, and now suffers from relaxed and cold genitalia, emissions, prostatic discharge at stool. His young and beautiful wife excites no erection, though only recently he had a clandestine success, and he has morning erections but no more.

Out of the above cause and condition come many distressing symptoms. Loss of memory, despair, suicidal thoughts, anxiety, fear and peevishness. These patients suffer from headaches, photophobia and nervous symptoms too numerous to mention. Formication of the skin. Tearing pains to head, face and teeth. All but the simplest food disorders the stomach, and he complains much of nausea. His muscles are flabby. He is anæmic, and his glands are enlarged, especially the spleen. He is growing increasingly flatulent. The abdominal viscera hang down as a weight. There is a growing weakness of the rectum and constipation, and he presses hard at stool, which often fails and slips back, like *Silica, Sanic* and *Thuja.* The stool is large and hard. Itching, smarting at the anus, noisy flatus of a urinous odor. Excoriated anus. He soon takes on a hacking cough and night sweats. The limbs are tired and cold. He is sensitive to cold, and wants to remain quiet. Exertion and motion intensify his complaints. He has been to many advisers, and they have told him he has *Neurasthenia.* He must have Agnus castus.

AILANTHUS GLANDULOSA

This medicine is especially suitable in the low zymotic forms of sickness, such as we find in diphtheria and scarlet fever, in blood poisoning and in symptomatic typhoids, especially those cases that are characterized by capillary congestion in spots, red mottled spots. Perhaps the most striking manifestation of such a low type of sickness is malignant scarlet fever. The regular rash does not come out, but in its place red spots, roseola-like, make their appearance; the usual uniform spread of the eruption has failed, or has been suppressed, and there is bleeding from the gums and nose, and dreadful tumefaction in the throat. The countenance is purple and besotted, the eyes are congested and there is even bleeding from the eyes. There is an appearance of great prostration, but it is really stupefaction; he Seems stupid and benumbed. If you look at the throat you see it is covered with little purple patches, intermingled with an edematous appearance similar to that found in *Baptisia.* It is a low depressed type of sickness. Decomposition of the blood is going on rapidly. The blood that oozes is black. The child is going into a state of stupor and it is with difficulty that he can be aroused. Sometimes blisters are formed on the ends of fingers, or here and there over the body. From the mouth and nose come fœtid odors.

The child is going as rapidly as possible into a form of malignant disease. Sometimes the disease comes on as a light febrile attack, but from taking cold and suppressing some of the natural manifestations the case takes on a low typhoid form and whereas you had at first only a simple remittent, the case has now assumed a state of prostration with a very rapid heart, fœtor, purpleness or blueness, a passive congestion with purple blotches of the skin, causing a mottled appearance. When a disease turns so suddenly blood poisoning is going on and a symptomatic typhoid state appears. A remittent that turns into a sharp zymotic state in the course of twenty-four hours, a diphtheria that takes on this form with stupidity and mottled skin are examples of such a type of sickness.

The mental symptoms accompanying this state are interesting. I read from some notes I have made. A continued dreamy state of mind though awake. Child cries all the time. Sees little animals like rats running around. Feels a rat or something small crawling up the limb and over the body. There seems to he constant loss of memory, even the things spoken of a moment ago go right out of the mind. Constant forgetfulness. All past events are forgotten. Past events are forgotten or remembered as belonging to someone else, or as matters read. That is in keeping with the dreamy state, it seems as though those things that are past appear as in a dream, as if he had dreamed them. Cannot concentrate the mind in any mental effort; cannot answer questions correctly; is as if in a semi-conscious state, and finally he goes into complete unconsciousness. There is in the earlier stages of this zymotic state great anxiety and restlessness, later there is stupor and indifference to everything. Continual sighing with depression of spirits; extremely irritable, semi-conscious, finally unconsciousness, stupor delirium and insensibility; muttering delirium with sleeplessness and restlessness. This mental state is such as occurs in zymotic sickness; the chronic illness has not been well brought out. Dr. Wells used this remedy in a number of cases, as it was at that time an epidemic remedy for scarlet fever, in Brooklyn, and many patients were saved by it. It seemed to be able to change the character of the malignant forms of scarlet fever into a mild type.

In addition to the symptoms of the text it has been observed that the hair falls out and flashes of light play before the eyes on closing the lids at night. "Pupils widely dilated; copious, thin, ichorous and bloody discharge from the nose." That is in the zymotic states in scarlet fever. "Nostrils congested. Great prostration and a countenance indicating much distress. Face dark as mahogany." That is in suppressed scarlet fever. Purple, bloated and puffed, besotted face. This remedy is one not very much used, and it is not very often indicated, but it is very useful when indicated. You will not very often see this particular type even in malignant scarlet fever. You will often see such a scarlet fever running to a number of other remedies, but this remedy corresponds to one or the most malignant types, and its commonest use will be in an epidemic in which the cases largely run to the malignant type. There are three common types of scarlet fever. In one season you find the cases are mild and simple, the typical eruption is present and comes on speedily without any great amount of fever. Such cases will often run their course with good nursing, a warm room and plenty of clothing without much medicine. The skin is bright red, smooth and shiny. The case is not serious. In other epidemics you will find only an isolated case of this kind, while the majority of cases present marked trouble in the throat; the rash is scanty when present, and congestion of the head and spinal symptoms come on with pain in the back of the neck. The throat is dreadfully swollen and inflamed, bright red and very painful. Then there is a third type in which the throat is severely swollen, all the mucous membranes are swollen, and the whole tendency is toward blood poisoning or zymosis with enlargement of the glands, puffiness of the skin and a great deal of fœtor; the skin is dusky and the eruption is scanty, sometimes hardly visible from beginning to end. These cases will almost all die if let alone; they are very serious. The old authors call these three forms "scarlatina simplex," "scarlatina anginosa," and "scarlatina maligna." In some epidemics you will see all three of the appearances, in some families you will see two forms. One child will have a mild type, and another will have it more severely with zymotic blisters here and there, on the ends of the fingers and these will be attended with foetor; as soon as the blisters break ulceration wilt take place if the child live long enough; but these are the deadly cases, the malignant type. Even when the rash does not come out in the low forms of scarlet fever, the impression of the finger makes a white mark which will be slow to fill up. The more marked that is, the lower the type. The more zymotic the type the more sluggish the circulation, and in this remedy especially is this state present. The congested condition of the skin is present even when there is no rash, a passive congestion of the veins. Quite a number of medicines have that, but *Veratrum viride* produces such a vaso-motor paralysis that a line upon the skin made by pressure will remain a long time. In all these zymotic complaints there is a fœtid odor that is sometimes cadaveric, sometimes like stinking meat; this will be found in the low types of disease where this remedy is indicated.

"Throat much swollen, dark red, almost purple in color. Diphtheria with extreme prostration. Throat livid, swollen; tonsils prominent and studded with deep ulcers." The throat and tonsils very often appear as if they would pit upon pressure like a dropsical state. In some of these zymotic cases where a reaction ought to take place a diarrhœa sets in that is horribly offensive; a critical diarrhœa. With these zymotic states there is pain in the back of the neck and head no matter what the name of the disease is.

"Breathing hurried, irregular, heavy. Burning in the palms and soles, hunts to find a cool place to put them. Feels a rat running up the leg. Feeling as if a snake crawled up the leg." These mental symptoms occurred in one of my provers. In low, adynamic forms of disease characterized by sudden and extreme prostration, "vomiting, pulse small and rapid, purplish appearance of skin." "Electric thrills from brain to extremities." "Chill at 8 A.M. with chill, heat and sweat." During the chill vomiting of food and piercing pain over the hip. Chill is preceded by malignant eruption, especially on the face and forehead. "During chill hunger, empty feeling, intolerable pain in back of neck, upper part of back and hip joint." That pain in the back of the neck is a common forerunner of low types of fever. It generally precedes a congestive attack of great violence characterized by fulness of the head with heat.

This miliary rash spoken of in the text, looking like measles, is when the scarlet fever rash or the measles rash does not come out in its uniform fashion, but in patches, little circles here and there and is dark. "Irregular, patchy, livid eruption, disappearing on pressure and returning very slowly; interspersed with small vesicles, worse on forehead, neck and chest. Eruption appeared scantily for two days with sore throat and mild fever." This eruption is like the petechiæ that we see in typhoid forms of disease. The record of this remedy in scarlet fever makes it worthy of further study; it ought to be reproved that we may have a fuller understanding of it. "Eruption plentiful, of a bluish tint. Typhoid scarlatina." "Eruption is slow to make its appearance, remains livid". "Body and limbs covered with an irregular patchy eruption of a very livid color." Here you see but one type of scarlet fever. This low type of fever sometimes needs *Sulphur,* or *Phosphorus,* or *Belladonna,* or *Baptisia,* or *Lachesis.* That you may be able to distinguish one from the other and keep the picture of each remedy clearly in mind requires a prolonged study of the Materia Medica. It is an easy matter to compare remedies for yourself after you have first studied each one separately. You can then bring out many comparisons, and especially in this case at the bedside. If you go to the bedside with a good knowledge of the generals of Materia Medica you will be surprised at the number of symptom pictures which will come into your mind, called up by the signs of the sickness. When you go to the bedside of scarlet fever you should not call to mind the names of these medicines you may have heard recommended for scarlet fever; let the appearance of the patient bring to mind such remedies as appear like this patient, regardless of whether they have been associated with scarlet fever or not. When you see the rash perhaps you will say that looks like an *Aconite* ram but there is such scanty zymosis in the nature of *Aconite* that it is no longer thought of. *Belladonna* is not suitable, for in that remedy the rash is shiny and smooth, the typical Sydenham rash. On the other hand, you will say *Pulsatilla* has a measly rash, and often associated with a low form of fever, but not so low as the typhoid type, so *Pulsatilla* goes out of your mind. You now think of the remedies that are typical of all zymotic states; the prostration, the aggravation after sleep, general stupor and delirium, and almost at a glance you see *Lachesis,* the type of such forms of disease. Its picture comes into your mind speedily. You see another case of scarlet fever where there is a scanty rash, the child before you keeps on picking the skin from the lips and nose, lies in a state of pallor and exhaustion, no rash to speak of, urine nearly suppressed; almost in a moment you think of *Arum triph.* It is the aspect of things that will call the remedy to the mind. In another case you have all the purple appearance I have spoken of in this remedy; horrible fœtor, a good deal of sore throat, and the child cannot get water cold enough, wants a stream of water running down the throat all the time; you may safely trust to *Phosphorus.* In these low types of sickness there is always something to tell the story if you will only listen, study and wait long enough.

ALETRIS FARINOSA

This most useful and neglected remedy has been frequently indicated in the complaints of women, especially in those predisposed to hemorrhages; uterine hemorrhages particularly whether it be after an abortion or in connection with menstruation. Copious bleeding from the uterus is characteristic; hemorrhages when the uterus fills with blood until it becomes distended, and its contents are expelled in large clots, followed by copious hemorrhage with or without painful contractions.

A copious menstrual flow followed by watery oozing during the intermenstrual period, now and then dilating into copious gushing flow with black clots; this remedy is useful at the critical period when it is attended with hemorrhage.

The hemorrhages of this medicine are particularly due to a relaxed or debilitated state of the uterus. Weakness of the reproductive organs may be said to be the guiding feature; atony. Weakness of the uterus with repeated abortion or hemorrhages with debility of the individual. Bruised feeling in the region of the ovaries, particularly in the right. Bearing down in the region of the uterus as if the contents of the pelvis would escape. Much worse while walking.

An attack of hemorrhage that came on with great violence in the middle of the night, the patient waking, unable to speak, so exhausted from the flow: was cured by Aletris 45m. This patient lost her urine when coughing, sleeping or walking, and this symptom which has been present many years was entirely cured by Aletris. This involuntary escape of urine was always brought on by catching cold.

Digest for food; nausea; obstinate indigestion.

The patient has a pale sickly chlorotic face, would like to lie down all day and do nothing but rest. Such debilitated patients when they become pregnant, suffer from vomiting and colic; the stomach seems to be in the same weak condition as the reproductive organs.

Most inveterate constipation.

Until this remedy was known, Kreosote was the most promising remedy for copious frothy eructations with vomiting; this remedy must take the place of Kreosote in the vomiting of pregnant women, when the symptoms agree.

There are violent pains in the rectum and anus. Stool very large and hard, most difficult to expel. Painful constipation.

ALLIUM CEPA

Allium cepa is used principally for "colds." There are various phases of these "colds," in the nose, in the throat, in the larynx, in the bronchial tubes. The patient and all the phases of his "cold," his coryza, his laryngitis, his cough, all his complaints, are aggravated by warmth, are worse in a warm room, excepting the tickling in the larynx, which is sometimes aggravated by drawing in cold air. In this way the cough is sometimes excited by cold air, but the patient himself is better in cold air and sensitive to heat. Most of the symptoms are worse in the evening, the symptoms of coryza, the "cold," and the general symptoms. These are the two most striking general features of Allium cepa.

It is not strange that the old ladies used to bind onions on the ear for earache and around the neck for sore throats, for onion is very frequently indicated in almost every climate for the effects of cold. Cold, damp, penetrating winds, in any climate, are likely to bring on Allium cepa complaints—coryza, la grippe, influenza or whatever they may be called, and usually there is a congestive headache. Rawness in the nose, copious flow of water from the eyes, which is always bland; copious watery discharge from the nose, which is always excoriating. Rawness in the larynx and throat, extending down into the chest. Rawness in the nose. In twenty-four hours it reaches the larynx. Cough, excited by tickling in the larynx and when lying down at night in a warm room. On going to bed in the evening Allium has its most troublesome aggravation. I have heard patients describe the pain in the larynx on coughing, saying that it felt as if someone was reaching down with a hook at every cough. Tearing in the larynx with every cough. Sneezing, rawness of all the mucous membranes and that tearing cough, all symptoms worse in a warm room and in the evening; it is astonishing how quickly the onion will break up that "cold.'

Now we will take up the particulars of the coryza. Among the earlier symptoms will be the sneezing, which comes with increasing frequency. A watery discharge drips from the nose constantly, burns like fire, and excoriates the upper lip and the wings of the nose until there are rawness and redness. Notice that the fluid from the nose is excoriating and the fluid from the eyes bland. Bear that in mind, for when we come to study *Euphrasia* we will find just the opposite. We will find just such a watery discharge from the nose and such copious lachrymation; but the lachrymation is acrid and the discharge from the nose bland. The nasal discharge of Cepa fairly eats the hair off of the upper lip. And there is so much congestion that the patient has a sensation of fulness in the nose, with throbbing and burning, and sometimes nosebleed. Pains through the jaws, in the face; and these pains extend into the head. Dull frontal headaches, occipital headaches; headaches very severe and the eyes cannot stand the light; tearing, bursting, throbbing in the head.

Now, there is another phase of this medicine. Why it begins on the left side and goes over to the right I do not know, but it usually does this. Stuffing up of the side of the nose, watery, acrid discharge from the left side of the nose—in another twenty-four hours the right side is invaded. "Profuse nasal discharge. Colds after damp north-easterly winds." That is, after damp, cold winds, for they may conic from different directions in different localities. Fluent coryza with headache, tears from the eyes, want of appetite, cough and trembling in the open air. "Every year in August, morning coryza, with violent sneezing, very sensitive to the odor of flowers and skin of peaches." That is one form of hay fever cured by Allium cepa. It will wipe out an attack of hay fever in a few days, when the symptoms agree. You may know that the true nature of hay fever is not generally understood. It is really only an explosion of chronic disease, that is, it is a manifestation of psora, and can be eradicated only by antipsoric treatment. Many a time have I seen hay fever wiped out in one season by a short-acting remedy, only to return the next just the same, and perhaps another remedy will be required. As soon as the hay fever is stopped you must begin with constitutional treatment. There will be symptoms, if you know how to hunt for them, that differ altogether from the acute attack. When the hay fever is on these do not appear. It is a difficult matter to find a constitutional remedy when the hay fever is at its height, for it resembles an acute disease; but it is a manifestation of psora, like any other manifestation of psora, as eruptions, cough, etc. The nose may manifest only a certain phase of chronic disease in one season which may, for instance, be suited to Allium cepa. I remember one time having occasion to prescribe Allim capa at long distance. It was near a homœopathic pharmacy. I wired the pharmacist to send my patient Allium cepa, and he labeled it. Well, the patient kept the bottle and used it next season, but it did no good. That is likely to be the case, even when the symptoms seem to agree. In a psoric condition a short-acting remedy is insufficient, it may help for one day only, and the deep-acting remedy that includes the patient as well as the hay fever and all the other symptoms will have to be administered. The best time to treat hay fever is after the acute attack subsides and until it begins again the next season. It will then occur in a greatly modified form, different from any the patient has ever had, and calling for a different remedy. That will be the case if the constitutional remedy has been properly selected.

In these coryzas the inflammation soon spreads to the ears, the throat and the larynx. The old mothers used to put onions on the baby's ear when it had earache. That is not surprising, when we see all the pains and aches belonging to this remedy. Jerking pains from the throat toward the Eustachian tube. Violent earache, even to the discharge of pus from the ear. Ringing in the ears. Stiches towards the ear from the forehead. Pain like thick threads drawing from deep within the head. Stitching, tearing pains in the ear, with whooping cough, with coryza, with laryngitis. In the household where a medicine case is kept *Pulsatilla* is the standard remedy for earache, and it is true that only occasionally has a doctor to be sent for. *Pulsatilla* has such a strong affinity for the ear that it will cure earache in almost all sensitive children who cry pitifully. But those who are snappish, who are never suited, who will throw away something they have asked for and slap the nurse in the face must have *Chamomilla.* With *Pulsatilla, Chamomilla* and Allium cepa you can cure the majority of earaches in children.

Further, as to the eye-symptoms that accompany the Allium cepa colds. Remember that the discharge from the eye is bland. Although there is burning in the eyes the tears do not excoriate as they flow down over the cheek. Profuse, bland lachrymation. Lachrymation in the evening in a warm room.

We all know what a flatulent vegetable the onion is. It is wonderful medicine for babies with colic. Cutting, rending, tearing pains drawing the poor little thing almost double. It screams with the violent cutting in the lower abdomen. "Stitching pains in the abdomen." "Colicky pains beginning in the hepatic region and spreading over the whole abdomen, worse around the navel; worse when sitting." Wind colic. Allium cepa is a wonderful remedy in whooping cough, and when it is indicated the child will often have indigestion, vomiting and flatulency; will pass offensive flatus, will be doubled up with colic. Allium cepa also cures a ragged, sensitive condition of the anus, with bleeding, in infants.

Acute complaints of the voice; catarrhal hoarseness; copious expectoration of mucus from the larynx. Violent inflammation of the larynx coming on very rapidly, with that cough I spoke of, and the tearing in the larynx. Some will describe it as a sensation as if something were being torn loose. Those who describe more accurately will say that it feels as if a hook were dragging up through the larynx with every cough. Tickling in the larynx with hoarseness. In the whooping cough there is this same painfulness of the larynx. The child shakes and shudders and you can see that it dreads the cough because of the tearing pain in the larynx. Cough and difficult breathing from inspiring cold air, yet a warm draft will so increase the tickling that it is sure to set the patient coughing. So the cough is aggravated both by cold air and a warm room. Colds sometimes travel down into the bronchial tubes and are attended with fever and rapid pulse. If the tickling in the larynx, the cough from inspiring the cold air, worse in a warm room and in the evening, with tearing pain in the larynx, are present, Allium cepa will cure. The cough is spasmodic and resembles croup or whooping cough. Cepa has a record for croupy cough. The old lady binds onion on the throat of the child with croup. and no doubt, out in the back woods. where there are no doctors, it was far better than Old School treatment.

Here is a fairly good description from the Guiding Symptoms: "Hoarse, harsh, ringing, spasmodic cough. excited by constant tickling in the larynx; cough produces a raw, splitting pain in the larynx, so acute and so severe as to compel the patient to crouch from suffering, and to make every effort to suppress the cough." "Severe, laryngeal cough, which compels the patient to grasp the larynx; feels as if cough would tear it." The child will reach up to the larynx and clutch it. This is wholly different from the *Aconite* condition, when the child, after exposure to a dry, cold wind, wakes before midnight with a hoarse. barking cough, and clutches the larynx. So *Aconite* cannot be substituted for Allium cepa.

Another affection over which this remedy has marvellous power is traumatic neuritis, often met with in a stump after amputation. The pains are almost unbearable, rapidly exhausting the strength of the patient.

ALOE

Aloe, much like *Æsculus*, has a peculiar engorgement of the veins, causing stiffness and fulness throughout the body, but the greatest disturbance is in the veins of the portal system, with great fulness in the region of the liver, and abdominal, rectal and intestinal fulness. This is associated with hæmorrhoids. It has abdominal pains that drive him to stool like *Nux vomica*, cutting, cramping pains around the navel. Pains about the navel that shoot down towards the rectum, cutting like knives. Dysenteric and diarrhœic troubles. In the attacks of diarrhœa there is gushing of thin. yellow, offensive, excoriating fæces, which burn like fire, and the anus is sore. He holds the stool with difficulty, does not dare take his mind off the sphincter because as soon as he does so the stool will escape. He cannot let the least quantity of flatus escape,. because with it there will be a rush of fæces. With the Aloe diarrhœa the abdomen is distended with gas, causing a feeling of fulness and tightness. and he must go often to stool, Little ones. soon after they begin to walk, will drop all over the carpet, involuntarily, little yellow drops of mucus and fæces. The mother sometimes punishes the little ones, but they cannot help it, they cannot hold the stool, as it is passed involuntarily. There is a lack of control of the sphincter. This state is not always confined to diarrhœa, because sometimes children will go around dropping, involuntarily, little, hard, round marble-like pieces of stool. They do not even know the stool has passed. There is relaxation about the rectum and protrusion of the anus, with bleeding piles. Every mouthful of food hurries him to stool; drinking water will often hurry him to stool. Diarrhœa from eating oysters out of season. You might be disposed to give *Lycopodium,* because in the text books poisoning from oysters is laid down under *Lyc.* I do not know that you would be justified in saying poisoning from oysters in season is *Lyc.,* and out of season is Aloe, but there is a tremendous poisoning effect about oysters in the hot weather and in the breeding season that is not found at any other time. A great many people become nauseated, bloat up, purge tremendously, vomit everything for several days after eating oysters. Now, when that group of symptoms is present *Lycopodium* will cure it and will remove the tendency to get sick from oysters. But if you notice those who get sick have a cholera-like trouble from eating oysters in the hot season, you will find that that is where Aloe is the remedy.

This remedy is not well proved hence I have first referred to the things it is used for clinically. It is more nearly related to *Sulphur* in its venous condition than to any other remedy. If you study together, side by side, *Kali bi., Sulphur* and Aloe, you will be astonished at their wonderful relation to the stomach and bowels.

Among the few mental symptoms we notice, "She knew she would die in a week." "Life is a burden." ¡Disinclined to move." Very little is brought out by which we can distinguish it; only a few things common to many remedies are given. The Aloe patient is extremely excitable when under the influence of pain, and the pains are generally in the abdomen. Colic-like pains, flatulent pains in the abdomen, that drive to despair; he becomes extremely irritable and excited in his attacks of colic. A little symptom that is somewhat striking is, "Hates people, repels everyone."

The head congestion, which occurs during the bowel disturbance, is a sort of venous stasis such as is found in the portal system. "Headache across forehead." "Headaches aggravated from heat, ameliorated from cold applications." Aggravation from heat and relief from cold runs through Aloe. He wants to be in a cold room; feels hot and flushed; the skin is often hot and dry; he wants to be uncovered at night in bed; burning of the extremities, hot hands and cold feet, or cold hands and hot feet; these alternate. The head feels hot and he wants something cool upon it. This is from the heat of the surface, not fever. Sensation of heat in the surface, feeling of congestion and fulness of the surface of the body; fulness and engorged veins all over the body. Bleedings are common in this remedy, venous oozings from the nose, the bowels, the bladder; bleeding in general. The veins become varicose and the skin is hot. Much heat in the orifices of the body; the eyes, mouth and throat are hot and burn. There is a sensation of dryness, burning and excoriation about the anus.

Under "Eating and Drinking" we find "Soon after supper growling in abdomen " There are colicky pains in the bowels from eating and drinking when there is no diarrhœa, even when there is a state of constipation.

This remedy is useful for the complaints of old beer drinkers. Diarrhœa brought on from drinking beer. In persons who have a diarrhœa every time they drink beer you will most likely find that Aloe will agree with the symptoms, but sometimes it will he *Kali bi.,* for these two remedies are very similar as to their stomach and bowel symptoms. "Belching with oppression of stomach." Here is another instance of the tendency to capillary and venous engorgement. "Vomiting of blood" and blood from the bowels.

There is much pain in the hepatic region, burning and heat, etc. Mostly in the right hypochondrium you will find distension and fullness. It is pre-eminently a liver medicine. It is not as deep in its action as *Sulphur.* You will often find that Aloe will serve as a palliative when it will have to be followed by *Sulphur, Sulph. ac., Kali bi.* or *Sepia,* the medicines that follow Aloe and are complementary to it, finishing its work. Aloe will make a good beginning in these liver troubles when there are great fulness, distension, stitching pains in the region of the liver and a dry, hot, burning skin, with no increase of temperature. Aloe has some fever, but this sensation of heat of the skin and dryness is without fever and is such as is found in psoric patients. The proving has not been sufficiently extensive to demonstrate whether Aloe produces eruption to any extent or not, but if such could be proved this would place it among the anti-psorics. It is not a deep long-acting constitutional remedy like *Sulphur,* and yet it is not so short-acting as *Aconite* or *Belladonna.* Complaints come on only with a moderate degree of rapidity. It may be associated very well with *Bryonia. Bryonia* does not go so deeply into the life substance as *Sulphur.*

Perhaps one of the most striking features of the abdominal state is the fulness, distension and rumbling. It seems as if the abdomen would burst and the rumbling is so great that it can be heard by anyone in the room. It keeps on one continuous gurgling. The stool gurgles out with a noisy rumbling, like water out of a bung-hole. The text of the earlier writers speaks of it as a sputtering, for while the stool is passing out it is accompanied by much flatus which gurgles and sputters. The abdomen seems to be as much distended as ever even after great quantities of flatus have passed. There is no relief. The pain is especially felt across the abdomen, about the hips. Great distension as if the abdomen would burst across the transverse colon, and also in the ascending and descending colon; pain; gurgling, rumbling, heaviness, and feeling of pressure outwards. "Twisting and griping pain in the upper abdomen, around the navel, compelling him to sit bent up which relieves." "Feeling of weakness in abdomen as if diarrhœa would result." The weakness is sometimes very great, so much so that he is compelled to go to bed with the diarrhœa, and you will often mistake it for. *Podophyllum,* so great is the exhaustion. *Pod.* has great distension, tremendous gushing, much flatulence, great rumbling in the bowel and the trouble comes on at 4 o'clock in the morning. Aloe is like *Sulph.* again, in that it drives him out of bed in the early morning with diarrhœa, and there are times when he puts the feet out from beneath the covers to cool them off; the soles of the feet burn and he uncovers them. Griping in the abdomen, feeling of weakness in the abdomen. "Painfulness in whole abdomen, especially in sides and along both sides of navel." So sensitive is the abdomen that he can find no comfortable position. "Dull, abdominal pain as after taking cold, morning and evening repeatedly."

Now here are abdominal symptoms that relate to the condition of the women and not to diarrhœa. "Feeling as if a plug was wedged in between symphysis pubis and os coccyges" "Labor-like pains in the groins and loins worse when standing." Aloe has cured prolapsus of the uterus of long standing when it was associated with fulness, heat of the surface of the body, tendency to morning diarrhœa, dragging down of the uterus and sensation of a plug wedged in between the symphysis pubis and coccyx. The outward pressure of the uterus causes that sensation. Dragging down as if all parts of the pelvis would push out. A funnelling sensation in the vagina, in the pelvis.

"Urging to stool, only hot flatus passes, giving relief, but urging soon returns." The idea is that it compels him to go to stool, but when upon the commode nothing but wind passes. It is useful also in old chronic sufferers from this trouble, those who suffer from constipation, who go many days without a stool, but feel every little while, or several times in the day, that they must go to stool, and then only a little wind passes. *Natrum sulph.* will very commonly overcome that state. "Lumpy, watery stool." That is a strong feature of Aloe; hard lumps mingled with a watery stool; the lumps are in the water or in the liquid fæces; little hard lumps looking like marbles or sheep dung. In the constipation the stool is lumpy, like marbles. Sometimes these little nodules remain in the rectum a long time without any urging to stool, and finally escape unconsciously, being found in the clothing. Entire loss of sensation in the anus, an anæsthesia; no feeling during the passage of the stool.

Much of the Aloe trouble is dysenteric in character, with a sharp, inflammatory condition of the rectum and lower portion of the colon; bloody discharges and yellow, jelly-like mucus. Sometimes the Aloe patient will pass nothing but large quantities of this catarrhal, jelly-like mucus. Don't forget Aloe for hæmorrhoids that form like a bunch of grapes. "Itching and burning in anus, preventing sleep." He is compelled to bore with the finger into the anus; so violent is the itching that the patient cannot let it alone; it seems it will drive him to distraction. He gets relief only from applying something cold. A common feature of Aloe is that ointments increase the burning. There is increased burning of the skin round about the ulcers after applying an ointment. The *Sulphur* patient also cannot bear any application; it is poisonous to him and he breaks out in eruptions.

Wherever a mucous membrane is inflamed there is formed a deposit of thick, jelly-like mucus. If there is an ulcerated spot or aphthous patch or inflamed surface, thick, jelly-like cakes of mucus may be peeled off almost as thick as leather at times. At times the lower portion of the rectum is in this state and the patient will say that the lumpy stools are caked in jelly. The lumpy stools in *Graphites* look as if embedded in coagulated white of egg. Sometimes the Aloe patient, before having a stool, will expel a teacupful of thick, jelley-like mucus which has occupied the lower portion of the rectum. Aloe cured a case of stricture of the rectum in which it was indicated by this symptom. The stricture prevented nearly all the fæcal matter from getting down to the anus, but the rectum would fill up three or four times a day and compel the patient to expel a quantity of jelley-like mucus. The fæces that could be forced through were scarcely larger than a pipe stem. It has been said that our medicines are not capable of curing strictures, but they sometimes do cure strictures. If they can cure the patient it is marvellous how nature will take up all that inflammatory tissue and the canal become normal. This thing has been seen many times in stricture of the urethra and stricture of the rectum.

ALUMEN

This medicine, like *Alumina,* seems to produce a peculiar kind of *paralytic weakness* of the muscles in all parts of the body, a sort of lack of tone. The extremities are weak. This weakness is felt especially in the rectum and bladder. The stool becomes impacted from want of ability of the rectum and colon to expel their contents. The bladder is also slowed down in its action, and it is with great difficulty that the urine is voided. After urinating, the bladder often remains half full. The urine is very slow to start, and when the patient stands to urinate the urine falls down perpendicularly, as in *Hepar.* From this we see the sluggish action. The paralytic condition extends also to the veins producing a vaso-motor paralysis.

Another peculiar condition running through the remedy is the *tendency to induration* wherever there is an inflamed surface. All remedies that have this in their nature relate more or less to cancerous affections, because in cancer we have as the most natural feature a tendency to induration. Ulcers are common in Alumen. and this induration underlies the ulcer; ulcers with indurated base. Or little scales may appear upon the skin where the circulation is feeble, over cartilaginous portions for instance, and a great thick indurated mass forms. Infiltration takes place under this crust, the crust keeps coming off, and a lack of healing follows because of the weakness of the tissues from a vaso-motor paralysis. Epithclioma is scarcely more than that, and so we have in this remedy features like epithelioma and other cancerous affections. What is the scirrhus but a peculiar form of induration? When the economy takes on a low type of life, a low form of tissue making, and the tissues inflame and upon the slightest provocation indurate we can see that this is a kind of constitution that is predisposed to deep-seated troubles, to phthisis, Bright's disease, diabetes, cancer, etc. We are on the border line of ultimates mid something is going to happen. This remedy leads the economy into such a state of disorder. a low type of tissue making is found, and many of these indurations will have cancer as an ultimate. This is a long acting antipsoric remedy.

There is also in this medicine a tendency to induration of the neck of the uterus and the mammary glands. Glands become slowly inflamed, and do not stop with ordinary congestion and hardness, but become as hard as bullets. This induration extends to the various glands of the body, but is especially noticeable in the tonsils. For those who have a tendency to colds which settle in the throat, especially singling out the tonsils and indurating these; those who keep on taking cold and the tonsils keep on growing and indurating, we have in Alumen a medicine that fits the whole process, the hardening and infiltration, and it cures these cases according to the law of similars— when the symptoms agree. It cures young children growing up with enormously enlarged and very hard tonsils, in whom every cold settles in the throat. Alumen is one of the cognates of *Baryta carb.,* which has the same tendency. In one patient there will be one kind of constitution, and, after thoroughly examining it, looks like *Baryta carb.* You may have a different constitution in another patient, and, after carefully examining it, see that it looks like Alumen; another you will see is *Sulphur;* another, if you look into it carefully, you find is *Calcarea carb.,* and another, *Calcarea iod.,*" and so on among those remedies capable of bringing about the conditions described. If we can find symptoms which picture the constitutional state we have no trouble. When the symptoms have been well gathered the case is as good as cured; it is easy then to find a remedy.

This remedy is imperfect from the fact that it is only partially proved. I do not care to dwell upon partially proved remedies, but when they have a number of striking features that fit into everyday life it is important to know them. The mental symptoms of this remedy are very few. The remedy should be proved in the higher potencies upon sensitive persons in order that the mental state may be brought out.

Some of the symptoms of the head are very striking and valuable. Pain on the top of the head with burning. The pain is a sensation as if a weight were pressing down into the skull. You will see a woman in bed with her hand on top of the head and she will say: "Doctor, it burns right there like fire, and it presses as if my skull would be crushed in, and the only relief I get is from pressing hard upon it and. from an ice cold cloth pressed upon it." She wants the cloth changed and made cold every few minutes. It is a queer thing that a pressing pain is made better from pressing upon the part. This is like *Cactus,* pressing pain on vertex relieved from pressure. The rubric of remedies with that symptom is very small, and hence this remedy fills a place. There are some strange, rare and peculiar symptoms for which we have a paucity of remedies, and we have to work in other channels and along sidetracks in getting the constitutional state of the patient. Alumen cured the pressing pain on the vertex in one patient in whom it alternated with the most troublesome chronic, irritable bladder.

"Vertigo lying on his back, with weakness in pit of stomach; > opening eyes, > turning on right side." There is another feature, however, in this remedy, the *palpitation* is brought on from *lying on the right side.* It would strike anyone as something very singular, because palpitation is generally worse lying on the left side. A heart that is fluttering, enlarged or disordered is generally worse while lying on the left, as the heart has less room then, but it is strange, rare and unique when these symptoms are worse lying on the right side. When this condition is present in a patient it is necessary to find a remedy having just exactly that symptom, and very often it will be seen that the rest of the symptoms of the case fit into the remedy that has produced this peculiar state.

There is one more feature that you must add to these things, viz.: *slowness and sluggishness of the muscles* throughout the body, a slowing down of all the muscles, a sense of weakness in the arms and legs.

In the *constipation* there may be some urging to stool without result or he may go several days without desire. There is no ability to expel the stool. He will strain a long time with no success, and finally after many days the stool is passed and is an agglomeration of hard balls, large masses of little' hard balls like marbles all fastened together. This is a very strong feature in an Alumen constitution. "Stool: less frequent, dryer and harder; large black, hard or in small pieces like sheep's dung; no relief afterwards." After stool there is a sensation as if the rectum were yet full. This peculiar feature comes with the weakness or paresis of the rectum, *i.e.*, the rectum is not strong enough to expel all of its contents, and hence the sensation of unfinished stool. In the rectum there is ulceration with bleeding from the ulcers. The hæmorrhoids ulcerate and they are very painful, so that after every stool he has prolonged suffering, a dull aching pain in the rectum.

Catarrhal conditions prevail throughout the remedy. In old scrofulous, psoric patients, who are subject to chronic yellow bland discharges from the eyes, with enlarged veins; chronic yellow discharges from the vagina and from the urethra in the male; chronic painless gonorrhœa. In addition to the catarrhal discharges there is a tendency to ulceration, so that there are little ulcerative patches in the vagina, little aphthous patches in the vagina and on the cervix of the uterus: When a patient is suffering from a chronic gonorrhoea, instead of the discharge becoming white as in a gleet it remains yellow, and there are little indurations along the urethra, which the patient will call the physician's attention to as "lumps." Discharge with "little hunches" along the urethra. These are little ulcers, and beneath the ulcers are indurations. When this state is present you have an Alumen gonorrhœa. In a little while the patient will have two or three strictures unless he gets this remedy, because these little ulcers will each end in stricture narrowing the canal. Another strange feature in the catarrhal states and in the ulcers is its tendency to affect the vessels. The veins become varicose and bleed, so that there may be bleeding from any of the inflamed or catarrhal areas and bleeding from the ulcers.

There are many neuralgic pains about the *head* of a nondescript character. These head pains come on in the morning on awaking. The *eye* symptoms are of an inflammatory or congestive character, with tendency to ulceration. Purulent ophthalmia; chronic sore eyes. "Sees things double by candle light." "Nasal polypus left side. Lupus or cancer on the nose. Face pale as a corpse, lips blue. Scirrhus of the tongue." See what a tendency it has to produce minute growths, little indurations and infiltrations. Bleeding from the teeth; the teeth decay and the gums recede from the teeth; the teeth become loose; scorbutic appearance of the gums. "Mouth burning, ulcerated; grey, dirty, spongy skin about a tooth, which is surrounded with proud flesh; offensive saliva." In the mouth we have the same general feature of ulceration, with dryness of the mouth, dry tongue and throat, and great thirst for ice cold water. "Uvula inflamed and enlarged. Predisposed to tonsillitis." "Vomits everything he eats." After that you can put the word "ulcer," because it especially refers to that state of congestion where there is easy ulceration.

Under *abdomen* we find flatulence. The intestines do not perform their work, they take on spasmodic action, and consequently the patient suffers from cramps and colicy pains; boring, rending, tearing pains. Retraction of the abdomen and drawing in of the navel. If you will compare *Lead* in its poisonous effects upon those who work in white lead you will see quite a counterpart of this remedy, and you will not be surprised to observe that *Plumbum* and this remedy antidote each other. They do so because they are so similar, they cannot live in the same house. Alumen is a great remedy to overcome lead colic in those who work in lead; it removes the susceptibility. There are many patients who have to give up their occupation on account of this susceptibility. Alumen will often overcome this tendency and enable them to go back to their business.

In the female we note "weight of uterus presses down collum; granu-lations of vagina; leucorrhœa copious; emaciation; yellow complexion; indurations of uterus, even scirrhus; ulcers of uterus." Sometimes you get evidence of this vaginal state by the woman saying that coition is so painful that it becomes impossible. It is not to be wondered at that the natural act cannot be performed when so much trouble is present.

"Voice entirely lost." Chronic loss of the voice from a low state of the economy and from always taking fresh colds. Expectoration of much yellow mucus; scraping of the throat all the time to get rid of a little accumulation of yellow mucus. "Dry cough in evening after lying down." "Chronic morning cough." Cough is not a very important thing in this remedy; it is the general state of the economy that is to be looked at. The cough will not interpret the nature of the disease to the physician, because when these little ulcers are present they must cause some kind of a cough. This patient may go into phthisis or be affected with any of the ultimates of disease.

Alumen has been very useful in the treatment of old people who suffer from copious, ropy, morning expectoration, catarrh of the chest, hæmop-tysis and great weakness of the chest, so that it is difficult to expel the mucus. In this it is similar to *Antimonium tartaricum*.

Because of its relation to *Alumina* further provings will undoubtedly develop that fact that it has many spinal symptoms. It is well known that it has a weak spine, with coldness of the spine, a feeling as if cold water were poured down the back. Pain in the dorsal spine on a line with the inferior angle of the scapulæ; weakness in this region and in the shoulders. Like *Alumina* it has the sensation of constriction, as of a cord or band around the limbs. Feeling as if a cord were drawn tightly around the upper arm. The clumsiness of the fingers, as seen in dropping things, the pain in the lower limbs at night, the lassitude and numbness, are other manifestations of spinal symptoms. Sensation as of a cord around the leg under the knee; soles sensitive to pressure on walking; feet numb and cold, although warmly covered; legs cold to knees. These are all further evidences of the action of the remedy on the spinal cord. Bruised pain in all the limbs. Crawling, tingling paralysis of all limbs.

He is kept awake at night by a sensation as if the blood rushed through the body. Many complaints come on during sleep. Nightmare. He is sensitive to weather changes and very sensitive to cold.

ALUMINA

This remedy comes in very nicely after *Alumen,* which has much Alumina in its nature and depends largely upon Alumina, which is its base, for its way of working. It occurs to me to throw out a little hint. When you have a good substantial proving of an oxide or a carbonate, and the mental symptoms are well brought out, you can use these, in a measure in a presumptive way, in prescribing another salt, with the same base, which has a few mental symptoms in its proving. For instance, you have a group of symptoms decidedly relating to *Alumen.* The mental symptoms of *Alumen,* however, have not been brought out to any extent, but still you have the mental symptoms of the base of *Alumen,* which is the oxide, so that if the patient has the mental symptoms of Alumina and the physical symptoms of *Alumen,* you can rationally presume that *Alumen* will cure because of the *Aluminum in* each.

We know the mental symptoms of Alumina fairly well. It especially takes hold of the intellect and so confuses the intelligence that the patient is unable to effect a decision; the judgment is disturbed. He is unable to realize; the things that he knows or has known to be real seem to him to be unreal, and he is in doubt as to whether they are so or not. In the *Guiding Symptoms* this is not so plainly expressed, but in the *Chronic Diseases* we have a record of this which is the best expression of it that occurs anywhere. There we read: "When he says anything he feels as if another person had said it, and when he sees anything, as if another person had seen it, or as if he could transfer himself into another and only then could see." That is to say, there is a confusion of mind, a confusion of ideas and thoughts. It has cured these symptoms. The consciousness of his personal identity is confused. He is not exactly certain who he was; it seemed at though he were not himself. He is in a dazed condition of mind. He makes mistakes in writing and speaking; uses words not intended; uses wrong words. Confusion and obscuration of the intellect. Inability to follow up a train of thought.

Then he enters into another state, in which he gets into a hurry. Nothing moves fast enough; time seems so slow; everything is delayed; nothing goes right. Besides this he has impulses. When he sees sharp instruments or blood, impulses rise up within him and he shudders because of these impulses. An instrument that could be used for murder or for killing causes these impulses to arise; impulse to kill herself.

The Alumina patient is very sad, constantly sad. Incessantly moaning, groaning, worrying, fretting and in a hurry. Wants to get away; wants to get away from this place, hoping that things will be better; full of fears. All sorts of imaginations. A sort of general apprehensiveness. When he meditates upon this state of mind he thinks he is going to lose his reason. He thinks about this frenzy and hurry and confusion of mind, how he hardly knows his own name, and how fretful he is, and he wonders if he is not going crazy, and finally he really thinks he is going crazy.

Most of the mental symptoms come on in the morning on waking. Sadness and weeping on waking in the morning. His moods alternate. Sometimes his mental state is a little improved and his mood changes into a quiet, placid state, and again he goes into fear and apprehensiveness. Some evil is going to take place and he is full of anxiety. Anxiety about the future.

The next most striking feature is the way in which the remedy acts upon the nerves that proceed from the spine. There is a state of weakness of the muscles supplied by these nerves; weakness over the whole body. There is difficulty in swallowing, a paralytic condition of the œsophagus; difficulty in raising or moving the arms; paralysis of one side of the body, or paralysis of the muscles of the lower extremities, or of the bladder and rectum. The paralytic state begins as a sort of a semi-paralysis, for a long time merely an inactivity, which grows at length into a complete paralytic condition.

Everything is slowed down. The conductivity of the nerves is impaired so that a prick of a pin upon the extremities is not felt until a second or so afterwards. All of his senses are impaired in this way until it really means a benumbing of the consciousness and appears to be a kind of stupefaction of his intellect, a mental sluggishness. Impressions reach his mind with a marked degree of slowness.

The paralytic state runs through the remedy and is observed in various parts in many ways. The bladder manifests it in the slowness with which the urine passes. A woman sits a long time before the flow starts, with inability to press, and then the stream flows slowly. The patient will say she cannot hurry the flow of urine. The urine is slow to start and slow to flow, and sometimes only dribbles. At times it is retained and dribbles involuntarily. This slowness is observed also in the rectum. Its tone is lost and there is inability to perform the ordinary straining when sitting at stool, and so paretic is the rectum that it may be full and distended, and the quantity of fæces enormous, and yet, though the stool is soft, there is constipation. In this remedy there is often a hard stool, but we notice that the remedy will do the best work where there is this paretic condition of the rectum with soft stool. If the mental symptoms, however, are present, such as I have described, with large, hard and knotty or lumpy stool, Alumina will cure. Now, so great is the straining to pass a soft stool that you will sometimes hear a patient describe the state as follows: When sitting upon the seat she must wait a long time, though there is fulness and she has gone many days without stool; she has the consciousness that she should pass a stool and is conscious of the fulness in the rectum, yet she will sit a long time and finally will undertake to help herself by pressing down violently with the abdominal muscles, straining vigorously, yet conscious that very little effort is made by the rectum itself. She will continue to strain, covered with copious sweat, hanging on to the seat, if there be any place to hang on to, and will pull and work as if in labor, and at last is able to expel a soft stool, yet with the sensation that more stool remains.

Of course a number of other remedies have this straining to pass a soft stool, but they have their own characteristics. Take for example an individual who cannot keep awake; she says that it is impossible for her to read a line without going to sleep; that she can sleep all the time; she suffers night and day from a dry mouth, and the tongue cleaves to the roof of the mouth. Now let her describe this state of straining and struggling to expel a soft stool, and you hardly need to go any further before you know the remedy. If that patient in addition to what she has said tells you that she is in the habit of fainting when standing any length of time, that she is disturbed in a close room and has all sorts of complaints in the cold air, it is *Nux moschata*. Now you see how easy it is for remedies to talk; they tell their own story. Suppose a woman should come to you who has been suffering from hæmorrhage, from prolonged oozing, who is pallid and weak and is distended with flatulence, with much belching and passing of gas, and the more she passes the worse she feels, and she has these same symptoms of straining a long time to pass a soft stool, tremendous effort with inactivity of the rectum. You could do nothing but give her *China*. By allowing remedies to talk and tell their own story individualization is accomplished. I have said all that to show that it is not upon the inactivity of the rectum that you are to decide upon the remedy. Individualization must be made through the patient. That is a principle that should never be violated. You may have twenty remedies all possessing a certain symptom, but if you have a few real decided things that you can say about the patient; the manner in which he does business, the manner in which the disease affects the entire man, then you have something to individualize by. You have seen the Alumina patient, the *China* patient and the *Nux moschata* patient. The sole duty of the physician is to treat the sick, which means to study the *patient himself* until an idea of the sickness is obtained.

This medicine is full of vertigo; he quivers, reels and "objects go round" almost constantly. It corresponds to the vertigo of tired-out people, old broken down patients, men worn out from old age. Vertigo also that comes on when closing the eyes, as is found in spinal affections, in sclerosis of posterior lateral columns. Alumina has produced affections analogous to locomotor ataxia. It produces numbness of the soles of the feet, the fulgurating pains, the vertigo when closing the eyes, and produces staggering and disturbances of co-ordination. It is true that in an early stage of locomotor ataxia Alumina will check the disease process by bringing into order the internal state of the economy. With *Aluminum metallicum* I have stopped fulgurating pains in old incurable cases, and improved the reflexes wonderfully, thus showing the general improvement of the patient.

Most of the symptoms are < on rising in the morning. In the morning, as I have mentioned it, the urine is slower to pass than after he has moved about and warmed up a little. His limbs are stiffer in the morning and in the morning he has to whip up his mental state. He wakes up confused and wonders where he is. You will see that in children especially—they wake up in the morning in a bewildered state, such as you will find in Alumina, *Æsculus, Lycopod* He has to put his mind on things to ascertain whether they be so or not, as to how things should look and wonders whether he is at home or in some other place.

There are many headaches with nausea and vomiting. The headaches come whenever he takes cold. This probably is due to the catarrhal state. The Alumina patient suffers almost constantly from dryness of mucous membranes, the nose is dry, stuffed up, especially on one side, commonly the left. Nose feels full of sticks, dry membrane or crusts, old atrophic catarrh, crusts in the posterior nares and in the fossa of Rosenmuller. Large green, offensive crusts all through the nose. Now comes the relation to the. headache. Every time he catches cold the thick yellow discharge slacks up and gives way to a watery discharge and he has pain in the forehead over the eyes, going through the head, with nausea and vomiting. So when it says headache from chronic catarrh that is what it means. The headache > lying down. He has sick headaches and periodical headaches. You will see that Alumina corresponds to a constitution that may be called psoric—old, broken-down, feeble constitutions, scrofulous constitutions, such as are inclined to tubercles and catarrhal affections.

The catarrhal tendency of this remedy is marked. Catarrhs are found wherever mucous membranes exist. Alumina affects the skin and mucous membrane extensively, *i.e.*, the external and internal skin, the surfaces of the body. The patient is always expectorating, he blows the nose much and has discharges from the eyes. There is much disturbance of vision belonging to this catarrhal state that may be spoken of now. Dimness of vision, as if looking through a fog, sometimes described as through a veil. A misty dimness of vision. There is also disturbance of the muscles of the eye, of the muscles of the ball and of the ciliary muscle. Weak and changeable vision. The paralytic weakness, such as belongs to the whole remedy, will be found in certain muscles, or sets of muscles, so that it is with great difficulty that glasses can be adjusted. The activity of the eye muscles is disturbed.

The catarrhal state extends over into the back of the nose and the posterior nares are filled up with tough mucus and crusts, and on looking into the throat you will see that the soft palate and the mucous membrane of the tonsils and pharynx and all parts that can be seen are in a state of granulation, are swollen, congested and inflamed. The pharynx feels dry and there is a chronic sensitiveness and soreness. When swallowing food there is stinging and sensation as if the throat were full of little sticks, especially after a moment's rest, better by moistening and swallowing. In the night air, after keeping still a while, there is an accumulation of ropy mucus. This extends into the larynx with soreness in the larynx and chest and chronic dry, hacking cough. The same catarrhal state proceeds down into the œsophagus, so that it becomes sensitive and clumsy. He swallows with difficulty. The bolus goes down with an effort and he feels it all the way down. There is soreness and clumsiness, paresis and difficulty of swallowing. This paralytic weakness reminds the patient that he must put on a little force in order to swallow and this swallowing is felt while the substance goes down as if the œsophagus was sensitive. It has a catarrhal state of the stomach, bowels and rectum, so that with the soft and difficult stool there is often an accumulation of mucus. There is also a catarrhal condition in the bladder, kidneys and urethra and an old gonorrhœa will be prologned into a catarrhal or gleety discharge. Sometimes it is not a gleet, but the discharge remains for many months and instead of its being a light milky white, such as is natural in most prolonged cases of gonorrhœa, it remains yellow and is painless. So it is with the vagina. The mucous discharge from the vagina is a thick yellowish-white discharge, sometimes excoriating. Thus we see, in the constitution we have described, that an extensive catarrhal state belongs to the remedy.

When we come to the skin we find that it takes on a similar state of affairs. The patient is subject to all sorts of eruptions. The skin withers, becomes dry and is subject to eruptions, thickening, indurations, ulcerations, cracking and bleeding. The eruptions itch worse in the warmth of the bed. The skin itches, even when there is no eruption, when becoming warm in bed, so that he scratches until the skin bleeds. This presents an idea as to eruptions that you will have to consider. A patient comes to you covered with crusts, and he says: "When I get warm at night I have to scratch, and I scratch until the skin bleeds." Now in Alumina it is very important to find out whether these crusts were produced by the scratching or whether the eruption came out as an itching eruption, for in Alumina in the beginning there is no eruption. but he scratches until the skin is off and then come the crusts. You must here prescribe not for the eruption, but for the itching of the skin without eruption. Now in *Mezereum, Arsenicum, Dolichos* and Alumina the skin itches and he scratches until it bleeds, and then he gets relief. Of course after this there is an apparent eruption because crusts form. As soon as the healing begins the itching begins, and he is only relieved when the skin is raw. With the bleeding and moisture of the skin there is relief of the itching. Now some of the books do not make the distinction between itching without eruption and itching with eruption, and hence mostly all young doctors get to thinking that itching of the skin must always be associated with eruption, and make a mistake in figuring out what kind of an eruption it is. The skin thickens and indurates and ulcerates, and there are indurations under the ulcers. There is a very sluggish condition of both mucous membrane and skin with a tendency to induration. Thickening of the mucous membrane will be found anywhere; after the thickening come little ulcerations, and in the course of time indurations are formed at the base of the ulcers. The same thing is true of the skin. Dryness and burning run through everything and may be said of all the mucous membranes and the skin in general.

Chronic granular lids. If we turn the eyelids down we will see that the mucous membrane is thickened. Sometimes this thickening or hypertrophy causes a turning out of the lids like ectropion. "The eyelashes fall out;" that is in keeping with the general state. The hairs all over the body fall out. Parts become entirely denuded of hair; the hair of the scalp falls out extensively. All sorts of sounds in the ears, buzzing. etc., and derangement of hearing; purulent otorrhœa:

"Point of nose cracked" is in keeping with the remedy. Induration here and there so that it favors lupus and epithelioma in one who is subject to these swellings and eruptions. Alumina and *Alumen,* like *Ars., Lach., Sulph.* and *Conium,* are medicines that relate to these troubles. Some of these have made brilliant cures where there is infiltration. Upon the skin of the face and other parts of the body there is crawling. Itching especially when getting warm. Sensation of tension. Peculiar sensation about the face and other parts not covered by clothing, a sensation of dried white of egg on the face, of dried blood or cobweb on the face. If you have ever been going through a place where there are cobwebs and a little cobweb has strung across your face you will know what a peculiar sensation of crawling it produces, and you cannot leave it alone until it is removed. That sensation particularly belongs to Alumina, *Borax, Bar. c.* Little crawlings and creepings in the skin. Itching of the face. These symptoms are so irritating that the patient will sit and rub his face all the time. You will think that he is nervous. He has the appearance of being nervous as he sits rubbing the back of his hands. It is well to find out whether he does this because he cannot keep his hands still or because of the itching. Because of this itching sensation in the face he carries the hand to the face as though to brush away something.

Perhaps I have not said as much as should be said about the throat. "Ulcers in the fauces, spongy, secreting a yellowish brown, badly smelling pus." It may be said that the patient is often a victim of chronic sore throat. There is this about Alumina, it has a special tendency to localize itself upon mucous membranes. You will find in an Alumina subject bleeding from all mucous membranes. He has catarrh of the nose and red eyes, and his nose becomes stuffed up and he has many acute colds; very severe throat trouble. Discharges from all of the orifices. It is not a medicine that would be selected for a cold settling in the throat, not a remedy for acute sore throat, but it is a deep-acting antipsoric and acts for months. Its greatest usefulness is as a remedy for taking cold. In this respect it is like *Sil.*, *Graph.* and *Sulph.* It effects tissue changes, and it does this slowly, for it is a slow-acting medicine. While the patient himself with these deep-seated psoric affections feels better generally after the remedy, it will be months before his symptoms go away. He may say: "I feel better, but my symptoms all appear to be here. I can eat better 'and sleep better." Then it would be unwise to change the remedy. You need not expect to get immediate relief of the catarrhs and pains in the back and other symptoms for which you gave this remedy. You may be satisfied if you get the results after many weeks. You will find the same thing in the paralytic weakness produced by *Plumbum.* There is a new drug that is coming into use, the proving of which is very full and rich; and it is analogous to the symptoms of this remedy. It is *Curare.* I wish we had a finer proving of it, but it is rich with a great many things similar to Alumina and *Plumbum,* and especially in the weakness of the hands and fingers of pianists. An old player will say that after she has been playing for some time her fingers slow down. The weakness seems to be in the extensors. Lack of ability to lift the fingers; the lifting motion is lost. *Curare* to a great extent overcomes that, causes quickness to that lifting power of the fingers. But this remedy also runs through in a general way such paretic conditions; while *Curare* is especially related to a paralytic condition of the extensors more than the flexors, the paralysis in Alumina is of both flexors and extensors.

This medicine is one of the few that have been found to he aggravated from starch, especially the starch of potatoes. Aggravation from eating potatoes. It has indigestion, diarrhœa, great flatulence and aggravation of the cough from eating potatoes. It has also aggravation from salt, wine, vinegar, pepper and from spirituous drinks. Alumina is a spinal remedy and aggravation from spirituous drinks is in keeping with some other spinal remedies. You find it in *Zincum*. The *Zincum* patient cannot drink wine, for all of his complaints are aggravated by it. This medicine is so sensitive and so easily overcome by a small amount of liquor that he is obliged to abandon it. He is not only intoxicated by it, but it aggravates his complaints.

Now the digestion has practically given out in this medicine. He is subject to catarrh of the stomach, to ulceration of the stomach, to indigestion from the simplest food. Sour and bitter eructations. Vomiting of food, mucus or bile. Nausea, vertigo, heartburn, much flatulence. Vomits mucus and water. Stomach is distended with gas. The liver is full of suffering. Both hypochondria are full of misery, but especially the right.

When going over *Alumen* I called attention especially to its antidotal relation to *Lead.* This remedy also will overcome the poisonous effects of lead and sensitiveness to lead. Colic and paralytic weakness in lead workers, painters and artists and in those who are so sensitive to lead that from using hair wash containing lead they are paralyzed. Not many years ago the acetate of lead was commonly used by women for leucorrhœa, but it was found that so many were sensitive to it that it was abandoned. Alumina is the most prominent antidote to the affections which have come about through that sensitive state.

There is so much under stool and rectum that belongs to the general state that there is scarcely anything left to be presented except some important particulars. As you might suppose, this remedy has fissures; you would naturally expect these when you consider what kind of mucous membranes and tissues this patient manufactures. He suffers greatly from constipation, he does much straining, the mucous membrane is thickened and swollen, and hence we have a fissure. When you see a remedy manufacturing and producing such a state upon the economy, growing that kind of mucous membrane that would favor fissures. you do not have to wait until you have cured a fissure with that remedy to find out if it will suit the case. You do not have to resort to the repertory to see what this remedy has done in fissure. From your general knowledge of the medicine, you will see that it ought to cure the patient, as it produces such a condition of the mucous membrane and skin as would be naturally found in one who has a fissure. The skin indurates and ulcerates and becomes clumsy and unhealthy and constipation is produced, and so, after studying the remedy in that way, you are not surprised if it cures a fissure. You can also think over what other medicines have this state of the economy and see what other remedies you would expect to cure a fissure with. If you look into the nature of *Nitric acid, Causticum* and *Graphites,* you will see why they have had a wonderful record for curing fissure. That is the way to study your Materia Medica; see what it does to the man himself, to his organs and tissues.

"Frequent micturition." "Urine voided while straining at stool, or cannot pass urine without such straining." That is a high grade symptom, it is a peculiar symptom, and may be called a particular of first grade. He must strain at stool in order to empty the contents of the bladder. "Urine smarting, corroding." "Feeling of weakness in the bladder and genitals." "Swelling and discharge of light yellow pus from urethra." "Burning with discharge of urine."

The symptoms of the male sexual organs are characterized by weakness, impotency and nightly emissions; suitable when the sexual organs are worn out from abuse or over use. There is fulness and enlargement of the prostate gland and various disturbances of the prostate, with sensation of fulness in the perineum. Unpleasant sensations and distress in the region of the prostate gland after coition. Complaints at the time of, or after ejaculation, or after an emision. The sexual desire is diminished and sometimes entirely lost. Paralytic weakness or paresis of the sexual organs; a state that is in keeping with the whole remedy. "Discharge of prostatic fluid during difficult stool." "Painful erections at night."

The female has a great deal of trouble that can be cured with this remedy, but her troubles are mostly catarrhal. An instance of this is the leucorrhœa; copious, acrid or excoriating, yellow leucorrhœa; leucorrhœa so copious that it runs down the thighs, making the parts red and inflamed. Ulceration about the os. The mucous membranes are weak and patulous and ulcerate easily. All the parts are in a state of weakness. There is dragging down from the relaxed condition of the ligaments. Sensation of weight; the pelvic viscera feel heavy. The discharges are commonly thick and yellow, but they may also be albuminous, stringy, looking like white of egg, copious and acrid; "transparent mucus". "Leucorrhœa, corroding, profuse; running down to heels." It is more noticeable in the daytime, because these complaints are generally worse when walking or when standing, which is not really an important symptom, but a common condition. After menstruation it takes the woman nearly until the next period to get straightened up. All her muscles are weak; there seems to be no tonicity about her. It is highly suitable to women drawing near the end of menstruation, about forty years of age; the menstrual period prostrates, the flow is scanty, yet prostrating; the sufferings are terrible and the patient is miserable at the menstrual period. After menses, exhausted in body and mind, is a strong feature of Alumina. It is a suitable remedy again when the woman has a gonorrhœa which has been prolonged by palliation. She has been made comfortable by partly suitable remedies, but it seems that no remedy has been quite deep enough to root out the trouble, for it keeps coming back. In a discharge that keeps returning, better for a little while on

Pulsatilla. and on this and that and the other thing, and even on *Thuja,* given more especially because it is gonorrhœa than because she is a sick woman. The patient is tired and worn out, and when you come to look at the whole patient and you see the paretic condition, the continued return of the discharge that has been palliated by remedies, think of this medicine in both the male and female.

The discharge is a painless one in the male. The gonorrhœal discharge has lasted a long time, going and coming, until now there is left but a few drops and it is painless. This remedy has cured many of these old cases. Threatening chronic catarrh. The mucous membrane everywhere is in a congested state and is weak.

A pregnant woman has some trouble as well. A woman, who is not naturally a sufferer from constipation, when pregnant becomes constipated, with all the characterizing features of Alumina, *i.e.,* the inactivity of the rectum, no expulsive force; she must use the abdominal muscles, must strain a long time. Again, the infant has a similar kind of straining. You will see the newborn infant, or the infant only a few months old, that will need Alumina. It is a very common medicine for constipation in infants when you can find nothing else; the child will strain and strain and make every effort to press the stool out, and upon examining the stool it is found to be soft, and should have been expelled easily.

It has hoarseness and loss of voice and paralytic weakness of the larynx. That is not strange; it is only in keeping with the general state, the broken down constitution. He has a weak voice and, if a singer, he is capable of singing only a little while, only capable of slight exertion. Everything is a burden. .A paralytic condition of the vocal cords, which steadily increases to loss of voice.

The most striking things we come to now are the cough and chest troubles. There is expectoration in some of the coughs, but the cough is usually a constant, dry, hacking cough, one of those troublesome lingering coughs that has existed for years. It competes with *Arg. met.* in its character of the dry, hacking cough, especially associated with weakness, but *Arg. met.* has the cough in the daytime, which is not so in Alumina. The Alumina cough is in the morning. Here is a symptom that about covers the Alumina cough: "Cough soon after waking in the morning." Every morning, a long attack. of dry cough. The cough is hard, a continued dry hacking, and she coughs until she loses her breath and vomits, and loses the urine. This symptom commonly occurs in the woman. "Dry, hacking cough with' frequent sneezing." It says in the text "from elongated uvula," but it should read "from sensation of elongated uvula." It is a sensation as if there were something tickling the throat; a tickling as if the uvula were hanging down a long distance, and he

will tell you that his palate must be too long. Another expression which is the
same thing is "cough from sensation as of loose skin hanging in throat."
Sometimes those who do not know about the palate will talk of something
loose in the throat, while those who know they have an uvula will generally
call it the palate. But it is the same idea. Tickling in the larynx, too. This is
always quoted in singers. We would think of Alumina when singers break
down in the voice from paralysis or from overwork of the voice. The voice
lets down and becomes feeble, and, when taking cold, there starts up a peculiar
kind of tickling. Alumina is very useful in these cases. *Arg. met.* was the
remedy used by the earlier homœopaths for singers and talkers with much
trembling and letting down of the voice before the value of Alumina was
known in such conditions. Let me tell you something here about *Rhus,* as I
may not think of it again. Many old singers, after taking cold, have a weakness
left in the voice, which they notice on beginning to sing. On beginning to
sing the voice is weak and husky, but after using it a little while it improves.
Give *Rhus* to all these patients, prima donnas, lawyers, preachers, etc. They
must warm up the voice and then they are all right, but they say: "If I go back
into the green-room and wait a little while, when commence to sing again I am
worse than ever." The voice is better if they stay in a very hot room and keep,
it in use. This fits into the general state of *Rhus.* There is a kind of hoarseness
that you may discover to be a little different from the paralytic hoarseness of
Alumina and *Arg. met.* This hoarseness of which I speak belongs to this
same class of people; on first beginning to use the voice it seems that they
must get rid of some mucus by clearing the throat until the voice can get to
work. The vocal cords on beginning to work are covered with mucus and on
getting rid of it they can do very good work, so long as they keep at it. That
is *Phosphorus.* In such cases the use of the voice becomes painful. The
vocal cords are painful after motion and the larynx is painful to touch.
Sometimes this is so marked that it is like stabbing with a knife on trying to
use the voice. So we must individualize hoarseness very extensively.
Homœopathy is a matter of discrimination.

Soreness of the chest, which is much increased by talking. There is
weakness of the muscular power of the chest. The lungs seem weak and the
chest has a sensation of weakness in it. Jar increases the misery of the chest.

The next most striking features will be in connection with the back and
limbs, and I have spoken of these in a general way. Burning in the spine;
much pain in the back. Burning and stitching pains in the back. He expresses
it as follows: "Pain in the back as if a hot iron was thrust through lower
vertebræ." In myelitis this medicine does wonderful work when there is a
considerable amount of spasmodic condition of the back as well, showing
that the membranes are involved. Another thing that belongs to this remedy

that is a well-known state in myelitis is the hoop sensation; sensation of bandages here and there about the limbs and body is a common symptom. A sensation of a tight cord around the body characteristic of the most marked state of irritation and myelitis. Irritation of the spinal cord with sensitive places. Burning places as if a hot iron were forced into the spine. Pain along the cord, rending, tearing pains in the cord with paralytic weakness, increasing paralysis and complete paralysis; paralysis of one side of the body.

"Pain in sole of foot on stepping, as though it were too soft and swollen." "Numbness of heel when stepping." "Trembling of knees," this is a mere matter of the general weakness. "Limbs go to sleep when sitting." Whenever the limb is pressed against anything it will go to sleep. Feeble circulation, feeble conductivity, feeble nerve action; everything is slowed down. Arms and legs feel heavy. "Pains in limbs as if bones were squeezed narrower, with pressure in the joints." Now I will read some of the nerve symptoms which will corroborate some of the things we have gone over. "Want of bodily irritability." "Great exhaustion of strength, especially after walking in open air." "One-sided paralysis, especially of the extensors." "Rheumatic and traumatic paralysis in gouty patients." Gouty patients with nodules in the joints; old broken down constitutions with paretic exhaustion. "Excited condition of mind and body." Tremblings here and there in the body. "Slow, tottering gait as after severe illness." He must make slow motions, he cannot hurry. "Involuntary motions."

There are all sorts of dreams and disturbances in sleep, so that the sleep may be quite disturbed and restless. Unrefreshing sleep, waking up with palpitation of the heart. "Many dreams and frequent awaking; starts in affright; muttering or crying." "During sleep cervical muscles drew head backward;" this is in cases of paralytic weakness; has to wake up, as the muscles of the back of the neck pull so. Jerks in the back of the neck during sleep.

Running through the remedy very often, there is a great lack of animal heat, coldness, and yet the patient wants to be in the open air; must be well clothed and kept warm, but wants to be in the open air. The patient takes cold continually from every change and draft. Sometimes the patient will go to bed as cold as a frog, and when warm in bed is so disturbed by itching and the warmth of the bed that there is no comfort. These are two extremes coming together. The circulation is so feeble over the extremities and backs of the hands that in cold weather the hands are constantly cold and covered with cracks and fissures that bleed.

The skin along the shin bone is rough, ragged and itching. It has been said that dry weather and dry, cold weather increase the complaints of Alumina, and that wet weather sometimes ameliorates.

The febrile condition of this remedy is not at all marked. There is not much chill and not much fever, but the passive, slow, sluggish, chronic elements and chronic symptoms are the ones that prevail most markedly In weak, broken-down cases there are some night sweats and sweating towards morning. Slight chill in morning. Chill with thirst.

A striking feature of the remedy is the chronic dryness of the skin. Sweat is rare and scanty. This is not especially suitable for those copious, exhaustive sweats. It is the very opposite of *Calcarea,* which sweats copiously, but this remedy, with spinal and paralytic affections, is tired out from exertion, very exhausted, but does not sweat. Pile on the covers to make him sweat if you will, but he only gets hot and itching and does not sweat. Scanty sweat. Entire inability to sweat. Chronic dryness of the skin with fissures. The skin becomes worn and ragged and fissured from its dryness. Great dryness of the thick skin over the back of the hands, and in cold weather the hands become cold and discolored.

ALUMINA PHOSPHORICA

The symptoms present aggravations, MORNING, forenoon, AFTERNOON, NIGHT; before midnight, after midnight. Strong desire for open air, open air ameliorates. Marked general anæmia. Single parts go to sleep. Catarrhal conditions generally. Chlorosis. The patient is sensitive to cold and cold generally makes the symptoms worse. He is sensitive to both cold and warm room in a general way; symptoms worse from cold air and from becoming cold; takes cold on slight exposure to cold. Constriction about the body like a band. It is marked for its convulsive action of muscles; its convulsions are clonic; epileptic; hysterical; inclined to fall; with marked stiffness; tonic contraction; convulsive movements. The blood vessels are distended. Symptoms are worse after eating and there is *marked aggravation from physical exertion.* Faint feeling and frequent fainting. General emaciation. Cold drinks and cold food, milk, potatoes and *warm foods* disagree. Formication all over the body. *Lack of vital heat.* A general feeling of heaviness. A lack of physical irritability. Symptoms worse by jarring and stepping. Jerking of muscles and limbs; FEELING OF EXTREME LASSITUDE; desire to lie down. Lying aggravates the breathing but ameliorates the headache; worse after lying long, worse lying on the back. Symptoms worse before, during and after menses; most, symptoms are worse from motion, but the pains in the back are better from motion. There is a marked aversion to motion and exertion.

There is numbness in the limbs and external parts. Congestion and orgasm of blood. The pains are boring, *bruised, burning,* cutting, digging, jerking, *pressing,* sticking and tearing. It is destined to become one of our most useful remedies in paralysis, especially of the lower limbs. It has paralysis of one side, of organs; the paralysis is painless. There is strong internal pulsation. It has fast, weak, irregular pulse. Great internal and external sensitiveness. General amelioration from pressure. The weakness and nervous prostration are as though from sexual excess. Electric shocks are very common and the symptoms are worse after sleep. Standing is a very tiresome position. Tension all over the body. Trembling and twitching. Walking and walking in the open air increase the symptoms, though the open air is grateful to the patient. Great weakness in the morning on waking; from a diarrhœa; from *exertion;* during menses; WALKING; nervous and paralytic weakness. *Extreme weariness.*

Aversion to answering questions and to company; anxiety in the morning on waking; evening; night; of conscience, with fear; about the future; about his health. He is absent-minded and it is impossible to concentrate the mind; confusion of mind in the morning. He is discouraged, discontented, contrary and sure he is going to die. Very excitable and forgetful. Fear in the evening; of death; of disease; that something will happen; of insanity; of misfortune; of people; on waking. It is a remedy to overcome the chronic effects of grief and follows IGNATIA. At times there is great hurry, excitement and his mind is full of ideas and this changes to dullness, heedlessness, deficiency of ideas and indifference much like imbecility. Irresolution is very marked and irritability is extreme. Insane actions, and speech. Aversion to work and laments constantly over his imaginary misfortunes. Spasmodic laughter, maniacal actions, wildly mirthful; moods change rapidly and mental state alternates; loathing of life; extremely obstinate; moments of reserve and absence of all imagination. Mental prostration is a strong feature of this wonderful remedy. Sadness in the morning on waking also in the afternoon; dullness of the senses; very sensitive to noise. Extremely serious at times. Inclination to sit in silence. Starting on falling asleep. It is a very useful remedy after *sexual excesses and prolonged mental efforts.* It is often suited to a mental breakdown at the end of college life. Indisposed to converse with friends; stupefication of mind; disposed to dwell on suicidal thoughts. Talking in sleep. Becomes very timid. Thinking of his symptoms makes them worse. Periods of unconsciousness. Weeping in the morning on waking; during the night; alternating with laughter; involuntary; in sleep VERTIGO in the *morning;* afternoon, evening; *on closing eyes;* lying ameliorates; with nausea; sitting; stooping; walking. Objects turn in a circle, tendency to fall forward.

This remedy will cure the particulars given below where the generals above strongly predominate.

Coldness of the head; occiput; rush of blood to head. Constriction of head; forehead. Empty sensation in head. Hair falls out. Heat in head morning and evening; after eating; in forehead. Heaviness of the head in the morning; on stooping. Itching of scalp; forehead. Numbness of scalp. Pain in head, morning in bed; on waking; noon; afternoon; evening; night; ascending; binding up the hair; *after eating* must lie down; before and during menses; moving head; pulsating; sitting; after sleep; from spirituous liquors; stepping heavily; stooping. walking; *warm room.* Pains are better in open air, better lying, better from pressure. Headaches are periodical, every other day. Pain felt deep in brain; pain in the forehead in the morning on waking; afternoon; evening; above the eyes. Pain in *occiput; after sleep;* on stooping. PAIN IN THE SIDES OF HEAD; in temples, evening. Pulsating pain in vertex in afternoon. Boring in temples. Bruised feeling in head. Burning in forehead and temples. Bursting, cramping in the head. Cutting in temples. Drawing pains in sides of head. Dull pain in the whole head. Pressing pain in head in evening; worse on pressure; in forehead; pressing outward in forehead, over eyes. Pressing in occiput; sides of head, temples, worse night; pressing inward in temples; pressing vertex. Shooting in occiput; vertex; sore pain in whole head; stitching pain in head on coughing; in forehead over eyes; sides of head; temples; right side; vertex; stunning pains in head, tearing in forehead; sides of head; temples; vertex. Pulsation in forehead; occiput; sides; temples; vertex Shocks in head.

Lids stick together during the night. Cracks in the canthi. Yellow, purulent discharges from eyes. The upper lids are heavy and seem paralyzed. Dryness of the eyes. Inflammation of the conjunctivæ. Itching of the lids and inner canthi. Lachrymation in the open air. Opening lids difficult from dryness, from weakness of lids and from being stuck together with discharge. Pain in eyes from reading. Burning in morning on waking and in *evening;* in the canthi. Pain as though a foreign body in the eye; *pressing,* as though, sand in eyes; sore, stitching. Photophobia and quivering of lids. Redness of the eyes. Swollen lids. Twitching of the lids. Styes on the lids. He sees bright colors; halo of colors around the light. *Vision is dim;* exertion of vision causes many symptoms. Flickering and foggy vision. Atrophy of the optic nerve. It has cured blindness from anæmia of the optic nerve.

Purulent discharge from ears. Eruptions on ears. Sensation of flapping in ears; they are hot and red. Itching of the ears and inside. Noises in ears, in morning; evening; with vertigo; buzzing; fluttering; humming; ringing; roaring; whizzing. Roaring in the evening. Pain in ear on blowing nose and swallowing. Boring, burning, stitching, and *tearing in ears.* There is pulsation and a stopped sensation in ears; swelling of the ears. Hearing is acute, later impaired.

Dry coryza alternating with fluent; with cough. Discharge bloody; copious; crusts; excoriating; *greenish;* offensive; purulent; yellowish-green; yellow; viscid thick. It cures most stubborn nasal catarrh. Painful dryness in the nose. The nose bleeds on blowing it. The nose is very red and it itches. One-sided obstruction of the nose. Pain in the nose and root of nose, worse on touch or pressure; soreness in nose; burning in nose; *smell lost;* nose swollen; ulceratic in nose; frequent sneezing.

Dry, cracked lips. Sickly, pale, bluish, red; alternating with pallor, red spots. Eruptions on cheeks, chin, forehead and nose; eczema and pimples; pimples on forehead; itching and heat of face. Pain in face worse in open air and from chewing; worse from motion of jaws; drawing, stitching and tearing pains; tearing in bones of face. Sweat on face; swollen face and lips; sensation of white of egg dried on face.

The gums bleed easily and the tongue is coated white. The mouth is very dry and the breath is offensive, even putrid. Pain in gums and palate; sore gums and palate; burning of the mouth. The gums are much swollen and the saliva is abundant. Taste is bitter, insipid, metallic, saltish, sweetish; taste is lost. Burning ulcers in the mouth; pain in teeth in evening, in open air, from masticating, from touch; pain boring, drawing, stitching, tearing.

Constriction of the throat from dryness in evening and on waking. Much hawking to clear the throat of tenacious mucus. Inflammation of the throat. Sensation of a lump in the throat. Pain in the throat in the morning, on *swallowing.* Burning, pressing, rawness, soreness; worse in morning; stitching on swallowing. Swallowing. is difficult, Swollen tonsils.

Appetite increased, even ravenous, without relish of food; hungry even after eating. Appetite wanting. Aversion to his accustomed beer and cigar; to food and meat. Coldness in the stomach. Constriction of stomach. Desires coffee, fruit and sour things. Distension after eating. Emptiness not relieved by eating; without hunger. Eructations in the evening; after milk; bitter; empty; sour; waterbrash; eructations give some relief. He suffers much from heartburn. Fulness and heaviness after eating. Hiccough after eating. He suffers much from indigestion. Nausea, in the morning, evening, night after eating, during headache. Pain in evening and night; after eating; better after warm drinks; cramping, cutting, drawing, gnawing, pressing, sore. stitching. Retching. Sensation of sinking. Extreme thirst. Thirstless during fever. Vomiting on coughing; after drinking water; bile; blood; food; mucus; watery.

Sensation of coldness and fulness of the abdomen. Flatulent distension. The abdomen feels heavy and constricted. Pain in abdomen morning and afternoon; after eating; before menses; when walking; better from warmth. Cramping, like colic. Pain in the liver. Burning, cutting and stitching pains; stitching in liver and sides of abdomen; rumbling; sensation of retraction of abdomen; jerking in abdominal muscles; sensation of weakness in abdomen.

Constipation with very difficult stools; no desire for stool and fruitless straining; constriction of anus during stool. Diarrhœa morning; afternoon, after breakfast; after eating; during menses. Abscess of the anus. Fistula ani. Flatus very offensive. Formication of anus. Hemorrhoids that bleed and protrude, worse walking. Itching and moisture of anus. Pain in anus and rectum. Burning during stool. Cutting during stool. Pressing pain. Soreness during stool. Stitching and tenesmus; paralysis of rectum. Stricture. Stool black, bloody; dry, *green, hard, knotty,* large, long and narrow, soft, *thin.*

Frequent ineffectual urging to urinate at night; tenesmus; retention of the urine; paralysis of bladder. Pressure in bladder. Urination difficult; *feeble stream, frequent at night;* involuntary on coughing; must wait long for urine to start; must press a long time before urine flows; an unsatisfied feeling after urination. A feeling of weakness in the bladder. Pain and inflammation of the kidneys. Enlarged prostate gland. Emission of prostatic fluid with stool. Gleety discharge from the urethra. It has cured chronic gonorrhœa with yellow discharge. Burning during the flow of urine. Cutting during the flow of urine. Swollen urethra. The urine is acrid, albuminous, burning, cloudy on standing, dark, *pale, copious;* cuticle on the surface; *scanty;* the urinary sediment is red, thick or white.

Erections very troublesome during the night; frequent, painful, violent, later impotency, inflammation of glands; itching of the genitals; soreness of testes; swollen testes; sweat on the genitals.

The woman has aversion to coition; coition without enjoyment. *Leucorrhœa excoriating,* bloody, burning, copious, thin, yellow, before menses, after menses. Menses irregular, too soon or too late; painful, pale, scanty, short; prolapsus uteri, ulceration of the os uteri.

Catarrh of larynx and trachea; dryness of larynx, mucus in larynx, rawness and soreness in larynx and trachea; itching in the larynx, hoarseness in the evening, with coryza worse from talking; the voice is rough, hollow and finally lost. Difficult breathing at night; asthmatic, rattling and wheezing; breathing arrested from coughing; desire for a deep breath.

Cough MORNING, afternoon, evening, night; before midnight; in cold air; asthmatic; dry evening and night; dry evening and loose morning cough; hacking in evening; from irritation in larynx, trachea; loose in morning; paroxysmal; rattling; short; from talking, tormenting; violent. Expectoration in the morning; bloody and copious; difficult; mucus, bloody; putrid; salty; sweetish; viscid; white; yellow.

Anxiety and constriction of the heart. Sensation of heat in chest. Inflammation of bronchia. Itching of skin of chest especially of mammæ. Oppression at night. Pain in chest at night; on coughing; after eating; on inspiring; in sides of chest; aching and burning; pressing; rawness on coughing; soreness on coughing; stitches on inspiring.

Palpitation in morning on waking; evening; anxious; after eating; during menses; on waking; tumultuous. Weak sensation in chest.

The back feels cold. Pimples on the back. Inflammation of the spinal cord. Itching of the back. *Pain in the back,* better by motion; rising from a seat; worse while walking. Pain in cervical region on moving the head. Pain between the scapulæ. Pain in the lumbar region; sacrum; coccyx when touched; spine. Aching in lumbar region during motion and walking; cutting pains in the back. *Sore, bruised pain* in spine; in sacrum. Stitching in back; scapulæ, lumbar region. Tearing in scapulæ; lumbar region. Stiffness of back; cervical region. Weak feeling in lumbar region.

While walking he staggers. Old chilblains came back. Coldness of hands, legs and feet. His corns smart and sting. Hands and fingers cracked. Cramps in the calf. Boils on nates and thighs. Eruptions on legs. Formication on upper limbs and feet. The hands are hot. Heaviness of *upper* and *lower limbs.* Ingrowing toe nail. Itching of limbs evening, worse after scratching; upper limbs and hands; *lower limbs.* Jerking in lower limbs. Numbness of limbs, upper limbs, lower limbs, legs, feet. Pain in limbs at night; in joints; pain in upper limbs. when they hang down; in left shoulder; elbow; pain in thighs, legs, feet and soles; aching in legs. Burning in upper limbs; soles. Drawing pain in limbs; arm; forearm; thighs; knees. Sore, bruised limbs; joints; lower limbs; legs. Stitching pain in limbs; upper limbs; arms; elbow; lower limbs; hips; knees; legs; soles; toes. Tearing pain in upper limbs; shoulders; arms; elbow; forearm; hands; fingers; *lower limbs; hips; thighs; knees;* legs, foot. Paralysis of limbs; *one-sided;* painless; *lower limbs.* Stiffness of lower limbs. Tension of thighs and legs. Tingling upper limbs; hands; fingers, lower limbs; feet; trembling of limbs, hands and knees. Twitching of the muscles of limbs. Weakness of limbs; upper limbs, *lower limbs; thighs; knees.*

Deep sleep. Dreams anxious; of death; of falling; of robbers; of vexations. Late failing asleep. Restless sleep. Sleepiness in morning; forenoon; evening; after dinner. Sleepless *before midnight.* After sleep he is unrefreshed. *Frequent waking.*

Chill forenoon; noon; afternoon; *evening in bed; night,* before midnight. Chilliness after eating; internal chill; coldness predominates. Shaking, quotidian chill; chill or coldness one-sided; warm room does not ameliorate the chill; desire for warmth which does not ameliorate.

Fever afternoon; evening; night without sweat; fever alternates with chill; heat goes from below upwards. Flushes of heat.

Perspiration morning and during night; during least exertion; from *least anxiety.*

Biting and burning. Anæsthesia. The skin is dry, burning or cold. Red spots on the skin. Yellow, as if jaundiced. Eruptions biting; boils; blood boils; burning; coppery, become moist with yellow discharge; dry; eczema. Herpes burning, corrosive, itching, scabby, stinging; eruptions itch in a warm room.

Pimples, rash and scabby eruption; smarting, sore, stinging eruptions. Urticaria, nodules after scratching. Vesicular eruptions. *Formication.* Itching at night in bed; biting, burning, crawling, worse after scratching; stinging; worse in warm bed; moisture after scratching. Pain in skin after scratching. Hyperæsthesia of the skin. Itching and stinging after scratching. A feeling of tension in the skin. Ulcers; offensive; with yellow pus; *indolent,* itching, sensitive, smarting, stinging, unhealthy. The skin refuses to heal where injured.

ALUMINA SILICATE

This valuable remedy is made from a species of rock known as andalusite and composed of aluminium sixty-three and silica thirty-seven parts. It was prepared by trituration in the usual way.

It has been proved and used clinically by the author for many years. It is a deep and long acting remedy and cures chronic complaints of the brain, spinal cord, bowels and the nerves, that have heretobefore been most stubborn.

Its complaints are sometimes noticed in the forenoon, but mostly in the afternoon and evening. Some symptoms come on in the night, even after midnight.

There is a desire for open air which is grateful, but cold air aggravates all complaints; much worse after becoming cold and a marked tendency to take cold. There is great coldness during pains and all pains are better from warmth and warm applications. The prover loses flesh, and it has cured patients markedly emaciated and anæmic. There is great weakness and many symptoms are worse going upstairs. Congestion of brain and cord and spinal nerves, with marked burning and stinging. It has cured multiple neuritis and locomotor ataxia. Constriction is a marked general symptom, also constriction of orifices, a sensation as if constricted. It has been of great service in epileptic and epileptiform convulsion; not when, the convulsion is on but as a constitutional remedy causing the attacks to diminish and come less frequently, and finally disappear. Stiffness and tonic contractions occur with provers. Distension of all the veins, and fainting spells. The symptoms are worse after eating and he is better fasting or eating very small quantities of food; worse from cold drinks, cold food, milk and very warm foods.

Formication of the skin, extremities along the *course of nerves* and in internal parts. A sensation of fulness throughout the body, with distended veins. Heaviness of the body and all the limbs. Induration of parts inflamed. Inflammation of the nerves, with burning, stinging, crawling and numbness; the brain, spine and abdominal viscera are extremely sensitive to a jar, as in riding in a carriage over rough roads. Jerking and twitching in muscles. The lassitude is so great that she was compelled to keep to the bed; she must lie down, a marked sense of spinal weakness. It cured a woman who had lain in bed many years from weakness. Straining of muscles from lifting, like Rhus tox. Yet some symptoms are worse lying in bed, but lying generally helps and rests the patient. She says, "I am so comfortable while lying." Some symptoms are worse lying on the back. She desires perfect rest, aversion to all motion and worse from all motion. The mucous secretions are increased. It has cured lupus. Numbness of single parts and of painful parts; numbness with neuritis. There is orgasm of blood, flushes of heat, even great rushes of heat to head from body.

The pains are worse from excitement and motion and better from external warmth and perfect rest. The pains are of all kinds, boring, *burning* and *stinging.* Constricting, cutting, digging, gnawing, jerking, paralyzing, pinching, *pressing.* The whole body is sore to touch and pressure, *stitching,* TEARING, *ulcerative* pain wandering from place to place.

The pains as well as many other symptoms show a marked periodicity. Pressure sometimes increases and sometimes helps the pains. Pulsation all over the body and in the head and abdomen. The pulse is fast, evening and night. The patient is better resting in bed and worse rising up from bed or chair. Sensitive externally and internally. Complaints all worse standing.

Extreme heat of summer takes her strength. There is swelling in affected parts and of glands. Throughout the body and limbs a feeling of tension. The limbs tremble and she trembles all over. Twitching all over. Complaints felt on waking. Walking is almost impossible; walking fast or any exertion brings out all symptoms; weakness from walking. Wet weather increases the symptoms. Close, warm room causes many symptoms.

It is very useful in nervous debility where there is great mental excitement and aggravations from anger and vexation. Absent-minded. *Anxiety,* evening, *night;* anxiety of conscience, anxiety about her health; worse after sleep. One prover felt that she would become insane and urged to have the 30th, which she had taken, antidoted. Wants this and that and never satisfied, she criticises everybody. She desires to be alone, but becomes worse when alone and better in company. She has much difficulty in concentrating the mind. Confusion of mind every morning, worse on waking. Worse from contradiction. Contrary and whimsical.

Several provers were timid and cowardly.

She thinks she is growing smaller and that she will fall if she rises to her feet; she sees visions; there is despair; she is discontented, discouraged and distracted; long periods of dullness of mind; dullness of mind after sleep.

There is marked exaltation of fancy. The mind is in a constant state of fear; wakes up with fear and frightened easily. There is a marked mental weakness forgetful, indifferent, irresolution, deficiency of ideas, so that it is easy to see the resemblance to imbecility or the borderland of insanity. She laughs much as in hysteria and many mental symptoms are hysterical in character. She is morose and obstinate and the memory is weak. Changeable moods. She makes mistakes in speaking and writing and uses wrong words. There is remorse; religious affections of the mind and great mental weakness bordering on insanity. It is useful in brain-fag after prolonged mental exertion. The mind is anxious and restless at night. There is great *sadness*. One prover said she was never so unhappy in her life, but she felt better after telling it to somebody. Great dullness of the senses. She is very sensitive to noise. She sits a long while without appearing to notice what goes on. She walks in sleep. Starting on falling asleep. She thinks much about suicide, loathes life and desires to die. She sits long, indisposed to talk; she talks in sleep; weeping in sleep. Will power very weak. Aversion to mental as well as physical work.

Vertigo morning and evening; while sitting; stooping; walking; turning the head suddenly; ameliorated while lying. Vertigo while closing the eyes, tendency to fall forward; on turning there is a tendency to fall in the direction turned; vertigo as if intoxicated, with nausea.

Rush of blood to the head, with boiling sensation and coldness of the occiput; constriction of the scalp, especially of the forehead. The head feels empty. Heat and *heaviness* of the head in the evening, especially of the forehead. Much itching and formication of the scalp. There is much pain in the head, *morning, afternoon, evening* and *night.* The headaches are worse from bending the head forward, binding up the hair, after eating; when biting the teeth together, before and during menses, while sitting; after sleep, after stimulants, stepping heavily, stooping. The headaches are better from binding up the head, *from cold applications, cold air, lying,* moving head, pressure standing and walking. There are intermittent pains day and night. Periodical headaches. Noise causes the headache to become pulsating. She wants the body wrapped up, but wants head in cold air. Sensation of crawling, as though ants in the brain, this sensation travels down the body and leaves at the toes. Pain in the *forehead,* over eyes afternoon and evening. Pain in occiput, temples, vertex and sides of head, worse on the right side. The pains in the head are burning, bursting, cutting, drawing, pressing, shooting, sore as if bruised, stitching and tearing. There is a dull pain in occiput, vertex and temples, worse from pressure and mental work. Pressing in forehead, pressing outward over eyes. Pressing in temples, vertex and occiput. The head is so sore during pain she cannot comb or brush the hair. Stitching pain in *forehead,* sides of head and temples. Many of the headaches were so severe that she was stunned by the pain. Violent, tearing pains in the evening; tearing in forehead in evening; tearing in frontal eminence; tearing pain in temples and vertex. Wandering pains in the head, better during rest and while sitting.

Pulsating headache worse from noise; pulsating in forehead and vertex. The brain seems to be sensitive to a noise. When something drops on the floor it seems to drop on her sore head.

The eyelids are stuck together during the night, and in the morning discharge thick mucus; dark rings around the eyes; eyes feel enlarged with dryness; catarrhal inflammation in the open air, with itching. Pain in the eyes; burning in the evening as from smoke; burning in lids and in the canthi; pressing pain in the eyes; soreness and pain as from sand in the eyes; stitching in the eyes. *Photophobia.* Redness of the eyes; styes and swollen lids. The vision is dim, worse at night by artificial light, and exertion of vision. The vision is foggy, weak, Hypermetropia.

Purulent discharge from the ears, with itching in the auditory canal. The ears are hot. Noises in the ears; humming, fluttering, ringing, roaring and whizzing. Pain deep in the ear; boring, stitching and tearing pains in the ear. Stopped sensation with pulsation. Hearing at first acute, later impaired.

The air feels cold in the nose on breathing. Catarrh of the nasal cavity and posterior nares. The discharge is BLOODY, containing crusts, *excoriating, greenish,* hard lumps; offensive, purulent, thick, sometimes watery, yellow or yellowish-green. Coryza with cough; dry, alternating with fluent, violent coryza; much dryness in the nasal cavity. Epistaxis on blowing the nose; the nose feels full, itching; in the nose. The nose is obstructed with thick mucus and crusts. Burning and tearing in the nose; much soreness in nose, root of nose and septum sore to touch; dull pain in nose on breathing transmitted upward to middle of vertex. Smell first acute, then diminished, later lost. Frequent sneezing, with and without coryza. Ulceration in the nose. The nose is greatly swollen.

Pain in the face; pain in malar bones, with pain in temples; pain from temples to malar bones and worse in open air and when chewing. Drawing stitching and tearing pains in the face. The face is purple.

Apthæ covering the mucous membrane of the whole mouth; the gums bleed and the tongue is coated white. Dryness of the mouth; when a chill or lacerating pain in head comes on the lips stick together. Mucus collects in the mouth, and the odor from the mouth is offensive; pain in gums and teeth from cold air, on biting, and after eating. Sore gums, palate and tongue; stitching and tearing pains in the teeth; *salivation,* swollen gums; the taste is bloody, metallic, sour or wanting. Food is *tasteless.* Ulceration of gums. Teeth very sensitive. Pain from roots of upper teeth to head, when biting teeth together.

Mild form of inflammation in the throat and tonsils. Hawks up much mucus; dryness of the throat on waking; sensation of a lump in the throat; tough, tenacious mucus in the throat; pain in the throat on swallowing; burning, rawness and soreness in the throat. Splinter sensation in the throat; stitching pain on swallowing; swallowing is slow and difficult; ulceration of the throat and the tonsils are swollen. Swollen cervical glands.

The appetite is increased, later ravenous, but the first mouthful causes nausea. The appetite is strong, but food is not properly relished; appetite for things not obtainable. Aversion to food, to meat, to coffee; thinks she cannot digest food; an empty feeling, which is not helped by eating. Eructations bitter, empty. sour, of food. after eating tasting like spoiled meat, waterbrash, eructations give relief. Fulness after eating, often only a mouthful. Weight in the stomach after eating; hiccough, heartburn and loathing of food. Nausea morning, evening and night; after eating, during headache. The sight and thought of food causes nausea. Pain in stomach, evening and night, aggravated by eating. Burning extending upwards, *cramping,* pressing, gnawing, cutting, stitching; pressing pain after eating, better by eructations. Soreness on pressure. Retchings. Sinking sensation. Sensation of a stone in the stomach. Water tastes as if spoiled. Some thirst, but no thirst during fever. Vomiting or *coughing after* eating and during headache; vomiting of bile, black blood, of food, mucus and water.

Obstructed flatulence in the abdomen, fulness, distension, hardness, heaviness, constriction; distension worse after eating. Pain in abdomen, worse after eating, before menses, during menses, worse walking and better by warm applications. Pain in region of the liver; burning in the abdomen. Cramping, colicky pains begin in the stomach and pass down into bowels, with urging to stool. Cramping all over abdomen, and then must run and pass a watery, fetid, yellow stool. Cutting and pressing stitching pains in left hypochondrium and in the liver; tearing pains in abdomen. Rumbling and tensions.

Constipation, very difficult stool; unsatisfactory, scanty stool; much straining, even soft stool is difficult. Constriction of the anus during stool. Diarrhœa driving out of bed at 5 a.m.; first undigested, then watery, clear, with much flatus, from fruit. Passes much flatus with stool; flatus offensive without stool. Crawling at the anus. Hemorrhage from external piles. Inactivity of the rectum; itching of the anus—worse by scratching; moisture around the anus; pain in anus during stool; burning during stool. Cutting, pressing, soreness and stitching. Tenesmus of the rectum; paralysis of the rectum. Ineffectual urging to stool. The stool is bloody, copious, dark, dry, hard, knotty. large, offensive, scanty, soft, thin, watery, undigested.

Paralytic weakness of the bladder. Retention of urine. Tenesmus while passing urine. Ineffectual urging to urinate. Frequent urging to pass urine, worse at night; urination in feeble stream, frequent during the night; must wait long fur urine to flow; unsatisfactory feeling in the bladder after urination; involuntary urination.

Emission of prostatic fluid during stool, the gland is enlarged, sore and painful; prostate gland inflamed.

Discharge of mucus and pus from the urethra; burning when passing urine; cutting during the flow of urine.

Urine copious, later scanty, burning, cloudy and red. Red sediment, specific gravity normal, no sugar, no albumen.

Troublesome erections of the male during the night, which are very strong and painful; the testes are swollen and hard; the glans penis is red and excoriated; the scrotum itches and perspires. Frequent seminal emissions, sexual excitement is strong during the evening and night.

The woman has tormenting itching and crawling; worse after urination, worse after scratching, better by cold applications. Leucorrhœa acrid, bloody, copious, purulent, thin, white or yellow; worse before and after menses. Menses in one prover too frequent, in several provers, too late, intermittent, offensive, painful, scanty. Suppressed menses has been cured. Burning pain in the genitals; prolapsus of the uterus; ulceration of the labia.

Irritation of the larynx, mucus in larynx and trachea. It cures catarrh of larynx and trachea. Rawness and soreness in larynx. Must scrape mucus from the larynx very often. Constant tickling in the larynx and trachea. Husky, rough voice. Hoarseness, worse in the morning.

The breathing is arrested by coughing, wheezing, asthmatic breathing; rattling breathing. Difficult breathing from coughing.

Cough in the daytime, morning, *evening* and *night.* Asthmatic cough. Dry cough morning and *night;* dry cough with expectoration only in the morning; the cough is worse in cold air. Dry, hacking cough in the *evening.* Much irritation in larynx and trachea from hard coughing. Loud cough in the morning with fever. Lying on the right side causes coughing spells. Racking, paroxysmal cough from tickling in the larynx. Violent coughing spells.

Expectoration daytime, *morning,* evening and night, *acrid,* bloody, copious, offensive, viscid, white or *yellow.*

Orgasm of blood or a feeling of congestion in the chest. Constriction of the chest; oppression, heat and blood spitting; inflammation of bronchial tubes; pain in chest during the night; during cough, in the sides of chest. Burning in chest. Crushing pain in chest; rawness in chest when coughing; sore, bruised chest-walls from coughing. Stitching pain in chest from coughing and inspiring. Weakness felt in the chest and palpitation of the heart.

On exposure to cold air the back is cold as if cold water were poured on it. Many eruptions on the back. Itching of the *cervical* and dorsal regions; pain in the back on motion, rising from a seat, *stooping* or *walking.* Lying perfectly quiet the pain is relieved, but turning or trying to help herself out of a chair causes pain in back near the spine. Pain in cervical and in the *whole spine;*

aching in the spine, but especially lumbar region and sacrum. Great burning in the spine, burning pain in the cervical region and between the scapulæ. Pricking like needles in the lumbar region on exertion; better during rest. Sore and bruised feelings in the spine, especially the lumbar region; sticking like needles in the lumbar region. Stitching pains in the back, in the cervical region, in the scapulæ and between the scapulæ. Tearing pain in the back. *Stiffness* of the back and of the *cervical* region; extreme weakness of the back compelling her to remain in bed.

Awkwardness of the limbs, more in the lower limbs. A blue painful spot on the hand where she had a wart removed many years ago. The nails became brittle; the hands are constantly chapped; coldness of hands. *legs* and *feet;* hands cold as ice and fingers blue. Cramps in the calf. Emaciation of all the limbs, numerous eruptions on the limbs, notably boils and red rash. *Formication* is extreme. The hands are very hot. Heaviness of *upper limbs,* of *lower limbs, hands and feet.* Violent itching without eruption, upper limbs, hands and fingers, *lower limbs, thighs* and *soles.* Painful itching in arms along the course of nerves. Jerking in all the limbs. Numbness of all the limbs, upper limbs in forenoon, numbness of hands and fingers, numbness of lower limbs, *legs, feet* and heels; numbness of first two toes of right foot while lying on the back. Pain in the limbs from excitement, worse from motion, worse during the night. Pain in the joints; pain in upper limbs, shoulders, elbow, forearm, hand and fingers; pain along the course of nerves. Pain in lower limbs from motion and excitement; pain in thighs, legs and feet, pain along the course of nerves. Pain travels from below upwards, worse on left side; pain goes to cardiac region and then to left temple. Aching pain in legs. Burning pain in limbs; burning pain in arms from *excitement;* burning in the soles. Crushing pain in the bones of legs, and in the muscles. Drawing pain in upper arm and in forearm; drawing pain in thighs, knees and ankles; pricking pain, thinks a knitting needle is thrust deep into muscle of right hip. Sore, bruised limbs. *lower limbs,* legs, tibia, SOLES; stitching pains in upper limbs, shoulder, upper arm, elbow and wrist; stitching pains in hip, knee, calf, sole, toes. Tearing in upper limbs, shoulder, upper arm, elbow, forearm, hands and fingers; tearing pain in *lower limbs, hip,* thighs, KNEES, LEGS, calf, ankles, feet; tearing pains along the course of nerves. Wandering pains of all kinds in the limbs. Painless paralysis of lower limbs, also pain in the paralyzed parts. Tension in the upper limbs and in the arms when lifting anything; tension in the calf and feet. Swelling of the fingers. Stiffness in the lower limbs. Tingling prickling in all the limbs, upper limbs, hands and fingers, lower limbs and feet. Trembling all over, in limbs, hands and knees. Twitching of limbs, in shoulder, lower limbs, legs, feet. Ulceration about the nails. Weakness in the limbs, *upper limbs,* LOWER LIMBS, *thighs, legs.*

He is unable to step up when ascending stairs; it seems to him that he cannot lift his body to the next step.

Sleep is disturbed by visions; dreams anxious, confused, amorous, of death, *nightmare,* pleasant, of quarrelling, vexatious. Sleep is restless and broken. Sleepiness in the morning, forenoon and evening, and after dinner. Sleepless before midight; unrefreshing sleep, waking too early, *frequent waking.* Yawning.

Chilliness in the forenoon, noon, afternoon, evening; chilliness in the evening in bed; chilliness in the open air, after eating, better after warm drink; external coldness; internal coldness. Chilliness on moving in bed. Shaking chill at 5 p.m. One-sided coldness. Chilliness during stool. Desire for warmth which ameliorates the chill.

Heat afternoon, *evening* and *night.* Fever begins between 8 and 10 p.m., with severe crushing pain in both legs; pain goes to heart and left temple. External heat with chilliness. Flushes of heat; during sleep.

Perspiration morning, night, with anxiety; perspiration on motion—profuse after waking.

Dryness of the skin, coldness, biting, anæsthesia, yellow spots. *Burning,* cracked. Eruptions, blisters, boils, burning; chapping. DRY eczema. Herpes, dry, itching, stinging. Itching eruptions worse by warmth. Painful eruptions. Nodular urticaria, vesicular eruptions. Marked eruption moist after scratching, smarting after scratching. Stinging and burning eruptions. Suppurating phagedenic eruptions. Nodular urticaria, vesicular eruptions. Marked formication of the skin all over body, itching worse in evening in bed. Biting, burning, crawling; better by keeping perfectly still. Itching better by scratching. Stinging burning in the skin all over, but worse on the back of hands, arms and feet. Moisture of the skin after scratching. Skin extremely sensitive. Much tension in the skin. Ulceration, with itching, soreness and stinging. The skin is slow to heal after injury.

AMBRA GRISEA

On looking over this remedy as a whole it will appear to you that you have been studying the characteristics of one *prematurely old.* You will often see symptoms coming on in one at fifty years of age that should appear at eighty, and after studying this remedy you will see that the same aspect is presented, a premature old age. We recognize trembling and a peculiar kind of feebleness that cannot be described by any expression but senility; it is not the confusion of mind belonging to sickness, but the peculiar state we recognize in old people, in declining life; trembling and tottering and a dreamy state of mind with forgetfulness. He goes on from one subject to another, asking a question, and, without waiting for it to be answered, asking another. And so he jumps about from one topic to another. It can hardly be said to be confusion, it is a dreamy state of mind, a state of senility. This remedy is useful when such a state is found in young persons, when the mind is not insane and yet it is weak. Especially is it indicated in those persons who manifest a momentary, fleeting inquisitiveness, *jumping from one subject to another.* Often a patient asks me one question after another, never waiting to have the first one answered, a flitting, flighty talker, who does not seem to realize that I have not answered his questions; that patient, I say to myself, needs Ambra grisea. That state of mind belongs to modern society women in such great frequency that you will be astonished to note it on all hands. A modern society belle that could not darn the heel of her stocking to save her soul will in a few years get into just that state, and even Ambra will not cure her. But there is a kind of nervous sickness manifested by these symptoms that Ambra grisea will cure. Alternation of depression of spirits with vehemence of temper is another feature. That naturally belongs to old age. A period of greatest excitability is often followed by depression, a state of indifference to all things, to joy, to grief, to people, etc., treating with indifference things that would naturally break the heart of a well-balanced person. He does not even wonder why he is not excited over these wonderful things, so decided is the state of indifference. Many of the complaints are *worse in the morning.* He gets up with confusion and dulness of mind and is in a dreamy state and towards evening he takes on symptoms of insanity.

Ambra is one of the most frequently indicated medicines in simple, nondescript *vertigo* of old men. So dizzy that they cannot go out on the street; so dizzy upon getting up in the morning that they must wait a while until they can get around on their feet. It is the dizziness belonging to senility and to premature old age. Now, when this man undertakes to meditate upon something his ideas are whisked away. It is a sort of confusion with *vanishing of ideas.* He has to make an unusual effort a few times to bring his thoughts back to the place before he can concentrate the mind to meditate upon some idea. But while concentration of the mind is difficult, he is compelled to sit and *dwell upon the most disagreeable things* that force themselves upon him and he cannot get rid of them. It is somewhat analogous to *Natrum mur.*, but the peculiar feature of *Natr. mur.* is that she delights to dwell upon past unpleasant occurrences and lies awake at night thinking about them. Ambra grisea is forced to dwell upon such things. Images, false faces, hideous imaginations, fancies and visions annoy him and keep him awake. In the semi-dreamy state he is kept holding up before his mind these grimaces. Such a state of mind may come on from business embarrassments with vertigo, congestion to the head and brain-fag.

One thing running through this remedy is that the *presence of other persons aggravates the symptoms;* also the *marked aggravation from con-*

versation. A woman, when attended by a nurse, is unable to have a stool without sending the nurse into another room. In spite of much straining she can do nothing unless alone. It is said that in *Natr. mur.* the patient cannot urinate in the presence of other persons. The urine will not start when anyone is around. That is a sort of general feature of this remedy. Confusion of mind and embarrassment in the presence of other persons. Embarrassment in company. As soon as he goes into company there is flushing, trembling, nervous excitement and the thoughts vanish. With these symptoms the patient imagines that he is going out of his mind, and finally he settles down into a state of *melancholy,* sadness and despair, and does not want to live. He loathes his life and wants to die, "Great sadness." "Melancholy, sits for days weeping." Such is the mental state of this prematurely old patient with broken down constitution. It is a picture of a wreck and the question will arise when you find a patient that looks and acts in this way whether you have received him in time to cure him. You readily see you have before you one who is going down hill and going into insanity of one form or another. A physician sees the forerunner of a great breakdown when he sees an Ambra grisea patient with the nervous mental state, the quivering, trembling, and excitement in one who was once a strong, vigorous man. Some great business or domestic shock has come upon this patient. it is not the aspect you see when phthisis is coming on; you do not see the cachectic condition, but it is a prostration of the nervous system, a mental prostration. A man goes through the trial of one death after another in the family and there seems to be nothing remaining; he cannot look at it philosophically; he has lost his business and his friends and then he takes on dreaminess and wonders whether life is worth living. Then it is you get the Ambra grisea aspect.

Many of the complaints come on *in the morning* and many come on *after eating.* "Vertigo with feeling of weight on vertex; worse after sleep," but especially in the morning. It is not mentioned in the text, but it is also worse after eating. "Had to lie down on account of vertigo and feeling of weakness in stomach."

Running through the nervous symptoms we have *music* is *intolerable;* music makes him tremble, aggravates his mental symptoms and gives him pain in the back as from a hammer. A number of physical symptoms are brought out by listening to music. The tones seem as if they were a material substance taking hold of him.

Complaints are often *one-sided;* perspiration on one side of the body or perspiration on the affected side. "On right side of head, a spot where hair when touched pains as if sore." The same sensation is in the skin, oversensitive to touch. "Scalp feels sore in the morning when awaking; this is followed by a sensation of numbness." The word *numbness* you will find running through the complaints. You will find a peculiar kind of numbness, such as belongs to old people. Diminished sensibility of the parts; feeble circulation.

Again, we find under the eye symptoms, "Dulness of vision as if from looking through a mist." There is dimness of vision coming on without any condition in the eye that would justify it. It is a nervous dimness of vision, a senile paralysis coming on. "Itching on eyelid as if a sty was forming." *Itching* is felt all over the body; itching in all the little openings.

Among the symptoms that are not in the text and that are decided symptoms belonging to this remedy are, "Pressing headache starting from both temples, drawing and tearing in the head, to and fro. Shooting through the head, lancinating, cutting pains, worse on exertion, better from quiet and lying. Headache when blowing nose. Pressing pain in the left frontal eminence and in the eye. Burning in the right eye and in the eyelids. Tearing in short streaks in and upon the right eye, pressure on the left eyebrow, shooting, aggravated after eating; lachrymation." These are in the original provings, but not in the text; they have been left out. This is the case all through the *Guiding Symptoms;* important symptoms were left out because it was necessary to cut down the work.

"Hearing decreases." Dulness of hearing without any organic affection of the ear. So perverted is his ability to hear that music aggravates his symptoms, that is through the nerves of hearing. "Listening to music brings on congestion to head." Music aggravates his cough. Think of one commencing to cough simply because he hears music! What a strange thing that is! *Calcarea* has such sensitiveness that the stroke of the piano is painful in parts, especially in the larynx.

This remedy is full of *bleeding.* Copious bleeding from the nose in the morning. There we get the morning aggravation again. We get the idea of the feeble circulation because of the easy oozings from mucous membranes. "Copious nose bleed early in bed." "Dried blood gathered in nose." "Long continued dryness of the nose, frequent irritation as from sneezing." In the nose an old, dry catarrh with atrophic condition of the mucous membrane The nose inside becomes shiny and withered.

Dryness of the mouth without thirst. Biting pain in the throat between the acts of swallowing. Rawness in the throat. The throat complaints are worse in the morning. Complaints are worse after eating and worse from warm drinks especially from warm milk. "After caring, cough and gagging." There is a peculiar combination of symptoms about the throat. Dryness and accumulation of mucus in the throat which he tries to expel, and when making an effort to cough out the mucus he gags and sometimes vomits. Vomiting from cough. Weakness at the pit of the stomach after every evacuation; an "all-gone" feeling in the pit of the stomach. Pressure deep in the region o the liver; worse in the morning; worse after eating; worse after stool. Distension of the abdomen with great flatulence, especially after eating. Some symptoms are worse after drinking. Sometimes these complaints come on in the middle of the night, rousing him up with rumbling and cutting in the bowels. The abdomen is cold; it feels as if the whole inside of the abdomen were cold. At other times the coldness seems to be on one side of the abdomen.

Inveterate *constipation* in old persons, and especially when it is impossible to have anyone near at the time of stool. "Frequent ineffectual desire for stool; this makes her very anxious; at this time presence of other persons becomes unbearable." After the normal stool there is pressure in the abdomen or a sense of emptiness and weakness in the abdomen which is better after passing flatus or eructation.

Bloody *urine* with red sediment in the urine. Urine when emitted is clouded, yellowish-brown and deposits a brownish sediment. "Sour-smelling urine." The urine is copious. "During urination burning, smarting, itching and titillation in the urethra and vulva." "Sore rawness between the thighs." "Voluptuous itching on scrotum." "Violent morning erections without desire," with numbness of the genitals. The symptoms are most erratic, as much so as in *Ignatia* and *Natr. mur.* Taken as a whole they can be reconciled, but taken a few at a time they seem wonderfully inconsistent. You must get the whole remedy in order to comprehend it.

Copious discharge of blood between the menstrual periods. "Discharge of blood between periods at every little accident." Discharge of blood from the vagina from pressing at hard stool; even from a walk that is a little too long or from too great exertion. "During menses left leg becomes quite blue from distended varices, with pressive pain in leg." "Lying down aggravates uterine symptoms;" quite an unexpected thing. Menses too early and too profuse. "Menses appear seven days before time," and then comes that horrible itching of the genitals; "soreness, and itching with swelling of labia."

Another marked feature of this remedy that you might expect with all this nervous excitement and prostration is dyspnœa with cardiac symptoms, difficult breathing, a sort of asthma. it comes on from any little exertion. Asthma on attempting coition.

"Itching, scraping and soreness in larynx and trachea." "Titillation in throat, larynx and trachea." Everywhere there is itching, and the itching is very often a form of crawling. "Asthma of old people and children," in feeble, tremulous, weakly ones. "Whistling in chest during breathing." "Spasmodic cough." *"Violent spasmodic cough with frequent eructations and hoarseness."* A good deal of this cough is of nervous origin. It is a cough with excitement, with nervousness, with trembling, which would make one of considerable experience wonder if that patient did not have brain and spinal cord trouble. Nervous cough, such as occurs often in spinal irritation. Cough from constriction of the larynx followed by copious flow of white mucus. This is a paroxysmal cough, much like whooping cough. Asthmatic dyspnœa from any little exertion, from music, from excitement. Cough with congestion of blood to the head. Cough from thinking and from anxiety.

It is not very long after these symptoms show themselves before this patient will emaciate and wither, until the skin looks like dried beef. With all he is a tremulous and shaky patient.

He complains a great deal of tearing pressure deep in the left side of the chest. Sensation of rawness in the chest and itching in the chest, Titillation and itching, moving about here and there if he tries to touch the place and scratch it.

You will not be surprised to know that this patient suffers from palpitation of the heart upon slight exertion, from excitement. from music, from any effort to put the mind on anything, with trembling and quivering. And this palpitation he notices even to the extremities; he throbs all over. His extremities pulsate. He is conscious of his arteries everywhere and the palpitation of his heart causes oppression of breathing.

The limbs easily become numb; pressed upon in the slightest manner they go to sleep; go to sleep on being crossed. Coldness, trembling and stiffness of the extremities. The finger nails become brittle and are shrivelled. The arms go to sleep when lying down. "Sore and raw between the thighs and in hollow of knees." Heaviness of lower limbs, paralytic weakness; the patient is growing old; senility is coming on. This remedy has cured the premature trembling that comes on in middle-aged persons. It has cured the "going to sleep" and numbness and feeble circulation with loss of muscular power. It is very suitable in children who are excitable and nervous and weak. "In lean persons." "Old persons and children."

AMMONIUM CARBONICUM

If we were practicing in the old-fashioned way and considered the wonderfully volatile nature of Ammonium carb. in some of its forms we would only look upon it as an agent to relieve fainting and simple affections and use it in the form of hartshorn to comfort old maids and some other women. But Ammonium carb. is a deep-acting, constitutional medicine, an anti-psoric. It effects rapid blood changes, it disturbs the whole economy and it establishes a scorbutic constitution. Its fluids are all acrid. The saliva becomes ,acrid and excoriates the lips, so that they crack in the corners and middle, and become raw and dry and scabby. The eye-lids fester and become dry and cracked from the excoriating fluids from the eye. The stool is acrid and excoriates. The genitals of the female become raw and sore from the acrid menstrual discharge and leucorrhœa, and wherever there is an ulcer upon the skin the fluids that ooze from it excoriate the parts round about, this excoriating character belonging to all of the exuding fluids and discharges.

This remedy has bleeding of black blood, often fluid blood, that will not coagulate, flowing from the nose, the uterus, the bladder and bowels. The blood is dark, showing that a great disturbance is taking place in the circulation. The skin has a mottled appearance intermingled with great pallor.

It produces a violent action upon the heart, in which there is audible palpitation, and every motion aggravates the pulsation. With this is associated great prostration. It is rather a strange coincidence that the ancients knew that Amm. carb. would overcome difficult breathing from cardiac attacks and that aqua ammoniæ or hartshorn is used to-day to a certain extent in indications similar to those mentioned. They use it as a stimulant, but when indicated the single dose very high is enough. The ancients knew enough, also, to use hartshorn in the low forms of pneumonia, at the turning point in the advanced stage; that is an old allopathic practice, but it had a homœopathic relation some of the cases. Once in a while they would cure a patient in the awful stage of prostration with heart failure at the end of pneumonia, and because they relieved such a one it was then established as a remedy for all future use.

Ammonium carb. has a state analogous to blood poisoning, such as we find in erysipelas and in the most malignant forms of scarlet fever, with prostration, great dyspnœa, so that it seems as if the heart were giving out. With this there is an unusual patchy condition of the surface, due to the paralytic condition of the blood vessels, enlargement of the glands, duskiness and puffiness of the face. Amm. carb. has been used allopathically in just such a state for centuries and it has demonstrated its homœopthic relations by its efficacy.

It belongs to the simple enfeeblement, weak heart, emaciation. There is quite an absence of symptoms and a lack of response to remedies. The patient must lie in bed because of the palpitation and difficult breathing on motion. It is a matter of mere weakness. Such a case furnished me much amusement for a year and a half. There was a woman in this city who answered just such a description; her state was one of peculiar cardiac weakness with dyspnœa and palpitation on motion. I had been treating the case, but had not fully studied it, and as she did not progress under my management she was taken out of my hands and taken to one of our most able neurologists, who put her upon the "rest cure" and promised that in six weeks she would be perfectly well. But at the end of six weeks she was worse than ever and a cardiac specialist was then brought to examine her. He said it was true the heart was not vigorous, but there was no organic affection and consequently the case did not belong to his branch. Then a lung specialist was brought in, and later she was examined by all kinds of specialists. All of her organs were fully investigated, and it was announced that nothing was the matter with them; but the poor woman could not walk because of her sufferings and palpitating heart. She had a little dry, hacking cough that did not amount to anything, but her chest was examined and there was nothing wrong with it. But after she had been in this continual fire for about three months, and was steadily failing, the side of the family that were my adherents prevailed against the others and I went to see her again. I continued to study the case, which was extremely vague, having nothing but those few symptoms, and finally I settled upon Ammonium carb., and she has been on this remedy for eighteen months. She now climbs mountains, she does everything she wants to do and is about ready to go to housekeeping. She has grown from a case of nervous prostration, brain-fag and any other diagnosis that might have been heaped upon her to a well woman, and under that one remedy. This shows you how deeply this remedy acts. One dose generally acts upon her for from six weeks to two months, steadily improving her each time.

Exhaustion coming at every menstrual period. An attack of cholera cr what one might mistake for cholera, coming the first day of the menses; a copious diarrhœa. Sometimes it is an exhaustion with vomiting, exhaustion as in *Veratrum,* with coldness, blueness, sinking, dyspnœa: The kind of dyspnœa that I have been speaking of up to this time is not an asthmatic dyspnœa; it is a cardiac dyspnoea, due to a weak heart; but this remedy has also asthma, and in the asthma there is this peculiarity: if the room is warm the dyspnœa increases until suffocation seems imminent; as if he would die for want of breath. He is compelled to go out into the cold air for relief. While the warm room increases the dyspnœa in asthmatic complaints the bodily state of the patient is worse from cold. The complaints of the body and the headaches are worse from cold.

A common thing running through this remedy is aching in the bones. The bones ache as if they would break. The teeth ache violently from every change of weather or from change of the temperature in the mouth. The jaws ache or the roots of the teeth ache. A prominent feature is falling out of the hair, the finger nails become yellowish, the gums settle away from the teeth and bleed, the teeth become loose, all in keeping with the scorbutic constitution.

This remedy has hysteria, and it is not surprising that nervous women carry a bottle of ammonia hanging to their chain. Many women do this because as soon as they go into a close place they faint and must use their hartshorn. This condition in the woman, if in a mild degree, is not hysterical; it belongs to the sensitive nature of women; but if carried to a more marked state it is hysterical. The hysterical fainting will be averted by the use of the hartshorn. Amm. carb. will stimulate the action of the heart and relieve.

The remedy is full of depression of spirits. She weeps much, has fainting fits, anxiety, uneasiness and exhaustion from motion. Oversensitive about what she hears other people saying. Complaints from listening to others talking. Complaints, both mental and physical, are worse in the wet weather, and she is sensitive to cold, raw, wet weather. The gouty complaints, nervous complaints, prostration, cardiac complaints, dyspnœa, headaches, etc., come on in raw weather. A congestive headache comes on in wet weather and from weather changes. Sensation as if the brain would ooze out through the forehead and eyes.."Pulsating, beating in the forehead as if it would burst." The headache is worse from stepping, especially the headaches that come at the menstrual period. Headache worse in the morning. This medicine in such headaches, with the symptoms I have described, shows its antidotal relation to *Lachesis,* because *Lachesis* produces all this state of prostration. In the old text-books you will notice this expression, "Inimical to *Lachesis.*" This means when *Lachesis* has been given in high potency and has acted curatively, Ammonium carb. is not likely to act curatively after it, and is sometimes capable of disturbing the case, confusing it and mixing up the symptoms. But when *Lach.* has been given in too low potency, and the patient has been poisoned with the crude medicine, this remedy then becomes an antidote, used in a high potency, because of the similarity in its action. It will overcome many of the poisonous symptoms of the case. If you will examine the appearance of people who have been bitten by snakes and then examine the pathogenesis of this remedy you will see a great similarity between them. It is well known that this remedy has had repeated use in snake bites. Evidently it did not save all of them, but it must have done something for these cases or it would not have established so great a reputation for itself. Give it not as an antidote *per se,* but when indicated in blood-poisoning and animal bites with zymosis, with a tendency to black liquid bleeding, as in *Elaps.* Running through the snake poisons there is a tendency to bleeding of black blood that will not coagulate.

It has many eye symptoms. Sparks before the eyes in connection with headaches; double vision; aversion to light. "Large, black spot floats before the eyes after sewing." When these symptoms have been present in such a constitutional state as I have described the remedy has cured cataract; it has cured the patient and finally the crystalline lens has cleared up. Burning of the eyes, smarting eyes, blood-shot eyes.

It disturbs the hearing, causing hardness of hearing and discharge of acrid fluid from the ears.

We have had scorbutic, catarrhal condition of the nose, such as described. Discharge from the nose acrid. "Severe pain as if the brain were forcing itself Out just above nose." "Nose-bleed when washing face or hands in morning." It has many complaints from bathing, and a prominent feature is that the skin is covered with red, mottled spots after bathing. Bathing produces surging all over, here and there, as well as nose-bleed. Palpitation is worse from bathing.

In the throat we have an appearance like malignant scarlet fever. diphtheria and other zymotic states; purple, swollen, ulcerated and bleeding, and gangrenous, accompanied by great exhaustion, with enlarged tonsils and glands. The glands outside of the throat and neck are enlarged and felt as lumps. In diphtheria, when the nose is stopped, the child starts from sleep gasping for breath. Here again we observe its relation to *Lachesis* and the ophidia, for soon after the patient drops to sleep he wakes up suffocating. In diphtheria, in chest troubles with great prostration, the patient is worse after sleep.

Menses too soon. "The menstrual blood is blackish, often in clots." The leucorrhœa is acrid. "Violent tearing in abdomen and vagina." "Irritation of clitoris." Swelling of the genitals. Now, let me tell you something not mentioned here, but important, and that is a sensation of soreness in the whole pelvic viscera; at times it seems as if all her inner parts were raw. It is a sensation of soreness; not always sore to touch. This sensation of deep-seated soreness is especially felt during menstruation. All through the menstrual period soreness and rawness. "Menses premature, abundant, blackish, often in clots, preceded by griping and colic."

The remedy is full of catarrhal symptoms and cough, with much rattling of mucus in the chest and air passages. Oppression of breathing, a catarrhal dyspnœa. Especially is this a remedy, when the symptoms agree, in hypostatic congestion of the lungs, a filling up of the chest with mucus which it is difficult to expel; great rattling in the chest and great weakness. It is a good palliative in the last stages of consumption. A dose of Ammonium carb. when there is great coldness, prostration and weakness in the chest. It is not unlike that sensation of weakness in the chest which is like *Stannum*. He can hardly cough out loud, and because of the weakness he cannot expel the mucus, like *Ant, tart.* Short asthmatic cough.

The complaints of this remedy come on especially at three o'clock in the morning. The cough comes on at that time. Old people who suffer from catarrh of the chest have an aggravation at three o'clock in the morning with the palpitation and prostration, waking up at that hour with cold sweat and dyspnœa. Almost pulseless; weakness of the heart. Face pale and cold.

"Great lassitude." Defective reaction with, or at the close of, severe zymotic troubles, typhoid, diphtheria, scarlet fever, erysipelas, etc. In those complaints that should come to a crisis, if the patient goes into a state of great exhaustion under remedies fairly well selected, you have an instance where this medicine competes with *Arsenicum* for the nervous prostration. You see "heart failure" spoken of in old school literature. They say the patient got along very nicely, but finally died of heart failure. In a great many instances if Ammonium carb. were given in time it would save life.

"Averse to walking in open air." "Children dislike washing." The warmth of the bed relieves the rheumatic pains, relieves the chill. "In a warm room the headache is better." "From washing reappearance of the symptoms; nose bleed; blue hands; swollen veins." "Worse in cold air."

We come now to the appearance of the skin: "Body red as if covered with scarlatina." "Putrid flat ulcers with a pungent sensation." "Malignant scarlatina with somnolence, starting from sleep." "Erysipelas of old people when cerebral symptoms are developed." Whenever treating a severe form of disease and an eruption comes to the surface, like a carbuncle or erysipelas, and does not give relief to the patient then there is danger. A remedy must be found soon. When a patient is coming down with severe internal troubles it is not a very uncommon thing for unhealthy looking boils to come out, or carbuncles or erysipelas blotches. It is always serious when these are not immediately followed by relief to the patient. It shows a pernicious state that has been pent up and cannot be held any longer and this violence is going to destroy. This is one of the remedies that you may look for to check the progress of such states. Any remedy, of course, which corresponds to the totality of the symptoms is the remedy to administer.

AMMONIUM MURIATICUM

The patient frequently feels a boiling throughout the body as if in the blood vessel. Sensitive to cold. Many complaints increase while in the open air. Flushes of heat, ending in sweat. Tearing pains and smarting prevail extensively. Burning and excoriation of mucous membranes. Drawing or sensation of shortening of tendons. It is a long-acting remedy. There are few reliable mental symptoms known. Anxiety, fretfulness and antipathy to certain persons. Neuralgic and rheumatic pains in the head. Tearing pains in the head. Stitching and tearing in the temples. Itching of the scalp and other parts. Rash all over body Like measles. It cures capsular cataract, when the symptoms agree. Yellow spots before the eyes. Burning of the lids and balls in twilight or dim light. Mist before the eyes in a bright light. Burning of the ears when walking in cold air. Difficult hearing. Catarrh of right car, throat and larynx.

Much sneezing, watery burning discharge, yet stoppage of nose. Coryza with burning in larynx. It has been used extensively in traditional medicine for coryza. Some sore throat and inflammation of the larynx. For these troubles in olden times the large chunk of sal ammoniac was produced, a few crystals shaved off with a common jack knife into a glass of water. All got the same thing, regardless of symptoms. Sonic were cured promptly of these bad colds, with or without fever. It is now an overlooked remedy. Its symptoms should be carefully studied.

With many of its complaints there is much pallor of the face. Tearing in the bones of the face. Swelling of the submaxillary and parotid glands with stitching pains. Burning and excoriation of mouth and lips, like *Am. c.* Tongue swollen. It is a very useful remedy for nondescript sore throat; but especially useful where there is marked burning and much viscid mucus, pulsating in the neck and glands of neck, great swelling, pale face, stitching in the throat, great pain on swallowing, with or without thirst.

Eructations of food as eaten, and vomiting. Sensation of hunger with fulness, which is a flatulent state. Empty feeling, gnawing in the stomach and spleen. Burning, stitching, tearing pains in the abdomen. Distension from flatus. Much grumbling in the bowels. Much pain in inguinal region. Pain in abdomen and back during menses. The abdomen is fat, relaxed and heavy, and the lower limbs are lean. Excoriation and burning of the rectum and anus during and long after stool. Stitching, tearing pains in the perineum. Hard, crumbling stool, most difficult to expel; must use the abdominal muscles. All the salts of ammonia, like this one, have painful hæmorrhoids. It cures diarrhœa when the stools are like scrapings, bloody and watery; also green, slimy stools in the morning. Diarrhœa and vomiting during menses, like *Am. c.* It has cured enlarged prostate, also enlarged uterus.

Menses too soon each month, with pain in back and abdomen. The flow is black and clotted, much like *Am. c.* During menses there is often hæmorrhage from the bowels or rectum with cholera-like symptoms.

Copious uterine hæmorrhage. Copious white painless leucorrhœa. With all the abdominal and menstrual symptoms there is copious flatus, with rumbling and colic.

These symptoms especially in pale, sickly, feeble women.

In catarrhal troubles that extend into the larynx and bronchial tubes, with stitching, tearing, burning. Hoarseness and loss of voice, with burning in the larynx. Constantly scraping white mucus from the larynx. Difficult breathing when using the arms or from manual labor. Weight on the chest in open or cold air. Dry cough from constant tickling in the larynx. Daily recurring suffocating cough. In weakly people going toward phthisis, with daily dry cough and fast pulse.

Violent backache at waist line, worse at night. Coldness between the shoulders.

Stitching, drawing, tearing in limbs. Drawing in the limbs. Tension in the muscles and tendons of the lower limbs. Tension in posterior part of thighs when walking. Cold feet at night in bed. Copious night sweats latter part of night. Flushes of heat and fever.

If the reader will take up the provings and study them carefully he should be able to use this remedy in the direction pointed out, and most likely would see uses not mentioned.

ANACARDIUM ORIENTALE

This remedy is full of strange notions and ideas. The mind appears to be feeble; almost, if not complete imbecility; seems as if in a dream; everything is strange; slow to comprehend. Marked irritability; disturbed by everything; cursing. Weak memory. Forgetful of things in his mind but a moment ago. All his senses seem to vanish and he gropes around as if in a dream. Change of states; alternate states. Dulness and sluggishness of the mind prevail. He is in a continuous controversy with himself. Irresolution marks his character. He cannot settle between doing this and that, he hesitates and often does nothing. He cannot decide, especially in an action of good or evil. He hears voices commanding him to do this or that, and seems to be between a good and an evil will. He is persuaded by his evil will to do acts of violence and injustice, but is withheld and restrained by a good will. So there is a controversy between two wills, between two impulses. When this is really analyzed by one who knows something of the nature of man it will be seen that the man is disturbed in his external will, but the internal will cannot be affected by medicine. His external voluntary is continuously excited by external influences, but his real will, in which is his conscience, restrains that and keeps him from carrying the impulses into effect. This can only be observed when its action is on a really good man. He has a controversy when his external will is aroused, but in an evil man there is no restraint and he will not have this symptom.

Hallucinations: a demon sits on one shoulder and an angel on the other. He is disposed to malice and has an irresistible desire to curse and swear. Laughs when he should be serious. So it is carried on until all things in the external will are inverted. Internal anxiety, i.e., the internal will is in a turmoil over this external disturbance. "Contradiction between will and reason" is an attempt to express what the individual knew nothing about. "Feels as though he had two wills." That is better. It finally destroys or paralyzes the external will, and when a man is naturally evil and is under the paralyzing influence of Anacardium he will do acts of violence. A wicked man is restrained, not by his conscience, but by fear of the law. Anacardium paralyzes the external will and places him in a position of imbecility, and he does acts of violence from his own natural perverted self. It has so acted on a portion of the mind that it teaches a great deal. I have learned much from Anac., *Aurum* and *Argentum* of the strange action of medicines on the human mind. Psychology must be figured out by the action of drugs on the human mind. By this means we get at facts and can lay aside many hypotheses.

Ideas as if nothing were real, all seems to be a dream. Fixed ideas. He thinks he is double. This comes from a vague consciousness that there is a difference between the external and internal will, a consciousness that one will is the body and another is the mind. Dwells on thoughts about salvation. That a stranger is by his side, is another recognition of the two wills. That strange forms accompany him, one to his right side and one to his left. This mental state drives him to madness. Alternation of his moods and understanding. One moment he sees a thing and another moment he does not understand it. One moment she sees it is her child and another that it is not. One moment it is a delusion and next moment it is an illusion. One moment thinks it is so and next moment has enough reason left to know that it is not so. Delusion is an advanced stage of illusion. In the Repertory we have the same remedies often in illusion and delusion, it is a matter of grade. When the intellect is slightly affected it is an illusion, and what he sees he knows is not so. He sees demons, and at first he knows from his intelligence that a demon is not there, but later he wants you to drive him out. It does not matter which, they are similar symptoms, and it is a matter of degree, and so, in the Repertory, delusions and illusions are not given separate places.

Anac., *Hyos., Stram.* and *Bell.* are important in bringing out the quality of the perverted human mind as to the intelligence and affections. Whenever a medicine makes a man desire to do something it affects his will, and when it affects his intelligence it is acting on his understanding. Medicines act on both.

Low-spirited, disheartened, fears he is pursued, looks for thieves, expects enemies, fears everything and everybody. Full of internal anxiety. No peace. He is separated from the whole world, and he despairs to do that which is required of him. Cowardly in the extreme. Fears some dreadful thing will happen. Morose, sulky, sullen. Unsocial; complains of weak memory. Slight causes make him excessively angry. A strong feature is that all moral feeling is taken out of him. He feels cruel. Can do bodily injury without feeling. Cruel, malicious, wicked.

Bad effects of mental excitement. Weak-minded. Consequences of fright and mortification. Suitable in religious mania when the conflict between the external and internal will is kept up. It is analogous to *Hyos.*

Many complaints are ameliorated by eating.

Sensation here and there of pressure, described as of a plug, all through, the body, in the head, eyes, in the navel and down the spine. Objects appear too far off. Things have a strange look, sometimes uncanny. Illusions of smell, burning timber, pigeon's dung. Chronic dry coryza.

The whole body has been well covered by symptoms; but it seems that the mind represents the principal aspect, and it will seldom be used excepting for such mind symptoms. Usually when the mental symptoms are strong the physical are also covered by the remedy.

Full of trembling and paralytic weakness. Tetanus; epilepsy. Sensations as of a hoop or band around the body, limbs or head; pressing as of a plug.

The eruptions are like *Rhus* in many respects; erysipelatous eruptions dark, dusky, and of malignant types. It is an antidote to *Rhus* poisoning. Eruptions all over. Yellow vesicles are common. Intense itching of eruptions. Warts on the palms like *Natrum mur*. Skin burns much. It seems closely related in its symptoms to all the *Rhus* family.

ANTIMONIUM CRUDUM

You will be surprised, when studying full provings of this substance, to notice that all the symptoms seem to centre about the stomach; it does not matter much what kind of complaints he suffers from, the stomach takes part in it. The pains disturb his stomach and bring on nausea; with his headache he is sick at the stomach; with all complaints his stomach is out of order, and, on the other hand, whenever he disorders his stomach he is sick all over. Complaints that manifest themselves through the stomach very frequently need this medicine.

First in importance are the mental symptoms showing the type of constitution likely to need this remedy. It produces a very serious state in the mind, an absence of the desire to live. It is well known to physicians that the case is a serious one if the patient has no desire to live; life is a burden. When I hear a patient say: "Oh, doctor, if I could only die." I do not like such a case; there is some deep-seated trouble in the economy that is hard to remove. Something is threatening, and when it comes it is a common thing to see the patient actually die. "Loathing of life." You will find this especially in a low, lingering, continued fever, such as typhoid. This remedy has all the prostration of typhoid, and it has the continued type of fever as well as the intermittent and remittent. The prostration is similar to *Arsenicum,* but *Ars.* has overwhelming fear of death, while this medicine has loathing of life; and so they both part company. *Ars.* has overwhelming restlessness, this remedy is seldom restless. *Ars.* has an intense thirst, this medicine is thirstless. So even though both these remedies have excessive exhaustion with continued fever, we see they have features dissimilar enough to make them wholly distinct.

Such a typhoid will sometimes be seen in young girls about puberty who are threatening to go into chlorosis. They have loathing of life, but it is a hysterical loathing of life. Moments of great exhaustion, sudden attacks of weakness and fainting. You will commonly find another feature with this, not coming at the same moment, but alternating with it, or only present at times, namely, these over-excitable, intense, nervous, hysterical, ecstatic young girls and women are overcome by mellow lights such as flow through stained glass windows or the mellow light from the moon in the evening. That is what is meant when it says in the text: "Sentimental mood in the moonlight." It is a hysterical state, a disorderly outburst of the affections, such affections as can be aroused only in one who is sick, or one who is unbalanced in the general nervous system. This kind of patient gives us the mental state and constitution of Ant. crud., and along with such mental states the physical conditions seem to strike to the stomach, as it were.

We have running through this remedy a general state that you should keep in mind, that is, a gouty or rheumatic state, in which the symptoms change with the changes of the weather; worse in cold, damp weather, worse from cold bathing, better from the heat of a hot bath, worse from taking sour wine, and worse from stimulants of any kind. When you use the expression "worse from wine," it is not only important to know that the patient is worse from wine, but also the character of complaints that are worse from wine. This patient becomes easily intoxicated, but the physical symptoms are more disturbed than the mental; his gouty symptoms are worse from sour wine; all the pains and aches of the body are worse from sour wine; headaches come from this cause and the gastric disturbances are greatly aggravated from sour wine.

This patient is worse at night, worse in damp weather, worse from damp cold, better from lying down quietly, better from applied heat, but much worse from over-heating and from radiated heat, and in a warm room. Many of the symptoms come on in the sun's rays and from the heat of an open grate. The open fire is wholly against the Ant. crud. patient. A child with whooping cough will cough more after looking into the fire. Such things are queer; they are so strange that there is no philosophical hypothesis to explain them, no theory that looks toward an explanation, but they are facts which we must accept.

The whole gouty nature of the case seems to change so suddenly that you wonder where the more exterior symptoms have gone to, for all at once in a night or a day the patient commences to vomit and you have persistent vomiting lasting days and weeks, until the gouty symptoms come back into the extremities. It is wonderful how quickly this old-fashioned metastasis will come on, this changing from one place to another. The gout suddenly ceases in the extremities and stomach symptoms come on, and you may call it gout in the stomach if you will.

There are catarrhal symptoms in this remedy; catarrh of the nose, stomach, rectum, etc., and an increased flow of mucus from any of these localities from drinking sour wine and from taking cold. A distressing feature of the catarrh is the stuffing up of the nose at night. As soon as he gets into an overheated room, his nose gets stuffed up. The coryza has a tendency to become chronic, because of the low and feeble circulation and the poor constitution. When it becomes chronic it is worse at night and is associated with headaches. As the catarrh slackens up and becomes dry the headache becomes worse; he has neuralgia in the head, crushing pains and dreadful sickness at the stomach with vomiting. He often has an attack of sick headache and it will be called by the family a gastric sick headache, but the condition just mentioned comes on from taking cold, which slacks up the thick discharge into a dryness of the nose and the inhaled air burns the nose like fire. Sometimes these troubles pass off after an intense vomiting spell; sometimes they do not, but the headache may remain for days not relieved by vomiting, or relieved only after prolonged vomiting. There are remedies full of headache and as soon as he vomits he feels better, but in this remedy he vomits long, and becomes relaxed and exhausted. The headache is worse moving about, worse at night, better from lying down, from keeping quiet, better in the open air, worse in warm room, worse from overheating, worse from radiated heat and light. You see now how the catarrh, the headache and gastric symptoms all belong together. It is because the patient is sick that you cannot take symptoms separately, you must prescribe for the whole man.

There is another feature belonging to the mucous membranes, and an important one; these membranes have a tendency to throw out a milky white exudation or deposit, and it is especially noticed upon the tongue. The whole tongue is covered with a milky-white coating. This you find in all diseases where the remedy is indicated. In the stomach disorders of children, in gastric fevers, in complaints with fever and much vomiting, great irritation of the whole nervous system and in irritation of the stomach in typhoids, the tongue looks white. Upon the slightest provocation he will retch and gag. Everything seems to disturb him. He has loathing of food; the thought and smell of food disturb him. This is like *Arsenicum.*

He takes a cold bath at night on going to bed and gets up in the morning voiceless; cannot speak a word. This has come on in an aparently painless manner; he does not know that it is present until he attempts to speak in the morning. This may be present with spasms of the larynx, clutchings of the throat. Colds sometimes go down into the throat and into the trachea, producing a bronchitis or pneumonia.

Dry, hacking spasmodic cough in diminishing paroxysms. I will explain that: The first paroxysm occurs with great violence, racking his whole frame, and lasting a longer or shorter period, to be followed by one with less violence and another with less violence; perhaps after a dozen or less paroxysms of diminishing violence, he ends up with a dry, hacking cough which is not a paroxysm. When this first cough shakes the whole body, whether it is a bronchitis or whooping cough, and the tongue is white, and there are more or less gastric disturbances, Ant. crud. is the remedy. It will change the whole aspect of the case at once. The chest remains sore, lame and bruised from the violence of the cough.

The stomach symptoms must be particularly considered. Constant nausea, lump in the stomach, feeling all the time as if he had an overloaded stomach, as if he had eaten too much, and that is when he had not eaten at all. The stomach feels distended although the abdomen is flat. He feels distended and vomits the contents of the stomach; he vomits slime after he has emptied the stomach of its contents; prolonged retching, nausea, sickening load in the stomach and it seems to go on and on. The vomiting does not relieve and there is increasing exhaustion.

Inflammation and hardness of the liver or any portion of it. Pain in the region of the gall bladder. Great pain in the region of the liver, rending, tearing pains in the liver. Jaundice is associated with these symptoms at times.

In the abdomen we have a group of symptoms; violent abdominal pains, burning, great distension; there appears to be an increasing distension as if by a screw, gradually forcing down upon something gradually increasing the tension. We find this state in the tympanitic condition of typhoid fever, we find it in cases of flatulence, we find it in summer diarrhœas. It will be associated with gastric symptoms and the white tongue, especially if such disturbance had been brought on by drinking sour wine, by taking a cold bath, in one who has a gouty constitution, where the nodules in the finger joints become painless and the stomach and bowels become distended and painful.

This remedy has a nondescript diarrhœa, but also a lumpy and liquid diarrhœa. Diarrhœa from sour wine. It seems to take a long time to empty the bowels. He burries to stool and passes a little lump and some liquid, and is soon hurried again to stool and more lumps and liquid are passed, and this goes on in summer diarrhœas until finally the bowel is emptied and then there is great tenesmus. It is a diarrhœa ending in dysentery; inflammation of the rectum and colon, with suffering, much tenesmus, prolonged efforts and great exhaustion.

Troublesome hæmorrhoids in old gouty constitutions. They are always soreand inflamed from a cold, wet day, from cold bathing and are always worse if he is foolish enough to drink sour wine or take sour food. The stomach, bowel, rectum and hæmorrhoidal complaints are all worse from disordering the stomach with sour wine, sour fruit or indigestible substances, from cold bathing and wet weather.

The pelvic viscera become greatly relaxed, especially in women, so much so that there is a dragging down in the pelvis. It seems as though the contents of the pelvis would be expelled, or would fall out. There is prolapsus of the uterus and a discharge resembling leucorrhœa. Disturbances of various kinds at the menstrual period. Irritable and painful ovaries, such as we find associated with hysterical girls; those who suffer from unrequited affections; dreamers.

This medicine produces sweating; copious, exhaustive sweats night sweats, such as we find in lingering diseases. Sweats from the slightest exertion. If he becomes slightly overheated he fairly boils with perspiration and then takes cold.

The skin is ulcerated and has a tendency to grow warts, callosities, bad nails and bad hair. Hard, horny excrescences grow under the nail and are extremely painful. From the ends of the fingers little horn-like excrescences appear. The slightest pressure will produce a callosity, or a sore place, and in working men you will find an unusual tendency to thickening of the skin on the soles of the feet. They are very sore to walk upon, because these callous places are sensitive and have numerous centres of little-corns. The tendency to build up and indurate belongs to the remedy. Warts grow upon the hands. The hair is unhealthy. Pustules form upon the skin with red areola. Pustular eruptions have an inflamed base that is red, and sensitive.

Now, if you will study the proving and get the particulars of the remedy, and fit them into this framework, you will understand something of Ant. crud.

ANTIMONIUM TARTARICUM

About the first thing we see in the study of an Antimonium tart. patient is expressed in *the face*. The face is pale and sickly; the nose is drawn and shrunken; the eyes are sunken and there are dark rings around the eyes. The lips are pale and shrivelled. The nostrils are dilated and flapping, and there is a dark, sooty appearance inside of the nostrils. The face is covered with a cold sweat and is cold and pale. The expression is that of suffering. The atmosphere of the room is pungent, more pungent than fœtid or putrid, and makes you feel that death is in it. The family is disturbed; they are going hither and thither, and the nurse is in an excited and busy state, and you enter upon this scene to make a homœopathic prescription. It is one of excitement and one that you cannot act rapidly in, but one in which you must make a very quick prescription. These things will interfere somewhat with your thinking at the time that you must do the best thinking and the most rapid thinking.

Now, in what kind of cases do we find this state and appearance, where all the features and symptoms conform to the nature of the remedy? First, in *catarrhal patients,* in broken down constitutions, in feeble children, in old people. Catarrhal conditions of the trachea and the bronchial tubes. Our ears being open we hear *coarse rattling* and bubblings in the chest. If you have ever been in the room of the dying you have heard what is called the death rattle. It is coarse like that. Now and then there is expectoration of a mouthful of light-colored, whitish mucus. The condition is one in which the chest is steadily filling up with mucus, and at first he may be able to throw it out; but finally he is suffocating from the filling up of mucus and the inability of the chest and lungs to throw it out. It is a paralytic condition of the lungs. It may occur in cases of grippe. At first it may be a case that comes on quite rapidly, running a rapid course. It may be a case that produces early prostration, that is, in three or four days or a week. The first few days of the sickness will not point to Antimonium tart. So long as the reaction is good and his strength holds up you will not see this hippocratic countenance, sinking, and coldness and cold sweat. You will not hear this rattling in the chest, because these symptoms are symptoms that indicate a passive condition. Antimonium tart. has weakness and lack of reaction. Hence we see that it is suitable in those cases that present this state, or in such patients as are so feeble, when they are taken down, that they at once enter upon a passive or relaxed state. In cases of bronchitis with pneumonia, inflammation of the trachea, inflammation of the air passages in general, the inflammation is likely to be attended with dryness or a scanty flow of mucus. If this be violent in a few days it will reach a state of relaxation and weakness. But the first state does not indicate Antimonium tart. Such medicines as *Bryonia* and *Ipecac.* come in for the first period, and your impression is, when administering those medicines, that they will be sufficient for the whole case, and they will he, except in those states wherein this weakness is present from the beginning, or where there is lack of ability to react sufficiently from your remedy to recovery under it. Then comes in a second remedy, and that is the time when this medicine begins its operation.

Ipecac. has some of this coarse rattling, but it is attended with great expulsive power of the lungs. This medicine has the coarse rattling that comes after many days. *Ipecac.* has it the first days of the sickness. This remedy has the coughing and gagging and retching, but in the stage of great relaxation, prostration and coldness. It seems as if he will die. When you hear him cough you are at once impressed with the idea that there must be some profound weakness in his lung power. We know that it is in the power of the lungs to produce an expulsive action with the deep inspirations. They have no such power in Antimonium tart. The chest is full of mucus and it rattles; the cough is a rattling cough, but the mucus does not come up, or only a small quantity comes up, but it does not relieve him. His chest is full of mucus, he is suffocating and he is really passing away, dying from carbonic acid poisoning due to a lack of expulsive power. In cases of pneumonia; when first coming down with a chill, it may be a very violent attack, such an attack as from its violence produced prostration early, that is, after three or four days. It is not indicated in the beginning during the chill, and during the high grade of inflammation, but during the stage of exudation. But the violence of the attack leads him to a state of prostration, or he is already feeble as if he were old, and therefore he becomes easily relaxed and prostrated from the disease. Altogether unlike *Aconite, Bell., Ip.* and *Bry.,* for they come down with violence—the very opposite is present in Antimonium tart. Little fever, cold sweat, coldness, relaxation, hippocratic aspect. So it is the remedy that closes out the scene with the severe cases of bronchitis, pneumonia; most of these cases die in an Antimonium tart. state. This patient is an old *gouty patient,* debilitated from long illness, always shivering, pale, with enlarged joints. Every spell of wet weather brings on a catarrhal state of the chest, larynx and trachea which runs into a state of copious secretion of mucus. He is in bed at once, prostrated, with coarse rattling. In children that have frequent attacks of bronchitis, from cold wet weather, from cold rainstorms in the autumn, in the spring and in cloudy weather. No sooner do they get over one cold than another cold comes on. The acute stage is never violent with them, but they keep having these passive rattling colds. Recurrent rattling in the chest. Chilly, and pale. Those florid children that do not look sick when they have a cold, are more or less vigorous, who have rattling in the chest, but do not come down with weakness and are not prostrated from it, but do not come down with weakness and are not prostrated from it, but keep on rattling, they call for *Kali sulph.* That is quite a distinguishing feature,—the weakness at once speaks for this remedy. In *very old people* this weakness occurs, old broken down people who have for years had *catarrh of the chest.* Every sharp cold spell in the winter brings on catarrh of the chest, with thick white mucus, and attended with great dyspnœa, driving him to bed. He must sit up in bed and be fanned; cannot lie down because of the difficult breathing, and filling up of the chest. Antimonium tart. will ease him over a number of these attacks before he dies. When the mucus is yellow and purulent in one of these old people, *Ammoniacum* will tide him over a good many winters. We see a good many old people that suffer from catarrh of the chest during the winter; they have had it for years, and do not expect to be any better. When the expectoration is yellow *Ammoniacum* will pull them through, and Antimonium tart. when it is white and attended with prostration, sweat, coldness, pallor and blueness of the face. These are the principal uses of this remedy in practice.

It has many pains and aches. To a great extent Ant. tart. builds upon the *Antimonium crudum* basis. It forms its chest symptoms to a great extent upon that basis. Many of the symptoms are like *Antimonium crudum; many* symptoms are worse when warmed up, and from too much clothing. You will see this patient sitting up in bed with no clothing around the shoulders or neck, and the night-gown wide open in order to breathe. Suffocates if the room is too warm. It gets that from the *Antimonium crud.* It is worse from bathing in cold water, like *Antimonium crud.* The mucous membranes are covered with thick white mucus, like *Antimonium crud.* Also he does not want to be meddled with or bothered. Everything is a burden. The child when sick doesn't want to be touched or talked to or looked at. Wants to be let alone. The infant is always keeping up a pitiful whining and moaning. Many times the respiration is a moaning respiration. Rattling and moaning. Always in bad humor, that is, extremely irritable when disturbed. Any disturbance seems to increase the breathing and is an annoyance and makes the patient irritable. No wonder the patient is wonderfully anxious, because from his appearance we would say that he must have the feeling that he is dying. He looks as if he were sinking, and if he does not get relief soon he certainly will die, for there is a filling up of the chest that is suffocating him, and the feeling is that of suffocation, dyspnœa, which is steadily increasing. The wings of the nose move as in *Lycopodium. Lycopodium* competes with it very closely and resembles it very much.

There are many headaches laid down under Antimonium tart., but *Antimonium crud.* is more likely to work out for Antimonium headaches, while this medicine is more likely to work out for Antimonium chest troubles. Both of these remedies have very decided gastric symptoms. Constant nausea, vomiting and indigestion. Antimonium tart. with its difficult breathing is sick at the stomach. Loathes everything, loathes food; vomits even water. He has also a docile state and if allowed to be quiet, in spite of all the sufferings, he will fall into a sleep, or go into a state of inability to feel. He will cough and sleep, and snore through the dyspnœa, so that it is in many ways like *Antimonium crud.,* but *Antimonium crud.* has nothing like the copious flow of mucus from mucous membranes that are inflamed. It has nothing like the passivs state of the whole economy. It is not so desperate in its provings, and not so dreadful to look upon.

Clinically Ant. tart. has been confined in its use mostly to the mucous membranes of the chest, but it has the same passive conditions of all the mucous membranes of the body, discharges of white mucus from the eyes. "Eyes prominent, glaring. Dim, and swimming. Gonorrhœal ophthalmia." But the rheumatic conditions furnish another form of this remedy, another phase of it like *Antimonium crudum.* The joints are affected, take on a passive, slow infiltration and become dropsical; dropsical swelling of all the joints. Gouty infiltration of the joints, and these are especially bad during the cold, wet weather. Eye symptoms of this gouty character. Eyes infiltrated along with the joints, so there is a gouty state of the eyes. The gouty state affects the whole body. The mucous membrane is pale instead of being red and inflamed; it is pale and relaxed, and it appears to ooze; mucus forms upon it very readily. This is the state that occurs in the chest. It is not that burning rawness found in *Ars.* and the more acute remedies, although there is a state of prostration and the anxiety and cold sweat which resembles *Ars.*

Then this gouty state affects the teeth. His teeth are all rheumatic. "Rheumatic pains in the teeth," with rheumatic pains in the joints. Teeth are sensitive. "Teeth covered with mucus."

With all the complaints the *stomach* gives out, and there is nausea, inability to digest and loathing of food. Vomiting of everything taken into the stomach; vomiting of even a spoonful of water. In most complaints this remedy is *thirstless.* It is an exception that it has thirst. Generally in these attacks of dyspnœa the friends of the patient stand around with a very strong desire to do something, if it is only to hand a glass of water. This patient is irritated by being offered a swallow of water. He is disturbed, and shows his annoyance. The child will make an offended grunt when offered water. Thirstlessness with all these bronchial troubles, with copious discharge of mucus and great rattling in the chest. Sometimes there is an irresistible desire for cold things in the stomach, but it is the exception. "Desire for acids or acid fruits," and they make him sick. Troubles brought on in the stomach from vinegar, from sour things, from sour wine, from sour fruits, as in *Ant. crud.* Aversion to milk and every other kind of nourishment, but milk especially makes the patient sick, causing nausea and vomiting. The stomach and abdomen are greatly distended with flatulence. The abdomen is tympanitic. With the stomach symptoms and bowel symptoms there is this *constant nausea,* but it is more than a nausea, it is a deadly loathing of every kind of food or nourishment, a nausea with the feeling that if he took anything into the stomach he would die; not merely aversion to food, not merely a common nausea that precedes vomiting, but a deadly loathing of food. The weakness takes on an increased anxiety, and he increasingly suffocates when he is offered food. Kind-hearted people very often want him to take something, for perhaps he has not taken any food all day, or all night; but the thought of food only increases the dyspnœa, increases his nausea, his loathing and his suffering. Vomiting is not an easy matter in this remedy. The vomiting is more or less spasmodic. "Violent retching. Gagging and retching and straining to vomit. Suffocation, gagging, through great torture." The stomach seems to take on a convulsive action, and it is with the greatest difficulty, after many of these great efforts, that a little comes up, and then a little more, and this is kept up. "Vomiting of anything that has been put into the stomach, with quantities of mucus." Thick, white, ropy mucus, sometimes with blood. "Vomits slime, with great

exertion. Vomiting large quantities of mucus. Vomits tenacious mucus."
"Vomiting of slime, with bile. A tough, watery mucus, then some food, then
bile." But the principal thing vomited is the thick, white, ropy mucus, flowing
from the mucous membranes everywhere. Tough and stringy; can be drawn
out in strings. The patient is often choked while this thick, ropy, white mucus
is expelled from the œsophagus and mouth. The mouth fills up with it. It is a
tremendous effort, a spasmodic effort, for this patient to rid the stomach of
its contents, which is mucus, or mucus and bile. Early in the vomiting it is
mucus, and after much straining there is a regurgitation of bile into the
stomach, and the continuing of vomiting is from bile. The great straining also
induces a flow of blood into the stomach, and the contents of the stomach
will be streaked with blood. *Ulceration* of mucous membranes everywhere. It
has ulcers in the nose and in the larynx, and ulcers that bleed. Bleeding
ulcers in the stomach, and so there is vomiting of blood.

Like *Antimonium crud.*, it has been useful in old drunkards. Old drunkards sometimes take on a debilitated form and take frequent colds. After
getting over a big debauch, having been many days on one of their times,
they become relaxed and cold, and take cold, and the chest fills up with
mucus, and they are vomiting, suffocating and vomiting. "Rattling of mucus
in the chest of old drunkards." Ant. tart. is sometimes required. *Ant. crud,*
when the trouble is confined mostly to the stomach. Ant. tart. when the chest
symptoms are present with growing anxiety and the coldness and the
prostration; prostration from long drinking. Old gouty patients, old drunkards;
old broken down constitutions. In children also that have broken down
constitutions, as if they had grown old. These take cold in the chest, with
great rattling of mucus, and require this remedy.

Very commonly there is anxiety in the stomach, it is not always described
as a pain, but an anxious feeling, a deathly sinking, an indescribable sinking
in the stomach as if she was going to die. "Anxiety in the stomach with
nausea." A passive congestion of the liver, with vomiting and bile.

The remedy is also full of cutting pains, cutting like a knife. Pinching in
the intestines. Colicky pains. Distension of the abdomen. The abdomen may
be distended with serum, or it may be distended with flatus. "Sharp, cutting
pains, as with knives. Most violent pains in the abdomen." Dropsy is one of
the natural conditions of all forms of Antimonium. I remember an energetic
horse doctor feeding all the horses *Black antimony* when the epizootic was
upon the land, going through all the stables. I learned that he was giving
Black antimony to all horses and I left instructions that mine should not
have any medicine except what I gave. Nearly all the horses that he treated
ended in dropsy, and were laid up for days and weeks with the legs wrapped
up. It was a proving of Antimonium. Ant. tart. is full of it. It was a common

thing, formerly, for old broken down constitutions to be put on Ant. tart. at the end of pneumonia and fevers, but they almost always had bloating of the feet for three or four months after getting up. If they did not have that, they had "fever sores." Antimonium is a common cause of the "fever sore," the lingering indolent ulcer that forms upon the legs following old fevers in broken down constitutions. Sometimes they never get rid of them. They certainly never get rid of them unless they fall into the hands of a prescriber of our school.

APIS MELLIFICA

This remedy has so many symptoms on the surface of the body we will study the outer aspect first. All over the body is found a thick rash, sometimes of a rose color. It is rough and can be felt as a rough rash under the fingers. The patient at this time is greatly distressed by heat and the skin is sensitive to touch with the rash or without it. Nodular swellings here and there come and go. Then comes an erysipelatous inflammatory condition, in patches, here and there, about the head, with great tumefaction about the face, eyes and eyelids. Erysipelas may occur anywhere, but it more commonly belongs to the face and runs to a high degree of inflammatory action, with stinging, burning and œdema. In the extremities we have a marked dropsy, swelling with pitting upon pressure. A general anasarca may appear. The face is greatly swollen at times, the eyelids look like water bags, the uvula hangs down like a water bag, the abdominal walls are of great thickness and pit upon pressure, and the mucous membranes in any part look as if they would discharge water if they were punctured. Puffing or œdema, with pitting upon pressure, is a general condition that may be present in any inflammatory state. There is a general amelioration from cold and aggravation from heat. The skin symptoms and the patient are aggravated from heat. This prevails also in the mental state, in inflammatory conditions; in cardiac conditions, in dropsy, in sore throat, etc. Sometimes this aggravation amounts to aggravation from warm drinks, warm room, warm clothing, warmth of the fire, etc.; if it is heat the patient is greatly disturbed. In brain troubles, if you put an Apis patient with congestion of the brain into a warm bath he will go into convulsions, and consequently warm bathing is not always "good for fits." It is taught in old school text-books so much that the old women and nurses know that a hot bath is good for fits, and before you get there just as like as not you will have a dead baby. This congestion of the brain, with little twitchings and threatening convulsions, makes them put the baby in a hot bath, and it is in an awful state when you get there. If the baby needs *Opium* or Apis in congestion of the brain the fits become worse by bathing in hot water. If the nurse has been doing that kind of business you have learned the remedy as soon as you enter the house, for she will say the child has been worse ever since the warm bath, has become pale as a ghost and she was afraid he was going to die. There you have convulsions worse from heat, pointing especially to *Opium* and Apis. That is the way with Apis all through. It is not laid down in the books that Apis is worse in the throat symptoms from warm drinks and wants altogether cold things, and will not take warm things which aggravate, but one of our graduates wrote me that by making use simply of the generals, as he had been instructed, Apis conforming to all the rest of the case, he made a beautiful cure of a case of diphtheria which had the relief from cold, which shows how generals are continued into particulars and how they can be made use of. The generals continue to build and enlarge our Materia Medica.

Upon the outer surface then we see that Apis is full of dropsy, red rash, eruptions, urticaria, erysipelas, which inflammations extend to the mucous membranes. The outer part of man is his skin and mucous membrane. When we are dealing with man from centre to circumference, we think of the inneremost as the brain and heart and internal organs that are vital, while their coatings and coverings are external. Apis affects the things that are external; it affects the envelopes, the coverings. You notice how frequently it affects the skin and the tissues near the skin, and it also affects the envelopes or coverings of organs; for example, the pericardium. It establishes serous inflammations with effusion. Apis produces an inflammation of the membranes of the brain. In the serous sac which encloses the heart, pericardium, and also in the peritoneum it produces the same kind of inflammation. Thus we see that the coverings are especially affected by Apis, viz., the skin and mucous membranes and the coverings of organs; and with these we get dropsy, catarrh and erysipelas. In all of these inflammatory conditions there is stinging and burning; burning like coals of fire at times, and stinging as if needles or small splinters were sticking in.

The *mental symptoms* of Apis are very striking, and the most striking thing throughout the mental state is the aggravation from heat and from a warm room. The symptoms themselves are great sadness, constant tearfulness without any cause, weeping night and day; cannot sleep from tantalizing thoughts and worrying about everything. Depression of spirits with constant weeping. Sadness and melancholy; extreme irritability; borrowing trouble about everything. Foolishly suspicious and jealous Absolutely joyless. Absolutely indifferent to everything that would make her happy or joyful. No ability to apply things that would make her happy to herself, they must mean someone else. Foolish, silly, childish behavior in a woman in confinement, in a woman in advanced years; talking foolish twaddle, such as a child would talk, on serious occasions. Another aspect of the mental state is the delirium, which comes on in serious forms of brain affections in children. The child gradually goes into a state of unconsciousness. Lies in a stupor, one side of the body twitching, the other side motionless, rolling head from side to side; head drawn back rigidly; pupils contracted or dilated, eyes very red, face flushed, a stupid state or state of semi-consciousness. Child lying with the eyes partly closed, as if benumbed. It is suitable in congestion of the brain, meningitis or cerebrospinal meningitis with opisthotonos when all the symptoms are aggravated from heat. The child puts on a more dreadful state if the room becomes overheated; becomes extremely death-like or pale if the room becomes overheated. If the child is able to do so it kicks the covers off. If it is in a position where it can look into a large open grate it will be much aggravated. I have seen Apis children who had to be removed from near an open fire. They will cry to get away from the heat that comes upon them from the register or open fire. The heat increases every symptom, and sometimes causes them to break out in a cold sweat all over the body, which does not ameliorate their fever nor the burning heat. Very often the head is rolling and tossing, the teeth gnashing, and the eyes flashing with threatening convulsions, the child carrying the hand to the head at times, a state of semi-consciousness, and the child screams out with that peculiar scream which is known to mean congestion of the brain—cri encephalique —the brain cry. The shriek is a very strong Apis feature. The child cries out with this shriek in sleep when going into brain troubles. It says in the text: "Sopor interrupted by piercing shrieks." We must be able to see in the general beginning of provings the disease which they resemble, for we do not always see the remedy in the advanced state. We see the disease in a state of progress, and must be able to see it in its beginning. As was the disease in the beginning so was the remedy in the beginning. Things that have similar beginnings may have similar endings.

Apis also has muttering, delirium and loquacity. All kinds of screaming and shrieking, shrill and otherwise, violent and less violent. Premonition of death, dread of death, fear of apoplexy. "Very busy, restless; changing kind of work, with awkwardness." Awkwardness is especially found under the fingers, toes and limbs in Apis. The whole nervous system shows a disturbance in co-ordination. This disturbance in co-ordination runs through the remedy, awkwardness, staggering with the eyes shut. Dizziness when the eyes are shut. "Ailments from fright, rage, vexation, jeolousy or hearing bad news." "After severe mental shock paralyzed on the whole right side."

The complaints of Apis are attended with violence and rapidity. They come on with great rapidity, rush on with violence, until unconsciousness is reached. It has been my fortune to see many violent cases of poisoning from the sting of the honey-bee. When the oversensitive patient is poisoned by the sting he is dreadfully sick. The majority of people in the course of their life have been stung by the honey-bee and a mere little swelling occurs in the region of the sting, a swelling as big as a robin's egg or a hen's egg at most, without constitutional states; that is, when the individual is not sensitive to Apis. He may have been stung in half a dozen places, and each one gives him a little lump. But you meet one who is sensitive to the sting of the honey-bee, and if he gets one little sting on any place in his body, he comes down with nausea and anxiety that makes him feel that he is dying, and in about ten minutes he is covered with urticaria form head to foot; he stings and burns and wants to be bathed in cold water; he fears that he will die if something is not done to mitigate his suffering, rolls and tosses as if he would tear himself to pieces. I have seen all these symptoms come on after Apis. The antidote for that is *Carbolic acid.* I have seen *Carbolic acid* administered in that state, and the patient described the sensation of the *Carbolic acid* going down his throat as a cooling comfort. He says "Why, doctor, I can feel that dose go to the ends of my fingers." When you administer an antidote under such circumstances listen to what your patient says. When you get the true natural antidote, and, at times, when you get the true curative medicine in a case, no matter how high the potency the patient will say: "I feel that to the roots of my hair and to the ends of my toes." Such is the feeling it gives when the true atnidotal medicine goes to the innermost portions of his economy, and that is the way we want to get our medicines always, to be guided by the symptoms of our patient that they will tell us what medicines to administer, and when the medicine is administered its highest reaction is of that sort.

If we are well acquainted with the symptoms of Apis we can many times get along without having a specialist to treat the eyes. They make more people blind with their lotions, caustic solutions, etc., than they benefit. The old fashioned way was to cauterize with copper and silver nitrate solution, and the modern things are not much better. At the present day the homœopathic physician who is not capable of taking eye symptoms as well as lung symptoms and symptoms of any part of the body is not competent to practice medicine. Eye cases can be prescribed for by the physician. In Homœopathy there is no such thing as treating the eye and other organs of the body, but the patient with all his organs, not the patient with one or two organs.

Apis is a great remedy for the eyes. It has deep-seated inflammatory complaints of the eyes as a result of disease. Inflammations that are erysipelatous in character, that leave thickening of the mucous membrane and lids and white spots over the eye; opacities. Inflammation with opacities very extensive or in patches. Enlarged blood-vessels. When the inflamamatory condition is active it is attended with œdema of the lids, both upper and lower and the whole face is sometimes in a state of œdema, such as you would expect to see after a bee sting. The swelling of the mucous membranes of th lids is so enormous that they roll out, looking like pieces of raw beef. The fluid will run out over the cheeks in great abundance. Burning and stinging like fire, better from washing, from cold applications, worse from heat. Chronic eye troubles that are worse from looking into an open fire, worse from radiated heat; wants something cold applied. Chronic granular lids. The results of chronic inflammation are numerous and extensive. Worse from looking at white things, worse from looking at the snow. Pain in the eyeballs, pain deep in the eyeballs, stitches, burning, stinging and shooting. Chemosis. Apis is often suitable for old scrofulous affections of the eyes. Vascular affections, the veins are enlarged. "Iritis." "Congestion to the eyes, blood-vessels injected;" whole conjunctiva inflamed. Photophobia. Rheumatic ophthalmia, that is, a high grade of inflammation of the eyes in rheumatic subjects. Catarrhal inflammation of the eyes; scrofulous inflammation of the eyes. Hot tears gush out of the eyes; burning in the eyes. Erysipelas of the eyes and sides of the face, *extending from the right to the left.* This direction is an Apis feature in many other respects. Erysipelas commences on the right side of the face, extends over the nose to the left side. Inflammation commences in the right side of the abdominal viscera and extends over to the left. In inflammation of the ovary the right is preferred to the left. The right side of the uterus is perferred. Pains in the whole right side of the pelvis extending over towards the left. Burning stinging here and there extending from right to left.

Inflammation of the middle ear in connection with or after scarlet fever.

Now we come to the throat troubles of Apis. We have much throat trouble. Apis cures diphtheria, especially when there is a high grade of inflammation and the membrane is scanty or comes slowly or insidiously, and it is somewhat of a surprise the gradual progress it makes; the parts are œdematous and the soft palate is puffed like a water-bag, and the uvula hangs down with a semi-transparent appearance like a bag of water. All around the throat and mouth there is an œdematous condition looking as if it would flow water if pricked. Burning, stinging pains in the throat ameliorated by cold and aggravated by heat. Aversion to all warm substances and drinks. The tongue swells until it fills the mouth, worse on the right half of the tongue, or involving the right side first. Raw beef appearance, denuded appearance of the tongue and buccal cavity and throat. Various kinds of swelling in the throat; benign swellings, with burning, stinging and redness. Ulcers in the throat that come as a result of this inflammation. Apis is suitable in the severest forms of sore throat accompanying scarlet fever. It cures scarlet fever when the symptoms agree, and it is not an uncommon thing for Apis to be suited to scarlet fever, though the rash is sometimes rough. The scarlet fever rash in not always smooth and shiny. When the rash does not come out at all the face is very pallid, with a high grade of inflammation of the throat; the scarlet fever is in the family, and the skin is red without any rash; in those cases that are worse from heat, want the covers off, and are sensitive to the heat of the room. The patient desires a low temperature in the room, is worse from heat, wants cool things, worse from radiated heat especially, or hot air that comes from a register or fire. He suffocates when a little warm air is radiating over the body. He is disturbed from heat even in the chill of an intermittent fever; if in a warm room when having a chill, he suffocates. So it is with the scarlet fever, with the sore throat, and in diphtheria; from the least whiff of radiated heat he suffocates. He wants the doors and windows open, wants something cold. Sometimes the scarlet fever patient will go into convulsions because the rash fails to come out. Apis is sometimes a suitable remedy and must be compared with *Cuprum, Zincum* and *Bryonia.* A warm bath will intensify the convulsion.

"Sensation of constriction and erosion in the throat in the morning." Throat sore and swollen; stinging pains. "Could not swallow solid food." With these complaints there is often shivering, shuddering, little chills intermingled with the febrile state. Many times you will think to comfort him by covering him up with a warm blanket, but it will make him worse, he will throw it off. A child will kick off the covers. An adult is shivering while covered up will kick off the covers. These strange and peculiar things are guiding features, things that cannot be accounted for.

In Apis there is vomiting, nausea, retching and vomiting, with great anxiety. Vomiting of bile and everything eaten. Vomiting of bitter and sour fluids.

Apis causes soreness and tightness throughout the abdomen and hypochondria. Sensation of tightness runs through many of the complaints of Apis. The abdomen is distended with gas. Meteoritic condition, great tension and fulness, hard and drum-like. In all inflammatory complaints, in peritonitis inflammation of the liver, inflammation of the pelvis, there is great tension, tightness; but this tightness is not always general, sometimes it is local; sometimes it is with little congestion, but tightness prevails throughout the abdomen, and this tightness makes it impossible for the patient to cough for fear something will burst. The cough makes him feel as if something would be torn. Cannot strain at stool. This is common in the abdominal and pelvic complaints of women. The woman will say she cannot strain at stool, because of the feeling that if she strains something will break loose. The same state exists in the chest. It seems that on coughing something will tear loose, as if the fibres are in a state of tension or stretching.

Hypersensitive state of the liver; inflammation of the liver and spleen. Pain under the short ribs, worse on the left side. "Pains from below the ribs spreading upward. Obliged to bend forward from a painful contracted feeling in the hypochondria." All the complaints are likely to make the patient bend forward and flex the limbs, because the state of tension is painful.

Sensitiveness of the stomach to touch. Over the whole abdomen she is so sore that touch is extremely painful; in all the inflammatory complaints of women the abdomen is very sore and painful. Soreness, distension and stinging burning pains through the abdomen. Burning heat in the stomach.

In the external abdomen there is an œdematous state. Dropsy, sometimes alone, sometimes with anasarca. Limbs swollen to the full extent. pitting upon pressure, the feet and limbs swollen, with burning, stinging and numbness in the limbs.

Feeling as if the intestines were bruised. Watery diarrhœa is common in Apis; yellow stools, green stools, olive green stools, watery stools, etc. Every day six to eight diarrhœic stools, which smell like carrion. It is especially useful in a peculiar kind of stool occurring in children and infants, an intermingling of blood, mucus and food, giving the stool an appearance like tomato sauce. The anus protrudes with stool and seems to remain open, an open anus like *Phosph.* and *Puls.* Chronic diarrhœa, dysentery, hæmorrhage from the bowels. In its constipation it is related more commonly to head troubles. He goes many days without a stool. The bowels seem to be perfectly paralyzed, with congestion of the brain and acute hydrocephalus.

The urinary troubles are numerous in Apis. The urine is scanty, coming only in drops. Much straining before the urine will start, and then only a few drops; dribbling a little hot urine, burning urine, bloody urine. As soon as a few drops collect in the bladder the urging comes, constant, ineffectual urging. Later the urine is almost suppressed. Infants go a long time without passing urine, screeching and carrying the hand to the head, crying out in sleep, kicking off the covers. Very often a dose of Apis will be found useful. It is often called for in scarlet fever when the urine is loaded with albumen. Urinary troubles, with swelling of the genitals, and the swelling is œdematous. Scanty urine in little boys, with the foreskin enormously distended, or in hydrocele. Every time the call to urinate comes he will shriek, because he remembers the pain he had the last time. Inflammatory complaints of the kidneys and ureters, bladder and urethra. The whole urinary tract is irritated, very much like *Cantharis,* and these two medicines antidote each other. If you are called to a child that has been drugged with crude Apis you can generally antidote it with *Cantharis.* If you go to a woman who has taken *Cantharis* for vicious purposes, you can very often overcome it with Apis. The violent frenzy that has been brought on by *Cantharis* will be overcome by Apis. The smarting, burning and stinging along the urinary tract will be found under Apis. "Flow of urine unconscious." Stitching pain in the urethra with enuresis. Morbid irritability of the urinary organs. "Strangury. Agony in voiding urine. Retention of urine in nursing infants." It is queer how the old women knew, long before Apis was proved, that when the little new-born baby did not pass its water they could find a cure by going out to the bee-hive and catching a few bees, over which they poured hot water, and of which they gave the baby a teaspoonful. Some domestic things like that have been known among families and among nurses, and it is consistent because it is just like what we give Apis for. "Urine scanty and fœtid, containing albumen and blood corpuscles." Especially in acute albuminuria. The acute inflammatory affection of the kidney with albuminuria, such as occurs in scarlet fever or diphtheria, or after these, such as occurs as a sequel of acute disease. Inflammation of the kidney closes up the case and kills off a good many in allopathic hands, never in homœopathic hands. It is closely related to the genital organs of both male and female. Swelling and œdematous state of the genitals. Apis is a great friend of the woman. It cures all of her inflammatory complaints it seems, when the symptoms agree. That is to say, it produces inflammation of the uterus and ovaries and dreadful sufferings in the external and internal parts, and we have only to discover when the symptoms agree to cure most of these inflammatory troubles. It even stops abortion. It will stop abortion after some miserable scoundrel has attempted to getrid of the offspring, and she has taken drugs and brought on pains, pains strong enough to expel the contents of the uterus, especially in the first, second and third months. A little hæmorrhage has come on, a mere threatening, the membranes are not yet ruptured, but they soon will be, and she has stinging, burning pains, and lies uncovered and suffers from the heat, probably from the overdose of *Ergot*. Apis will overcome this greatly to her regret. This kind of villainy prevails. But women have accidents and weakness, whereby, in spite of the fact that they desire to hold their offspring, they are threatened with abortion, and Apis is a great friend to the prospective mother. Burning and stinging pains in the ovaries, especially the right; when greatly enlarged and even cystic, Apis has proved a curative remedy, has often cured tumors, and has caused cystic formation to stop growing or to disappear. The right ovarian region is very sensitive. Pain in the uterus and ovaries before and during menstruation. Stinging, rending, tearing pains cutting like knives, worse from heat. It is a very easily got symptom, because in most painful symptoms heat or the hot water bag are tried with the natural hope of relief, but with this remedy it aggravates. She throws it aside, for the pain is worse from heat. "Ovaries enlarged," etc. Dropsy of right ovary. Ovarian tumor.

APOCYNUM CANNABINUM

This remedy comes in as a good one to contrast with *Apis*. You will find in analogous in its symptoms and much like the complaints cured by *Apis*. You will be astonished in going over the dropsical condition, the rheumatic condition, the tumefaction of the cellular tissues, the dropsy of the sacs, the scanty urine resulting in dropsy; the inflammatory swellings with œdema, at the great resemblances; and if you were to start in with two cases and work them out from their particulars, and if one feature were left out, the aggravation and the amelioration, the cold and the heat, in many cases you would not be able to distinguish between *Apis* and Apocynum, so near alike are their swellings, their bleedings, their distensions, and their disturbances. Both are remedies for dropsy: routinists will try first *Apis*, and then they try Apocynum, and then they will try something else that is good for dropsy.

But all the way through this medicine is *aggravated from cold,* the patient himself is aggravated from cold. His complaints are worse from cold applications. In his distended, dropsical state, he is chilly, sensitive to air. He is sensitive to cold drinks. He has a pain in the stomach, and even vomits, from cold drinks. Pain in the abdomen from cold drinks. Uneasiness here and there in the body when cold things are in the stomach; you see at once how different that is from *Apis.* Anyone who follows symptom hunting and does not distinguish between circumstances that relate to the patient and modalities that relate to symptoms cannot appreciate these two grand distinctions, where the one patient is aggravated from heat and the other one ameliorated by heat, in all complaints.

The *excretions* are all *diminished.* The urine is scanty. The skin is dry. No matter what his complaints are, he cannot sweat. He feels if he could only perspire he would get well. There is no outthrow of water. He drinks plentifully, and it goes into the cellular tissues to distend them, and he becomes dropsical. He has a water constitution, one that takes in water and lets out none. He passes little water, and he perspires scantily or none at all; his skin in dry, sometimes hot, yet he is chilly. The skin feels husky and rough, but he is chilly. *Apis* suffers dreadfully from dry skin, from scanty urine; yet *Apis* is aggravated everywhere from heat and ameliorated from cold. That is the grand distinguishing feature in the dropsies and rheumatisms and many internal complaints. "Dropsy of serous membranes." Dropsy of the brain, pericardium, pleura, peritoneum; all of these are distended with serum. And there is great suffering, great uneasiness. The inflammatory rheumatism is again like *Apis*, in that it takes on dropsy with it. Inflammation of the joints, of the ankle-joints, of the toes, of the fingers, inflammation of the joints all over the body. The swelling about the joint pits upon pressure like *Apis.* But with the scanty urine, want of sweat, with the febrile condition, he is all the time chilly, and wants the parts well wrapped where *Apis* wants them uncovered. One might say, "Why, that is only one symptom." All who do not perceive the difference between symptoms predicated of the patient and symptoms predicated of the parts will see that as only one symptom with the rest of them. When he takes up a case and works it out in the Repertory he will use it as one symptom. Yet that feature will sometimes rule out all the rest, because it is predicated of the patient and not predicated alone of his parts. We have many remedies where the patient himself is ameliorated from heat. He wants to be in the heat, he wants to be warm, and yet he wants cold applied to the part. But that which is the general is the ruling feature, and if we do not know and distinguish the things that are general from the things that are particular, we get our Materia Medica mixed up. We must distinguish the things that belong to the patient himself from the things that belong to his parts. "Dropsy, with great thirst."

This is a great medicine for the low forms of disease, such as typhoid and scarlet fever, and is useful after lingering sicknesses. Patients become greatly prostrated, very chilly, very anæmic, have great thirst, the urine becomes scanty, the skin becomes dry. It is a bad convalescence; he has not recovered. Dropsy sets in; dropsy after scarlet fever, dropsy after typhoid fever. A low form of disease, like typhoid fever, has kept him in bed for four or five weeks, and he is emaciated and prostrated, and now he does not again gain flesh, he has no appetite, but he drinks copiously; he seems to want nothing but water. His skin commences to distend, fills up, and becomes dropsical. That is like *Apis,* and *Apis* would be indicated provide he was always hot, and wanted to be uncovered, and wanted cold things.

The mental symptoms of this remedy have not been brought out. We only know a few clinical symptoms, and they are of little importance. It has cured that peculiar kind of stupor belonging to hydrocephalus, but we do not know what kind of a primary case of brain disease this remedy would fit, because of lack of provings. We only know the condition after it has existed for a long time, that is, for weeks; rolling the head and tossing about, and he is greatly emaciated. The little one has chills and fever along with it, and his skull is beginning to distend, the fontanelles are growing wider; then we begin to think of some of those remedies capable of curing dropsy in the shut sacs, and this is one of them. But we do not know the beginning. We do know the beginning of *Apis,* but not of this remedy. Hahnemann's provings are full of particulars. He cross-examined his provers as to their modalities, the time their symptoms began, and where they ended. Many of the symptoms he felt upon himself, because he proved many remedies. Hahnemann had a sensitive constitution and deep perception, and his provings gave him an insight into medicines that he could not have obtained in any other way. Those who prove medicines properly, conscientiously, prudently, learn more about Materia Medica than anyone else. They become inured to hardship, and live longer therefrom. They are hardened to their environments, to their atmosphere, to their associates, and their surroundings. They are made better, and they may be able to perceive something of what Hahnemann perceived. But now-a-days provings are made and nothing recorded but common symptoms, that is, stomachache, nausea, headache, pain in the back, cold feet. Many of our remedies are not proved much further than that. What, when and how much, are left out. The modalities are left out. The finer sensations are not described, because they are considered emotional. "Low-spirited and bewildered. Feels as if she could do nothing but cry." We do not know the affections of either the male or the female. We do not know the desires or aversions, mental or physical; and hence it may be said that this is only a partial proving and suitable only for those complaints that show themselves upon the surface.

"Hydrocephalus, with great stupor." That is the last stage of it where there is great prostration, loss of flesh, stiffness of all the limbs, with dropsical swellings. Many times in hyrocephalus pains shoot along the nerves and attack the joints. Then it is that such remedies as *Apis* and *Calc. carb.* and this one take hold with wonderful depth. The first permanent and substantial indication that the remedy is working in a hydrocephaloid case is that it increases the flow of urine, which has been scanty all the time. For hydrocephalus study *Tuberculinum*

The expression of the face is that of anguish. "Flace bloated, puffed, swollen. Bloating under the eyes. Pitting upon pressure. Tongue dry; great thirst." There is another remedy that comes into this sphere that will be very often misunderstood, too, and will be likely in most instances to be given before this remedy. It is *Ars.* It has all the dropsical conditions of *Apis* and Apocynum. It has all the coldness and distension of the abdomen and of the shut sacs. It, too, is ameliorated in all of its symptoms, and the patient himself is ameliorated, from heat, and intense heat is required for that purpose. He wants to be in a very hot room, but it has something else. It has a deathly prostration, a deathly anxiety and terrible restlessness, not found in either of these remedies. It has also such a cadaveric odor, discovered on entering the room, which is not common to either of these remedies. In this way we have to take up our medicines and study them only one at a time, but we have also to study them by comparison. The medicines that are similar in generals have to be compared, as to heat and cold. In that way we get a list of those that are ameliorated by cold, and a list of those that are ameliorated by heat; and another nondescript list not ameliorated by either. That is the starting point, and we have to divide and sub-divide these, and so on.

"Thick, yellow mucus in the throat. Great thirst. Stiffness in the thoracic region. Fulness. A sense of distension." You will think a moment and see that filling up the pleural cavity does not cause very much outward distension, because the ribs prevent it. They form a wall, and hence the growth or distension is towards the lungs and downward towards the diaphragm. By this means we get increasing dyspnœa, with cough. This medicine, like *Apis*, must sit up; cannot lie down. You will find it is a common feature in hydrothorax for the patient to be compelled to sit up, because lying down increases the pressure upon the lungs and narrows the breathing space; and hence, he must sit up in order to let this heavy waterbag, the pleural sac, hang down, against the diaphragm, and that produces pressure in the abdomen and distension of the bowels. "Thirst on waking. Thirsty all day. Great thirst but water disagrees." He likes cold water, but it so disagrees with his stomach, causing pain in the stomach, or causing him to vomit before it even gets warm, or causing distension, or causing uneasiness, so that he dreads to take cold drinks. He is more comforted by hot drinks. Warm drinks warm him up, make him more comfortable, cold drinks aggravate. Yet his thirst is for cold.

Then come distension and vomiting. You will find patients so distended in all their cellular tissues with a general anasarea that it seems that no more water can be taken from the stomach into the blood. He is full. The blood vessels are distended, his stomach is distended and he must vomit; and with this distension of his whole body he drinks and vomits. It is with difficulty he can eat; cannot keep it down; it will not digest. From this comes a part of these symptoms. "Sense of pressure in the epigastrium, in the chest," so that it is almost impossible for him to get breath enough to move. Very little food makes him feel distended. He wakes up and wants something in his stomach. There is a gnawing hunger, but every little thing, even a mouthful, makes him feel distended. His stomach is already full of water and he vomits up great quantities of water, of bile, and of undigested substances that he has swallowed. The stomach finally, in dropsical conditions, becomes very irritable. It seems as if nothing passes through him. He finally becomes paralyzed in the bowels. The kidneys are not acting, and scarcely any urine passes. The tongue becomes inflamed. The mucous membranes are all inflamed, and probably the stomach is. Abdomen very much distended; dropsy of the abdomen.

Then another phase comes on. It seems that one by one each organ ceases to perform its functions. The ovaries and uterus fail to perform their functions, and amenorrhœa comes on with dropsical conditions. Many times this seems to be the beginning of such troubles; a failure of these organs to perform their functions, and then dropsy sets in. A woman passes along to a low state of weakness and nervous excitement, no menstrual flow, tenderness of the abdomen, distension of the abdomen, and then distension of the limbs.

Apocynum has been a curative remedy in diarrhœic conditions alternating with dropsy. Sometimes a diarrhœa will set in and all the other troubles go away. The diarrhœa is copious, yellow, watery and involuntary. I once knew large doses to be given in a case of dropsy, and it established its own peculiar diarrhœa, and while that diarrhœa lasted the enlarged spleen and the dropsical condition of the body all went away apparently, to the doctor, in a natural manner. It was brought to my observation, and I said, "Wait." Finally he was brought to stop the poisoning by Apocynum, and heart failure followed at once. A similar effect is to be seen from the allopathic use of *Digitalis*. The time comes when the doctor will be compelled to stop *Digitalis*, and the patient dies of heart failure; *Digitalis* is never charged with the death, and the doctor never seems to learn that *Digitalis* will kill.

Everywhere the functions are impaired, in the skin, the kidneys, bowels, uterus, and all tends toward the formation of dropsy. Urinary troubles are exceedingly troublesome. Scanty urine accompanies many complaints among the early symptoms. Retention of urine; painful micturition; urging to pass urine constantly. The bladder is sometimes only partially full, but he cannot pass urine. "Retention with great urging." "Paralysis of the extremities. Urging to urinate." Numbness, tingling in the extremities, and finally entire loss of power. Some patients remain this way for a while, and finally dropsy will set in. It has alternating conditions, as I have mentioned; dropsies, alternating with copious discharges. The dropsy may be relieved with copious watery discharges from the bowels or by copious spasmodic action of the kidneys, the urine being so profuse that he can hardly realize where so much water comes from. All at once it ceases. The urine becomes scanty, and then the tissues fill with serum, and the dropsical condition progresses. These conditions cease after a while, and the heart fails. "Urine diminishes to one-third its usual amount, without pain or uneasiness about the kidneys or bladder. Urine suppressed. No urine at all in brain affections." It was a routine medicine once, given to all children for wetting the bed, and as it cured many it must have that symptom, but that is a clinical symptom. It is not surprising, seeing its action is so marked upon the bladder, that it has cured involuntary passage of urine. "Dropsy of the genital organs."

I have mentioned the suppression of the menstrual flow, the amenor-rhœa, but it has also marked hæmorrhagic tendency. It will establish hæmorrhage anywhere, but especially from the uterus. Copious hæmorrhage. The menstrual flow may become copious, too frequent, last too long; but it will also establish a uterine hæmorrhage at another time. It will cause the patient to bleed so copiously that she becomes anæmic from uterine hæmorrhage; and then will follow dropsy. The old practitioners were in the habit of giving *China* in most instances where dropsy followed a hæmorrhage. It was so generally useful, and so commonly relieved, that they seldom used any other remedy. But Apocynum is also a remedy for dropsy following hæmorrhage. Many times it will fit the symptoms clearly in dropsy following hæmorrhage. "Prolonged menorrhagia, or hæmorrhage from the uterus for six weeks. Blood expelled in large clots, sometimes in a fluid state." Moderate flow for a day or two; suddenly sets in with such violence that she cannot be out of bed. Compels her to lie quietly. "Shreds, or pieces of membrane with the fluid blood. Menorrhagia continuing, or paroxysmal," that is, a continuous flow until the patient is exhausted. That is like *Phos.* and *Ipecac.* and *Secale.* In most instances, a uterine hæmorrhage will cease after about so much blood has been lost. In medicines where the flow is so liquid as it is in this medicine that tendency to cease does not come until a state of profound exhaustion has come on. Then the dyspnœa, as has been described, will not permit the patient to lie down. This is commonly from hydrothorax. It has also a hypostatic congestion of the lungs in patients that have been sitting up a long time, so that it fills up from below, gradually creeping up so that a large portion of the breathing space is destroyed. "Great oppression about the epigastrium. Difficult breathing. Gasping for breath.

Wheezing and coughing." It has all the rattling that is found in *Tartar emetic* and *Tartar emetic* has a similar filling up of the chest, cannot lie down.

Pulse small and irregular; almost pulseless. Disposed to faint whenever she attempts to raise her head from the pillow. Small weak pulse. Dropsy of the pericardium. Palpitation very troublesome.

ARGENTUM METALLICUM

We will take up the study of Metallic silver. No wonder that this is a very deep acting remedy, for it has been used symbolically, and medically throughout all history. It has been a valuable substance throughout all history. It is an anti-psoric, and from its symptoms I believe it to be an anti-sycotic. It goes deep into the life. Especially affects the nerves, nerve sheaths. Has complaints along the nerves. All cartilages in the body are affected by it. It produces a hypertrophy of cartilages, a thickening of the cartilaginous portions of joints, of the cartilage of the ears, and of the nose. Produces cartilaginous growths and tumors; infiltrations. It affects the nerve substance, it is a deep organic remedy. It is more than an ordinary remedy, for it affects all there is of man. In those nerve fibers especially that carry messages. It affects the brain in a very profound manner, bringing about changes and a gradual softening. A strange feature about it in its general action upon man is, that it singles out mostly the intellectual faculties. It scarcely disturbs his affections; only makes slight and vague changes in his voluntary system. But the memory, the intellectual part of man is disturbed increasingly to imbecility. In great sufferings—and it is full of suffering—it affects his ability to reason. In nearly all the headaches and pains in the back, and the rending, tearing pains that it produces over the body, it disturbs his memory and reasoning faculties. Disturbs his ability to think. And it comes on in persons who are in the habit of laboring with the intellectual faculties. Business men, students, readers, and thinkers. Reasoners come to a point when they can no longer reason, and the slightest mental effort brings on vertigo. He is fatigued. All symptoms are worse after sleep. Instead of being rested for the day, he wakes in the morning with mental fatigue and weakness, so that he can hardly move, and it is with great difficulty that he gets himself together for a mental or physical effort of another day. If he undertakes to do any more mental work, he gets a headache. Headache mostly in the front of the head, but also in the occiput.

Another strange feature about it, it is full of rending, tearing pains along the nerves, predominantly of the lower extremities. Tearing, as if the nerves would be torn in pieces *during rest*. Cold, damp weather, stormy weather will bring on rheumatism—not so much with swelling, although it has that, but pains apparently in the cartilages, and pains along the nerves. And these pains are so severe that he cannot keep still. Hence, it has a rheumatic state from cold, damp weather, from becoming chilled, in the joints and in the nerves, so that he walks and walks. Many symptoms are better from motion and especially walking. So tired and exhausted, but the pain is so severe that it drives him to walk. These pains are many times palliated by copious drafts of coffee, and this will suppress the sickness, and leave upon him all sorts of difficulties, under which he is threatening with break down, and in time he becomes almost useless. "Mental weakness. Physical prostration." Rending, tearing pains. Affections of the joints, the cartilages of the joints. Tearing pains along the bones—and he is really a wreck, an old broken down constitution when he is yet young. "A man of forty is like one of eighty." All these pains are better from motion.

Again, it is full of infiltrations. Inflamed cartilages infiltrate and form into hard knots. A superabundance of cartilaginous tissue, so that round about the joints the cartilages are thickened. In the ear and nose the cartilage is thickened. The infiltration that belongs to epithelioma. It has been a wonderful palliative in scirrhus, and in epithelioma. It has cured epithelioma. It is on record as curing an epithelioma of the cervix uteri.

Ulceration everywhere; but ulcers that have their beginning in the cartilaginous tissue, and break out through the cellular tissue, and copiously discharge. The ulcers infiltrate at their base, and become hard.

Another marked feature is that it affects both testes, but it has a predominant action in the right. The left ovary and the right testis. Such things are singular, that in one sex it should produce symptoms in one side of the body, and in the other sex on the opposite side.

It has cured all sorts of tumors, enlargement of the ovary, and infiltrations of the tissues. It is a chilly remedy. Wants to be kept warm, and its pains are ameliorated by heat. Its headaches are ameliorated by heat—are ameliorated by pressure, by bandaging. I have many times cured these symptoms in headaches when the patient had the head wrapped up.

Now, in this medicine we class the patient as one having a lack of vital heat. He wants to be warm. Likely to be lean, growing increasingly lean, increasingly nervous, increasingly sensitive. Takes on all sorts of whims. Women needing Silver very often do such strange and unaccountable things in (compare *Argentum nitricum*) their nervous states that they bar out all sympathy of their friends, and are called hysterical. Deep seated trouble of the nerves. Growing increasingly sensitive to surroundings.

Now, the mental state of Argentum met. is just such as is aroused by confusion, just such as is aroused by the emotions, just such as the loss of balance from fear, from anger, from fright, from disturbance of the mind. Because this patient is so sensitive to his surroundings and so disturbed by annoyances. With his pains he becomes delirious, and it is not that involuntary delirium that we see in low forms of fever, but he becomes wild and full of rage. He takes on mental excitement, rage and a state in which he talks nonsense with great rapidity. Sometimes there is a stage of unusual excitement in his conversation all mixed up about the character of his thought. All of the time looks as if he were intoxicated, and he flies from one subject to another, and prattles. For a moment appearing to be very intense and active in mind, and forgets all that he was talking about.

"In society indisposition to talk." Because he is incompetent. He is tired mentally and he forgets what he is talking about. Loses the thread of his discourse; and he dreads to talk because he gets complaints while talking. If compelled to answer, he becomes dizzy, and feel strange all over, and has nervous shakes or shocks. And shocks go over him when tired like an electric shock. It comes suddenly, but the most favorable time for that to come is just when he wants to go to sleep. He thinks, now he is away from all the troubles of the day and can rest, and the instant sleep comes over him he is roused from head to foot by a shock, and another one, and another one, sometimes the whole night he jerks from head to foot. His limbs jerk up, his lower limbs twitch and jerk, then he gets out of bed and walks—tries to walk it off. This comes out in the proving of *Argentum nictricum,* but it belongs as much to Argentum met., and Argentum met. has long cured it. In Hahnemann's study of the remedy he lays down the importance of shock on going to sleep. Shocks in the limbs. But it is an electric shock that causes the whole body to jerk. "Anxious about the health. Thinks he is certainly breaking down," for he is growing weaker. He cannot walk, though he is growing increasingly restless. He cannot exercise mentally or physically without distress. From meditation or as soon as he enters a warm room he becomes dizzy—and that is an exception belonging to a few of the head troubles and the sensorium; he usually is sensitive to cold. In the house when the room is close he becomes dizzy.

It has been an astonishing feature in this remedy that precisely at the hour of noon a great many troubles come on, and the pains and aches. Chills. Headaches. Pains in the ovary at noon. Dizziness with vertigo as if intoxicated. The headaches are frontal and occipital. One-sided brain affections. One-sided headaches. Violent neuralgia in the head upon one side at a time, as if deep in the brain, as if involving one-half of the brain. Mostly the headaches have been on the right side—the one-sided headaches. Those broken down patients that have become prostrated and overwrought by exposure to the sun. Upon the scalp, the ears, here and there upon the body, itching places. Itching and burning, like frost bites. It has an itching and burning like *Agaricus,* in the toes, in the ears, and he scratches the part, and scratching does not relieve it until the skin is off, until it oozes, but no relief from scratching. Rawness in the ears, kept up by constantly boring and scratching in the ears. Scratching the skin off because of the tingling, itching and burning.

Another strange feature is that about the eyes Silver affects the lids more than the globe. It affects the sight, producing dimness of vision, and loss of vision; but it produces infiltration of the lids, thickening of the lids until they are almost as hard as cartilage. The mucous membrane is infiltrated and hard, and the eyelids cannot be opened. They spasmodically close, they cannot be pulled apart except by violence. It is a blepharitis, with thickening and infiltration. Copious discharges. Now, as we strike this as a catarrhal region, let me say that all through the remedy we will find passive catarrhal discharges. In some instances thick and yellow, but at the same time passive, a passive state of the mucous membrane. But the characteristic, the principal discharge of Argentum met. is gray, thick, tenancious mucus. He expectorates from the lungs—and from the air passages, from the trachea and from the larynx, gray mucus. Gray mucus from the vagina, gray mucus from the urethra, gray mucus from the eyes. Only in a few instances does it have yellow discharges. When ulceration takes place, as in the larynx and on the eyelids, we have from this ulceration thick, yellow discharges; but from the ulcerated mucous surfaces it will generally be found to be gray, except in the urethra. It has cured old cases of chronic gonorrrhœa. If we get the general character of the remedy we know what to expect when it goes to each region. If we do not know the general character of a remedy we do not know what to expect; and if we get into a region where we have the very opposite of it we know then that that is a particular, and does not conform to its generals. But first of all we have to single out what is general, what may be expected, what belongs to the nature of the remedy, so that when we see its opposites we may recognize it and know it as an opposite, as a particular, and as an exception. Here is one of the characteristic features of Argentum itching. "Scratching until bleeding, in the ear." Now, this itching involves the whole outside ear, and extends into the ear, so he scratches the ear until it is red, and swollen, and bleeds. The cartilage of that ear is lumpy and nodular; is infiltrated. The cartilages of the nose are also infiltrated. Argentum met. cures many of these cases that are operated on when they have some portion of the inside of the nose removed by the surgeon, so that the patient can breathe better. "Thickening of the bones in the nose, the thickening and building up of the mucous membrane and the cellular tissue in the nasal passages." Argentum met. is often indicated in such cases. This remedy has a very decided action. Infiltrations go on thickening and hardening, and then we have serum in joints. This is one of the most important remedies to know in the necrosis of cartilages everywhere in the body. But with it must go such nervous and mental symptoms as the remedy has, such as I have described. The patient looks sickly, pale, careworn, tired. A broken down patient. An Argentum met. patient is a sickly one who should have had a homœopathic doctor years ago, but one who can be patched up and benefited now if he has not gone too far.

"Painful tension and drawing in the throat. Throat feels raw and sore during expiration." This is extended into the larynx. "Painful soreness from breathing. Rawness from coughing in the larynx. Great quantities of gray mucus expectorated easily. Tension in the fauces on the right side."

Argentum met. has abdominal troubles. Bruised, sore feelings in the abdomen. If these progress from a catarrhal inflammation of the mucous membranes to a general congestion of all the tissues in the abdomen, diarrhœa comes on, or constipation of the most inveterate character, tuberculosis of the mesenteric glands, emaciation, weakness, trembling. Paralytic feelings here and there in the body. Painful soreness in the whole abdomen in connection with the urinary troubles. It has a low form of tissue making, such as tuberculosis, cancerous affections, infiltrations, such as we have mentioned. Dry stool, like sand. Undigested stool; very offensive. Catarrhal inflammation of the mucous membranes of the urinary passages, the whole urinary tract. It cures albuminuria; it cures diabetes, with sugar in the urine; and many of the broken-down conditions of the kidneys. Low, broken-down constitutions. Enormous quantities of whey-like urine. A copious flow of urine.

Children lose the urine in sleep. Broken-down, nervous constitutions lose the urine in sleep.

It has a very decided action upon the genitalia of both male and female. In the male it especially affects the testes and the mucous tract. It infiltrates the testes, producing hardness. In the text it reads, "crushed pain the right testicle." "Clothing increases pain on walking." Inflammation with infiltration. Chronic orchitis. It has cured a very suspicious testicle believed to be a cancerous affection, which began in the epididymus, following a gonorrhœa. Inflammation, great hardness, pain, swelling, burning and stinging.

Another symptom here is of great importance: "Yellowish-greenish gonorrhœa of an indolent character from the beginning, of eight months' standing." That clinical symptom has been verified. Now, it is a natural feature of gonorrhœa for the discharge to be yellow, or yellowish-green, and thick in the early stage, for it then to become lighter and lighter until it is whitish thick or thin, growing lighter in character until it becomes white and gleety. Argentum met. is the remedy when the discharge remains yellow. The pain has all ceased, and generally when the pain ceases the discharge soon begins to be lighter, but in the Argentum met. cases the pain ceases, it becomes a passive discharge, the urethra loses its sensitiveness to pain, and the mucous membrane loses its sensation to a great extent, but the thick greenish or yellowish discharge remains. Now, in these thick passive discharges that are long-standing, old cases, we are very much troubled to find remedies. These old stubborn cases that still remain yellow, and still remain thick. They will not yield to ordinary remedies—they come under a peculiar class of remedies. Argentum met., *Alumina, Alumen, Sulphur.* Ones not usually thought of in the early period, but the general constitutional state of the patient forms the character of his symptoms.

In the female we have ovarian troubles, infiltration, hardness, cystic troubles, cystic ovaries, that are cured by this remedy; ovarian tumors; very large, hard indurated ovaries—especially the left. The right testicle, the left ovary. Pain in the left ovary and back. Prolapsus, with pain in left ovary. Pain in the small of the back while sitting. The cures have been predominantly of the left ovary, although it cures complaints of both.

Another grand feature found in this remedy is weakness, relaxation of muscles through the whole body; trembling; and now, if that thought is applied—if that feature of the remedy is observed in the pelvic organs—it will be seen that those muscles that hold up the uterus, the broad ligament, etc., are in a state of relaxation, they allow the uterus to sag. In other words, we get prolapsus. You will be astonished to know that homœopathic remedies are wonderful in their ability to create tonicity, and thereby restore the prolapsed uterus to its normal position, and to remove the dragging down feeling women generally describe, a sensation as if the inner parts were being forced out. All of these are sensations that accompany a prolapsus. Argentum is one of the medicines. In fact, the whole pelvic system is engorged, increased in weight; tissues infiltrated, likely to be hardened. Cervix congested and indurated. Takes on ulceration. Greatly enlarged, congested. It has been a palliative medicine in epithelioma of the cervix, with burning, stinging pains, copious, putrid, yellowish-green and bloody discharge. It has cured a tendency to menorrhagia, copious menstural flow; the relaxation that must be present in hæmorrhages will soon be overcome when the symptoms agree, when the general state is present. Ulcer of the uterus; discharge purulent, ichorous. "Sometimes bloody water, with unbearable stench." It is a medicine of great use in horribly offensive leucorrhœa (*Kali ars., Kali p.*). "Neck of the uterus very much swollen, presented a spongy mass, deeply corroded with ulcers in different directions." Where it was given in case of scirrhus of the uterus it says. "In less than three days foul smell was lost entirely." When a remedy acts in that manner it actually stops the growth. In fact, a cancerous state that would go on to its termination in fourteen to sixteen months will go two or three years and the patient remain comfortable. The remedy that is indicated stops the ulceration, it checks the destruction, and keeps the patient comfortable and with her friends for years. In cancerous affections the state of life is very low. The state of order is generally beyond restoration.

Then we come to a state of the larynx. It is a wonderful laryngeal medicine. Loss of voice with inflammation, from overuse of the voice, such as occurs in singers and talkers. One who is compelled to use the larynx much. It is then a paralytic weakness of the vocal cords. Running all through this remedy there is aggravation from any little prolonged exertion—a paralytic tendency with aggravation from exertion. So it is in the lungs—in every part of the body. And then comes the loss of voice. Now, apply all that we know of its ability to infiltrate. We have tuberculosis of the larynx. Singers, public speakers, who are broken down, nervous, of poor digestion, bad inheritance, take on tuberculosis of the larynx, and the voice is lost. Ulceration follows. And this trouble finally goes into the lungs. They emaciate and get night sweats. "Loss of voice." Generally of a painful character.

Again, colds settle in the larynx. "Cannot speak a loud word; constant tickling in the larynx, provoking cough." Rawness and soreness in upper part of larynx. Laughing aggravates the coughing—laughing will cause tickling in the larynx, and he will scrape out *quantities of gray mucus.* If the irritation is in the smaller air passages, in the lungs, laughter will set him to coughing, and he will scrape out gray mucus. "Over the bifurcation of trachea, a raw spot; when using the voice, talking, laughing, or singing." In the middle of the chest a raw sensation. "Roughness and hoarseness of the voice. Phthisis of the larynx;" in those withered young people; a young man when he is not more than twenty-five looks to be fifty. Many wrinkles as though he had had many cares. Has a dry cough; gets up a little gray mucus. Yet he may be somewhat wiry, getting about fairly well. Has inherited phthisis. The cough is a deep cough, is aggravated from laughing, talking and in a warm room. Laughing causes cough and causes mucus in the larynx. This remedy will turn aside this threatening phthisis, this dry teasing cough. A little dry, hacking cough especially comes under this remedy. In no instance are we likely to have those violent spasmodic shaking coughs, such as we find in *Bry.* When coughing a sore feeling in the larynx. "The cough is accompanied with an easy expectoration." He does not usually cough so much to get up the mucus as he does to relieve a little irritation; but when there is mucus it generally comes up easily. It is not so difficult to detach as we find in many remedies. "Easily detached mucus in the larynx." He simply scrapes it out by an effort of the larynx. Cough and scraping of the larynx during the daytime and evening, worse in a warm room and better in the open air and from motion.

It has a sense of weakness of the chest. There are two remedies having this weakness of the chest and you cannot easily tell them apart. Weak voice, weak chest; a feeling that it is so difficult to breathe, and so difficult to talk, and so difficult to cough, because the muscles of the chest feel so weak. These two medicines are Argentum met. and *Stannum.* Great weakness of the muscles of the chest. The patient dwells upon it much, and it is a weakness far beyond what can be accounted for in tuberculosis, a sense of muscular weakness in the chest. A paralytic weakness of the chest. Of course, this is wholly different from the *Antimonium tart.,* which has a dreadful weakness of the chest, but in that remedy you will remember it is in the acute affections. It is suitable in lingering complaints, sickness of long standing, so that "great weakness of the chest" means that which I have tried to describe and it is that which patients will often fail in their efforts to describe. "Doctor, I feel so weak in the chest."

Now, this remedy is full of cardiac disturbances. Palpitation when lying on the back. "A sense of trembling in the chest." A sense of quivering, fluttering, or trembling, as it will be described by the different patients, trembling in the chest. That tremulous weakness of the whole body, hands and feet; palpitation with general trembling is strong in this remedy. "Frequent palpitation. During pregnancy, palpitation. Palpitation at night, Palpitation associated with headaches." With general weakness. Gradually increasing weakness. From his general weakness the knees knock together when walking. Trembling in the knees with palpitation and general weakness. The limbs become stiff. "Numbness in the limbs, as if asleep." Loss of power. *Many of the complaints are increased during rest.* Pain in the back and limbs while sitting, better while walking. All the nervous excitement that is possible in remedies comes up in this remedy.

ARGENTUM NITRICUM

We shall find by examining the symptoms of this remedy that the intellectual feature predominates, as in the metal; that the affections are disturbed only in a limited way. There is a predominance of mental symptoms. First of all, disturbance in the memory, disturbance of reason; he becomes most irrational in his explanations of his actions and methods. He is irrational and does strange things and comes to strange conclusions; does foolish things. He has all sorts of imaginations, illusions, hallucinations. He is tormented in his mind by the inflowing of troublesome thoughts, and especially at night his thoughts torment him to the extent that he is extremely anxious, and this puts him in a hurry and in a fidget, and he goes out and walks and walks, and the faster he walks the faster he thinks he must walk, and he walks till fatigued. Strange notions and ideas and fears come into his mind. He has an impulse that he is going to have a fit or that he is going to have a sickness. A strange thought comes into his mind that if he goes past a certain corner of the street he will create a sensation, will fall down and have a fit, and to avoid that he will go around the block, he avoids going past that corner for fear he will do something strange. He is so reduced in his mental state that he admits into the mind all sorts of impulses. There is inflowing of strange thoughts into his mind, and when crossing a bridge or high place the thought that he might kill himself, or perhaps he might jump off, or what if he should jump off, and sometimes the actual impulse comes to jump off the bridge into the water. When looking out of a window the thought comes to his mind what an awful thing it would be to jump out of the window, and sometimes the impulse comes to actually jump out of the window. There is fear of death, the over-anxious state, that death is near, and often at times like *Aconite* he predicts the moment he is going to die. Looking forward to times he is anxious. When looking forward to something that he is about to do, or that he has promised to do, or in the expectation of things, he is anxious. When about to meet an engagement he is anxious until the time comes. If he is about to take a railroad journey he is anxious, full of fear and anxiety and tremulous nervousness until he is on the car going and then it passes away. If he is about to meet a certain person on the street corner he is anxious and breaks out often in a sweat from anxiety until it is over with. Not only is this particular symptom present, but the symptoms come on as a result of his anxiety. He is excitable, angers easily, and as a result of this pain comes. When he becomes angry he becomes vehement and pain in the head comes on; cough, pain in the chest and weakness follow this anger. The anxiety he has from these circumstances will bring on complaints. When he is going anywhere, going to a wedding, or to the opera, or any unusual event, it is attended with anxiety, fear and diarrhœa. So it is we have in this a wonderful medicine. It says in the text that he gave a sorts of queer reasons for his strange conduct, endeavoring to cover up, as it were, his foolishness which he himself realizes. Sadness, melancholy and confusion. Defective memory. The sight of high houses makes him dizzy, and his vertigo is increased or comes on from closing the eyes; with the vertigo there is buzzing in the ears, great weakness and trembling.

Constitutional headaches from brain-fag, from exertion of the mind. In such mental exhaustion, headaches, nervous excitement and trembling, and organic troubles of the heart and liver in business men, in students, in brain workers, in those subject to long excitement, in actors who have kept up a long time the excitement of appearing well in public. This state of mind progresses until there is a general state of weakness; with trembling, paralysis, numbness, disturbed functions, palpitation, throbbing all over the body, with the mental state. The nervous state continues until there is disorder of all the organs of the body. The stomach refuses to digest, everything taken seems to go into gas, and he becomes distended and suffers with pain. The circulation seems to be greatly disturbed in addition to the palpitation. Fulness of the blood vessels and throbbing all over the body. The blood vessels become diseased. Atheromatous degeneration and dilatation of the veins, varicose veins. Upon the mucous membranes and skin ulceration, and this progresses and the heart becomes increasingly feeble, and the extremities become cold and blue and the lips are cold and blue, with aggravation of all these complaints from mental excitement, from going to the opera, from meeting a friend, from keeping an engagement. The medicine is pre-eminently a nervous one, full of spinal symptoms, rending, tearing pains down the extremities; such pains are found in locomotor ataxia, fulgurating, shooting pains. There is one grand feature running through this patient modifying most of his symptoms, with few exceptions, and that is that he is like a *Pulsatilla* patient; he wants cold air, cold drinks, cold things; he wants ice, ice cream; wants the head in the cold air; suffocates in a warm room. He suffocates from warm clothing, wants the door and windows open; cannot breathe in a stuffy room, suffocates if other people are in the room; cannot go to church or to the opera, cannot go to places of amusement or gatherings, must stay at home. He dreads a crowd, dreads certain places.

Everywhere we find ulceration, but particularly upon the mucous membrane. The throat has ulcers in it; ulceration of the eyelids, and of the cornea; ulceration of the bladder. Ulcers of the uterus, of the vagina and of the external soft parts. This tendency to ulcerate seems rather strange, peculiar that it should have in its pathogenesis such a tendency, when the old school has been using it to cauterize ulcers and yet it heals them up. We know that

Phosphorus will burn and it intensifies the tendency to ulcerate, makes the ulcer go deeper, while Argentum nitricum sets it healing. Upon mucous membranes we find red elevations, granulations, enlargement of vessels, purplish aspect. Sensitive ulcers. The complaints in women come on *before* and *during* the menstrual period. It is a favorable time for all her complaints to be aggravated; if she have Argentum nitricum symptoms they are likely to be at their worst at this time. She suffers from most violent dysmenorrhœa, from nervous excitement, from hysterical manifestations, and an unusually increased flow. A tendency to hæmorrhages belongs to this remedy. The ulcers bleed; there is bleeding from the nose, bleeding from the chest, the urine is bloody; leucorrhœa copious, menstrual flow copious; menorrhagia; bleeding from the mucous membranes generally, from the uterus. Vomiting of blood. It has cured prolonged and most inveterate ulceration of the stomach, when there has been vomiting of blood.

The aggravation at the menstrual period is a strong feature and she is free from symptoms during the interim. The palpitation, the trembling, the coldness of the surface, though desiring cold open air, blueness of the lips, coldness of the extremities, blueness and coldness of the lower extremities to the knees and of the hands and arms to the elbows, and yet the patient wants cool things, wants something cold. This may not be seen at any other time. Here is a striking feature. "Patient cannot lie on the *right* side because it brings on so much palpitation." We have plenty of remedies with palpitation worse from lying on left side, but remedies with palpitation worse lying on the right side are rare (*Alumen, Badiaga, Kalmia, Kali n., Lil. t., Platina, Spong.*). It is uncommon, strange, rare and peculiar. It is such a strong feature in this remedy that to a great extent it becomes quite general, because it is a *heart* symptom and is intermingled with the general symptoms. With this sensitiveness he is compelled to get into some other position; must get up and walk, because of lying on the right side. The patient will say he throbs from head to foot while lying on the right side; he throbs all over, a general pulsation when lying on the right side. Do not forget in this medicine all these general things when we come to apply them in their particulars and the particulars in the generals. Do not forget that this medicine is one of the most *flatulent* medicines in the books. He is distended to bursting; gets scarcely any relief from passing flatus or eructations.

He is possessed with the distressing idea that all his undertakings must fail. When walking he becomes faint with anxiety which makes him walk faster. Everywhere you will find the intellectual symptoms predominant.

The headaches are of a congestive character; considerble throbbing, ameliorated by cold, and tight bandaging. Headache from mental exertion, from excitement, with vertigo, nausea and vomiting. Pains in the right side of the head, jagging, cutting, stitching, pulsating. Head feels much enlarged.

The eye symptoms are too numerous to mention. They are of a general character such as we find in catarrhal conditions with ulceration, relieved by cold. All of the eye symptoms are worse in a warm room, worse from sitting by the fire. Wants cold applications, cold washing. Intense photophobia; aversion to light, and this is worse in a warm room; wants it cold, wants it dark. There is much swelling and tumefaction of the blood vessels of the eye, and redness, and it has a raw denuded excoriated appearance. "Chemosis with strangulated vessels." "Cornea opaque." "Ulceration of cornea in new-born infants; profuse purulent discharge from the lids," and this is what the "Regulars" in former days and almost up to date have been using for the eyes, treating them with Argentum nitricum. Photophobia: after long looking at fine sewing, fine print. In one who has suddenly taken on far sightedness, it has come on as a congestive condition; not of old age but something that should be cured. All at once he cannot see print at the usual distance but must hold it away off; if it occurs in some one twentyfive years of age or in a child. At close distance it is indistinguishable. Such a disturbance of accommodation producing far sightedness it has caused and cured. "Œdema of lids," etc.

Œdema is a word which runs through the remedy. That is to say, it has a dropsical state wherever dropsy may occur.

The face is the next place we find particulars worthy of note. "Face: sweat stood in drops on his face." "Face sunken, pale, bluish." "Looks prematurely old." "Face blue, heavy breathing, pulseless."

Then come the throat symptoms. Another feature of this remedy is its general tendency to produce warts. There is a tendency to favor the growth of warts and in the throat there are little wart-like growths; polypoid growths in the throat and about the genitals and anus; hence its great use in sycotic constitutions. It has all the discharge necessary to its use in the sycotic constitution.

"Felt as if he had a stick in the throat when swallowing." At once you will see its close relation to *Hepar.* In inflammatory conditions of the throat with ulceration. In Argentum nitricum he wants to be in a cold room, wants cold air, and to swallow cold things. In *Hepar* he wants warm things to drink, a warm clothing, warm room, and cannot put even his hand out of bed or his throat will begin paining him. Things, you see, just exactly opposite, but they both have "sticks" in the throat. In dry chronic catarrh *Alumina* and *Natrum muriaticum* have "sticks" in the throat; but in red throat with tumefaction and pain these two remedies give no relief, the former two are better. "Sticks" in the throat like fish-bones. *Nitric acid, Hepar* and Argentum nitricum are the most striking remedies for the fish-bone sensation. Many remedies have sticking in the throat, but these are the most prominent. We know how

Argentum nitricum has been used for ulceration in the throat, and here it comes in as one of the most useful remedies in congestion of the throat of long standing. Catarrhs with loss of voice. Warty growths, condylomata, etc. Loss of voice, tumefaction of the mucous membrane round about the vocal cords and paresis of the vocal cords. Condylomata on the vocal cords.

"Loss of appetite" and refuses drink. This is another feature. *Desires sugar.* He feels that he must have it and it makes him sick, brings on eructations, increased flatulence, sour stomach. He cannot digest it; it acts like a physic and brings on a diarrhœa. So marked is the aggravation from sugar that the nursing infant will get a green diarrhœa if the mother eats candy. Then is it astonishing that the baby can get a dynamized dose from the mother, when the dynamized dose can travel like lightning, and sugar takes all day to be digested and dynamized and fed as poison to the baby? I remember a case that I figured and figured on. The baby had *Mercurial stools,* sure enough, they were grass green. Well *Chamomilla* has grass green stools and *Arsenicum* and *Mercurius* and lots of remedies have grass green stools. Routinist that I was in those days I could not get anything but *Mercurius* out of it, and although the baby had gotten *Merc., Ars.* and *Cham,* there was no relief, until I found that the mother had been eating candy. When she was asked if she ate sweet things, sugar, etc., she said, "Oh, no." "Why, yes, you do," said the husband; "I bring you home a pound of candy every day. What do you do with it?" "Oh, that was nothing," she replied. But the baby did not get well until it got Argentum nitricum and the mother stopped eating sugar. *"Irresistible desire for sugar."* Quite a number of medicines have craving for sweets, but many of them can eat sweets with impunity. It is always a peculiar thing when one of the articles of diet, such as milk, sugar, salt, stareh, etc., and the things of the table make sick. When it is said that "I cannot eat a teaspoonful of anything with starch, egg or sugar in it without being sick," it is always strange and peculiar, because it is not something that comes in only as a craving and affecting the stomach, but it affects the whole patient. The patient says: "I become sick," and hence it becomes a general. When the patient gets a diarrhœa from eating sugar it is not merely a local and particular symptom, because the whole patient is sick before the diarrhœa begins; the diarrhœa is the outcome. Hence as it is a general it is necessary that it should be examined into.

"The vomited substances tinge the bedding black." Incessant vomiting of food. He sometimes spits up food by the mouthful until the stomach is empty. Eructations of air accompanied by a mouthful of undigested food, like *Phosphorus* and *Ferrum.* Spitting it up; welling up in mouthfuls.

"Eructations relieve." "Flatulence passes upwards, in quantities." Frequent eructations. Eructations do not always relieve. It is more like *China* in its eructations. The eructations of *Carbo veg.* relieve for some time and he feels better. This is the way with *Carbo veg.;* he is distended almost to bursting and he cannot get up any wind, but finally after much pain and distension it wells up in empty eructations and then he gets relief. With *China* he is distended, and every little while getting up gas, but with no relief. It does not seem to help, and sometimes patients will say they seem to get worse after it. So it is with Argentum nitricum at times. It evidently has both. "Most gastric ailments are accompanied by belching." 'Belching difficult; finally air rushes out with great violence." "Nausea after every meal; nausea with troublesome efforts to vomit." I have seen these Argentum nitricum patients vomiting and purging in the same moment, not vomiting one second and purging the next, but gushing out both ways with great exhaustion like cholera morbus, so relaxed, prostrated and weak. "Vomit; streaked brown, flocculent, like coffee grounds."

The stomach, liver and abdomen are full of pain. The abdomen distended with all this troublesome flatulence. Inflammation of the stomach, ulceration of the stomach, most troublesome diarrhœa. Diarrhœa with copious flatus. Stool with copious flatus in nursing children, with tormina and viscous sanguinolent stools and tenesmus. "Diarrhœa of children after weaning." Another feature in connection with the diarrhœa and dysentery is that casts are passed with the stool, like diphtheritic membrane or deposit; casts like the rectum, strings of membrane, come with the stool. Stools of green, fœtid mucus with noisy flatus at night.

"Urine passed unconsciously and uninterruptedly." "Urging to urinate; the urine passes less easily and freely." "Bleeding of the urethra; painful erections; gonorrhœa." It has most painful gonorrhœa with painful erections in the male. In the female the vagina is extremely sore, and the external soft parts are swollen; tumefaction. Vagina feels sore on urinating; bloody discharge. In the male, orchitis from suppressed discharge. In the female, ovaritis, inflammation of all the pelvic organs. Great soreness all over the pelvis. Bleeding from the vagina. Ulceration of the uterus. Coition is painful or impossible. "Pains like sticks or slivers in and about the womb," etc. This sensation prevails wherever there are ulcers. "Prolapsus with ulceration of the os or cervix." Hæmorrhage of short duration; shooting pains through abdomen and stomach. Metrorrhagia. Complaints of nervous women and at the menstrual period. Menses suppressed or scanty. Complaints during pregnancy.

Under the symptoms of the heart and pulse: "Anxiety with palpitation and throbbing through the whole body;" "Violent palpitation from the slightest mental emotion or sudden muscular exertion. Palpitation obliges her to press hand hard against heart for relief. Heart's action irregular, intermittent," etc.

Pain in the lumbar region comes on while sitting, but is better when standing and walking. Pain in the back from flatulence. Sore pain in the spine. Pain in back at night. Great weight in the lumbar region. It is a very useful remedy in locomotor ataxia.

Great restlessness. The nervous symptoms are very numerous. Periodical trembling of the body. Chorea, with tearing in the legs. Convulsions preceded by great restlessness. Nervous, faintish, tremulous sensation, etc.

The sleep symptoms are quite general. Distressing nightmares. The dreams are horrible. Wakens in excitement and with starting. All sorts of strange, horrible things in sleep. Dreams of vicious and violent things, and that everything is going to happen to him, Dreams of departed friends, etc.

On waking in the morning limbs feel bruised; aching in the chest, etc. Cannot sleep at night because he is so nervous.

Erysipelatous bed sores. While riding, palpitation and anxiety compelling him to get out of the wagon and walk, and that real fast.

Purplish rash, such as appears in the most serious forms of scarlet fever and zymotic diseases.

Its most natural antidote is *Natrum muriaticum.* When you have the ulceration where the throat has been cauterized or the cervix uteri or eyelids have been cauterized by Nitrate of Silver study *Natrum mur.* and see if the symptoms of the case would not justify its administration. It is the most common natural antidote for these vicious practices.

ARNICA MONTANA

The Arnica patient is morose, wants to be let alone, does not want to be talked to, does not want to be approached. He does not want to be approached, both because he does not wish to enter into conversation, a mental state, and also because he does not wish to be touched on account of the great bodily soreness. These are the two most striking things in this medicine. Irritable, morose, sad, fearful, easily frightened, imagines all sorts of things, especially that he has heart disease, or that he will mortify, or that some deep-seated trouble is upon him. Full of nightmare, dreadful dreams, dreams of muddy water, robbers, etc. Horrors in the night. He frequently rouses up in the night, grasps at the heart, has the appearance of great horror, fears some dreadful thing will happen. A sudden fear of death comes on at this time, rousing him up in the night; he grasps at the heart, and thinks he is going to die suddenly. He is full of dreadful anguish, but finally he comes to himself, lies down and goes off into a sleep of terror, jumps up again with the fear of sudden death and says: "Send for a doctor at once." This is repeated night after night in persons who are fairly well in the daytime, who have no sympathy because there seems to be no reality in their sickness, only a mental state. It is also seen in persons who have gone through a railroad accident, or through some shock, who are sore and bruised from injury. They rouse up in the night with a fear of sudden death, with an expression of terror; the horrors they really went through are repeated. This is similar to *Opium,* only the *Opium* fear remains, even in the day time. Arnica dreams of it.

When sick in bed afflicted with a zymotic disease, with violent fever, or with fever after an accident or injury, he becomes greatly prostrated, stupid and unconscious. He can be aroused and will answer a .question correctly, but goes back into a stupor, or he hesitates about a word and is unable to find correct words when trying to answer and goes back into the coma. When roused up, he looks at the doctor and says: "I do not want you; I did not send for you; I am not sick; I don't need a doctor." He will say this even when he is seriously ill. I have seen an Arnica patient lie back upon his pillow after emptying the stomach of a black fluid like blood, seriously ill, with the face mottled, in zymotic sickness or such as threaten malignant chill, that one would think he was almost going to die, look up and say: "I am not sick; I did not send for you; go home." Yet when in a state of health he was friendly, kind-hearted, knew me well, glad to shake hands with me; but now he is irritated at seeing me there and insists there is nothing the matter with him. Such is the "shock" state, almost a delirium. After finishing such a sentence he will lie down in a stupor, will lie in bed drawn up in a heap and merely groan when spoken to. He wants to be left alone, does not want to be bothered, does not want to be talked to. That state ushers in complaints after a shock that has shaken the whole system, that has disturbed the circulation. When a symptomatic typhoid is coming on, *i.e.,* when an intermittent or remittent is taking on symptoms that are typhoid in character, when the tongue becomes shiny, and sordes appear about the teeth and lips, when there is sinking, and soreness all over the body, there are times when this mental state that I am describing will appear and the patient must have Arnica. Arnica will interrupt the progress and prevent a typhoid state. Arnica is sometimes suitable to the scarlet fever, when the eruption does not come out, in those severe forms when the body is dusky, mottled and covered with red spots; the patient is constantly turning and that mental state is coming on with moroseness, and stupidity. It is a wonderful remedy, a misunderstood remedy, a misused remedy, because it is almost limited to bruises. It is one of the sheet anchors in certain seasons, in the malarial valleys of the West, for intermittent fever. In congestive chills, in those dreadful attacks with prostration, stupor, mottled skin, with congestion that comes on suddenly, with anxiety. The doctors know these fevers, they dread them, and can only cope with them by using such remedies as Arnica and *Lachesis* and other deep-acting medicines. It is not true that these patients must have *Quinine.* For many years I practiced among these cases, and I have seen numerous congestive chills and had no need for *Quinine.* I would rather have my repertory and a few potencies than all the *Quinine* in the drug stores. The sugar pills cure safely, permanently and gently, while the *Quinine* never cures, but suppresses, and there is nothing in the after history of that patient drugged with *Quinine* and *Arsenic* but congestion and violence so long as he lives.

"Horror of instant death, with cardiac distress in night." From that it spreads on throughout the system, but that horror of instant death is a striking feature and it comes on regardless of heart disease. A horror in the night when there is nothing to come upon the patient; a horrible congestion, which affects especially the cerebellum and upper part of the spinal cord.

"Stupor with involuntary discharges." "Coma, insensibility." "Lies as if dead." These symptoms come in the low forms of disease, in the typhoid type of disease. Many of the remittent fevers, if badly treated, or permitted to run their course under bad nursing, will turn into a continued fever. While the true idiopathic typhoid comes on after many weeks of gradual decline, a symptomatic typhoid may come on suddenly, and it has symptoms of graver form than the ordinary typhoid. The idiopathic typhoid will seldom kill and will generally run to a favorable termination, if the doctor stays at home. This remedy is full of delirium in these low types of fever, even delirium like delirium tremens. "Hopelessness; indifference." "Hypochondriacal anxiety, peevishness." "Fears being struck by those coming towards him." That is both bodily and mental.

Now, with this mental state thoroughly in mind, we are prepared to take up the general physical state, which has in all complaints, all over the body a feeling as if bruised. It is not strange that Arnica is used for bruises, but it is very foolish to put it on the outside and to rub it on in the form of the tincture. It produces in its pathogenesis mottled spots, like bruises. If you take Arnica internally, in large doses, you will have mottled spots, bluish spots, which become yellowish, due to ecchymoses, from extravasations of the smaller capillaries. This is, to a certain extent, what takes place in bruising. It is an extravasation of blood from the capillaries, and sometimes from the larger vessels. But all over the body he is sore and bruised, as if he had been beaten. If you watch an Arnica patient in order to get the external manifestations of his state, you will see him turning and moving. You will at once ask yourself, Why is he restless? and if you compare remedies in your mind, you will say, He is like *Rhus tox.;* he stays in a place a little while and then he moves. No matter if he is only semiconscious, you will see him make a little turn, part way over, and then a little further over, and so on until he is over on the other side. Then he commences again, and he will shift a little and a little, and so he turns from side to side. The question is, why does he move so, why is he restless? It is an important matter to solve. We notice the awful *anxiety* of the *Arsenicum* patient that keeps him moving all the time. We notice the *painful uneasiness* felt all over the body with the *Rhus* patient so that he cannot keep still. The Arnica patient is so *sore* that he can lie on one part only a little while, and then he must get off that part or to the other side. So if we ask him, "Why do you move so?" he will tell us that the bed feels hard. That is one way of telling that the body is sore. A more intelligent individual will say it is because he is so sore and feels as if bruised and beaten, and he wants to get into a new place. This state of soreness is present if it be a symptomatic typhoid, an intermittent fever, a remittent fever, or after an injury when he is really bruised all over. You get the the same continual uneasiness and motion, moving every minute. He moves and thinks that now he will be comfortable, but he is comfortable only for a second. The soreness increases the longer he lies, and becomes so great that he is forced to move. With *Rhus tox.* the longer he lies the more restless he grows and the more he aches, until he feels as if he will fly if he does not move. With *Rhus tox.* the uneasiness passes off after moving, and with Arnica the soreness passes off if he gets into a new place. With *Arsenicum* you see him moving about and look wild, and he is anxious, and this anxiety forces him to move, and he gets no rest, for he keeps going. The *Rhus tox.* and Arnica patients get better from every little motion.

The Arnica patient bleeds easily; his blood vessels seem to be relaxed, and extravasation is easy. Blue spots come easily upon the skin, and internally the mucous membranes bleed easily. The parts that are inflamed bleed. He is subject to catarrhal conditions, and if he has a cough he bleeds easily. The mucus that is hawked out of the chest and throat is streaked with blood, or dotted with tiny pin-head blood clots. His urine contains blood and there is bleeding from the various orifices of the body. There is not sufficient tone in the fibres of the vessel to hold the blood within the vessel walls and they ooze.

All over the body there is a lameness, and soreness, and a feeling as if bruised; a rheumatic lameness; the joints are swollen, sore and lame. If an acute disease becomes more severe, we shall find the mental symptoms as described, and there will be an increasing soreness in the muscles. Arnica is very suitable for that sore, bruised condition of the body, therefore Arnica is a very important remedy in injuries, bruises and shocks, injuries of joints, injury of the back with lameness and soreness. In such conditions Arnica becomes one of the first remedies, and unless there are general decided symptoms calling for other remedies it should be the first remedy. Arnica will very often take all the soreness out of a sprained ankle and permit him in a few days to go walking about, to the surprise of everybody. The black and blue appearance of sprained joints will go away in a surprisingly short time, the soreness will disappear, and he will be able to manipulate that joint with surprising ease. I have seen a sprained ankle when it was black and blue, so swollen that the shoe could not be put on, but after a dose of Arnica, the swelling disappeared in an astonishing way, the discoloration faded out and the patient was able to stand on the foot. No such result can be obtained with the use of Arnica lotion externally. A high potency of Arnica is most satisfactory in bruises, and when no decided contra-indication is present Arnica is the first remedy; but for the weakness of tendons that follows such a condition Arnica is not always sufficient, and then *Rhus tox.* is its natural follower. If the weakness and tenderness remain in the joints, follow the *Rhus* with *Calcarea.* One will not, of course, give these remedies all on the same day, and not in the same glass, but will wait until all the good has been gotten out of the Arnica before following with *Rhus.* It is quite a common thing for aching and restlessness and weakness to come into a part that has been injured, and *Rhus* is then a suitable remedy; and it is quite common for a joint that has been badly treated to remain sore and weak, and then *Calcarea* comes in as a natural follower of the *Rhus.* Now and then we have to resort to *Causticum, Staphisagria,* and other remedies, because of some peculiar feature in the case, but these remedies are all related more or less to Arnica, *Rhus* and *Calcarea.* For another class of injuries compare *Ledum* and *Hypericum.*

Arnica is useful in some chronic cases; especially in old cases of gout. It is quite a common thing for old cases of gout to rouse up into a new soreness of joints, with great sensitiveness. You will see the old grandfather sit off in a corner of the room, and if he sees little Johnnie running towards him, he will say, "Oh, do keep away, keep away." Give him a dose of Arnica and he will let Johnine run all over him. He does not want to be touched or approached; he feels that anything that is coming towards him is going to hurt him. He is extremely sensitive, his joints are sore and tender, and he is afraid they will be hurt.

This medicine has erysipelatous inflammation. If you have an erysipelas of the face with the mental state described, with soreness, and sore, bruised feeling all over the body, you need not wait longer before prescribing Arnica. The sore, bruised feeling all over the body, and the mental state, would decide in favor of Arnica against any medicine. In inflammation of the kidneys and bladder, of the liver, and even in pneumonia, the mental state and the sore, bruised feeling all over the body would enable you to do astonishing work in such cases, even though Arnica has never produced pneumonia. It has all there is of the rusty expectoration, with all the soreness of the chest and catarrhal state, the coughing and gagging, and sore, bruised feeling all over the body, and then add to this the condition of stupor and the mental state that belongs to the inflammatory condition of any organ and is especially strong in this medicine. We do not have to worry about any particular fineness of diagnosis to settle upon Arnica.

Arnica has aversion to meat, broth and milk. There is great thirst at particular times; for instance, *during the chill* of intermittent fever he has thirst, while at other times he is thirstless. "Vomiting of dark-red coagula, mouth bitter; general soreness." Vomiting of black, inky substances.

Arnica is a useful remedy in inflammatory conditions of the abdomen, liver, intenstines, with tumefaction, tympanites, prostration, tendency to uneasiness, and so sore that he cannot be touched. This state also comes with typhoid. Do not forget the symptoms of Arnica in appendicitis. You do not need to run for the surgeon for every case of appendicitis if you know *Bryonia, Rhus tox., Belladonna,* Arnica and similar remedies. The homœopathic remedy will cure these cases, and, if you know it, you need never run after the surgeon in appendicitis except in recurrent attacks. If you do not know your remedies, you will succumb to the prevailing notion that it is necessary to open the abdomen and remove the appendix. It is only deplorable ignorance that causes appendicitis to be surrendered to the knife.

Offensiveness is a feature of Arnica; there is offensiveness of the eructations, and of the flatus. The stool is horribly offensive. "Nightly diarrhœa." "Stool involuntary during sleep." "Stools of undigested food, purulent; bloody, slimy, mucus." Dark blood, very fœtid stool. Here we see the tendency to oozing from the mucous membranes. Black watery stools with black vomit. "Retention of urine from exertion," from overwork, from injury, from concussion of the brain, from some violent accident. The urine is brown, or inky, dark. "Piercing pains as from knives plunged into the kidneys." "Urine very acid, with increase of specific gravity."

Another feature of Arnica occurs in pregnant women. The extreme sensitiveness, soreness or tenderness throughout the whole body is especially felt in the abdominal viscera, in the uterus and pelvic region. Sensitiveness to the motion of the fœtus, sore and bruised; the motions of the fœtus are very painful and keep her awake all night. Arnica will remove that soreness and she will not distinguish the motion of the fœtus. It is not an increased motion of the fœtus, but that she is sensitive to it. "Constant dribbling of urine after labor."

A general feature also of the remedy is that the body is cold and the head hot; the whole body and the extremities are cold, but the head feels hot. This is a marked condition in sudden congestive attacks, in congestive chill and congestive intermittent fevers. This, sometimes, is the very beginning of a severe attack when there has been almost no warning except a night or two of bad dreams and distress, fearfulness and stupefaction, with soreness in the body. If he comes out of this, an increased soreness in the body comes on, which grows worse and worse until he is sore and bruised all over. Children going into severe attacks of infantile fever may threaten convulsions, the head is hot and the body cold. Most physicians will think of *Belladonna,* which has such cold extremities and such a hot head. Do not forget Arnica, especially in those children who seem to have an aversion to being touched, and scream out every time the mother takes hold of the leg or arm. Look into the history a little and you will see that this is a soreness, and if you strip the child you may observe dusky spots, which give an added indication of Arnica.

This is a whooping-cough remedy; you can easily conjure up what the indications are for whooping-cough; aggravation from touch, sore, bruised condition, spasmodic cough with expectoration of blood, or dark blood-streaked mucus, or little tiny pin-head dots all through the mucus. Vomiting of food with black mucus. The mental state of the child can easily be imagined. The child is cross and fretful. "Cough excited by cries in children when accompanied by anger and tossing about." "Paroxysms of cough at night." "Whooping cough; child cries before paroxysms as though in fear of soreness." You can easily apply that which we have seen in the remedy to the various diseases that come on. Stitching pains in whooping cough, pleuritic pains with catarrh of the chest, with pneumonia or pleurisy, inflammatory conditions. It has also more lingering complaints, "fatty degeneration of the heart." Stitches in the cardiac region, stitches from left to right. "Weary, bruised, sore, great weakness, must lie down, yet bed feels too hard."

It will be well to read over all these symptoms; there are numerous particulars in the remedy, many little symptoms that are of great interest.

It follows well after *Aconite* and is complementary to *Aconite, Ipe-Cacuanha* and *Veratrum.*

ARSENICUM ALBUM

From the time of Hahnemann to the present day Arsenicum has been one of the most frequently indicated medicines, and one of the most extensively used. In the Old School it is most extensively abused, in the form of Fowler's solution.

Arsenic affects every part of man; it seems to exaggerate or depress almost all his faculties, to excite or disturb all his functions. When all our medicines have been as well proved we will effect wonderful cures. It is a substance easily proved because of its active nature, and from its very abuse we have learned much of its general nature. While Arsenic impresses the whole economy and disturbs all the functions and tissues of man, there are certain prevailing and striking features in it. *Anxiety, restlessness, prostration, burning* and *cadaveric odors* are prominent characteristics. The surface of the body is pale, cold, clammy, and sweating, and the aspect is cadaveric. In chronic sickness with great debility, anæmia, from long exposure to malarial influence, in the poorly fed and from syphilis this remedy is of great service.

The *anxiety* that is found in Ars. is intermingled with fear, with impulses, with suicidal inclinations, with sudden freaks and with mania. It has delusions and various kinds of insanity; in the more active form, delirium and excitement. *Sadness* prevails to a great extreme. So sad that he is weary of life; he loathes life, and wants to die, and the Arsenic patient does commit suicide. It is a remedy full of *suicidal tendencies*. The anxiety takes form also in the restlessness, in which he constantly moves. If he is able to get up he goes from chair to chair; the child goes from nurse to mother, and from one person to another. When in bed, unable to sit up, the patient tosses and turns from side to side; if he is able, he climbs out of bed and sits in the chair, keeps moving from one place to another, and, when thoroughly exhausted, he gets back into bed again. The restlessness seems to be mostly in the mind; it is an anxious restlessness, or an anguish, with the idea that anguish is a deathly anxiety. That is an effort to express it in the extreme. It seems that he cannot live, and it is not pain that drives him to anguish, but it is an anxiety intermingled with restlessness and sadness. This state prevails in all diseases intermingled with prostration. An uneasiness comes in the early stage of disease, and lasts but until the prostration becomes marked. While lying in bed, at first he moves his whole body, moves himself in bed and out of bed; but the prostration becomes so marked that he is able to move only his limbs' until at last he becomes so weak that he is no longer able to move and he lies in perfect quiet in extreme prostration. It seems that prostration takes the place of anxiety and restlessness, and he appears like a cadaver. So remember that these states of anxiety and restlessness go towards the cadaveric aspect, towards death. This is seen, for instance, in the typhoid, where Arsenicum is indicated. At first there is that anxious restlessness with fear, but the increasing weakness tends towards prostration.

Running all through the remedy there is the *burning* mentioned as one of its most marked generals. There is burning in the brain, which makes him want to wash his head in cold water. This sensation of heat in the inner head with pulsation is ameliorated by the cold bathing, but when there is a rheumatic state that affects the scalp and outward nerves, and there is burning, the burning then is ameliorated by heat. When the headache is of a congestive character, with the sensation of heat and burning inside the head, and there is a feeling as if the head would burst, and the face is flushed and hot, that headache is better from cold applications and in the cool open air. So marked is this that I have seen the patient sitting in the room with clothing piled on to keep the body warm and with the window open to relieve the congestion of the head. Therefore, we say a striking feature belonging to this medicine is relief of all the complaints of the body from wrapping up and from warmth in general, and relief of the complaints of the head by cold, except the external complaints of the head, which are better from heat and from wrapping up. The neuralgias of the face and eyes, and above the eyes, are better from heat.

The burning is felt in the stomach; there is burning in the bladder, in the vagina, in the lungs. It feels as if coals of fire were in the lungs at times, when gangrenous inflammation is threatened, and in certain stages of pneumonia. There is burning in the throat and burning in all the mucous membranes. The skin burns with itching, and he scartches until the skin is raw, and then it burns, but the itching ceases; as soon as the smarting lets up a trifle the itching commences again. All night the itching and burning alternate, burning for a minute, when he scratches it until it is raw, but soon the itching begins again and it seems that he has no rest.

The secretions and excretions of Arsenic are *acrid;* they excoriate the parts, causing burning. The discharge from the nose and eyes causes redness around the parts, and this is true of all the fluids from the various orifices. In ulcers there is burning, and the thin, bloody fluid discharged excoriates the parts round about. The *odor* of the discharge is *putrid.* If you have ever discovered the odor of gangrene, of mortified flesh, you know the odor of the Arsenicum discharges. The stool is putrid, like decomposed flesh, putrid blood. The discharges from the uterus, the menstrual flow, the leucorrhœa, the fæces, the urine, the expectoration, all the discharges are putrid. The ulcer is so putrid that it smells like decomposing flesh.

Arsenic produces a tendency to *bleeding.* The patient bleeds easily and may bleed from any place. There is vomiting of blood; bleeding from the lungs and throat. Bloody discharge from the mucous membrane, at times, when inflammation is running high; hæmorrhage from the bowels, kidneys, bladder and uterus; anywhere that mucous membrane exists, there may be hæmorrhage. Hæmorrhage of black blood and discharges that are offensive.

Gangrene and sudden inflammatory conditions like gangrenous and erysipelatous inflammations are common in Arsenic. Parts suddenly take on erysipelas, or parts that are injured suddenly take on gangrene. Gangrene in internal organs, malignant inflammations, erysipelatous inflammation. No matter how you look upon the condition, no matter what it is called, if it is a sudden inflammation that tends to produce malignancy in the part it belongs to Arsenicum. Inflammation will go on in the bowels for a few days attended with a horribly offensive discharge, vomiting of clots of blood, great burning in the bowels with tympanitic condition. You may almost look upon this as a gangrenous inflammation, so violent, sudden and malignant is it, and it has the anxiety, prostration, fear of death, and chilliness, the patient wanting to be covered warmly. When with this inflammation of the bowels the patient is relieved by heat, it means Arsenic. You should remember that *Secale* has a similar state; it has all the tympanitic condition, all the ulceration and prostration, all the offensive odor and expulsion of offensive clots, and all the burning, but the *Secale* patient wants to be uncovered, wants things cold, wants the windows open. The only distinguishing feature between these two remedies in a case may be that *Secale* wants cold and Arsenicum wants heat, but this is the way we individualize in our homœopathic prescribing. When there is gangrenous inflammation in the lungs, we find the patient has been taken with a chill, there has been restlessness, prostration, anxiety and fear; as we enter the room we detect a horrible odor, and on looking into the pan we see the patient has been spitting up by the mouthful, black, foul expectoration. Look and see if the patient wants to be covered warmly; if he is easily chilled, and heat feels good; then it is a hard thing to cover that case outside of Arsenicum. The prostration, the vomiting, the anxiety, the restlessness, the cadaveric aspect are present, and where will you find a remedy with that totality outside of Arsenic? I have many times gone a long distance to detect, from the very aspect of things, these symptoms that could be gotten while walking from the door to the bedside. Every symptom is Arsenic; he looks like it, acts like it and smells like it. You may go to a patient with high grade inflammation of the bladder, with frequent urging to urinate, straining to urinate, and there is bloody urine intermingled with clots. It has been found by the attending physician when he introduces the catheter to draw off the urine that clots dam up the catheter, a little is drawn off and then it stops. We have a history of restlessness, anxiety, fear of death, amelioration from heat, great prostration. You must give Arsenic, not because there is inflammation of the bladder, but because it is a rapidly progressing inflammation, and because it is gangrenous in character. The whole bladder will be involved in a short time, but Arsenic will stop that. So it is with all the internal organs, the liver, lungs, etc.; any of them may take on violent and rapid inflammation. We are not now speaking of the particulars. but only illustrating the general state of Arsenic, in order to bring out what runs through the whole nature of it. We shall find when we take up the remedy and go through it in a more particular way these features will stand out everywhere.

The *mental* symptoms show in the beginning anxious restlessness, and from this a continuation towards delirium and even insanity with all that it involves; disturbance of the intellect and will. "He thinks he must die." I went to the bedside of a typhoid patient once with all the general aspect I have described; he was able to talk, and he looked up at me and said: "There is no use of your coming, I am going to die; you might as well go home; my whole insides are mortifying." His friend was seated on one side of the bed, giving him a few drops of water, and just about as often as he could get there with it he wanted it again. That was all he wanted; his mouth was black, parched and dry. He got Arsenic. One of the characteristic features of Arsenic is *thirst for small quantities often,* just enough to wet the mouth. It is commonly used as a distinguishing feature between *Bryonia* and Arsenic for the purpose of memorizing, that *Bryonia* has thirst for large quantities far apart, but Arsenicum little and often, or violent unquenchable thirst.

"Thoughts of death and of the incurability of his complaints." "Thoughts crowd upon him; he is too weak to keep them off or to hold on to one idea." That is, he lies in bed tormented day and night by depressing ideas and distressing thoughts. This is one form of his anxiety; when tormented with thoughts, he is anxious. In the delirium he sees all kinds of vermin on his bed. "Picks the bed-clothes." "Delirium during sleep, unconscious mania." "Whimpering and gnashing teeth." "Loud moaning, groaning and weeping." "Lamentations, despair of life." "Screaming, with pains." "Fear drives him out of bed, he hides in a closet." These are instances of insanity that take on first a state of anxiety, restlessness, and fear. Religious insanity, with the delusion that she has sinned away her day of grace, the biblical promises of salvation do not apply to her, there is no hope for her, she is doomed to punishment. She has been thinking on religious matters until she is insane. Finally she enters into a more complete insane state, a state of tranquility; silent, and with aversion to talk. So we see one stage enters into another; we have to take the whole case together; we have to note the course that the case has run in order to see it clearly and note that in one stage there were certain symptoms and, in another stage, other symptoms. For instance, we know that in the *acute* conditions of Arsenicum there is either thirst for ice cold water, and for only enough to moisten the mouth, or there is thirst for water in large quantities and yet it does not quench the thirst; but this thirsty stage goes on to another in which there is aversion to water, and hence we see that in *chronic* diseases Arsenicum is thirstless. So it is in a case of mania; in the chronic state he is tranquil, but in the earlier stages, in order to be an Arsenicum case, he must have gone through the Arsenicum restlessness, anxiety and fear.

Fear is a strong element in the mental state, fear to be alone; fears something is going to injure him when he is alone; full of horror; he dreads solitude and wants company, because in company he can talk and put off the fear; but as this insanity increases he fails to appreciate company and the fear comes in spite of it. He has a violent increase of his fear and horror in the dark and many complaints come on in the evening as darkness is coming on.

Many of the mental troubles, as well as the physical troubles, come on and are increased at certain times. While some complaints, pains and aches are worse in the morning, most of the sufferings of Arsenicum are worse from 1-2 P. M. and from 1-2 A. M. after midnight, very soon after midnight sometimes, his sufferings begin and from 1-2 o'clock they are intensified. Extreme anxiety in the evening in bed.

"Averse to meeting acquaintances, because he imagines he has formerly offended them." Great mental depression, great sadness, melancholy, despair, despair of recovery. He has dread of death when alone, or on going to bed, with anxiety and restlessness. He thinks he is going to die and wants somebody with him. The attacks of anxiety at night drive him out of bed. This is an anxiety that affects the heart, and so the mental anxiety and cardiac anxiety almost seem to coincide. A sudden anxious fear comes over him at night; he jumps out of bed with fear that he is going to die, or that he is going to suffocate. It is full of dyspnœa, cardiac dyspnœa, and varying forms of asthma. The spells come on in the evening in bed or after midnight; from 1-2 o'clock he is attacked with mental anxiety, dyspnœa, fear of death, coldness, and is covered with cold sweat. "Anxiety like one who has committed murder." This is one form of his anxiety; he finally works up to the idea that the officers are coming after him, and watches to see if they are coming in to arrest him. Some unusual evil is going to happen to him; always looking for something terrible to happen. "Irritable, discouraged, restless." "Restlessness, cannot rest anywhere." "As a consequence of fright, inclination to commit suicide."

The Arsenicum patient with this mental state is *always freezing,* hovers around the fire, cannot get clothing enough to keep warm, a great sufferer from the cold. Chronic Arsenicum invalids cannot get warm; they are always chilly, pale and waxy, and in such invalids, after they have had several unusual weak spells, dropsical conditions come on. Arsenicum is full of puffiness and dropsy; œdematous condition of the extremities; dropsy of the shut sacs or of the cavities; swelling about the eyes; swelling of the face, so that it pits upon pressure. Arsenicum in these swellings is especially related to the lower eyelid rather than the upper, while in *Kali carb.* the swelling is more in the upper eyelid than the lower, between the lid and the brow. There are times when *Kali carb.* looks very similar to Arsenic, and little features like that will be distinguishing points. If they run together in generals, then we must observe their particular peculiarities.

In the *headaches* we have a striking general feature of Arsenicum, brought out in their periodicity. Running all through this remedy there is *periodicity,* and for this reason it has been extensively useful in malarial affections which have, as a characteristic of their nature, periodicity. The periodical complaints of Arsenic come on every other day, or every fourth day, or every seven days, or every two weeks. The headaches come on these cycles, every other, or third, or fourth, seventh or fourteenth day. The more chronic the complaint is, the longer is its cycle, so that we will find the more acute and sharp troubles in which Arsenic is suitable will have every other day aggravations and every fourth day aggravations: but, as the trouble becomes chronic and deep-seated, it takes on the seventh day aggravation, and in the psoric manifestations of a long, lingering and deep-seated kind there is a fourteenth day aggravation. This appearing in cycles is common to a good many remedies, but is especially marked in *China* and Arsenic. These two remedies are similar to each other in many respects, and they are quite similar in their general nature to the manifestations that often occur in malaria. It is true, however, that Arsenic is more frequently indicated than *China*. In every epidemic of malarial fever that I have gone through I have found Arsenicum symptoms more common than those of *China*.

These headaches bring out the interesting point that we mentioned above. Arsenicum has in its nature *an alternation of states,* and this carries with it certain generals. Arsenicum in all of its bodily complaints is a cold remedy; the patient sits over the fire and shivers, wants plenty of clothing, and wants to be in a warm room. So long as the complaints are in the body this is so; but when the complaints are in the head, while he wants the body warm he wants the head washed in cold water, or wants the cold air upon it. The complaints of the head must conform to the generals that apply to the head, and the complaints of the body must be associated with the generals that apply to the body. It is a difficult thing to say which one of these two circumstances is most general, and it is sometimes difficult to say which one is the general of the patient himself, because he confuses you by saying: "I am worse in the. cold," but when his headache is on he says: "I am better in the cold, I want to be in the cold." It is really only the head, and you have to, single these out and study them by the parts affected. When things are so striking you must examine into it to see what it is that brings about the modality. You will see a similar state running through *Phosphorus;* the complaints of the stomach and head are better from cold, *i.e.,* he wants cold applications upon the head with head sufferings, and wants cold things in the stomach with stomach complaints, but in all the complaints of the body he is ameliorated from heat. If he steps out into the cool air, he will commence to cough, if he have a chest trouble. So we see that the modalities that belong to the part affected must always be taken into account. For instance, you have a patient suffering from neuralgia or rheumatic affections and these same pains extend to the head, then he wants the head wrapped up because they are ameliorated from heat. But when it comes to cases of congestive conditions of the head, he then is better with his head very cold. Now, as I have said, there is an alternation of these states in

Arsenicum. I will illustrate by mentioning a case. Once a patient had been dragging along with periodical sick headaches. The sick headaches were better from cold water, cold applications to the head, could hardly get them cold enough, and the colder the better. These headaches came every two weeks, and so long as they were present he desired cold to the head. Then these periodical headaches would be better, for long periods; but when they were away he was suffering from rheumatism of the joints, which was also periodical, and also more or less tenacious, and when this rheumatism of the joints and extremities, with more or less swelling and œdema, was present he could not get warm enough; he was at the fire and wrapped up; he was relieved by heat, and wanted warm air and a warm room. This would last for a period and then subside, and back would come his sick headaches and last for a while. That is what I meant by the alternation of states. Arsenicum cured that man, and he never had any of them afterwards. The alternation of states sometimes means that there are two diseases in the body, and sometimes the remedy covers the whole feature in alternation of states. I remember another case, which will illustrate this peculiar nature of alternation of complaints, which is shared by other remedies besides Arsenic. A patient suffered from a pressure in the top of the head, such as I recently described to you under *Alumen*. She would suffer for weeks from that pressure on the top of the head, and the only relief she could get was from hard pressure; she tired himself out with hard pressure and would contrive all kinds of weights to put upon the head. That would go away in the night and she would wake up the next morning with constant urging to urinate. The irritable bladder alternated with pain on top of the head. *Alumen* cured. In many of these antipsoric remedies we have an alternation of states. This illustrates the necessity for getting the symptoms of all the states that present themselves for cure, otherwise you will many times prescribe in a chronic case of psoric character and temporarily relief it, when back comes another aspect of it. You have only hastened the disease a little faster than it would go if let alone. But that is not homœopathic prescribing. Be sure, when a remedy presents one state, that it is as clearly indicated in the other state, otherwise that remedy is not the simillimum. You must hunt until you find the remedy that has both states, or you will be disappointed. We sometimes do not discover this alternation of States until we have brought it back two or three times by incorrect prescribing. Some people are so reticent and so difficult to get symptoms from that we do not always get these symptoms But you examine your record and you find where you have made a foolish prescription, that you drove a new condition away and back came the first trouble, and you kept on with this see-saw business. Now remember in doing this your patient is not improving, and that you must re-study the whole case, taking the alternating states into account. In Arsenic, the head symptoms alternate with physical symptoms. You will find running through certain remedies, as a part of their nature, that mental symptoms alternate with physical symptoms; when the physical symptoms are present, the mental symptoms are not traites the necessity for getting the symptoms of all the states that is determined it is a good point, but sometimes you do not find a remedy, because many of our remedies are not well recorded; they have not yet been observed in their alternations and marked as such. We find in *Podophyllum* the peculiar feature that the headaches alternate with diarrhœa; he is subject to sick headaches and to diarrhœa, and one or other will be present. In *Arnica* the mental symptoms alternate with uterine symptoms. The uterine symptoms, when observed, look like *Arnica,* but these go away in the night and mental symptoms come on, the mind being heavy, gloomy and cloudy. When we have remedies that have these manifestations it requires a greater depth of vision to see the alternation of states, because these things are not always brought out in the proving; for the reason that one prover had one group of symptoms, and another, another. Yet a remedy that is capable of bringing out the two groups of symptoms is sufficient to cure this alternation of states.

The periodical headaches of Arsenic are found in all parts of the head. They are the congestive headaches with throbbing and burning, with anxiety and restlessness; hot head and relief from cold. There are headaches in the forehead, which are throbbing, worse from light, intensified from motion, often attended with great restlessness, forcing him to move, with great anxiety. Most of the headaches are attended with nausea and vomiting. The sick headaches are of the worst sort, especially those that come every two weeks. In some of these old, broken-down constitutions you will find he is cold, pallid, sickly; he is always chilly and freezing except when the headache is on, and it is better from cold; the face much wrinkled, great anxiety and no desire for water. Remember that it was said in the acute state of Arsenic there is thirst, thirst for little and often, dry mouth and desire for water enough to moisten the lips, but in the chronic states of Arsenic he is generally thirstless. There are headaches on one side of the head involving the scalp, one-half of the head, worse from motion, better from cold washing, better from walking in the cold air, though very often the jar or stepping starts up a feeling as of a wave of pain, shaking, vibration or looseness in the brain; such are the sensations and these are conditions of pulsation. Then there are dreadful occipital headaches, so severe that the patient feels stunned or dazed. They come on after midnight, from excitement, from exertion; they come on from becoming heated in walking, which produces determination of blood to the head. *Nat. mur.* is a medicine analogous to this in its periodicity and in many of its complaints. It has congestive headaches from walking and becoming heated; especially from walking in the sun. The Arsenicum headaches are generally worse from light and noise, better from lying down in a dark room, lying with the head on two pillows. Many of the headaches commence in the afternoon from 1 to 3 o'clock, after the noon meal, grow worse into the afternoon, lasting all night. They are often attended with great pallor, nausea, prostration, deathly weakness. The pain is paroxysmal; violent head pain during the chill of an intermittent fever; headache as if the skull would burst during an intermittent fever. Arsenicum has this head pain of a congestive character in intermittent fever, as if the head would burst. A peculiar feature of the thirst is that there is no thirst during the chill except for hot drinks; during the heat there is thirst little and often for water enough to moisten the mouth, which is almost no thirst, and during the sweat there is thirst for large drinks. Thirst begins with the beginning of the heat and increases as the dryness of the mouth increases; he desires only to moisten the mouth until he breaks out in a sweat, and then the thirst becomes a desire for large quantities very often, and the more he sweats the more desire he has for water. The headache is during the chill; it increases, so that it becomes a congestive, throbbing headache during the chill and heat; this grows better towards the end of the heat as the sweat breaks out, it is ameliorated by the sweat.

In chronic headaches, congestive headaches and malarial complaints, a *tendency* to *shrivel* is observed upon the skin; a prematurely old, wrinkled appearance of the skin comes on. The mucous membrane of the lips and mouth often shrivels and becomes wrinkled. This is also found in the diphtheritic membrane of the throat as a peculiar feature of Arsenic, and belongs, as far as I know, to no other remedy. The exudation in the throat is leathery looking and shrivelled. A shrivelled membrane is not a sure indication for Arsenic, but when Arsenic is indicated you would be likley to find this kind of membrane; such cases as are very malignant in character, very offensive, putrid, those with a gangrenous odor.

At times the head is in constant motion when there are complaints in the body, because parts of the body are too sore to be moved; then the motion of the head comes on because of restlessness and uneasiness, and he keeps it in motion even though it does not ameliorate. The face and head are subject to œdema; dropsy of the scalp and erysipelatous inflammation of the face and head. The scalp pits upon pressure and there is a little crepitation under it from pressure. The scalp is subject to eruptions and is very sensitive. So sensitive is the scalp that the hair cannot be combed; it seems as if the touch of the comb or brush when rubbing over the scalp went into the brain.

Sensitiveness is a feature of Arsenic; sensitiveness to smell and touch; oversensitiveness of all the senses. A peculiar feature that perhaps I have not brought out is the oversensitiveness to the circumstances and surroundings of the room. The Arsenicum patient is an extremely fastidious patient. Hering once described him as "the gold-headed cane patient". If this is carried out in a woman who is sick in bed she is in great distress if every picture on the wall does not hang perfectly straight. Those who are sensitive to disorder and confusion and are disturbed and made worse until everything is placed in order have a morbid fastidiousness which has its simillimum in Arsenic.

The eye symptoms of this remedy are very prominent. In old cases of suppressed malaria, in broken down constitutions, in pallid, sickly people who are subject to general catarrhal conditions, and such catarrhal conditions as localize more especially in the nose and eyes, the eye symptoms will be troublesome. There are discharges from the eyes. It may be a conjunctivitis, in a general way involving the lids and the globe, going on sometimes to ulceration with thin, bloody discharge, increasing to thick, acrid discharge that excoriates the eye, making the canthi red and causing granulation with burning. The burning is better from washing in cool water and also better from dry heat. Very often ulcers appear on the globe of the eye, often upon the cornea. It has various kinds of hypertrophy beginning in patches that will form scars, and in old ulcerated patches little growth similar to a pterygium growing towards the centre of the eye and threatening blindness. The inflammations are sometimes attended with swelling, burning and excoriating discharge; this swelling is bag-like in character, and so we find "baggy" lids and little bags forming under the eyes. The face is waxy and pale, presenting the appearance of a broken down constitution or a dropsical condition.

The catarrhal state involves throat and nose, and it is sometimes difficult to separate the nose symptoms from the throat symptoms. The Arsenicum patient is always taking cold in the nose, always sneezing from every change in the weather. He is always chilly and suffers from drafts, and is worse in cold, damp weather; always freezing, chilled through. These pale, waxy, broken down constitutions with catarrhal discharges from the nose on looking at a bright light become blind. Sneezing and coryza with inflammatory conditions through the whole nasal cavity, throat, larynx and chest. The cold begins in the nose and goes down into the throat, very often causing hoarseness with dry, tickling, hard, rasping cough. It is a difficult matter to find remedies for a coryza that begins in the nose and extends into the chest with bronchial troubles; very often you require a change of remedy, as the chest symptoms often run to a different remedy. It is difficult to find a remedy that covers the symptoms of both nose and chest.

Arsenicum is the remedy for old, chronic catarrhal troubles of the nose where the nose bleeds easily, and he is always sneezing and taking cold, always chilly and pallid, tired, restless, full of anxiety in the night and has troublesome dreams. The mucous membrane is easily inflamed, producing patches of red and ulcers that bleed easily. Great crusts form in the back of the nose. There is a striking tendency to ulcerate in Arsenicum. If it is a sore throat it ulcerates; if colds settle in the eyes, they may end in ulceration; catarrhal troubles in the nose end in ulceration; and this ulceration tendency, no matter where the trouble locates, is a very strong feature of Arsenicum. It is the remdey for catarrhal complaints of the nose and other places in broken down constitutions from syphilis or malaria, or a constitution that has gone through blood poisoning of some kind, either poisoning from a dissecting wound, or from erysipelas or typhoid fever or other zymotic states improperly treated, or poisoning with quinine and like substances that break down the blood and establish a state of anæmia. If an ulcer comes upon the leg, if a leucorrhœa comes on, if any discharge is established the patient is relieved thereby. Now let some of these discharges slack up and you have a chronic state apparently from retained secretions, but it is a form of blood poisoning. So it is with suppressed ear discharges, suppressed throat discharges, suppressed leucorrhœa and ulcerations. Arsenicum is one of the medicines that will conform to the anæmic state that follows each suppression. At the present day it is fashionable to use the cautery, to make local applications to stop Ieucorrhœa and other discharges and to heal up ulcers. Now, when these external troubles go there is an anaemic state established in the economy, the patient becomes waxy and pallid, sickly looking, and these catarrhal discharges come on as a means of relief because of the suppression of some other condition. For instance, since the suppression of a leucorrhœa the woman has had thick, bloody or watery discharge from the nose. It is frequently suitable to the constitution when an ulcer has been dried up by salves, or an old ear discharge has been stopped by the outward application of powders. The doctor thinks he has done a clever thing in stopping such discharges, but he has only succeeded in damming up the secretions which are really a relief to the patient. Such medicines as *Sulphur, Calcarea* and Arsenicum are suitable for the catarrhal discharges that come from these suppressions, in broken down constitutions. Arsenic is also like unto the condition that has been brought about from the absorption of animal poisons. It goes to the very root of the evil, as it is similar to the symptoms brought on from a dissecting wound. Arsenic and *Lachesis* are medicines that will go to the cause at once and antidote the poison, establishing harmony and turning things into order.

The nose symptoms, then, of Arsenic are very troublesome and furnish an extensive part of the symptom image of an Arsenicum patient. They always rake cold easily, are always sensitive to cold and the catarrh is always roused up on the slightest provocation. When an Arsenicum patient is at his best he has discharge more or less of a thick character, but when he takes a little cold it becomes thin; the thick discharge that is necessary to his comfort slacks up, and then he gets headache and on comes thirst, restlessness, anxiety and distress. This goes on to a catarrhal fever of two or three days' duration, and then the thick discharge starts up again and he feels better; all his pains and aches disappear. It has been of great service in epithelioma of nose and lips

Inflammation of the throat and tonsils with burning, increased by cold and better by warm drinks. There is redness and a shrivelled condition of the mucous membrane. When there is blood poisoning going on, as in diphtheria, an exudate appears upon the mucous membrane and it becomes gray and shrivelled, ashy colored, and this sometimes covers the whole of the soft palate and the arches. It looks withered. He is prostrated, anxious, sinking, weak, not a great deal of fever, but much dryness of the mouth.

The catarrhal state goes down into the larynx with hoarseness, and into the trachea with burning, worse from coughing, and then comes constriction of the chest, asthmatic dyspnœa and dry, hacking cough with no expectoration. This teasing cough is attended with anxiety, prostration. restlessness, exhaustion and sweat, and the cough does not seem to do any good. The cough is the early part of it and keeps on as a dry, rasping, harsh cough for several days without doing any good; and then asthmatic symptoms come on, when he expectorates great quantities of thin, watery sputum. There is constriction about the chest, a great sense of tightness and wheezing, and he feels he will suffocate. Bloody mucus is expectorated at times, but the symptoms are more generally of a catarrhal character. Symptoms of pneumonia sometimes appear with the rusty expectoration. The expectoration is excoriating. There is in the chest a sense of burning, as if coals of fire were in the chest, and it goes on to bleeding and livercolored expectoration.

Arsenicum is a bleeding medicine, one that predisposes to hæmorrhage, and bleeding takes place from all mucous membranes; commonly of bright red blood, but in this region the parts take on a gangrenous state and the hæmorrhages become black and there are little clots like portions of liver. The same are found in the vomited matter and in the stools. The expectoration is horribly offensive, so much so that you soon get the idea that there is a state of gangrene. The patient is at this time going into a state that perhaps cannot be any better described than a gangrenous inflammation; there will be signs to indicate the inflammatory condition, and there will be the smell of the expectoration which you will detect as soon as you open the door. The expectoration is a thin, watery fluid intermingled with clots. In the pan you will find this watery expectoration looking like prune juice, and in the midst of it will be clots of blood; the offensiveness is horrible. He has gone through the period of restlessness and is now prostrated, sinking, pallid, and likely enough covered with a cold sweat.

When we come to the stomach we find everything that may be called a gastritis, vomiting of everything taken, even a teaspoonful of water, extreme irritation of the stomach, great prostration, horrible anxiety; dry mouth; a very little hot water will sometimes comfort him for a minute, but soon it must come up; cold fluids are vomited immediately. The whole œsophagus is in a state of inflammation; everything burns that comes up or goes down. Vomiting of bile and blood. Extreme sensitiveness of the stomach is present; he does not want to be touched. Heat applied externally relieves, and there is a temporary relief from warm drinks; the heat is grateful. In the bowels we have much trouble; this remedy has all the symptoms of peritonitis; distension of the abdomen, a tympanitic state; cannot be handled or touched, yet he will keep moving because he is so restless, he cannot keep still, but finally he becomes so weak that exhaustion takes the place of restlessness. Dysentery is likely to come on, with involuntary passages of urine and fæces, one or both, with hæmorrhage from the bowels and bloody urine. As the bowels move, we get the cadaveric odor to the stool, a smell like putrid flesh. The stool is bloody, watery, brown like prune juice, or black and horribly offensive. Sometimes dysenteric in character with dreadful straining and burning of the anus; every stool burns as though there were coals of fire in the rectum; burning in the bowels, burning all the way through. The pain in the abdomen is better from the application of hot things. The tympanitic condition is extreme. Sometimes there is a gastro-enteritis that takes on a gangrenous character that in olden times used to be talked about as gangrene of the bowel, a mortification that always ended in death. A thick, bloody discharge is passed with a horrible odor, all substances are vomited, the patient desires to be in a very warm room, wants to be well covered, wants hot applications and warm drinks, looks cadaveric and smells cadaveric, with a dry, pungent odor that penetrates everything, but if he wants the covers off, wants a cool room and windows open, wants to be sponged with cold water, and wants ice cold drinks then he must have *Secale*.

I want to warn you against the too promiscuous use of Arsenic in the summer complaints of young babies, for dysentery and cholera infantum. It has so many little symptoms that are so common to these complaints that if you do not look out and are not warned yon will be likely to give your patient Arsenic, suppress some of the symptoms, changing the aspect of the case so that you cannot find a remedy for it and yet not cure the case with Arsenic. There is a strong tendency to be routine and give Arsenic without a sufficient number of generals being present; *i.e.*, if you give it on particulars and not on the generals of the case.

This medicine is full of diarrhœa and dysenteric symptoms; in these conditions there will be the pallor, the anxiety, the cadaveric aspect and the cadaveric odors. In the dysentery there is most distressing and frequent urging to stool, scanty, slimy, black, fluid, inky stools with cadaveric smell, great prostration, restlessness and pallor. In the bowel troubles, in low forms of disease, the stool becomes involuntary. This is a condition of the rectum, a relaxation of the rectum, great prostration. Involuntary stool generally indicates either local or general exhaustion, and in this remedy there is terrible exhaustion, so that there is involuntary diarrhœa in typhoid and in low forms of zymotic disease; involuntary urine.

Purging is sometimes present in Arsenic, but generally he does not have much purging, such as we find in *Podophyllum, Phos. ac.* Usually there will be little, frequent gushes, little spurts with flatus and the great exhaustion that occurs in cholera, little spurts with mucus, slimy, whitish stools. Arsenic is not so commonly indicated in cholera, *i.e.*, during the gushing period, but sometimes after the gushing is over and the vomiting and purging have passed, leaving a state of extreme exhaustion, we have a state that appears like coma, the patient looks almost as if dead, except that he breathes. We find, then, that Arsenicum will establish reaction. Cholera infantum with great prostration, sinking and cadaveric appearance, great coldness, covered with cold sweat, cold extremities, cold as death; cadaveric, sickly, foul, pungent, penetrating odor in the room from the fæces and urine and even of what is vomited. The passages from the bowels are acrid, excoriating, causing redness and burning. Very often the burning extends into the bowels. The rectum and anus burn, smarting all about the anus. It has tensesmus, painful, unbearable urging, great distress in the lower bowel, in rectum and anus, terrible state of anxiety of the patient and the pain is so violent and the suffering so intense, the anguish so intense, that he can think of nothing but death; the fearfulness and frightful feelings are such as he has never experienced in his life, and he feels confident these mean he is going to die. This, like all other complaints, is attended with restlessness, and when not at stool he is walking the floor, going from bed to chair and from chair to bed. He will get on the stool and then back to bed, then he is hurried to stool again, sometimes he loses it. Sometimes there is a chronic hæmorrhoidal state with burning, and the hæmorrhoids protrude when at stool, he is much exhausted after getting back into bed after a stool, with these protruding lumps which are like grapes and feel like coals of fire. They are hot, dry and bleeding. Fissures of the rectum that bleed at every stool, with burning. Itching and eczematous eruptions about the anus with burning.

This kind of pain may be felt anywhere in the body; burning is characteristic of Arsenic, stitching is characteristic of Arsenic. Now, put these together and the patient often describes it as being stuck with red hot needles all over him. This red hot sensation, which is a common feature all over, is felt at the anus, and especially when there are hæmorrhoids. burning and sticking like hot needles in the hæmorrhoids.

At times when a patient is coming down with the early stage of a violent attack he will have all rigor and chill that it is possible to find in the Materia Medica and that can be found in disease. Rigors and chills of violent character, and at such times he describes a feeling as if the blood flowing through the vessels were ice water. He feels a rushing through the body of ice cold waves. When the fever comes on and he is intensely hot from head to foot, before the sweat has appeared, he feels that boiling water is going through the blood vessels. Then comes on the sweat and dyspnœa and all complaints in which he is prostrated and becomes cold. While the sweat sometimes relieves the fever and pains, yet it is prolonged and attended with great exhaustion and does not relieve his exhaustion. Many of his complaints are increased with the sweat; for instance, thirst is increased, the drinking is copious and does not relieve, it seems he cannot get enough and patients will say: "I can drink the well dry," or "Give me a bucket of water." Such things are indicative of the state of thirst During the fever he wants little and often; during the chill he wants hot drinks.

Arsenicum is a very useful medicine in the eruptions of the genitals with burning. In little ulcers that burn, even when they are syphilitic; herpetic vesicles that appear upon the foreskin and upon the labia; chancre or chancroid with burning, smarting and stinging, but especially in those that are weak, that offer no willingness to heal, but that do the very opposite, that spread, those that we call phagedenic, those that eat from their outer margins, become larger and larger. Arsenic and *Merc. cor.* are the two principal medicines for spreading ulcerations such as eat in every direction, very offensive. Such ulcerations as follow the opening of a bubo in the inguinal region where there is no tendency to heal. A little, watery, offensive discharge keeps coming and extending, ulceration keeps spreading round about the opening, no tendency to heal. Or the patient has been in the hands of a surgeon who has passed his knife down the threatening suppurating bubo and it has been followed by red, angry, erysipelatous appearance and shows no tendency to heal. The edges have been removed by ulceration, and now the surface has cleared off, leaving a surface the size of a dollar; sometimes becoming serpiginous. These ulcers are sensitive to touch and burn like fire.

In the male and female sexual organs there are many symptoms of importance. In the male organs a dropsical conditions, dropsy of the penis, œdematous appearance, so that the penis is enormously swollen and looks like a water bag; the scrotum, especially the skin of the scrotum, greatly swollen and humid round about the parts. In the female the labia are enormously swollen with burning, stinging pains, hard and swollen. Erysipelatous inflammation of these organs, ulcerations of a syphilitic character; these when such symptoms as burning, smarting and stinging are present. In the female, violent, burning pains in the genitals with or without swelling, burning that extends up into the vagina, with great dryness and itching of the vagina. The leucorrhœal discharge excoriates the parts, causing itching and burning with great suffering. Whitish, watery, thin discharges that excoriate; so copious sometimes that it will run down the thighs. The Arsenicum menstrual flow is very often excoriating in character. Copious leucorrhœal flow intermixed with menstrual flow, very profuse and very acrid. Suppressed menstruation going on for months; amenorrhœa in prostrated, nervous patients, wrinkled, careworn, haggard faces. Of course, Arsenic has a wonderful reputation in the old school for anæmia, and it is said to be as good as *Ferrum* for anæmia; *Ferrum* and Arsenic are the strong drugs for anæmia, so that it is not to be wondered at that these pallid mortals find benefit from Arsenic. "During menstruation stitches in the rectum." "Leucorrhœa acrid, corroding, thick and yellow," etc. After parturition the woman does not pass the urine; no urine in the bladder; suppression, or the bladder is full and it does not pass. In connection with this subject you will find *Causticum* the most frequently indicated remedy when you go back, and the woman has not passed the urine and it is time that she should; you will frequently find it indicated when you have no other symptoms to go on. *Aconite* will be more frequently indicated than any other remedy if the infant has not passed the urine. This is keynote practice and is to be condemned when there are other symptoms to indicate a remedy. If there are no other symptoms study *Aconite* and *Causticum* and see if there is any reason why they should not be given. Another feature in connection with the woman, Arsenic is a wonderful palliative in cancerous affections, such as occur in the uterus and mammary glands. Burning, stinging pains have entirely disappeared, in incurable cases, of course. It becomes one of the palliatives.

Arsenic has loss of voice, laryngitis, with dry teasing cough; a cough that does not seem to do any good; hacking constantly, dry, hacking cough. Study its relation to asthma and difficult breathing, dyspnœa. Arsenic has cured some long-standing cases of asthma of a nervous character; asthma that comes on after midnight, in patients who suffer from the cold, those who are very pallid, dry wheezing cough, must sit up in bed and hold the chest, anxious restlessness with prostration.

The heart symptoms are troublesome to manage when they get to be like Arsenic; the symptoms correspond to a state of great weakness, great palpitation, palpitation from the least exertion or excitement, great anxiety, anguish, weakness; he cannot walk, he cannot go upstairs, he can hardly move without increasing the palpitation; every excitement brings on palpitation. "Severe paroxysms of palpitation or attacks of syncope during endocarditis." Arsenicum corresponds to most serious complaints of the heart, corresponds to many of the incurable complaints of the heart; *i.e.*, when you see Arsenic corresponding in all of the symptoms with these marked cardiac affections, dropsy of the pericardium, etc., you have a class of cases that are very serious, "Angina pectoris," etc. "Rheumatism affecting the heart," etc. "Hydropericardium with great irritability," etc. "Pulse frequent, small, trembling." "Pulsation through whole body," etc., etc. Again this goes on to another state when the heart becomes weak, pulse thread-like, patient pale and cold, covered with sweat, pulse very feeble. When this is not a state of the heart itself then Arsenic becomes a wonderful remedy; that is, it is capable of cure.

I want to say a few things concerning a few essentials, some few things most general to the Arsenicum type of intermittent. You can read the general state of intermittent fever and fevers generally and apply what has been said. Arsenic has all the violence of the chill that you can find in any remedy, with excitement, headache, prostration, dry mouth, desire for hot drinks and to be covered up warmly, with all the anxious restlessness and prostration that you can find in any medicine; but the time of the Arsenic case is an important thing. A striking feature of the Arsenic time of chill is its irregularity, coming not twice alike, coming at any time. It has afternoon chill and after midnight chill, sometimes in the morning, sometimes at 3 or 4 P.M., sometimes at 1 P.M. It has a striking periodicity in its nature. Hence it has an intermittent nature. It has a striking feature of thirst. During the chill, while there is sometimes great thirst, he has aversion to cold things, hence can take only hot drinks, hot teas, etc. During the fever the thirst increases because he has dry mouth, and he drinks little and often, just a teaspoonful to wet his dry mouth. Water does not quench his thirst, for he wants but a tablespoonful, little and often. This runs on into the sweat with prostration, increased coldness, desire for copious drinks, unquenchable thirst for cold drinks. The chill is attended with great aching in the bones, likely to commence in the extremities, and during the chill there is a great head congestion with purple fingers and toes. Put these things together and the prostration that occurs with the awful anxiety, and you can most always in a general way pick out the Arsenic case. But it has so many details in its chill, fever and sweat that if you take the details of symptoms and leave these general features out you will be likely to be able to cover almost any case of chills, *i.e.,* you may think you will, but unless some of these general states are present that stamp it as Arsenic you will fail. It is one thing to stamp the whole case as Arsenic and another thing to say that these are Arsenicum symptoms. So it is with *China* and *Quinine;* they have numerous particular symptoms, and yet to make the case a *China* or *Quinine* case the striking general features must be present.

ARSENICUM IODATUM

From a study of the elements making up this agent, it may be known that it is a deep-acting constitutional remedy. Its complaints come on in the MORNING, afternoon, *evening,* NIGHT, after *midnight.* In hectic conditions, with many abscesses. Extreme anæmia, such as belongs to tuberculous subjects. The patient craves open air when not too cold; wants the windows open, is sensitive to a close room. Marked general *physical anxiety.* The hands and feet tingle as if asleep and the limbs feel as if tied with a band. Complaints are worse from bathing; takes cold from bathing. It has been of the highest use in cancerous affections and has cured lupus and epithelioma. Its symptoms are often found in chlorotic girls; it has cured choreic action of muscles in girls. Some are very sensitive to cold, like *Arsenicum,* and others to heat, like *Iodine;* it is sensitive to both heat and cold; cold wind and cold wet weather make the patient worse and bring out symptoms. Always taking cold, which brings on coryza and increases his catarrhal troubles. Many constrictions, internal and external, and constrictions of orifices are found in this remedy. Convulsive movements of limbs. Dropsy, external and internal, like *Arsenicum.* He is worse when hungry and, like *Iodine,* better after eating. Increasing loss of flesh and weight in phthisical patients; emaciation in children, extreme aggravation from slight physical exertion.

In women who are subject to faintness and fainting spells. Formication all over the body. Hæmorrhage from any mucous membrane. A sensation of being too warm, must have fresh air. Feeling of heaviness of the whole body. Induration is a strong feature; sometimes in glands, in ulcers, in skin affections. The glands are swollen and hard. Inflammation, external and internal, in many parts, glands, bones and serous membranes. He has symptoms as though he had lost fluid. Extreme lassitude; lack of reaction, lying in bed and lying on the painful side makes the symptoms worse. She is worse during the menses; worse from motion, but *desire to move.* Mucous secretions generally increased, copious, catarrhal discharges, thick, yellow, or yellowish-green and honey-like. Numbness of the limbs and painful parts, flushes of heat and surging of blood in the body; pain in the bones and glands. Bruised sensation in the body. Burning internally and in outer parts; paralyzing pains, pinching, pressing, stitching and tearing pains. Predisposition to phthisis and complaints in the consumptive diathesis. There is much soreness, and pressure increases his suffering. Pulsation internal and external, like *Iodine;* the pulse is frequent and small, full, hard, intermittent, irregular. Burning is a strong feature, like *Arsenicum.* It has been very useful in all scorbutic conditions when the symptoms were similar. Very sensitive to pain. The symptoms predominate on the right side; he is sensitive to the summer heat and the cold in winter. Dropsical and inflammatory swelling; swelling in affected parts and in glands. It has been curative in *all stages and forms of syphilis.* Trembling and *twitching* of muscles, walking makes him worse, especially walking fast; worse from warmth, warm air, warm bed, warm room and warm wraps. Weakness, like a vital prostration, in the morning, when ascending, on *exertion,* during menses, and on walking; worse in wet weather, worse from the warm south wind.

Anger and irritability during all complaints; aversion to answering questions; extreme anxiety, restlessness and fear; worse in a warm bed; confusion of mind morning and evening; delirium during the night; illusions of fancy and delusions about dead people. Sadness, even to despair; discontentment, and he is often in a state of great excitement; mental exertion increases many of his symptoms; there is marked mental weakness; fear of insanity, of misfortune, of people, and he is generally timid. He is impatient and in a constant state of hurry; he becomes indifferent to his friends, to happiness and to his surroundings. Aversion to work. He seems to be going toward insanity. He is unable to decide between two opinions. He suffers from a sudden impulse to kill somebody. Very talkative at times; mirthful; changeable moods and alternating conditions of mind; a degree of mental prostration prevails continuously. He is over-sensitive, especially to noise. Inclination to sit; averse to being spoken to and he starts during sleep. Persistent tormenting thoughts; wandering thoughts; stupefaction of mind. In the woman there is much weeping. Vertigo while walking. It will cure the particulars given below when the generals above mentioned strongly predominate.

Although there is hyperæmia of the brain, the scalp feels cold. Eruptions crusty, scurfy; eczematous; the hair falls out and the head feels heavy; itching of the scalp, with and without eruptions. Pain in the morning and afternoon; better in open air; worse in warm room; better after eating and worse when hungry; worse from motion, noise, walking; pain in head from catarrh of nasal passages, with coryza; periodical headaches from malaria, with heart troubles and from syphilis; pain in forehead in the evening; above the eyes, over the *root of* the nose; pain in occiput, sides of head, temples and vertex; pressing pain in forehead, with sleepiness; pressing pain in occiput and temples; sore, bruised pain in the head; stitching in head, in temples; tearing pain in head. The head pains are stunning. Perspiration of the forehead; pulsating in the head, forehead, temples.

Inflammation of the conjunctiva, and of the iris; chronic catarrhal condition of the eyes in psoric and syphilitic subjects; easy lachrymation, worse in cold air; pain in eyes when reading; soreness of the eyeballs; stitching pain in eyes; protrusion of the eyeballs; pupils dilated: redness of eyes.

Staring look. Sunken eyes. The lids are swollen and œdematous; twitching of the lids. Wild look in the eyes; the eyes are jaundiced; vision is dim, flickering, foggy and weak. Sparks before the eyes.

The ears discharge an excoriating fœtid pus; buzzing, humming, ringing and roaring in ears. Catarrh of Eustachian tubes and middle ear; the pain is aching, stitching and tearing. Stopped sensation in ears; hearing is impaired.

Most stubborn nasal catarrh with bloody, acrid, copious, *excoriating, greenish, purulent,* thick, yellow or yellow-greenish discharge; honey-like discharge; coryza with watery discharge; coryza in open air with cough. It has been a most useful remedy in *hay fever.* Dryness in nose and *epistaxis. Obstruction of nose,* pain in nose. Smell lost. Much sneezing. Swelling inside of nose; ulceration in nose.

The face becomes cold. Bluish lips and bluish circles about the eyes; brownish, earthy, or pale face; again the face is red and there are circumscribed red cheeks; the face is sallow and jaundiced; yellow spots on the face; sickly look; the face looks drawn and emaciated; eruptions on face and nose; acne, eczema, pimples, pustules, expression sickly and old; pain in the face. Swelling of the glands of the lower jaw. Swelling of the *submaxillary glands.* Twitching of the face.

In the mouth there are aphthæ; the gums bleed easily, and the tongue is cracked. The tongue is coated brown or white; mouth and tongue are dry at night and during sleep, the tongue feels enlarged; inflammation of the gums. Mucus in the mouth in the morning; the mouth is offensive, even putrid. Pain in the gums; sore, burning tongue; *salivation,* scorbutic gums. Speech stammering. Swollen gums. The taste is bad; bitter, putrid, saltish, *sour,* sweetish; teeth feel elongated; pain in the teeth after eating; tearing pain in the teeth.

Much choking in the throat; dryness in the throat; membranes form in the throat; burning in the throat; constantly scraping the throat. Swallowing difficult. Swollen throat; ulceration of the throat from syphilis.

The appetite is increased, even ravenous; aversion to food, constriction of the stomach; the stomach is distended. He desires stimulants. Sensation of emptiness; eructations empty, sour; waterbrash; sensation of fullness in the stomach. Frequent attacks of heartburn; load in the stomach after eating; indigestion and much hiccough; chronic gastritis; loathing of food; nausea after eating. Pain after eating; burning, cramping, cutting, gnawing, pressing and stitching pains in the stomach; pulsating, retching when coughing; sensation of tightness in stomach; thirst, evening, extreme; thirst during meal; unquenchable thirst. Trembling in the stomach. Continuous vomiting; vomiting with diarrhœa, after drinking, after eating, after milk. violent vomiting; vomiting of bile, blood, food; vomiting yellow, watery substance.

The abdomen is distended with flatus; the flatulency is obstructed and there is much rumbling. Enlargement of liver, spleen, mesenteric glands, glands of groin. Inflammation of the intestines, liver and spleen. It has many complaints of the liver. Pain in abdomen after eating; during menses; during stool; better by external warmth. Pain in hypogastrium, hypochondria, groin, liver, spleen and umbilical region; burning, cramping, drawing pain in abdomen; cutting in abdomen during stool; cutting pain in liver; pressing pains and soreness in liver. Stitching pains in hypochondria; pulsating in abdomen; restless feeling in abdomen; pain and soreness in spleen.

Very troublesome constipation; diarrhœa alternating with constipation; stool hard, knotty and light colored. The diarrhœa comes in the morning and after eating; in old people, excoriating stool. Dysentery with bloody, mucous stools and tenesmus; diarrhœa with brown, copious, frequent, offensive, yellow or white watery stools; ineffectual urging to stool; urging after stool; offensive flatus. External piles. Itching of anus. Burning in anus after stool.

It acts deeply upon the bladder and kidneys. It has been most useful in Addison's disease. Retention of urine; constant or frequent urging to urinate; worse during the night; urination is dribbling and *involuntary;* suppression of urine; the urine is albuminous, cloudy, dark, red, copious or scanty and offensive.

The genital organs present many symptoms and complaints. Erections, strong toward morning; later incomplete and wanting. It cures hydrocele and induration of the testes. Itching of the penis and glans; perspiration of the genitals; seminal emissions; swelling of the testes; ulcers on the penis; chancres and chancroids with bubos.

It has been a great comfort to the women in many complaints. It has restrained the progress of cancer of uterus in a notable manner; the burning and odor are removed and the ulceration is lessened. Life has been prolonged to four years in several cases. Sexual desire is increased. It has cured enlargement and induration of the ovaries; it has cured inflammation of the ovaries. *Leucorrhœa, acrid, bloody, burning, copious,* after menses, thick or thin, yellow; menses absent or suppressed, copious, frequent, late, painful, short. Hæmorrhage from the uterus; pain in ovaries, especially the right; sore, bruised genitals and ovaries. Prolapsus of the uterus; swollen ovaries. It has stopped the growth of ovarian tumors.

Croupous condition of the larynx. Dryness in the air passages. Inflammation of the larynx and trachea; much mucus in the larynx and trachea; spasmodic conditions of the larynx like laryngismus; burning rawness and soreness in larynx and trachea; phthisis of the larynx. The voice is hoarse, rough and weak and finally lost; respiration is fast and *asthmatic;* respiration is difficult at night, on ascending, on exertion and motion, with palpitation; respiration is irregular, rattling, short, suffocative and *wheezing.* Asthma from 11 P.M. until 2 A.M. The cough is in the morning, evening and after midnight; the cough is asthmatic, croupy, deep, dry, exhausting, during fever; cough from irritation and tickling in larynx and trachea; the cough is loose, spasmodic, suffocative; worse from motion and talking; worse in a warm room. It cures whooping cough. Expectoration most in the morning; is bloody, copious, greenish-yellow, difficult; mucous and bloody; mucus offensive, purulent, tough, viscid, yellow, tasting putrid, saltish, sweetish.

There is marked anxiety in the region of the heart. Catarrh of the bronchial tubes; constriction of the chest, of the heart; fatty degeneration of the heart. Enlarged and painful mamæ. Heat in the chest. Inflammation of the bronchial tubes, endocardium, pericardium, lungs and pleura; murmurs of the heart; stitching of the skin of chest; oppression of the chest and heart in a warm room; pain in the side of chest; in the heart; burning in the chest; cutting pain in chest and in the heart; pressing pain in chest; rawness in chest; stiching pain in chest on coughing; palpitation from excitement, from exertion; tumultuous palpitation. Paralysis of the heart, of the lungs. It is a very useful remedy in ulcerative conditions during phthisis; swollen axillary glands; tremulous heart; tumor of the axilla. Great weakness of chest and heart.

Pain in the back during menses; pain in the lumbar region during menses; pain in sacrum and coccyx.

Coldness of hands, legs and feet; cramps of upper limbs, lower limbs, thighs, legs and feet; scaly eruptions, eczema and vesicles; heat of hands; heaviness of the limbs as though tired; heaviness of the feet. Hip joint disease. Itching of all the limbs; numbness of all the limbs, fingers, legs and feet; pain in all the joints, gouty and rheumatic; rheumatic pain in upper limbs; pain in elbow, forearm, hip, thigh, knee. foot; drawing in lower limbs, thighs, knees; stitching pain in shoulders, wrists and knees; tearing in joints, elbows, fingers; paralytic weakness in upper limbs; paralysis of lower limbs. Cold perspiration of hands and feet. Stiffness of limbs, of fingers. Dropsical swelling of hands, legs and feet; trembling of hands and lower limbs; twitching of upper limbs and legs; weakness of upper limbs and knees.

Dreams amorous; anxious; of dead people; distressing; vivid; nightmare. Restless sleep; sleepiness in the evening; sleepless after midnight, waking too early.

Chill at night in bed; chill external and internal, worse from motion. Quartan, tertian shaking chill; periodicity marked; warm room does not ameliorate the chill. Fever afternoon and night; fever alternates with chill; fever and chill intermingle; dry, external heat; flushes of heat; chronic intermittent fever; internal heat with external coldness; fever with no sweat, and desire to uncover. Hectic fever. Perspiration morning and night; cold sweat; exhausting sweat; sweat on motion, or on slight exertion; profuse night sweats.

Anæsthesia of the skin; burning skin; the skin is jaundiced; liver spots and red spots. The skin is cold to touch; dryness of the skin with inability to perspire. Many eruptions on the skin; boils, pustules, rash and scales; moist eruptions, eczema, itching eruptions; herpes; psoriasis. It has cured ichthyosis. Dry, scaly, burning eruptions; urticaria. It cures all syphilitic eruptions where the symptoms agree, where eruptions have been .suppressed by local treatment. Excoriation; erysipelas; formication, indurations; itching, burning and stinging; rough skin; purpura hæmorrhagica. Dropsical, spongy swelling of skin; ulcers with bleeding or bloody discharges, with corrosive watery, yellow discharge. Cancerous ulceration. Indolent and indurated ulcers; sensitive and suppurating ulcers; ulcerative pain in ulcers; in old syphilitic ulcers.

ARSENICUM SULPHURETUM FLAVUM

This is one of our deepest remedies and is to be used against psora and syphilis, especially in old broken constitutions. The Encyclopedia and Guiding Symptoms furnish valuable fragmentary provings. This study is based also upon new provings and extensive clinical observations. It is a most useful medicine in old cases of malaria, in great weakness following the abuse of quinine. When eruptions have been suppressed from local treatment, and there is great weakness and lack of reaction.

The symptoms are worse in *morning,* forenoon, *afternoon, evening,* in twilight, NIGHT, *before midnight, after midnight.* It has a marked tendency to form abscesses. Aversion *to* open air. Aversion to open air alternating with a desire for open air. Extremely sensitive to a draft. Open air makes some symptoms better and some worse. ANÆMIA and PHYSICAL ANXIETY. Weakness and suffocation from going up stairs. Parts feel constricted as with a band. He takes cold from bathing and all symptoms are worse. It is a most useful remedy in combating the symptoms of epithelioma, lupus and scirrhus, even where ulceration is far advanced. The appearance of the face and skin is much like chlorosis. Choreic action of the muscles all over the body. In general the patient is cold, worse from cold air, from becoming cold, from cold, wet weather; takes cold easily. Convulsions, abdomen puffed up; offensive bilious diarrhœa, slimy vomiting. Discharges from all mucous membranes and outlets *very excoriating, offensive, thin and yellow.* Dropsy of the extremities and in abdomen. The symptoms are worse before and AFTER EATING. There is marked emaciation of the body. Slight exertion increases all conditions and symptoms. Faintness from many causes, but *especially after stool.* Worse from cold drinks, sour food, cold food, fat food, fruit and milk. Formication all over the body. The mucous membranes bleeding easily. The body feels heavy and loggy. Sometimes he is too warm and sometimes chilly. Inflamed parts and base of ulcers indurate. Inflammation of organs and glands. Lassitude and lack of reaction. He always desires to lie down. He feels worse lying, worse after lying awhile, worse lying on back, yet he feels better in bed. Symptoms all worse during menstruation. Motion in general ameliorates, yet motion aggravates some symptoms. The patient dreads motion. Old people much broken down, seem to rally under its action. Pains are cutting, BURNING, internal and external, PRESSING, *stitching,* tearing; tearing downward, tearing in muscles. *Thrusting pains.* Periodicity is very marked. Perspiration gives no relief. Complaints after suppressed sweat. Pulsations all over the body. The pulse is fast, irregular, intermittent, small, weak. Running or fast walking increases all symptoms. Extremely sensitive to pain. Shocks felt throughout the body; many symptoms worse on right side of the body. Complaints worse sitting. Symptoms before sleep, on going to sleep and during sleep. Standing aggravates. Stiffness in body and limbs. Dropsical swelling and swelling of glands. Affected parts sore to touch. Trembling of body and limbs. Twitching of muscles. Varicose veins. Many symptoms worse after sleep. Walking ameliorates, walking in open air aggravates; walking fast aggravates. Warmth of bed ameliorates. Extreme weakness, weakness in morning, during menses, after exertion, after eating. from perspiration, after stool, from walking in open air.

Absent-minded and he is greatly affected from anger. Aversion to answering questions and when he does answer his mind works slowly. ANXIETY, *morning,* EVENING, EVENING IN BED, *during the night.* Anxiety of conscience, with fear, during fever, about salvation, after a swoon, during stool, on waking. He is very critical with his friends and desires things which are not useful to him. Confusion of mind in the morning on waking. Over-conscientious about small matters. Longs for death. Delirious and raving during the night. His mind is full of delusions. A general feeling of despair. He is discontented and very excitable. His mind is full of *fear at night;* fear of a crowd, of *death,* of evil, of ghosts, of people, of *solitude.* Memory at first active, later he is forgetful *Easily frightened or startled,* starting on going to sleep and during sleep. It has been useful during fevers when he picks the bed clothing. Hurried feeling and always hasty in actions. Many hysterical symptoms. Impatience, indifference, indolence. He seems to be growing weak-minded. It has been used in insane conditions, in drunkards. *Extremely irritable* during chill; in the morning on waking. Loathing of life. Sometimes he is lamenting and again he is laughing. At times very talkative and again very malicious, almost maniacal like one intoxicated. It has been used in mania-a-potu. Mental work is impossible after eating. Great liveliness, then muttering. Extremely unreasonable and obstinate. Offended without cause and quarrelsome followed by insane fury. Religious affections remorse. Great mental fatigue. Restlessness evening, *night,* tossing in bed, during fever, during menses. Sadness evening, during heat, during sweat. Extremely sensitive and touchy, Inclined to take all matters seriously. Speech incoherent and wandering. Aversion to being spoken to, indisposed to converse on any subject. Suspicious of all his friends and his family. Periods of stupefication, vanishing of thought. Weeping at night. Weeping in sleep. Extremely timid, bashful, feeling of weakness in head.

Vertigo evening, as if dancing up and down. Inclined to fall to the right. Vertigo with headache. Looking downward, with nausea; walking in the open air.

Whenever the general symptoms given above strongly predominate in any given case, the following particulars will yield to this remedy.

The head is cold during headache, especially the forehead. A feeling of tightness of the forehead and marked hyperæmia of the brain, moist crusts and scales on the scalp. *It has been very useful in eczema.* Pulstules on the scalp. Inflamed patches much like erysipelas. Much heat in the head and especially in the forehead. Great weight in forehead morning and evening. Itching of the scalp. The head is painful in the morning on waking. Pain in the afternoon. Pain at 4 p.m. and 5 p.m. Pain in the head evening and *night.* Pain worse in cold air on coughing, after eating, from exercising, in bright light, moving head, riding in a carriage, in a warm room, shaking the head, after sleep, from stimulants, from stooping, from walking in the open air. Pain comes during chill, during menses, comes periodically, every two weeks. Pain is violent and pulsating. Violent pain deep in the brain, in frontal region and right ear. Pain in forehead worse in right side, better after sleep. Waking often with dull pain above the eyes extending to the top of the head. Pain in the occiput extending to sides of head 7 to 11 a.m. Pain in sides of head. Pain in vertex. Sore, bruised pain in whole head, in forehead. Burning in head. Drawing pain in forehead. Pressing pain in forehead, occiput and temples. Dull pain in right frontal region, which increases in severity and becomes a sharp, pulsating and shooting pain extending to occiput on the right side, worse from motion and stooping, 4 p.m. Stitching pain in the head, in temples, worse on coughing. Tearing pain in occiput. Cold sweat on the forehead; temples worse on coughing. Pulsation in the head. Shocks in the head.

Eyelids stuck together in the morning. Discharges from eyes acrid, bloody, yellow. Dryness of the eyes. Dullness. Eruptions about the eyes. Excoriation of the lids. Glassy look of the eyes. Gum in canthi. Granular lids. Chronic inflammation of eyes, of conjunctiva, cornea, iris, lids. The veins of eyes are injected. Lachrymation. Half open eyes. Opening lids difficult. Pain in eyes evening, on moving eyes, when reading, aching in the eyes. Burning in evening when reading. Burning in margin of lids. Pains are drawing, pressing, sore, bruised, stitching, tearing, paralysis of optic nerve. Photophobia in sunlight. The eyes feel as if protruding. Redness of lids, of veins, spots on the cornea; sunken eyes. Swollen lids. The tears are acrid. Twitching of the lids. Ulceration of the cornea. In the field of vision there are sparks, flickerings and dark colors. Objects look yellow. Foggy vision. Dim vision.

Discharges from ear fetid and offensive. Eruptions on and behind ears. Formication. Heat of ears. Sensation of fulness in ears. Itching of ears and in ears. Noises; buzzing, humming, ringing, soaring, rushing, snapping. Pain in ears in evening. Pain behind ears. Pain in ears; burning, drawing, pressing outward, stitching, tearing. Pulsation in ears. Ears feel stopped. Tingling of ears. Tensive feeling behind right ear on stroking the hair. Hearing impaired.

Cold nose. Fluent coryza. Nasal discharge bloody, burning, crusty, excoriating, greenish, offensive, thick, white, yellow. *Dryness in nose.* Bleeding from the nose. The nose is obstructed with thick mucus. Offensive odor from nose. Burning inside of nose, Smell at first acute, later wanting. *Frequent sneezing.* The nose is swollen. Ulceration high up in nose.

It has cured epithelioma of the lip. The face is chlorotic and cold. The lips are cracked. The face is bluish and there are dark circles under the eyes. Earthy, pale or sallow. Jaundiced face. Circumscribed red cheeks. Red spots. Redness of the face. Dryness of the lips. Eruptions, acne, pimples, pustules, rash scurf, vesicles. It cures eczema when the symptoms agree. The expression is *anxious, sickly,* suffering. Heat and itching of the face. Inflammation of the submaxillary gland. Pain worse in open air and better from warmth; comes on periodically. Pain in the submaxillary gland. Pains of face are BURNING, drawing, *tearing.* Cold sweat on face. The face looks sunken. Swelling of the face and *submaxillary gland.* Twitching of the face. Ulceration of the lips.

Copious aphthæ in mouth and on the tongue. Bleeding of the gums. Cracked tongue. The tongue is red or coated brown, white or yellow. Mouth and tongue very dry. Inflammation of the tongue. Much frothy mucus in the mouth. The mucous membrane of the mouth and tongue is inflamed and excoriated, offensive odor from the mouth. Burning mouth and tongue. Copious saliva. Scorbutic gums. Shining tongue. Speech difficult. Taste is bad; better in morning on waking; bloody, insipid, putrid, saltish, sour, sweetish, ulcers in the mouth and on the tongue. The mouth is full of vesicles.

Choking in the throat and constriction of the œsophagus. The right tonsil is enlarged. Dryness, redness and heat in the throat. Inflammation of throat and *tonsils.* Sensation of a lump in throat. Much mucus in throat. Pain in throat in evening on swallowing. Burning, rawness, soreness and stitching. Scraping in the throat, swallowing difficult. The throat is swollen. Ulceration of pharynx. It is a very useful remedy in stubborn syphilitic ulceration of throat with rapid destruction of tissue.

A feeling of anxiety in the stomach. Appetite ravenous, with easy satiety. Appetite wanting for the evening meal. Aversion to fats, to food, to rich food, to meat. Sensation of coldness in stomach. Constriction of stomach. Craves stimulants. Coffee, fruit, sour things, sweets, warm things, warm drinks. The stomach is disordered from milk. A sensation of emptiness. Eructations acrid, bitter, empty; of food, foul, SOUR. Gnawing in the stomach. Fulness in stomach after eating, especially after breakfast. Heartburn. Weight in stomach after eating. Hiccough after eating. Indigestion from all heavy food. Loathing of food. Nausea after cold water, after eating, during headache, during stool. Pain in stomach after eating. Burning, cramping, cutting, pressing and stitching pains. Burning after cold drinks, pressing after eating. Extreme tenderness of the stomach. Pulsation. Retching when coughing. Sensation of a stone in the stomach. Thirst morning, evening and *night.* Burning thirst. Thirst after chill. Extreme thirst during heat. Unquenchable thirst. Vomiting worse nights; on coughing, after drinking, after eating, during headache, after milk; vomiting bile, black substance, food, mucus; *sour,* watery substances.

A feeling of anxiety in the abdomen after stool. Bluish spots over the abdomen and thighs. Cold abdomen during chill. Distension after eating. Tympanitic abdomen. Dropsy of peritoneum. It has cured enlarged spleen. Eruptions on the abdomen. Flatulence, fulness and *gurgling. Fulness in the hypogastric region.* Itching of the skin. The abdomen feels heavy and the liver is hard. Pain in the abdomen at night. Pain as though diarrhœa would come on. Pain in abdomen after coughing; after eating, during menses, while walking; better by external warmth. Pain in the liver and in the hypogastrium. Burning in the bowels. Cramping before and after stool. Cramping and vomiting. Cutting pain before stool, worse walking, better by pressure. Great tenderness in the abdomen. Strong pulsations in abdomen. Rumbling in abdomen; worse before stool. It has cured painful and swollen spleen in old malarial cases. Sensation of tightness in the abdomen. Ulceration of the navel.

Constipation alternating with diarrhœa. Stools hard and knotty. Difficult. Diarrhœa in the morning after rising, daily at 8 a.m., afternoon, NIGHT, AFTER MIDNIGHT. Stools acrid, black, pure bile, bloody mucus, offensive, mushy and yellow, undigested, thin. Diarrhœa after drinking, after eating, after fruit, during menses. The diarrhœa is generally painful, but sometimes painless. Dysentery with bloody mucus, scanty stool. Excoriation of the anus and around it. The antis is fissured. Flatus copious and offensive. Hemorrhoids worse during the night, external, large; worse walking. Itching of the anus. Moisture that excoriates. Pain in rectum and anus DURING STOOL, and after stool, during straining to stool. During urination. *Burning during* and after stool. Cutting during stool. Soreness and stitching pains. Tenesmus with dysentery and after a yellow mushy stool. Paralysis and prolapsus of rectum.

Fulness of the bladder. Inflammation of the bladder. Pain in the bladder. Paralysis of bladder. Retention of urine. Urging to urinate worse at night, constant ineffectual, sudden, must hasten. or will lose the urine. Urination dribbling, painful, difficult, involuntary at night, unsatisfactory. Inflammation of kidneys; urine suppressed. Burning in urethra when passing urine. The urine is albuminous, bloody, burning, cloudy on standing, copious or scanty, offensive, with purulent sediment; thick; specific gravity is high. *Specific gravity low.* Gonorrhœa with terrible pains; discharge copious, yellow, constant burning day and night along the entire urethra with restlessness.

Stitching of glans penis and scrotum, perspiration of genitals, drawing pain in left spermatic cord. Seminal emissions. Ulcers on prepuce. Itching of the vulva. *Leucorrhœa; excoriating, bloody,* burning, *copious,* thick, *yellow* after menses. Menses copious; dark, too frequent, protracted, burning in the vulva.

Catarrh with viscid muscus. Itching in the larynx, causing coughing. Dryness in larynx, causing choking. Soreness, burning and rawness in larynx. Hoarseness. Voice lost.

Asthmatic breathing during the night. Dyspnœa evening and during the night. Dyspnœa worse ascending stairs, after eating, from least exertion, while lying. Respiration is rattling, short, singing, *suffocative,* wheezing.

Cough MORNING, afternoon, *evening in bed,* NIGHT, from cold air, open air, asthmatic, on becoming cold, after eating, *lying.* Dry cough from tickling in the larynx. Hacking cough; loose cough; racking, spasmodic cough; suffocative cough. Whooping cough. Expectoration; *bloody,* copious, frothy, offensive mucus; *purulent,* thick, viscid, *yellow.*

Anxiety of the chest. It has been of great service in cancerous ulceration of the breast. It is a most useful remedy in bronchial catarrh. The chest feels cold, sensation of tightness of the chest. Effusion in the pleura and pericardium. Eruptions of many kinds on the chest. Hemorrhage of the lungs. Inflammation of the lungs, pericardium and pleura. Oppression of the chest on ascending, when coughing, after eating, when walking. Pain in the chest when coughing, worse from motion and from breathing. Pain in the sides of chest and in regions of heart. Burning in chest. Cutting in chest, worse from motion; 5 a.m., between fifth and sixth ribs. Cutting *in heart;* worse from respiration. Pressing pain. Sore, bruised chest from coughing. Stitching in chest on coughing. Stitching in sternum and heart. *Violent palpitation;* worse during the night and from exertion. It is a most useful remedy in phthisis in all stages, when incurable it is a great palliative. Feeling of weakness in chest, with weak voice.

The back is constantly cold. Many eruptions on the back. Pain in back evening and night; during chill and fever; during menses. Pain in back of neck and *between the scapulæ.* Pain in lumbar region and sacrum. Pain in coccyx to anus, morning on rising. Aching in lumbar region. Burning, drawing and tearing in back. Drawing in lumbar region. Sore, bruised pain in lumbar region. Tenderness of coccyx. Perspiration of the back. Stiffness of cervical region. Weakness of lumbar region.

Cold hands, legs and *feet.* Cramps in *calf,* feet and sole. Blueness of fingers and nails *during chill.* Eruptions; boils; *pimples; pustules;* vesicles. Desquamation of limbs. Excoriation between the thighs and nates. Formication of limbs. Heat of feet. Heaviness of lower limbs; *of feet.* Itching of limbs worse after scratching; of lower limbs at 1 p.m., of thighs and toes. Jerking of lower limbs. Numbness of upper and lower limbs; of feet; of heel and outer side of foot. Pain in limbs evening; night; *after midnight;* during chill; rheumatic in cold weather; wandering; relieved by external warmth and warmth of bed; in wet weather. Pain in *joints, bones.* Pain in upper limbs, as though in the bones relieved by warmth; rheumatic worse towards morning; wandering, *lower limbs;* sciatica; right thigh; knee; leg. Pain in lower third of tibia relieved by motion. Burning hands and feet. Bruised pain in limbs. Stitching pains in limbs. Tearing pain in all limbs; upper limbs; shoulder; arm, elbow, forearm, fingers. Tearing in *thighs, legs* and *feet.* Paralysis of limbs; hemiplegia; painless; upper limbs; right for three days; lower limbs. Perspiration of hand cold; of *feet offensive and cold.* Restless limbs, legs, feet. Stiffness in knees. Stiffness in all the joints after recovering from the poison. Swelling dropsical and inflammatory; joints; upper limbs; hands; fingers; knees; legs; ankles; feet. Trembling of body and limbs, upper limbs and hands; lower limbs and feet. Twitching of thighs. Ulcers on legs. Weakness of all the limbs; of *joints;* upper limbs; *lower limbs;* knees; legs; ankles; feet.

Deep sleep, even comatose. Dreams; amorous; anxious; of death; of the dead; frightful; of misfortune; nightmare; vexatious; vivid. Falling asleep late. *Restless sleep.* SLEEPLESSNESS *afternoon* and *evening.* Sleeplessness before midnight; after midnight; after 3 a.m. If he wakens cannot get to sleep again. Unrefreshing sleep. Waking easily and frequently.

Morning on waking; FORENOON, noon, *afternoon,* evening in bed; *night,* midnight. Chill in open air; in cold air; walking in cold air. Chill alternating with sweat. Chill ascending the body; the back. Chilliness with sweat. Creeping chills in the evening. Chill after drinking cold water; after eating: worse from motion. External and internal coldness. Congestive chill. Chill followed by sweat. Quartan, quotidian and terian chill. SHAKING chill afternoon and evening. Trembling with the chill. Warm room does not relieve the coldness nor the chill, but is grateful. Specific times of chill; 1 a.m., 10 a.m., 1 p.m. 2

p.m., 4 p.m., 5 p.m., 6 p.m., 7 p.m., 8 p.m., 12 p.m.

Morning, afternoon and *evening* heat. Evening fever with chilliness. Fever *during night with* chilliness. Fever after midnight. Fever alternates with chill and with perspiration. Burning fever afternoon, evening and night. Fever without chill at night. Fever and chill intermingled. Continued fever worse during the night. Long lasting *dry heat.* External heat with chilliness. Flushes of heat. It has done excellent service in hectic fever. It should become one of the best remedies in intermittent fever. It has fever with sweat and without sweat. It is suitable in remittent fevers as its fevers are afternoon, evening and night and there is a remission in the morning and forenoon. During the fever he wants to be uncovered. It is a strong remedy in zymotic fevers.

It has morning sweat and again during the night. Sweat from the least excitement or anxiety; from the warmth of the bed; on coughing; while eating; from least exertion; on motion; *during sleep* and *after waking.* The sweat is cold, clammy, debilitating, offensive, sour. Profuse night sweat. Sweat of single parts. His symptoms are not relieved while sweating. *If he becomes cooled while perspiring he suffers much.*

Burning of the skin after scratching. Burning in spots. Marked coldness of skin of body and limbs. Discoloration of skin; blotches; blue spots; liver spots; pale, red spots; white spots; periodical dry burning skin. Eruptions; blisters; bloody after scratching; boils; burning; carbuncles; desquamating; *dry;* ECZEMA; fetid; herpes; itching; moist with corrosive yellow discharge; painful petechia; painful pimples; psoriasis; PUSTULES; rash; SCABBY after *scratching;* brain-like scales; stinging; *suppurating;* URTICARIA that is nodular and worse after scratching; vascular, worse after scratching, with yellow fluid. All eruptions *worse after scratching* and the itching without eruption is also *worse after scratching.* Inflammation of the skin like erysipelas. Excoriation of the skin. Formication, inactivity and marked *induration.* Itching, burning, crawling and stinging, worse after scratching. Moisture *after scratching.* Pain in the skin after scratching. Purpura hemorrhagica. The skin is very sensitive to touch. Sticking, stinging and swelling of skin in places and spots. Ulcers bleeding; *burning;* CANCEROUS; crusty; DEEP; indolent; inflamed; *painful, phagedenic; pulsating;* RED; STINGING; stinging margins; SUPPURATING. Ulcers discharging corrosive, offensive, thin, watery, yellow pus.

ARUM TRIPHYLLUM
(Indian Turnip)

Many boys have wandered in the low grounds where this wild turnip grows, and have taken a nip out of it, and probably remember the sensations in the mouth that they received at that time. I distinctly remember making an endeavor to enjoy a piece of wild turnip. The tingling that is left in the lips and tongue and from the throat to the end of the nose, and wherever sentient nerves come to the surface, is astonishing. The prickling and tingling is painful. It is a sensation that cannot be let alone. It requires a continued manipulation, and from this we gather the sensations that must be present in children when they are suffering from acute diseases and this remedy is indicated. For, in spite of the rawness and bleeding and smarting of the parts, they will insist on pinching and scratching and picking the lips and pressing around the mouth and boring into the nose. It has been a guiding feature in acute diseases, scarlet fever, many throat affections, diseases that take on a low type, such as continued fever and eruptive fevers. Among other complaints, sore throats, zymotic affections, delirium and excitement, even maniacal manifestations. It is manifested to a great extent in these associated symptoms. It must be that there is in the nose and lips painful tingling that the patient persists in boring the fingers into the nose. Manipulating and pinching the lips, picking the lips. It is altogether a different symptom that occurs in delirium of a low, muttering type, which we call carphologia, picking the bedclothes, picking all the time, picking and handling the clothing, a busy, low form of muttering, must be doing something all the time, groping around with the fingers and feeling for something. This is the carphologia and it is a mental symptom. While "pickng the lips" is given under the "mental" symptoms in the repertory, it is not intended to mean that it is a mental symptom like carphologia. Now, you will find two expressons in the repertory, and it is necessary to have two—the one is that "the nose itches," and the other is "he rubs the nose," he does something; that is what an individual would do if his nose itched. One's mind is not always directed towards the two —one is a direct and the other is an indirect expression.

This remedy has not been sufficiently proved to bring out the nature of its chronic manifestations. It has undoubtedly something of that kind, but it has been used in a limited way among acute affections of a zymotic character. It has not been used to any great extent for chronic sick headaches, but it has cured some headaches that are worse in the heat, worse in a warm room and from warm clothing, worse from becoming warm, worse from wrapping up the body. Heat in the head, determination of blood to the head. It has also cured eruptions upon the scalp like eczema. It has also been found useful in catarrhal affections of the nose, eyes and lids. About the nose its affections have been mostly of the acute kind. It has most dreadful coryza. The nose is stopped up, and more stopped up on the left side. Must breathe through the mouth. Sneezing worse during the night; fluent acrid coryza. The discharge of saliva flowing over the lips produces rawness, smarting and burning of the mucous membranes, and the lips bleed. The fluid from the nose as it flows over the skin leaves red streaks.

"Acrid ichorous discharge excoriating the inside of the nose, the alæ and upper lip." That is expressive and occurs in diphtheria, in various forms of sore throat, in scarlet fever, when this remedy is indicated.

Inflammation of the tongue, with acrid discharge from the nose. Inflammation of the root of the tongue, of the throat and soft palate, of the tonsils. The glands of the neck are swollen. This inflammatory condition is followed by paralytic weakness, making it impossible for him to swallow liquids or food, and when the mouth forces food into the pharynx the œsophagus refuses to operate, and then fluids and liquids are forced up into the nose and run out of the nose. This has been clinically observed many times in diphtheria and sore throats. The sneezing is like an ordinary coryza, with repeated chills over the body, and aching in the bones as if the bones would break, like *Nux, Eupator., Arn., Rhus, Bry.* and *Ars.,* that have aching all over during "cold". This is one of the most striking medicines as an illustration of the keynote system, that is, with those who prescribe on one symptom and give this medicine whenever the patient bores his nose or picks his lips, notwithstanding that *Cina* bores the nose and picks the lips. *Cina* has more of the congestive and nerve symptoms. The nostrils are really so sore from the acridity of the fluids inside of the nose that it feels as if the nostrils were filled with fire. This is the language of the patients who narrate their symptoms in an Arum triphyllum case. They come into the office with a sore, raw nose, and it tingles and tickles and he cannot let it alone. Fluids run down over the lip and excoriate. The glands of the neck are often enlarged. When he takes cold in the nose there is soreness of the neck and parotid gland. Desire to bore into the nose. This boring into *the side* of the nose is another symptom and differs from the one "boring the nose". You will see children boring in the nose, inside of nose. It is an inflammation of the nasal duct, the duct that leads from the eye to the nose, and accompanied by a discharge of tears over the cheeks, with the tickling that extends up there which they cannot reach, but they undertake to reach it. Can hardly talk on account of phlegm in the back part of the nose. He talks through the nose. The nose is filled with mucus and there is great tumefaction of all the mucous membranes, which gives him a nasal tone. "Swollen, bloated face." If you observe the nose and face you will be surprised to see that so much of the trouble is on the *left* side of the face, left nostril, left lachrymal duct, etc. There is bleeding of the lips, upper and lower. The under lip especially is denuded and drops of blood stand upon it, and the patient is constantly picking and pinching the lips, and when you request of the little one to stop it or take his hands away he yells with a sort of sepulchral yell. "Children will often pick and bore into raw surfaces, though it gives them pain and they scream with it, but they keep on boring." That is a striking symptom. Fluids make the lips raw and then this tickling comes on and he cannot let it alone, he must keep at it. "Appearance of raw bleeding surfaces on the lips, buccal cavity, nose, etc." Great itching tingling describes it. In typhoid, where you would hardly expect much swelling of the parotid. these glands are enlarged. In diphtheria, scarlet fever and sore throat enlargement of the salivary glands. This inflammatory condition with soreness and swelling of these glands; the glands are hard and tender to the touch. The tongue is red, the papillæ elevated; the tongue appears to be almost denuded. It is raw and bleeding, sometimes does bleed in a few places, and sometimes, after this has gone on for a few days, when the tongue is projected it looks like a big red straw berry, and for that reason has been called "Strawberry tongue". "Tongue cracked, bleeding, burning, painful; smarting on tongue and fauces." Putrid odor from the mouth. Mouth foul, so sore that he was unwilling to drink. All this points to tingling and raw condition of the buccal cavity far back into the throat. If you look into the buccal cavity you will see the parts raw, denuded and bleeding. Excessive flow of saliva, which is acrid. Mouth burns and is sore. Cries when anything is offered. Buccal cavity covered with diphtheritic ulcers, also with aphthous patches, which cover the whole mouth and tongue. It says "stinging," but it is a painful tingling, stinging like the sting of a bee, stinging pains in the throat, and the parts are ulcerated, raw and bleed.

It has a diarrhœa, such as occurs in idiopathic typhoid. If you have ever seen the yellow corn-meal mush when it is dropped on a plate, it has the appearance of the typhoid yellow stools. When this medicine is suitable diarrhœa is yellow like corn-meal; freuent, fæcal, thin, mushy, yellow, is the description of this typhoid stool. There are other times that the stool is dark brown, watery, thin. As is usual, the fæces are acrid. The thin fæces escape from the anus and keep the parts raw and burning. With other complaints, in typhoid especially, in the groin where the thigh bends upon the abdomen an excoriation takes place with acrid moisture. Again, we notice rawness over the coccyx. A moisture and rawness from acrid fluid in the posterior part of the fissure back of the anus so that over the coccyx and back of the anus there is rawness and acrid moisture.

The voice comes in for an extensive part of the trouble. It has been found especially to relate to singers and public speakers. At times when a lawyer has had a long case and he is making a final effort, and has been speaking three or four hours, and while in a sweat has got into a draft or gone out, he finds himself hoarse and cannot finish his speech, a dose of Arum triph. will enable him to go on with his speech in a clear voice. It clears up the hoarseness. In public speakers and singers who have been compelled to strain the voice and have taken a little cold and the voice is hoarse after prolonged exercise; this is the most striking feature of the Arum triph. voice. "Voice hoarse; from over-exertion of the voice in speaking or singing." "Voice uncertain, uncontrollable, changing continually, now deep, now hoarse, etc."

It manifests itself in this way. A person starts in a certain pitch and he cannot talk to you, but he tries another pitch and can talk. It is a queer thing that on certain notes they are voiceless, which shows that there is an irregular and patchy inflammation of the vocal cords; it is not a uniform inflammation or the voice would be uniformly affected. "Clergyman's sore throat," is not a good expression, because it is clergyman's hoarseness that is meant; hoarseness and rawness of the throat of public speakers when talking. Of course you would say any voice that is hoarse is aggravated when talking, but it is not always so. The *Rhus* hoarseness carries with it its characteristic relief from motion, and the use of the voice is motion of the larynx.

When the *Rhus patient* commences to use the voice he finds that he is hoarse, but after using the voice a little it loosens up, becomes freer, or, in other words, it is better from ,motion. This may be so either in acute or chronic hoarseness. Now, in this remedy as in *Phosphrous,* the voice is ameliorated from clearing the vocal cords of a little mucus. It is not so in *Rhus tox.,* for it is a weakness and paralysis from cold. It is well known under *Rhus tox.* that the tendons and muscles that are rheumatic become weak, they are stiff on beginning to move and are ameliorated when they are warmed up; so it is with the voice.

Now, in the chest there is burning and rawness when coughing; this extends to the pit of the stomach. "Raw feeling in chest." "Lungs feel sore." "Soreness in l. lung." You will notice that many times patients and provers state sufferings are in the lungs, which may not really be the region affected. Most likely from what is known of other symptoms this burning is in the trachea, although it says in the lungs. This remedy does have burning in the trachea, the whole length of it, during an attack of coughing, and burning in the larger branches of the bronchial tubes. The catarrhal state is largely confined to these parts, the trachea and bronchi, but this medicine has cured pneumonia. It has been found useful as a palliative in phthisis. It is used in crude form among the farmers as a domestic medicine for coughs and colds and as a palliative in consumption. In many of the farm houses you will find the wild turnip hung up in strings like beads to be dried and grated and used with sugar and cream.

I mentioned the fact that it seems to favor the left side of the head, the left nostril, the left side of the face. It also prefers the left chest and the left lung. It has soreness in the left side of the chest and left arm. It has a sensation of fulness in the thorax and soreness extending down and involving the left lung.

Here is a clinical picture of fever: "Typhoid forms of fever; picking ends of fingers and dry lips till they bleed, etc."

In most of these complaints the urine is very scanty and is sometimes suppressed. You will very commonly note a good action of this medicine in these complaints by its immediately starting up a copious flow of urine. It is a sign of relief.

It has upon the skin all the scarlet rash that you would expect to find in scarlet fever, and it has also the typoid petechiæ.

ASAFŒTIDA

This remedy in olden times was frequently abused for man and beast. Our grandfathers supposed it was a protection against disease, and hence they used it in the stables. Lumps of "fœty," as they called it, were put in the corn for the horse, to keep off distemper. What it has accomplished I am unable to say, but it is certain that these farmers looked upon Asafœtida as a great protective against disease. It has been used also by the laity as a medicine for fainting, for hysteria, and all sorts of nervous symptoms and complaints. The use is justified by the proving. These things are scarcely worthy of note, but it shows the general use among the people, as a domestic medicine, in crude form. It has been used more extensively in this form than in professional practice in a legitimate way.

There is one class of patients you will find who will trouble you. Those cases that come into your office with puffed, venous, purple faces; they have an appearance of plethora; the face looks puffed, bloated and dropsical at times; it is a dark red, dusky face; such a face we shall cure sometimes with Asafœtida. *Carbo an., Aurum, Carbo veg.* and *Pulsatilla* are also related to this kind of face, but it is a very troublesome face, it shows more or less cardiac disturbance and venous stasis. The venous side of the heart will often be involved, or be about to be involved, when you have this kind of face. I never like to see them come into my office, for they are hard cases to manage. They have deep-seated troubles, with bleeding, they are subject to sudden inflammations, and they do not rally quickly. In this constitution we have ulcerations; a little place will ulcerate and suppurate, and the ulceration will burrow; this is just what this remedy does. Another thing this kind of constitution will do is to set up an inflammatory condition of the periosteum with swelling, periostitis of the tibia for instance, where the circulation is not very active; inflammation of cartilages with tumefaction and purple skin, stitching pains and dropsy, ulcerations and fistulous openings. This medicine is good for just such states. "Ulcers with extreme sensitiveness."

Patients often say, "I get no sympathy when I am sick because I look so well;" fat, flabby and purple. This remedy will seldom be thought of in lean persons; they seem to be free from complaints like those of Asafœtida, but in fat, flabby persons, extremely nervous, extremely sensitive to pain, full of hysteria. Purple when out in the cold, purple when excited. In other words, you see before you the venous constitution, and these people get the worst kind of hysteria; they go off almost from no cause into fainting; from a close room, from excitement, from any disturbance; sometimes cramps come on, but more especially fainting. They are subject to stitching pains from the bone to the surface; that is, from within out. The periosteum becomes irritated, and glands become swollen. Syphilis sometimes produces this kind of condition. Vascular disturbances in the body; periostitis, necrosis, induration of glands, nerve syphilis and head pains. In old syphilitics with this kind of venous face, subject to bleeding, ulcers turn black or become purple. In this there is a similarity to *Lachesis*. Old scars turn purple, threaten to suppurate, take on a venous aspect, become painful and turn black. Ulcers form at the site of old scars in old syphilitic patients and sometimes in psoric patients. Most complaints come on during rest and are better by slow motion.

There is another grand feature running through this remedy; it is full of discharges, catarrhal discharges, discharges from ulcers, watery discharges from different places, and even watery stool; and all these discharges are horribly offensive and ichorous. Deep, flat ulcers from bone and periosteal affections give out a watery, bloody discharge that is horribly offensive, with pains shooting outwards. Get the idea of the venous stasis well fixed in your mind and with this syphilitic state added to it.

There are many pains running through the remedy and they are night pains like those of syphilis, nightly bone pains, and pains in the periosteum. The ulcers are deep, with bluish edges. Varicose veins surround the ulcers. Inflammation of the bone and periosteum, with blueness all around the ulcers. When there has been an inflammatory condition of the periosteum, somewhat passive in character, the skin adheres to the bone, glues down to it by adhesion. It is too feeble to ulcerate, it does not get up a likely inflammation, but only a passive state. The glands all over the body are hot and throbbing, with shooting, jerking pains, in syphilis or old psoric and scrofulous complaints.

The bone pains that are felt in the head are sometimes very distressing. Old syphilitic bone pains in the head, stitching, penetrating. It seems where there are lumps and nodules, about the head, this medicine seems to hurry things. Shooting, stitching, tearing pains under left frontal eminence. This stitching pain is sometimes described as if a nail or plug were driven into the head. These nervous headaches are syphilitic, hysterical or scrofulous; hysterical pains described as rending, tearing, stitching. All over the head there is stitching pain, but in the frontal eminence, in the temples, there is a sensation as if a nail or plug were driven in, and most of the pains seem to bore, as if they extended from the bone to the surface, and hence are said to be from within out.

It is useful in old syphilitics who are subject to eye complaints, ulcers on the eyeball, ulcers on the cornea, ameliorated in the open air, with a sensation of numbness in the eyes; inflammation of the iris, with ragged appearance of the iris; they are subject also to severe, sharp stitching pains that come from within out. The remedy is full of burning, and so the eyeballs burn, better in the open air. Iritis, but the inflammation sometimes involves the choroid, the retina, and mucous membrane, making a general inflammatory condition of syphilitic character. There are tearing pains in various places around the eyes; stitching, stitching pains, worse at night. Ulcers, with stitching pains, worse at night. Burning, stitching in the eyes with dryness, so that the lids stick to the balls of the eyes, pain worse at night.. There is a misty appearance before the eyes, dullness as if looking through a fog. It also seems as if the atmosphere were filled with little floating black flies. "Muscæ voliantes". You have looked into the air and seen little gnats and mosquitoes; well it appears to these patients as if these were there when they are not there. The discharge from the eyes is ichorous, bloody and often offensive.

This same syphilitic miasm may attack the ear and the bones of the ear. These bones may decay and the hearing be lost. "Burning in the ear with discharge of fœtid pus." Stitching pains in the *ears from within out.*

A horribly offensive discharge comes from the nose; ulcers high up in the nose; caries of the bones of the nose; syphilitic ozæna. Putrid old catarrhs. "Feeling as if the nose stopped high up, as if he could not breathe through it, with fulness of the head, when riding in a carriage." (*Aurum, Aurum mur.*)

Numbness is a great feature of this remedy, numbness of the scalp, or deep in the head; numbness here and there; numb, dead feeling associated with the pain; numbness after pain; often numbness after sleep. Other nervous manifestations occur besides those that are hysterical. It has choreic motions. You would expect such a peculiar nervous constitution to have almost everything among its nervous symptoms. "Constantly chewing and working frothy slime out of mouth, with swollen tongue." "Speech unintelligible." "Grinding of teeth; starting at night." Swelling of the lips, and of the whole buccal mucous membrane, especially the lower lip, with burning in the mouth.

There are syphilitic symptoms in the throat, attended with the usual burning, darting, stitching in ulcers; pain when swallowing; a sensation of a ball rising in the throat, such as occurs in globus hystericus; choking, must constantly swallow. Hysterical and choreic affections of the œsophagus and trachea. Spasms of the œsophagus. This lump in the throat, or suffocation, is a sort of hysterical spasm of the œsophagus. "Dryness and burning in the œsophagus."

In the stomach troubles, if you have ever seen a typical case of Asafœtida, you will wonder where all the air comes from; it comes up in volumes. "Hiccough-like contractions of the diaphragm." Choreic jerkings of the diaphragm, with expulsion of wind like the sound of a pop-gun going off almost every second. It is a condition that the patient has no control over. It is like the shooting off of little guns forcing loud belching, loud eructations of wind from the stomach. There are a few symptoms mentioned in the text just here that are worthy of note. "Pulsation in pit of stomach; perceptible to sight and touch." "Pressing, cutting, stitching pains." A queer observation has been made that flatus was not passed downward, but all upwards. "Eructations; smelling like garlic; tasting rancid, sharp or putrid." Always horribly offensive. Offensiveness is a characteristic of the remedy. And then there is a "gone empty feeling in the pit of the stomach," not a pain. "Pulsations after eating." "Meteorism of the stomach." The remedy has many gastric and abdominal complaints; full of bellyache; stitching pains, colic. The diarrhœa is more or less troublesome. These patients are afflicted with diarrhœa from the slightest indigestion, after any indiscretion in diet, a painful, watery diarrhœa. "Liquid stools of most disgusting smell." "Blackish-brown papescent offensive stools, which relieve."

"Bearing down in genitals, worse when riding in a carriage." "Uterine ulcer sensitive and painful." This medicine has been very useful in palliating uterine cancer in such constitutions as described; those with purple faces, never the very pallid ones. Women of feeble, flabby, venous constitutions are subject to hæmorrhages and miscarriages. Women who are not pregnant sometimes have the breasts fill up with milk, a wonderfully annoying thing, and but few remedies have it; this is one of the few. It has also deficiency of milk. "Then days after delivery milk diminished."

These patients sometimes get hysterical asthma; all sorts of disturbance in breathing, dyspnœa. "Asthmatic feeling in trachea." "Asthmatic attacks at least once a day all her life, brought on by every bodily exertion, coition, especially by every satisfying meal." Attacks of dyspnœa after coition, like *Ambra.* "Obstinate titillating cough < at night." Many of these complaints are worse at night; nightly aggravations. Syphilitic complaints are commonly worse at night and such antisyphilitic remedies as *Mercurius, Staphisagria, Hepar, Nitric acid,* etc., are all worse at night. Among the other chest complaints, I will read a few of those that are marked here prominently and are striking ones. "Pressure and burning of the sternum." "Compression of chest as from a heavy weight." "Stitches in chest." "Single, violent stitches from within outward, at short intervals."

This remedy is full of rheumatism and gouty symptoms; gouty affections in general, in nervous constitutions. When such a nervous constitution finally produces gouty formations, the nervousness often disappears; for it has been relieved by the deposit in the joints; a transformation scene has taken place.

AURUM ARSENICUM

The symptoms of this remedy present themselves in morning, in forenoon, evening, during the night, after midnight. The symptoms are worse in the open air, worse in cold air. He desires open air. Worse on ascending. Asleep-feeling in single parts. A sensation of a band around parts. It is a most useful remedy in cancerous affections; in epithelioma; in caries of bone; worse, in cold, wet weather. It is a useful remedy in many kinds of convulsions; clonic spasms with consciousness; epileptiform; hysterical. Dropsy of the extremities and of cavities. The symptoms are worse during and after eating. The body emaciates, complaints come on after slight exertion and after cold drinks. Formication all over the body. The body and limbs feel heavy. Induration is a common feature; in glands; cancerous induration. Inflammation and congestion in many parts; in mucous membranes; bones; glands; periosteum; serous membranes. Marked physical irritability. Desire to lie down, but lying brings on great restlessness and many symptoms are worse lying. Worse after lying awhile. Lying in warm bed ameliorates many symptoms. Motion aggravates in general. He is restless and desires to move. The mucous membranes are much affected. Numbness of many parts; in suffering parts. Orgasms of blood. There are pains of all kinds in all parts of the body; pains in bones and glands; boring; bruised; burning; cutting; pressing in internal parts; stitching; tearing. Painless paralysis. It is useful in broken down as well as in plethoric people. Strong internal pulsation. The pulse is fast, irregular, small, weak. Any exertion or hurry like running is impossible. General sensitiveness; sensitive to pain. The symptoms resemble persons much debilitated by sexual excesses and vices. The symptoms are predominantly right-sided. Symptoms come on going to sleep and during sleep. He is better in summer and worse in winter. The glands are swollen. It is one of our most useful remedies in advanced stages of syphilis; in nervous syphilis. General aggravation from touch. Trembling in all parts. Ulceration of glands with marked induration; in cancerous conditions. Symptoms appear after sleep; worse from uncovering the body; while walking. Worse walking in open air; walking fast; walking in the wind. Marked general weakness; in the morning; from mental exertion; from physical exertion; weariness. Worse in windy weather and in winter.

Absent-minded. Easily angered and complaints from anger; anger with silent grief; from contradiction. He suffers from anguish. Anxiety day and night; of conscience; with fear; about salvation. Inclined to criticise and find fault with everybody. Confusion of mind in the morning. Over-conscientious. Contrary. Desires death. Delirious at night. Delusions; about animals; thinks he has done wrong; illusions of fancy. Despair; during chill; with pain;

periodical; of recovery, religious. Excitable and discontented. Excitement during chill. Symptoms are worse from mental exertion. Exaltation of fancy. Fear; evening and night; in a crowd; of death; of evil; of people, when alone. Forgetful and easily frightened. He suffers from grief and lasting complaints come on after grief. Always excited and in a hurry. Hysterical disposition and conduct; disorderly methods and perverted desires. Neglects the household and children. It is a many-sided remedy. Ideas abundant, clear minded. Imbecility, impatience, idolent, even marked aversion to work or industrious and loves activity. Insanity of fanatics; of drunkards; religious. Irresolution. Extreme irritability; alternating with cheerfulness; during chill; when spoken to. Lamenting, loquacity and laughter. Loathing of life. Malicious. Mania. Memory active; weak. Obstinate and easily offended. Mental prostration. Quarrelsome. Remorse. Reproaches himself for having done wrong. Reproaches others for imaginary injury. Insane reserve. Restlessness, night; anxious. Sadness in the evening; from suppressed menses; during perspiration. Oversensitive; to noise; to voices. Mental symptoms from sexual excesses and from secret vice. Shrieking; prolonged periods of silence. Wandering speech. Aversion to being spoken to. Suicidal disposition, during perspiration; wants to jump out of window. Indisposed to talk. The symptoms are worse when he thinks of them. Timid. One moment he is tranquil, the next he is violent. Weary of life. Weeping; during chill, in hysteria, in sleep. Vertigo during headache; while walking in open air.

Hyperæmia, fulness and heat of head from mental exertion. Eruptions on the scalp; crusts; pimples. The hair falls out. Heaviness in the head in the morning on rising. Hydrocephalus. Itching of the scalp. Pain in the head; morning; afternoon; evening; in cold air; in cold weather; rheumatic; from binding up the hair; on coughing; hammering; hysterical; lying; from mental exertion; from motion; nervous; periodical; pulsating; on rising from lying; after sleep; in windy weather; heat ameliorates. Pain in forehead. Pain in one side, either side or in both sides. Pain in temples; in temple and forehead; Bruised pain in head. Burning pain in head;. in forehead. in vertex. Drawing pain in head. Pressing pain in head; in forehead; in occiput; in temples. Stitching pain in head. Tearing pain in head; in forehead; in occiput. Pulsation in head; in forehead; on sides of head. Uncovering head brings on complaints.

Discharge of mucus and pus from eyes and the lids are stuck together in the morning with yellow pus. Granular lids. The lashes fall out. The eyes feel hot. Inflammation of eyes; catarrhal; scrofulous; of the cornea; of the iris; from syphilis. Lachrymation. Unable to open the eyes. Pain in the eyes; morning; night; from light; when reading; warmth ameliorates; aching; burning; pressing; core; as from sand; stitching; tearing. Paralysis of the optic nerve. Photophobia. Protrusion. Pulsation. Pupils contracted. Redness of the eyes; of lids; staring. A stye near the inner canthus. Swollen lids. Ulceration of the cornea. Vision blurred; bright colors before the eyes; dim; foggy; hemiopia, upper half lost; sparks; vision lost.

Mastoid caries. Discharge from the ear; fetid; offensive; purulent; thick; yellow. Sensation of flapping in ears. Itching in ears. Noises in ears; buzzing; crackling; humming; ringing; roaring; rushing. Pain in ear; behind ear; inside ear; burning, stitching. Hearing acute at first; for noise; later impaired; finally lost.

Caries of the bones of nose in old cases of syphilis. It is a most useful remedy in old stubborn catarrhs. The nose is red. He has frequent attacks of coryza, fluent or dry. Discharge from nose; bloody; crusts; offensive; fetid; greenish; purulent; suppressed; thick; watery; yellow. The nose is obstructed and there is itching and bleeding. It is a useful remedy in ozæna. Pain in the nose; in the bones; boring; burning; sore inside; ulcerative pain. Smell at first acute, later lost. Frequent sneezing. The nose is swollen. Ulceration in nose.

Epithelioma of face and lips. Lupus. Cracked lips; discoloration; bluish; bluish like; earthy; pale; red spots; eruptions: nose; acne rosacea face and forehead; comedones; coppery eruptions; pimples on face and forehead; pustules; scurfy eruptions. Suffering expression. Erysipelas. The face is hot. Inflammation of the parotid gland. Pain in face; in parotid gland; in submaxillary gland; burning lips; drawing pain in face; stitching; tearing. Perspiration of face; cold. Swelling of the face; lips; parotid; sub-maxillary ulcer on lip.

Apthæ in the mouth. The gums bleed easily. Cracked tongue. Brown tongue, red tongue, dry tongue. Heat in the tongue, mucus in the mouth. Odor from the mouth offensive; putrid. Burning tongue, soreness of gums. Speech difficult. Swollen gums; tongue. Taste: bitter; insipid; metallic; putrid; sour; sweetish; wanting. Ulcers in mouth syphilis; on gum; tongue; vesicles in mouth. Caries, sensation of elongation and loosening of teeth. Grinding of teeth in the night. Pain in teeth; night; when masticating; on touch; tearing.

Inflammation in throat. Lump in throat, mucus in throat. Pain in throat on swallowing; burning; stitching; scraping and swelling. Swallowing difficult.

Appetite is ravenous. Aversion to food; to meat; desires alcoholic stimulants; bread; coffee; cold drinks; milk; distension, emptiness and bitter eructations. Nausea with headache. Hiccough. Pain in stomach; violent; burning; cutting; pressing; stitching. Extreme thirst. Vomiting bile.

Atrophy of the liver. Suppurating bubo in groin. Distension of abdomen. Enlarged liver. Fulness and great flatulence. Hardening of the liver. It has cured numerous liver conditions and complaints. Itching of the skin of the abdomen. Pain in abdomen; night; colic; on coughing; after eating; during menses; warmth ameliorates; in right hypochondrium; in inguinal region; cramping; cutting in right hypochondrium; soreness in abdomen; in hypogastrium. Stitching pain in hypochondria; in hypogastrium. Rumbling in abdomen. Swelling of mensenteric glands; inguinal glands.

Constipation; alternating with diarrhœa. Diarrhœa in morning; night. Offensive flatus. Bleeding from anus. External piles. Moisture at the anus. Pain in the anus; during stool. Burning pain in anus with diarrhœa; during and after stool. Soreness and stitching pains. Urging in the rectum and prolapsus ani. Stool: copious; green; green mucus; hard; knotty; large; offensive; thin.

Retention of urine. Urging constant; ineffectual. Urination dribbling; dysuria; involuntary at night; seldom; unsatisfactory. Suppression of urine. Inflammation is urethra with burning. Urine albuminous; bloody; burning; cloudy on standing; red; copious; offensive; scanty; mucus sediment; sand; thick; watery. Inflammation of glans penis; testes; sore pain in testes. Perspiration of genitals. Swollen testes; Ulcers on the penis; chancres.

It is a very useful remedy in cancer of the uterus. The desire is increased. Eruptions on the vulva. Inflammation of ovaries and uterus. Itching of the vulva. Leucorrhœa; acrid; copious; thick; white; yellow. Menses absent; copious; too frequent; scanty; suppressed. Pain in ovaries and uterus. Burning in the vulva. Prolapsus of uterus.

Mucus in larynx and trachea. Hoarseness. Respiration is rapid. Asthmatic at night; difficult at night, on ascending, while lying and while walking; irregular; short; suffocative.

Cough: morning; night; in cold air; dry at night; short; spasmodic at night. Expectoration: morning; evening; bloody; mucus; offensive; purulent; tasting sweetish; tough; yellow.

It is a most useful remedy in heart affections. Angina Pectoris. Anxiety in chest; in the heart. Constriction of chest; of heart. Fluttering of heart. Heat in chest. Oppression of chest, from rapid motion; when lying; while walking; of the heart. Pain in chest; on coughing; on inspiration; in sides of chest on inspiration; in heart; burning in chest; pressing in chest; in sternum; in heart. Stitching pains in chest on inspiring; in sides; in sternum in heart. Palpitation: at night; anxious; on least exertion; during menses; on motion; tumultuous; on walking; trembling of the heart, weak heart.

Coldness in the back. Pain in the back on inspiration; in lumbar region; sacrum; spine; pressing pain in lumbar region; sore in lumbar region; stitching in lumbar region. Weakness in lumbar region.

Chilblains on the feet and toes. Cold hands; icy cold; legs, feet, during headache. Blueness of nails. Heaviness of upper limbs; of feet. Itching of limbs; palms; lower limbs; feet. Numbness of limbs; during rest; upper limbs;

lower limbs. Pain in limbs; at night; during chill; in joints; gouty, rheumatic, wandering; in upper limbs; shoulders, rheumatic; forearm; knees; heel; aching in legs; burning in toes. Drawing pains in limbs; upper arms; knees; feet. Gnawing pain in legs. Stitching pain in limbs; in shoulders; in wrist; knee; foot. Tearing pain in limbs; joints; upper limbs; upper arms; elbow; wrist; fingers; thigh; soles. Painless paralysis of limbs. Sensation of paralysis in fingers. Restlessness of limbs; of lower limbs. Stiffness of the joints, of lower limbs; of knees. Swelling of the joints; dropsical swelling of limbs, forearm and hand, lower limbs, legs and feet. Ulceration of nails. Weakness of joints; of upper limbs; lower limbs; knees.

Deep or comatose sleep. Dreams amorous; anxious; of dead people; of death; frightful; vivid; restless sleep; sleepiness in afternoon. Sleeplessness before midnight; after midnight, after waking. Unrefreshed after sleep. Waking too early; waking frequently.

Coldness in evening. At night in bed. Chilliness when undressing. Shaking chill. Fever at night. Burning hot in blood-vessels; intense heat; aversion to uncovering. Perspiration in morning; in night; profuse; aversion to uncovering.

Burning skin. At times marked coldness of skin. Discoloration; blue; liver spots; spots yellow. Eruptions: blisters; boils; burning eczema; herpes; painful, pimples; psoriasis; red; scabby; scaly; bran-like; smarting; syphilitic; urticaria; vesicular; erysipelas. Formication, itching sensitive; sore feeling in skin. Dropsical swelling of skin. Tension in skin. Ulcers; bluish, burning; cancerous; deep; discharging. Green, ichorous, offensive, yellow pus; fistulous; foul; indurated; painful; sensitive; suppurating; syphilitic. Warts that are syphilitic.

AURUM IODATUM

The symptoms are prominent in morning, afternoon, evening and night. *Strong desire for open air and feels better in open air.* Asleep feeling in single parts. A sensation of a band around parts. It is very useful in cancerous affections and in caries of bones. The patient feels better when cool and worse when in warm air. Congestion of blood to glands and organs. Dropsy in cavities and limbs. Exertion increases all complaints. Induration is characteristic and especially in glands. Inflammation of organs; bones; glands; serous membranes.. *Lying aggravates,* especially lying in a warm bed. Motion increases the suffering. Numbness in many parts, especially of painful parts. *Orgasm of blood.* Pain in bones; in glands; bruised feeling internally; internal burning; pressing internally and externally; stitching pains, tearing pains, internal pulsation. Pulse is fast. It is one of our great heart remedies. Running brings on many symptoms. The symptoms are strong and *right-sided.* Sitting increases the suffering. Swollen, painful glands. It is a most useful remedy in syphilis. Trembling. Walking fast aggravates. Slow walking ameliorates. Warmth in general aggravates; warm air; becoming warm in open air; warm bed; warm room; warm wraps. Weakness in morning.

Anxiety day and night. Spells of unusual cheerfulness. Aversion to company. Want of self-confidence. Confusion of mind in the morning. Over-conscientious about small matters. Despair of her salvation and of recovery. *Excitement. Worse from exertion of mind.* Fear of evil and of people. Feels hurried and seems hysterical. Fretful and impatient. Dread of all work. Indolence. Insanity with enlarged heart, orgasm of blood, red face, full veins, bloated appearance. Irresolution. irritability and mania. Mirthful without cause. Moods alternate and changeable, Mental prostration. Extreme sadness; restlessness, sensitive to noise. Timid, weeping and dizziness.

Heat, heaviness and rush of blood to head. Itching of scalp. Pain in the head in the morning; better in cold air and by cold applications; in forehead on left side; one-sided. Pressing pain in head; in forehead; occiput; temples; vertex. Stitching pains in head. Tearing in head; in temples. Pulsation in forehead.

Inflammation: conjunctiva; catarrhal; scrofulous; syphilis; iritis. Lachrymation. Pain in eyes, pressing, stitching. Protrusion of eyes. Redness of eyes and swollen. Bright colours before the eyes. Dim vision, diplopia; foggy vision; sparks.

Purulent fetid discharge from ears. Noises in ears; buzzing; humming; ringing; roaring. Stitching pain in ears. Hearing acute for noise. Impaired.

Post-nasal catarrh. The nose is red. Fluent or dry coryza. Discharge from nose; bloody; greenish; hard chunks; *offensive;* PURULENT; *thick; yellow.* Dryness in nose. Epistaxis. *Obstruction in the nose.* Pain in the nose, boring pain. Smell lost. Much sneezing. The nose is swollen. ULCERATION in NOSE.

The face is pale. Sometimes red. Eruptions on face and nose; pimples. Pain in the face. Pain in submaxillary glands; in lymphatic glands.

Aphthæ in mouth, and bleeding gums. Redness of gums. Brown tongue. Dryness of tongue. Putrid odor from mouth. Burning pain in tongue. Salivation, swollen gums. Taste putrid, sour, sweetish. Ulceration of gums. Drawing, tearing pain in teeth, and the teeth feel too long.

Much mucus in the throat and burning pain. Swallowing is difficult. The throat is swollen and ulcerated. It has cured goitre. It has cured enlarged thyroid with fast pulse and protruding eyes. The goitre is right-sided like *Lycopodium.*

The appetite is INCREASED; RAVENOUS. Aversion to food. Desires alcoholic stimulants. Distension of the stomach. A sensation of emptiness in the stomach. Eructations which ameliorate. Hiccough and nausea. Pain in the stomach; burning; cutting; pressing; stitching. *Thirst :* burning; *extreme.* Vomiting bile.

It is a very useful remedy in a variety of liver affections. The liver is enlarged but it is of great service in atrophy of the liver. Obstructed flatulence. Pain in the abdomen. Colic; after eating; during menses; in the right hypochondrium; in inguinal region; burning in the liver; cramping; cutting in right side. drawing; pressing in right hypochondrium. Rumbling in abdomen. TABES MESENTERICA.

Constipation alternating with diarrhœa. Difficult stool; inactivity of the rectum. Morning diarrhœa. Much flatus. External piles. Burning in the rectum. Stool copious; offensive; hard; knotty. Retention of urine. Urination dribbling, frequent. Urine is *album nous;* cloudy; *copious;* offensive.

Atrophy of the testes. Erections troublesome at night; later impotency. Hydrocele. *Induration of testes. Pain in testes;* ACHING. Perspiration of the genitals. Sexual desire increased. *Swollen testes.*

In the female the desire is also increased.INDURATION OF THE OVARIES; UTERUS; cervix uteri. Inflammation of *ovaries* and *uterus. Leucorrhœa;* acrid; copious; *thick;* YELLOW. Menses absent; copious; late; suppressed. Pain in ovaries and uterus. Prolapsus uteri. *Sterility.*

Hoarseness., Respiration is fast; asthmatic; difficult at night with cardiac affections and when ascending; irregular; short; suffocating.

Cough: dry; short; spasmodic. Expectoration in the morning. Bloody with cardiac affections: difficult; mucus; offensive; tough; yellow.

Anxiety in region of heart. Congestion to chest. CONSTRICTION OF CHEST; *of heart.* Heat in chest. *Hypertrophy of heart.* Inflammation of heart; endocardium. Milk suppressed. Cardiac murmurs. Oppression of chest; OF HEART. Pain in chest; during cough; sides of chest; in heart; burning in chest; cutting pain in chest; stitching pain in chest. Palpitation of heart; *at night; anxious; on least exertion;* on motion; TUMULTUOUS; when walking. Swelling of axillary glands without any tendency to suppurate.

Pain in sacrum; stitching pain in lumbar region.

Cold hands with hot head. Cold legs and feet. Heaviness of feet. Hip joint disease. Itching limbs. Lower limbs. Pain in limbs; *joints;* gouty rheumatic; elbow; hip; drawing pain in knee; stitching in shoulder and wrist; tearing pain in limbs; upper limbs; fingers; finger joints; joints of thumb. Dropsical swelling of limbs; hands; legs; feet; weakness of limbs upper; lower; knees.

Dreams: amorous; *anxious;* distressing; frightful; vivid. Restless sleep; *sleepiness.* Waking too early.

Chill in warm bed. Shaking chill. Perspiration morning and night; profuse.

Skin burning. Coldness of skin. Eczema of neck, chest and forearms. Herpetic eruptions. Itching and burning. Ulcers; cancerous; discharging; yellow pus; sensitive.

AURUM METALLICUM

The general features of the remedy are such as relate to the mind and such as relate to the tissues of the body in general. If you run through the mental symptoms, taking them all in as one great whole, you will see that all the affections, natural to healthy man, are perverted. So great in extent is this that one of the fundamental loves, which is the love of living, of self-protection, is perverted and he loathes life, is weary of life, longs to die and seeks methods to commit suicide. No love of life. The affections pre-eminently are deranged, the intellectual sphere is only secondarily changed. Of course insanity runs through the remedy, but it is an insanity that begins in the will and proceeds to the intellect; it is first observed as a perversion of the affections. It is astonishing that one could get into such a state of mind, such horrible depression of spirits that there is an absolute loss of enjoyment in everything. You take away a man's hope, and he has nothing to live for, he then wants to die. Such, it seems, is the state in this medicine. Self-condemnation, continual self-reproach, self-criticism, a constant looking into self; she does nothing right, everything is wrong, nothing will succeed, hopelessness. "Imagines he cannot succeed in anything, and he does everything wrong; he is in disunion with himself." Imagines he sees obstacles in his way everywhere. He is all the time imagining that he has *neglected something, that he has neglected his friends.* He imagines that he deserves reproach in consequence of *having neglected duty;* he has neglected something, he is wrong, is wholly evil, has sinned away his day of grace, is not worthy of salvation; this is the train of thought that constantly runs through his mind. The thought really becomes uncontrollable; he is absorbed in himself and sits and broods over it, and by brooding over it he only intensifies his present state and hatches new grievances, continues to worry over himself, thinks he is wholly unfit for this world, and then he longs to die. He looks on the dark side of everything.constantly expecting bad news, looking for everything to go wrong. The future looks dark to him, and he wants to die; he never will succeed, for everything goes wrong that he turns his hand to. His business is dark, his family troubles him, his friends annoy him; he becomes *extremely* irritable, easily angered, is worried over trifles, and easily excited. Every little thing rouses him into anger and turmoil, he is always in a vexation. The Aurum state of mind is an insanity dreadful to look upon because of its turbulence and melancholy. It is suitable in the most profound states of melancholy and depression where the patient sits silent and says nothing. When disturbed he is aroused to great vehemence, anger and violence. "Melancholy, feels hateful and quarrelsome." "Terrible melancholy after abuse of *Mercury.*" The causes of this state of insanity are prolonged anxiety, unusual responsibility, syphilis and loss of property. Persons who have been repeatedly drugged with *Mercury*, have established upon themselves a mercurial disease, with enlargement of the liver, and this is almost always attended more or less by melancholy and sadness and such hopelessness as we find in Aurum. Aurum produces such affections of the liver as are associated with cardiac affections, endocarditis, dropsy of the heart and rheumatic affections that have gone to the heart. You will notice that wherever the *affections* are pre-eminently disturbed in mental disease that there is either cardiac weakness, endocarditis, enlargement of the heart, or some organic or functional disease of the heart. You will very often find a history of taking *Mercury* that has superinduced a rheumatic state that has been rubbed away with liniments until the heart is affected, and with this comes hopelessness, insanity of the will, disturbance of the affections. Then it appears to spread in this remedy from the will to the understanding, and the intellectual portion of man becomes involved. Think what a state it is for a man who has been in good condition of health, respected in his business circles, to have a desire to commit suicide. You will see other kinds of insanity and a breaking down or a state of feebleness of the intellect, he cannot think nor reason; his affections are practically intact, but he finally goes into a state of imbecility, or he becomes wild and commits suicide from impulse. That is an instance where the intellect has been affected first and spread to the will. Sometimes this state comes on, and no disturbance in the man's intellectual nature has been observed; it is intact, it is sound. He has been sound in his business affairs, he has been a good father, he has been observed by those around him to be intelligent, but he has silently brooded over his state and his hatred of the world; he has told nobody of it, and then he has been found hung in his room. The man's intellectual nature keeps the man in contact with the world; but his affections are largely kept to himself. A man can have affection for all sorts of things and perversion of the affections, but his intellect will guide him not to show his likes and dislikes to the world. The affections cannot be seen, but man's intellect is subject to inspection. He cannot conceal his intellect. We shall see that the affections are interior, they are covered with a cloak, they are his innermost and are hidden from inspection; but the understanding is the outermost garment, it surrounds and hides his affections, just as does the garment he wears over the body hide the body. The affections that Aurum resembles are those like unto the very innermost nature of man.

"Ailments from grief, disappointed love, fright, anger, contradiction, mortification." "Pain makes her desperate so that she would like to jump out of the window." He meditates upon death, upon suicide; he wants to get out of the world, wants to destroy himself, has no love for his life which he thinks is worthless.

The remedy is full of rheumatic affections, not unlike such as are found in old mercurial cases; rheumatic affections with swelling of the joints; affections of the cartilages and bone, inflammation of the periosteum: thickening and induration of the periosteum. Indurations of glands; induration of the cartilages about the joints. These are all of syphilitic and mercurial character. It is useful in old syphilitics when the bones are breaking down in any part of the body; the shin bones, nose bones, ear bones, any of the small bones. Like syphilis and mercury, the complaints are aggravated at night, coming on in the evening and keep up all night. The pains are violent, they tear, the bones ache as if they would break, not in acute fevers but in old syphilitic bone troubles. Knife-like pains in the periosteum. Pains in the joints rendering them immovable. Inflammation of the bone itself with caries. It is not strange that the vascular coating of the bones, the periosteum, should be greatly affected because there is a strange vascularity, all over the economy, in this medicine. The veins are enlarged, in a state of congestion and inflammation, and friable. The veins become thickened and tumefied. The blood vessels pulsate all over the body. "Erethism or vascular fulness characterizes nearly all complains." Fulness of the veins of the extremities; this goes on until swelling appears with weakness so that dropsy is prevalent throughout the remedy. Œdema of the extremities, with pitting upon pressure, which occurs in heart and liver affections. A false state of plethora seems to exist in the body and finally turmoil and excitement occur. Violent orgasms in the body, sometimes demonstrated as violent heat, coming in flushes with excitement. Fidgetiness, feeling as if something dreadful were going to happen throughout the economy. Then it settles into a state of quiescence for awhile and then this repeats itself. These violent orgasms come preparatory to the localization or establishment of some breakdown in the economy. At times it is a cardiac affection, with marked oppression behind the sternum with dyspnœa on walking fast or going upstairs. Endocarditis will have this turmoil in the body; by and by look for albumin in the urine, look for enlargement of the liver, look for signs of cancer of the uterus, and deep-seated affections.

"Boring in bones." "Pains drive to despair." The pains drive the patient out of bed at night and make him walk. This is seen in old syphilitic bone pains, and old mercurialized patients. The patient has been taking *Mercury* all his life and his liver is enlarged, and his joints are enlarged. He goes to every doctor, with an endeavor to get relief from his distressing sufferings. *Mercury* and disease are so mixed up that a great turmoil will result from your first prescription. He will go through these stages of violence and periodical attacks. You will have to know such medicines as Aurum, *Chelidonium* and *Staphisagria* to get this patient over these awful attacks which he is obliged to go through.

This medicine wonderfully affects the glands, the parotid glands, the glands about the groin, the lymphatics in the abdomen; in fact, the glands everywhere. The mammary glands, the testes and ovaries, are involved, and undergo states of hardness, infiltration, etc. Aurum cures chronic enlargement of the testes, and lumps in the mammary glands. Tumors in these glands, of cystic character, have been cured by Aurum. Hahnemann potentized Aurum and gave some of it to a patient, and it did not work, but he thoroughly triturated it until he got it to the fifteenth potency and then it worked and restored that patient to the bosom of his family. Hahnemann says that in the earlier triturations the dose was yet too large to cure; so he went higher until it was sufficiently small to cure, sufficiently attenuated to go into the interior of the economy through the various envelopes of man.

There is one grand feature running through the Aurum state; it is the manner in which he is affected by temperature, and by the weather. Here are some symptoms that relate to the whole man, which must be examined in this connection. "Desire for open air." This patient ranks along with *Pulsatilla* as to temperature; but Aurum is not mild, gentle and yielding, he is obstinate, irascible, the very opposite of the *Pulsatilla* patient. "Generally > growing warm." This is in connection with the headaches. "Cold water ameliorates pain in eyes." "Averse to uncover," hut he desires open air like *Pulsatilla.* "Warm air, asthma <." Many symptoms disappear after washing, especially cold washing; but whenever the patient is suffering from great excitement, turmoil and vascularity, constitutional orgasm, pulsations, he wants the doors and windows open, wants to get out in the cool air; wants the clothing thrown off. This state of excitement and pulsation is ameliorated by the open air. It has those flushes of heat so common to women at the critical period, and these are followed by sweat, sometimes by chilliness.

Most that we have said of the remedy is about its general aspect, for everything about the mind is general.

In Aurum the pain in the head is very intense, maddening, often accompanied by a sensation as if air were blowing upon him; he looks around to see where the draft comes from when there is none; extremely sensitive. Often has to have the head wrapped up, although it feels hot, with a good deal of congestion and rush of blood to the head. The head is sore and feels bruised. Stitching, burning, tearing pains in the head; much throbbing in the head. The face is bloated, flushed and shiny with the congestive headaches. These headaches are often found in syphilitic subjects; often associated with cardiac disease. Pain in the back of the head associated with cardiac disease, with sluggish circulation, purple face, duskiness of the skin. Exostoses as in syphilis. The skull bones are sensitive to touch; the periosteum is tender to touch. In old mercurialized cases with bone affections and necrosis of the skull, as in syphilis and mercury, the hair falls out copiously; the head becomes bald. Baldness due to syphilis; the scalp is left shiny and the hair will not grow in again. In acute diseases there is falling out of the hair, but it grows in again. But young syphilitics often lose the hair and remain bald all the rest of their life.

There are disturbances of the eye, of a catarrhal character, even to the extent of ulceration and infiltration of the various coatings of the eye. Iritis; great disturbance of the whole visual apparatus; some of the striking features I will read from the book, but remember the constitution that we must always have in view; remember the mental state, the mercurial and syphilitic states, the gouty tendency, and the complaints that belong to joints, remember the cardiac disturbances. As we review the eye symptoms we thus see the constitution with which they are likely to be associated. "Photophobia." Weak sight and eyes. "By gaslight a number of bright, floating specks and dots are seen." "Eyes ameliorated by moonlight:" "Large letters cannot be distinguished." "Yellow, crescent-shaped bodies floating obliquely upward in field of vision." "In upper dark section of field of vision occasional showers of bright, star-like bodies." In *Calcarea* there is a queer symptom; he sees a sudden flash arise from the lower portion of the field of vision; it shoots up and divides, and then he sees stars in every direction. It is the appearance you will see sometimes in the shooting off of one of those rockets that explode and come down in a shower. That has been observed in *Calcarea.* "Hemiopia of the left eye." And so it goes on with many of these peculiar things that can hardly be described except in the language of the text. "Protruding eyes." Protrusion of the eyes, such as occurs in exophthalmic goitre, with enlargement of the heart, has been cured by Aurum. Enlargement of the thyroid gland with rapid and full pulse. Exophthalmic goitre has been cured by Aurum, *Natr. mur.* "Staring, dreary look." "Iritis marked by much pain around eye, which seems to be deep in bone." Such a state would be likely to be produced by syphilis that had been treated with *Mercury* and Aurum would come in as an antidote to both the syphilis and the *Mercury.* "Pupils irregularly dilated." It has catarrhal states of the eye. It has inflammation of the conjunctiva, choroid, iris and retina. Well, syphilis does this, taking hold of the eye in just this way and causing great infiltration. Pains round about the eye; the thin plate bones, and the skull bones are all sensitive to pressure; the bones seem tender; periostitis; opacity of the cornea.

Syphilis often takes hold of the ear, affecting the bones of that organ. "Caries of mastoid process, obstinate otorrhœa." Caries of the bones of the ear. "Parotids swollen, painful to touch." "Oversensitiveness to noises; but music relieves." "Humming, buzzing and rushing in ears." Rushing like the rushing of wind and falling water. "Annoying dryness in ears and nose." This is all like the complaints of syphilis, which are cured by Aurum, but Aurum also corresponds to and has cured many times otorrhœa following scarlet fever where there is even entire loss of the drum of the ear and loss of the bones. Of course it does not restore hearing. Patients will come to you for ear troubles, and you may find that the whole ear apparatus is destroyed; the mucous membrane and bones of the ear are all in a state of ulceration and necrosis and the discharge is fœtid. The patient consults you in order to have the hearing restored and it may not be possible; stop that ear discharge and restore the hearing are the only two things he thinks about. If you go to-day to our ear specialists and speak about curing the patient, they would not know what you were talking about; the only thing that would be thought of would be the stopping of that ear discharge as quickly as possible. They would examine the ear to see whether it is intact or not; and if it is not, the hearing is of course gone and the stopping of the discharge is then all that is taken into consideration. Homœopathy teaches that the *patient* should be treated and the patient only, after which the organs and tissues become normal. The whole duty of the physician is to restore health to the patient. We have the nose specialists with their local applications. These things will only bring on bone disease, and tubercular troubles; they stop the discharge from the nose, and of course nature must have a vent somewhere and so she establishes a discharge in the chest; the trouble progresses from the mucous membranes into the lung, into the parenchyma of the lungs, and is often of a tubercular character, and then these men tell you the bacilli have come. This is spurious science. Clean, healthy tissues are the only safeguard.

Aurum is full of nasal troubles, with fœtid discharge. The bones of the nose necrose; syphilitic necrosis, the nose flattens down; the bones are discharged. You see these people walking about with flattened-down nose and if you get near enough to them the stench will be observed. They are nearly all syphilitics. A few remedies have the power of curing this syphilitic nose condition; Aurum, *Mercury* and *Hepar* are three of them. I have cured this state a number of times with *Hepar.* I once cured a man after the bones were completely softened, so that when the nose was handled it would bend right over; only a sort of cartilaginous structure held the nose in place. I gave that patient *Hepar.* It cured him of syphilis after he had been filled in vain with *Mercurry.* "Coryza, thick discharge, like white of egg." "Mucous discharge from posterior nares in morning." Tip of nose knobby, red, like *Lach.;* strawberry nose. Little knobs on the nose composed of varicose veins in heart cases, with disturbance of the right side of the heart; sometimes found in old drinkers and in heart affections generally. Face red and swollen. Aurum has cured epithelioma of the wing of the nose and lip. Remember the horribly offensive odor from the nose, loss of smell following pains in the nasal bones; nasal catarrh. "Ulcerated, agglutinated, painful nostrils." "Crusts in nose." "Nose feels obstructed as in dry coryza." With nearly all of these nose affections, the patient is bowed down with sorrow, full of grief; black clouds hang over him and he wants to die. Loathing of life and wants to find some way to commit suicide.

"Puffy under eyes." "Blue about nose and lips." "Face glowing red." "Violent boring in right zygomatic process when walking." "Carious teeth." "Toothache at night." "Foul breath." "Syphilitic ulcers in palate and throat." "Boring in hard palate." This medicine has cured craving for alcohol, the craving of dunkards.

Another marked feature of this medicine is its ability to harden, enlarge and inflame the liver; induration with cardiac affections; enlargement of the heart and liver. When you take into consideration the venous system, the portal system and its close association with the heart in establishing the circulation of blood in the abdomen, and the work that it does in the abdomen as a great receiving apparatus, you will not be surprised to find that heart and liver affections are associated with hopelessness and despair. Notice, on the other hand, something that will set you to thinking perhaps, in cases of phthisis, none of them is hopeless, they think they are going to get well; the lungs are almost gone with tubercles, but he knows if he could only get up that little something out of the throat he would get well. Notice then that peculiar relation between the lungs and the understanding, and between the heart and the will. With every little trouble located in the heart there comes hopelessness, but when the manifestation of disease is in the lungs there is hopefulness.

Dropsical conditions of the abdomen. "Inguinal hernia." "Tabes mesenterica." All of the glands of the body are involved more or less. All sorts of disturbances of the sexual organs. "Testes indurated." "Frequent nightly emissions." Complaints as the result of vices. "Hydrocele." "Ulcers on scrotum after gonorrhœa." "Burning and stinging in perineum." "Condylomata around anus." "Induration of uterus." "Menses too late and scanty" "Uterus prolapsed and indurated." "Leucorrhœa thick white." Complaints in the uterus and region of the pelvis from straining and reaching up the arms; abortion from reaching up at the windows and fixing a curtain, etc. Aurum is a medicine that is suitable for induration of the uterus and ulceration of the uterus as a result of repeated abortions. When you study the loss of affections that is involved in such a state and the affections or lack of affections that are found in Aurum you can see a deep well-grounded similitude in the symptoms, and that is the way to, hunt for a remedy. It is in the sphere of the physician to examine into this state of mankind in which he can destroy his offspring and to examine into the nature of remedies producing such a state. We see in Aurum this entire perversion of all the loves of mankind, and finally their entire destruction.

The symptoms of asthma and of difficult breathing you would naturally expect to be associated with the cardiac affections. Notice this also, that the difficult breathing is of two kinds, such breathing as involves the lung, and such breathing as involves the heart. So it is we have an asthmatic condition of dyspnœa that is cardiac in character, and dyspnœa that is purely respiratory. These are entirely distinct in character; one belongs to such remedies as have a predominance of action on the affections, and another belonging to those having a predominance of action on the intelligence; one will involve the lung and finally bring on emphysema; the other one is entirely different in its character, with irregular heart action, and only secondarily associated with emphysema. Study your pathology with these things in mind and you will be able to perceive the nature of sickness and its results. These things are not mere observation, whims and theories, but are the outcome of studying things from internal to external.

In this remedy the pains wander from joint to joint and finally locate in the heart. Angina pectoris is often the ending of an old rheumatism that has wandered from joint to joint. "Difficult breathing." If the case goes on a little while, there will be blood spots, and if he lie on the right side the lower part will be dull on percussion and the upper part will be resonant. Palpitation with great agony. Extreme oppression in the region of the heart on walking fast and going upstairs with œdema of the lower limbs.

AURUM MURIATICUM

This remedy exercises a profound action upon the mind and body. The patients suffering from latent syphilis are over-sensitive to it, and often require it in their complaints. It has many bone symptoms and pains and they are worse at night. Its catarrhal condition is very much like that found in old cases of syphilis, such as had long treatment with *Mercury* and *Iodides*. It is a rheumatic constitution also and is useful in acute and chronic rheumatism. It has cured rheumatic fever where the joints have been mostly affected but are now better and the heart is the principal seat of suffering. Many complaints are associated with cardiac disease. Dropsical states from heart disease, from liver affections, with albumin in the urine after scarlet fever or with intermittent fever. Where old syphilitics continue to lose flesh. The glands and parts inflamed become indurated. It has been useful in cancerous glands. Inflammation of the bone and periosteum; caries, exostosis after *Mercury* in latent syphilis. Caries of the joints with nightly boring and gnawing pains. It has *burning pains in many parts.* The pains are tearing, drawing, pressing and stitching. Many symptoms come on during rest and some during motion. Cold, wet weather ameliorates. Warm air, warm bed, warm room, warm wraps, becoming warm, even in open air, and warmth in general aggravates the general feeling. Exertion and walking increase many symptoms. The palpitation, suffocation and great weakness come from walking and exertion. While open air ameliorates he is even in the open air incapable of exertion. Fast walking is impossible. The nervous symptoms are very marked. Excitement, sensitive to noise, starting when spoken to, starting in sleep. When the above symptoms are concomitants of heart and liver diseases this remedy will most likely be useful. Fullness of the veins all over the body is a strong feature of this remedy. It is a most useful remedy in patients suffering from the chronic effects of gonorrhœa and syphilis, where fig warts and syphilitic ulceration are present together.

The mental symptoms are largely such as are found in Aurum. It has the same suicidal disposition. His mind dwells upon his broken health until he becomes low-spirited and desires death. He loathes his life. Weeping and aversion to his occupation. *Indolence.* The melancholia of old syphilitics. Extremely anxious with palpitation.

Said to be "full of whims and notions." Extremely irritable. Nothing can be done to please him. Constant fretting. Extreme mental and physical restlessness. He walks the streets slowly, to be in the open air which ameliorates; he is much worse in the house, and in the warm room. Thinking about his complaint caused the heart to beat strong and fast. Symptoms worse after fright, vexation and mortification. When the general symptoms mentioned above strongly predominate it will cure the particulars in the various parts below.

It cures violent syphilitic headaches with vertigo. Violent left-sided headaches. Intense ache in forehead. Burning in occiput. Cerebral congestion. Pulsating in the head. Pain ameliorated by cold application. His forehead is hot. Heat of the head and cold extremities. Great soreness of the periosteum and exostoses of the skull. Tearing pains in the skull. Worse nights.

It cures chronic eye troubles due to syphilis. The mucous membrane of the lids and ball is red, thickened and very vascular. The lids stick together in the morning. Dim vision in the evening by artificial light. Loss of vision after syphilis, and after scarlet fever. Very slow accommodation. Amaurosis, chronic inflammation of margin of lids. Burning pain in the eyes.

Buzzing, ringing and roaring in the ears followed by deafness. A sensation as if the ears were wide open. Music relieves the ear symptoms. Eczema behind the ears. Burning and itching behind the ears at night.

It is one of the most useful remedies for catarrh of the nose in patients who are sensitive to the warm room. It classes with *Pulsatilla* and *Kali sulphuricum,* as both of these are better in the open air. The discharges of the remedy are thin or thick like pus, very offensive and sometimes bloody, and there are many hard crusts in the nose. Bleeding of the nose on blowing out of the crusts. Yellow, greenish discharge. It cures the most stubborn syphilitic catarrh. The nasal bones become sensitive to pressure. Caries of the bones of the nose. Red, swollen nose. Deep cracks about the wings of the nose. Lupus of the wings of the nose. Infants with inherited syphilis with snuffles and indented nose.

The circumscribed red face with pallor of face and neck in heart complaint, palpitation on slight exertion, pressure behind the sternum when walking, suffocates in a close room, wants cool air, ameliorated by gentle motion and we have a combination that this remedy often cures. The pale face with red spot on each cheek is not that which is found in consumption, but in heart complaint. The infant's face looks old. Acne on the face. There is often a red, healthy look on the face of very sickly people. Red faced from venous stasis; it is a false plethora, like that described in *Aurum*. Caries of the lower jaw like *Phosphorus* and exostosis of right cheek bone. Burning and swelling of the lips. Indurated lips. Cancerous ulcer of the lips. Painful swelling of the submaxillary gland.

It has been useful in cancer of the tongue. Inflammation of the tongue followed by induration. Dry, red, excoriated tongue. Warts on the tongue. Metallic taste and salivation.

Pains in the throat and ulceration. Ulceration of the tonsils. Inflammation with dryness in throat.

The stomach is very weak and digestion is slow. Nausea, distension and diarrhœa after eating. Coffee, tea and wine disagree. Eructations putrid. Nausea in the morning, better after breakfast. Vomiting of green fluid. Gastritis, cramps in stomach. Sharp pains in the stomach with burning, intense thirst.

Enlargement of liver and spleen. Chronic inflammation of the liver. The liver is large and hard. Burning in the liver. Tight feeling in the region of the liver. Liver troubles associated with heart disease with albumin in the urine and dropsy of the limbs.

Abdominal dropsy. Drawing pains and distension from gases. Great tenderness of abdomen.

Frequent fluid stools, grayish, white, bileless. Diarrhœa with liver affection, or with Bright's disease. Diarrhœa worse at night. Hæmorrhoids with bleeding at stool. A heavy ring of warts around the anus with copious moisture. Marked excoriation around the anus. It has cured fistula in ano. Fig warts of the anus with ulceration.

Frequent urination day and night, but worse during the night. Urine dribbles. Increased flow of urine. Urine turbid, reddish sediment. Gonorrhœa in old syphilitic subjects where they have been badly treated. Chancre on the prepuce and scrotum. Fig warts on the penis, scrotum or anus. Bubo in left groin. Surceased sexual desire. Induration of testes.

Enlargement and great hardness of uterus. Indurated cervix. Chronic inflammation of uterus and ovaries. Menses frequent and profuse, flow excoriating. Leucorrhœa copious, yellow. Uterus prolapsed and heavy. Inflammation of vagina and labia. Gonorrhœa and swelling of glands in the groin. Heat, burning and itching of the vagina and labia.

Suffocation in a warm room, from the clothing, from ascending stairs and from walking fast. Dyspnœa at night. Dry paroxysmal cough at night. Heart cough. Loose cough with thick yellow expectoration. Most distressing pressure under the sternum as if it would burst on walking fast, ascending steps or on any exertion, with palpitation. Palpitation on exertion and from excitement. Palpitation if suddenly spoken to. Sharp pains in the chest, going from place to place. Pain in the heart. Drawing and cutting in the heart. Violent pressure in the region of the heart. Cardiac anguish. Angina pectoris. Endocarditis. Enlarged right side of the heart. The palpitation keeps her from sleeping. Rheumatic heart. Palpitation from mental exertion. Pulse small, weak and fast. The heart is feeble. Pulsation strong in neck and temples. Violent, irregular heart.

Trembling of the hands in the morning. Shocks in the arms. Burning, shooting pains in the forearms. Drawing in the shoulders. Worse in the warm bed and during rest. Tearing pains in the shoulders. Stiffness of arms and fingers.

Dropsical swelling of the lower limbs. Exostoses on the tibia. Periostitis of the labia. Extreme sensitiveness of the tibia. Pain in leg at night. Burning feet. Pain in feet worse from warmth and motion. Cutting in the toes when walking. Burning, redness and swelling of the toes. Limbs cold and covered with a cold sweat. Drawing, tearing in all the limbs. Venous engorgement of the lower limbs.

Sleeplessness from palpitation and from excitement, wakes with a start. Violent dreams, tormenting dreams of sadness.

AURUM SULPHURICUM

The symptoms of this remedy appear in the MORNING, forenoon, after noon, *evening,* and DURING THE NIGHT. DESIRE FOR OPEN AIR. The open air aggravates many symptoms. Ascending brings on many symptoms. Asleep feeling in single parts; a sensation of a band around parts. Cancerous affections. ULCERS. Worse from cold in general; from cold air; from becoming cold; after becoming cold. Congestion of blood. Hysterical convulsions. Dropsical tendency. Worse during and after eating and from exertion. Formication. Fulness of the veins and a feeling of distension; lack of vital heat. Induration of glands and other parts. Inflammation of internal organs; of bones; of glands; of serous membranes. Desire to lie down, but lying aggravates some symptoms; worse lying in bed. A most useful remedy in cases abused by mercury. Motion intensifies most symptoms. Mucous secretions much increased. Violent orgasm of blood in chest and head. Pain in bones and glands; aching, *boring,* cutting, *pressing,* stitching, tearing pains in many parts; bearing downward in bones and muscles; paralysis of organs. It is most useful in red-faced, full-blooded people. Pulsation in internal parts; the pulse in *small,* FAST, *irregular and weak.* Marked aggravation follows hurried actions, like running. Oversensitive to pain, in glands. Complaints are predominantly right-sided. Sitting erect aggravates some symptoms; standing aggravates many symptoms. Swelling of affected parts; of the glands.

A feeling of tension all over the body; symptoms are worse *from touch.* Trembling in body and limbs. Walking ameliorates; walking fast aggravates; walking in open air aggravates. Warm bed increases some symptoms, in some cases worse from both heat and cold; worse in warm room and from warm wraps. Marked general weakness; weariness. Complaints worse in winter.

Absent-minded; irascible, even violent; ANXIETY; of conscience; with fear; about salvation. Very critical with all her friends; morbidly cheerful and gay; *aversion to company.* She has lost all confidence in herself. Confusion in the morning, worse from mental exertion; very timid, even cowardly. Loathing of life and *desires death.* Delusions about animals. *Despair of recovery* and salvation; EXCITEMENT and discontentment; exertion of mind makes all the mental symptoms worse. Marked increase in her imaginative powers. Fear on going into a crowd; of death; of evil; of people; of robbers; very forgetful and easily frightened. It is a very useful remedy for chronic complaints that date back to grief. Hysterical and in a hurried state of mind; at first mental activity, later dullness; imbecility. He is becoming weak-minded and indolent; will not work, becomes like a tramp. These states change to excitement and a mania for work. It should become an excellent remedy for insanity, irresolution and *extreme irritability;* moaning and lamenting. Maniacal conduct and loquacity, weakness of memory; insane mirth; moods constantly changing; morose, obstinate and easily offended; MENTAL PROSTRATION; quarrelsome. Great restlessness, worse during the night. Extreme sadness in the morning but worse in the EVENING and during perspiration. Generally oversensitive. Desire to sit and brood. Averse to being spoken to; SUICIDAL THOUGHTS occupy his mind; suspicious; indisposed to talk; weeping, worse at night; alternating with laughter.

Vertigo in the open air; with headache; must lie down; when standing when stooping; walking in open air.

Fulness of head; constant hyperæmia of brain. *The hair falls out.* Heat in head; burning scalp. Heaviness in moving or rising; in occiput; hydrocephalus, itching of scalp worse at night. Nodding of head like paralysis agitans. Pain in head; morning in bed; afternoon; evening; better in open air, worse from binding up the hair; from coughing; worse lying; from motion; from strong odors; from warm room; after sleep; from straining the eyes; from talking; in windy, stormy weather. Aching pain in forehead, worse from motion, in occiput; in occiput and forehead; in sides of head; in temples; in temples and forehead. Boring in head; in forehead; in vertex. Drawing pain in head; lancinating pain in occiput. Pressing pain in head; *in forehead;* in occiput; in temples; in vertex. Stitching pains in head; in forehead; in sides of head. TEARING PAIN IN HEAD, in forehead; in occiput; in sides of head; in temples. Pulsating in head on coughing and on motion, in sides of head.

The eyelids stick together in the morning; discharge of yellow mucus from the eyes; heat in eyes. Inflammation of eyes; catarrhal; SCROFULOUS; *syphilis;* of chancroid, with ulceration of cornea; of iris. Itching of lids; of canthi. Much and easy lachrymation; OPACITY OF THE CORNEA. Pain in the eyes; from motion; when reading; aching, burning in the eyes and canthi; *cutting, pressing;* as from sand; stitching. *Paralysis of the optic nerve.* Photophobia, protrusion and *pulsation in* eyes. The pupils are contracted. *Redness of eyes;* of *lids. Scrofulous affections of eyes.* Spots on the cornea; stye near outer canthus; swollen lids. Floating black specks in the field of vision; DIM VISION; *diplopic.* All the eye symptoms are worse from any exertion of vision. FOGGY VISION. Hemiopia; can see only the lower half of objects. Vision lost from paralysis of the optic nerves; vision smoky; sparks; stars.

Discharge from the ear; fetid; offensive; purulent; sequelæ after *sup-pressed eruption;* the ears are red; dryness in ears; scanty wax; stitching of the ears; noises; buzzing; crackling; fluttering; *humming; ringing; roaring;* rushing sounds. Pain inside the ear; stitching in, and behind ears; tearing in ears. The ears burn. Hearing acute; for noise; *impaired; lost.*

Catarrh of nose; discharge *bloody;* dry crusts, worse on right side; greenish; HARD; OFFENSIVE; PURULENT; THICK; YELLOW. The nose is red and swollen; most marked at tip. Coryza fluent and dry; dryness in nose; epistaxis on blowing nose; itching of skin of nose and inside. The nose is obstructed; offensive odor from nose; œzena. Pain in nose at night; in bones of nose; on touch; burning; soreness; ulcerative pain, right side; polypus in nose. Nose very sensitive to touch. Smell acute, later lost. Frequent sneezing. *Swollen nose.* ULCERATION in NOSE.

Epithelioma of lip; cracked lips. Discoloration of face, earthy, pale, red, red spots. Eruptions on face; forehead; *nose;* acne rosacea; comedones; crusty, crusty on nose; pimples on face and forehead; pustules; scurf. Pain in face; right side; worse in cold air, in parotid gland; in *submaxillary gland; burning pain in lip;* drawing in face; stitching tearing; tearing in cheek bones and lower jaw. Perspiration of face; cold. Swelling of the face, cheeks, glands in general; lips; *parotid gland;* submaxillary gland; ulceration of lip.

Apthæ in mouth and on tongue; Bleeding gums. The tongue is cracked. The mouth feels hot. Offensive, even putrid odor from mouth. Speech is difficult. The gums are swollen. Taste: bitter, insipid, metallic, putrid, sour, sweetish, lost. Ulcers on gums and tongue. Vesicles in the mouth. Caries of teeth. Sensation of elongation of teeth. Grinding teeth in sleep. The teeth become loose. Pain in the teeth, worse from touch; drawing, stitching, *tearing.*

Inflammation of throat and *tonsils,* with elongation of uvula. Sensation of a lump in throat; much mucus forms in the throat. Pain in throat on swallowing; burning, stitching, scraping. Suppuration of tonsils; swallowing difficult. Swelling of throat and *tonsils;* swelling of thyroid gland. Ulceration of throat, tonsils, uvula, *syphilitic.*

The appetite is ravenous. Aversion to food, to meat. Desires stimulants, coffee, cold drinks, milk. Distension of stomach. Digestion very slow; *a sensation of emptiness.* Eructations watery, bitter, tasting of food, ameliorate. Fulness in the stomach; flushes of heat. HICCOUGH. Nausea after eating; during headache. Pain in the stomach; burning, cutting, *pressing.* stitching. Thirst burning; extreme. Vomiting bile.

Atrophy of the liver; *enlargement of liver.* Abdomen distended with gas; with serum. Bubo in groin. Flatulence obstructed. Fulness and heaviness. Pain in abdomen; night, after midnight, *from colic;* on coughing; after eating; during menses; in hypochondria; in inguinal region as though a hernia would appear; burning in right hypochondrium; cramping, cutting, pressing pain in abdomen; in hypochondria; in hypogastrium. Rumbling in abdomen; swelling of *inguinal glands.*

Condylomata of anus. *Constipation; alternative with diarrhœa; difficult stool;* inactivity of rectum, during menses. Diarrhœa; morning; night, with burning in anus. Fistula in ano. Flatus passed from rectum; *offensive,* which ameliorates. Bleeding piles; external piles. Itching in anus. Moisture at anus. Pain in anus during stool; burning in anus with diarrhœa; soreness at anus; stitching pain in anus; prolapsus ani. Urging in rectum. Stool: gray, green-mucus, thin mucus, hard, KNOTTY, LARGE.

The bladder symptoms are very numerous and important. Pressing in the bladder. Retention of urine. Urging to urinate constant; ineffectual. Urination dribbling, difficult, *frequent, involuntary at night;* unsatisfactory. Suppression of urine. Prostatic discharge. Burning in urethra when passing urine; stitching and tearing in the urethra. Urine: *albuminous, bloody,* burning, cloudy on standing, copious, offensive; sand in the urine; SCANTY; mucus sediment; thick, yellow.

Condylomata of the glans penis. Impotency. Hydrocele in boys. Indura
tion of the testes. Inflammation of glans penis; of testes; of epididymic Itching
of the scrotum. Pain in the TESTES; ACHING IN TESTES;drawing pain in testes;
lancination in penis; PRESSING IN TESTES. PERSPIRATION OF GENITALS. *scrotum.*
Seminal emissions. Sexual desire increased, with relaxed penis Swelling of
testes; especially the right. *Chancres on penis; in* syphilitic cases that have
had much mercury; cancer of uterus. Sexual desire increased in women.
Inflammation of the uterus. Itching of the vulva. Leucorrhœa: worse in the
morning, acrid, *copious, thick, transparent, white* YELLOW. Menses absent;
copious; irregular; first menses delayed in girls too frequent; late; scanty;
suppressed. Pain in ovaries, in uterus, bruised bearing down in uterus,
especially during menses; burning in genitals and vagina. Lancination in
vulva. PROLAPSUS UTERI. The vulva is swollen.

Mucus in the larynx and trachea; hoarseness. Respiration is rapid; asthmatic; dyspnoea at *night;* on ascending, while lying, while walking; respiration is irregular, short and suffocative, worse at night.

Cough in the morning; nightly paroxyms; worse in cold air; short, dry,
hard, racking; short, spasmodic. Expectoration in morning and evening;
bloody, difficult; scanty, greenish, offensive, *purulent,* yellow.

Congestion of chest with anxiety; spasmodic constriction of chest.
Cracked nipples. Fluttering of the heart. Heat in chest. Milk disappearing or
is suppressed. Oppression of chest worse at night. Pain in chest; on coughing;
on inspiration; in sides of chest on deep inspiration; aching in heart; burning
in chest; cutting in chest and in heart; pressing in chest, sides and sternum;
soreness in chest; stitching pain in chest; on inspiring; in sides of chest on
inspiring or deep breathing; in sternum; in heart; in nipples. Palpitation at
night; on *ascending;* anxious; from least excitement; on slight exertion; during
menses; on motion; tumultuous; visible; when walking. Swollen mammæ;
swollen *axillary glands.* Trembling of the heart.

The back is cold; heat in lumbar region; itching of the back. Pain in the
back in the morning; on breathing; in dorsal region; lumbar region, worse
while sitting; in sacrum, in spine; aching in sacrum; bruised in lumbar region;
drawing in cervical region; pressing in back and in lumbar region; stitching
in lumbar region. *Stiffness in back,* weakness in lumbar region.

Gouty nodosites in the finger joints; caries of bone. COLD HANDS, LEGS
AND FEET. Cracked skin of hands. Blueness of finger nails. The feet feel heavy.
Hip joint disease. Itching of the upper and lower limbs. Numbness of the
limbs while lying and on waking; lower limbs. Pain in limbs while lying and on
waking; lower limbs. Pain in joints; in shoulder, upper arm, elbow, forearm;
hip; bruised pain in all the limbs; drawing in all the limbs, but especially in
knees and feet; stitching in shoulder, wrist, feet, and toes; tearing in the

limbs, joints, upper limbs, upper arms, *fingers,* FINGER JOINTS, thighs, toes. Painless paralysis of limbs. Staggering gait. Stiffness of knees. Dropsical swelling of legs and *feet.* Tension of thighs; weakness of limbs; of joints, upper limbs, lower limbs, knees.

Comatose sleep. Dreams: amorous, anxious, of assassins, of dead people, of de: .a, *distressing, frightful,* of thieves; pleasant, VIVID. Sleep is very restless; sleepiness afternoon; after dinner. Sleepless before midnight; after midnight. Waking easily.

Coldness in evening in bed; chilliness; shaking chill. Fever of a mild nondescript type. Perspiration in the morning; during the night; profuse.

Burning of the skin, cold skin. Eruptions; blisters; boils; burning; eczema; *herpes;* pustules; scabby; urticaria; vesicles, Erysipelas; excrescences. Formication. Itching, itching burning, itching creeping, itching stinging. Sensitive skin. Sore feeling in the skin. *Ulcers;* burning, *cancerous, deep,* offensive, discharging yellow pus; fistulous, sensitive, suppurating, *syphilitic.* It has cured *syphilitic warts.*

BAPTISIA

Baptisia is suitable for acute diseases. It is principally a short-acting medicine, suitable for complaints that are not long lasting. So far as we know it is not an antipsoric, does not go deep into the life. All of its acute diseases and complaints have the appearance of zymosis, like scarlet fever, diphtheria, typhoid, and gangrenous complaints. There is one thing that is unusual about it, it brings on this septic state more rapidly than most other remedies. The zymotic complaints of *Ars., Phos., Rhus,* and *Bry.,* are much slower in their pace. But Baptisia is suitable for typhoid that come on rapidly, and hence it is not so often suitable in idiopathic typhoids. When an individual comes down suddenly from cold, from malaria, from drinking poisonous waters, and from any zymotic or septic cause he is hurled into bed in a few days, instead of going through a period of four, five or six weeks. The old idiopathic typhoid fevers come on slower. Baptisia is suitable for those blood poisons that are highly septic, such as the puerperal state, such as scarlet fever. He comes down perhaps with the appearance of a sudden violent break down, with a remittent fever. But all at once it turns continued, and takes on. septic symptoms. So much for its progress and its pace. Every medicine must be observed as to its velocity, as to its pace, as to its periodicity, as to its motion, and its wave. We get that by looking at the symptoms. You take an individual who has been down in a mine, in the swamp, down in the mud, in the sewers, who has inhaled foul gases, who goes into bed with a sort of stupor, from the very beginning he feels stupid. It is not gradual, but he goes down very suddenly, and he is stupid. He is prostrated. His face is mottled. Sordes begin to appear on the teeth much earlier than in the regular typhoid. The abdomen becomes distended much earlier than in a regular typhoid; that is, one who is accustomed to observing those things knows they are postponed for a number of days; while with this remedy the third day the abdomen is distended, his mouth is bleeding, and is putrid. His odors are horrible; and he is in a marked state of delirium, such as would not be expected until the typhoid is out for many days. So it has rapid running diseases. It has velocity. That is, he is going down toward death rapidly. He is increasing in his prostration more rapidly than usual. It is not a gradual decline of days and weeks. He goes into a state of stupor. When aroused he takes on delirium. It does not matter whether it is scarlet fever, or typhoid fever, or a septic surgical fever, or a puerperal fever, or what. He has fever, and if you look at him, and talk to him, and turn him over, and rouse him up, and make him realize that you want to say something to him— which is difficult—he gives you the impression that he has been on a big drunk. That is the first thought you will have in a Baptisia case. His countenance is besotted. It is bloated and purple and mottled. Blood oozes from the mouth. You have seen the besotted countenance of drunkards, and it is like an old drunkard.

His mind seems to be gone. He does not know what he is talking about. He is in confusion, and when aroused he attempts to say something, and utters a word, or two and it all flits away, and he is back in his state of stupor again. No matter what disease that comes in, no matter what inflammation is present, no matter what organ is inflamed, if that state of the blood that can give rise to such symptoms and such sepsis is present, if that state of the mind is present, it is Baptisia.

All of the discharges are putrid. The odor is cadaverous, pungent; pene-trating. His perspiration, if he has any, is sour, fœtid, pungent, and pene-trating. If he has no sweat the body gives off an odor that is unaccountable. The odor is so penetrating that on going into the front door the whole house, if the room is open, is filled with the odor. The odor from the stool is putrid and so penetrating that it can be detected on first going into the house.

Now, a strange thing that runs through the remedy is a peculiar kind of mental confusion, in which he is in a constant argument with his parts. He seems to feel that there are two of him. He realizes a dual existence whenever he is roused up. He will begin talking about the other one in bed with him. It is said clinically that "his great toe is in controversy with his thumb." Or, "one leg is talking to the other leg." Or, one part is talking to another part; or, he is scattered around over the bed; fumbles and you ask him what he is trying to do—"why, I am trying to get those pieces together." He never succeeds; he is in delirium, of course. These are only examples; you will get a new phase every time you get a Baptisia case. Most of the time he is unconscious except when roused. Sometimes mutters. You will see his lips go, and you rouse him to see what he is about, and he is trying to get the pieces together. "Confused as if intoxicated." There are stages when he is not quite so stupid, and he is sleepless and restless. That is the exception. Most generally you will find him lying upon one side curled up like a dog, and he does not want to be disturbed. Again, when the stupor is not so great he is restless and turns and tosses. In that case he cannot sleep, because he cannot get the pieces together. He feels if he could once get matters together he could go to sleep, and these parts that are talking to each other keep him awake. His mind wanders as soon as his eyes are closed. Dullness, especially at night. Indisposition to think. Mind seems weak. There you find the whole picture of the mental aspect in all complaints, in all acute diseases—but they all come on in a hurry. They are zymotic, of a low form such as scarlet fever, such as malignant diseases; and yet it takes on a continued type of fever. These patients will die in from ten to twelve days if let alone. Whereas, ordinary typhoid will run for weeks, and sometimes die at the close of four weeks in a crisis. The bleedings are black and offensive. The putridity is marked. In the mouth, the mucus from the throat and nose is bloody and putrid. It has a diarrhœa. Thin, fæcal, watery, yellow. It has a typical typhoid discharge; the most typical typhoid stool is like yellow corn-meal mush, coming on many times a day, but soft, pappy, just about the consistency of soft mush. This remedy has that stool, but it is not the commonest form—but the black, the brown, the dark. In treating a good many cases of typhoid it was my fortune to observe a large number of Baptisia cases, which the remedy cured promptly. The stool where the Baptisia did the most service was like ground up slate, slate colored, brownish. The odor was penetrating. In addition to that I have seen this medicine cure that kind of diarrhœa when it was slate colored, even thin as water, if it was horribly putrid like decomposed meat; like the cadaver, attended with great prostration—I have seen it cure that diarrhœa when there were none of the elements of typhoid fever present. A simple prostrating form of diarrhœa. Exhaustion. Exhaustion comes rapidly. In three days he has a deathly sinking coming over him.

The headaches are nondescript. Only those congestive attacks, frontal headaches—violent pains in the head, and especially in the occiput, such as occur in the low forms of disease. I hardly ever go into the details of headaches. Baptisia is not a headache remedy. It is not a remedy that we would single out to treat headaches with, except such violent pains in the head of a congestive character that are associated with this low form of fever.

It has characteristic eye symptoms. Congestion. Redness. Pains in the eyes, and back of the eyes. So it has with hearing. So it has with nasal symptoms. But associated with fevers. But as soon as we come to the face we begin to realize the Baptisia symptoms, that besotted expression. The countenance shows that. The eyes show it, the face shows it. And these are the symptoms: "Dark red with besotted appearance. Hot and perceptibly flushed; dusky." That tells the whole story. Burning; heat in the face. "Critical sweat on forehead and face. Anxious, frightened look." On rousing from sleep looks as if he had a horrible dream.

And then comes the mouth, and the teeth, and the throat, and the tongue, all show marked Baptisia features. The tongue is swollen, painful, offensive. Covered with black blood. Raw; denuded. Stiff and dry as leather. Described as if it was made of wood, or burnt leather; ulcerated. Ulceration runs all through the remedy. Aphthous patches. These little ulcers that start no bigger than a pin-head become black and are so offensive and run together so that the whole surface of the mouth will be in a state of ulceration; raw and denuded, oozing a thick saliva that is putrid: The throat takes on ulceration; is raw and bleeding. There may be diphtheritic exudations in the throat. But round about it there are those low, dark, offensive surfaces. The throat is greatly swollen, and it is with difficulty that he can swallow. Baptisia has been a very useful remedy in gangrenous sore mouth. and sore throat. "Cancrum oris." The ulcers spread rapidly and eat rapidly. They are really phagedenic. Sordes form rapidly on the teeth. And when he is roused from sleep after a few hours of stupor there is a building up on the lips and around the corners of the mouth ridges of dry blood; very offensive. Bleeds much from the mouth, throat and nose. Thick oozing. Putrid. "Tongue red, and dry in the middle. The roof of the mouth swollen and feels numb. Foul or bitter nauseous taste in the mouth. Tongue of a dark hue. Tongue dry, brown down the centre. Tongue covered with a thick, brown crust. Tongue yellowish white, deeply furred." Ulcers all over the mouth. Baptisia has cured the ulcerated sore throat of young mothers—and nursing sore mouth in children, when the parts become dusky and the ulcers spread, and the mouth is putrid, and prostration is coming on rapidly. The child or the mother is growing weak with great rapidity, is becoming prostrated. Now, all this without fever. Many of these ulcerative states in Baptisia arc not attended with fever. It seems sometimes as though there were not life enough to get up a fever. Aphthous appearance in typhoid, in children, and with nursing mothers. Canker sores in the mouth. "Putrid ulceration of the whole buccal cavity." Now, with all this trouble saliva pours into the mouth, is thick and ropy and runs all over the pillow; like we find in *Mercury*.

The sore throat may be gangrenous. A strong feature of it is that the ulcers are rapid and painless, as if numb, without sensation. But it has a painful sore throat. "Fauces dark red; dark, putrid ulcers; tonsils and parotids swollen. Putrid sore throat. Tonsils and soft palate swollen, not accompanied by pain."

Great swelling; great tumefaction; purplish. The darker it is the more likely would I be to think of Baptisia—but never a bright red. I have never seen the Baptisia mental state associated with a bright red appearance. That low form of mental state is associated with blood decomposition, with duskiness, with a dark appearance of the skin, and of the mucous membranes. Not bright red, not pink, as we find in *Bell. Bell.* is more commonly bright red, although it has duskiness, but nothing to the extent of Baptisia. There is nothing like the putridity in *Bell.* that there is in Baptisia. "Œsophagus feels as if constricted from above down to stomach." Now, we have another phase of it. From the sore throat the trouble extends into the œsophagus, and the œsophagus is at first in a state of spasm. Later it is paralyzed. Fluids will at first go down the throat, but he cannot swallow a particle of solids. The bolus of food will go into the upper end of the œsophagus and there it chokes him and feels like a lump, and he chokes and struggles and gags and throws it back, and then takes water or fluids. He can swallow fluids but he cannot swallow solids. Every particle of solid food gags; but he can swallow liquids. *Natr. mur* and quite a number of other remedies have spasms of the œsophagus coming on with nervous complaints, but in this low state I know of no other medicine having that one symptom, having these features, and the paralysis, and the spasmodic condition of the œsophagus. "The œsophagus feels as if constricted from above down to the stomach." Constrictive feeling causing frequent efforts at deglutition; throat sore, feels constricted. *Can swallow only liquids.* Children cannot swallow solids. The smallest solid substance causes *gagging,* thus he cannot use anything but milk; sometimes, thin, watery, offensive passages day and night; associated with putridity, with the offensiveness, with the duskiness and with the prostration. You need to know no more, if it is diphtheria, or scarlet fever, if it is typhoid fever, that will lead you to a certain remedy. "Paralysis of the Organs of deglutition." To draw out from every remedy that which is positive, to get the associations that make up a particular remedy, and that only is the duty of every clinician.

The abdomen is distended; the stomach is distended. We may have these symptoms in inflammation of the liver, when this remedy would be useful. Along with the diseases that I have mentioned, tympanitic abdomen. Great soreness in the right iliac fossa; so sore and tender, no bigger than a fist; but all of this putridity, I am sure, would prevent you from using a knife to cut off that little appendix.

"Fœtid, exhausting diarrhœa. Aphthous diarrhœa;" which means that the parts of the anus that roll out are ulcerated, little aphthous patches inside of the margin. "Involuntary diarrhœa." Involuntary urine and Stool in these low forms of disease. "Dark brown, mucous and bloody stools. Fœtid stools." It has dysentery. After confinement the lochia stops. Great tenderness of the abdomen. All these putrid signs—breaking down of the blood, the appearance of the face, the sudden prostration, suddenly becoming stupid; and add to that the mental symptoms—these are all signs for Baptisia in puerperal fever. Now, intermingled with this after the case has been running on a few days the limbs become helpless and tremulous. The tongue when it is put out is tremulous. The hand when it is raised is tremulous, and the limbs are tremulous. Quivering all over the body. Prostration increases. The jaw drops and he lies upon the back unconscious, with the mouth wide open. He gradually slides down toward the foot of the bed. A peculiar sort of paralytic weakness. This is how the prostration increases with the disease; but even yet when he is as low as this, with the signs present, Baptisia will break that fever. Baptisia will stop the typhoid fever, when it is indicated. Prostration and trembling. Huddles down in bed, feels as if sinking away. Lies in a semi-conscious condition when she appears dying. Excessive drowsiness. Delirious stupor. Lies in a semi-comatose state. "Discharges and exhalations foetid." Breath, stool, urine, ulcers; all putrid. Ulceration of mucous membranes.

BARIUM IODATUM

Complaints come on in the morning; afternoon; evening; night; after midnight; strong desire for open air; better in open air; better in cold air. Takes cold easily; worse in cold, wet weather. Congestion of many parts. Convulsive action of muscles. Feels worse before eating and when fasting; worse after .eating; some symptoms are better after eating. Emaciation. Exertion aggravates most symptoms. Fainting spells. Formication all over the body. General sensation of fulness. Easy hemorrhage. Induration in many parts; in glands. Inflammation or congestion in internal organs; in glands. Lassitude; continued lying rests him. Lying on the back aggravates. Lying in bed increases some symptoms. Worse before and during menses. Motion increases the symptoms. Pain in bones and glands. Pressing, sore, stitching pains. Tearing in many parts; downward; in muscles. It suits the complaints of plethoric people. Pressure aggravates many symptoms. Pulsation all over body. Pulse fast; full; hard; small. Very sensitive to pain; glands sensitive. Swelling and inflammation of affected parts and of glands. Tension all over body. Touch aggravates. Trembling and twitching. Walking aggravates all symptoms. Worse from warmth in general; in a warm room; on becoming warm. Weakness; during menses. nervous; while walking.

Anger, anxiety and aversion to company. Concentration of mind difficult. Confusion of mind. Timidity even cowardly. Delusion; thinks he sees dead people. Illusions of fancy. Marked dullness of mind. Fear of evil and of people. Memory weak; very forgetful. She feels hurried and hysterical. Impatience. Irresolution; indolence; indifference. Talkative and irritable. Mental weakness marked. Alternation of moods. Marked restlessness. Sadness and weeping. Oversensitive to noise. Desire to sit and brood over events. Vertigo while lying, stooping; walking.

The head feels cold. Heat and hyperæmia of head evening and night. Heaviness of head. Pain in head; morning on rising; forenoon; afternoon; better or worse in open air; worse binding up the hair; from noise; while walking; warm room. Pain in forehead; right side; evening; above eyes; occiput, sides of head; temples. Bruised pain in head. Pressing pain in head; in forehead; over eyes; in occiput; temples; vertex. Shooting in occiput; stitching in head; occiput; sides of head; temples. Stunning pains. Tearing in vertex. Perspiration of scalp. Pulsation in forehead and temples.

Inflammation of conjunctiva. Tubercular iritis. Itching of eyes. Opacity of the cornea. Pain in eyes worse from light; aching; burning; pressing; as from sand; tender feeling. Photophobia; protrusion; pupils dilated. Redness of eyes and lids. Swollen lids. Vision dim; diplopia; flickering; foggy; sparks; weak.

Discharge of pus from ear. Sensation of flapping in ears. Noises in ears; when chewing; buzzing; fluttering; ringing; roaring. Tearing pain in ears. Stopped feeling in ears. Hearing acute for noise; impaired.

Catarrh of nose; discharge bloody; copious; hard mucus; thick; yellow; post nasal. Redness of nose. Dryness in nose. Fluent coryza with cough. Epistaxis on blowing nose. Obstruction of nose at night. Pain in nose; in root of nose. Frequent sneezing. The nose is swollen and red.

Coldness of face. The face is congested and red; the lips are blue; face sometimes pale and sometimes circumambient redness. Face looks drawn and shrunken. Emaciated. Eruption on face and nose; boils and pimples. Pain in face; in submaxillary gland. Swelling of glands of lower jaw; parotid glands; submaxillary gland.

Bleeding gums, cracked tongue. The gums are detached from the teeth and the teeth become loose. Dry mouth in morning; dry tongue. Mucus in mouth which is offensive, even putrid. Burning tongue; sore gums. Salivation. Swollen gums. Taste bad; bitter; sour. Drawing and tearing in teeth.

Throat dry and constricted. The tonsils are enlarged. Inflammation with marked swelling of tonsils. Membranous exudation in throat. Pain in throat on empty swallowing; burning. Swallowing difficult: Swollen and indurated glands of neck.

Appetite diminished; increased, even ravenous with emaciation; without relish of food; wanting, aversion to food. Emptiness. Eructations: empty; sour; waterbrash; ameliorate. Fulness and heartburn. Flashes of heat in stomach. Heaviness after eating. Indigestion with hiccough. Nausea and loathing of food. Inflammation of stomach. Pain in stomach after eating; cramping; gnawing; pressing; soreness; stitching. Retching. Feeling of tension in stomach. Thirst extreme; unquenchable. Vomiting bile; watery.

Distension of abdomen; enlarged mesenteric glands. Flatulence; rumbling. Pain in abdomen; after eating; before and during menses; in hypochondria; inguinal region; umbilical region; cramping; cutting; drawing; pressing in hypogastrium; stitching in hypochondria and sides of abdomen. Distension of abdomen.

Constipation; difficult stool; inactivity of rectum; insufficient stool; hard; knotty stool. Diarrhœa with yellow, watery stools, much flatus, external piles. Itching anus. Pain in rectum; burning after stool; tensesmus. Ineffectual urging to stool.

Retention of urine; constant; frequent. Urination frequent at night; involuntary. Enlarged prostate gland. Urine copious.

Induration of testes. Erections wanting. Seminal emissions. In the female the desire is increased. Leucorrhœa bloody; before menses. Menses copious; frequent; painful; short; suppressed.

Mucus in the trachea. Voice: hoarse; lost; rough, weak. Respiration fast; asthmatic; difficult at night and on ascending; rattling; short; suffocative.

Cough morning; evening; asthmatic; dry in morning; from irritation in larynx or trachea; rattling; spasmodic; suffocative; as talking; from tickling in larynx and trachea. Expectoration in morning and evening; difficult; mucus; purulent; salty; viscid; yellow.

Catarrh of chest. Constriction of chest. Inflammation of bornchial tubes; of lungs. Oppression of chest. Pain in chest; stitching in chest and in mammæ. Palpitation of heart; night; tumultuous. Paralysis of lungs. Swollen axillary glands.

Pain in sacrum; stitching pain in back and in lumbar region.

Cold hands, legs and feet. Hot hands. Heaviness of limbs. Itching limbs. Numbness of arms and fingers. Pain in joints; gouty; in hip; thigh; knees. Stitching in knees; tearing in knees and legs. Perspiration of hands; palms; feet. Weariness of knees.

Dreams: amorous, anxious; vivid.

BARIUM SULPHURICUM

The symptoms of this remedy appear in the *morning; forenoon;* afternoon; evening; *night;* after midnight. Desire for open air which ameliorates; the mental symptoms are better in the open air. There is a marked physical anxiety. Many symptoms show themselves or are worse on *exertion and ascending stairs.* Single parts become numb and prickle. Generally worse from bathing; in a close room; from cold; from cold air; from becoming cold; symptoms are worse after becoming cold; takes cold easily; there is a lack of vital heat; worse in cold, wet weather. Constriction of many parts. Clonic spasms and epileptic convulsions. The blood vessels are distended. Symptoms come on during and after eating; worse after eating to satiety. Emaciation; faintness and the muscles become flabby. Formication and a sensation of fulness. Induration of glands. Heaviness and lassitude. Inflammation of glands. Lack of reaction. Jerking in muscles. Desire to lie down. Symptoms come on before and during menses. Aversion to motion. Most symptoms are worse from motion. The patient feels worse from motion. Orgasm of blood in body. Pain in the bones; in glands; boring; burning; gnawing; jerking; pressing; stitching; tearing. Tearing in glands; tearing downwards. Paralysis, *one-sided;* of organs; painless; pressure aggravates the pain and many symptoms. Pulsation all over the body. Pulse feeble on motion. Rising up aggravates. Sensitiveness in external parts; to pain. Electric shocks felt in the body. It is a one-sided remedy; mostly *right-sided.* Sitting erect and standing cause some symptoms. Stiffness of muscles and joints. Swelling of glands. Tension felt all over body. Trembling in body and limbs. Walking brings on many symptoms. Walking in open air ameliorates. Weakness after eating; during menses; while walking.

Anxiety in the evening in bed; during the night; before midnight; with fear; WITH FEVER; about the future. Desires things which are not needed and soon put aside. She is very critical. Aversion to company. Concentration of mind impossible. Confusion in the morning; in the evening; better in the open air. Fear in the evening; in a crowd; of death; of evil; of people. Forgetful especially of words. Easily frightened. Always in a hurry and becomes hysterical after grief. Mentally weak like imbecility. Impatience, indifference, indolence and *loss of will power.* Irritability is very marked, but worse in the evening. Memory weak. Moaning and lamenting. *Suspicious* and dread of conversation. Bashful Talks in sleep. *Fainting spells;* unconscious. Weeping. worse at night. Aversion to mental work. Vertigo; objects turn in a circle; when standing; when walking.

The head is sometimes cold, again there is marked hyperæmia with cold feet. Constriction of forehead and occiput. Empty feeling in the head. Eruptions on the scalp; crusts; moist; pimples. Formication of the scalp and the hair falls out. Heaviness of the head in the evening; of the forehead; of the occiput. ITCHING OF THE SCALP. A feeling of looseness of the brain. A sensation of motions in the head. Pain in the head in the morning in bed; in the forenoon; in the afternoon; *in the evening;* better in the open air; worse from coughing; after eating; from becoming heated; from a jar; when lying; moving head and eyes; from *pressure;* shaking the head; after sleep; from sneezing; *when stooping;* in the summer; from heat of the sun; violent; when walking; worse in a warm room; better while walking in open air. Pain in forehead; in the evening; worse on the right side; above the eyes; in the occiput; in. the SIDES OF THE HEAD; in the temples; boring in forehead and temples; bursting in head and forehead; drawing in forehead, sides of head and temples; dull pain in head; jerking pain in head. Pressing pain in head; as though in a vise; *in forehead,* outward; over eyes; occiput; sides of head; temples; vertex. Shooting pain in head; in vertex. Sorebruised pain in head. *Stitching* pains in head; in *forehead;* in frontal eminence, in temples; in vertex. Stunning pains in head. Tearing pains in occiput. Perspiration on scalp. Pulsation in temples. Electric shocks in head.

The eyelids arc stuck together in the morning. It has cured cataract. Dryness of eyes. Inflammation of the conjunctiva, of the lids. Itching and lachrymation. It has cured opacity of the cornea. Pain in eyes on exertion of vision; WORSE FROM LIGHT; aching; burning on using eyes; burning in canthi; pressing; pain as from sand; tearing. Paralysis of optic nerve. *Photophobia.* Protrusion of eyes. It has cured exophthalmic goitre. Pupils dilated and insensible to light. Redness of eyes. Swollen lids. Black spots;. specks and flies before the eyes. *Dim vision. Exertion of vision aggravates. Foggy vision.* Sparks before the eyes. Weak vision.

Bloody discharge from ear. *Eruption behind ears.* Formication of ears; *Itching in ear.* Noises in ears; *buzzing;* cracking; crackling; fluttering; reverberations; *ringing.* ROARING. Pain in right ear; behind ear; drawing behind and in ear; *stitching in ear;* tearing pain in ear. Pulsation in ear. Twitching of ears. HEARING IMPAIRED.

Constant inclination to blow the nose. Fluent coryza with cough. Catarrh of the nose with discharge bloody; copious; crusts; hard lumps; offensive; thick; yellow. DRYNESS IN THE NOSE. Epistaxis on blowing the nose. The nose is often obstructed. Smell is acute. Much sneezing. The nose is swollen.

The face is cold. Convulsive twitching of face. The lips are dry and cracked. The face is pale or red. Eruptions on the face; forehead; nose; acne; boils; crustry; eczema; herpes; pimples. The face is red and hot. Pain in face; in *submaxillary gland.* Drawing pains in face. Swelling of face; *parotid gland;* SUBMAXILLARY gland; PAINFUL.

Bleeding gums. Cracked tongue. The gums are detached from the teeth. The tongue is coated white. Dry mouth and tongue in the morning. Mucus in the mouth. Offensive, even putrid odor from mouth. The tongue burns. Salivation. Speech difficult., Swollen gums. Taste is bad, bitter or sour. Burning vesicles in mouth and on tongue. Pain in teeth worse from cold things; cold drinks; after eating; from warm things; boring; drawing; stitching; tearing. Constriction in throat. Dryness in the throat. Enlarged tonsils. Hawking mucus from throat. Chronic inflammation of throat and tonsils. Liquids are forced into nose. Sensation of a lump in throat. The membrane of throat is covered with exudate and throat is full of viscid mucus. Pain in throat on *empty swallowing;* burning, stitching on swallowing. Roughness in throat. Spasms of the esophagus on swallowing. Swelling and suppuration of tonsils. Swallowing difficult; of solids. Induration of cervical glands. Pain in external throat. Swollen cervical glands. Tension in neck.

Appetite is variable; diminished; *ravenous;* easy satiety; *wanting.* Aversion to food. Sensation of coldness in stomach. Craves sweets. A sensation of *emptiness.* Eructations; after eating; bitter; empty; sour; watery; WATER-BRASH. Fulness in stomach even after eating so little. Heaviness after eating. Heat felt in stomach. Heartburn. Hiccough. Weak and slow digestion. Loathing of food. Nausea in the morning. Pain in stomach; after 'eating; cramping; gnawing; PRESSING AFTER EATING; tenderness; stitching; severe retching. Tightness. Thirst in the evening; unquenchable. *Vomiting;* bile, mucus, *sour,* watery. The abdomen is distended and flatulence and feels full. The abdomen is large and hard; the mesenteric glands are enlarged. Pain in abdomen in the morning, after eating; during menses; on motion; on pressure; after stool; in inguinal region; cramping; cutting; before stool; stitching in inguinal region and sides of abdomen; tearing; rumbling and tension. Constipation; inactivity of rectum; difficult stool; unsatisfactory stool; *hard, knotty stool.* Diarrhœa; worse at night from taking cold; yellow watery stools. Offensive flatus. Crawling and itching in rectum and anus. Bleeding from anus; from piles. *External piles.* Involuntary stool. *Constant moisture at anus.* Pain during and after stool; pressure; soreness; stitching; tenesmus. Constant or frequent ineffectual urging to stool. Ascarides in the stool.

Retention of urine. Urging to urinate; constant; *frequent;* sudden, must hasten to urinate or lose it. Dysuria. Urination frequent at night. Involuntary during the night. Urine copious at night. Discharge from urethra gleety; purulent. In the male there is no sexual desire and erections are wanting. Induration of testes. Sweat on the scrotum. *Seminal emissions.*

In the female desire is also absent. *Leucorrhœa;* smarting; copious,. before the menses. Menses *scanty;* frequent; protracted; suppressed. Burning of the vulva. Catarrh of the trachea with copious mucus. Voice: hoarseness; lost, rough; weak.

Respiration: accelerated; asthmatic; difficult at night and on ascending; *rattling;* suffocation.

Cough; morning after rising; evening; night; in cold air; in open air; in damp cold air; asthmatic; dry morning and evening; from irritation in larynx and trachea; rattling; spasmodic; suffocative; worse talking; from tickling in larynx and trachea; tormenting; whooping cough. Expectoration morning and evening; difficult; mucus; purulent; scanty; viscid; yellow.

Catarrh of chest with marked constriction and oppression. Pustules on the chest. A feeling of fulness in the chest. Chronic inflammation of the bronchial tubes. Itching of chest; of mammæ. Pain in the chest in evening. Soreness in the walls of chest. Pressing and stitching pains in chest. *Palpitation; night;* anxious tumultuous. Sowllen axillary glands.

Feeling of weight in the back. Itching of the back. Pain in the back; before and during menses; while sitting; in cervical region; in lumbar region in evening and before and during menses; in the sacrum; aching in back and especially in lumbar region; burning in spine and in lumbar region; drawing pain in lumbar region; stitching in back, in cervical and lumbar regions. Pulsation in lumbar region. Stiffness in the back; in cervical regions. Tension in back; in cervical region, lumbar region; sacrum. Weakness in lumbar region.

Cold hands and feet. The corns sting and burn and are sore and painful. Cracked hands and fingers. Cramps in the calf. The hands are very dry. Painful eruptions on the limbs; pimples. The hands are hot. Heaviness of upper and lower limbs. Itching limbs; upper; lower; thighs. Jerking of the lower limbs. Numbness of the upper limbs; hands; fingers. Pain in limbs; joints; upper limbs; shoulder; hands; hip; thigh; knee; leg; bruised limbs and joints; drawing in upper limbs, LOWER LIMBS; thighs and legs; stitching in knees; tearing pain in all the limbs; forearm; wrist; lower limbs; thighs; KNEES; legs; feet. Painless paralysis of upper limbs. Perspiration of hands, palms; offensive sweat of feet; suppressed foot sweat. Tension of thighs. Ulcers on legs; weakness of lower limbs.

Deep sleep. Dreams; anxious; frightful; of misfortune; vivid. Falling asleep late. *Restless sleep.* Sleepiness in afternoon; evening; after dinner. Sleeplessness before midnight with sleepiness.

Chill in the morning; forenoon; noon; afternoon; evening; night; chilliness in the open air; in the least draft; coldness in bed; external coldness; daily spells of coldness; shaking chill; one-sided chill; generally left-sided; coldness relieved in a warm room. Fever evening and night; alternating with chilliness; burning heat; flushes of heat. Perspiration after midnight; cold; while eating; offensive; on single parts; during sleep; on waking.

Burning skin at times; otherwise coldness; cracked skin. Pale skin; red spots Dry burning skin. Eruptions; burning, with yellow moisture; DRY; herpes; ringworm; itching; painful; eating; pimples; rash; scabby; worse after scratching place bare; after scratching; smarting; stinging; suppurating; tubercles; nodular; urticaria; vesicular; vesicles after scratching. Excoriation of the skin. *Formication.* Itching at night; itching; burning; *itching crawling;* unchanged by scratching; *itching stinging, in a warm bed.* Moisture of the skin after scratching. The skin is very sensitive. Stitching in the skin after scratching. Stinging in the skin. Tension. Small wounds slow to heal and often fester. WARTS; small stinging.

BARYTA CARBONICA

Baryta carbonica is an interesting study, because it is fully proved and a constitutional remedy. Such remedies are always more interesting than the short-acting, superficial ones. They take hold in deep-seated, long-lasting, miasmatic troubles. This remedy looks towards the development of the young. You will see in the text commonly expressed under this medicine, "dwarfishness". That does not always mean small in stature as it is spoken of in this remedy. Dwarfishness in body and mind; mental dwarfishness, and dwarfishness of organs. You realize what precocity means; young persons who arc unusually brilliant; well advanced mentally. We say they are beyond their years. They are precocious. Get this in mind first, and think what it means; and then in the Baryta carb. constitution we have the very opposite state. That is what we mean by dwarfishness. Children are late coming into usefulness; or activity; late with their studies; late learning to talk; late learning to read; late learning to make the combinations that enter into life; late learning to take in images, and form perceptions; to take on their activities; to do their work. We say sometimes that *Calc. carb.* is late in learning to walk, but Baryta carb. is also late learning to walk, although it has an entirely different cause. To express it in a common, old-fashioned way, Baryta carb. is late learning how to walk, even with pretty good limbs. *Calc.* has miserable, weakly limbs, flabby muscles, poor bones, and hence he is late learning to walk. "Late walking" is *Calc.* "Late learning to walk" is Baryta carb. It competes also with *Borax* and *Natium mur.* All three of these medicines have a peculiar kind of tardiness in the development of the brain, so that they are late learning to do things; late in developing. But Baryta carb. leads them all in this late coming into the activities and uses of life.

You will have patients to treat, where this slow development manifests itself in girls 18 to 25 years of age, who do the things they did when they were children, and say things as they said them when they were children. "Childish manner of doing things, and childish behavior. Playing with dolls and saying foolish things." They have not come into womanhood. They are late in taking on the activities and uses of the woman. They lack the prudence of the woman. They have not become circumspect, and say things just as a boy or just as a little girl would say them. That is the dwarfishness of the mind. To appreciate that late development, and to see it in Baryta carb. from all of its symptoms and peculiar features, leads to a remedies as *Graph.*, *Sulph.* and *Calc.*, but nothing compared to this remedy. This seems to suspend the development that makes the child into a man or a woman. It is not a small person that makes me think of Baryta carb., but the dwarfishness that is mental, and that is of organs. Oargans, as it were, become paralyzed, or one organ does not develop. It stops, and the others go on. That would make me think of this remedy. A single organ fails to mature, and the others go on; onesidedness, a partiality of development.

The next grand feature of this remedy is its affinity for the lymphatic glands all over the body. The glands all over the body enlarge and indurate; the glands of the neck, the glands of the groin, the lymphatics in the abdomen are all affected—knotty chains form in the neck. With a few other things that we will put together shortly we will see in this patient a peculiar figure It has emaciation—gradual dwindling in persons who have been fat, who have been well nourished. It has an enlarged abdomen. It has been found suitable in marasmus, for children with enlarged glands, enlarged abdomen; emaciation of the tissues, emaciated limbs and dwarfishness of mind; you have there the whole Baryta carb. marasmus.

The patient himself is chilly; sensitive to cold; wants to be well wrapped. Marked weakness with feeble pulse is a strong feature and he must lie down; he is worse standing and sitting. The weakness is worse after eating. His pains are better from motion and in the open air. His complaints are aggravated by cold. The enlarged glands take on tenderness and congestion from being exposed. The tonsils gradually increase. The glands of the neck increase in size, and in hardness, from every cold and from becoming chilled.

"Swelling and induration of glands. Inflammation of glands with infiltration." Infiltration belongs to the remedy. The glands become harder and harder. Ulcers become indurated in their base. Open surfaces become indurated in their walls. When a child has almost any disease, measles, scarlet fever, mumps, or even a bad cold, or a malarial attack, the development ceases and dwarfishness results, a state in which he was not born, but a state that he has acquired, arrest of development. It brings on emaciation and dwindling of the whole body, except the abdomen, which gradually enlarges. These are phases not to be overlooked in the very beginning, because the symptoms only help to establish this basis and these troubles and tissue changes come on as ultimates.

Another grand feature in this remedy is the application of these things to more advanced years. We say this is a childhood state, this is the state of youth and arrested development. Now it does not matter whether we have this arrested development in youth, in childhood, or at the advanced age of fifty. From some strange circumstance which we are not able to fathom we say the individual is taking on the appearance of old age. We call it premature old age. Baryta carb. has cured lingering complaints that have resulted from malaria, overwork, mental or physical, prolonged mental strain, when the appearance of premature old age was a prominent feature. Old age creeps upon him too soon. There is but little difference between childhood and old age, and hence old age is called second childhood; but we always regret to see a man under seventy becoming childish, and yet we do see many becoming simple and childish. It does not mean merely imbecility, but childlike behavior. Doing and saying things like a child. So in premature old age these symptoms lead us to think of Baryta carb.

Baryta carb. has cured fatty tumors, encysted tumors, lumps, outward growths of tuberculous character, sarcoma; and it has mitigated the pains and sufferings, and has prolonged life in cancerous affections.

Mentally it is worthy of careful study, and we will see cropping out in the mental symptoms all of the phases intermingled with tissue changes. The Baryta carb. child will be seen hiding behind the furniture when strangers come in; will hide as for shame of something, or as if afraid. It imagines all sorts of strange things, that it is talked about, or laughed at. It does not seem to advance. It does not seem to do any good to teach it, for it does the same things over and over and remains untrained. They either cannot comprehend, or they cannot memorize, or they cannot maintain a thought, and you go over it and over it, and the mother wonders if that child is ever going to learn something, and the teacher reports that the child lacks capacity. The teacher cannot comprehend it, the mother cannot comprehend it, but the homœopathic physician should know all about it at once. If he knows his Materia Medica he should he well up in the development of a feeble child; those who are going towards rickets, who are feeble, who are always depending on somebody, fitted only for menial places. The homœopathic physician does well when he trots the little Johnnies and the little Susies on his knee and takes a good, fair observation of their ability, and of what they lack, and understands how to build up what is lacking. Is not that in itself worth working for? It requires all of the potencies that have ever been made to master constitutions. Some will require medium potencies, some very low, some very high. Let us not deprive our little ones of anything they need. Only so we look forward to the highest use, to develop them into their fullest capacity.

There is an expression here in the text, "Want of clear consciousness." Do we not see from what I have said what that must mean in this remedy, and that it is different in this remedy from what it is in a good many others? And yet if you had read that symptom first you would not have appreciated it. "A want of clear consciousness." Especially in old age has that been useful. It is not that confusion of mind that we know to be dizziness. But he is not clear in his intellect. We see how this medicine takes hold of the intellect. It takes hold of his memory. It begins with a feeble state, and it gradually travels toward imbecility. You press it to its extreme and it has imbecility, and up to this we have degrees all along the line from the very beginning, from a mere matter of cloudiness in his thoughts to imbecility.

When the Baryta carb. babies appear in the clinic they will keep the hand up over the face and peek out through the fingers. Bashful. Timid. Easily frightened. Afraid of strangers. Other remedies have similar features, but it is a strong feature of this medicine. Withered face. Sickly countenance. It is the idea of hiding, the idea of timidity. The child does not want to play, and it sits in the corner. Does not pay any attention to its hammer, if it is a boy; or its doll, if it is a girl. Sits and sits. Does not seem to be thinking; a lack of ability to think. Children grow up without any distinctiveness, without any ability to perceive, and therefore fail to develop. Always borrowing trouble. Like *Caust.*, fear of something going to happen. Full of imaginations; imaginary cares and worries. Hatching up all sorts of complaints and grievances that may happen. A good deal like *Ars.* Children in a constant whining mood; always whining. Running through the complaints will be the sufferings of the parts, or the mental symptoms. "The more he thinks about the complaint the worse it gets." If he thinks about his troubles, his sufferings, they at once grow worse. Premature old age and brain-fag from prolonged mental work.

Troublesome headaches. "Pressure in the brain." A feeling of looseness in the brain, as if the brain fell from side to side or was rising and falling. A sensation of motion in the brain when moving the head or from sudden jar. Seems as if the brain moves to and fro to correspond to the motions of the head when the head is turned from side to side. "Pressing headaches." Headaches ameliorated in fresh air, in the open air, and aggravated from heat. That is the opposite of its general state. The Baryta carb. general state is agravated from cold; he is sensitive to cold, and his complaints wale on from becoming cold; but his headaches arc ameliorated in cool air. The Baryta carb. patient is often sensitive to the extremes of heat and cold. Hot weather will bring on complaints. Hot weather will cause the blood to mount to the head, and favors apoplectic conditions. It has many complaints of the head like unto the stupor of apoplexy. It has some of the paralytic conditions analogous to the complaints in old apoplectics, and it has been very useful in re-establishing the supply and flow of nerve force along the nerves. It parallels *Phos.*, and is an excellent remedy for old paralytic conditions that have come from a rupture of a blood-vessel, and therefore pressure upon the nerve supply. The headaches are congestive. pressive headaches; a feeling of pressure in the brain.

These puny infants, such as we have described, have eruptions upon the head; eczema upon the head; and those who are born for better things have the eruption driven back by ointments and applications. "Moist crusts upon the scalp." "Dry eruptions upon the scalp. Falling off of the hair. Baldness." Head complaints and a dwarfish state of mind. an intellectual defect, as results of suppressed eruptions.

It is full of eye symptoms. "Granular lids. 'Thickening of the eyelids; thickening of all of the membranes and tissues about the eyes. Opacity of the cornea." Infiltration of the various coverings. It has cured cataract, it has cured various kinds of dimsightedness, hut especially in those that have a hazy cornea, a slight opacity of the cornea (*Bar. iod.*) so that things look hazy, "looking as through a fog, or through smoke." Ulceration of the cornea. Little white spots, causing defective vision. "Lids agglutinated in the morning." Styes. "A sensation of weight in the upper lids." A sensation of weight in the brow with headaches as if the forehead was pressing down over the eyes. Like *Carbo veg., Carbo an.* and *Natr. mur.* The patient will often grasp the whole forehead with the hands, and say, "I feel as if the forehead was pressing down over the eyes."

It has many noises in the ears, but especially cracking and flapping when breathing, swallowing and chewing; better while lying. If affects the right ear most. Rushing sounds in the ears when breathing. "Eruptions about the ears. Glandular swelling and eruptions about the ears." Inflammation of the parotid glands, with hardness. First it may be called swelling, but it is finally a permanent enlargement and induration, and it means a great growth sometimes. Other glands about the neck are affected in association with the ear troubles. Knots of lymphatic glands down the neck under the ear (*Bar. m., Tub.*). Sometimes the sub-maxillary gland is affected, being enlarged and indurated. Sometimes the tonsils enlarge and indurate. All these glands inflame and become sensitive, and get a little larger, after any exposure to cold, and from sudden changes of the weather. It is a wonderful medicine for the cure of enlarged glands. Clinically it is laid down in the books for suppuration of these glands, but all my life I have failed to find it a good remedy for suppuration. The inflammation is more likely to turn into an increased infiltration. It is laid down in the books here for suppuration of the tonsils, but from long experience it is one of the last remedies I would think of for suppuration of the tonsils. It may have done so, but it has not been my observation that it runs that way, and I am very much in doubt about the great value and high marking of that observation. But it certainly has infiltration gradually increasing from becoming cold. The enlarged tonsils will redden up and inflame and become painful, and the acute inflammation and pain will subside, but the tonsils arc a little larger than with the last cold. In that way the tonsils keep growing. In children these are often cut out. There are instances in which I might admit it was necessary to cur them off, when there is a wonderful superabundance, creating much disturbance in swallowing and in speaking. Two or three times I have absolutely failed to cure with remedies selected to the best of my ability, and they have gone to the surgeon and he has cut them off; but I believe these tonsils ought to be all cured. One thing in Homœopathy taught in Hahnemann's Organon is that unless there are symptoms to indicate the remedy, no great things should be expected from the administration of the remedy. The enlargement of the tonsils alone is not a symptom upon which a remedy can be selected, and it necessitates guessing a dozen times, and perhaps not hitting at all. That is the worst sort of practice, guessing at a remedy; yet there are children having enlarged tonsils that appear to us without any symptom whatever to select a remedy by. The symptoms to prescribe on are such as represent the patient, not the glands; not the changed tissue. We must always regret that the surgeon must come in, for in cutting off anything it may be done to the constitutional detriment of the patient. Yet there are things that have to be done that we know are to the constitutional detriment of the patient. We have to keep servants on their feet to earn their living, and operations have to be performed upon them, because they cannot lie up a year or two to be cured. The surgeon will always have a place with us, but let us do our part as physicians first.

Eruptions upon the face. The face is sickly, often purple, red and bloated, or lean and emaciated, looking old and withered. The infant looks like a little old person, like the state we find in *Nat. mur.* and *Calc.* With face troubles, with teeth troubles, and especially with throat troubles, enlarged glands under the jaw and down the neck. Ear diseases following scarlet fever. Enlargement and induration of the parotids and of the sub-maxillary glands after scarlet fever. Scarlet fever often stirs up much trouble in the economy, especially when it has not been properly treated, when it has been treated by the allopath, or by a nervous homœopath. A nervous homœopath is one who does not wait for his own convictions to be ultimated, does not wait for his remedy to work, and he gives another and another, and by the time the scarlet fever runs its course the patient becomes dreadfully sick, ends up with ear troubles, enlarged glands and sometimes kidney affections. When it runs into ear troubles and enlarged glands of the neck this is one of the several remedies to be studied.

"Paralysis of the tongue in old people. Weakness of the tongue in old people. Hardness of the tongue in old people." Premature old age and giving out of muscles.

There is a catarrhal state in this remedy, an accumulation of mucus in the nose, throat, larynx and trachea. It is very suitable for old people who have rattling in the trachea. On every cold change of the weather, and on every exposure to the cold, he gets an additional aggravation of the rattling. Rattling respiration. There are a few remedies that have, in such high degree, this coarse rattling in the chest of old people, that it is well to emphasize it. Baryta carb. is one of them. *Senega, Ammoniacum* and *Baryta muriatica* should be compared. When there is coarse rattling in the chest all the time in an old person, an octogenarian, who is pretty comfortable in summer, but miserable all winter from the coarse rattling in the chest, and there are no other symptoms, *Ammoniacum* will keep him comfortable.

The sore throat in this remedy has numerous symptoms. "Inflammation of cellular tissues of fauces and tonsils." This remedy is one in general catarrhal' symptoms of the throat. Granulations of the throat, so that the pharynx looks shiny, studded with coarse granules becoming inflamed with every cold spell, or from being chilled. Every cold change inflames the tonsils, and in children they very soon enlarge. Children with enlarged tonsils, and with enlarged glands in other places, somewhat dwarfish intellectually, slow to learn—Baryta carb. will cure the enlarged tonsils. But these, you see, are constitutional symptoms. You are not selecting the remedy purely on enlarged tonsils. "Inflammation of the tonsils." The inflammation is not so violent as that which comes in *Bell.*, it does not come on in a night, it does not go on rapidly to suppuration; but it is a very sore throat, has come on slowly after many days of exposure and there is gradual growth and gradual development. That is the character of the Baryta carb. tonsillitis; while that of *Bell.* comes on with great rapidity. *Hepar* is also rapid and goes on to suppuration. There is a remedy for inflammation of the tonsils where the ear is involved and is ameliorated by heat, that very few use, but it is of great value, it is *Chamomilla,* and it is especially indicated if the patient is irritable. The pain is ameliorated by heat and comes on with great violence. It might he mistaken for a *Bell.* inflammation, but *Cham.* cures it permanently. "Sensation of plug in the throat;" that is, the tonsils are so large they feel like a great ball or great lump in the throat. They change the character of the voice, cause difficulty. "Much burning in the throat. Inability to swallow anything but liquids." This irritation keeps up a constant choking and spasmodic constriction in the throat; contractions, and drawings, and crampings in the throat. It also has a spasm in the œsophagus when swallowing, especially in old nervous, or prematurely broken-down people. "Spasm in the œsophagus. Difficulty in swallowing." The bolus of food goes down a little way, and then causes spasms, and he gags and chokes. This gagging and choking with a little food is a very strong feature in *Kali c., Graph.* and *Merc. cor.* This is also a strong feature of Baryta carb., but much stronger in *Merc. cor.*

The troubles of eating and drinking and appetite and stomach can all be run together. *There is weakness* of *digestion.* All sorts of disorders and disagreeable sensations in the stomach after eating. Sometimes gastralgia; sometimes distension. "Stomach aches after eating." Extreme weakness after eating. Abdomen hard and tense. "Mesenteric glands swollen and hard; with a big belly; abdominal muscles sore to touch." It has cured, in the early stages, tabes mesenterica. It has cured the enlarged abdomen of children, when there was emaciation of the limbs, emaciation everywhere, knots of enlarged glands and a dwarfed intellect.

Baryta carb. has an inveterate constipation. "Difficult, knotty stools. Stool hard, and insufficient." A lack of action in the rectum, and hæmorrhoidal protrusion during stool and urination.

Of the male sexual organs we have some strange features. This medicine takes away all sexual desire and ability, leaving the genitals relaxed, and in a state of impotency. "Relaxed penis. Impotence. Diminished sexual desire. Hypertrophied prostate. Atrophied testicles." It cures old gleety discharge from the urethra. An old, painless, whitish, gleety discharge that has been in existence a long time. It is an offensive discharge and there is no inflammation. "Numbness of the genitals."

The female has many troubles. Sterility. Dwindling of the ovary. Dwindling of the mammary glands, and yet the lymphatics become enlarged and infiltrated. A passive leucorrhœal discharge, whitish, thick, persistent, often copious, worse about a week before the menstrual period.

With some a constitutional weakness takes hold of the larynx; a paralytic weakness. Voice entirely lost. Or, "hoarseness and huskiness." Low, deep voice. Aphonia from constitutional weakness, and from paralysis. Feeling in the larynx all the time as if inhaling smoke, or pitch, or sulphur fumes, or dust. With the hoarseness there is a chronic dry, hoarse, barking cough; not a hard cough, but it comes every night. Suffocative cough of old people. It says here, "impending paralysis of the lungs." That is in keeping with the general nature of the remedy. Chest full of mucus, but unable to expectorate it. You observe from the effort made in the cough that there is a weakness somewhere, a lack of power. It is not a strong effort. "Night cough, with asthmatic breathing." Cough excited by irritation in the larynx and trachea. There is a cough in Baryra carb. where he coughs and coughs. and gets no relief until he lies on the abdomen; and so long as he lies on the abdomen he is free from cough. Palpitation from slight exertion when lying on the left side when thinking about it, with anxiety and orgasm of blood, with strong pulsation in the head, rapid pulse. Palpitation in chlorotic girls.

"Tension in the muscles of the back. Swelling of the glands of the back of the neck." Swelling of the cervical glands. "Fatty tumors upon the back." A number of times a patient has said, "Doctor, did you intend to take away that fatty tumor I had on my back?" The chances are I did not know he had one. That is generally the way such things appear in the practice of the homoeopathic physician, for he does not prescribe for the tumor, and the chances are he thinks little about the tumor in his prescription; he gives the constitutional medicine, and they often disappear after a while, and then the patient thinks the doctor has done a wonderful thing. He gets more glory and more credit for curing a wart than he does for curing the patient. The doctor who prescribes correctly turns the vital state into order. He cures the patient, and the patient, being in a state of order, commences to repair his body, and the tissues go through a general house cleaning, and such things as are not needed are dispensed with; and the physician is considered a wonderful man. So this remedy cures tumors and warts. Warts upon the limbs, and upon the back, and upon the hands.

The pains are of a gouty, rheumatic character, worse from becoming cold and from cold weather. Paralytic weakness and trembling and numbness of the feet. Offensive perspiration of the feet which causes soreness of the soles, ulcers on the feet, checkd foot sweat. Trembling of the feet while standing and tottering while walking. Tearing, drawing pains in lower limbs. Sudden sharp pains in knees.

BARYTA MURIATICA

This is one of our deep acting constitutional remedies and one much neglected. It was much used by the earlier men in our school with great effect. In mental weakness, insanity, enlarged glands and sexual excitement we have a group of symptoms hard to cure without Baryta muriatica. Add to this profound increasing muscular weakness and we must have this remedy sometime during the case or die cure will be slow. Its complaints are prominent in the *morning,* forenoon, afternoon, evening, *night* and after midnight. In the diseases most amenable to this remedy are the affection of the lymphatic glands and other glands. The patient desires the open air, yet the open air often increases the symptoms. Many cases of aneurism have been benefited by it. General physical anxiety is a strong feature. Complaints are worse ascending stairs such as dyspnœa, palpitation and weakness. Dread of bathing, like *Sulphur.* The symptoms are often worse in cold air and from becoming cold. The convulsive tendency is a very important feature; convulsions with headache, deafness, vomiting and burning in the stomach; convulsions with full consciousness with electric shocks; clonic spasms. It has cured most stubborn cases of epilepsy. Distension of the blood vessels; emaciation, fainting spells. Complaints worse in fall and spring. Formication all over the body. Sensation of internal fulness. Bleeding from mucous membranes and from ulcers. Heaviness externally and internally as from weakness and relaxation. Induration of glands; inflammation and swelling of glands. Extreme lassitude, compelled to lie down. Symptoms come before and during menses. Some symptoms are better from motion; bruised feeling internally; burning in many parts; cutting pains in internal parts; digging pains are not uncommon; gnawing in external parts. Painless symptoms predominant and pain is the exception. Convulsive jerking in the limbs; stitching in glands and along nerves; downward tearing as if in the muscles; one-sided paralysis; left side. Many parts are tender to pressure. Pulsation in abdomen and limbs. Pulse fast; 120; full, hard, small. Rising up brings on many symptoms. *Electric shocks with convulsions.* Complaints left-sided—worse while sitting; must lie down. Symptoms come on during sleep—worse while standing. Painful swelling of glands, Dropsical swelling after scarlet fever; tension, trembling, twitching; weakness in whole body. can hardly move a limb; while walking; general muscular weakness; paralytic weakness; weariness. Complaints and symptoms grow worse in wet weather. It is the natural complement of *Conium* in glandular affections and it is very similar, but much deeper acting.

Easily angered. Anxiety in the evening; about the future; with nausea; retching and pressure in the stomach. It is useful in children who are slow to learn or understand; children do not desire to play like other children. Concentration impossible. The locality around him seems strange, transformed; timid and cowardly; delusion that he walks on his knees. Dullness of mind. Thinks she is going to die. Fear: of evil, of men; foolish behavior; idiocy; imbecility, indifference, insanity; erotic insanity. Insanity where the sexual excitement becomes strong. Irresolution. Irritable in the evening. *Mania in every form when sexual desire is increased;* nymphomania. Sadness in the morning; sits in silence. Children sit in the corner and give confused answers. Easily startled; suspicious; indisposed to talk; talks in sleep; unconsciousness; fainting; vertigo when walking; things turn around.

The scalp feels constricted. It is a remedy of great usefulness in eruptions of the scalp. Thick, offensive crusts; eczema of the whole top of the head, extending to sides and occiput; suppurating with copious pus. Crops of pimples. The head feels so heavy he cannot keep up; heaviness of forehead and occiput; sensation of looseness of the brain; a feeling of movement in the head. Pain in the head in the morning on rising; afternoon evening, worse in open air; from binding up the hair; after eating, while lying; on moving the eyes; from noise; from pressure; on stooping; while walking; in the forehead, occiput, sides of head, temples; boring in temples; bruises in head; burning in head; pressing in head and in forehead; outwards; stitching in forehead, occiput, sides of head, in temples stunning pain in head; tearing in occiput, sides of head; shocks in head, ulcers on scalp.

Agglutination of the lids in the morning; discharge of mucus and pus from the eyes; inflammation of the eyes in scrofulous patients. Itching and smarting, pressing pain in eyes; paralysis of upper lids; photophobia; pupils dilated and immovable. Redness of the eyes; of the lids; veins injected; stiffness of the eyes; ulceration of the cornea; swollen lids; complaints of the eyes and head from exertion of vision, much like Corium; dim vision with flickering.

Abscesses behind both ears; discharge from both ears; copious; offensive; like spoiled cheese; purulent; after scarlet fever. Eruptions on ears; recurrent inflammation of the ear; auditory canal; itching in the ear; noises in the ear on chewing and on swallowing; catarrh of the Eustachian tube; buzzing, ringing and roaring; pain in both ears; deep in; worse in the right ear; pain in the ear with sore throat; worse lying on the painful side; better from cold drinks; drawing, stitching, tearing pain in ear; tearing behind ear; pulsation in ear; tingling of the ears; twitching; hearing impaired, finally lost.

Catarrh of the nose with copious, thick, yellow discharge; coryza fluent with fever; dryness in the nose; epistaxis. Itching in the nose; the nose is obstructed; rawness in the nose. A red nodule on the side of the top of the nose; stitching pains in the nose. Frequent sneezing; sneezing in sleep without waking.

The face is red with fever, otherwise pale. Drawing and spasms of the face. Dryness of the lips. Enlarged and indurated submaxillary gland with otorrhœa; eruption on forehead and nose; crusty, pimples, expression is anxious and the face is hot. Inflammation of the right parotid gland after scarlet fever; swelling of the glands of neck and jaw; very hard; right parotid; submaxillary. Tension of the face with nausea and diarrhœa.

Bleeding gums. Cracked tongue; white tongue. Dryness of the mouth in the morning, of the tongue; coated tongue; viscid mucus fills the mouth and covers the tongue; odor from mouth offensive; putrid; like from mercury. Burning in the mouth; the gums are sore. Paralysis of the tongue. Salivation with every paroxysm. Speech difficult. Swollen gums and palate. Taste is bitter; putrid, sour, sweetish; food tastes putrid. Ulceration of tongue. Looseness of the teeth with salivation; pulsating pain in the teeth. Compelled to sit up in bed; worse after midnight and after sleep; jerking; stitching, tearing.

Inflammation of the throat and tonsils; recurrent tonsillitis from taking cold; dryness in throat. Enlarged tonsils; elongation of the uvula with sore throat; viscid mucus in the throat; pain in the throat and ear, worse on right side; with salivation; worse on swallowing; burning in the throat. Suppuration of the tonsils. Swallowing very difficult. Swollen tonsils. Varicose veins in the throat. Swelling and induration of the cervical glands.

Appetite ravenous; wanting; aversion to food. Desires dry wheat bread. Distension of the stomach. A feeling of emptiness in the stomach. Eructations after eating; bitter; water.

Flushes of heat rise from the stomach to the head. Fullness and weight in the stomach after solid food; heartburn, hiccough. He can eat only the simplest food, as digestion is slow and the stomach is feeble; inflammation of the stomach; loathing of food; nausea. Pain in the stomach; cramping; pressing after eating; sore; stitching. Retching. Tension. Thirst with dry tongue; during chill; extreme. Vomiting in the morning; with headache; incessant, bile, blood, mucus, watery, with purging and great anxiety.

Distension of the abdomen. Enlarged and hard liver and mesenteric glands.
Flatulence; fullness: hard abdomen. Pain in abdomen in the morning, after
eating; before stool, in hypochondria, burning, cramping, cutting, stitching
in hypochondria and inguinal region. It has been of great benefit in abdominal
aneurisms. Swollen liver; swollen inguinal glands after suppressed
gonorrinœa. Abdominal tension. Ulcers in the inguinal region.

Constipation; difficult stool; no desire for stool; stool hard and covered
with mucus; generally painless. Diarrhœa which is also generally painless.
Dysentery, bloody mucus; jelly-like stools; frequent; generally painless. Much
offensive flatus. Hæmorrhage from rectum and from intestines. External piles,
protrude during urination; itching of the anus; involuntary stool; moisture
about the anus; some pain in the rectum during stool; burning during and
after stool; pressing pain; soreness, stitching; tenesmus. Paralysis of the
rectum and of the sphincter ani. Stool bloody, jelly-like, hard, green, fœtid,
soft, thin, watery, white and hard; yellow and slimy; worms with stool.

Inflammation of the bladder. Retention of urine. Urging to urination;
constant, frequent, ineffectual, violent. Urination difficult; frequent at night;
frequent during perspiration; involuntary during the night. Gleety urethral
discharge. It has cured chronic gonorrhœa. Pain the urethra during urination.
The urine is hot, copious, offensive, with whitish sediment; watery, yellow,
with great stench.

Enlarged testes. Induration of testes; inflammation of testes from suppressed gonorrhœa; seminal emission; sexual passion greatly increased, even
violent. Induration of the ovaries. Leucorrhœa. Menses copious, too often,
painful. Pain in the uterus. Sterility.

Catarrh of the larynx and trachea; irritation in larynx and trachea; tickling
in the larynx. Voice is hoarse, husky and weak. Respiration is fast, anxious,
asthmatic, deep, difficult, with cough, and she must sit up; rattling short.

Cough in daytime, morning, evening, night, before midnight; asthmatic,
dry, *chronic dry cough of scrofulous children; from irritation* in larynx and
trachea; rattling, whooping cough. Expectoration in the morning; mucous;
copious; muco-purulent expectoration from bronchial tubes; yellow. It has
cured phthisical conditions of the chest with herpetic eruptions and indurated
testes. Marked palpitation. It has been a very useful remedy in spinal
curvature.

Cold hands and feet; cramps in the toes; drawing up the limbs ameliorates. Eruptions on the limbs; pimples. Hot hands. Heaviness of the whole
body, must lie down. Itching of the limbs; the thighs. Painless jerking of the
arms at night. Violent periodical jerking of the limbs with convulsions.
Lassitude; numbness of the fingers. Pain in the upper limbs and thighs.
Paralysis of the left side; paralysis of the lower limbs. Perspiration of the

feet; suppressed foot sweat. Pulsation of the shoulder. Swelling of the hands,
lower limbs, knees, feet. Tension in knees. Trembling of the limbs Twitching
of the upper limbs, thighs, feet. Ulcers on the legs. Weakness of the limbs.

Dreams; amorous, anxious, frightful, of misfortune, pleasant, vivid.
Restless sleep; sleepiness; afternoon, evening, after dinner; sleepless before
midnight; frequent waking.

Coldness in the morning; evening; in bed; chilliness; external chill; shaking chills every third day. Fever in the evening and during the night; burning
heat; heat with chilliness; dry heat all day; dry heat during the night.

Dryness, biting and burning in skin; cold skin; eruptions; eczema; herpes
all over body; pimples; scabs, yellow scales; stinging, urticaria; erysipelas,
formication, horripilation. Inflammation of skin. Itching. Swelling and tension.
Whole body covered with small ulcers. Unhealthy skin. Burning ulcers.

BELLADONNA

Belladonna is a remedy that takes hold of the system with great violence.
It is especially suitable to plethoric, vigorous individuals and intellectual
people. Brainy people have complaints coining on suddenly, providing they
are in a substantial state of health, and are reasonably plethoric and vascular.
The complaints of Belladonna come on suddenly, run a regular course, and
subside suddenly. The pains and suffering conic on suddenly and with great
violence, and subside suddenly. Colds ultimate rapidly, run a sharp course, a
course of great violence, and subside suddenly. Belladonna especially affects
the whole vascular system, the heart, lungs, brain and nervous system.

Among the earliest conditions to examine is the heat. It has inflammations of all the organs, especially the brain, lungs, and liver. The intestines
are also involved as well as the other organs. These inflammations arc always
attended by *violent heat;* the heat is something unusual. It is more marked in
Belladonna than in almost any other remedy. When you put your hand upon
a Belladonna subject you will suddenly withdraw it, the heat is so intense.
The memory of the heat is carried in the hand and fingers for some time.
Pains, inflammations, and sufferings, nightly attacks of delirium, violent
attacks inflammatory in character are attended with that kind of heat. No
matter where the inflammation is, there is that same intense heat. There are
times, though, when that kind of heat is present, and it is not Bell., and that
is when the fever is of the continued type. Bell. has no continued fever in it.
It is true the older books tell you about Bell. for this violent heat in typhoid
and some other continued fevers, but if you examine Bell. from beginning to
end you will find nothing continued in its fever. Its fever is remittent. It never

comes on in its complaints gradually like typhoid. It has not the gradual rise
and the gradual fall like a continued fever. I only mention that so that you will
not be lost. Our lamented Hering, one of the ablest teachers the world ever
had, classes Bell. for typhoid fever when the delirium and the heat are
somewhat like Bell. but let me tell you just what will take place. When you
give Bell. for the delirium in typhoid fever—for such a delirium as looks like
Bell.you may subdue the delirium, but other manifestations will rise in that
fever. You will not subdue the fever, but you will subdue the patient. The
patient will be sick longer, will go into a greater state of prostration than if
you had let that delirium alone. But *Stramonium* fits perfectly Hering's
description of a case in which he says Bell. should be given. The idea of that
heat must be well fixed in the mind. *Heat, intense heat, violent heat.*

There is another phase of Bell. that runs all through these inflammatory
complaints and its fevers. The inflamed parts, and very commonly the skin,
are *very* red, and, as the inflammation advances, grow dusky, as the fever
advances the face becomes mottled; but the first representation of Bell. is
bright red, and the skin is shiny. An inflamed part that can be seen will be red.
In inflammation of glands the skin over the glands will be bright red in spots.
Hence red spots in the neck over inflamed glands. Inflammation of the parotid
glands, inflammation of the sub-maxillary glands, inflammation of the glands
of the neck—there will be a spot as red as fire over each. The throat is as red
as scarlet. The mucus membrane is inflamed, and red as scarlet. After a little
it grows dusky, finally mottled; showing the character and direction of the
Bell. constitution. It travels gradually towards a zymotic state, such as we
see in scarlet fever, in low inflammatory conditions; at first intense congestion,
but vaso-motor paralysis follows. Intense congestion and blueness, or purple
and mottled.

Another grand feature of Bell. is present in its inflamed parts, and in its
painful parts. Whenever Bell. brings out anything like a decided action, it
has *burning;* intense burning. The burning in the throat with a Bell. sore
throat is like a coal of fire. Inflammation of the tonsils, burning like fire. The
skin burns, and it is burning hot to the sensation of the patient, and intensely
hot to the doctor. The skin burns in scarlet fever. He says, "It burns so,
doctor, it burns so;" in bilious or remittent fever. In inflammation of an organ,
the skin burns, there is a burning fever,, and the part itself burns. Inflammation
of the bladder, with burning. Congestion of the brain, and the head burns.
Congestion of the throat, and the throat burns. It is hot locally, and it also
burns subjectively. In gastritis there is burning. In inflammation of the liver,
the liver burns. Congestion of the liver with jaundice, and the liver burns.
Now, we have three leading features: do not call them "key notes," for that is
not what I mean; *heat, redness and burning.* We will see how they modify

the whole feature of the sickness, how they permeate and ramify, and how they take meaning.

But, that is not all. We have much *swelling* in Bell. The inflamed parts swell rapidly; are extremely sensitive to touch; are very painful, with the sensation as if they would burst, with pressive pains, stinging and burning. There is heat, redness and burning in these inflamed parts, as well as swelling. Swelling, stinging, burning, throbbing. All over he *throbs*. With all congestions and inflammations he throbs. The part itself throbs, and his carotids throb. When children are sick in bed with congestion of the brain, they have an intensely hot head. If old enough to talk about it, they will say "it burns." But then we will notice the throbbing. The temporal arteries and the carotids pulsate, with great violence. A turmoil is going on. An earthquake is taking place. Everything is being shaken when the patient needs Bell. It is one of the most painful of remedies. It is so sensitive to Pain. So sensitive that he suffers more than ordinary people do from the pain. And, remember, *the pains come suddenly,* they remain longer or shorter, and *they go suddenly.* They do this in neuralgia; they do this in inflammatory conditions; they do it in inflamed organs; they do it wherever they come. Pains, tear, shoot, burn, and sting, and press, and smart, all at once. All of these characteristics are bundled up into one bundle, so that he suffers. All of his pains are worse from motion, worse from light, worse from a jar, worse from cold. He wants to be wrapped up warmly, and is worse from any exposure or a draft. The headaches are like many of the other pains; it feels as if the brain was going up and down, tearing and burning at every step he takes, and from every motion of the eyes, or turning the eyeballs, or going up stairs, rising from his seat, or sitting down; all motion creates violent pains; feels as if the head would burst, as if the eyes would be pressed out. If he moves he starts the heart to pulsate on his sore parts and he calls them "hammering pains." Wherever that pain is he cannot have it touched. If it is touched it will throb. If uncovered it will become worse. If some one walks across the floor, the jar makes him worse. *The jar of the bed,* if he is in bed, is a common aggravation of Bell. If he is so sick that he is in bed, *the jar of the bed* makes all of his complaints worse. You go to the bedside of a patient suffering from an inflamed liver, and he will not let you put your hand on the bed, for the jar makes him worse. If the pain is in the abdomen; if it is an inflamed uterus; if it is in confinement, it is the same. This aggravation from the jar is such a marked feature that it is not always confined to inflammations. It is often a modifier in a state of nervous hyperaesthesia. A woman in confinement, when there is no inflammation, and none threatening, is in such a state of hyperaesthesia that she wants the windows closed to keep the air out; she does not want to be touched; she does not want the bed moved, any little jar aggravates; she is so sensitive to a jar, even when there is no sensitive part. You go to , such a case, and you will realize in time that you are going to have a difficult and painful labor, without Bell. But with a dose of Bell. all of these complaints pass away quickly, so quick is the action of this medicine. The jar of the bed will often reveal to you the nature of the remedy. If you walk to the bedside of a patient suffering from gallstone colic, with violent pains, he cannot have the bed touched. His face is red, his skin burns, he cannot be touched, he is in excruciating agony, and he tells that before you have crossed the room. You see it all. He says, "Don't touch the bed, doctor." That is a special feature; the aggravation from a jar is marked.

Spasms—general spasms and local spasms. Spasms of little canals, of the circular fibres, of tubular organs, like that I have spoken of in the gall-stone colic. In the ductus communis choledochus there is a clutching—or it may be in the cystic duct that the circular fibers clutch that little bit of stone and will not let it through. The passage is large enough to admit it and it has started to go through—but the irritation of the part causes a spasm and it clutches that little stone. You put a dose of Bell. on his tongue, the spasm lets up, stone passes on, and there is no more trouble; in fifteen minutes the gallstone colic is gone. There is never a failure in homœopathic prescribing in gallstone colic. The symptoms are not always Bell., but in this instance, where that horrible sensitiveness is present, it is Bell.

"Convulsions in infants." They are violent and are usually associated with cerebral congestion. The skin is always in a state of fever. They are brought on from light, from a draft of cold air, from the infant becoming cold. Nervous, brainy children, those with a good sized head and plump, large-headed boys; boys especially, but also girls that have boys' heads, when exposed to the cold have convulsions. Light, motion and cold will bring on these convulsions. The Bell. subject as an individual, like *Bry.,* is worse in all his complaints from motion. Motion brings on convulsions, motion brings on pain; motion increases the action of the heart and brings on throbbing; motion brings on many complaints and increases the sufferings. Now think of these generals whenever you come to Bell. This idea of Bell. must prevail. No matter how many little symptoms you accumulate, get at these first.

The mental symptoms of Bell. are delightful to study, but dreadful to look upon. The mental symptoms are such as come on in intense fevers, such as are observed in maniacal excitement, in delirium. Excitement runs all through. Violence runs all through the mental symptoms. The mental symptoms are all active, never passive. There is no passive delirium in Bell. It is a wild state. He is wild; striking, biting, tearing things; doing unusual things; doing strange things; doing unexpected things. He is in a state of excitability. These mental symptoms that come on during fevers, the delirium and excitement, are very commonly ameliorated by eating a little light food. That is not generally known in Bell., but it is quite a strong feature. But remember the violence, and with it, if you go to the bedside where there is this violent delirium, keep in mind the *heat, redness and burning.*

Full of imaginations. Sees ghosts, and spirits, and officers, and wild things. In the early part of the fever the delirium is very violent and excitable; but as it passes on he goes into a sleep, a sort of half-slumber, a semi-comatose state. Apparently in a dream, and he screams out. Dreams horrible things. Sees in his dreams the things that he talks about. When he has real sleep, or resting, as near as it is for him to rest, he has violent dreams; night-mare. Sees things on fire. He is in a delirium, and in torment. He becomes stupid at times, appears to lose consciousness. Loses the memory of all things and then becomes wild. His delirium goes on when he appears to be sleeping. These symptoms often occur with cerebral congestion, the violent cerebral congestion of the infant. If they are old enough to talk they will talk about the hammering in the head. in Bell. the infant also commonly remains in a profound stupor, the profound stupor that goes with congestion of the brain; pupils dilated; skin hot and dry; face red, throbbing carotids. Finally the child becomes pale as the stupor increases and the neck is drawn back, because as it progresses the base of the brain and spine become involved, and the muscles of the neck contract, drawing the head backwards, and he rolls the head; eyes staring, pupils dilated. This mental state is associated with scarlet fever and with cerebrospinal meningitis.

Again, these mental states take the form of acute mania, when the patient will bite the spoon; will bark like a dog; will do all sorts of violent; things; even jump out of the window. He has to be restrained, put in a strait-jacket. The face is red and the skin is hot, and the patient at times says that he burns all over, or that the head burns, and the head is very hot. During all this time the feet are cold. Head hot, feet cold, or feet and hands cold as ice. It seems all the blood is being hurried to the head. All sorts of delusions and hallucinations are mingled with the acute mania; ghosts; horrid monsters; strange things, and deformed subjects. Fear of imaginary things, and wants to run away. In the delirium of Bell. he wants to jump out of the window, wants to run, wants to get away from his attendants. He thinks they are doing him injury. Throughout the acute mania, and throughout the delirious state, all the manifestations partake of violence. Destructiveness. The Bell. patient in the most acute state must be watched, controlled, handled, and sometimes tied. In the text it describes these states as "rage, fury." He wants do violence. "Moaning. Instead of eating, bit wooden spoon in two, gnawed plate, and growled and barked like a dog. A boy violently sick, ran around the room laughing immoderately." It has an insane laughter. A loud, boisterous laughter. "A piece of bread, which he took to be a stone, he threw far from him. He turns and rolls in bed in a perfect rage. Aversion to noise and company." Aversion to light; is better in the dark. At times a more passive state intervenes between these attacks of violence. The active time is always that of violence; but there is sometimes a more passive state when the patient will sit or lie in bed and tear the bed clothing, or break anything that she can get hands on. If it is a stick, she will break it up.

Running all through the complaints, whether delirium, fever or pains, there is *starting*. Starting in sleep like an electric shock. Just as soon as he falls asleep a sensation like an electric shock throughout the body. "Starts in fright at approach of others. Fear of imaginary things, wants to run away from them." *"Great anxiety"* runs through the remedy. As a patient comes out of these attacks of delirium, as he comes out of convulsions, fear is depicted upon the face. The patient is in great excitement; the circulation is in a state of great excitement; the heart is in great excitement; motion and emotion increase the bearing of the heart.

It may have been gleaned that Bell. is a remedy that is *oversensitive;* a state of hyperæsthesia; extreme irritability of tissues. This is said to be an increased irritability of the nerve centres. This develops a state of increased ability to taste, and to smell, and to feel; excitability of the sensorium. Sensitive to impressions. *Sensitive to light, to noise, to touch, to jar.* The sensorium is violently excited. Excessive nervous irritability stands out, perhaps, as one of the most prominent features of Bell. in contrast with medicines like *Opium* that deprive the patient of all sensitivity. The more congestion there is in Bell. the more excitability. 'The more congestion there is in *Opium* the less excitability. And yet they are very similar in many respects; very similar in aspect; in the appearance of the eyes and face; similar in pathological states. If I were to prescribe on the pathological state, the congestion of the brain, the appearance, without taking in the intensity of the one or other, I would not be able to distinguish between *Opium* and Bell. They often antidote each other. But we do not prescribe on pathology, but upon symptoms, after careful individualization.

"Vertigo," with this intense excitability. Turning in bed, or moving the head makes him dizzy. "Things go round." "Vertigo with pulsations". Moving the head increases the pulsation, and the vertigo. The patient lies in bed cannot hold the head up. This increased sensitiveness especially applies to the scalp. We notice it particularly in the woman. She cannot have the hair bound up. It is often the case that Bell. patients will not have the hair combed or brushed. "Lets the hair hang down the back;" so sensitive is the scalp. "Hair feels as if pulled. Does not want the hair touched." There are some remedies that correspond to extreme irritation in very sensitive natures; like *Hepar*, where she faints with the pain; like *Nitric acid*, when cannot hear the-noise of vehicles going along the street, because it creates such violent sufferings; like *Coffea*, where footsteps aggravate all the complaints; he was so sensitive to pain that the noise of one entering the door when he was on the third floor aggravated his sufferings intensely, though no one else could hear it. In *Nux vomica*, even the sound of footsteps increases the pain all over the body. Bell. has in its nature all this sensitiveness to pain. It is a part of the general sensorium; the whole bodily state is intensified. The *Chamomilla* patient is oversensitive to pain, but we do not need to sympathize with the *Chamomilla* patient, he will fight it out himself. But you will pity the Bell. patient, you will pity the *Pulsatilla* patient, and the *Nitric acid* patient.

A strange part of it also is the reactive excitability. The reaction to medicine is so quick and so sudden that I have many times heard a patient say, before I had turned my back away from the bed, "That medicine has relieved me," so quick is• the reaction. In many medicines reaction is slowed down, but in Bell. it is intensified. So it is in *Nux vomica* and in *Zincum*. When the case is very acute, but sometimes also when the case is somewhat chronic, this sensibility is marked. *Cuprum* is so sensitive all over. It has sensitive skin, sensitive polypi, everything sensitive; and it is so sensitive in its reaction that, when it is needed, partially indicated remedies will not work, because the patient is so oversensitive to everything that everything overacts. The smallest dose, the mildest dose, the simplest dose overacts and everything aggravates. Odors aggravate; well selected remedies disturb instead of cure. *Cuprum* tones down, relieves that sensitivity, and wellselected remedies will then act curatively and long. *Cuprum* lacks it in that high state of congestion—it is not like in that; *Cuprum* does not have that sensibility along with the active fever and congestion, the throbbing and disturbance of the circulation; but it has it in a chronic state. Women and children are so sensitive that they get no sympathy—and it is not suitable for hysterical ones either, but those that are not able to control themselves perfectly. Such is *Cuprum*. We have medicines that are suitable to sensitive people, and especially sensitive women. Sensitive to odors, sensitive to every conceivable influence. The doctor who will go out and take care of these poor sick little mortals, who understands their nature, perceives their quality, and relieves them of their suffering, will command the whole community, in spite of the reputation of all the doctors that are there before him. He must not be one who measures everybody by his own sensorium; he may be a pachyderm, but he will find patients that are sensitive.

This sensitivity is present in most of the Bell. headaches. There are stabbing pains, throbbing pains, shooting pains, all in connection with congestion. They are all sensitive to motion, to every jar, to light, even to the winking of the eyes; sensitive to draft. Bell. will be indicated when the head is rolling—the patient rolling the head because the pain is so severe he cannot keep still, although the motion increases the headache. A child lies and turns and tosses its head with congestion of the brain, screaming out with the brain cry, a sudden shriek. After awhile it wakes up and commences to toss the head, and every few minutes it shrieks with that brain cry; it is going into a stupor, the neck is drawn back, the face is flushed, it is now becoming pale. There are times of stupor, and in that stupor the child cries out. In all brain troubles we must be careful about feeding much, or overloading the stomach, because the stomach is very feeble. It will not digest much, but the food should be well selected and light.

Great heaviness of the head. The head feels like a weight, and is drawn back. Sometimes we see the head drawn back from contraction of the muscles of the neck when the membranes of the upper portion of the spine are involved. Again, we see the Bell. patient drawing the head back himself, because drawing the head back often ameliorates the violent headaches. This amelioration is kept up so long as he holds the head back. Aggravated from bending the head forward when sitting, from bending the head forward when standing, or stooping. It feels as if the brain would fall out or push forward. This increases the headache so much that it sometimes turns into knife-like, or hammering pains. These are the expressions used. Sensation of nails and hammers, jagging and tearing; but with all, pressure and throbbing. When rising from a seat these sensations are all intensified. Throbbing; pulsation, like hammers hitting the inside of the sore skull, described by patients as if the inside of the skull was one continuous sore and was being pecked by hammers with every pulsation. Sometimes it will settle down while sitting still, or while lying; but rising up from a chair will set that hammer going. "Expansive" is an expression that is often used by the patient, and it was used by the provers. Expansive sensation, as if the head was enlarged; pressure from within out. All these headaches are relieved by pressure upon the outside. Sudden touch or pressure will aggravate; but pressure that is gradually increased and brought to bear carefully upon the head will ameliorate, like the pressure of a bandage, or a tight-fitting cap. Again, all of these headaches are brought on by exposure to the cold air; from standing in the cold air with the head uncovered. Sometimes a severe headache will come on from merely having the hair cut. Congestion of the head lasts for days, with throbbing and pulsating; from having the hair cut. Ear troubles, chest complaints, rheumatic complaints come on from having the hair cut, or from standing in the cool air with the hat off; so sensitive is the head to cold. It may be said of this remedy that complaints of various parts of the body come through the head and go downwards. Complaints in the lower extremities, rheumatic complaints of the joints, with great redness and swelling, come on from uncovering the head, from exposure of the head, or from getting the head wet, or from being caught in a shower. There is one complaint which will puzzle you if you ever meet it and you do not know just what I am going to tell you. The complaints of Bell. in a general way are ameliorated from rest, and aggravated from motion; but there is a kind of restlessness with tearing pain from the hips down, most troublesome to observe, that keeps the patient walking all of the time. The instant there is rest the pains come on. They sometimes shoot downwards, they sometimes tear up and down the nerves; and this comes on from exposure of the head, and not from getting the feet wet. Complaints of *Aconite* and *Pulsatilla* come on from getting the feet wet, and these complaints rise upwards, come on through the feet and go upwards and affect the head. Bell. complaints come on from exposure of the head and go downwards; sometimes affect the head, sometimes the chest, sometimes the stomach. sometimes centre in the abdomen, sometimes centre in the uterus .and ovaries. *Rhus* has complaints from getting wet, but the complaints are in the parts that are wet. If he gets the legs wet he will have rheumatism in the legs. There is a vast distinction, and this distinction has to he made in almost every prescription you will make. Homœopathy is a matter of individualization as to how complaints spread. Some complaints begin on the right side of the body and spread to the left. Some complaints begin in the top of the body and go downwards. That is the way this remedy acts. In some remedies the exposure of the feet to an ice cold draft will bring on headache (*Silic.*); but in Bell the exposure will bring on a headache, or neuralgia of the lower extremities. Now that pain that comes on from rest is an exception in Bell. That illustrates again the importance of distinguishing very decidedly between generals and particulars. Without knowing "generals" and "particulars" you will never do accurate   prescribing. The lower extremities here are the particulars. The patient and the general condition of the patient are ameliorated by rest; the symptoms of the patient are ameliorated by rest. All of those symptoms that can be predicted of the patient himself are ameliorated by rest, but the pains of the lower limbs, as described, those neuralgic pains are ameliorated by motion, and come on in rest. That does not mean that *all the* pains in the lower extremities are ameliorated by motion, because the pains in rheumatism are invariably ameliorated by rest, and aggravated by motion. Those tearing pains, from the hips downwards, with no swelling, come on during rest. All remedies are full of freaks, and it is the figuring out of these peculiarities that enables us to do good prescribing.

   With all the complaints of Bell. do not lose sight of the congestion upwards.

"Rush of blood to the head. Cold extremities." Cold feet, cold hands; hot head.

Inflammatory conditions of the eyes. "Glistening eyes. Dilated pupils. Flushed face, Intense redness of the inflamed part." Inflammation of all the tissues of the eyes, the lids, and all the parts of the eyeball, with most violent pain. Heat, redness, and burning. These three strong features that run through the remedy will be found in the eye sufferings. Pulsation, tumefaction, lachrymation; intense pains; sufferings all worse from motion, and worse from light. Most intense photophobia. "Flashes of light and flickerings before the eyes." When reading, lines appear crooked. "Dimness of vision, or actual blindness." Intense congestion and fulness of all the parts. "Apoplexy of the retina. Half-opened, protruding, staring eyes." You will see that in the infant when the child lies in a stupor; eyes half open; congestion of the brain; face flushed and intensely hot; rolling the head from side to side; if it has been going on for several days the face will later become pallid, and the neck drawn back. In these congestive troubles, lying with the eyes half open; almost no winking. "Orbital neuralgias. Protruding eyes, with dilated pupils. Inflammation of the optic nerve. and retina. Eyes congested and red." Another feature belonging to the eye is strabismus. Not those cases coming on gradually, such as will need the surgeon, but those that come on with congestion of the brain, with this state of congestion and dilated pupils and rolling the head from side to side, flushed face, throbbing carotids and intense heat. After a day or two the eye begins to turn in, and the little one is cross-eyed. That is an additional indication for Bell. Sometimes, coming out of a severe congestion, the strabismus remains and Bell. is sometimes the suitable remedy. All of these cases coming on from the circulatory conditions should be cured with remedies. They should never be sent to the surgeon. Though they remain some time, even months, they will be cured by well-selected remedies, while those that come on gradually, and those that are born so, will not be relieved by remedies. Only those spasmodic ones that are associated with, and come on from, congestion of the brain. In connection with congestion of the liver and duodenal catarrh there is yellowishness in the eyes.

In inflammations of the ear which go on to suppuration Bell. is rarely useful. We have to look to deep acting remedies. We may have the pain, tenderness, oversensitiveness, all inflammatory conditions; but cases requiring Bell. rarely go on to suppuration.

Now we come to the mucous membranes, the nose, mouth, throat, larynx, chest, the mucous membrane extending into the ear through the Eustachian tube, and we have another strong feature of Bell. which characterizes most of its conditions. *Great dryness;* a sensation of dryness. Dryness in the nose;

mouth; of the tongue; in the throat; in the chest, and such evidences as dry cough and spasmodic conditions. These are so general that with the nose symptoms, the coryza, the throat symptoms, the cough, this is intensified; dryness of mucous membranes will generally be found. It is that way with *Phos.* When *Phos.* has a sore throat it will have dryness of the mouth, tongue and air passages. This is general as to the respiratory tract. Then there is coryza with much sneezing. "Pricking, burning in the nose." Hot sensation in the nose. The general states present much redness of the face, much heat with the coryza; hot head, cold extremities; marked headache, because there is dryness. The very dryness itself is sometimes causative of pain, because the natural flow from the mucous membranes is dried up. Whenever we have checked secretions we have fever, and in Bell. this is marked. Checking of the discharge with fever, with heat, redness and burning; red face, burning face; heat in the face and head, and cold extremities. It says in the text, "maddening headache, with suppressed catarrh."

Now, in such a climate as this most people during winter and cold weather and the changes have more or less mucous flow from the nose, and eyes, and air passages. They are better when this takes place. All at once it stops, and all the parts become dry; then look out. An awful, maddening, throbbing headache comes on. It is not so suitable for those old catarrhs where there is a copious flow of thick, yellow mucus. The catarrhal state wherein Bell. is useful is simply the exaggeration of the whitish mucous flow. Where it has been thick and yellow, and then stops suddenly from a cold, and a coryza comes on, Bell. is worthless. Always bear in mind that you select for suppressed catarrh a medicine that is within the sphere of the symptoms that have been suppressed. Hence, the medicine for thick, yellowish-green discharges might he *Merc., Sulphur,* or *Pulsatilla;* then you are within the range of medicines capable of re-establishing the flow, and at the same time beginning a curative effect on the state of the tissue, leaving the patient in a much better state.

Violent faceaches. Rending, tearing pains in the face; throbbing pains in the face. Pains in the face worse on the right side; worse from a jar; with much heat; throbbing carotids; hot head; brought on from exposure to cold wind, and riding in the cold wind. Bell. has cured paralytic conditions, but *Causticum* is generally the remedy for paralysis of the face from riding in a cold wind. Spasms of the muscles of the face. Extraordinary twitchings of the face. Erysipelas in the face; a bright red gradually becoming purple if there is a fever accompanying it. In the neuralgic pains there is always more or less congestion of the face with violent pains, and the face will be bright red. With the zymotic state, as the febrile condition becomes more profound, and as the blood becomes more zymotic, the face grows from duskiness into a mottled state, as you will see in *Baptisia*, more marked in *Baptisia* than in Bell. "Red face, with burning heat." The teeth are full of pains, congestions, and aches of a similar character. Very sensitive teeth.

The tongue should be a dry tongue, as that is general with its mucous membranes. Dry mouth; dry tongue; swollen tongue; protruding tongue, dry and hard, feels like leather. Loss of sensation, loss of taste, loss of power of the tongue and loss of speech are all Bell. features. "Paralytic weakness of the tongue; trembling of the tongue when it is protruded." It comes out weak. In a very few days the Bell. fever patient is greatly reduced, is greatly exhausted, has almost a paralytic weakness. When he raises the hand and holds it a moment it trembles in the same way. That which is found in the tongue is only a part of the general state. Trembling from congestion of the nerve centers. The papillæ of the tongue are erect, and the tongue is bright red. Bright red tongue in scarlet fever. Bright red tongue in congestion of the brain, with the erect papillæ. When going over *Arum triphyllum* I told you it had been pronounced "strawberry tongue". It is the same with 'Bell. The tongue looks as red as a strawberry, and the papillæ stick up like seeds. "Red streak in the middle of the tongue, wide and broader towards the point. Tongue, white centre with red edges." White tongue with brain affections is not uncommon. It has thick, milk-white, delicate fur all over the tongue in brain troubles. "Dryness of the mouth, with thirst." "Dryness of the mouth, with no thirst." Bell. is full of thirst, we will find when we come to study the stomach symptoms. Sometimes Bell. wants large quantities, sometimes water constantly to wet the mouth, like *Ars.* It is a common feature in Bell., Like *Ars.*, to want water little and often. Just enough to wet his parched tongue, mouth and throat. Dryness in posterior nares, and the mucus that he drags down from the posterior nares is tough and stringy, and very scanty, and it is white; or, if changed at all from white, it is bloody. Yet I have not said anything about this remedy for bloody discharges and for bleeding. We will find before we finish that it is a hæmorrhagic remedy, that parts bleed easily. There is bleeding from the eyes, bleeding from the nose, bleeding from the throat, bleeding from the larynx, bleeding from the chest, bleeding from the bladder, bleeding from the uterus. Ulcers bleed. Little fine ulcers in the throat no bigger than a pin-head. Little aphthous patches bleed. An aphthous inflammation of the throat; but the most of the complaints of the throat are dry and red. Great tumefaction. Extremely sensitive; much swelling; inability to swallow. Great pain on swallowing, with' all the sensitivity of the surrounding parts, with the sore throat, and with the inflamed throat. Inflammation and swelling of the tonsils, with red face, intense heat, throbbing carotids, high fever, coming on from cold. Fauces and pharynx deep red. Soft alate and tonsils swollen. Swallowing painful, particularly of fluids. Speech hick. "Feels like a lump in the throat" that is from the swollen tonsils. Constant craping and hawking in the throat. The pharynx and larynx are very commonly n a state of spasm; partly from dryness, partly from extreme sensitiveness of he nerves of the part. Clutching of the throat on going to sleep, clutching of hroat on coughing. Spasms of the œsophagus. "Spasmodic constriction on he throat." Constrictions that are spasmodic. Constrictions of the larynx, of he pharynx, of the throat. Bell. has constrictive pains in parts that feel like he clutch of fingers. That sensation of clutching is felt in the uterus; it is a pasm. It is felt in the liver; it is felt in the brain; it is felt in the throat. Jerking nd twitching of muscles, with violent pain, in painful parts. That is a strong Bell. feature. Patients sometimes in their inability to describe their feelings vill say, "Doctor, I feel a clutching in there."

This constriction that comes in the sore throat occurs just in the act of wallowing fluids or solids, and that action will force the food and fluids up nto the nose, and sometimes out of the nose. Some remedies have it as a aralytic conditions because the muscles of deglutition are paralyzed and hey do not favor the natural contracting actions to force the food down the esophagus, and in that way the food is forced up into the nose and causes trangling. In Bell., in its acute states, its inflammatory conditions and its pasms would distinguish it from *Lachesis,* where it occurs as a paralytic ondition after diphtheria, and from *Alumina,* which has a spasm of the esophagus. These are slow in coming on, Bell. is early. The early part of the ever is the time of its irritation. The latter part of the fever is the time of its elaxation. Rapidly forming aphthous patches upon the tonsils. With the sort hroat such as we have described you will nearly always find an enlargement nd inflammation, or soreness of the glands, under the jaws about the neck. enderness along with a Belladonna sore throat is a natural concomitant.

A strange feature running through the Bell. fevers of all sorts is an nconquerable craving for lemons, and lemon-juice. Lemonade seems to agree ometimes. In acute diseases when they crave lemon it is good for them. hey often crave things to eat. You must not be so violently temperate and in avour of prohibition that if a patient longs for beer in acute sufferings you vill not give it. "Thirst for water changed into thirst for beer." Thirst for ings that could not be endorsed in health, even.' "Excessive thirst for cold vater."

In the stomach and bowels we have inflammatory conditions which can ll be grouped as one. Pain, burning, distress, distension; sensitive to a jar, nd to the slightest motion, and to the slightest pressure. Sensitive to a jar, nd sensitive to motion. "Pain in the stomach extending through to the spine." nflammation of the stomach from becoming chilled, with intense heat; with

much burning. It has violent colic, intense cramping pain in children. Fac
red and hot; pain relieved only by bending forward: There are exceptiona
instances where it has been relieved by bending backward, when it is simila
to *Dioscorea*. The mother finds that by holding the child on her hand it wil
relieve the colic. That is like *Colocynth;* but *Colocynth* is without muc
fever, without much thirst, a pain in one spot, an intense colic in the abdome
ameliorated by doubling up, ameliorated by bending across something hard
is *Colocynth.* In that instance *Colocynth* can he prescribed on that on
group of symptoms.

"Great pain in the ileo-cœcal region; cannot bear the slightest touch
even the. bed clothes." There are instances where Bell. is the remedy i
appendicitis.

Belladonna has dysenteric troubles. Diarrhœa, with scanty fluid stoo
marked straining, but with it the face is flushed. Heat, redness and burning i
the face and head. Cold extremities, with hot head. Much straining, but passe
scanty stool. "Spasmodic constriction of sphincter ani; with hæmorrhoids.
Hæmorrhoids that are violently painful, that are intensely red, that are greatl
swollen and inflamed, a high grade of inflammation; cannot be touched; mus
lie with limbs wide apart, the hæmorrhoids are painful and there is muc
burning.

No remedy has a greater irritation in the bladder and along the urinar
tract than Bell. The urging to urinate is constant. The urine dribbles, and
burns intensely along the whole length of the urethra. The whole urinary trac
is in a state of irritation. Bell. has cured inflammation of the bladder. With th
irritation and the congestion there is all the sensitiveness to pressure we fin
in any other part where Bell. is indicated; sensitive to a jar. Irritable state *of th
mind,* irritable state of the whole nervous system. "Tenesmus of the bladde
After passing urine sits and strains," in torment. The urine is diminishec
bloody, sometimes pure blood, or little blood clots. A considerable quantity c
blood in the bladder comes away in little clots. "The urine looks as if mixe
with brick dust, or streaks. Strongly acid." There is a spasmodic retention c
urine and there is involuntary passing of urine. Dribbling of urine in brai
troubles. During sleep, dribbling of urine. Dreams that he is passing urine
and involuntarily passed it. Retention of urine after shock, or from congestio
of the brain, or after confinement. Bladder full; great pain; great sensitivenes
Involuntary dribbling while standing and walking; or sometimes from mer
motion the urine spurts. The urging is violent and sudden. When a little urin
has collected in the bladder he has a sudden, painful urging. Much of th
trouble is at the neck of the bladder, and it is spasmodic. He feels the spasmod
clutching. At the time of the urging, and at other times, he has spasm of th
neck of the bladder, from shock, from cold, from anxiety, from menta

isturbances. When becoming old, or chilled, or in very cold air, women lose
1eir urine, like *Dulcamara* and *Causticum*. Starts in sleep, and wets bed.
)reams of a fright, which causes a starting, and she wets the bed. On going to
leep, a sudden electric shock goes through the whole body, and she wets the
ed. Bell. is rich with such strange little peculiarities; but it only shows the
eneral spasmodic condition and the general irritability of the whole
3elladonna constitution. We see those strange conditions and states, the
rritability in all parts of the body, especially where there are sphincters, where
1ere are circular fibers clutching in the neck of the bladder; clutching at the
1outh of the vagina; constriction of tubes. Constriction of the uterus. Here
ve see a special marked feature of it in the neck of the bladder. It has more
roubles in the woman than in the man; that is in the symptoms and conditions
1 relation to the female sexual organs, and to parturition, and to the breasts,
nd during the period of gestation there are many conditions where Belladonna
vill he needed. It is really an important remedy for the nervous sensitive
voman, the woman of irritable fiber.

In the male genitals we have scarcely any important symptoms; but with
1e female there are many, and some very distressing ones. They have
ymptoms of great suffering, of great excitability. The parts are sensitive;
1e uterus and ovaries are congested, sore to touch, sensitive to jar. Irritable
terus, until it has become enlarged and painful, and sore to the touch.
ometimes it remains in this state after parturition. Or, after every menstrual
eriod it is a little larger, and remains. It does not return to its normal state,
ut remains congested, and the woman feels all through the interim as if she
vas 'menstruating. Bruised feeling; sensitive to a jar. The flow is copious
nd clotted. But the most striking feature here is the uterine hæmorrhage.
Jterine hæmorrhage from congestion, with spasms, with great sensitiveness.
he uterus contracts with violence, hence, a spasmodic contraction. Great
oreness, with a *copious flow of bright red fluid mixed with clots, is the
haracteristic of the Belladonna flow.* It is like *Sabina* in that respect. Those
wo medicines have that in a high grade. The uterus fills with a clot, and then
omes a contraction like a labor pain and expels it; for a while a copious flow
f fluid; and then contractions like labor pains come on again, expelling the
lots, and then comes the flow. The blood clots soon, and the hæmorrhage is
ttended with great exhaustion. Now this occurs almost without any
rovocation. This hæmorrhage occurs also in connection with abortion.
3elladonna is a great remedy to check the hæmorrhage in connection with
bortion or from any cause whatever where the symptoms of sensitiveness
re present. Sensitive to touch, sensitive to a jar; the patient herself is in that
tate of irritable sensitiveness, great nervous excitement manifested both

when awake and in sleep; often with fever. Hæmorrhage, with febrile condition
but usually the hæmorrhage takes the place of the fever, and commonly
there is hæmorrhage it will relieve the fever.

It is also a great remedy for hæmorrhage after confinement. *The bloo
feels hot.* Hæmorrhage, with hour-glass contraction. It is not an uncommo
thing for the placenta to be grasped in, its middle by a contraction like a
hour-glass tearing it loose here and there, and from below comes the bleeding
a copious flow of blood. Bell. relieves this hour-glass contraction

It has also the most violent dysmenorrhœa. Pains like labor-pains. Spas
modic labor-pains. Circular contractions are the commonest forms in Bell. A
of the fibers should take part uniformly and do their work uniformly, an
thereby gradually bring to bear a tightening upon the contents. In Bell. it i
just like a cord going around the body of the uterus, tightening it, and
interferes with labor. That is the way it is in its dysmenorrhœa. Violer
contraction of the circular fibers, and hence, a woman will often describe it a
feeling as if the uterus was clutched with a string. As if it were tightenec
Bell. is rich in spasmodic conditions, in hæmorrhagic conditions, in states c
irritation, and in soreness, and the parts are sensitive to pain, and the woma
herself is dreadfully wrought up and shocked by pain. In addition to tha
pains in the ovary. Belladonna acts in many instances on the right side. It i
common for the right ovary to be more painful than the left, or the right to b
entirely affected and the left not at all, in Belladonna. So it is with the righ
side of the throat. So it is sometimes in the right side of the body. "Pains i
the ovaries with the appearance of the menses. Pains in the pelvic regior
which come on suddenly, and cease as suddenly." The characteristi
Belladonna pains come on suddenly, sometimes stay a few seconds, sometime
a few minutes, and leave suddenly. Pains from uterine congestion. Acut
inflammation of the uterus. "Enlargement of the uterus, and periodicall
spasmodic bearing down." It has a relaxation in the parts as well. The uteru
has been congested and is enlarged, and heavy, and the little suspensor
attachments have become relaxed, and tired, and weak, and have stretche
and elongated, and the already distended and overweighted uterus keep
pulling on them, and this creates the sensation that women so often describe
a bearing-down sensation as if the uterus would escape. It is sometime
described as a funneling sensation. These are the expressions of wome
when they suffer from prolapsus. That relaxation is common in a great numbe
that have been poisoned with *Ergot.* The uterus comes down and is partl
exposed between the labiæ Prolapsus as if the whole inner parts were comin
out is a common feature, and with this she is worse from a jar. There is a grea
sensitiveness in the parts. There is a great soreness in the uterus, and
sensation of heaviness, I have seen women sit with their limbs wide apart, s

sensitive is the neck of the uterus that is protruding from the vulva. "Must sit; cannot lie down:" Many of the Bell. cases cannot lie down, because of the stretching of the abdominal muscles. When they lie down they must draw up the limbs to relax those muscles. Must sit, or take a flexed posture. Great sensitiveness in the parts. Pressing and urging towards the genitals. There are all sorts of positions, and aggravations, and ameliorations in Belladonna, in accordance with what particular muscles are involved. Some patients can lie better than they can sit. Almost all are worse standing. Some are made better by sitting with the limbs wide apart. Most are aggravated by bending forward too much. Sitting in a chair she cannot bend forward too much, neither can she bend backwards without increasing the suffering. So sensitive, and so much swelling in these parts. She is worse from motion, worse from jar, worse from excitement, worse from the slamming of the door, because that makes the muscles twitch. All this illustrates how sensitive the irritated parts are. Then in the external and internal genitals and ovaries there is burning, and twitching, and much heat. Often tearing pains; the tearing pains are generally an exaggeration of those clutchings and constrictions, and such are known as spasms especially of the circular fibers.

Belladonna is well suited to pregnant women who are extremely sensitive, who are plethoric, who have congestion from taking cold, who have soreness, where there is threatened abortion, or during or after abortion when there are haemorrhages. Then again Bell. is useful in red-faced plethoric, vigorous women who have married late in life and become pregnant, and when the day of delivery comes the muscular fibers are in a state of tension. The uterus will not relax. She is flushed and has heat, and is in a state of excitement, sensitive to touch, sensitive to jar. Relaxation will soon follow. It is not to be expected that she will have an easy labor, because women who marry at 28 or 30, or later, suffer from prolonged labor.

There is one strong feature of the haemorrhages, and of the discharges; the flow of blood feels hot. During confinement gushes of blood that. feel hot. After abortion, gushes of blood that feel hot. A lochial discharge that feels hot, along with the sensitiveness and soreness of the parts. Tenderness to pressure. There are inflammatory conditions of the breasts accompanying confinement. Milk fever. When the breasts become red, extremely sensitive to touch. She cannot turn over in bed; she cannot have the bed jarred, the face is flushed, and the carotids are throbbing; there is fever; the sensitivity is aroused throughout the economy. Great induration; hard as a stone. Bell, will stop the pain in the breast in a few hours. It will stop that congestion, and will relieve all sufferings.

When the mammary glands are inflamed without any general symptoms, but merely an inflammation of the glands give *Phytolacca*.

Inflammation of the larynx. There is that clutching again, and choking. It begins with a rawness in the throat, a smarting and scraping, and the formation of a little mucus. After much scraping and hawking it extends up the throat a little; but before he begins to cough it is quite dry. There is smarting, and loss of voice. As soon as he attempts to go into a sleep, that clutch comes on and wakes him up. Hoarseness and rawness and clutching in the throat. Laryngitis with sensitiveness. "Sudden attacks of hoarseness;" every motion, or the slightest attempt to talk, the slightest effort to move the larynx or to touch it causes suffering. Moving the head backward, or moving the head from side to side, causes pain and cough. Swallowing aggravates. As the bolus goes down behind the larynx he feels a great big sore place, it is the larynx. The voice changes. One minute it is one key, and in another it changes. Sometimes it is hoarse and sometimes it is squeaky. And then, there is complete loss of voice, unable to utter a sound. "Croup-like spasms in the larynx. Spasms of the glottis. All the symptoms of croup," but no membrane It is simply a dry, denuded larynx, with rawness and scraping; an inflamed condition. And this is the form of the acute laryngitis; it comes on very suddenly. His respiration is short, rapid and painful. Often asthmatic Asthmatic condition, with spasmodic breathing. And again, these symptoms seem to involve the whole chest. Oppression of the chest. Asthma in ho damp weather.

The Belladonna cough comes on from clutching in the larynx. As if a little speck of something had crept into the larynx; a little dust, or a little food, o a drop of water had gotten into the larynx, and he coughs. "Dry, spasmodic cough." An intense cough. Cough at night. Cough when lying down, more a night than in the daytime. The cough is spasmodic, barking, short. It is a remedy for whooping cough, with spasms of the larynx which cause the whoop and difficulty of breathing. Finally after long coughing, the expectoration of a little blood, or a little thin white mucus, is the result of the violent turmoil going on in the air passages from coughing. The Belladonna cough is peculiar. As soon as its great violence and the great effort have raised a little mucus he gets peace for a little while, and stops coughing. Bu during the restful period the larynx and the trachea and the air passages grow drier and drier, and finally they commence to tickle, and then comes o the spasm, as if all the air Passages were taking part in it, and the whoop an the gagging, and sometimes vomiting. Then he gets up a little mucus and the cough subsides. Another little interval and he has another spell. That is the way it goes on, like whooping cough, but during all of the interim there i constant dryness. Hence the cough is called paroxysmal.

Tightness in the chest. Painfulness in the chest. Soreness in the chest. I Bell. the child will cry the instant it feels that urging to cough, because knows what a great suffering is going to take place. The chest is so painful, the child dreads the cough and screams. By the child's cry we know that it is going to have a coughing spell. Just like *Bry., Hepar* and *Phos.*, which have that feature more than other remedies. There is burning in the chest; violent congestion in the chest. With all of these chest complaints there is that dry, harassing, spasmodic cough; worse at night.

This remedy cures pneumonia and pleurisy. I am sure every one here could picture a Belladonna pneumonia, or a Belladonna pleurisy. I am sure you know the *patient* so well that I need not describe the patient, the head, the congestion; the red face, or the burning; but in pleurisy I will tell you its secret. Bell. prefers the right side. Great pain; extreme soreness of the part; *cannot lie on it; worse from the jar of the bed—and* you have the Bell. pleurisy. *Bry.* also prefers the right side, but the *Bry.* patient must lie on that side; must have pressure, and is not so sensitive to a jar; he has not the intense heat, he has not the great throbbing, and the burning. Every kind of sickness that you go to you have to individualize in that way. There is no other way to practice Homœopathy.

Remember, with all the inflammatory conditions there will be throbbing, heat, redness, burning, soreness to touch, and sensitiveness to a jar. With Bell. it means he cannot lie on the inflamed part; while with *Bry.* he is ameliorated from lying on the inflamed part.

Throbbing in all the arteries. Great congestion. Vascular excitement. These are present with all the congestions, and inflammations.

Belladonna cures inflammatory rheumatism, when all the joints are swollen, or a great number of them, and they are hot, red, and burn. We have in the rheumatism the heat, redness and burning running through; with the same sensitiveness of the whole patient, and a sensitiveness of the joints to the jar of the bed. He wants to lie perfectly still, is very much worse from motion and has considerable fever. Sometimes when the fever in inflammatory rheumatism runs pretty high there is delirium. But the striking features are, the swelling of the joints with the redness, and great sensitiveness to motion and to a jar. It is especially suitable to those that are very sensitive to cold, who cannot bear the least uncovering, cannot bear a draft, very sensitive to the motion of the covers, and ameliorated by heat. The very stamp and character of Bell. is in its rheumatic state, like it is in all of its other complaints. It is the *patient* that has given Bell. that character in the provings; it is the patient that gives disease that character when he has it, and it is only the fulfilment of the Law of Similars when these come together, and the remedy annihilates the sickness.

Inflammation of the joints, coming on from sudden exposure of that articular joint. Or from a severe attack of cold on joint becomes inflamed.

A trouble that is localizing itself: It may be any joint of the body, for Bell affects all the joints. The sudden exposure to cold, in plethoric individuals, is one of the most prominent causes of the Bell. sickness. In chronic cases the taking of cold generally locates, or creates, a disturbance, and increases disorder, that manifests itself in the weakest place. Vigorous people take cold in the nose, where they throw it off easily. You can often say to sickly patient that "your cold now affects you in the weakest place. If you have liver trouble your cold will settle in the liver," and so on; "but when you get well you will take cold like other people, in the nose." Absolutely healthy people seldom take cold, but we do not have many such, they are so rare that we do not often seen them; and the snuffles, and sneezing, and the running at the nose are simply throwing off of the cold of ordinarily healthy people.

In the limbs; again, we have convulsions, which is a part of the generals In all the muscles in the limbs, and throughout the body, convulsions. Children go into convulsions with head troubles, with congestion of the brain, with irritation of the brain. Convulsions from taking cold, in plethoric children and the limbs are most likely to show forth those convulsive efforts of the muscles. Violent cramping. All the limbs are in a state of convulsive movements. Sometimes the spasms are clonic, and sometimes tonic. The convulsions in the limbs are sometimes such as draw them up suddenly throw them out suddenly; sometimes convulsions that throw the body backward, called opisthotonos, and sometimes throwing the body forward called emprosthotonos. The most of the complaints in Bell. are ameliorate by keeping still. The drawing pains, the pulsations, the inflammatory conditions drive the patient into a desire for perfect rest, are aggravated from motion. The disinclination and aversion to the slightest motion is common in Bell., and as strong in Bell. as in *Bry.* Bell. is so sensitive in parts that the motions of talking are painful; so sensitive that the concussion of the voice is painful in the sore spots. A person with a strong voice, a bass voice hardly thinks of the concussion that take place; and much less is that of the female voice, and yet I have seen that aggravation from motion, and that aggravation from jar so marked in the female that her voice was like the pounding of hammers. In inflammation of the uterus, and ovaries, and the bowels, she refrains from talking, because her voice creates a concussion in the sore parts. That only illustrates the extremes of this great sensitiveness to motion, and to jar. Jar is only an exaggerated form of motion, bringing out that sensitiveness.

If you will study the nerves you will find the greatest array of peculiar nervous manifestations, such as sensitiveness of the nerves, aggravated from shock; spasms; various disturbances of the whole nervous system; twitching jerking; trembling; subsultus tendinum, etc. Cramps, and spasms, and convulsions in children. Convulsions come on with great suddenness. They come on entirely unexpected. In most instances of convulsions in the long acting remedies and medicines of the zymotic type, the patient has not been prospering in the last days of her gestation; but with Bell. she goes on part way through the labor, or finishes it, and little is expected. Perhaps her face is a little too red, but she goes into a convulsion unexpectedly, a violent one from head to foot. Congestion of the brain, with excitement. Intense heat; everything is intense, violent, sudden and unexpected. The pains sometimes leave in confinement suddenly, and a convulsion comes on. But look and see that all the sensitiveness that I have described runs through the patient. The pains cease suddenly. The blood seems to mount to the head. *The face becomes red.* Congestions come on suddenly. Convulsions epileptiform in character. Bell. is not suitable for those numerous recurrent complaints, even though the single attack should be mitigated with Bell. Take any of these attacks; whether they are convulsions or headaches, or congestion of the brain, they are running down and become excitable, take on congestive attacks of the head, go right to bed, and roll the head. You treat those with Bell.; the attack is relieved. Take notice, I start out by saying this is only one of a series. You may not know it. This may be the first one. You reduce that one, and when that same exposure comes again, that same attack comes back; but Bell. does less this time than it did before. After two or three attacks Bell. will do no more and you are worse off this time than you were before. When it has broken the first one the physician should see that this is one of a series, and that Bell. is not suitable. Often it is a case that needs *Calc.,* I say often, not always. All the symptoms should be examined between the attacks, so that the child may be elevated above these attacks because the acute remedy will do no more than suit the first, or second, or third at most. It has not the depth of action. It has not the length of action. It does not affect the economy profoundly enough. It passes away after a few days; has to be frequently repeated. The patient should be followed up and watched in all these recurrent spasmodic and periodical complaints. Bell. is not a good remedy for recurrent complaints for it lacks periodicity, just as it lacks continuance of complaints. Even if the first attack looked like Bell. the next attack would come back just the same. Belladonna is suitable in those complaints that if conquered have no tendency to recur; those complaints that end in death or recovery. It will only *mitigate* those complaints that are periodical.

Its sleep is a congestive sleep, a stupor; full of dreams; full of violence. Wakes with fright from a horrible dream, a nightmare. Jerks and twitches in sleep. "Restless sleep." Moaning and groaning in sleep. Doing all sorts of violence. Delirium in sleep. "Starts in sleep as if frightened." In sleep sometimes the patient will commence to talk, will talk faster and louder, the head becomes hot, and the feet cold, and he ends with a shriek. "Restless tossing in sleep. Feet becoming icy cold in sleep. Head getting hot in sleep.

Wakes up in a fever, and excitement."

It has symptoms so much like a typical old-fashioned Sydenham scarlet fever that it has been useful in scarlet fever, Perhaps it is one of the most frequently indicated medicines in that disease. In some seasons, at least, it will run all through, and the majority of cases will be Bell. cases, with the bright red face and glossy appearance of the skin. Bright red, intense heat, great congestion; after a short time if Bell. is not administered it will grow darker. But running through all this are those three words, *heat, redness and burning*. Burning everywhere. The temperature I described among the generals as being so marked, so intense that you will carry it with you on the ends of your fingers for hours after you have touched a Bell. scarlet fever. It differs wholly from the *Apis* case, which has a rough rash. Bell. is smooth and shining. *Apis* wants to be cool, wants to be uncovered; Bell. wants to be warm, wants a warm room; *Apis* has no thirst, to speak of; in Bell. it is the exception to have no thirst, generally very thirsty for water, little and often. The intense dryness of the mucous membranes and skin. Coldness of the extremities with hot head. In *Arum triphyllum* there is a constant picking of the mouth, with suppressed or scanty urine; pale surface, only here and there a little rash; the itching of the fingers, toes, nose and lips will lead you to prescribe *Arum*. You remember the *Baptisia* case, with that mental state where he is feeling all over the bed "to get the pieces together." On the other hand, where there is no rash to speak of, now and then a patch enough to make a diagnosis, or the diagnosis is made from the fact of some one else having the disease in the family, the child is swallowing ice water, but vomiting it up when it gets warm in the stomach, who would not give *Phos?* So it is at the bedside we pick out the distinguishing things and see that these remedies are not at all alike. Bell. stands out with its heat, its redness, its turmoil. Remember it has not continued fever; it is not suitable in typhoid. Bell. in a night will bring down the fever, will allay the delirium; but how is it the next night? On comes the fever, and the patient is worse than he was before. Simply because Bell. cannot hold what it starts with. It is not suitable. It has not that continued feature in it. We are led to a medicine that corresponds to continuous fevers, and such must be selected when we go into the typhoid state. Our earlier practitioners often only thought of what they saw at the time. It was only after our school had considerable experience that it was found that periodicity constitutes a symptom. Every remedy has its pace, its times of aggravation and its times of amelioration. So it is with Bell. Its time is 3 o'clock in the afternoon, commonly. Its complaints are generally worse in the night. Its complaints commonly start about three o'clock in the afternoon and run till three in the morning, or until after midnight. So that during the night its fever is highest. The fever comes on, and rises rapidly, to a very high temperature, sometimes 104 or 105, and runs down again to almost normal; but not with complete apyrexia. It is not suitable in complaints with complete apyrexia, for that marks complete periodicity which Bell. has not.

The heat, the redness and the burning characterize most of the skin symptoms. It has a fine rash; not the coarse rash, but the fine, scarlet red, smooth rash. It has inflammation of the skin, phlegmonous, a deep inflammation. First bright red, gradually grows bluish or purple, or mottled; and in this there is the heat, redness and burning. It is not suitable generally for the erysipelatous inflammation of the skin and deeper tissues, covered with vesicles, like *Rhus*. Vesiculation is sometimes present, but it is the exception, while in *Rhus* it is the general character. *Rhus* begins with inflammation; it has heat, redness and burning; but whenever *Rhus* begins an inflammation, just that instant it throws out a great blister, and it fills with serum. Almost any Bell. surface that is inflamed is likely to throw out a red rash. In intense fevers, where there are not scarlet fever or any of the common rashes, a red, fine, glossy eruption is likely to come out. It is not an uncommon thing in congestion of the brain, and in bilious fevers, for this rash to appear, and it sometimes deceives the physician into making a diagnosis of one of the eruptive diseases, whereas it is a mere hybrid. The Bell. skin, while it turns red, has such a passive redness that you can write your name, almost, on the skin. As you take your finger and make a line on it, it leaves a white line behind your finger. That was an old diagnostic phase of scarlet fever, and it shows that Bell. produces upon the surface that peculiar passive congestion very much like the scarlatina. So we have in the Bell. provings a symptom that is even a pathognomonic symptom of scarlatina. But we do not prescribe on a symptom. Of late years no homœopathic physician ever thinks of giving a medicine simply for the purpose of bringing the pulse down, or bringing the fever down. He prescribes for the *patient*. It is true that the temperature does come down, if we get the right remedy; but to prescribe a remedy to bring the pulse down is going at it wrong end to. One who thinks homœopathically never prescribes to remove a symptom; but guided by the symptoms he selects the remedy, no matter what follows. It is true the symptoms subside. Others might say he prescribed to remove the symptoms, because they subside. Learn to keep the ideal of Homœopathy in mind, and think rationally; in order to do that you will have to rid yourselves of a tremendous amount of inheritance. We have inherited the way to think wrong end to.

"Yellowness of the skin from congestion of the liver, and catarrh of the duodenum." When persons have been over-medicated with quinine until they take cold on every occasion, and a sudden attack of congestion of the liver comes on, with the great soreness, and the skin becomes yellow with all the sensitiveness of this remedy, Bell. will cure such cases.

There are conditions that follow Bell. that relate to its chronic state. Where Bell, has been suitable for the acute conditions, the congestions, but there is that periodicity that I have mentioned, it has its natural followers, and *Calcarea* is one of them. In boys that are big-headed, plump, plethoric, precocious, that take cold easily, and come down with headaches, and congestion; school children that get headaches which Bell. at first helped; very commonly if you look carefully into the case it will turn out to he a *Calc.* case. It is so common for *Calc.* to relate in this way to Bell. Now-a-days we frequently find the dry, hacking cough in the hands of doctors who have given too much *Lachesis. Lachesis* is commonly given to over-sensitive women, and it produces many of those conditions; it sometimes cures great troubles, but it leaves behind for weeks a dry, hacking cough that keeps her from sleeping. Sometimes it comes on after the first sleep which is commonly about 11 o'clock; a dry, hacking cough from lying down. Bell. will cure this old effect of *Lich.,* the nervous state and excitability and the cough. Bell. will be suitable as an antidote for *Lach.,* that is, for the acute symptoms. *Calc.* is an antidote for the more chronic effects of *Lach.* After the abuse of Bell., *Calc.* comes in as one of the natural antidotes.

BENZOIC ACID

Whenever we see in the nature of a remedy a well-defined state and condition of the human system pointed out by certain distinctive groups of symptoms we may know that there is such a *diseased* state in the human family. They have not the power to create by themselves any diseased state except there is first such a state in the economy of the human race to be aroused. They simply call up in a single individual something that the individual has, and that something belongs to the human race, and so whenever we see a diseased state in the remedy we know that it exists in correspondence to something in the human race. Things are so adjusted that everything is for use. There may be conditions in the human race that we, as yet, know no remedy for. We see certain groups of peculiar symptoms frequently repeat themselves and we know they are repre-sentatives of a state of the economy, but up to this day we may not have seen in the Materia Medica their counterpart. In medicines we have the exact counterpart for the diseases of the human race.

Now this remedy has a state and condition that is sometimes called the *gouty* constitution, the uræmic or the lithæmic constitution, and these cases are very difficult to manage, as the state is so persistent. It is one of the manifestations of Psora. These patients suffer more or less from irregularity in the action of the kidneys; sometimes the urine is scanty and then they suffer from bodily complaints; again the urine is copious and then they arc relieved of their complaints. They are subject to rheumatic attacks and pains in the joints, showing the gouty constitution, and then they have relief when the urine is copious and heavily laden with deposits; but on comes an attack when they have more or less urine, but it is light in specific gravity, and then they arc full of pains; in that way they fluctuate. Now, the young prescriber will sometimes see the patient when he is passing large quantities of uric acid forming the red pepper deposits and he thinks he must stop that; his main idea is to check that one particular thing. But the patient is a great deal better off while he has it. To check it is like suppressing a skin eruption, or restraining any other manifestation of disease.

It will he noticed, as one of the foremost things in this remedy's manifestations, that it has strong smelling urine; the urine is pungent, and it sometimes becomes so strong that it smells Iike hippuric acid, and so it is said *urine smells strong like that of a horse.* The odor in this remedy approximates that of hippuric acid.

The complaints, then, of Benzoic acid are such as are changeable, and we know why they are changeable; when the urine is copious and plenty of uric acid is being passed, and the urine is full of deposits, then the patient is at his best; when the urine is scanty or of light specific gravity he suffers from backache and pains in the joints, he suffers from atmospheric changes, is sensitive to cold drafts and to the air; but let the urine start up again, which it does in a sort of alternating way, light urine alternating with heavy urine, and the patient is comfortable again. Then, there are complaints in which the urine smells strong and pungent; this often occurs in children. It is astonishing that these little ones manifest the uric acid diathesis in early life. Mothers often describe it as intensely urinous. It smells like intensified urine; it is not the smell, so much, of decomposed urine nor of fœtid urine, but urine intensified. it has cured many times wetting the bed, involuntary urination in sleep, when the bed that has been wetted several times becomes uncleanable. You can smell it almost as quick as you go into the room; the children all smell like urine, strong urine; the house smells like urine. If two or three of these little fellows wet the bed at night, the urine is so strong it tells the story at once.

This medicine needs reproving; details have not been brought out, yet its nature is known. We have a good many medicines having this nature, but this is perhaps as intense as any. This remedy does not, of course, fit all these patients, because it does not fit their special symptoms; but it has the nature or general state which, of course, precedes everything, and when it relates to all the particular: as well it does make wonderful changes.

There are a few mental symptoms. "Inclined to dwell on unpleasant things; if he saw anyone deformed, it made him shudder." Alternation of profound sleep with prolonged periods of wakefulness. In the period of wakefulness, he dwells, during the night, upon all the unpleasant subjects that he can think of. This state alternates with nights of stupid sleep for weeks, and this fluctuates in accordance with the fluctuation of the state of urine. "Sadness." "Anxiety while sweating." "Child cross."

There are many headaches; they are uræmic in character and come in many regions with many details. "Fearful pain in occiput or cerebellum." "Rheumatic pains in head." That is well described, because these headaches of uræmic character take on a similarity to rheumatic pains. "Pain and heat in region of organs of reverence and firmness." "Tearing pain in vertex." The headaches are very numerous; the remedy is full of dull, aching occipital headaches, coming on in the night from change of weather. Pains located in the base of the brain after pains have existed for some time in the joints, and they are passing but little urine. Every time he takes a little cold the urine becomes scanty and he is full of dull aches, and pains in the head and especially in the occiput.

Perversion of smell. "Sense of smell diminished." "Pain in nasal bones."

Another form of transformation scene takes place in this remedy, when all the gouty symptoms of the body cease and inflammation of the tongue comes on. The pains in the joints cease suddenly from taking cold, from stormy weather and on comes a sudden swelling of the tongue. *Mercury* also has this state. "Extensive ulcerations of tongue, with deeply chapped or fungoid surfaces." Then, again, peculiar kinds of sore throat take place from this same cause. Sudden stoppage or slacking up of the quantity of urine; it becomes scanty, high colored, and pungent, smelling like that of a horse (*Nitric acid*), along with acute inflammation and swelling of the tonsils and throat; inflammation of the tonsils with scanty, strong, pungent urine smelling like that of a horse. Another feature that seems almost like metastasis. Take an individual who is going around with more or less rheumatic aches in the joints; he takes cold and all this ceases, but the next day he comes down with inflammation of the tongue or sore throat, or *inflammation* of *the stomach;* so that he vomits everything he eats. The gout goes to different parts and in this instance it goes to the stomach; and then Benzoic acid, *Antimonium crud.* or *Sanguinaria* is likely to he useful. When it goes to the throat or is followed by swelling of the tongue *Mercury* and Benzoic acid should be thought of. Whenever this gouty condition goes to the stomach, of course it must conform to those symptoms that are in the nature of this remedy. In this remedy we have "loathing, sickness at stomach," "nausea with gagging," "vomiting of a salty substance; bitter." 'When we think of Benzoic acid for the stomach symptoms, it is important that we have in mind its whole nature, how it brings about its complaints and what characterizes a Benzoic acid patient. We would not be able to distinguish from the stomach symptoms alone; we must carry with them the character of the remedy.

It has much disturbance of the liver, and many liver symptoms. As to the bowels, the stool, the rectum, anus and urinary organs, it is very rich in symptoms. Its striking ones I will call your attention to, but remember its migrating, metastatic nature, its complaints going from one part to another, which will accompany these symptoms. "Stools, copious, watery." This is true in summer diarrhœa, that has come on suddenly, "excessively offensive." The white stool, like soap-suds, is so strong a symptom that the remedy does not fail to cure even when the gouty constitution is not present. "Excessively offensive, scenting the whole house." "Putrid, bloody." "Watery, light-colored, very offensive stools (in children)." So we get the idea that the stools are white and that the first passages are like soap-suds, but later the soap appearance subsides and leaves a white stool. it is well, often, when a stool is passed that is of a light liquid, to bear in mind a few remedies that produce this state and ascertain whether it is like soap-suds or filled with bubbles of air. "Diarrhœa of children." The urinous odor of the body, and especially that peculiarly pungent, intense smell of the urine. "Slightly elevated, wart-like, round surfaces around anus."

The urinary symptoms are too numerous to read. "Fœtid urine." "Urine of a very repulsive odor." "Effervescing with hydrochloric acid." The odor is somteimes like hartshorn; it is pungent; these are only efforts to describe the strong smell. "Urine dark brown." It is true that normal urine after, standing a while will get a fœtid odor, but, in this remedy, that just passed is properly described as being intensely urinous. "Urine contains mucus and pus." "Morbid condition of urine." "Renders urine acid." It says in the text "hippuric acid," but this is a rare condition. "Brown urine smells sour." "Too frequent desire to evacuate bladder." "Nephritic colic." "Urine dark, urinous odor highly intensified." Gouty troubles of the liver; rheumatism; nephritic colic; it has cured such states after gonorrhœa, but it is not much of a gonorrhœal remedy. When the rheumatic states and these symptoms are present there are more or less pains in the kidney. "Sore pain in the back; burning in the kidney." "Prolapsus uteri with fœtid urine." "Retention of urine in infants." "Asthma with inflammatory rheumatic complaints." "Cough followed by expectoration of green mucus."

The organ that is most commonly affected in these rheumatic complaints is the heart. No organ is so likely to be affected when rheumatism leaves the outermost parts as the heart. Pains in the heart. So in this diathesis, with the strong smelling urine and the gout, we may expect affections of the heart.

"Pains change place incessantly." "Palpitation of the heart." The rheumatism, of course, is affecting the heart. "Awakens after midnight with violent pulsations of the heart." Think a moment and you will see in what kind of a case you will need Benzoic acid. The constitution of the remedy comes to mind at once with the heart symptoms, the dyspnœa, pain in the heart with rheumatic symptoms; "cannot go to sleep." Think of the alternation of sleeplessness with sleep; think of the strong urine, of the fluctuating complaints, of the erratic constitution. "Palpitation worse at night." "Rheumatic pains in extremities relieving heart." There we get relief; complaints going back to the extremities with relief to the heart. The heart will relieve when the urine becomes copious or when the rheumatism goes back to the extremities, into the fingers and knees, especially the knees in Benzoic acid. Rheumatism alternating between the extremities and heart. This medicine has cured affections of the heart when the rheumatism has a long time ago disappeared from the extremities and has ever since been affecting the heart; after Benzoic acid has been admi-nistered a very good sign of its action is that the extremities become painful and the urine becomes copious; free urine and solids increased; the urine becomes heavy, whereas it was light. "Hard, frequent pulse.'

The extremities are full of rheumatic affections. "Lassitude in lower limbs." "Swelling of knee." All gouty affections belong to this remedy. "Gouty concretions." "Nodes on joints." Benzoic acid is often an excellent palliating remedy in old gouty constitutions; they want to be relieved of the pains in their fingers and in the nodes and joints. The fingers crack and are clumsy and painful. But often the pain has been relievd and gone to other parts. This is one among the remedies that will drive the complaints away from the internal organs and generally increase the pain in the extremities, which they will scold about. "Trembling with palpitation of heart." "Extreme weakness; sweat and comatose condition." Note that comatose condition with sweat; the Benzoic acid patient sweats without relief. Copious, exhaustive sweat and profound sleep, but there is no relief. "Awaken with difficulty of breathing." Pulsation all over.

"All sorts of catarrhal states; gouty diathesis, gout with arthritic nodo-sites, syphilitic rheumatism, etc." These patients arc getting low down in the scale of life, the tissues become feeble. Ulcers form upon the skin and mucous membranes.

BERBERIS

When we have finished the study of Berberis we will see that it is not a very extensive remedy, but it is a very important one. Like *Benzoic acid;* it fits into the gouty and rheumatic sphere. It corresponds to such gouty conditions as do not determine to their proper places. A low state of the economy is present; anæmic condition; feeble constitution; pallid and sickly, old and worn out; prematurely old and wrinkled men and women. They are too feeble to determine the gouty deposits to the finger joints, where they naturally belong, and the trouble is yet, as it were, wandering around through the economy. Wandering pains in the nerves, and nerve sheaths. The wandering, stitching, tearing, twinging pains that run through Berberis are found in old gouty constitutions, and that is where we get the greatest benefit from Berberis. Its proving would lead us to see it is similar to the wandering, twinging and tearing pains of old gouty constitutions, in persons who are pallid, and sickly, and chilly, where the deposits have not been so marked in the joints; but where the twinging in the fingers and in the toes are just such as are found where the deposits do exist. Of course in all of the gouty states we must look to the liver and kidneys for pains and various distresses; they are centers of observation, because these organs are more or less disturbed. And very often cardiac troubles go along with them. The kidneys, liver, and heart are more or less disturbed in their functions and we see that Berberis takes hold of these organs. We have the uræmic state, and the state of disorder that ends in these conditions. We will have twinging pains along with kidney disturbances.

Irregularities of the urine. Copious discharges, alternating with scanty discharges. Light urine,, and heavy urine, excessive deposits of uric acid and urates. It is changeable, like *Benzoic acid.* These two remedies run very much together, yet their symptoms are wholly unlike. We find among these sensations that stitching pains are found in almost every region of the body, and they are all the time changing. Wandering and stitching pains; little twinges. As you sit by his side and talk to a gouty patient—"Ow," he will say. What does he mean by it? He has had one of those twitching pains. The next thing he knows it is in his knee; then it is in his toes; then it is in his head, all over him. Finally the gouty deposits become prominent in the fingers, and after the gout has determined itself, then we have sore fingers; but these correspond more particularly to *Ledum, Sulphur, .AEsculus* and *Lycopodium,* where the disease has become marked and has located in the joints. In Berberis these twinging, tearing, stitching, burning pains are everywhere, they never remain in one place, but are always moving, and they are not often affected by motion. Whether he moves, or keeps still, they keep coming. In a few instances we have pains aggravated by motion, but a very few in proportion to the many pains in Berberis. He moves many times, because he cannot keep still. He moves, because he suffers. There are also many pressing pains. But the burning, stinging, tearing, stitching, wandering pains are the main feature, the grand feature of Berberis. If you single them out in places, in a given joint, from that one joint they will radiate in every direction. If it is the knee joint, they will go up, and down, and every way; if it is the finger joint, they will run in every direction. If it is the kidney, they will go down the ureters; if it is the liver, they will *go* down into the abdomen in every direction. "Radiating from a particular point," is a distinguishing feature, and it puts Berberis almost alone for radiating pains. This is such a strong feature that Berberis has cured renal colic in many instances because of its well known ability to shoot out in every direction. It cures gall-stone colic when these little twinges go in every direction from that locality. We see these twinging, shooting pains in gouty constitutions are associated with urinary troubles, and with liver troubles, and we begin to lay a foundation for the study of Berberis.

The joints sometimes swell. "Enlargement of the joints." But the swelling is not so common as the pains without swelling. Soreness, lameness in the joints, with these radiating pains. There will be burning, stitching, tearing, and the pains will radiate and appear in one part of the body then in another. "A pain in the heel as if it were ulcerating," and then the pain shoots off in every direction. Numbness. Lameness.

As to the heart, the pulse becomes slow. Very often it is slowed down astonishingly.

The mental symptoms are very defective, that is, we do not know the mental symptoms. There are a few. We know this, that the mind is weak, that he is unable to sustain a mental effort, and that he is forgetful. "Defective recollection and weak memory. Terrifying apparitions in twilight." It is not a strange thing for a child in the dark to imagine all sorts of things, because they have heard graveyard stories from old people; but with this remedy between the daylight and darkness he sees ghosts, imaginary forms coming round him. It has melancholy, apathy, prastration of mind. Some dizziness. The headaches are of the same character as the general pains in uræmic subjects, where there is plenty of sand in the urine, red pepper deposit. The head comes in for its share of these wandering pains. Stitching, tearing, twinging in the scalp; in the skull; in the eyes, ears, back of the head. Burning pains. "A feeling in the head as if it was becoming larger," is a peculiar symptom; a puffy sensation. Always putting the hand to the head; it feels as if he had on a skull-cap. It fits down over the brow, and it is not an uncommon thing with such patients to put the hand to the head to take off the cap. "Feels as if he had a cap on the head," when there is none there. This symptom is not always described like a cap on the head. It is convertible into numbness of the scalp; many patients describe a sensation of numbness in the scalp, as if they had on a cap. Sometimes patients will deny that it is a sensation of numbness, and say it is just a cap. At one time I fully believed the "cap" belonged to two sensations. If it was painful I placed it under "pressure." If it was not painful it was supposed to belong to "numbness;" but I have now made a new rubric, "the sensation of skullcap," which I now think is entirely distinctive from numbness; but they both have to be compared.

Then the eyes take on that same gouty condition, with stitching tearing pains, twinging pains, shooting pains. Shooting off in various directions. There is one grand feature about Berberis, that it has no particular direc-tion; it has all directions. Most remedies have pains taking a direction from one part to the other, pains going from the eye to the temple, etc., but in Berberis it cannot be said the pains go to any place in particular. They are wandering pains and they radiate. Pains in the ears of the same character. In every part of the body we have these twinging, tearing, burning, shooting pains coming and going, causing the patient to scowl and make a sharp noise.

The patient has a sickly look; face pale, earthly complexion, with sunken cheeks and hollow, blue-encircled eyes. That is a description of a sick face. Berberis has been very useful in phthisical conditions; and in the pains, and twinging, and sufferings in persons who have been operated on for *fistula in ano*. When the fistula has been closed, these pains will come if it is a Berberis case. The kidney manifestations will come on, or the liver manifestations, or the enfeebled heart, or these wandering pains. At one time feverish, full of pains, with violent thirst; alternating with the very opposite state. Prostration and aversion to water. Want of appetite at one time; canine hunger at another. The stomach is disordered, digestion is slow and feeble, and we have manifestations usually known to patients as "bilious". Eructations that are bitter and of bile.

The liver is full of suffering. In the liver we have these pains, and added to them sudden stabbing like a knife puncturing the liver. Shooting, tearing, burning, stitching, twinging pains, wandering from one place to another. "Gall-stone colic." These pains with jaundice. The liver seems to slow down in its actions, and the patient becomes jaundiced. The stool becomes white, bileless. "Sharp, pinching pains in the liver, which come suddenly and with great severity. Violent stabbing pain in the region of the liver, taking his breath away. Had to bend double." These pains last a moment and pass away. In gall-stone colic pains are spasmodic, increase in intensity and diminish, but do not let up entirely. Berberis when it is indicated will let the little gall-stone loose, and it will pass through, and the patient will take a long breath and wish he had sent for the doctor sooner. Anything that is spasmodic can be relieved instantly.

Pains through the abdomen. Copious, thick, mushy stools, and these are yellow, like yellow corn meal mush. "Diarrhœa; mush-like yellowish discharges." "Clay-colored." From what we have seen it is not surprising that it is clay-colored, that it is bileless, that it is white. The action on the liver does that. When you have these symptoms associated with radiating pains, and with wandering pains in broken down constitutions, persons who are suffering from cold, who are pallid and sickly, you have a Berberis case.

Then the patient becomes constipated, but the stool is white, or very light colored. "Burning, stinging pain before, during, and after stool." Enlargement of the prostate gland, which causes a constant pressure in the perineum. Pressure as if there were a lump, or as if something was pressing down." "Tearing extending around the anus. Herpes around anus. Fistula in ano." Now the surgeons nearly all advocate that if there is a fistulous opening around the anus it must be operated upon. Homœopathy cures such cases. I have not operated on one for twenty years. The remedy that is indicated for the *patient* will cure the *patient,* and the fistula. Above all things, they should not be operated on. To close up that fistulous opening, and thus neglect the patient, is a very dangerous thing to do. Knowing all that I know, if such a trouble should come upon me and I could not find the remedy to cure it I would bear with it patiently, knowing I was keeping a much less grievance. Nor could I advise my patient to have a thing done that I would not have done upon myself. It is a dangerous thing to operate upon a fistula in ano. It is a very serious matter. If it is closed up, and that patient is leaning towards phthisis, he will develop phthisis; if he has a tendency towards Bright's disease, that will hasten it; if he threatens to break down in any direction, his weakest parts will be affected, and he will break down. Occasionally time enough elapses so that the physician who is ignorant does not see the relation between the two. But now that you have heard it, you can never forget it.

And then the kidneys and the urinary organs come in for their troubles. There is such a soreness in the lumbar region, in the region of the kidneys, that he can bear no pressure. He cannot step down from a carriage to the pavement without letting himself - down very carefully. A jar is a great shock to him, and sometimes the soreness is so great that he almost faints. Soreness in the back; in the muscles of the back, and in the region of the kidneys; and this associated with all sorts of disturbances in the urine, with excessive deposits. The kidneys radiate in every direction. Pains run up into the kidney, and they become worn out if he does not get relief, he will have some serious disease. Hence we have these symptoms. "Burning and soreness in the region of the kidneys. Burning stitches, single or several in succession, in region of loins and kidneys. Much pain, soreness and tenderness in back, in the region of the kidneys. Sensitiveness in the region of the kidneys so great that any jarring motion, riding in a wagon, jumping from it, was intolerable. After kidney complaints, a foul, bitter taste, rush of blood to the throat. Great urging, with pain in the neck of the bladder, with burning, scanty urine. Voilent, cutting, tensive pain, deeply seated in left side of bladder, at last becoming a sticking, obliquely in female urethra, as if in its orifice; lasting a few minutes." Now we see how these symptoms manifest themselves. Sore, inflamed, sensitive kidney, one or both. And then, the formation of little calculi in the pelvis of the kidney—little stones like pinheads; and every now and then one of them takes a start down the ureter to the bladder, and, oh, how he suffers. Then it is that the pains in the kidneys radiate in every direction. Pains run up into the kidney, and down into the bladder. In the male they appear as if they ran down the spermatic cord into the testes, and he is a great sufferer. You will be astonished to know how quickly Berberis will relieve this particular kind of renal colic. Burning pain in the bladder; burning pain in the kidney. "Urine dark, turbid with copious sediment. Urine very slow to flow. Constant urging." The bladder becomes very irritable. Catarrhal conditions of the bladder. Smarting, burning, stitching pains. Many troubles, pains and aches in the spermatic cord and testes in gouty constitutions. Burning pains along these regions.

Berberis especially fits a woman who is tired, with a gouty constitution; though not old in years she is physically tired, so that all of her domestic affairs fret and tire her. Coition becomes painful, and she has an aversion to it. The orgasm is delayed, or is entirely absent, and she is prostrated by it. In all the affairs of her innermost life she is a drudge. Full of twinging pains in all of her nerves. "Burning in female urethra, Burning pain in the vagina." A lack of sensation normal to these parts in the woman.

BORAX

Borax is one of those domestic remedies that has been long used for local conditions as a soothing substance and for a healing purpose. In "nursing sore mouth" of mother or child Borax has been used in the families of old, in the form of Borax and honey, as a wash. The extensive use that has been made of it would make the homœopath wonder if the people had not hit upon something, and it is a fact that Borax will rapidly heal up a sore mouth. It is not strange that it does so, for Borax, in its proving, produces aphthous conditions of the mouth, which extend to the throat and even into the stomach. It cures where the genitalia and anus are covered with these aphthous appearances.

Anxiety, fidgetiness, and sensitiveness are prominent in Boarx. He is anxious about trifles. He starts at every noise, on hearing unexpected news, from music, from excitement. This anxiety or nervousness, this indescribable feeling that is within him, is aggravated from upward or downward motion. Such a motion as going up in one of our elevators nearly drives him to distraction, but he is made worse going down. All complaints are aggravated from downward motion. It has been said in routine practice, that in all cases of sore mouth in children, when the child is worse from downward motion, Borax is the remedy. When the mother is in the act of laying the child down on the bed it often rouses up in its sleep and cries out in fright. The anxiety may be better appreciated if you will go to the top of one of these high buildings and go down in the elevator. It is natural for every one to feel, with the rapid motion, an anxious feeling in the stomach, a sensation of falling; that is natural to the healthy man, but if you exaggerate that intensely you have the Borax condition in which the slightest downward motion, of even riding down hill or walking down stairs, or, in the child, when being carried down stairs in the mother's arms, produces a violent aggravation. All the nerves are in a fret.

We notice that Borax has an intensified activity throughout the body; all of his senses are made more acute. His hearing is intensified, he is oversensitive to his surroundings, over-anxious. He has an excitable spirit throughout. Riding down hill produces vertigo. On nervous excitement, fear and apprehension. This is a strong feature of Borax. It has many such symptoms, but the nervous elements partake of this type. As we go through the remedy many other things will be called out; but this may be said to be the principal feature of the mental state, and it is to a great extent the key to Borax cases. "Anxious feeling during downward motion or rocking." The diarrhœa will be cured when that state is present. Aphthæ will be cured when that state is present. The rheumatism, menstrual troubles and numerous other complaints will disappear upon the administration of Borax, when this key is present.

It has hysterical manifestations. "Changes from one work to another." It has a restless, nervous, anxious, excitable state that runs through his body. The child screeches and screams when it is dandled and tossed up and down. The motion of the brain, the upward and downward motion, as in swinging, rocking, etc., makes the patient lose himself, he hardly knows where he is; confusion and vertigo come over him. If one rocks the child, it has an anxious expression of face. "Very anxious on riding rapidly down hill." "Anxiety increased until 11 P.M." That I have noticed in Borax as a peculiar time of aggravation of the anxiety. I have noticed it in women who had periods of insanity, whose nervous trouble and mental state would keep up until 11 P.M. You will notice sometimes in insane people that it seems as if they were possessed of the devil; and at once a lucid interval will come and they will talk just as if nothing had happened. So it is in Borax, that a great change may occur at 11 P.M.; this state of anxiety and nervous excitement may stop at that hour. "Fretful, ill-humored, indolent" state increased until there is a stool and relieved by stool. "He starts on hearing an anxious cry;" on hearing an unexpected noise, on hearing something drop from a chair to the floor, or if a door opens unexpectedly. This is all in keeping with the nature of Borax. If you compare Borax with other *Natrums* you will find an astonishing likeness in the nervous excitability; *Natrum carb.* and *Natrum mur.* Aggravation from noise, oversensitiveness to noise and overexcitement of the nerves run through all the *Sodium* family They are wonderfully intense people.

"While engaged in thinking at his work, strong nausea." Borax has many times cured this kind of trouble. I have seen it come up in this way; from any sort of meditation he becomes nauseated and excitable and must leave his work and rest a little while, and then he goes at it again until he becomes sick at the stomach and so must rest again. With the aggravation from mental exertion, from noise, from excitement, from downward motion, we get the mental aspect of Borax.

A further examination of the sensorium shows: "Vertigo and fulness in head on descending a mountain or stairs." This is a form of the same anxious feeling. This remedy has a good deal of vertigo, sometimes constant vertigo, which is made so intense on downward motion that he must sit still, and do nothing. It has many congestive headaches, pressive headaches and much heat in the head.

There are many eye symptoms. "Granular lids." "Lashes turn inward towards eye and inflame it, Entropion." Granulation and thickening of the mucous membrane of the lid; contractions and scars and drawing inward. "Difficult opening of lids."

Like all the salts of *Sodium* the nose suffers from chronic inflammation of the mucous membrane, a catarrhal state, with copious discharge, and crusts in the nose; stoppage of the nose. The whole *Natrum* family has these dry crusts in the nose, and copious discharges from the nose. *Natrum mur.* predominantly produces *white* discharge, and so does Borax; *Natr. sulph.* produces *yellow* discharge, and so does Borax; *Natr. sulph.* produces *yellow* discharge from the nose, even yellowish-green. Borax is laid down as producing greenish discharge; it characteristic discharge, which is a general of the remedy, is a white discharge.

The face of the infant is pale, and clay-colored. "Children have small vesicles around the mouth, and on the forehead." *Natr. mur.* produces herpetic eruptions around the mouth in all of its febrile states, and when the patient takes cold. Borax is sometimes forgotten, and *Natr. mur.* is thought of because it is better known. When the *Natrum* constitution is present, then it becomes a process of individualization to determine which one of the *Natrums* is indicated.

"Aphthæ in mouth and on tongue." "Aphtllæ on tongue and inside of cheek." This alone is not an indication for Borax, although Borax is one among many medicines when the mouth is so sore that the child lets loose its hold of the nipple or bottle. Many prescribers give Borax on that indication alone; but the constitutional state ought to be hunted up, so that there may be constitutional foundation for the remedy. *Sulph. ac.* is more frequently indicated. "Red blisters on tongue." "Vomiting after drinking." This leads one to expect that this aphthous state has travelled down the *œsophagus* into the stomach. There are many stomach symptoms present that are likely to be the result of some such condition. "Buccal mucous membrane highly reddened." The sore mouth, such as mothers have and such as infants have, can be cured with Borax. "After every meal flatulent distension." Constant vomiting." "Vomiting of sour slime." The Borax patient with stomach aphthæ will gag and retch and cough, and that is what is called a "stomach cough". Mothers say, "It is a stomach cough," because the child gags and retches with it. "Stomach cough with pain extending into region of spleen."

Little ones often get summar complaints when they need Borax. All around about the anus you will see the aphthous appearances. Great slimy stools are passed day and night; the child keeps up a pitiful crying; the mouth is aphthous, child is emaciating, and holds its head back. "Stools; frequent, soft, light yellow, slimy." Quantities of fluid like boiled starch are emitted from the anus; Borax has that as well as *Argentum nitricum.* There are also conditions of the rectum producing thickening of the mucous membrane, with stricture, growing smaller and smaller until finally a long thin stool is passed, no larger than a pencil. This inflammatory stricture has been cured by Borax.

In this oversensitive child when the catarrhal state is general the urine burns so when it passes that with the first urging (which causes the child to realize it must soon urinate) it screams out; screams with the desire to urinate. That is what it means when it says "Worse before urination." It is not that the state of the urinary organs is worse before urinating, but the child in realizing that it must urinate screeches and screams. "Frequent urination preceded by cries." The urine burns and you may know that the child must soon urinate because it commences to cry. "Orifice of urethra pains as if sore, after urinating." "Desire to urinate without being able to pass a drop."

This remedy has cured gonrrhœa. Wherever there is mucous membrane you may expect to find the aphthous patches. There is another feature like *Natr. mur.* and *Natr. carb.,* in both male and female it takes away sexual desire; it benumbs the patient; and hence the mind and sexual organs are in a state of indifference.

Then we come to the most striking feature of Borax in regard to the female sexual organs; in the menstrual flow will be found *membrane.* Borax cures the most violent forms of membranous dysmenorrhœa, when there are violent labor-like pains before and during the flow and it seems as if the uterus would expel itself from the vagina. The flow starts slightly, but the same violent pains keep on, until the expulsion of the membrane. I have known Borax to cure when the membrane was a cast of the uterus. Such patients are easily startled from downward motion; let that be your guide to Borax in membranous dysmenorrhœa. She dreads downward motion, and motions like swinging and rocking. "During menses; throbbing in head and rushing in ears." "Pinching and griping in adbomen;" that word does not describe it exactly, for it is like the pain in labor; "pain extending from stomach." Pain like the stabbing of a knife in the groin,. and that may occur either before or during menstruation. "Tired; sweat after midnight." But, remember, with such things you must have the mental state, the nervous, excitable state and then Borax will cure this dysmenorrhœa. Another grand feature of Borax I read in the next sentence. "Leucorrhœa like the white of eggs." It has albuminous leucorrhoea which feels like a hot fluid, and flows down the legs. "White albuminous or starchy leueorrhœa." "Acrid leucorrhœa appearing for two weeks." "Leucorrhœa white as mucus, without any other ailment." Now from this acrid leucorrhoea, from the menstrual state, this false membrane forming and being thrown off, it is no wonder that women are sterile. All these women are sterile, all who have such symptoms are sterile and Borax has cured sterility when this condition was the cause. You will find routinists prescribe Borax for all women who are sterile, regardless of the state. When a remedy is given for sterility, the *state* must be looked into which is peculiar to the remedy given such a state as that remedy can produce upon the healthy woman.

Another feature. Many times I have used Borax when the mother could not nurse the child, she talks about always having a little, thick milk. "The milk is too thick and tastes badly." This condition of the milk prevents the mother from nursing her child. This is a constitutional state, and Borax, if given in the beginning of pregnancy, to a Borax patient will so change the milk as well as the rest of the constitution that the mother will he able to nurse the child. I have a number of times, when a mother has brought forth several children that she was unable to nurse, given Borax and it has so affected the case that she could nurse the next child. This remedy also has loathing of the breast in infants, due to the fact that the milk tastes bad and not due to any defect on the part of the child. You might think of prescribing for the infant, but if you examine into the case you will find that the child will not take the milk because it is loathsome. The mother needs a dose of Borax, which will cure the child of its diarrhœa and loathing of milk. "The infant becomes pale, nearly earth-colored." "The child throws up its hands when an attempt is made to put it down." If the mother was a Borax mother, the child very likely is a Borax child; it is not an uncommon thing for the mother and baby to need the same remedy; many times I have medicated the child through the mother's milk if both needed the same remedy. Another peculiar feature is that when the child is nursing, there is *pain in the opposite breast*. Borax is not necessarily 'limited to the state of confinement; there is a practical use for Borax among nervous women in all states of life.

Borax has cured pleurisy that very much resembled *Bryonia,* especially on the right side like *Bryonia;* stitching or darting pains from without inward as if through the upper right lung posteriorly; the stitching pains might make you think of *Bryonia.*

"Wilted, wrinkled skin." "Skin pale or livid." Emaciated; flabby child becomes emaciated. Children become marasmic along with the aphthous condition; they cannot digest. They vomit or have diarrhœa; aphthous condition that extends the whole length of the intestines; involving all mucous membranes. Oversensitive child screams from downward motion. The aphthæ involve a good many other symptoms; crying before urination, because the bladder is involved. The aphthous condition and worse from downward motion; the oversensitiveness to noise, easily startled, anxious feeding, etc. are the most striking and characterizing features.

BROMIUM

Bromium is one of the routine medicines. It is one of the medicines that the neophyte will make use of for every case of diphtheria and croup, and laryngitis he comes across; and when it does not work he will "try something else". All who prescribe on the name use Bromium as one of their routine medicines; but Bromium is so seldom indicated that most homœopaths give it up as a perfectly useless medicine. The reason is that they do not take the symptoms of the case and prescribe in accordance with the individualizing method. They do not prescribe for the *patient,* but for the disease. You may see very few cases of diphtheria calling for Bromium; but when you see a Bromium case you want to know Bromium. There is one underlying feature of the Bromium conditions, they are found especially in those individuals that are made sick from being heated. If there is a diphtheria epidemic and the mother bundles up her baby until she overheats it, and keeps it in a hot room and it happens to be a child that is sensitive to being wrapped up, and on whose complaints are worse from being wrapped up, look out. You are going to have a Bromium diphtheria. It is indicated also in complaints that come on in the night after a very hot day in the summer.

Now, this is as near as you can come to being routine in croup and diphtheria. If the mother has the baby out in a dreadfully cold, dry day, and along towards midnight it wakens with spasmodic croup, you know that it is more likely to call for *Aconite* than any other medicine. But if the mother has had the baby out in a hot day in the summer, and that baby has been overheated, with too much clothing, and it is a plethoric child, and towards midnight you are called up, and the child has a red face, and your examinations reveal a membrane in the throat, we will see as we study the remedy that this may be a Bromium case.

"Hoarseness coming on from getting overheated. Loss of voice coming on from getting overheated." A turmoil in the whole economy; with headaches, coming on from getting overheated. That runs through Bromium. So it is in the hot weather, and being confined to a hot room, and after going from the cold into the heat. But after the complaint comes on, no matter where it is, he is so sensitive to cold that a draft of cool air freezes him; but he cannot be overheated without suffering.

Bromium has running through it a tendency to infiltrate the glands. The glands become hard, but seldom suppurate. They generally remain hard. The glands of the neck, the parotid, the sublingual, the submaxillary, are enormously enlarged and very hard. The processes of inflammation are slow; they are not that rapid, violent kind like we find in *Bell.* and *Merc.* "Parts that inflame infiltrate, becoming hard" Inflammation with hardness is the idea. It has been very useful in ulcers with this infiltration; very useful in enlarged glands with great hardness, without any tendency to suppurate. Glands take on tuberculosis, and tissues take on tuberculosis. Glands that inflame for a while begin to take on a lower form of degeneration, a lower form of tissue making. It is very similar to these enlarged, hard, scrofulous glands that we find in the neck; enlargement of the parotid and submaxillary. It has cured enlargement and great hardness of the thyroid gland.

Again, we have emaciation, and when we see the tendency to infiltration it is not strange that it has been a curative medicine in cancer and tuberculosis. There is weakness in this remedy. The legs become weak. Growing prostration, with tremulous limbs. Twitching; tremulous weakness; fainting. In the catarrhal affections there is a formation, more or less, of membrane. Membranous exudate is a natural course of events. A natural feature of the mucous membrane is infiltration, so that the mucous membrane appears to exude little grayish-white vegetations, and beneath them is induration. That is true in ulcers, it is true in mucous membrane. An ulcer will form upon the mucous membrane and eat in, and build beneath it a hardened stratum of tissue. It has febrile conditions along with these catarrhal states. Great nervous excitement. "Icy coldness of the limbs." "Heat of the head." "Dyspnœa, with great sweating." Croupy manifestations.

Running through most of the complaints there is palpitation. Palpitation with nausea, palpitation with headache, palpitation with various kinds of nervous excitement. So weak is he gradually becoming that he has an 'aversion to every kind of work; to reading. Takes no interest in household duties." Becomes indifferent. Very tired. "Great depression of spirits. Low spirited. Sad and discouraged." Anxiety with most complaints. Headaches from becoming overheated. "Noise in the ears. Throbbing and burning in the ears." And then the complaints of the glands that are so closely associated with the ears. With ear troubles, enlargement of the glands; the parotid becomes enlarged and hard. Ear affections following scarlet fever, with discharges from the ears. Pains and aches; inflammation; abscess of the ear. Suppuration of the parotid gland occasionally, but it is an exception. "Swelling and hardness of the left parotid gland." The ovaries, testes, etc., are all affected by Bromium.

Bleeding of the nose. Ulcerations in the nose. Catarrhal affections of the nose. Much sneezing. Acute coryza, violent, with much burning in the nose, and a sensation of coldness, as if the mucous membrane of the nose were cold from inhaling cold air. It is useful for June cold, with the first hot weather in June, or if the first hot weather comes in July. Violent coryza once a year, during the hot season. Fluent coryza, with headaches. "The nose is sore and the wings of the nose swell. Scurf forms on it, with pain and bleeding on wiping it." Rawness round about the nostrils. A Bromium patient is one that is likely to have flushed face, especially those due to acute Bromium conditions. "Flushed face." He becomes heated easily. But this is entirely the opposite of the chronic constitutional Bromium condition. That is true with a good many remedies, especially many of the antipsorics. The old sickly broken-down constitutions, those needing Bromium for chronically enlarged glands, for goitre, for cancerous affections, will have the "gray, earthy color of the face. Oldish appearance." It is a sickly face, an ash-colored face. "Face ashy gray." Then again we 'have children that are plethoric, with red face, easily overheated. Of course, when the acute condition is on and the breathing has been that of dyspnœa for several hours or many days, then the patient becomes cyanotic, gasping for breath, and choking, the face becomes ashy pale, as it is in diphtheria, in croup, and in laryngeal affections.

"Stony, hard swelling of glands, especially of the lower jaw and throat." We find that repeated in many divisions of the subject. Many of the throat complaints that are laid down in Bromium begin in the larynx and creep up into the throat. Some of them begin in the throat and go down into the larynx; but the two are so closely associated in Bromium that both are likely to be affected; so that diphtheria spreads from one to the other. Diphtheria begins in the throat and goes into the larynx. Bromium fits the most malignant type of diphtheria. The membrane grows like a weed, shuts off breathing, closes up the larynx. So severe are the cases, that though he has been sick but two or three days, and even when Bromium has mastered the case, the patient is left with great prostration. All those that belong to Bromium are of that type. Great violence; great prostration. Extremely sick, and with deathly weakness. A great many of the cures that have been performed in the throat have been left-sided diphtheria, yet it has cured both sides. You will very seldom see Bromium develop in cold dry weather; but in hot damp weather Bromium cases come on; affections in the spring, and in the fall and summer.

The chronic cases that will need Bromium are such as have ulcers of the stomach. Suspicious ulcers in the stomach, and suspicious symptoms about the stomach. Vomiting like coffee grounds, and vomiting with signs of ulceration. Aggravation after eating; either vomiting, or diarrhœa. Cannot take acids. Diarrhœa or cough worse after eating, or after acids. "After eating oysters, diarrhœa, and a disordered stomach. Worse from the slightest inhalation of tobacco smoke. Vomiting of bloody mucus. Eructations." Foul stomach. Pain in the stomach from warm things, from hot tea, hot drinks. It is a common feature when there is ulcer in the stomach or when the mucous membrane is about to ulcerate, that hot drinks are intolerable. "Pains from taking hot foods."

In studying the stool and rectum symptoms we find exudation. Membranous formations pass in the stool. Diarrhoeic stool with membrane. "Black, fæcal stool." Diarrhœa; must go to stool after eating.

We have running through the remely enlarged veins. These are found also in the rectum. Hæmorrhoids protrude from the rectum, burning. Smarting day and night. "Blind, intensely painful varices, with black, diarrhtric stools. Blind, painful hæmorrhoids," and hæmorrhoids that protrude. "Hæmorrhoids during and after stool." During the stool the rectum is painful from hæmorrhoidal tumors.

Swelling and induration of the left testicle. Notice the left-sidedness, the left side of the throat. and the left testicle. Then, again, dull pain in the region of the *left* ovary. "Constant dull pain in the ovary; with swelling and hardness." There is the same induration of the left ovary. It does seem strange that some medicines single out more particularly the left organs and the *left* side of the body. Like *Lach.* in many instances it picks out the left side of the body. A great many remedies show a preference for one side of the body; the glands in this remedy are more affected upon the left side of the body than the right. "Swelling of the ovarian region before and during menses." Suppression of the menses. Loud emission of flatus from the vagina.

In the larynx it has produced more symptoms than in any other part of the body. It produces a raw, sore feeling in the larynx from inhaled air. "Rawnes in the larynx. Loss of voice. Hoarseness from overheating." From too much clothing on a warm day, or from keeping on an overcoat in a room that is heated; coming out into the air he cools off. He has laryngitis. "Tickling in the larynx," keeping up a constant coughing. Scraping and rawness in the larynx. Scraping mucus from the larynx, scraping and coughing. It is not a hawk, because that noise clears the throat. Every medical student should go through all the noises he hears others make, and try and observe as much as possible what feeling is accompanied with that noise, so that he can put himself in the other's place. Each one is accompanied with its own sound, and the instant you hear it you realize the exact place he is drawing mucus from and just where the irritation is. If you allow the patient to describe it he always calls it by the wrong name. The patient knows very little about this part except that it is the throat, and if he is drawing mucus from the throat, or scraping it from the larynx, he always calls it the throat. But the physician must waive all that and observe as to sound. So let each one go alone by himself and make all these noises that he hears people make, and then realize for himself what part it is he is scraping. It may seem ludicrous, but how else will you learn about it? It is just as important to figure out these sounds as it is to figure out what a child needs by its sounds and motions. It is impossible to get the symptoms and wants of a child except by interpreting its motions. Every motion it makes indicates something. An astute observer, one who has been watching children for a number of years, will understand the child; and will hardly have to ask the mother a question. He will know at once where the child is sick by what it does. The child is like the animal. You never have to ask a horse or dog where he feels pain, because he will always tell by his motions. So does the infant.

The hoarseness comes on after being overheated. Remember that. "Rough, dry cough; pain in the larynx." Jumping up for want of breath. "Gasping and suffering for breath, with wheezing and rattling in larynx. Sensation as if air passages were full of smoke." Now we have all these rough sounds; rough breathing; croupy breathing; rasping breathing—. different ways of describing different forms of croup. You cannot individualize a remedy by these because one child will croup in one pitch, and another will croup in another; but to get at the constitution of the child and the mother is the important point. "Voice hardly audible." "Spasm in the glottis." In the croupy condition it is really a membranous formation upon the inflamed surface, very often extending downward through the trachea into the bronchial tubes, and producing a croupous pneumonia. Bromium has that in its nature. But without any membranous formation at all Bromium constricts the larynx. It has constriction of the larynx, just like a clutching, a spasm. "Tickling in the larynx, with irritation to cough. Scraping and rawness in the larynx. Sensation of coldness in the larynx." That is a very peculiar symptom with Bromium. In laryngitis, where the patient says the feeling is as if it was *covered with down*. I have heard them describe it as if it was covered with velvet , but it feels so cold. The air breathed feels cold, just like it was the air blown off from snow or ice. Sensation of coldness in the larynx. "Constant sore pain in the larynx." This means that the larynx is painful to touch. *Phos.*, *Bell.*, and *Rumex* have soreness in the larynx, sore to touch; but the Bromium soreness is commonly below the larynx and in the throat pit as well. "Sensation as if the air tubes were full of smoke." Some patients will describe that as sulphur fumes, or as of smoke from tar. After the first few hours mucus begins to accumulate in the larynx and trachea, and a constant expectoration keeps up, of a whitish thick mucus, and he coughs and scrapes the larynx constantly, and there is no peace. This is often present in laryngitis without any membranous formation. Bromium is not given as often as it is indicated in voicelessness, in irritation of the larynx, in rawness of the larynx, because it is uncommon for persons to have laryngitis and hoarseness in the larynx from being overheated. Many of those cases would be cured promptly by Bromium. But where it is thought of by the routine prescriber is where there is croup or diphtheria. That was never taught by Hahnemann. "Much rattling of mucus in the larynx. Inspiration very difficult. Larynx drawn down." This would take place in croup, after the formation of the membrane. "Cough hoarse, crowing, suffocative; breathing sawing, whistling. Spasms of the larynx; suffocative cough. Membranous formation in larynx and trachea. Croupous inflammation formed by exuberant growth of fungi." "Asthma of sailors as soon as they go ashore;" relieved again as soon as they are at sea. Difficult breathing with rattling throughout the chest. Bronchitis and pneumonia. Bromium is often the remedy when whooping cough is prevailing in the spring, towards the hot weather, and membranes form in the larynx. The cough gets immediately worse from dust. Handling old books from the shelf aggravates. Sneezing, hoarseness, irritation in the respiratory tract from picking up and handling dusty things. "Cough, with sudden paroxysms of suffocation on swallowing." Bromium is full of catarrhal conditions, especially of the breathing apparatus. It has hepatization of the lungs; infiltration is one of its most natural features.

BRYONIA

Every medicine has a sphere of action, a peculiar nature whereby it differs from all other medicines, and hence it becomes suitable to complaints of one class and not suitable to those of another. It is like the nature of human beings, as they differ from each other, and also like the nature of diseases, which differ from each other in character. We study a remedy also in regard to its velocity and continuance, its remittence or intermittence. The symptoms of some remedies come on suddenly, with great violence, with great rapidity, stay but a short time in their paroxysm, and go off as if nothing had happened. Others come on slowly, are deep acting and continuous, like the continued fevers. We notice the complaints of *Ignatia,* how flitting and intermittent and unexpected everything is; we notice in *Aconite* how complaints come on with violence, and in *Belladonna* with what suddenness they come on. When we come to the study of Bryonia we find it is a most persistent remedy; its complaints develop slowly, *i.e., slowly for acute conditions.* Its complaints are continuous, remittent, and only occasionally intermittent. They increase into violence, but the violence is not the first flash as in *Aconite* or *Belladonna,* and hence it conforms to a type of disease with *continued fever;* to *rheumatisms* that come with gradually increasing severity, gradually increasing and involving one joint after another, until all the *white fibrous tissues* are in a state of inflammation, pain and distress. It has inflammatory conditions anywhere about the body, but particularly of the fibrous tissues, serous membranes, ligaments of joints and aponeuroses. It also affects the coating of nerves with its congestions, and these gradually increase in severity.

From the beginning there are present the characteristic features, and it may be seen that this patient is coming down with a Bryonia sickness. The patient has several days of preparation. He does not feel very well, is languid and tired, does not want to be spoken to, does not want to move, and this gradually increases; pains begin to flit over the body, they move around here and there over the fibres in one place and another, and every time he moves the pains increase, until they end in a steady and continuous pain. The parts become hot and inflamed, and at last he is down with rheumatism. The complaints come on *after taking cold,* not the first few hours, as in *Aconite* or *Bell.,* but the day after an exposure he begins to feel uneasy and he sneezes and the nose discharges, there is rawness in the chest, and in a day or so he has a chill and comes down with some inflammatory trouble, pneumonia or pleurisy. Its inflammatory complaints include inflammation of the membranes of the brain, sometimes extending into the cord; the pleural membranes, the peritoneum and the heart covering, these are the most common; it also has inflammation of organs. When these conditions come on there is noticed, very early in the case, even before the pains begin, an aversion to motion, and the patient does not know why, but finally he observes that his symptoms are made worse if he has to move, so that the slighest inclination to move is resisted with a feeling of anger, and when he does move he finds he is aroused to great suffering, and that all the aches and pains of the body come on. Thus we have the well-known Bryonia *aggravation from motion.* This runs all through the remedy.

This medicine is suitable in a great many diseases, diseases of a *typhoid nature,* diseases that take on a symptomatic typhoid, diseases that start out as remittents and run into a continued fever, as in pneumonia, pleurisy, inflammation of the liver, of glands, of the bowels, etc. It may be a gastro-enteritis or peritonitis, or inflammation of the bowels, with the sensitiveness, the aggravation from motion and the desire to keep perfectly still. Inflammation of joints, whether of rheumatic character or not, whether from cold, exposure or injury. Bryonia is often indicated in injuries of joints where *Arnica* would be a failure.

There is an extreme state of *irritability* in Bryonia; every word which compels him to answer a question or to think will aggravate him. The effort to talk will be attended with horror. At the beginning of complaints you go to the bedside of a patient who has been grumbling a few days; something is evidently coming on; the family meet you at the door and say, "The patient is almost unconscious;" you look at him, the face is puffed and purplish, he seems to be dazed, there appears to be a sort of venous stasis all over the body, but especially about the face; his countenance is almost that of an imbecile, yet he is perfectly capable of talking, although he has an aversion to it and appears to outsiders to ignore everything that is said. This sometimes comes on apparently in a short time; the patient awakens in the morning with a dull, congestive headache and a stupid feeling in the head; dulness of mind so that he cannot work, and this feeling gradually increases; such a state is sometimes the forerunner of a serious illness We find, when a pneumonia or inflammation of the liver, or some slow insidious inflammation is coming on somewhere in the body, but not yet located, that this state will begin in the morning. This is peculiar about the aggravation of Bryonia—its troubles commence many times early in the morning. On waking, with the first move, he realizes that things are not all right, there is a state of stupidity bordering on unconsciousness. Those who have been grumbling for a week or ten days wake up in the morning feeling miserable, some time that night or the next day they have to send for the doctor. If this is watched for a few days, a continued fever is observed. Or at night a chill will come on, with much pain in the chest, rusty expectoration, short, dry cough and other symptoms that will be spoken of under Bryonia later, showing that the trouble is going towards the chest; or the condition may gradually increase as a congestive, dull headache. This will be seen when congestion of the brain is coming on. Bryonia sickness often picks out *plethoric* subjects, those who are venous in their make up, those who, when suffering with cold, come down with catarrhal congestions. *Catarrhal fever* may be covered by Bryonia. This *sluggish* state of the mind then is the state of Bryonia, not an excitable state, as in *Coffea, Nux vomica, Ignatia,* but sluggish, aggravated from motion, aggravated from being talked to, wants to lie still in bed; very great irritability, which is as extreme as that found in *Nux* or *Chamomilla.* It also has acute complaints aggravated from anger, from being aroused, from being disturbed, from controversy. Following the early sluggishness, there is later a state of complete stupefaction in Bryonia, in which he becomes quite unconscious, as in typhoid. He goes from a state of partial unconsciousness to one of complete unconsciousness, as in hydrocephalic children.

In rheumatic complaints, in pneumonia, and in typhoid conditions, when he is aroused from this stage of stupefaction he is confused, sees images, *thinks he is away from home and wants to be taken home.* Sometimes he will lie and say nothing but that he 'wants to go home". The delirium is of a low type; it is not the flashing wild excitement of *Bell.* or *Stram.;* it is the very opposite; he talks and wanders and does not say much unless he is disturbed. You disturb him and he says, "Go away and let me go home," and if you let him alone he will relapse into a perfectly quiet state and seldom speak. "Irrational talk or *prattle of his business,* aggravated after 3 P.M. Usually you will find the *delirium* commencing *about* 9 P.M., and keeping up all night like the fever. *The acute mental state* you will find manifesting its symptoms *or rising in the morning,* but as the febrile state advances and takes possession of him the symptoms will take on a 9 P.M. aggravation; those who have chill will have it at 9 P.M.; in those who have a fever, the fever will come at 9 P.M. If mental symptoms are uppermost they increase and spread over the night. It has a 3 P.M. aggravation. *Bell.* will begin at 3 and run on towards midnight, but Bryonia will begin at 9 P.M. and run on through the night. The aggravation of the *Chamomilla* patients, who are also extremely irritable, is at 9 A.M. Sometimes we go to the bedside and can hardly distinguish between Bryonia and *Cham.* because they are both so spunky, but the *Cham.,* baby is worse at 9 A.M. and the Bryonia baby is worse at 9 P.M.

In Bryonia there is a key-note which really applies to a dozen or more remedies, "he wants something and he knows not what." It is a very important symptom of Bryonia. It is a symptom that calls for Bryonia only when the rest of the symptoms agree. You go to a child who is being carried in the arms of the nurse and wants one toy after another; you get the toy he wants and he does not want it and will throw it back at you. When that case is looked into thoroughly it may be covered by *Kreosote;* another is never satisfied with anything and rejects everything he asks for; you look into that case and it may be covered by *Chamomilla.*

"Desire for things that cannot be had which are refused, or not wanted when offered." "Apprehensiveness; fearfulness." "Anxiety in whole body compelled him to do something constantly." There is a feature worthy of consideration because it sometimes makes a case appear inconsistent. It is due to his anxiety that pervades the whole body. In Bryonia as in *Arsenic* there comes an anxious and uneasy feeling which compels him to move, but he is worse from motion, yet so uneasy and anxious that he must move. There are pains so violent that he cannot keep still, and yet when he moves he screeches from the pain. So it is really not an inconsistency but simply due to the great violence of the pain. Even though he knows that the motion is going to make him worse, he cannot keep still, for the pain is so violent. Early in the case he was able to keep still, and found that he was better from keeping still, and that the mental state was better from keeping still, and that the anxious restlessness increased the more he moved, until finally a reaction comes and he is obliged to move. You would think, looking at the case superficially, that that patient is better from motion as in *Rhus tox.,* but in *Rhus* you find that the patient moves and in moving he gets feeble, and when he sits down the pains begin to come on again. There is the distinction between the two, and yet they look alike if not examined into carefully. It is common for Bryonia to be ameliorated from *cool air,* and from *cool applications.* Now, if he moves, he gets warmed up, the pains are worse, but there are rheumatic complaints of Bryonia which are better from heat, and under these circumstances he is better from continued motion. It is another form of relief, and another of the modalities. I sometimes wonder whether Bryonia has a greater element of relief from heat, or greater element of relief from cold. Most of the *head complaints* that are of a congestive character are better from cool applications, from cold air, etc. Yet there are some of the Bryonia head complaints that are relieved by hot applications, and these seem to have no accompanying cerebral congestion. So that Bryonia has opposite modalities, but in all its opposite states there is still a grand *nature* running all through, sufficient to detect it.

In a damp climate Bryonia is one of the most frequently indicated remedies, but in the clear climates, where the thermometer runs low, *Aconite* will be indicated more than Bryonia. Still further South, the complaints assume more of the constitutional state of *Gelsemium* in inflammatory conditions. We know in the far North the sudden, violent cold brings on violent colds like *Aconite,* while here the complaints are more insidious, like Bryonia, and further South. These atmospheric changes should be thoroughly considered in relation to our Materia Medica.

The mental state of Bryonia is usually relieved from cool air, he wants the windows open. Anxiety, confusion of mind, fear, etc., are ameliorated from being cool. Sometimes the delirium, and the congestive fulness of the head affecting the mind, will increase if the room becomes very warm, or from the heat of the stove, from becoming heated, or from warm covers. In children this will be noticed, whereas if the window be thrown up to relieve the stuffiness of the room the child will sleep quietly. Such remedies as Bryonia, *Apis, Pulsatilla,* and many others, come in here. If you go into a room and find the child raging with delirium, turning and tossing, and the mother is trying to keep the room warm because *she* is chilly, and you say, "Why, how stuffy it is in here!" and you open the window and then notice that the child goes off to sleep, do not overlook that; because that relief was caused by something. There should be nothing that can possibly occur to a patient, but that you should solve the meaning of before you leave the room. Settle in your mind as to what it was that caused it.

"Fear of death." Full of fear, anxiety, despair of recovery, great despondency. Both mental and bodily quietness is required, that is, he wants to keep still. Often he wants the room dark. It has complaints from getting excited. Bryonia patients are nearly always worse from visitors. "Morose." Do not cross a Bryonia patient for it makes him worse. "Bad effects from mortification." "Ailments arising from chagrin;" these are headaches usually. Violent, congestive headaches that come on a few hours after altercation of controversy, or little misunderstandings with somebody that he cannot talk back to, will be covered by *Staph,,* but Bryonia also has that. *Staph.* is suited to irritable, violent, nervous, excitable people, that get into violent altercation or dispute. If a headache comes on, such a patient may need Bryonia. If in a chronic state a patient says, "Doctor, if I ever have a dispute with a man over anything I come down with nervous excitement, sleeplessness, headaches;" you do not have to work long upon that case, because more than likely *Staph.* will be suitable.

Bryonia has *dizziness;* the dizziness is worse in a warm room. You will notice, as I go through, that in everything of a nervous nature, nervous excitement, and commonly the bodily state, the patient is worse from a warm room, worse from too much clothing, worse from the warmth of the bed, wants the windows open, wants to breathe fresh, cool air. He suffers more than ordinary persons, from a stuffy room. Persons who are subject to Bryonia conditions suffer in church, at the opera, in close warm rooms, like *Lycopodium.* Girls that faint every time they go to church are relieved by *Ignatia*

We commence now with the study of the head. The head complaints may be looked upon as striking features of the remedy, because there is pain in the head with almost every acute complaint. Headaches are associated with inflammatory and congestive complaints. The mental dullness and confusion of the mind is spoken of with the congestive headache, and bursting headache. The head feels so full she wants to press it with the hand, or tie it up; tight pressure, over the whole skull, is grateful. The headaches are worse in a warm room and commonly worse from heat. Sometimes superficial neuralgias have relief from local heat, but a warm room or a close room is very distressing to the Bryonia headache. Headaches as if the skull would split open; the pains are worse from every motion, even the winking motion of the eyes, the motion necessary to talking, and the effort of thinking, so that all exertion of body or mind becomes impossible with a severe headache. Must keep perfectly quiet. Sometimes lying down and keeping perfectly quiet in a dark room will give some relief. Light aggravates; if you think a moment you will see that the accommodation to light and shadow of a room involves motion; it is said that the light aggravates, but even here it is the motion that is carried on by the muscles of accommodation. The headaches of Bryonia are very commonly the forerunner of other complaints, congestion of the lungs, bronchitis, or congestion of some other part of the body; he wakes up in the morning with headache; if it be coryza that is coming, he has the headache in the morning and through the day he commences to sneeze; or if the trouble is in some other part of the body, before the symptoms develop, he wakes up in the morning with this congestive headache over the eyes or in the back of the head, or both; it seems as if the head would burst; better from pressure, worse from the warmth of the room, and worse from every motion. Headache over the eyes, sometimes like the stabbing of a knife, worse from the first motion. He realizes it on waking, upon moving the eyes, with soreness in the eyeballs, with bruised feelings all over. The motion of the arms, doing work with the arms, as in various kinds of business that are carried on with the use of the arms and hands, is generally accompanied by complaints of the upper part of the body and especially the head, so that one of the old keynotes in the time of Hering was "complaints from ironing". You know that ironing is commonly carried on in a warm room, it involves the motion of the arms, and thus brings in two most striking features of Bryonia, so that this keynote is no longer an abstract statement; it is not to be considered apart from the general nature, but only serves to bring it out. Splitting, violent congestive headaches; headaches as if everything would burst out of the forehead. Pressure pain in the forehead, fulness and heaviness in the forehead as if the brain were pressed out. This fulness or congestion of the head is accompanied by what was described as sluggishness of the mind, and it will often be noticed that the countenance is somewhat besotted. The patient looks as if he were an imbecile. The face is mottled, and purple, with congestion in a marked Bryonia state. The eyes are red and congested; he is listless, does not want to move, to speak, or to do anything, because all these things are motion, are efforts, and they make him worse. You will see this is also true in *Bell.;* it has all of this congestion and pressure; but remember Bryonia is slow, sluggish, passive and insidious in its approach and progress, while in *Bell.* the mental symptoms and everything in connection are marked by activity. With the headaches there is more or less burning, and sometimes throbbing. The throbbing is seldom felt until he moves. After any movement, like going up stairs, walking, or turning over in bed during the headache, he feels the violent throbbing; on keeping still a moment it settles down into a bursting, pressing pain as if the skull would be pressed open. There are many other pains in connection with the Bryonia headache; in the text it is described "tearing and stitching pains", "Shooting pains," sharp pains. Some of the pressing pains are described as if a great weight were on the head, but the same idea prevails; it is an internal pressure; a sluggishness of the circulation in the brain, a stasis as if all the blood in the body were surging in the head. "Stitches in the head." "Splitting headache." "Rush of blood to head." Threatened apoplexy. "Headache after washing himself with cold water when face was sweating." That is, raking cold from suppression of perspiration. "Always on coughing, motion in head like pressure." The headache is so bad in many cases of pneumonia or bronchitis, in fact in any of the inflammatory or congestive conditions, that very often you will see the patient grasp the head when he knows he is going to cough. He holds his head because it hurts so from the action of coughing. Many remedies have this, but it is in keeping with the general aggravation of Bryonia from motion, from jar, from any effort. "The headache is expanding, aggravated by the slightest motion; after eating." The aggravation after eating is in keeping with the Bryonia state in general. The patient himself, in all complaints, feels worse after eating. It hardly matters what the trouble is, it is worse after eating;. the cough is worse after eating, the gouty state is increased by eating. The Bryonia patient will finally sum up the whole subject and say, "I am always worse after eating;" so that it becomes a general. The headaches are often accompanied by nose-bleed. "Obstinate headache with constipation." Bryonia is particularly suitable in venous, sluggish constitutions, with sluggish heart, poor circulation, yet apparently plethoric, apparently rugged, but subject to gouty exacerbations from change of weather.

Dandruff is common; sensitiveness and great soreness of the scalp; worse from the slightest touch of the scalp, feels as if the hair were pulled; women must always have the hair hanging down. In the Bryonia headaches, as well as rheumatic attacks, if he can perspire freely, he will get relief. Bryonia is ameliorated in all its complaints as soon as the perspirations becomes free and general.

Catarrhal conditions of the eyes are found in Bryonia; it is not so often thought of as an inflammatory remedy for the eyes when there are no other symptoms, but eye symptoms will be found, redness, inflammation congestion, heat, enlargement of the veins, burning and smarting, associated with headaches, with coryza, with troubles in the air passages, bronchitis, etc. Sore aching in the eyes, the eyeballs can hardly be touched, so tender to touch, as if bruised, increased from coughing or pressure. Such conditions come with chest complaints with colds and headaches. "Soreness and aching of eyes when moving them." "Pressing, crushing pains in eyes." "Inflammation in eyes and lips, especially in new-born infants." Think of Bryonia when gouty conditions have left certain parts and all at once the eyes are affected, tumefaction of the lids, the conjunctiva looks like raw beef, so highly inflamed is it, red and oozing blood. You find out that a few days before the patient, an old gouty subject, had rheumatic attacks of the joint, and now he has sore and inflamed eyes. "Rheumatic iritis, caused by cold." Rheumatic inflammation of the eyes, *i.e.*, in inflammatory conditions and congestion with redness, associated more or less with gouty affections. In olden times it was described as "arthritic sore eyes," which means sore eyes in a gouty constitution.

Many of the complaints of Bryonia commence in the nose; sneezing, coryza, running at the nose, red eyes, lachrymation, aching through the nose, eyes and head the first day; then the trouble goes down into the posterior nares, the throat, the larynx, with hoarseness, and then a bronchitis comes on, and if not checked it goes into pneumonia and pleurisy, so that the trouble has travelled from the beginning of the respiratory tract, the nose, to the lung tissue. This is a field for the complaints of Bryonia. All are worse from motion, all parts are subject to a good deal of burning and congestion; more or less fever, sometimes intense fever; the patient himself worse from the slightest motion and wants to keep still; dullness of mind, pressive, congestive headaches; sore, lame and bruised all over, often worse at 9 o'clock in the evening; increased dullness of the mind after sleep or on waking in the morning. The cough comes on with great violence, racking the whole body and increasing the headache, and with copious discharge of mucus from the respiratory tract.

"Frequent sneezing." "Sneezing between coughs." "Loss of smell." Bleeding from the nose in these congestions, or with coryzas. During menstruation there is epistaxis. Congestion of the head is present at the menstrual period. Epistaxis appears as a vicarious flow in case of menorrhœa. If the menstrual flow should be checked suddenly from cold, nose-bleed comes on. Dryness in the nose.

The aspect of the face is important; the besotted, purple, bloated countenance is not dropsically bloated, although it has the œdematous face sometimes, but puffed from vascular stasis, not pitting upon pressure; swollen and puffed, purple, with a doltish state of the mind, as if he were drunk. He will look at you and wonder what you were doing, and what you said; a stupefaction of the intellect; the eyes do not look at you intelligently. When a patient is about to come down with some Bryonia complaint, with a remittent, or with head congestions, or pneumonia, or some other respiratory disease, the family will notice when he awakes in the morning that he has that besotted expression, and he says he has to make such an effort to think or do anything, and his head aches hard, and is worse from motion. Or the face is red and burning, "red spots on the face and neck;" "hot, bloated, red face."

In children, as well as adults, there is gradually increasing cerebral trouble, dilated pupils, besotted countenance, and continual lateral motion of the lower jaw. This motion of the jaw in a congestive attack is a strong feature of Bryonia. It is not the grinding of the teeth so much that I refer to now, although that is found in Bryonia, but a lateral movement of the jaw as if chewing, but the teeth do not come in contact, and they keep it up night and day. A great many remedies have grinding of the teeth. When intermittent fever comes on with marked congestion, stupefaction of the intellect, violent rigors, even to a congestive chill, the patient lying in stupefaction or a semi-conscious state, without grinding the teeth, yet wagging the jaw back and forth by the hour, Bryonia is often suitable. Constant motion of the mouth as if the patient were chewing, in brain affections of children; it occurs in little ones when there are no teeth; but they keep up a chewing motion.

In regard to the lips and lower part of the face, that bloated, swollen condition, the sluggish circulation, a venous congestion or stasis will be found in Bryoina, making the aspect as of one long intoxicated; it is not so marked as in *Baptisia* and is not accompanied by so low a state, so advanced a stupor, as in *Baptisia*. Great dryness of the lips; the lips parched and dry. "Children pick the lips." "Lips cracked and bleeding." Lips parched, dry and bleeding, such as will be seen in typhoid states, where the whole mouth is dry and brown, cracked, parched and bleeding; dry, brown tongue. Sordes on the teeth. In *Arum triph.* there is marked picking of the nose and lips; they pick and pick and bore the finger into the nose.

Bryonia has toothache, worse from warmth. "Tearing, stitching toothache while eating;" from warm drinks, from warm foods, worse in a warm room, wants cold foods in the mouth, wants to be in cold air, but worse from motion. "Toothache > by cold water or lying on painful side." Pressing hard upon the painful tooth ameliorates it "Toothache < from smoking." You see how the relief from cold and aggravation from heat go along with us; we shall keep reiterating these modalities that affect the patient as a general state and we shall see as we go through that nearly all his symptoms are worse from motion, worse from heat, etc. He keeps on telling us they are better from pressure in each region we go over, until finally we come to the conclusion that they are general. We may have in two remedies the same set of symptoms, and yet they are all made worse from the opposite things. Thus you see modalities indicate and contra-indicate remedies. This is the studying of remedies by their modalities, for modalities sometimes constitute strong generals.

You will not be surprised to know that Bryonia loses his sense of taste, so that if he has a coryza nothing tastes natural. Not only is there mental sluggishness, but there is a slowing down of his sensations, his whole state is benumbed. "Taste flat, insipid, pasty." His intelligence is so affected ,that he does not know where he is even, thinks he is away from home, and even his tongue is no longer intelligent; so that something that is sour tastes as though bitter; his senses deceive him. "Tongue thickly coated white." In typhoid, in cerebral congestion, in sore throat, in pneumonia, in all diseases of the respiratory apparatus, in rheumatic affections, the tongue is thickly coated. "Dry and bleeding and covered with crusts." Such a tongue is found in typhoid fever, a dry, brown, cracked, bleeding tongue. When he takes a cold the mouth becomes dry. It is very common for the Bryonia patient to have great thirst; he is apt to drink large quantities of water, at wide intervals. With this dry, brown tongue, however, he loses his taste for water and does not want it; dry mouth and thirstless like *Nux moschata*. "Aphthæ." "Bad odor from mouth."

Bryonia has nondescript sore throats, with stitching pains, with dryness, with parched appearance of the throat, and thirst for large quantities of water at long intervals. "Constitutional tendency to aphthous formations in the throat," little white spots in the throat.

Then we come to the desires and aversions that relate to the stomach, and they are greatly perverted. He is worse from eating. The stomach has lost its ability to digest, and hence he has an aversion to all food. "Desires things immediately, and when offered they are refused." He is changeable, does not know what he wants. He craves in the mind the things he has an aversion to in the stomach. When he sees it he does not want it. His intelligence is in a state of confusion. He craves acids. "Great thirst day and night;" he wants cold water. "Thirst for large quantities at long intervals." Many remedies want to sip water all the time. In Bryonia the large quantities relieve the thirst immediately. In *Arsenic* the drink does not relieve, he wants a little and wants it often.

The stomach complaints of Bryonia are relieved from warm drinks; that becomes a particular because his desire is, for cold drinks, but his stomach is better from warm drinks. In his fever and head complaints and febrile states he wants cold things, which often bring on and increase the cough and pains, but the hot drink, which he does not crave, relieves the stomach and bowel complaints. In the chill, Bryonia often has desire for ice-cold water, which chills him dreadfully; and hot water relieves. "Desire for cold and acid drinks." Aversion to rich fat food; all greasy things. "Desire for things which are not to be had."

When patients are under constitutional remedies, they need caution about certain kinds of foods that are known to disagree with their constitutional remedy. A Bryonia patient is often made sick from eating sauer kraut, from vegetable salads, chicken salad, etc., so that you need not be surprised, after administering a dose of Bryonia for a constitutional state, to have your patient come in and say she has been made very ill from eating some one of these things. It is well to caution persons who are under the influence of *Puls* to avoid the use of fat foods, because very often they will upset the action of the remedy. It is well to say to patients who are under *Lyc.*, "See that you do not eat oysters while taking this medicine." These medicines are known to produce states in the stomach inimical to certain kinds of foods; certain remedies have violently inimical relation to acids, lemons, etc. If you do not particularly mention the fact, and say, "You must not touch vinegar or lemons, nor take lemon juice while taking this medicine," you will have the remedy spoiled, and then wonder why it is. The medicine often stops acting and the patient gets a disordered condition of the stomach and bowels; a medicine that should act for a long time ceases action and you do not know what the trouble is. Homœopathy will rule out such things as are inimical to the remedies and inimical to patients in general, or do not agree with a particular constitution. To have an iron-clad rule is not correct practice; the only iron-clad rule is to be sure that the remedy is similar to the patient when you administer it, and the things that he is to have are to be in agreement with that remedy. It is not an uncommon thing for a patient who has been under the influence of *Rhus tox.*, and has been doing well up to a certain time, after he has taken a bath, to have his symptoms return in the form of a *Rhus* state; the action of the remedy stops right there. He must of course take a bath, and yet it is true that some constitutional cases under *Rhus* must stop taking their ordinary bath in order to keep themselves under the influence of *Rhus*. It is the same with *Calcarea*—a bath will often stop the action. I only speak of these things to impress upon you the importance of feeding and treating your patient in accordance with the remedy; in accordance with a principle and not by rule; do not have one list of foods for your patients; do not have a list of things for everybody. There is no such thing in Homœopathy.

The patient himself in all the strange and peculiar things is worse from eating; the cough is worse from eating, the complaints of the head, the headaches, are worse from eating, and the respiration is worse from eating. The stomach is distended with wind after eating, but especially after oysters.

Oysters are not, as a rule, a dangerous article of diet, yet some are poisoned by oysters. "Worse after eating or drinking." When the case is one of whooping cough, the cough is worse, the paroxysms are more violent and all the symptoms are worse a little while after eating, but later, when digestion is finished and the stomach is empty, he is much relieved. The Bryonia patient is ordinarily relieved from drinking, but if, when overheated, he drinks cold water, all of his rheumatic symptoms are worse, the cough is worse, and the headache is worse. He will have a violent headache after drinking cold water when heated. In *Rhus* patients complaints are worse from drinking cold water when heated. The headache increases into a throbbing and bursting pain tenfold greater than it was before drinking.

The Bryonia patient is subject to hiccough, to belching, to nausea and vomiting, so that disordered stomach is the general term. Bitter eructations, bitter nauseous taste. He vomits bile. After eating all these things are increased. In the stomach and abdomen we have a great many symptoms resulting from disordered stomach, or from taking cold, or from becoming overheated, or from drinking ice water when overheated. Disordered stomach; irritation of the stomach so that he cannot eat without extreme pain, and this increases until the inflammatory condition involves the whole stomach and abdomen, and there is sensitiveness to pressure, and it can be diagnosed as a gastro-enteritis, with the soreness and tenderness, stitching, burning pains, all worse from motion; nausea and vomiting, diarrhœa, tympanitic abdomen; unable to move because it so increases the pain.

With the exception of the abdominal and stomach pains, the Bryonia *pains are better from pressure.* The Bryonia patient with the inflammatory conditions will often be seen lying perfectly quiet in bed with the knees drawn up; lying with the limbs flexed in order to relax the abdominal muscles; he does not want to be talked to, does not want to think; every movement is painful, and increases the fever and often cause alternation of chilliness with heat; high fever.

The Bryonia patient, when lying perfectly quiet, is sometimes quite free from nausea, but the instant the head is raised from the pillow the dreadful sickness returns, so that he cannot sit up. He cannot be raised up in bed because of the nausea, and if he persists in rising up the nausea comes on more than ever, with burning in the stomach. With every motion up in bed because of the nausea, and if he persists in rising up the nausea comes on more than ever, with burning in the stomach. With every motion he gulps up a little mucus and slime, which is putrid.

All sorts of pains are felt in the stomach and bowels, but most particularly stitching and burning pains; feels as if the stomach would burst, as if the abdomen would burst. Peritoneal exudations. Awful soreness. Sen-

ovaries, with sensitiveness to touch. The sensitiveness at the approach of every menstrual period, in both groins, will he spoken of by the patient, increasing as the menstrual period comes on, until the soreness proceeds across the abdomen and meets, and then the whole abdomen is painful during the menstrual period. The uterus is sore, the hypogastrium is tender. Inflammation of the uterus. Burning pain mostly in the body or fundus of the uterus. The Bryonia patient is subject to amenorrhœa, or the flow is suppressed upon the slightest provocation. If she becomes overheated from exertion, such as from ironing or washing a few days before the menstrual period, it will be suppressed, and the next time she will have a harder time than ever. in young plethoric women, after violent exertion, these complaints come on in that way. Violent exertion then scanty urine. Soreness of the abdomen, but the flow does not come, or is postponed a good many days after violent exertion; scanty urine and suppression of menses in plethoric girls.

From overexertion and becoming overheated, threatened abortion. In inflammation of the breasts and stopping of the milk flow in the lying-in period, Bryonia must be consulted. In milk fever and pains and swelling of the breast Bryonia must be studied. During confinement a woman becomes overheated and naturally perspires; just at the close of it as the delivery takes place, if the nurse and the doctor do not observe and throw more clothing over her, or at least keep the room warm enough, there will be sudden suppression of the sweat, and this will bring on milk fever and other febrile symptoms which will need Bryonia. Threatened peritonitis, from such causes, gonorrhœal troubles, old rheumatic troubles, pains or aches, if made worse from the slightest motion. If due to septicæmia rather than to suppression of the sweat, very commonly a deeper acting remedy is required. In inflammatory conditions of the breast one of the most striking things is the stony hardness of the breasts, hardness and heaviness. Bryonia is often suitable for inflammation of the breasts at other times; heaviness and hardness of the breast prior to menstruation.

Then we come to the respiratory tract again, which we have only hinted at, and here we have a tremendous study before us. Very commonly the Bryonia conditions commence with a cold ; it may be at first loss of voice, with rawness in the trachea and great soreness in the chest; dry, hacking cough, as if the chest would burst from coughing. The Bryonia patient sits up and holds the head, or holds the chest; presses both hands upon the chest when coughing, feels as if the chest would fly to pieces when coughing; pains in the chest on both sides, but mostly the right side. Bryonia prefers the right side when the condition is *pneumonia.* We see a patient who had first a cold, and the cold has travelled down the air passages, with hoarseness and rawness in the chest and cough; the cough shakes the whole body, then comes a hard chill. He is now down in bed, and when the physician sees him he sees the state of inflammation and knows the meaning of it, and listening confirms the diagnosis of pneumonia. The patient cannot move hand or foot; the pain is mostly in the right lung, and he is compelled to lie on the right side or back and dreads motion. Sometimes the pleura is involved and we have the sharp pains; every respiration causes intense pain, .whether it be pleuro-pneumonia or a simple pneumonia. But we see the Bryonia patient lying upon the side that is affected, upon the painful side, in order to diminish the motion that respiration causes; and very often he will have a hand under it to see if he cannot hold it still. With Bryonia the expectoration is of a reddish tinge, is rusty, and if you have this symptom and the right side affected it is all the more strongly Bryonia. There are a few medicines that look somewhat like Bryonia; take, for instance, a case with high fever, intense heat, great excitement, and consider the rapidity with which the trouble has come on, involving the *left* side and in the pan you see the sputum consists of bright red blood, *Aconite* will be the remedy. If the liver is involved, there is fulness in the side, stitching pain over the liver, and the face is yellow, it is not impossible for Bryonia to be indicated, for it has such things, but with pain very severe, continually going from the front to the back through the right shoulder-blade, *Chelidonium* is more likely to cure than Bryonia. These comparisons may be carried out indefinitely, but the study of Bryonia as to the respiratory apparatus is a wonderful one. With these colds that end in loss of voice, it has burning and tickling in the larynx, constant cough. Hoarseness and loss of voice in singers. Great soreness in the trachea; rawness and tightness in the trachea, even suffocation, like *Phosphorus*. The Bryonia breathing is panting and very rapid, little short rapid breaths, due to the fact that deep breathing increases the pain, the Bryonia patient desires to breathe deep, wants deep breathing, needs deep breathing, but it hurts him so. "Constant disposition to sigh," but cannot because it hurts him so. Shortness of breath, suffocation, asthma. Asthmatic attacks from becoming overheated. Asthma worse in a warm room, wants cool air to breathe. "Dry, spasmodic cough, whooping cough, shaking the whole body." Cough compels him to spring up in bed involuntarily, painful cough with difficult breathing, cough that shakes the whole body. Tough, difficult expectoration. "Cough evening and night, dry cough."

A great deal of the rest of Bryonia, as we go over it, is repetition. If you will only read the text carefully and make application of what has been said, you see the general character and idea of the remedy, you see its image and you will fill it out for yourselves, if you have a full text-book.

another will be an epileptic. Bufo underlies such a constitution; it is an antipsoric, it is a deep-seated, vital remedy; it goes to the very heart and interior of man's physical nature, and from this mental state it may manifest itself in his ultimates, the fingers and toes, eyes, ears, etc., so that even the touch is disordered. There are patches upon the skin that have loss of sensation and others with increased sensations. Spasms of various muscles, sometimes local spasm and sometimes complete epileptic spasms with bleeding at the mouth, unconsciousness, falling down. Besides such grave state, it has milder states that may be called mere dizziness or vertigo. The milder conditions of dizziness have gone on to sudden falling and collapse, a sudden state of unconsciousness with spasms and biting of the tongue. In the proving we find attacks of apathy and partial coma; numbness of the brain. So we see in the text that we have conditions ranging from mere dizziness to a complete and profound epilepsy. The study of this remedy may reveal to you something of the nature of epilepsy. From the allopathic treatises on epilepsy you will only get the appearance of the fit, and the fit is treated as epilepsy. They hunt for remedies to subdue and control the fit, thinking when they have done that they have cured the patient. They feed these patients Bromides in large doses and now and then they branch off into some side issue, but go back to the Bromides and stupefy and make imbeciles of their patients. Prescribing for the fit has never cured the patient.

"Congestive headaches." Again, its action on the circular fibres of the abdominal aorta furnishes a keynote in epilepsy. An awful sensation of anxiety is felt in the abdomen and then there is a sudden loss of consciousness; the aura or warning is first felt in the abdomen. Some writers have described it as in the solar plexus. The awful sensation occurs as an anxiety and then be falls.

"Cannot bear the sight of brilliant objects:" "Amaurosis," etc. "Pupils largely dilated and unaffected by light before attack." "More acute vision."

It has spasmodic conditions of the eye, but increased vision and diminished sensation, and lastly a tendency to 'profound trophic disturbance. Little blisters form upon the eye. These little blisters also form upon the skin, and the integument is thrown off and there is no healing. Ulcers will form upon the cornea. "Eyes become highly injected." Paralytic conditions of the lids and muscles of the eye. There is disturbance of all the senses. "Music is unbearable." One who is in a natural state is expected to enjoy beautiful music, whereas in this remedy music brings about a state of anxiety. The sense of hearing is so violently exaggerated that every little noise is distressing. "Purulent otorrhœa." "Swelling of the ears, of the parotids." "Phlegmonous erysipelas about the face." "Falling out of the teeth" in the peculiar disease known as Rigg's disease.

"Stuttering and stammering; gets angry when incoherent speech is not understood." "Biting the tongue." "Tongue cracked, bluish black." "Mouth wide open before an attack," showing that the spasm is coming on; and this condition increases so that when the attack is not on, he drops the jaw and looks stupid as if he had forgotten everything. Bufo often corresponds to lesser attacks resembling vertigo. In this state people do not fall, and for a few seconds everything is blank, or sometimes they do things automatically in these moments. A person, in this mild form of epileptic vertigo, will hardly show anything, but he will sometimes come to a perfect standstill and then go on as if nothing had happened. What occurred during that attack he knows nothing of. Sometimes he will continue right on doing what he was doing, and nobody will know of the spell. Sometimes when driving he will turn his horses around, and when he comes to himself he will know by this that he has had one of his attacks. Quite a number of medicines have produced that condition of the mind, a state in which he goes on doing things automatically.

"Vomiting after drinking." "Yellow fluid in vomit." "Vomiting of bile or blood." "Spasms end by convulsive movements in abdomen." It says in the text, "The attack originates in abdomen;" that is, he has a feeling of anxiety in the abdomen previous to the attack.

"Hæmorrhoidal tumors." "Urine passes involuntarily." The urine passes involuntarily in such as are becoming imbeciles from the epileptic attacks, in approaching softening of the brain, which is really what is taking place, a form of softening, a lowered form of integrity.

As you might suppose, there is great disturbance of the sexual organs, this is usually the case in insane people. Sometimes the sexual organs are in a state of excitement and sometimes in a state of impotency, but the patient is low-minded; inclination to carry the hand constantly to the genital organs. "Semen is discharged too quickly without pleasurable sensation." Spasms or epilepsy comes on during coition. It has also inflammation of glands, especially about the groins, such as are found in syphilis.

In the female sexual organs burning is the most striking feature; burning in the ovaries and uterus. It is one of the most troublesome symptoms you will have to contend with, when a case of dysmenorrhœa has burning in the ovaries and in the pelvis, at the coming on of or during menses. Burning in the genital organs, in the ovaries, and rending, tearing pains that extend down the thighs. This forms a troublesome kind of dysmenorrhoea, especially when there are cysts and hydatids about the ovaries. Some will tell you that these cannot be cured. All these conditions are curable! "Burning heat and stitches in ovaries." "Distending, burning pains or cramps in uterus." This remedy has been a great palliative for these awful burning pains that

contractions of circular fibers everywhere. When this comes in places where it can be felt, and realized by the senses, it is felt as contractions, as if caged in wires, and this gives us the key to Cactus. Where contractions cannot be felt, where there is no sense of feeling, we know that it goes on as a spasmodic condition of circular fibers; but these contractions that are felt are more upon the surface of the body, and in organs having circular fibers—tubes and canals. They constrict, and this constriction is felt like a spasm. It has a sensation of tightness and constriction about the head, about the chest, about the attachments of the diaphragm, all over the abdomen. Contractions about the heart that are tonic in character, like a tight clutching; constriction. "Constriction felt about the heart." These constrictions are felt about the throat, in the œsophagus, causing a spasm; in the vagina, causing vaginismus and preventing coition. In the uterus it produces the most violent cramps. Clutching and constrictions, as if the uterus were grasped and held tightly, like a spasm. But at these times, when these constrictions take place, there are congestions. "Rush of blood to the part, with constriction." "Violent congestion of the uterus, with constrictions. Rush of blood to the chest, as if the chest was filled with hot gushes of blood, with constrictions, and constriction of the heart." These peculiarities run through Cactus more markedly than any other remedy. Many remedies have similar things now and then, but in Cactus it is common; it is the nature of Cactus to constrict, to cause constriction in places where it has never been felt, and never been thought of. Constrictions of the whole body, as if the body was held in a wire cage. Constrictions of the scalp, of the skin, growing tighter and tighter. Violent congestions that come on suddenly. Congestion of the brain, with hot head, flushed face. At the beginning of complaints, at the beginning of pneumonia; congestive chill with hot head and cold body (like *Arn.*) with violent constrictions and tightness, as if the head were pressed, as if the membrane of the brain were too tight, as if the brain were covered with a tight cloth, and were being screwed tighter and tighter. Uniform tightness of an organ, as if it were being bound tighter and tighter. But in tubes and canals it is a constriction of a particular part, many times like as if tied with a string. Constriction, like hour-glass contraction, in the uterus. It has inflammations, congestions, rush of blood to the part, gradually progressing to inflammation, and infiltration. Inflammation of various parts.

It has rheumatism. It is a remedy very useful in gouty constitutions; very useful in acute inflammatory rheumatism; and in this instance the congestion is in the joints that happen to be affected. And then again the constriction, as if tied with a tape, or as if bandaged. Tightness, tension, pressure, are involved in that thought. It has such a prolonged determination of blood to the heart that the heart finally becomes disturbed in its function, disturbed in its tissues; and it has a profound curative action upon the heart and even cures organic heart diseases, such as are produced from this cause, conditions coming on from congestion, or coming on through congestion in rheumatic constrictions, where the rheumatism has left the joints partially and the heart has become involved, and there is constriction of the heart. Various efforts have been made by provers, and by patients, to describe the constriction of the heart. It is sometimes described "as if grasped with an iron hand." It is only to illustrate the tenacity of the constriction. In these rheumatic troubles when the joints have ceased to be affected and the heart becomes affected with this chronic congestion and enlargement, we have enlargement of the valves so that there are murmurs, the head is hot, and the patient gradually emaciates. Kidney troubles will come on; the heart grows weaker, and then dropsical conditions set in, that is the course of Cactus. Towards the last, cardiac affections, along with kidney affections, with emaciation, and then swelling of the hands and feet. That is the very nature of Cactus, and you will not find any medicine in the whole Materia Medica that reads like it. There is nothing to compare with it in the intensity of these symptoms. All these things that I have described seem to turn upon these words, congestion, constriction and contraction.

The pains in Cactus are violent, no matter where they occur. They compel the patient to cry out, and the pains are clutching pains, constricting pains; they often feel like tearing pains; but there is always that idea of clutching. Suppose you should tie a tape round a violently congested organ, and tie it tighter and tighter. It seems to me that is about the kind of suffering the patient has with that constriction of a congested organ. Pains in congested parts; pains in sore parts. Tearing; constricting; cramping, when pains occur in the intestines they are constricting, but when the pains are in the long muscles they are not the constricting pains, for it is not the circular fibers then but the long fibers that contract, and we call them cramps. Cactus produces some spasmodic conditions in long muscles, but not to any great extent. In *Bell.* especially, and also in many of those medicines that have this nature of cramping, and constricting and contracting of circular fibers, there is convulsive tendency. The violent congestion of the brain in *Bell.* will commonly be attended with cramps in the extremities and convulsions of the muscles all over, or in parts. Not so with Cactus. Violent congestion, and he grows stupid under it. Congestion of the brain, first with very red face, then darker from the venous stasis, and then stupor. He grows sluggish under the cerebral congestion.

The mental state is that of fear and distress, because of the intensity of the suffering. The patient has never felt such suffering, and he does not see what it can all mean. So much suffering, such violent suffering, such sudden

and it would be quite in the nature of it to bleed. It has hæmorrhages of two kinds. Hæmorrhage from vascular relaxation accompanying cardiac and vascular conditions, and hæmorrhage from violent congestion of a part. The rush of blood to the head is of such violence in the moderately plethoric patient that he bleeds from the nose, and hawks blood from the throat. Congestion of the chest so violent that he expectorates blood from the chest. Bleeding from congestion, rather than from tuberculosis. Congestion of the uterus with bleeding. Congestion of the bladder and kidneys, with blood in the urine, with discharges of blood from violent congestion. In old cardiac conditions, where relaxation is present in most marked degree, hæmorrhage from relaxation.

Strong pulsations felt in strange places, in the stomach, and in the bowels; sometimes in the extremities, the feet and hands, as well as in the head. Throbbing all over. Around the attachment of the diaphragm feeling as if a cord was tied tighter and tighter; round the lower part of the chest. This is a strange symptom; it clutches him so tightly around the waist line that it takes his breath away, and he struggles for breath, and wants to do something. It clutches him tighter and tighter. Cactus produces congestion of the bowels; inflammation of the uterus. Gastric inflammation and with it the clutchings.

It is a remedy for the cure of haemorrhoids; the relaxation of the great portal system, and the lower veins in the rectum, the hæmorrhoidal veins. The veins are in such a state of relaxation that tumors will form, and bleed copiously. Bleeding hæmorrhoids. Constriction of the anus. It has a very troublesome constipation; constipation in connection with hæmorrhoids. It has a paralytic weakness of the bladder. It has retention of urine. Such a constriction of the neck of the bladder that the urine cannot be passed for a long time, and there is retention. In the kidneys such a congestion as favors suppression of the urine. Bloody urine; blood in clots. It is a remedy that favors the formation of clots speedily. The blood that flows clots so rapidly and so densely that it blocks up the way. Bleeding into the bladder blocks up the way. Bleeding into the vagina causes a clot difficult to expel, and pressing upon the urethra of the female that it is impossible for her to pass urine. It is like an immense tampon. And hence it reads, "urination prevented by clots," clots in the vagina, as well as clots in the bladder. Inflammation of the ovaries; inflammation of the uterus. It is a medicine that you will need to know when a young, plethoric, vigorous woman comes down violently with congestion of the uterus at the menstrual period, and she screams because of the violent clutching and cramping of the uterus. Before the flow starts, or just at the beginning, there is violent spasm. The circular fibers clutch; and she describes it accurately as if a tape were tied around that sore and congested uterus. The uterus fills with blood clots, and the spasm to expel that blood is like a labor-pain, and she screams again, and it is some time before the flow becomes free enough to give relief. if this condition is met with in rheumatic diathesis, where there is more or less rheumatism of the joints, clutching pains and constriction in other places, we have a remedy in Cactus. The excitement and the sharp scream can be heard by the neighbors. Suffocative attacks with these pains, because the heart suffers, and constriction of the heart will commonly go along with the constriction of the uterus. In cardiac conditions it seems as if he will die for want of breath. Constrictions of the chest. Oppression as if a great load was on his chest, crushing the life out of him, so great is the constriction, and the congestion. A sudden congestion, and it comes on and ends without inflammation in many instances. A violent rush of blood to the chest, with awful dyspnœa and constriction of the heart—and it passes away without inflammation. At other times Cactus has conditions like pneumonia, inflammation of the lungs, and congestion ending in inflammation, with the usual expectoration, bloody or blood streaked. Cactus is also a remedy for hypostatic congestion of the lungs. He cannot lie down, must sit up in bed, and there is a dullness of the lower part of each lung, gradually growing higher and higher from an effusion of serum into the lower portion of the lungs. This hypostatic congestion is due to a cardiac weakness. Cactus will often relieve this a few times when it occurs in old broken down cases towards the end of Bright's disease, and at the end of dropsical conditions and heart troubles. It will postpone death. "Could only breathe with shoulders elevated and lying on back." Lies leaning back or sitting quite upright "Periodical attacks of suffocation, with fainting; cold sweat."

"Feeling as if heart was compressed or squeezed by a hand. Cardiac rheumatism. Heart seemed to be held by an iron hand for many hours. Pain in the cardiac region. Great pressure at heart, going round under left axilla to back." Often this pain shoots down the left hand, is attended with numbness, and sometimes with swelling. Numbness, tingling, swelling. "Dull pain in the heart. Heavy pain in the heart, aggravated from pressure. Contractive pain in the region of the heart going down to left abdomen. At times felt as if some one was grasping the heart firmly. Paroxysms of pain in the heart," that is, this kind of constriction comes in periods of violent paroxysms. "Acute inflammation of the heart. Chronic inflammation of the heart. Palpitation of the heart, continued day and night; when walking, and at night when lying on the left side."

Another thing running through the remedy is, that chest complaints often come on or are exaggerated at 11 o'clock. Eleven o'clock in the morning, or eleven at night. Its intermittent fever will bring on a chill with violent congestion to the head at 11 o'clock. Regular Paroxysms at 11 A.M. and 11 P.M., or sometimes at 11A.M. and sometimes at 11 A.M. A daily chill at 11 A.M. It has cured intermittent fever of the congestive type, when the congestions

occur at the beginning of the fever, with heat and restlessness. This medicine comes in after the fever, and with his anxiety he wants to keep still. *Arsenic* has anxiety and wants to move from bed to bed, and from chair to chair, and he fears death. In this medicine he seems to say: "Don't speak to me; don't bother me; let me die in peace." He wants to be perfectly quiet, and the state occurs at the close of a febrile disease. Many of these patients die because they cannot eat, but this remedy will save them. When you have a case of cancer, with burning, prostration, and vomiting, Cadmium sulph. will relieve these symptoms for weeks. I have seen them where the pains have been relieved by anodynes until nothing would stay on the stomach, and this medicine would relieve. It is a great remedy *in the gastric irritation of carcinoma,* a great palliative; *coffee ground vomiting.*

Burning and cutting pains in the stomach. Gastric symptoms, such as occur in pregnancy, in old drunkards. Burning in the stomach extending up into the œsophagus; fluids burn all the way up into the mouth and throat; sour, acid fluids. Cold sensation in the stomach. Cholera infantum with irritation of the stomach.

Pain in the abdomen with vomiting. Lancinating in the abdomen. From these pains we see it is a medicine which profoundly affects the liver, spleen, stomach and other abdominal viscera. Gangrene threatens. The main remedy in the hands of good prescribers.

Relapses in fever, with vomiting, diarrhœa, and great prostration. At times a case of yellow fever gets along fairly well, but a draft causes a slight cold and on come sudden prostration, black vomit, death. In that state it competes with *Carbo veg.,* which used to be the main remedy in the hands of good prescribers.

CALADIUM

Caladium is a wonderful remedy; perhaps some of you have read it endeavoring to understand it; it is a difficult medicine to understand, because it is quite evident from the provings that the prover did not understand how to describe and report symptoms; did not know how to tell his sensations because they were so strange; he could not relate his mental state.

An individual puts his mind to bear upon something which seems to have taken place during the day, but he is not quite sure whether it took place or not; he thinks the matter over, and yet he cannot be really sure whether it took place or not, until he actually goes and puts his hands upon the object thought about; proves to, himself by actual contact and observation that his vague impression was so, that it was true, then he goes away and again he is undecided as to whether it was so or not. This relates to things that actually happened. "Very forgetful, he cannot remember," etc. This led to the use of Caladium for a good many different kinds of mental affections, loss of memory where there is that vague state of mind. It might be bordering upon imbecility, it might be the borderland of insanity. All day long he finds himself looking into the things that should have been done; they have simply escaped his mind; he has forgotten them. So the mind is worn through in places. A state of absent-mindedness. It may come on in an acute state, with unconsciousness. There is a good deal of congestion of the brain, more or less excitement, but more important is prostration of the mind, weakness of the mind; feeble-minded; inability to perform intellectual work, it is impossible. He cannot think; the more thought he puts upon a thing the more fatigue he has and the further away that thing seems to be; the more he attempts it the less concentrated is the mind upon a subject. It is not strange, then, that the provers themselves were unable to put these ideas into speech so as to give us an intelligent idea of proving. It is only by reading between the lines, using the remedy and studying it that we can straighten out this tangled skein. "Very thoughtful, absent-minded." There is in acute states delirium, excitement of mind, unconsciousness, stupefaction. As the febrile state is continued, we have this mental state. This remedy is useful in fevers that are continued.

One of the most important things to decide when we are going into the mental state of a remedy is whether we shall use this remedy in hysteria, in the delirium of the various phases of fever, or in insanity, and to ascertain this we turn to that part of the proving which gives us the pace of the remedy. If we want to understand the delirium of *Belladonna* and *Bryonia* to see which one would be suitable in a certain case, we turn to the febrile action of the remedy and see what the nature of that is; the pace tells us largely what kind of delirium, if we do not know from the delirium itself. So we will see that in *Belladonna* there is no continued fever, and as a remedy must, in its very nature, be adapted to the very nature of the disease, it would be useless to follow the many injunctions that are written in our books telling us to give *Belladonna* in the acute form of delirium in typhoid fever; but *Bryonia* has just that condition; hence we will see that *Bryonia* is useful in such cases which present symptoms similar to it, because the pace of the disease *is* similar to the pace of *Bryonia,* which has continued fever. *Belladonna* has intermittent and remittent fever, particularly remittent, and hence the acute delirium of *Belladonna* is similar to the acute delirium of remittent fever. Now to bring this point to bear; this remedy's fever is a continued fever; it has no great amount of fever in it, but it is a continued fever, we shall see that there is coma and stupor from fever; "delirium, unintelligible murmuring", mental prostration. This remedy is suitable in low, murmuring, exhaustive cases of

spasms. Weakness, or vertigo, or momentary blindness. Convulsions with valvular disease of the heart. Evening and night aggravations are common. The patient is sensitive to cold—a lack of vital heat. Aversion to the open air. General physical anxiety. Many symptoms from ascending stairs. It has many burning pains like *Arsenicum.* It has cured many cases of albuminuria in the early stages. It is a useful remedy in chlorosis. Dropsy is a strong feature, as it is in *Arsenicum* and *Calcarea.* Complaints are *worse from slight exertion,* faintness, palpitation, dyspnœa and weakness come on. The left side of the body is most affected.

The following mental symptoms are often a guide to its use. Anger and complaints from anger and vexation. Anxiety in evening, at night, in bed, and during a chill, and on waking. Apprehensiveness; about the future, about his salvation, at night. Inclined to criticise. Desire for company. Confusion of mind on waking. Inability to concentrate the mind. Delusions. Sees dead people, phantoms, images. Illusions of fancy. Sees visions of fire, worse at night, and on closing the eyes. Despair of recovery, of salvation. Discontented. Excitable. Fear of death at night, of solitude, or insanity. Becomes indifferent to pleasure. Insanity. Irresolution. Irritable. Lamenting. Loathing of life; weary of life. Weakness of memory. Mischievous. Obstinate. Sensitive—easily offended. Extreme restlessness, especially at night, tossing about in bed; during heat; and during menses. Extreme sadness in evening, and during fever. Easily startled. Timidity. Weeping, at night.

There is violent rush of blood to the head with vertigo and general spasm. It has caused and cured many chronic headaches. A very peculiar feature of the pain in the head is that it moves from the side lain on and goes to the side not lain on, and continues to change about by changing position. Not all of its headaches do this way. It has many peculiar little symptoms. Pain in the head ameliorated during mental exertion, but much worse afterwards. Œdema of face, lids, temples and ears. Eczema of face and scalp. Coldness of head. Pale, sickly, bloated face. Fluent coryza. Sneezing. Loss of all desire for food, but thirst for cold water. Eructations and vomiting after food. Stomach easily disordered, especially after milk and cold food. Pain in stomach after drinking cold water, Load in stomach after eating. Pain in groin after drinking wine. Waterbrash and sour stomach. Anxiety and burning in stomach. Stitching pain in stomach. Gnawing pain in stomach. Distension of stomach and abdomen. It has cured gastric ulcer.

Much soreness in region of kidneys. Scanty, burning urine, contain albumin and casts. Pain in the spermatic cords, after exertion, and after drinking wine.

Excoriating yellow leucorrhœa. Offensive, bloody leucorrhœa. For offensive leucorrhœa it compares with *Kali ars.* and *Kali phos.* It is useful in cancer of the uterus when there is burning and acrid offensive bloody flow. It restores the menstrual flow, when the symptoms agree. Copious menstrual flow, or scanty flow, too frequent and protracted. Pain at the approach of the menses. Metrorrhagia. Burning pain in uterus and vagina.

Drawing as with a thread from larynx backward. Dryness in larynx. Loses the voice before an epileptic convulsion. Suffocation and palpitation at night in bed. Burning heat in chest and pain in region of heart before an epileptic convulsion. Orgasm of blood in region of heart. Throbbing in the blood vessels, especially in head and back; it drives him out of bed. Pain in heart with palpitation. Angina pectoris. Grasping pain in heart. Palpitation, with heat of face. Palpitation from least excitement or exertion; worse evening and night. Every fourth beat of pulse omits. Rapid pulse.

Violent headache between scapulæ and sacrum. Pain in back extends to arms. Pain in chest extends to arms. Œdema of the hands and feet. Weakness of lower limbs.

The sleep is disturbed by violent dreams. Palpitation and suffocation. Latter part of night wakeful, and much sweat.

If this wonderful remedy is studied with the mind on *Arsenicum* and *Calcarea,* a broader knowledge will be gained. It needs further proving in potencies.

CALCAREA CARBONICA

If you were about to produce a Calcarea subject to order you could do so by feeding him lime or lime water until the digestive organs were so debilitated that they could no longer digest lime, and then the tissues would be increasingly deprived of what they need, and give us the lime subject, the "bone salt inanition" case, for that is really what it is. Infants that are fed lime water in the milk will in a little while be lime subjects. They will soon get in such a state that they cannot take the lime from their natural food, and the result will be a Calcarea subject, such as we are about to describe. But the natural lime cases are those that have a natural sickness, are born so, born with an inability to digest the lime that is in their natural food, and they grow fat and flabby, and produce deficient bones. There is a greater proportion of cartilaginous material in the bones than lime, and the bones bend, and take on diseases and destructive troubles. Deficient teeth, or no teeth at all. The bones simply stop growing, and the patient goes into marasmus. What a foolish notion it is to feed that infant lime water because he cannot digest lime! Is it not just as reasonable as anything else in allopathy? and yet our homœopaths use allopathic medicines. They use the lowest potencies they

care of the abscess (when the symptoms agree), and it will not break. I have many times seen an abscess disappear when fluctuation was most positive. I have seen those abscesses disappear when pus was shown to be present by the needle; I have not only seen the abscesses go away, but also the pyæmic state which was prior to it. We have but a few medicines that will do that. There is something singular about this. Why does Calcarea favor the resorption of that fluid and encourage the part to become calcareous? It is more than I am able to explain, but it does it—when the symptoms agree. But *Sulph.* and *Sil.*, when their symptoms agree hasten suppuration. But Calcarea has that peculiar action of concentrating and contracting. One may be indicated in one case, the other may be indicated in the other. There are times when *Sil.* is indicated and the abscess is in such a dangerous place that if Sil. is given the result that naturally belongs to the spreading of that abscess is dangerous; in such an instance the surgeon must be called to drain the abscess in a safe manner, even when we know that if that abscess were located in a safe place, it would be far better for that patient to have the remedy he needs. Sometimes the periosteum is injured by a hammer striking it through muscles, injuring or contusing the periosteum. Inflammation will set in, pus will form rapidly, and if Calcarea is indicated by the constitution of the patient the surgeon's knife is entirely useless, and a most detrimental thing. But in thinking from the old standpoint, the physician who knows nothing about Homœopathy, and the wonders of our homœopathic remedies, would hold up his hands in horror. "Why, if you produce a resorption of that pus into the system you will have blood poisoning and death." But under Calcarea this resorption does take place in some manner, and the patient improves every moment, he stops his sweating, his rigor has disappeared, he becomes perfectly comfortable, his appetite improves, he is stronger by the time it is over, and remains well. Judging from the old standpoint, we cannot conclude anything about the problems that will come up under Homœopathy. We can only judge from our standpoint, and from what we know. And if you hear that somebody has tried this and tried that without success, remember that somebody has only demonstrated his own failure. Homœopathy is capable of demonstrating itself in all intelligent hands; wherever the physician has intelligence and makes use of the law and applies the remedy in accordance with the symptoms he will see the case turn out as described.

Another grand feature running through this remedy is its ability to grow *polypi*. Those who need Calcarea will grow polypi in the nose and ears, in the vagina, in the bladder, and here and there. Cystic growths also and strange little papillomata.

Another strange thing that it does is to cause *exostoses*. This state of disorder comes from the irregularity in the distribution of the lime. You would think that nature would try to distribute it around evenly where it can do the most good. But when this bone salt inanition has commenced the lime may be piled up in one place, and almost absent in another. One bone will be cartilaginous and another will have bony growths on it. Softening of the bone. Defective formation of bone. A keynote has grown out of this, viz: "Late learning to walk," because the legs are so weak. It is not late learning to walk, but it is late walking. It knows how to walk, but it can't walk. *Natrum mur.* has brain trouble, in which the child is late *learning* to do things. "Tardy development of bone tissues. Curvatures." Muscles flabby. Joint affections, like hip-joint disease. It is full of *rheumatism.* Rheumatic and gouty conditions of the joints.

The Calcarea patient is a *chilly* patient. Sensitive to the cold air. Sensitive to the raw winds. Sensitive to the coming of a storm; sensitive to the coming of cold weather, and when the weather changes from warm to cold it seems impossible for him to keep warm; he wants the body kept warm. The head is sometimes congested; and it is hot to the touch; but it often feels cold to him. His scalp feels as if it were cold. But the body is nearly always cold to the touch and he feels cold, and he wants plenty of clothing. The feet are cold. He sweats in various places, sweats in spots. Sweats upon the forehead, or upon the face, or upon the back of the neck, or the front of the chest, or his feet. Sensitiveness to cold and *weakness* run through the remedy. Weakness in the legs. Inability to endure. Worse from every kind of exertion. Out of breath. Fat, flabby amæmic subjects, sometimes they look plump, often flushed in the face, but they have no endurance, and if such a patient undertakes a little exertion he is down sick with a fever, or a headache. Calcarea is full of complaints brought on from lifting, from exertion, from walking, from walking enough to get into a sweat; and these come very suddenly, because he cannot stop that perspiration by keeping still without getting sick. If he gets into a sweat, and stops long enough to be comfortable, the perspiration will stop so suddenly that he will have a chill, or he will have a headache. Weak, tired, anxious. Difficulties of breathing. Weak heart. Weak all over. No ability of the muscles to sustain prolonged effort, and it is the same way with the mind. No ability of the mind to sustain prolonged mental effort. Calcarea is *a tired patient.* He is suffering from want of lime. He has been unable to digest lime, and he goes into a state with enlarged glands, emaciation of the neck and of the limbs, while the fat and the glands of the belly increase. Especially is this noticed in children. A big-bellied child, with emaciated limbs and emaciated neck. Enlarged glands. Pale, and flabby, and sickly. Those that take on flesh without any increase of strength. They take on flesh and grow flabby. Remain feeble. Those that get up from sickness take on flabby flesh, and in a little while they become dropsical. The Calcarea patient can't

overwrought, dreadfully excited from a loss in the household by death. The
mother loses her child, or husband; or a young girl loses her intended. She is
broken-hearted, and greatly excited. It is a hysterical state. And yet I have
seen the same in men. I remember one. It came upon him from business cares
He had that same feeling; he would walk up and down the house, he said he
felt as if he must fly or jump out of a window or do something. That is
analogous to the mental state found in hysteria, or a great state of nervous
excitement. "She thinks and talks of nothing but murder, fire, rats, etc." That
is that same idea of talking about little things and foolish things. Things that
are not interesting to anybody. And yet I have seen these things in patient
and I would ask them why they did it. It is generally said, "I tried a good while
to stop it, and when I could not I just kept right on at it, for it seemed to do m
good." "She thinks and talks of murder, fire, rats, etc." Your patient may talk
about other foolish things, but it is only to illustrate the idea that she sits
and talks about foolish things, and cannot control herself; thinking, thinking, or expressing it, talking, talking, talking. Violent screaming spells. And
then the Calcarca patient will refuse to talk, will say nothing. She may talk to
herself when alone, but will decline to enter into conversation, and will s
perfectly silent. A Calcarea patient sometimes takes an aversion to work, an
quits work. He will quit a most thriving business, and go home and do nothing
after being fatigued in carrying on the business until it reaches a most thriving
condition. He says business is not good for him. He is tired of business, an
when he goes to his business again it seems as if it would drive him crazy. He
does not want to see it, he does not want to know anything about it. Of
course, you can readily see that it is not so much in the Calcarca patient that
he is driven to weakness and fatigue from distress in business, although
has that, but that which I am speaking about is that he has overworked unt
he has given out, and right in the midst of his success he quits his busines
and goes home, and leaves all—it looks just as if he were lazy. If you look
him you come to the conclusion that he is lazy. Yet it is an insanity; not th
laziness that belongs to tramp nature, though that also might be cured mar
times. He has been industrious, and all at once takes a turn. A great chang
occurs in the mind, and he takes on symptoms. It is not such persons as we
born that way, born lazy, never would work; but those that become lazy. It
like the symptom in a pious upright man, whose talk and conversation h
been upright, but all at once he turns and commences to swear. Of course v
know that indivi dual is insane. On the other hand, we have patients th
have been only ordinarily industrious that develop an insanity for work, an
it seems they have ability in that insane industry to work almost night a
day; they are up early and late. It is a sick state. So when we see in t
Repertory "Industry" it does not mean an ordinary industrious state but o

that is exaggerated into a symptom. He has become so industrious that he has a mania for work.

"Whimpering. Low-spirited and melancholy." It is a strange thing to see a bright little girl of 8 or 9 years old taking on sadness, melancholy, and commencing to talk about the future world, and the angels, and that she wants to die and go there, and she is sad, and wants to read the Bible all day. That is a strange thing; and yet Calcarea has cured that. *Ars.* has cured that state, and also *Lachesis.* They are a little inclined to be precocious, and they have attended the Sunday-school, and they have taken too seriously the things they have learned. Children sad and unhappy, and old people who take on a loathing of life, become weary of life. That is a good deal like *Aurum.* In going over *Aurum* I explained that, and dwelt upon it, that the highest love is the love of life; and when an individual ceases to love his own life, and is weary of it, and loathes it, and wants to die, he is on the border line of insanity. In fact, that is an insanity of the will. You have only to look with an observing eye to see that one may be insane in the affections, or insane in the intelligence. One may remain quite intact, and the other one be destroyed. We find in Calcarea both equally disturbed. One patient may be insane in his voluntary system, so that all of his loves are perverted; he has no affection that is like what it used to be, like it was when he was well. Antipathy to his family or some member of his family. Or, he may have the affection fairly intact, but no intelligence, and does all sorts of strange things.

He is full of fear. Weary of life; hopelessness, anxiety. The world is black. "Fear that something sad or terrible will happen. Fears that she will lose her reason, or that people will observe her confusion of mind." "Fear of death; of consumption; of misfortune; of being alone." Fear abounds, especially when the voluntary system is disturbed. She is startled at every noise. He can't sleep so that the body rests or the mind rests. He is disturbed in his sleep with horrible dreams. His sleep is a restless one. "Great anxiety and oppression. Restlessness and palpitation. Despairing; hopeless." These symptoms have to be coupled and connected with that leucophlegmatic, pale flabby, sickly individual. "Child cross and fretful. Easily frightened." Many complaints after exertion of the mind. Many complaints after excitement, chagrin or fright.

He is so weak in his circulation, so much disturbed in the heart, it palpitates from every excitement. He is out of breath from every physical exertion; and these take part so much in the circulation of blood in the body, have so much to do with circulation of blood in the brain, have so much to do with the intellect, with the sensorium, that we see at once vertigo on almost all occasions, intermingled with all sorts of symptoms. Fear, anxiety, and vertigo. If his emotions stir him up he becomes dizzy From going upstairs the blood mounts to the head, and he becomes dizzy. Confusion of mind and vertigo from mental exertion. If he becomes shocked, or has bad news, or has an mental excitement or chagrin, this vertigo will come out. Confusion of mind determination of blood to the head, cold extremities, covered with sweat with vertigo. "Vertigo, when climbing into high places;" that is the effort o going up. The blood rushes to the head and he becomes dizzy. "On goin, upstairs or up a hill. On suddenly rising, or turning the head, even when a rest."

One of the most striking symptoms of *the bead* of the Calcarea patient i the sweat; the sweat of the head upon the slightest exertion. He will sweat o the face when he sweats nowhere else, and his head is covered with col sweat when he is comfortable in other places about the body. The same thin; is true about the feet. When his feet become very cold they will sweat. Whe they are warm they will sweat. You would naturally think that a person goin; into a cold room would stop his sweating, but sometimes the Calcarea patien will break out in a sweat, upon the head. and upon the feet, in a cold room. H sweats upon the forehead, so that every draft of air makes him chilly, and thi brings on headache. Coldness of the whole scalp, so he has to wrap up th head. Yet during congestions, the head is hot. So it has at times great heat in the head. The Calcarea headaches are stupefying, they are benumbing; they bring on confusion of mind. The Calcarea patient has a catarrh in the nose with more or less discharge; at his best he has considerable discharge. Bu he goes into a cold place, the discharge is slacked up, and he gets a headache Headache over the eyes. Congestion of the head; back of the head. "Tearin; headache above the eyes down to nose," is a strong symptom of Calcarea. I seems sometimes as if a great wedge were in there. This is relieved by very hot applications. It is relieved in the dark; it is aggravated in the daylight. H must go into a dark room and lie down for relief. Sometimes this headache i: ameliorated by lying down in the dark. This headache continues to grow worse during the day, until in the evening it becomes so severe that it i: attended with nausea and vomiting. It is one of the forms of constitutiona headache, it is a headache that sometimes occurs in two weeks. Head ache every seven days, or headache once in two weeks. Periodical head aches. Sick-headache, the old-fashioned American sick-headache. There i: commonly a periodicity belonging to it, of seven to fourteen days, but again it comes on whenever he is exposed, by riding in the wind, for he is a very chilly patient; if he becomes really chilled or very cold, he gets a headache, a sick-headache. Then, again, it has pain in the Left side of the head. One-sided headache. Headache worse from noise, from talking, but ameliorated in the evening, from lying in the dark. It has headache in the temples, and this headache seems to draw through to the root of the nose. The headaches from the supraorbital region draw through to the nose. Headaches in the temples seem to produce a feeling of tightness, a feeling of great tension in the forehead. Headaches worse from motion, from walking, from talking. Most of the Calcarea headaches, as soon as they become severe, are attended with pulsation. The pulsation is so strong that the patient is not satisfied by merely saying it is a pulsation, he describes it as hammering. Most of the pains are pressive, or tearing. "Concussive headaches." Stitching, pulsating pains in the head, as if it would split. Headaches worse from walking, and from a jar. Sometimes he feels a coldness in the head, it seems as if the cold head is numb, cold as if made of wood. He sometimes feels this numbness, and describes it as if he had a cap, sometimes as if there were a helmet, on the head. Now, all of these sensations are difficult to describe, but sometimes they are one and the same thing. All the headaches of Calcarea are more or less congestive. It is a peculiar feature of Calcarea, that the more marked the congestion of internal parts, the colder the surface becomes. With chest troubles, and stomach troubles, and bowel troubles, the feet and hands become like ice, and covered with sweat; and he lies in bed sometimes with a fever in the rest of his body, and the scalp covered with cold sweat. That is strange. You cannot account for that by any process of reasoning in pathology, and when a thing is so strange that it cannot he accounted for, it becomes very valuable as descriptive of the remedy, and is one that cannot generally be left out when prescribing for a patient. That is almost a general state, it is so marked. It has burning in the vertex, and this is often present with coldness of the forehead, or the whole head may feel cold, except a burning spot on the vertex. Calcarea will again have cold head and icy cold feet when walking in cold air, or in very cold weather; but as soon as the feet get warm, they go to the other extreme, and burn so that he puts them out of. bed. This has often led inexperienced prescribers to prescribe *Sulph.,* because that is a keynote of *Sulph.* All keynote prescribers give *Sulph.* whenever the patient puts the feet out of bed, but a number of remedies have burning feet, hot feet, so we are not limited to *Sulph.* Calcarea has affections of the bones of the skull, the outer part of the head. Slow formation of bone. The fontanelles remain open a long time. It has hydrocephalic conditions, effusion in the membranes, and the bones do not grow and keep pace with the growth of the head, and hence the sutures commence to separate and the head grows wider and larger all the time with hydrocephalus. In hydrocephalic children this sweating head is a common feature. The child lies at night upon the pillow, and the sweat pours from the head and wets the pillow all around; especially sweating at night. In persons suffering from softening of the brain, the pillow is wet all around the head. Children going through difficult dentition have dreadful times in their dreams, they screech out in the night, and the pillow is wet all around their head. Old plethhoric patients, broken down constitutions, fat, flabby, lymphatic patients, with enlarged glands, with sweating of the head, cold sweating of the head. The hair falls out, not in the regular way such as occurs in old age, but in patches here and there. You see a bald spot on the side of the head, or the back of the head; a tuft of hair has come out, or in two or three places. Then it has eruptions upon the head and face; eczema that we find in children and infants. "Thick scabs on the head, with yellow pus." Offensive eruptions.

The *eye* comes in for a share of troubles, and Calcarea is one of the best friends the oculist has, if he knows how to use it. It is not especially suitable for every inflammation, but in those fat, flabby constitutions, where every cold settles in the eyes, and produces an inflammation, and this goes on for a few days, and ulceration begins, then study Calcarea. Vesicles are formed and break and spread into an ulcer. From exposure of the feet in water, from riding in the wind, from cold, damp weather he gets eye troubles. Ulceration of the cornea. In all of the complaints of the eyes and of the head the photophobia is so marked that the Calcarea subject when he is at all disturbed cannot even stand ordinary light, and to be out in the sunlight is extremely painful, and many times inflammations are started from merely going into a bright sunlight, from steady looking, and from straining the eyes. All kinds of exertions bring on headaches and eye troubles. Tension, because one muscle is weak. There is a disturbance of accommodation. Worse from every exertion of the eyes; you see that is like its generals, that is, aggravated from exertion. He cannot endure any prolonged exertion; you see that is just as true of his parts as of the whole. You know that reading, writing and looking at one thing all are marked exertions. With Calcarea, the part itself is worse from exertion, and the whole body is worse from exertion. Calcarea has cured cataract. Calcarea has other disturbances of the eyes, in connection with head troubles, in connection with fevers, and when he is out of sorts from great exertion; he so easily gets into a fidgety state, confusion of mind that is almost a delirium, and on closing the eyes he sees the most horrible visions, spectres, ghosts. Long before any disturbance can be observed in the tissues, or in the retina, or any disturbance of the eye by looking into it with the ophthalmoscope he will complain of seeing smoke, or steam in the air before his field of vision, as if looking through a veil, as if looking through a cloud, all meaning the same thing. "Dim vision." His vision is weak. The muscles are weak. He suffers from dim vision, which is going on gradually to blindness as he grows increasingly weak. All of his eye symptoms, and his headaches, and his nervous symptoms are aggravated from reading, from looking steadily at one thing. He is very much exhausted after such an exertion and will have tearing pains over the eyes, behind the eyes in the head. That is a peculiar kind of a headache, such as he is in the habit of having. It may be in any part of the head. Called eye-strain. It is a wonderful remedy for eye-strain (*Onosmodium*). Calcarea has cured many cases of opacity of the cornea (*Bar. iod.*). In an old case a cure can never be promised. It is one of the results of disease, and we never know when we are going to remove the results of disease, because the intelligent homœopath never prescribes for the results of disease. He prescribes for the patient. An opacity itself, when it is present, is not a symptom, but a result of disease. Often when a patient is prescribed for on his general symptoms, such a state of opacity of the cornea will, after a while, begin to pass away. The patient grows better, feels better himself. His symptoms commence to subside, and after the symptoms have subsided pathological conditions will commence to subside. Do not be discouraged in prescribing if the pathological conditions do not go away; but if all the symptoms of the patient have gone away, and the patient is eating well, and is sleeping well, and doing well, do not feel that it is impossible for that opacity of the cornea to go away, for sometimes it will. I have known patients to come back, years later, even after I had given them up as cured, as their symptoms had all disappeared, and I was foolish enough to say to the patient, "Well, I do not suppose this condition will ever go away but you are all well. there is nothing to prescribe on there is not much use of your taking any more medicine," but in six months from that time the patient would come back to me and say "Doctor, do you suppose the treatment you gave me had anything to do with this trouble going away? It has nearly all disappeared." I only tell you this to give you an idea how long it takes to restore order, for nature herself to replace the bad tissue and put healthy tissue in that same place, to restore an organ. It takes time, and it is best that we should not be surprised. It may be that the medicine has done all it can do. Here is another thing I have seen: even when there were no symptoms left, and after waiting a considerable time and there were no symptoms, I have seen another dose of the same medicine that was given on the last symptoms give the patient a great lift, and pathological conditions commence to go away. So Calcarea is a great friend to the oculist, and every physician ought to be just as good a prescriber as the oculist can be, for he prescribes for the patient. So must the oculist. In prescribing I am in doubt whether there can be any such thing as a specialty, because the homœopathic physician prescribes for the patient. He prescribes for the patient, whether he has eye disease, or ear disease, or throat disease, or lung disease, or liver disease, etc.

In the ear we have a great deal of trouble. It produces thick yellow discharge from the ears. Cold, chilly weather brings on ear trouble; quite likely from becoming cold or chilled, from an exposure, or from a sudden change of cold damp weather he has additional complaints in the ears. While he is at his best the idea holds good here as in other catarrhal conditions, there is copious discharge. But from exposure and cold this slacks up a little, and when it does there is a little inflammation, and like enough throbbing, and headache. That occurs every time from exposure. Whether the catarrh is in the nose, the eyes, or the ears, there will be headache. The Calcarea patient is so easily disturbed from cold weather and exposure, he is so sensitive to the cold, that it is next to impossible for him to dress and protect himself. He is flabby and soft, easily disturbed, sensitive to his surroundings. If it is an ear trouble, he may have difficult hearing, abscess of the middle ear, catarrh of the Eustachian tubes, etc., but all of these bring on headaches; and around about the ear the glands are all affected.

The catarrh of the *nose* is extremely troublesome. Old lingering stubborn catarrhs, with thick yellow discharge; great crusts from the nose. In the morning he blows out enormous blackish, bloody chunks. He breathes part of the night through the nose, and then his nose clogs up so that he breathes through the mouth. It has cured a great many times polypi of the nose. The homœopathic physician, trusting so much to his symptoms, knows so well the remedy after studying the case, that he very likely will prescribe for the patient on the symptoms alone. He says: This patient needs Calcarea, there is no doubt about it. He prescribes for him and sends him away. After three or four weeks the patient comes back with a gelatinous looking tough thing on a handkerchief, and says: "Doctor, look there at what came out of my nose. Do you suppose your medicine had anything to do with that?" Perhaps you did not know he had polypus, it does not make any difference, your prescription cannot be any different if he has polypi in the nose, and you do not know it is there; you cannot by any process of torsion remove it before you prescribe, so you will have to leave that torsion to those that do not know about Homœopathy; and hence the examination is not so important as it is to those who prescribe for the polypi, and forget about the patient. Affections of the bones of the nose. That is, the catarrhs go on so long, and they are so deep-seated, that the bones of the nose and the cartilage of the nose are infiltrated, and they break down. Then operators cut out bones, remove cartilage, and perform operations too numerous to mention; and every one must have the same operation; but in order for him to be cured, he must even after that go to an homœopathic physician. He should first be cured and then if there is anything to be removed let him be operated on.

The *face* is sickly, cold, covered with sweat. Sweats on the slightest exertion, and sometimes it sweats in the night, on the forehead. "Cold sweat on the face. Face pale and cachetic," such as we see in advanced cases of cancer, and consumption. Face sallow, pale, sickly, dropsical. Eruptions on the face. Eruptions about the lips; and the lips are chapped and the mouth is raw. The lips are cracked and bleeding. Painful swelling on the parotid glands;

painful swelling of the sub-lingual and sub-maxillary glands. The glands all take part in the Calcarea troubles.

Calcarea is a medicine for *chronic sore throats*. The throat appearance itself is not always sufficient to prescribe on, but the complaints in the throat are those that come on in persons taking cold so frequently that the patient has not time to get over one before he goes into another, and this engrafts upon him a chronic sore throat. It may in the beginning be a *Bell.* throat, which is quite likely, but before he gets over it he has taken another cold. Remember that this is a part of the Calcarea patient, that he takes cold so easily; he takes cold from *every* draft, from every exposure, and from damp weather. When getting over a *Bell.* sore throat— about the time he thinks he is over it he takes a new cold. Perhaps it has been relieved two or three times with *Bell.,* and then it settles down into a chronic state, and there are little red patches, perhaps little ulcers, in the throat; this extends all over. It extends to the roof of the mouth, with a sore tongue, and a constant dry, choking feeling in the pharynx, covering the tonsils and extending up into the posterior nares, filling with thick, yellow mucus. Chronic inflammation. The uvula may be puffed; swollen. "Parts swollen, red, tumid," but in patches. The throat very painful on swallowing; dry, choking feeling.

The *stomach* in Calcarea is slow in its action. "Food taken into the stomach remains." It does not digest. It turns sour. "Sour vomiting." Milk sours. Milk disagrees; the digestion is also slow, feeble. He has a feeling of tumefaction and fulness; enlargement after eating; and everything sours in the stomach; everything disorders the stomach. Weak digestion. The Calcarca patient has a very strong *longing for eggs.* Little children crave eggs; at every meal they will eat eggs, and eggs will digest better than anything else. It is very seldom that little children naturally long for eggs; children with cold feet, emaciated extremities, large heads, enlarged abdomen; stomach distended like an inverted saucer, rounded out; bloated abdomen, and slender extremities; cold and sensitive to cold; pale skin; pale, waxy surface. Then, there is complete loss of appetite; no desire for any kind of food. If any desire at all, *it* is *for eggs.* Aversion to meat; aversion to warm food. This with enlarged glands, with goitre. Flatulency. Sour vomiting; sour diarrhœa; that is, it has a pungent, sour odor, especially in children. In infants living on milk, the milk passes in an undigested form; the stool is so sour that it is pungent. It excoriates the parts, and keeps the nates raw in infants where the diaper comes in contact with the parts. There are times when the abdomen is emaciated; the gases go out and the abdomen sometimes becomes flabby; but most of the time it is distended with flatulence. When it is flabby it can be observed that there are nodules in the abdomen. The lymphatic glands are hard, and sometimes can be felt through the emaciated abdomen. There is a *tubercular* tendency, and tabes mesenterica is one of the natural endings of the lime constitution, with this we get the glandular affections of the bowels. Tubercular deposits in the mesenteric glands. Diarrhœa comes on, sour, watery diarrhoea; gradual emaciation, especially of the extremities. Every cold brings on more indigestion, and more sour vomiting. Diarrhœa that can't be stopped, because every time he gets a cold it renews the diarrhœa. When it is an acute attack *Dulc.* often relieves it, but when it has recurred several times *Dulc.* can no longer relieve it, and Calcarea then becomes one of the remedies.

Again, it is one of the most useful medicines in old, lingering, stubborn cases of *constipation.* When there is only a moderate diarrhœa the stool is white; and when this constipation is present, the stool is white, or like chalk. In infants taking milk you can account for the white or pale stool, because of the milk; but when the patient does not live on milk, and lives on ordinary substances, the stool becomes bileless and is very light colored; is yellow or white; and in the constipation, often the stool is very light colored and hard.

Calcarea has a kind of indigestion, a fermentation that favors the formation of worms, so that Calcarea babies are sometimes wormy. Pass worms in the stool, and vomit worms. Calcarea so corrects this indigestion, when the symptoms agree, that worms no longer hatch out. The symptoms disappear, and we really wonder what becomes of the worms. The idea with the homœopathic physician is not to give vermifuges, but to so correct the digestion that worms will not thrive; and it is true that worms will not thrive in the healthy stomach and intestines. Whether they leave by expulsion or whether they are destroyed, or what becomes of them, I do not know. To remove them by physicking them out, and by vermifuges, only makes a bad matter worse, because it increases the indigestion, it increases the turmoil. So it is with all worms in the stomach and rectum; all those worms will come if they are favored with just exactly the right kind of fluids to hatch out in. They come, and they grow. I suppose at least twenty-five times in the last twenty years have I known Calcarea to bring away tape worm, and in most instances I did not know it was present; but I simply prescribed for the patient. I was not aware of its existence. It is so with many remedies, but this more than others.

The Calcarea patient is weak sexually, with general relaxation and weakness. Sometimes an inordinate craving, sometimes an overwhelming desire keeps him awake at nights. But weak; weak in this way, that any indulgence is followed by weak back, sweating, weakness in general, so that he is compelled to abstain because of the sufferings.

The woman is affected in a similar way. You need not be surprised, when you hear all of the constitutional weaknesses, that it is a common thing for Calcarea women to be sterile. So tired, so relaxed; wholly unfit for reproduction.

And the same as in the male, she suffers from lassitude, sweating, wakefulness, and weakness in general after every coition. The parts feel relaxed. The uterus drags down. Sensation as if parts would be forced out. State of general weakness and general relaxation of the sexual organs of both male and female. Calcarea has a tendency to grow warts and polypoid growths, pedunculated growths, that bleed easily, that are soft and spongy.

The woman flows too much at the menstrual period; too long, and, of course, this naturally brings her around too soon. Often every three weeks, lasting a week, with a copious flow. Menstrual period *too soon, lasting too long, and profuse*. Calcarea is not always indicated; not unless all of the symptoms go together to make up the Calcarea patient. Sometimes it may occur to your mind to say, that with five or six key-notes, certainly you would give Calcarea; but suppose you did have five or six key-notes of Calcarea, and the patient should be a *Puls.* patient, would you expect to cure her with Calcarea? Suppose the patient always avoided warm things and much clothing, and wanted the cold open air, and still had a dozen key-notes, you would find every time that Calcarea would fail. Unless you combine the particulars with the things that are general, and the generals with the particulars, unless the remedy fits the patient from within out, generally and particularly, a cure need not be expected. That is why I say, do not prescribe on key-notes, but upon the symptoms of the patient.

This great state of relaxation which we always have in every Calcarea patient is also manifested in *leucorrhœa*. Copious, thick, constant leucorrhœa, discharging day and night. Leucorrhœa that is acrid, keeping up an itching, and smarting, and burning. "Leucorrhœa thick and yellow," from one menstrual period to another, and sometimes it intermingles with the menstrual flow. "Vaginal polypi. Burning soreness in the genitals" from leucorrhœa. "Itching and rawness" from leucorrhœa. Hæmorrhage of the uterus from over-lifting; from excitement; from shocks; from anything that greatly disturbs; from fear, from any great emotion, or from straining the muscles. Such are the conditions of relaxation and weakness. Inability to strain the muscles, or to exert herself mentally or physically.

The complaints of *pregnancy* are generally those of great relaxation and weakness. Threatened abortion. After delivery, weakness and prostration; sweating. Weakness from nursing.

The Calcarea voice is that of *painless hoarseness*. The vocal cords are tired, and cannot endure strain; almost a paralytic weakness. Sometimes a copious flow of mucus from the larynx. Much irritation in the larynx, but weakness. Not that burning and rawness that we find in *Bell.* and *Phos.*, but painless hoarseness. In *Phos.* it is painful, in *Bell.* it is very painful. He cannot speak without pain. But in Calcarea he wonders why he has so much trouble in the larynx, because he has no feeling in it. This goes on from bad to worse, and with the tubercular tendency, look out for tubercular laryngitis. Given early it may keep off such a tubercular tendency. It has cured tubercular laryngitis. Much rattling of mucus; rattling breathing; coarse rattling; that is, much mucus in the trachea, in the larynx, in the bronchial tubes, in the chest. Great dyspnœa. The dyspnœa comes on *from going up stairs,* from walking against the wind. Anything that has any exertion in it will bring on the dyspnœa. We find this in asthma, weak heart, weak chest and in threatening phthisis. That state of the lungs you will know very often by the kind of breathing; because all that are going into phthisis, are tired and weak. He is too tired to make any effort at breathing, and he tires very easily, so that he has difficulty in going up stairs, climbing a hill, walking against the wind.

The *chest* trouble furnishes one of our best fields for Calcarea. We have spitting of blood; prolonged cough; copious expectoration of thick yellow mucus, or even pus; ulceration, or abscess. Tickling cough. We have, in threatening chest trouble, the beginning emaciation, the pallor, the sensitiveness to cold, changes, and to the cold air, and to wet weather and to winds. He takes colds and they all settle in the chest; gradual emaciation in the limbs; always so tired. It corresponds to just such constitutional weakness as precedes, or is present in the first stages of phthisis. It stops the patient taking cold, which is the very beginning of it. The patient will begin to feel better after taking Calcarca, and it improves his general state, and it will even encyst tubercular deposits. It turns them from a caseous into a calcareous form, and cysts have been found in the chest long afterwards. Patients have lived a long time and improved, and gone into a general state of health, when quite well advanced with tubercular deposits. Of course, when any person is well into a tubercular condition, it may be expected that he will go. Do not believe or think favorably of cures for consumption. Every little while we have some one coming out with something or other that cures consumption, a new cure. Every one who knows much about the real nature of phthisical conditions, cannot have much confidence in such things, and I certainly lose respect for an individual who has a consumption cure. He must either be crazy or something worse. Generally he is after the money that may be in it. Hardly anyone who knows anything about it can conscientiously present a consumption cure to the world. To prevent those things is what we want to do, and this is the great sphere of Calcarea. The expectoration is sweetish very often, like *Phos.* and *Stannum.* White, yellow, thick. We might go over all the general symptoms here, the soreness, the tenderness, the kind of pains, the lassitude, and a great many symptoms of that sort, they are too numerous to mention, but they are not descriptive, for the reason that after you get these pains and study them carefully, you are not better off. You must study the *constitution* of Calcarea, the nature of Calcarea, its character.

There are spine symptoms; plenty of them. Weak; all degrees of weakness. The Calcarea patient is so weak in the back that he slides down in the chair while sitting; cannot sit upright in his chair. Rests on the back of his head. The back of his chair and the back of his head come in contact. A weak spine, a sensitive spine, and the glands of the neck are swollen. Again, a marked condition of the spine is where the lime element is deficient, and we soon get deformity; curvature. It may be surprising to you to hear that Calcarea is a great help, and has sometimes cured that without any brace or support whatever, when taken early. You take infants manifesting a weakness of the spine, let them lie flat on their back in bed, put them on the indicated remedy— it is sometimes Calcarea—and in a little while that knuckling will cease, and the little one will sit up straight. Such wonderful things occur under the use of Calcarea, when the symptoms agree.

In the extremities we have all the *rheumatic* conditions that it is possible to describe. Gouty affections of the joints, with enlarged joints; gouty conditions, especially of the small joints, of the toe and finger. Rheumatic complaints of the joints from every exposure, from every change of the weather to cold, especially if it is cold and damp. The feet are always cold, or cold and damp, except at night in bed after piling clothing upon the feet more than any other part of the body, then the feet begin to get warm, and then they often go to the other extreme and burn; and so they burn at night in bed. But the feet are so cold that the patient has to put more clothing on the feet than the body will endure. Cold, damp feet. Late waking. Clumsiness; awkwardness; stiffness. Rheumatic conditions. Stiffness belongs to Calcarea all over. Stiff on beginning to move; stiff at night on rising from a seat. Stiffness in all joints on beginning to move; and if it turns cold or there is a cold rain, the Calcarea patient always suffers; suffers from coldness, stiffness, rheumatism; has rheumatism in every cold change in the weather.

The sleep is greatly disturbed. Late going to sleep, sometimes not till 2, 3 or 4 o'clock. Full of ideas; when closing the eyes horrible visions. Grinding the teeth. A child in sleep, chews and swallows and grinds the teeth. Sleeplessness a good part of the night. Cold feet at night in bed.

CALCAREA FLUORICA

This chemical union of lime and fluoric acid gives us a remedy with a new nature and properties. However conversant one may be with either or both of these elements, he could not predict the curative powers held in this double remedy. I refer to its ability to cure indurated infiltrations of glands, cellular tissues and bony formations. A nodule in the course of a tendon, an exostosis, a stony hard gland, bony infiltration in the periosteum, rice bodies in cartilages have been cured by this remedy wonderful to tell, when there was a paucity of symptoms. It will cure of course when symptoms agree, but it needs proving in order that individualization may be oftener possible.

A recurrent fibroid in the hollow of the knee was removed once by the knife, but returned, and grew to the size of a fist. The leg was drawn up to forty-five degrees, and the knee became immovable. This wonderful remedy was prescribed on the symptoms of the case and the hardness of the tumor. The tumor gradually dwindled, the limb became normal and as good as ever; this patient has given birth to a healthy child—is still perfectly free from the trouble. It is now ten years since she was cured.

The patient is sensitive to cold, to drafts, to changes in the weather, and to damp weather. The symptoms are ameliorated by heat and by warm applications. The symptoms are worse during rest.

This is a useful remedy in gout, with copious pale urine and diarrhoea. The patient is sad and miserable. This remedy has cured a fluctuating tumor on the cranium of infants known as Cephalæmatoma. Blur before the eyes after exerting the vision. Cataract. It cures ulceration of the cornea if the edges are hard; also hard, small spots and conjunctivitis. It has cured adenoids and thick, yellowish green discharge from the nose. Offensive catarrh of long standing. Scanty enamel of the teeth.

Pain, ulceration and granulation of the throat, worse from cold, and better from warm drinks. Pain worse at night. Large indurated tonsils will be cured after *Baryta carb.* has failed.

Pain in the liver at night, worse lying on the painful side, better from motion. Cutting pains in the liver, better walking.

Diarrhœa in gouty subjects. Itching of anus and hæmorrhoids, painful and hard bleeding. Fissure of anus. Constipation.

Copious watery urine. Strong smelling urine. Urine causes smarting when passing.

Indurated testes. Nodular testes. Varicose veins of the vulva. Uterine fibroid.

Hard nodules in the mammæ.

Dryness and tickling in the larynx. Desire to clear the vocal cords. Hoarseness after reading aloud. Hacking cough after eating, and in cold air, from tickling in the larynx. Spasmodic cough.

It cured an exostosis at the angle of the eighth rib.

It cured a lumbago, worse during rest, and better from heat, after *Rhus* had failed. Pain in back, extending to the sacrum.

Indurated cervical glands.

Vivid dreams, and unrefreshing sleep. Jumps out of bed in a dream. It is similar to *Silica* in suppuration.

CALCAREA IODATA

The symptoms appear or are worse in the morning; afternoon; *evening;* NIGHT; *after midnight.* It has produced abscesses. Strong desire for open air; open air excites and also ameliorates symptoms. The tendency is towards anæmia. There is general physical anxiety; asleep feeling in single parts; choreic movements. Becoming cold ameliorates many symptoms, but there is a tendency to take cold; cold weather aggravates. It is a most useful remedy in tuberculosis. It has cured convulsions; clonic; epileptiform; with falling. Convulsive movements. Many symptoms come on before eating and are better after eating; some symptoms are worse before and after eating. There is marked loss of flesh. Exertion is impossible. There are fainting spells, fainting in a warm room. Fasting brings on many symtpoms. Feeling of fulness internally. Internal hemorrhage. It is a most useful remedy in induration, especially following inflammation. Great lassitude; lying ameliorates, but lying long in bed aggravates, as the patient is worse from the warm bed. There is urging of blood in the body; pains are numerous but mild and flitting. Burning, cutting, jerking, pinching, pressing, stitching, tearing; there is more weakness than pain. He perspires easily and; becomes chilled during sweat. Pulsation all over. Many of the symptoms are right-sided. Swelling of affected parts and glands; swelling that suppurates. *Trembling and twitching.* The symptoms as well as the patient are worse from warmth, warm air, warm bed, warm room, 'warm wraps. GREAT GENERAL WEAKNESS; in the morning; during menses.

He becomes very angry over small matters. Frequent spells of anxiety; anxious over trifles. Aversion to company; confusion of mind; delusions; sees dead people. Despair; discontented; discouraged. Dullness of mind. Worse from mental exertion. Fear of insanity; of misfortune; of people. Impatience; indifference; indolence; irresolution. Irritability; during headache. Symptoms like insanity and mania. Mirthful. Mental prostration. Restless and anxious. EXTREME SADNESS. Dullness of the senses; starting in sleep; *weeping.* Vertigo in the morning on rising; while walking; with headache.

The head feels cold. There are congestion, heat and heaviness of the head; especially during menses. Crusty eruptions on the scalp. The hair falls out. It has cured Hydrocephalus. Itching of the scalp. Pain in the head; in the morning, binding up the hair makes the pain worse; with coryza and catarrh; compelled to lie down; before the menses; moving the head; noise; riding against a cold wind; stooping; talking; walking; warm room; wrapping up the head. Pain in the forehead above the eyes; in the *occiput;* pain in occiput before menses; sides of head but mostly in the right; temples, vertex. Pressing pain in forehead, occiput, sides of head, temples and *vertex*. Sharp pain in right temple. Shooting in head; in the occiput. Sore; bruised pain in head. Stitching pains in head, in the occiput, in sides of head, in temples, in vertex; stunning pains in the head; tearing pains in the head; in the temples. Perspiration on the scalp; on the forehead. Pulsation in the head; forehead; temples.

Dullness of the eyes; inflammation of the conjunctiva; scrofulous inflammation of the eyes. Lachrymation. Pain in the eyes; burning in the eyes. The ball of the eye is tender to touch. Protrusion of the eyes, exophthalmus *Pupils dilated*. Redness of the eyes; of the lids; sunken eyes; swollen lids twitching lids. Weak eyes. Vision foggy, dim. Colors before the eyes; sparks

Catarrh of the eustachian tubes; discharge from the ears. The ears are hot. Noises in the ears; buzzing, humming, ringing, roaring. Pain in the ear pressing, tearing. Hearing acute; later impaired.

Catarrh of the nose, also of the posterior nares; redness of the nose Coryza FLUENT and dry. Discharges from the nose excoriating; fetid; greenish purulent; thick; watery; yellow. Dryness in the nose. Epistaxis. The nose is obstructed and smell is lost; much *sneezing*. The nose is swollen.

The face is cold and sunken and the muscles twitch. The face is discolored, earthy *pale,* red, *yellow*. Scaly eruptions on the face. Pain in the face. Swollen submaxillary gland.

Aphthæ in the mouth; the gums bleed easily; the tongue is fissured dryness of the tongue. Offensive odor from the mouth. Pain in the gums teeth, and tongue burns. Salivation. Swollen gums and tongue. Taste astringent, bad, sour, sweetish. Ulceration in the mouth.

Dryness and constriction of the throat; enlarged tonsils, honeycombed with small crypts; viscid mucus in the throat. Pain in the throat on swallowing pressing pain. External throat swollen; many hard glands. It has cured GOITRE even exophthalmic goitre.

Appetite INCREASED ravenous or *wanting;* aversion to food, Desire stimulants. Eructations empty; sour; waterbrash; heartburn. Fulness in the stomach; flesh of heat in the stomach. Hiccough. Nausea at night and after eating. Pain in the stomach after eating; burning, cramping, cutting, *pressing* SORE, stitching. *Pulsating* in the stomach. Thirst extreme, unquenchable Vomiting on coughing, after eating, bile, blood, food.

Distension of the abdomen, tympanitic, Enlarged abdomen, mesenteric glands, spleen. Flatulence; obstructed. Hardness of the liver, mesenteric glands. Pain in abdomen; during menses, in hypochondria, in liver; burning cramping, *cutting,* pressing in the hypogastrium. Pulsation in abdomen Rumbling.

Constipation; inactivity of the rectum; difficult stool; hard stool. Diar-rhœa; evening, after eating. Exhausting; stool bloody, copious, watery, white, yellow; passing of copious flatus. Hemorrhoid. *Itching* of the anus; burning after stool; tenesmus after stool; ineffectual urging to stool.

Retention or suppression of urine; much urging at night; frequent urina-tion during the night; involuntary urination. Frequent paroxysms if busy; stinging pain in neck of bladder with frequent urging to urinate. It has been useful in Addison's disease. The urine is acrid, albuminous, cloudy, dark, pale, red, copious, with offensive odor and cuticle on the surface.

Erections wanting; seminal emissions; sexual passion increased without erections. Pain in the testes; induration of testes; swollen testes.

Sexual desire increased in the woman; congestion of the uterus. *Leucor-hœa* acrid, bloody, copious, yellow. Menses absent, *copious,* frequent, irregular, painful, suppressed. Metrorrhagia. Pain in ovaries and uterus. Sterility. Tumors on ovaries. Pain in both ovaries before menses.

Catarrh of the larynx and trachea; constriction, croup. Inflammation of the larynx; mucus in the air passages; pain in the larynx; phthisis of larynx; tickling in the larynx, HOARSENESS.

Accelerated respiration, asthmatic, difficult at night and on ascending steps; rattling, short. Suffocation.

Cough morning; evening, after midnight, asthmatic, DRY; from irritation in the larynx and trachea, short, *spasmodic;* from tickling in the larynx. Expectoration: morning; bloody, greenish, mucus, offensive, purulent, viscid, yellow. Violent, hard cough after pneumonia.

Anxiety in chest and heart; catarrh of the bronchial tubes; constriction of the heart. Induration of the mammæ. Inflammation of the bronchial tubes, of the pleura; oppression of the chest; pain in the chest on coughing; in the heart; burning, cutting, pressing, rawness; stitching on coughing; stitching in mammæ. Palpitation of the heart warm during the night. PHTHISIS. *Trembling of the heart.* It has cured nodular tumors in mammæ, tender to touch, painful in moving the arm.

Pain in the sacrum; soreness in the spine; stitching pain in back and lumbar region.

Enlarged points of the fingers; coldness of the upper limbs, hands, legs, feet; cramps in the feet; heat of the hands; heaviness of the limbs; of the feet; itching of the limbs; numbness of the hands, fingers, lower limbs, legs; pain in the limbs, in the joints; in gouty joints; in the thighs, in the knees. Itching pain in the shoulders, in the knees. Tearing in the joints, in the upper limbs, in the elbow, in the knees. perspiration of the hands, of the palms, of the FEET; stiffness in the limbs; swelling of the hands, legs, knees, feet; œdematous; trembling of upper limbs, of the hands, lower limbs;

twitching of the upper limbs, thighs, legs; weakness of the upper limbs, of the knees.

Dreams amorous, anxious, of dead people; nightmare vivid. Restless sleep; sleepiness in the evening; sleeplessness, waking too early.

Chill, external, internal; *shaking chill;* tertian; warmth does not ameliorate.

Fever in the afternoon; fever alternating with chill; *flushes of heat;* hectic fever.

Perspiration in the morning; during the night; in bed; cold; on SLIGHT EXERTION; on motion; profuse.

Burning of the skin; coldness. Red and yellow spots. Dry skin; eruptions, boils, herpes, rash, scaly. Erysipelas.

CALCAREA PHOSPHORICA

During the growing period many children need this remedy. If the head bones are slow in forming, or do not keep pace with the growth of the child this remedy is often called for. Where the child is losing flesh, slow learning to do things, slow learning to walk, or the legs are not strong enough to support the body, or it is behind in mental development, this remedy is one to be examined (like *Baryta carb., Borax, Ph. ac., Nat. m., Calc.*). Flabby shrunken, emaciated children. Non-union of fractured bones, swollen condyles, are symptoms accepted by all text-books as strong symptoms of this remedy. It has cured polypi of nose, rectum and uterus. It has cured enlarged glands of the neck, groin and abdomen. Rachitis, with fontanelle open, and diarrhœa, in emaciating children. Rheumatic pains in the joints and limbs, worse from cold weather, or in every cold change of weather. Pale waxy skin; anæmia. Growing pains nights in fast growing children. Phthisical subjects. Diseases of bone. Easy ulceration. Itching, burning eruptions. *Sensitive to cold.* Sensitive to a jar.

The pains are shooting, drawing, aching, burning, pressing. It has shaking chill that spreads downward. Dry heat in evening. Copious night sweats.

The complaints of this remedy are generally better during rest, come on during motion, and are greatly aggravated by exertion. Stiffness on moving in bed. General bodily weakness. Numbness of many parts. Trembling. Fear brings on complaints; palpitation.

Electric shock, so severe that the patient could not remain standing. Epileptic spasms. Convulsions of children; but the remedy must be given when not in the convulsion to secure the best effect. The mind shows above all a tired and weak brain. Feeble memory, and inability to sustain mental effort. Suffering in the head from mental exertion. Dreads mental exertion. Sluggish mind. Imbecility. Feeble minded children. The child grasps the head with the hands and screams. Thinking of complaints causes them to appear or increase. Extremely fretful. Ailments from bad news, grief, unrequited affections, vexation. She seeks solitude to commune with her thoughts and to shun the exertion of society. Discontented with his own surroundings and goes from place to place.

Vertigo in cold wind, from mental and physical exertion. when rising from sitting, when walking in cold air.

The head symptoms are still more striking. The dull headaches of school children—always come home from school with headache. The head is sensitive to a jar, to pressure, to the hat; wants it washed in cold water; wants to be quiet and alone. Throbbing and burning in the head. Rheumatic headache, seems to be in the whole head, in cold weather, being out in the cold wind; worse from walking, worse from exertion, worse at night. It has many times prevented hydrocephalus. Frontal headaches, and forehead and eyes worse from pressure of the hat. Perspiration of scalp; forehead cold to touch. Tearing pain in bones of head. Cold occiput. Eczema of scalp. Ulcers of scalp.

In children when coming out of brain congestion if there is strabismus, diarrhœa, and losing flesh. Glittering fiery circles before the eyes. Pain in eyes from reading in artificial light. Eyes blurred. Soreness in eyeballs. Pains worse thinking about them. Ulceration of cornea. Eyes feel hot. Easy lachrymation.

Rheumatic tearing in the ears when the weather changes to cold. Ears very cold. Aching deep in ear. Enlarged, painful parotid plands. Eruption about the ears. Noises in ears after stool. Dry catarrh of the middle ear.

This remedy is useful in chronic catarrh of the nose when the general symptoms agree. Polypi in the nose. Icy cold nose. Fluent coryza in a cold room, stopped in a warm room. Epistaxis.

Pale, waxy face, dirty skin. Rheumatic faceache in every cold spell of weather. Cold perspiration on face. Neuralgia of face at night, in cold air; worse from exertion, ameliorated by heat; sensitive to pressure (*Mag. p.* is better by heat and pressure). Dark blotches and pustules on the face. Swollen upper lip, painful, hard and burning.

Teeth late coming in or decay soon. Teeth sensitive to touch, pressure, or when masticating. Complaints of teething children. Foul taste in mouth. Bitter taste in the morning. Tongue coated in the morning. Tongue swollen, numb and stiff.

Growing children suffer from chronic throat troubles. Enlarged tonsils. Every cold settles in the tonsils (*Baryta c., Alumen*). Much mucus in throat. Dryness in throat at night.

Craves salt bacon and smoked meats. Strong appetite. Infants want to nurse all the time. Easily disordered stomach. Cold drinks, ice cream, fruits disorder the stomach, causing pain or diarrhœa. Pain in stomach after food. Eructations and nausea. Soreness in the stomach. Sour eructations, nausea and vomiting. Burning in the stomach. Nausea from scraping the larynx or throat. Vomiting in infants, in children, and in pregnancy. Violent pain in the stomach; diarrhœa aggravated by the least food. Gnawing, empty feeling in the stomach.

After becoming chilled, pain in the liver, soreness, aggravated after eating and by motion; wants to keep quiet. Stitching pains in the liver from breathing or sudden motion. Pulsating in the liver. Cutting pains in the spleen. Sinking sensation in abdomen. Burning in the abdomen, rising up into the chest. Pain in the abdomen ameliorated by passing flatus Colic, followed by diarrhœa. Ulceration of navel in infants. Motion in abdomen from flatus as from something alive. Abdomen large and flabby.

Tabes mesenterica with diarrhœa.

Green mucus and hot watery stools; white, mushy stools, copious, offensive flatus. Diarrhœa from fruit, ice cream, cold drinks or vexation. Diarrhœa in the morning in phthisical patients. Very offensive stools.

Constipation, with difficult, hard stool. Bleeding from the rectum and anus during stool. Protruding piles so painful that he is kept in bed for weeks; the pain is intense standing, walking, from touch; ameliorated by heat; with general sufferings, every sudden cold change of the weather. Piles itch and burn and discharge yellow pus. Itching of the anus in the evening. Stitching pain in the anus, with or without hæmorrhoids. Boils and abscesses about and near the anus, discharging blood and pus. Fistula in tuberculous subjects. Fissured anus, with burning stitching pains.

Weak and irritable bladder. Catarrh of the bladder. Frequent urging to urinate. Copious flow of urine. Pain in the neck of the bladder. Cutting in urethra. Stitching in prostate gland. Pain in neck of the bladder before and after urinating. Aching in the empty bladder. This remedy has cured diabetes mellitus. Violent pain in the region of the kidneys.

Sexual desire increased. Painful erections. It has cured many cases of chronic gonorrhœa when the discharge is gleety and there are sharp pains in the urethra and prostate gland. Gonorrhœal rheumatism when of long standing and worse in every cold change in the weather (*Med.*).

The woman has no better friend than Calc. p. Her sufferings at puberty when she is slow in maturing are often met by this medicine. From taking cold at first menstrual period often comes a painful menstruation that lasts during menstrual life, unless cured by this remedy. Violent cramping in uterus and groin several hours before the flow starts, relieved after the flow has been fully established. The pains make her cry out. Intense sexual excitement (like *Platina, Gratiola, Origamum*). Weak, sinking sensation in the pelvis. Prolapsus of uterus during stool and micturition, Uterine polypus. Labor-like pains at the beginning of menstruation. Copious menstrual flow, with very dark clots and membranes. Leucorrhœa like white of egg day and night. Throbbing, titillating in external genitalia. Burning in the vagina and uterus during menses. Child refuses mother's milk. It may be given to a woman who has brought forth one or two children that may be considered Calc. p. babies. The next child will be stronger and have a better constitution.

It is often observed that this patient scrapes mucus from the larynx before he can talk or sing. Hoarseness, dry, hacking cough day and night. Tubercular laryngitis.

Suffocation on slight exertion, or on ascending stairs. In thin, pale, sickly people with dry, hacking cough worse in cold, damp weather in rheumatic constitutions. Yellow expectoration.

Stitching pains in the chest. Emaciation of the chest. Difficult expectoration. It is a very useful remedy in phthisis and bloodspitting. Much sweat on the chest. Rattling in the chest with difficult expectoration, like *Caust.* Soreness of the chest to touch. Palpitation, with trembling of the limbs.

The back pains are worse in cold, stormy weather, attended with stiffness, and worse in the morning. The back is sensitive to draft. Pain in the back from lifting or straining. Curvature of spine. Tearing, shooting; tenderness and aching in the spine. Soreness in sacroiliac symphysis. Pain in lumbar region and sacrum at the menstrual period.

Rheumatic pains in the limbs in cold weather, worse from motion, better during rest and from heat. Trembling in all the limbs. Stiffness after resting, and in the morning. Aching in the bones, like growing pains. Gouty fingers and toes that become painful in cold weather. Ulcerative pains in the roots of the nails.

The most severe tearing, shooting pains are in the lower limbs. The probable reason for this is that the lower limbs are always cold to the knees, and the cold parts are always the suffering parts in this remedy. Sharp pains in tendons of the lower limbs. Intense aching boring pains in the knees, and long bones. Pains in the tibia with soreness. Drawing pain in the tibia. Cramp in the calves. Ulcers on the legs; weak, chronic; no granulation. Rheumatism of the ankles. Caries of the os calcis. Stinging and shooting in the toes.

Sleepy daytime and evening. Sleepless after going to bed until midnight or later. Very sleepy in the morning. Vivid dreams. Children cry out in sleep. Frightful dreams cause him to awaken with a start.

CALCAREA SILICATA

The silicate of lime is a very deep-acting remedy. The symptoms come on during all parts of the day and night—*morning,* forenoon, afternoon, EVENING NIGHT, *after midnight.* It acts profoundly upon the skin, mucous membranes, bones and glands. Abscesses, catarrhal discharges, ulcers, are marked with *thick, greenish-yellow pus.* Thick, greenish-yellow expectoration. Aversion to the open air. Extreme sensitiveness to drafts. One prover felt better in open air; very sensitive to wine and alcoholic stimulants. Marked paleness as in anæmia. Weakness and out of breath ascending stairs, like *calcarea.* Aversion to bathing and worse from bathing; especially cold bathing makes worse, in a prover who had always enjoyed cold bathing. Complaints worse after breakfast. It has cured epithelioma and lupus. From what is known of both calcarea and silica it ought to be a remedy in caries where the symptoms agree. Change of weather, from warm to cold, makes all symptoms worse. Many symptoms are worse after coiton. Worse from cold in general, cold air, becomnig cold and after becoming cold; worse in cold, wet weather. Takes cold in cold weather; seems to be constantly taking cold; many internal congestions. Contraction of orifices, a convulsive tendency. It greatly mitigates the constitutional condition in patients suffering from epilepsy, making the fits lighter and farther apart. The veins are greatly distended and a sensation of fulness in many parts. The symptoms are worse during and *after eating.* Emaciation is marked and especially in children who have inherited phthisis. Weakness, night sweats and seminal emission. The least exertion prostrates and increases many symptoms. Faintness creeps over her The muscles become flabby. He is more comfortable on low diet or when fasting; cold food, cold milk, and cold drinks make many complaints worse. The mucous membranes bleed easily. Hemorrhage from throat, nose, larynx and chest. He is cold all the time; marked lack of vital heat. One chilly prover became warm after the proving, curative action. Great aggravation from being overheated. The body feels heavy and the organs drag down. Inflammation in external and internal parts; in *bones* and *glands.* Extremely sensitive to a jar in all internal parts. Lassitude day and night, but worse evening and night; must lie down all the time.

The muscles, tendons and joints are weak and easily strained. The weakness is much like arsenicum and china, or as though from loss of fluids. He is most comfortable when lying in bed on the back; lying helps most symptoms; after lying a while he seems very well, but as soon as he walks about all the lassitude returns and he must lie down. Many symptoms come at the menstrual period—before, during and after. All symptoms are worse from motion. Mucous secretions increased and greenish-yellow. Numbness of single parts, of parts lain on and of painful parts. The weakness suggests it in complaints following onanism. The blood seems to rush from body to head with great flushes of heat.

The pains are boring, burning, CUTTING, jerking, pressing, bruised, *stitching, tearing*. Burning in internal parts. The function of organs and glands much impaired and slow. Slow digestion, slow action of bowels and liver. Periodicity is marked in many symptoms. When perspiring a slight draft or cold air will suppress the sweat and he becomes lame and the symptoms in general are worse. Pulsation all over the body—internal and external.

Sensitive all over, sensitive to pain; some internally. The bones are sore to touch. Its symptoms are like those that have come on from sexual excesses. The weakness and many other symptoms are worse standing. Stiffness in body, back and limbs when cold, after exertion and after sweating. It has swelling from dropsy and from inflammation; swelling of affected parts, of *glands with* hardness. Touch aggravates many parts and he dreads being touched. Trembling all over and in limbs, much twitching of muscles. It is most useful in restraining malignant ulceration in the mammary glands. Symptoms worse from uncovering. Walking fast and walking in cold air makes him worse. Great weakness, especially in the morning on waking, after least exertion, from mental exertion, walking in open air. Great nervous weakness. *He is always so weary*. Wet weather brings out all his sufferings. It seems that he can hardly get through the winter, so much are his symptoms increased, and he is correspondingly improved in the summer.

He is absent-minded and excitable and easily angered and his symptoms are worse after anger. Symptoms worse when alone. Anxiety in evening in bed and during the night about her health, worse during menses and on waking in the morning. Wants many things and soon tires of them; desires the unobtainable; nothing suits and he is very critical. Inability to concentrate the mind on what he is reading or listening to. He has lost all confidence in himself. *Confusion* of mind in the morning on waking and in the evening, after eating, after *mental exertion* and while sitting. Consolation irritates him; contrary and timid, even cowardly. She sits long in one place and looks into space and does not answer when spoken to. Passive delirium; talks and acts like one insane; talking to imaginary people who have long been dead. Talks nonsense and foolish things; talks coherently, but about impossible things. Answers questions correctly and goes off into muttering. Wants to go out of the window. Thinks her husband, long dead, is in the next room, and grieves because they will not let her go to him; her living son she calls by the name of one long dead. Mutters foolish things and sees dead people. She wanders all night in her room without sleep. She seems to see and converse with dead friends, with her dead son and her dead husband; wants to get dinner for her dead husband. She

imagines her husband will starve if she does not find him. Many delusions
about dead people; sees dead people and corpses; she sees dogs and images
nights. Horrible visions; sees disagreeable persons when half awake. Illusions
of fancy; she hears voices and answers the voices of the dead. Discontent and
despair; discouraged about her disease and thinks it proving an incurable
disease. Dullness of mind; imaginary fears and vexations after mental exertion
Emotional and easily moved to laughter or tears; exaltation of fancy. Exertion
of mind aggravates all mental and many physical symptoms. Great fear at night,
fear of brain lesion with headache in the morning; fear about family matters
also about financial matters; fear or dread of work or any exertion. Complains
from fear. He is so forgetful that he cannot recall the sentence just spoken
Easily frightened, all the time in a hurry. Many hysterical manifestations, and
at night his ideas are abundant, but in daytime deficient. Many of the mental
symptoms and his appearance are like one approaching imbecility. He is very
impatient with everything and everybody. "Utterly ambitionless," no desire for
physical or mental work and aversion to exercise. Irresolution. Marked irritability
in the morning and evening, after coition, from consolation, during headache
about trifles. Lamenting and wailing. Lascivious. Loathing of life. Memory
very weak. Mistakes in speaking; misplaces words. Changeable mood, morose
generally better when occupied; during the proving mild and yielding. Extreme
prostration of mind; restless and anxious during the night; sadness in the
morning and during the day; sadness during heat. *Mental depression* without
cause. Dullness of the senses; very sensitive to noise and to mild rebuke from
a friend. The mental symptoms are worse from sexual excesses. Shrieking during
sleep. Easily startled. Starting during sleep. Stupefaction and disposition to
suicide; indisposed to talk or to he talked to, and inclined to sit in silence
Timid and bashful. She is unconscious and her conduct is automatic; weary of
life. Weeping at night, in sleep; almost impossible to keep from, bursting into
sobs from imaginary fears and worries; sits and weeps by the hour; the will is
almost lost; great aversion to mental work.

Vertigo, morning on rising, after rising, in evening, tendency to fall
backward during headache. *Vertigo,* looking upwards, while lying, from mental
exertion, with nausea, on rising from stooping, while sitting, on stooping
while walking in the open air.

Coldness of the head, especially of occiput, and on vertex; congestion of
the head at night, and when coughing; constriction of the forehead; eruption
on the scalp; crusts, eczema, pustules; the head inclines to fall forward
marked sensation of fulness in the head. There is bristling of the hair; the hair
falls out. Heat in the whole head, worse in forehead, in the evening. Heaviness in
the head in the morning; heaviness in forehead. *Hydrocephalus* Itching scalp
itching occiput. Sensation as if the brain was in motion.

The head pains are severe and in all parts of the head. Worse *morning,* but felt also afternoon and evening, lasting all night; worse *from cold air* and a DRAFT; ascending steps; binding up the hair, in women; after coition; becoming cold, from taking cold; from cold, damp weather; wtih coryza; after eating; also worse from becoming overheated, and during heat with hammering; *worse from a jar; from light;* must lie down; worse before and during menses; *from mental exertion,* worse from moving about the room, from moving the head, *from noise.* The pain comes in paroxysms. It cures periodical headaches that come every day or only once each week; pulsating headaches. Pain is worse *after sleep,* from stimulants, stooping and stepping heavily, and from taking cold. Headache from *eye strain.* Head pains from touch, walking, wine, writing. The pains extend to occiput and nape of the neck. Aching deep in the brain, with pulsation on motion. Hard pain in forehead in the morning; steady dull heavy pain, better after eating and occupation; worse from mental exertion, *motion.* and waking and writing; better from perfect rest. Headache morning on waking; worse lying, worse rising from bed, better by occupation, better standing and walking. Severe headache in the forehead; pain over the eyes, pulsating; worse walking, worse from motion, better from lying, heat and pressure. Hard pain in occiput, and sides of the head, worse in right side. Severe pain in temples and vertex; burning pain in head; bursting pain in head, mostly in vertex; cutting in head; drawing pain in forehead and occiput; dull pain in wohle head in the morning. Jerking with the pain like a jerking pain. Pressing pains in forehead; *occiput,* sides of occiput, *temples* and *vertex.* Pressing-out pain in forehead. Shooting pains in whole head. Shooting in occiput. Scalp is sore to touch and while brain is sensitive to motion and jar, as if bruised. Stitching pains in forehead, occiput, sides of head and temples. The pain is so violent that *he feels stunned;* tearing in the forehead and frontal eminence, *occiput* and temples. Perspiration of the whole scalp; perspiration of *forehead.* Pulsating in forehead and whole head. Shaking or undulating sensation in brain. Twitching of muscles of head.

The eyelids are agglutinated with pus. It has cured *cataract.* Discharges from the eye of thick, greenish-yellow mucus and pus. Heaviness of the lids. Inflammation of the conjunctiva with thick discharges, also of lids. Injected, dark veins. Itching of the eyes. Lachrymation in open air, lachrymation of right eye with coryza. It has cured opacity of the cornea. Very severe pain in the eyes, worse from light, before and during a storm, with redness., The pains are burning, cutting, pressing, as though sand in the eyes; sore, bruised, stitching, and *tearing. Paralysis* of the optic nerve; *photobhobia;* pulsation in the eyes and the pupils are contracted; marked redness in eyes, especially inner canthi, of lids, of veins; spots on the cornea; swollen lids; twitching of the lids. It has cured ulceration of the cornea. The eyes look weak.

Colors before the eyes, spots, floating spots, dark colors. Dazzling. Cannot see to read with the usual glasses. He thought he was going blind. Hypermetropia. Exertion of vision causes headaches and many nervous symptoms; flickering and foggy visions before the eyes; dimness of vision; sparks before the eyes.

From the ear there is an offensive, *purulent, thick,* yellow and greenish-yellow discharge; watery, offensive discharge; bloody, watery discharge. Flapping in the ears. The ears are hot. Itching deep in ears. Noises in ears. cracking in ears when chewing. Fluttering in ears. Humming, ringing, roaring and whizzing in ears; violent drawing, jerking, stitching, tearing pain in ears. There is pulsation with and without pain; swelling inside with stopped feeling increased wax in ears; twitching in the ears. Hearing first acute, later *impaired.*

It causes vicious catarrh of nose and posterior *nares,* extending to fronta sinuses in tubercular constitutions, chronic coryza with cough; *coryza* with discharges fluent in open air, but patient feels better himself. It has cured many cases of hay fever. Copious discharges in morning after rising; albuminous and shiny in the daytime. Crusts blown out of nose. Hard crusts, excoriating, greenish *offensive, purulent, thick* and *yellow* or *yellowish-green;* copious, bloody, thin or watery discharges. Extreme dryness inside of nose. Epistaxis, bright red blood on blowing nose; itching inside of nose; obstruction at night and in morning or rising. It is a most useful remedy in *ozoena.* Much pain high up in nose, in roo of nose; soreness inside of nose; stitching pains in nose; polypus in nose has been cured by this remedy. Sense of smell at first acute, later diminished and finally lost. Sneezing, ulceration in nose; swelling of the nose.

The face is very pale, an earthy color; lips bluish and cracked; red face during headache; circumscribed red cheeks; dryness of the lips. Eruptions o the face, cheeks, chin, forehead, lips, on the nose, and around the mouth *Acne,* boils, comedones, *eczema,* herpes, pimples; scurfy eruptions on the face; the face is hot and red. Inflammation and suppuration of the parotic gland. Pain in face from cold, better by *warmth.* The pains of the face are boring, drawing, stitching and tearing. Perspiration of the face and scalp Swelling of glands; swelling of the parotid and *submaxillary* glands.

Mucous membranes of mouth covered with aphthæ and the gums bleed the tongue is coated white; the mouth is very dry, but at times copiou mucus; offensive, even putrid odor from the mouth. The tongue is very sore saliva is copious and speech is difficult. Swollen gums and tongue; ba taste, alkaline, bitter in the morning, metallic, putrid, sour. Taste is sometime wanting. Ulceration of mucous membrane, lower lip, on left side; stinging smarting, splinter-like pain, spreading, painful to pressure, lardacious inflamed edges; small ulcer appeared on right side. The teeth become loose and feel as though too long; caries of the teeth. Pain in the teeth at night. Th teeth are very sore when masticating; pain worse from cold air, from anything cold in the mouth; while eating, after sleep, better from external warmth and warm things in the mouth. The pains are boring, digging, drawing, *jerking, piercing, pressing, stitching* and tearing.

Inflammation of the throat, pharynx and tonsils with dryness and redness; constant effort to clear the throat, worse in the morning. Tenacious mucus in the throat; lump in the throat. Much pain in the throat on becoming cold, on coughing, on swallowing. Some pain and burning; splinter-like pain on swallowing. Stitching pain on swallowing; swallowing is difficult. Tonsils and uvula swollen; ulceration in the throat. Pain and swelling in cervical glands. Induration in the glands of the neck. It has cured goitre.

A feeling of anxiety in the stomach. The appetite is at first increased, then ravenous, and finally wanting, with aversion to food, especially to meat and milk. Some provers desire sour things and milk. Sensation of coldness in the stomach; sensation of emptiness not relieved by eating; sinking sensation in the pit of the stomach; eructations in the morning, after eating; bitter, empty, tasting like food eaten; *sour. Waterbrash, Heartburn.* Hiccough. Fulness in stomach after eating; loathing of food. Nausea in the *morning,* afternoon, evening, night; while eating, after eating, better after empty eructations, during headache, while walking. Pain in stomach, evening and night; after cold drinks, on coughing, after eating, while walking in the open air. The pains are burning, cramping, *cutting, pressing, bruised* and stitching; pressing pains in evening after eating, like a weight. Pulsation in the stomach; sensation of a stone in the stomach; marked sensation of tension. Thirst afternoon and *night; burning thirst; extreme thirst.* Vomiting morning and night; on coughing after drinking, after eating, during headache, after milk; vomiting bile, bitter substance, black *blood, food,* mucus, watery substances.

Distension of the abdomen after eating; dropsy of the abdomen, enlarged liver. Flatulence with much rumbling and fulness. The abdomen is very hard, the liver is hard. Inflammation of the peritoneum. Sensation of movements in the abdomen from flatus. Pain morning and *night;* pain before menses; pain in right hypochondrium; pain in liver and in the inguinal region. The pains are burning, *cramping,* cutting, *pressing,* stitching, tearing, twisting, stitching pain in sides of abdomen and in liver. Marked tension in abdomen; tympanitic abdomen.

Extreme constipation, with inactivity of the rectum; *difficult* stool, paralyzed feeling in rectum; constriction of anus; constipation, with dry stool, *hard, knotty, large* and soft, *light colored,* with much straining. Diarrhœa painless, with stool copious, lienteric, *offensive,* even putrid, sour, pasty, thin and watery. Dysentery; with bloody, scanty stools. Copious, offensive flatus. It has cured fistula in anus. Itching and crawling of anus. Hemorrhoids protrude during stool, sore to touch, worse when walking. Bleeding from rectum and anus with stool; itching after stool. Moisture about the anus, pain during and after stool, burning during and after stool. Pains are pressing, stitching and *tearing* marked soreness of anus. Paralyzed feeling in rectum. Stricture of the rectum not allowing feces to pass larger than a pencil, was cured. Tenesmus. Much urging to stool, urging during stool; ineffectual urging.

Tenesmus of bladder and retention of urine, pressing pain in the bladder catarrh of the bladder with much mucus in the urine; urging to urinate a night, worse moving about, better lying. Sudden urging, ineffectual urging Frequent urination during the night; involuntary urination during night i sleep; unsatisfactory urination. The urine is scanty.

The prostate gland is enlarged and tender; emission of prostatic fluid when straining to pass stool.

Urethral discharge purulent, greenish, yellow; cutting and burning urination. It has cured stricture of the urethra. The urine is copious, late scanty, red, cloudy, burning, containing mucus, with sediment purulent and sandy. It has cured diabetes mellitus.

Erection at night without thought or dreams; eruptions on the genitals o the male, on the prepuce. It has cured hydrocele and induration of testes. Marked redness of glans penis; itching of glans penis and scrotum; stitching pain in penis. Foul sweat on the male genitals. Sweat on the scrotum. *Seminal emissions* Sexual passion increased, sexual desire strong without erections. Swollen testes

In the female the desire is increased; eruptions on the vulva with much itching. Heaviness of the uterus and prolapsus. Leucorrhœa excoriating bloody, copious, before and after menses, milky, white or purulent and yellow or yellowish-green. Menstrual flow acrid, bright red, copious, too soon protracted or scanty; menstrual flow absent or suppressed, painful and irregular. Flow of blood between the menstrual periods; pain in the uterus aching, burning, labor-like and tearing; soreness in the genitals; ulceration of labia, vagina and os uteri.

Chronic irritation of the air passages, larynx and trachea; catarrh of th larynx and trachea, with copious yellowish-green mucus; rawness in laryn and trachea; phthisis of the larynx. He constantly scrapes the larynx. Ticklin in the larynx and trachea. Respiration fast, *asthmatic,* deep; difficult durin cough and when lying, rattling, short, sighing and suffocative.

It is one of our greatest cough remedies in phthisical subjects. The coug comes at *night,* but also morning after rising, and in evening in bed. Coug from cold air, from cold damp air, asthmatic, from cold drinks. It has a dr cough at night, with much expectoration in the morning; cough during fever hacking, hoarse cough; cough from irritation of larynx and trachea; hoars cough, especially in the morning; paroxysmal, spasmodic cough in the evenin racking the whole body. Cough worse lying, talking; virulent cough afte waking in the morning. Expectoration in the *morning, bloody, greenish-yellow, copious,* offensive, *purulent,* thick, viscid—sometimes white. It has cured abscesses of lungs and axilla. It has restrained cancerous ulceration of mammæ. It has cured desperate cases of catarrh of the bronchial tubes, constriction of chest, eruption of chest and excoriation of the nipples. Hemorrhage of the lungs. Chronic inflammation of bronchial tubes and lungs. Oppression of the chest. The milk is suppressed or absent. Pain in both lungs. Pain in chest during cough, on inspiration, on deep breathing. Pain in the sides of chest. The pains in the chest are burning, *pressing,* soreness, stitching and rawness in chest. Stitching pains on inspiring, in sides of chest, and in the mammary glands. Palpitation of the heart *at night,* after eating, from *exertion,* and even from slight motion. Perspiration all over the chest. *Phthisical conditions.* Extreme weakness of chest.

The back feels cold and there is a sensation of coldness in back of neck and sacrum. Eruption in the cervical region, pimples and pustules. Itching of the back. *Much pain in the back,* especially *at night.* Pain in back *during menses,* on motion, rising from sitting and while sitting. Pain in the cervical region, capula and in the spine between the scapulæ; pain in lumbar region when *ising from a seat;* pain in coccyx. Hard aching in the back, in lumbar region when rising from a seat, and in the sacrum. Drawing pain in the lumbar region, pressing pain in the lumbar region. The spine is sore to touch in many places. Stitching pains in the cervical region, scapulæ, lumbar region and sacrum. Tearing pains in the cervical region. Perspiration on the back, worse on the back of the neck. *Stiffness of the back, especially of the cervical region; stiff neck.* Tension in the cervical region. *Weakness of the back.* Weakness of the lumbar region.

It is a remedy for gouty nodosites of the fingers, awkwardness of the limbs, caries of the bone, chapped hands; chronic jerking of muscles; coldness of all the limbs, hands, palms, lower limbs, LEGS, FEET, *evening and night.* Contractions of tendons of hands and fingers. Many corns, painful, *sore* and *stinging. Cracked hands* and *fingers.* Cramps in hands, lower limbs, *calves, feet, soles, toes.* Eruptions, vesicles, boils on the upper limbs, vesicles on the upper limbs and fingers; eruptions on lower limbs, itching, pimples. Boils on the thighs; felons on the fingers. Heat of hands, palms, of the feet. Heaviness of all the limbs, especially of *legs and feet.* It has been of great service in hip joint disease; inflammation of all the joints. Intense itching of all the limbs, thighs and legs. The nails have ceased to grow for two years; the nails are hard and brittle. Numbness of all the limbs; upper limbs numb when lying on them; numbness of *hands* and *fingers;* numbness of lower limbs, legs and feet when sitting. Rheumatic and gouty pains in limbs, *joints* and *bones,* evening and night. Pain in upper limbs at night, worse from cold, motion and taking hold of anything; pain in shoulders, upper arm, elbow, forearm, fingers and finger joints; pain in the lower limbs, pain in the sciatic nerve; violent pains in the hip joint; pain in the hip joint as if an abscess were forming; pain in thigh, knee calf, foot and toes. Aching in all the limbs, with stiffness in cold, damp weather aching in the shoulder, worse from motion. Burning feet and soles. Drawing pain in upper arm, forearm, wrist and hand; drawing pain in the knee and leg Sore, bruised pains in upper limbs and thighs. Sensation as if sprained in wris and ankle. Stitching pains in the *joints.* Stitching pains in the shoulders, uppe arm, elbow, wrist and fingers. Stitching pains in hips, knees, calf, ankle, foot sole, heel, toes, especially the *great toe.* Tearing pain in shoulder, upper arm elbow, forearm, wrist, hand, fingers and finger-joints; tearing pain in thighs knee, *leg,* calf, *foot,* soles, toes, and especially the great toe.

Sensation of paralysis in upper limbs and in the hands; paralysis in lowe limbs. Cold sweat on all the limbs; cold sweat of *palms,* of hands; cold swea of *feet; offensive cold sweat of feet.* Stiffness of all the limbs, *joints, hands* and *fingers;* stiffness of lower limbs, knees. Swelling of hands, *knees,* legs, *ankles* feet. Tingling of the fingers; trembling of the upper limbs, of the hands, of the lower limbs; twitching of the upper limbs, thighs and legs. Ulceration of *lowe limbs, legs.* Varicose veins. Warts on the hands; on the dorsum of the thumb on the ball of the thumb; large, hard seed warts. Weakness of all the limbs and especially the *joints.* Weakness of thighs, *knees, legs,* calves and feet.

Dreams of anger, *anxious,* of business, confused, amorous, of the dead of death, of disease, fantastic, fire, *frightful, horrible,* murder, nightmare vivid, vexatious, visionary; dreams of sick people and caring for sick peo ple; a hideous old woman's face appeared in her dreams. Sleep is restless sleepiness in the morning, forenoon and *evening, after* dinner, *after eating* sleeplessness *before midnight;* sleeplessness with sleepiness; sleepless from much thinking; after once waking cannot sleep again; unrefreshing sleep Waking early and frequent. Yawning.

Chill in morning, forenoon and evening, in the open air, in the cold air even in bed, after eating, external and internal, shaking chill; chill with trembling from uncovering, warm room does not relieve, desires warmth, but it does no relieve; chilliness during stool. Fever forenoon and afternoon, but marke fever in *evening and night;* fever alternating with chill; dry heat at night i bed; external heat with chilliness; flushes of heat. It is useful in hectic fevers Mild fever *evening* and night. Heat with moist skin. Perspiration in the mornin and latter part of the night; perspiration with great anxiety. Cold sweat mostl on the extremities; sweat from coughing, during and after eating, from exertior from mental exertion; sweat from motion, from walking. *Profuse* hot swea Sweat of single parts; sweat during and after sleep; offensive, sour swea uncovering while sweating brings on many symptoms. If the perspiratio becomes suppressed from uncovering, or from a draft, he suffers much.

Burning of the skin after scratching; the skin is cold to touch; the skin of hands and fingers cracked; the skin is discolored; bluish, liver spots, pale, red, red spots, *white spots,* yellow Dry, burning skin and inability to perspire. Eruptions are biting, *burning, itching,* painful, *phagedenic,* stinging. Boils and chapping and desquamating. *Eczema* and herpes. *Dry, itching, crusting,* stinging herpes, eruptions discharge a white, pus-like substance. There are pimples, *pustules,* and red rashes; eruptions *scabby* and *scaly* after scratching. Suppurating eruptions, nodular urticaria after scratching. *Vesicles* in many places. Erysipelas with swelling, worse from scratching. Excrescences form upon the skin; formication and goose-flesh. Indurations. Intertrigo. Itching with and without eruptions, itching, biting, burning, crawling and stinging, worse after scratching. The itching is ameliorated by radiated heat. It has cured lupus. The skin becomes moist after scratching. The skin is very sensitive, sore feeling, and sore, raw places on the skin; sticking and stinging after scratching. Ulceration of the skin and ulcers bluish, burning, cancerous, *crusty, deep, corrosive,* offensive with yellow pus, *fistulous, foul, indolent, indurated,* stinging, and *unhealthy.* Warts painful, *hard,* inflamed, stinging, suppurating and withered. It has cured wens and other cystic growths.

CALCAREA SULPHURICA

Many years ago Schuessler introduced this remedy, and it has been used extensively upon the bio-chemic theory. Many excellent cures have been made in this way that most of us are able to recognize as homœopathic cures, though it is a sort of crude homœopathy. By studying these cures many symptoms may be obtained not supposed to be of importance by these reporters. These symptoms often furnish a basis for further consideration or further clinical observation. Many fragmentary provings have also been made, furnishing many of the symptoms recorded in this article. The author frequently made use of Schuessler's 12th potency, later the 30th and 200th; at present much higher potencies. From all of these many valuable symptoms have been obtained. Some of these symptoms have come out upon the sick while under the influence of this remedy, and have been since confirmed, so that the following symptoms must now furnish the best basis that we have to prescribe on. The best consideration that this remedy has ever received will be found in Boericke and Dewey's Materia Medica of the Tissue Remedies.

The tendency to the formation of abscesses in the body in any place is a strong feature of this remedy, and is quite similar to *Pyrogen.* An abscess that has ruptured and is slow to heal with a continuous discharge of yellow pus, is a strong indication for this remedy. The patient desires the open air; is sensitive to drafts: takes cold easily. It is very useful in the management of malignant growths after ulceration has set in. It is under such circumstances an excellent palliative. It is a deep acting constitutional remedy, an anti-psoric, and if given early enough will prevent a malignant growth terminating in its usual way. It is useful in the affections of bone, caries of bone. While the patient is cold in general, he often requires to be uncovered because of particular conditions. For instance, in croup and in headaches he feels the heat too much, but the pains of the body are often relieved by heat. He is sensitive to both cold and heat. After becoming cold, complaints come on. Tendency to take cold in drafts, or on slight occasions. He is sensitive to cold, wet weather. It cures the underlying basis of epilepsy, epileptiform and hysteric convulsions. The patient is aggravated from exertion. His muscles are flabby; he is disposed to hæmorrhages. When well selected remedies act only a short time, and the symptoms agree, this remedy is one that should be thought of along with *Sulphur, Psorinum* and *Tuberculinum.* Complaints from straining muscles and tendons, from overlifting, etc. Lame back from such causes. Throughout the chest and head, and sometimes extending into the limbs, there is a violent orgasm of blood, flushes of heat and pulsations. Onanism and sexual excesses reduce the economy to a state whereby they feel their constitutional disturbance, and this is one of the remedies that elevate the body to a better state of order in such conditions. Pain in the bones day and night. Pulsating all over the body. Standing aggravates many complaints, but especially the joints. Swollen and indurated glands. Twitching of the muscles all over the body. Many of the symptoms are aggravated on waking. Many symptoms are aggravated walking and especially walking fast and becoming heated. Aggravation from being over-heated. Wants to uncover. Aggravation from the warmth of the bed. A warm room aggravates. Warm wraps aggravate. Great bodily weakness. Thick yellow discharges from the mucous membranes. Thick bloody discharges. Purulent exudations in serous sacs. Bloody pus from abscesses, ulcers and mucous membranes. Prolonged suppuration. Wants to keep still.

Now, it will be found that the above general symptoms prevail throughout the particulars in many instances, and it will appear that the bodily state is more or less penetrated with these symptoms.

The patient is absent minded; irritable; easily angered. He becomes weak after anger and vexation. Aversion to answering questions. He is easily made anxious, especially in the evening in bed, during the night and when lying. Anxiety with fear during fever. Anxiety about the future. Anxious about his heart and his health in general. His anxiety is ameliorated in the open air. He has anxiety about his salvation. He has anxiety in the morning on waking. Many changeable moods and capriciousness. Aversion to company. Confusion of mind in the morning on waking and again in the evening. This is also ameliorated in the open air. Confusion of mind from mental exertion. Contrary and contradictory moods. He has many little delusions, whims and strange fancies. Frightful images in the night when trying to sleep. Has visions. Great despair of recovery during heat. Craves stimulants to overcome his tremulous weakness. He is discontented at all times. Great sluggishness of mind. Continuously in a state of apprehension. Fear of death. Fear that some evil will befall him. Fear of insanity and fear of misfortune, and this comes on at night. Forgetful. Full of hatred of people who do not agree with him. Always in a hurry. Hysterical. Impatient. Feeble minded, even to imbecility. Indifferent as to his surroundings. Irresolution. Extreme irritability in the evening. Irritable after coition. Lamenting because he is not duly appreciated. Loathing of life. Malicious. This remedy is especially useful in broken-down constitutions from drunkenness. Weakness of mind, of memory and of body. Some of the mental states that are aggravated in the morning with sadness, on waking become mirthful in the evening, even to hilarity. He stumbles in speaking and misplaces words. Changeable moods. Morose. Obstinate. Easily offended or insulted. Prostration of mind. Quarrelsome. Restlessness. Mental depression in the morning, with mirthfulness in the evening. Sadness during perspiration. Dullness of the senses. Sits and meditates over imaginary misfortune. Does not want to be talked to. Easily startled. Stupefaction. Suspicion. Suspicious. Indisposed to talk. Tormenting, persistent thought. While busily engaged thinking, his thoughts vanish. Becomes timid, bashful and apprehensive, and in his conversation is extremely wearisome. Weeping during perspiration. An aversion to mental and physical work. Real indolence.

Vertigo is a common feature with this patient. In the morning on getting up, or again in the evening; but this is ameliorated in the open air. Vertigo with nausea. Vertigo with a tendency to fall. Epileptic vertigo. Vertigo on moving the head quickly, on stooping and on walking fast. Coldness of the head, especially of the vertex. Hyperæmia of the brain, aggravated in the evening and at night. Aggravated after stimulants; especially on coughing; during menses; with suppressed menses, and in a warm room. Ameliorated in the open air. The head feels constricted, especially the forehead and occiput. Much dandruff forms upon the scalp. Eruptions upon the scalp with thick yellow crusts. Eczema, also pimples. Coldness in the head, especially forehead. Formication of the scalp. The hair falls out. Heat of the head morning and evening. Flushes of heat. Heat in the forehead and in the vertex. Heaviness in the forehead and occiput. Itching, burning of the scalp. Many inveterate chronic headaches and periodical headaches have been cured with this remedy. Headaches in the morning on waking. Headache coming on in the afternoon, lasting through the evening and at night, ameliorated in the open air. Catarrhal headaches. Pain in the head on coughing, after eating or disordering the stomach. Headache from becoming heated, and the pain is aggravated from jarring. Compels him to lie down. Aggravated looking upwards. Headaches in women before and during menses. The headaches are aggravated from mental exertion, from moving the head, from motion, from noise. Periodical sick headaches with nausea and vomiting. Pressure ameliorates. Pulsating with nearly all the headaches. Reading aggravates. Rising from lying causes pulsating and increases the pain. Shaking the head aggravates. He wakes up out of sleep with the headache. The headache is aggravated from spirituous liquors, from standing, from stooping, from the heat of the sun, from talking, from walking, from washing. Aggravated in cold weather. The headache comes on from becoming cold, and yet the headache when on is ameliorated in the cool air. Many of the headaches are in the forehead in the morning on waking, or come on in the evening after dinner. These are aggravated on stooping and walking. Severe pain above the eyes. It has occipital headaches; pain in the vertex and sides of the head. Many of these headaches are pressing and are aggravated from mental exertion. Stitching pains on coughing. Stitching pains in the forehead and temples. Tearing pain throughout the head. Tearing pain around the head, ameliorated from lying. Pulsation in the head and temples. Sensation as if he had his hat on at 4 P.M.

There are numerous eye symptoms, catarrhal and psoric. The lids stick together in the morning. This remedy has partly cured several cases of cataract. It has produced and cured double vision. Chronic inflammation of the eyes, with thick yellow pus. Ulceration of the cornea. Itching and burning, aggravated in the morning. Pressing pain in the eyes in the evening. Soreness to touch. Photophobia. Redness of the eyes, like raw beef. Redness of the canthi. Fissures of the canthi. Twitching of the lids. Dim, often foggy, vision. Flickering before the eyes.

Discharge from the ears, offensive and purulent. Cases dating back to scarlet fever, with thick and bloody pus. soreness and enlargement of the right parotid. Eruptions behind the ear. Itching in the ear and behind the ear. Buzzing, humming, ringing, roaring and singing, in the ear. Aching pain in the ear. Stitching, pulsating, stopped sensation. It cures catarrh of the Eustachian tube when the symptoms agree. Swollen parotid gland and swelling behind the ear.

Most inveterate catarrh of the nose has been cured by this remedy. Coryza, with discharge, ameliorated in the open air. Dry coryza. The discharge from the nose is bloody, excoriating, offensive, purulent, thick, yellow and greenish yellow. Clinically it has cured the one-sided cases best. Crusts form in the nose. Crusts form upon the margins of the nose. A sensation of great dryness in the nose. Epistaxis in the morning. Offensive odors from the nose. Itching in the nose and of the end of the nose. Obstruction of the nose, so that it is impossible for him to breathe through it. Keeps the mouth open. Caries of the bones of the nose. Loss of smell. Sneezing, ameliorated in the open air. Swelling of the nose.

Cracked lips and flushes of heat of the face. Pale, sickly, face. Many eruptions upon the face, boils, eczema, herpes; itching; pimples; pustules; scurfy eruptions; vesicles. Itching of the face. Pain in the face from becoming cold. Cutting pain. Cold sweat on the face. Swelling of the glands. Swollen submaxillary.

Dryness of the mouth and tongue. Hot mouth. Inflammation of the mucous membranes of the mouth. Inflammation of the tongue, with swelling. Much mucus in the mouth in the morning. Offensive odor in the mouth. Rawness and burning inside of the lips. Burning of the tongue. Flow of saliva from the mouth. The speech is difficult on account of the stiffness and swelling of the tongue. Swelling of the mucous membranes of the mouth. Gums swollen. Taste bad, bitter, metallic, sour, sweetish. Ulceration of the mouth, tongue and throat. Vesicles in the mouth. Thick yellow coating at the base of the tongue.

Choking is a characteristic of this remedy as it is of *Hepar.* Redness and swelling of the throat. Dryness and inflammation of the mucous membranes of the throat and of the tonsils. A sensation of a plug in the throat. Mucus in the throat. Mucus drawn from the posterior nares, thick and yellow. Pain in the throat on swallowing. Pressing pain. Rawness in the throat. Soreness of the throat. Stitching pains in the throat. Scraping mucus from the throat. Swallowing is difficult. Swelling of the tonsils, with suppuration. Ulcers in the throat. The external throat is swollen; the glands are enlarged and painful.

Increased appetite. Ravenous appetite. Or, appetite entirely wanting. Aversion to coffee, to meat and to milk. Desires fruit, cold drinks, acids, salt things; sweets. Thirst extreme. Distension after eating.

Emptiness in the stomach. Eructations after eating. Empty eructations. Eructations acrid, bitter, foul, sour. Eructations of food. Waterbrash. Fullness of the stomach after eating. Heartburn. Heaviness in the stomach, as of a load. Subject to indigestion on the slightest provocation. Nausea in the evening. Nausea with headache and with vertigo. Pain in the stomach in the evening. Pain in the stomach after eating. Burning pain, cramping, cutting, gnawing, pressing, after eating. Tenderness to pressure. Stitching pains. Throbbing in the stomach. Sensation of a stone in the stomach. Vomiting at night after eating, with headache. Bile, bitter, blood, food, mucus; sour vomiting.

In the abdomen there is great coldness, with distension, after eating Fullness after eating. Heaviness. Many of the pains in the abdomen are like colic and come on at night. Burning pain. Cramping, cutting, dragging, drawing. Soreness. Stitching. There is pain in the liver. pressing, soreness, stitching. There is pulsating, rumbling and distension of the abdomen.

Inveterate constipation. Difficult stool. Insufficient stool. Fistula in ano. Painless abscesses of the anus. Like *Sulphur,* it has cured morning diarrhœa. but has also an evening diarrhœa, and is very useful for diarrhœa in children. Aggravated after eating ever so little. It has a painless diarrhœa. In the rectum there is formication and intense itching. Hæmorrhage from the rectum and anus. External piles. Inactivity of the rectum. Involuntary stool. Moisture about anus, causing smarting and itching. Pain during and after stool. Burning pain during stool. Pressing, stitching and soreness in the anus. Tenesmus at stool. Prolapsus of the rectum. Ineffectual urging to stool. The stool is bloody, dry, hard, knotting, large; lienteric, soft, white, yellow and purulent.

This is a valuable remedy for catarrh of the bladder, with copious yellow pus. It has cured chronic inflammation of the kidney. It is a valuable remedy in urethral discharges, when the discharge is yellow, bloody, and often gleety. Burning in the urethra during urination. It is an excellent remedy for impotency, when other symptoms agree. In women who have had several abortions, when the symptoms agree. Excoriation of the labia. Inflammation of the labia, with suppuration. Itching of the genitals from leucorrhœa. Thick, yellow, bloody leucorrhœa. Itching of the labiæ during menses. Itching after menses. Itching high up in the vagina. The leucorrhœa is excoriating, bloody, burning, copious, thick and yellow. Leucorrhœa before and after menses. Absent menses. The menstrual flow is copious, dark, too frequent or too late. Irregular. Sometimes pale, protracted, scanty, suppressed. Delayed first menses in girls. Hæmorrhage from the uterus. Pain in the uterus during menses. Dragging down in the pelvis during menses, as if there were prolapsus. Burning in the genitals. Prolapsus of the uterus. Swelling of the labia. Fibroid tumors of the uterus. Ulceration of the genitals and os uteri.

Catarrh of the larynx and trachea. Dryness and inflammation. Copious expectoration of mucus, which is yellow and sometimes bloody. Rawness and soreness. Patients threatening to go into phthisis. Much scraping of the larynx. Obstinate hoarseness. It has now long been a valued croup remedy. Croupy cough, where there is much choking, when an experienced practitioner might well think of *Hepar*—but it will be remembered that in *Hepar,* uncovering a hand or throwing off the covers from the chest will increase the croupy tendency and aggravate the croupy cough, and that the patient in *Hepar* is very sensitive to a draft and to the air. In this patient uncovering is grateful. The patient throws off the covers and wants the air and seems to breathe better and croups less. It may seem strange that such a great difference should come between the sulphide and the sulphate of lime.

Respiration is difficult in the evening and night; aggravated on ascending, lying and walking. The respiration is rattling, is short. There is suffocation, and even wheezing. This is an excellent asthmatic remedy, when, the symptoms agree.

The cough is aggravated in the evening and night. Ameliorated in the cool air—unlike *Hepar.* Asthmatic cough, croupy in morning on waking and after siesta. Dry cough at night. Hacking cough. Hoarse cough. Loose, rattling cough. The cough racks the whole body. Short dry cough. Spasmodic cough and cough coming in paroxysms. The expectoration is copious in the morning. The expectoration is bloody, greenish, purulent, thick, viscid and yellow.

Abscess in the axilla. Anxiety in the region of the heart. Catarrh of the trachea and bronchial tubes. Hæmorrhage from the lungs. Badly treated pneumonia or results of pneumonia. Hepatization of the lungs. Oppression of the chest. Rawness in the chest. Soreness in the chest on coughing, or inspiration. Burning pain in the chest. Cutting in the chest. Palpitation at night; anxious; aggravated ascending, in persons going into phthisis. Suppuration in the chest. Weakness in the chest. Itching, burning of the external chest. Sensation of coldness in the back. This has been a valuable remedy in the treatment of curvature of the spine in the lumbar region, making it difficult for him to sit up.

The symptoms of the extremities make a gouty constitution. Gouty joints. Awkward, clumsy fingers, from gouty finger joints. Coldness of the extremities, of the hands, legs and feet. Cramps in the calves. Eruptions, pimples and vesicles. Heat of the hands. Heaviness of the lower limbs. This remedy has been of great service in many cases of hip joint disease. Itching of the skin of the extremities. Often itching and burning. Burning of hands and feet; burning palms and soles. Numbness of hands and also of the lower limbs and of the feet. Pain in the extremities during chill; rheumatic pain. Pain in the joints, gouty and rheumatic. Pain in upper limbs at night. Pain in the shoulder, elbow, wrist and fingers. Pain in the lower limbs; sciatica; rheumatic pains. Pains in the hip, thigh and knee. Burning pains in the feet. Pains in the lower limbs; drawing, stitching and tearing. Paralysis of the limbs, upper and lower. Perspiration of the hands and feet. The perspiration of the feet is cold and offensive. Stiffness of the arms. Stretching out the lower limbs aggravates the pain. Rheumatic swelling of the knees and legs. Œdematous swelling of the feet and legs. Tingling in the fingers, as if asleep. Trembling of the hands and of the lower limbs. Ulcers on the legs. Burning, itching scales. Varicose veins, Weakness of the upper limbs. Weakness of the lower limbs, knees, legs and ankles.

Sleep restless. Dreams anxious and frightful. Sleepiness in the evening. Sleepless before midnight and after 3 A.M. Sleepless from thoughts. This remedy has cured many cases of chronic intermittent fever with evening chill. Chill beginning in the feet. Shaking chill. Fever evening and night. Evening fever intermingled with chilliness followed by fever, but no sweat follows fever, with pain in lower limbs, better by walking. Flushes of heat. Hectic fever. Perspiration at night. Cold. Slight exertion brings on the perspiration. The perspiration is profuse and sour.

There are numerous skin symptoms, as might be expected from a study of *Sulphur* and *Calcarea.* Burning and itching. Desquamation. Cracked skin. The skin is cracked after washing in winter, especially of the hands, like we find in salt rheum. Liver spots; pale skin and yellow skin, even to marked cases of jaundice. Dryness of the skin. The eruptions are boils, burning moist or dry eczema, herpetic pustules, scabby scaly vesicles. Itching, burning eruptions. This remedy cures psoriasis when the symptoms agree. Rash. Suppurating eruptions. Tubercles. Urticaria. Excoriation and intertrigo. Formication. Itching in bed; itching, burning; itching, crawling. Itching, ameliorated by scratching. Sensitive skin. Ulceration of the skin. Wounds heal slowly. Unhealthy skin. Ulcers bleed, burn; are scaly, crusty and deep.

Ulcers discharge bloody pus, offensive, thick, yellow. Fistulous ulcers. Foul indolent ulcers. Indurated ulcers. Pulsating ulcers. Painful ulcers. Warts.

CALENDULA

The proving of Calendula is so nearly worthless that we cannot expect at present to use it as a guide to the internal administration of the remedy. There are only a few things that I have ever been able to get out of it. In injuries Calendula cannot be ignored, in cuts with laceration, surface or open injuries. Dilute Calendula used locally will keep the wound odorless, will reduce the amount of pus, and favor granulation in the very best possible manner, and thus it assists the surgeon in healing up surface wounds. Calendula is all the dressing you will need for open wounds and severe lacerations. It takes away the local pain and suffering. You may easily see we are not now dealing with a condition that exists because of a state within the economy, but because of something that is without. There is nothing that will cause these external injuries to heal so beautifully as the Marigold. Some will say it is not homœopathic, but these are the individuals who "strain at a gnat and swallow a camel". If there are constitutional symptoms suspend all medicated dressing entirely and pay your whole attention to the constitutional symptoms. Sometimes there are no constitutional symptoms to prescribe on, but when they are present resort locally to cleanliness and nothing else. Do not suppress symptoms that you will need to guide you to a remedy.

onCAMPHOR

CAMPHOR

The camphor bottle is a great mischief in the house as camphor antidotes most of our remedies. Camphor in potentized form will cure many complaints. It is suitable in some acute complaints attended with nervous excitement, even to frenzy, with spasms and convulsions and finally exhaustion. The Camphor state is one of convulsions or coldness. In the most acute period of the Camphor excitement, the excitability and frenzy of the patient are extreme, or he goes into the other extreme, in which the irritability is lost and there is loss of sensation, unconsciousness and coldness. The two extremes may be seen in one patient, one earlier and the other later. He may go from the extreme of mental excitement and violence to one of prostration and exhaustion, in which the body is blue and cold and yet must be uncovered. In the mental state there is anxiety and extreme fear; fear of persons, of strange spheres, of the dark, the dark is filled with imaginary spectres; he dare not get out of bed in the dark; everything that moves is a spectre and the inanimate things of the room become alive and terrify him. Frenzy. Coupled with this, there is kidney and urinary trouble, like that of *Cantharis,* and because of this similarity, the two remedies are both complementary and antidotal to each other. If a woman has poisoned herself with *Cantharis,* and there is present the frenzy and excitement, Camphor will act as an antidote.

The details of the mental symptoms are worthy of much consideration. The patient goes into a state not unlike imbecility, and the appearance is as if it had come on slowly. The mind and memory are gone. He closes the eyes, seemingly asleep, and answers no questions. Delirious with the heat, rage and mania, wants to jump out of bed or out of the window. Screams and calls for help. Tosses anxiously in bed. Anxiety and almost loss of consciousness. These symptoms will indicate Camphor in puerperal fever, in congestion of the brain, or in shock from violent inflammation of organs. Confusion comes from the shock and comes with violence. The more violently the patient suffers, the sooner he is cold, and when he is cold, he must uncover even in a cold room. This is somewhat like *Secale.* In *Secale* the patient, when cold, wants to uncover and to be in a cold room, and it also has frenzy, and so there is nothing in what we have yet seen to distinguish *Secale* from Camph. But there is another thing that runs through Camph., by which a distinction can be made. The coldness, frenzy and heat very often intermingle. When the Camphor patient is becoming cold, he has spells of heat which come over him; flashes of *heat* intermingle with rending, tearing, burning pains, either in the inflamed organ or along the nerves. The patient is a most troublesome patient to nurse; nobody and nothing suits. If an inflammation of the bladder

comes on, there is intense pain and tenderness, and from the shock of the
suffering the mind is in a state of frenzy. Coldness then comes on and the
patient wants to be uncovered, wants cold air, wants the windows open, but
before all this can be done, a flash of heat comes on and then he wants the
covers on, and the register turned on, and wants a hot iron and hot bottles;
but this stage now passes off, and while the nurse is bringing the hot irons
he wants her to open the windows and have everything cool. You will see at
once that these are serious cases. This occurs with opisthotonos,
convulsions, inflammation of the brain, liver, kidney, bladder, coming on from
violent shock and cold with great exhaustion. You will see this in one who
has worked for hours for his life, and when the excitement is over reaction
sets in and it is like a whirlwind; he has worked until he is exhausted and now
he is prostrated, cold and blue; here is the sphere where the old woman with
her Camphor bottle has established a reputation, but potentized camphor will
do more for him than the Camphor bottle, it will put him into a refreshing
sleep.

It is useful in the climacteric period with flushes of heat and sweat in a
warm room; the limbs and abdomen are very cold and she suffers from cold
when uncovered and sweats copiously when covered. She cannot endure
covering to warm her limbs though she suffers from cold.

The head is full of pain; throbbing pain. Contractive feeling as if laced
together in the cerebellum. The whole back of the head and neck throb like
hammers; worse from bending head forward; burning and stinging. Frontal
headaches.

We have heard about Camphor in cholera, which is a disease that brings
the patient down quickly. The face is cold, blue and shrivelled, without much
sweat, in the cases that would make one think of Camphor. There is not much
discharge from the bowels, not much vomiting and not much sweat; but
suddenly he becomes cold, blue and collapsed, as it were paralyzed and goes
into a stupor.

Convulsions with frothing at the mouth. Blue lips, lock-jaw, tetanus. Cold
sweat on the face with vomiting. Erysipelatous appearance of face.

There is a desire to drink without thirst. There is also insatiable thirst; he
is not satisfied with incredible quantities of cold water. Cannot get it cold
enough, and cannot get enough, but he soon vomits it up.

The gastric irritation is marked. Everything is vomited. The tongue is blue
and cold and the breath is cold. Everything coming out of the body is cold.
The air as it leaves the chest feels like that from a cellar, like *Carbov.* and
Verat. The tongue is cold and trembling. Such states are found in cholera. All
through the cold stage there is burning. The inside of the body seems to

burn, or there is a sense of internal smarting like a rawness or a sense of burning without heat.

The pain in the stomach in gastritis is so violent that the anguish on the face is equal to that in *Arsenic;* a deathly anguish is felt in his stomach and he feels that he must die. Burning, rending, tearing pain in the stomach with retching and vomiting. Cramps in stomach and bowels and spreading to other parts of the body until there are convulsions and opisthotonos. Anguish at the pit of the stomach drives him to despair. Heat in the stomach. Cold feeling in the stomach. Abdomen is full of colic and burning. Cold feeling in the abdomen.

Cholera stools; rice water discharges, with anxiety, restlessness, spasms of the muscles, cramps of the chest, prostration, increasing coldness and blueness; wants to be uncovered and he is going into collapse. The old Camphor, *Cuprum* and *Veratrum* still hold together for Asiatic cholera. In Camphor there is prostration, blueness, coldness and yet he wants to be uncovered and the body is cold and dry.

The other two remedies have all there is in cholera, but in *Cuprum* there is not so much coldness, more cramping, more convulsive tendency and not so much prostration. The more cramping there is the more it is *Cuprum.* The more copious the discharge from the bowels and the more profuse the vomiting and sweat, the more we would think of *Veratrum.* Cold and dry—Camphor. Cold and copious discharge—*Veratrum.*

After taking cold there is cutting, with involuntary discharge of dark brown fæces like coffee grounds. Tenesmus. At times the cholera patient, with the coldness and blueness, is retching and straining to vomit and suffering with horrible tenesmus to get rid of a little stool and has convulsions here and there. These bowel symptoms gradually increase until there is no ability to strain at stool, a paralytic condition. The rectum seems contracted and painful.

There is suffering in the urinary and sexual organs. Burning urination. Strangury. Frequent urination. Frequent desire, with difficulty. The same state arises in the bladder as in the rectum, and there is retention with horrible torture. The patient sits on the commode and strains to pass the urine, but there is a paralytic condition of the bladder. The urine is red, bloody, and comes by drops like *Canth.* Tenesmus of the neck of the bladder.

Camphor increases the sexual erethism to an unbearable degree. In some cases from large doses this is seen in the extreme, and in other cases the reverse takes place. It has both sexual erethism and impotency in its provings. I once knew a French woman who had an insane desire to keep her boys always at home with her, and she thought she could accomplish this if she could only keep them away from the girls; and to destroy their sexual desire she kept a bag of camphor under their pillows. All of them were made impotent. But in some provers it establishes sexual erethism. It has this like *Canth.*

Camphor produces a coryza, with a profuse discharge from the nose and from the air passages, from the nose to the bronchi. Bronchitis of children and old people. Old withered up people take cold at every exposure to weather and become cold and chilly. *Ant. crud., Am. carb.* and Camph. are wonderful remedies in octogenarians. Every cold seems threatening. Old people don't come down with cold the same as young people; they are prostrated, sinking, have rattling in the chest and the family think it is the death rattle and that it is grandpa's last spell. These three remedies fit the case, they are like the advanced stage of pneumonia. *Ant. t., Ant. c., Am.c,* and Camph. cover these cases in which the hot stage is omitted. Camph. has very little heat; it has the sensation of heat; but not a marked hot stage. There are other symptoms in this medicine such as you will find in old people.

Jerking of the muscles, trembling and jerking. Spasmodic conditions with trembling. Trembling of the tongue.

The general *constitutional* state of a Camphor patient is coldness and extreme sensitiveness to cold. In acute inflammatory conditions he is cold and wants the covers off. In acute complaints there is violent thirst, in chronic complaints thirstlessness. It is the same in *Arsenic,* in the acute thirsty, but in the chronic thirstless.

In Camphor an important thing to recall in the acute is that during the heat and when the pains are on he wants to be covered up. The coldness is relieved by cold, he wants more cold.

CANNABIS INDICA

A strange ecstatic sensation pervades the body and senses. The limbs and parts seem enlarged A thrill of beatitude passes over the limbs. The limbs tremble. Great weakness spreads over the body. The symptoms resemble catalepsy. Anæsthesia and loss of muscular sense. Complaints ameliorated by rest. Exaltation of spirits with mirthfulness. Wonderful imaginations and hallucinations. Wonderful exaggerations of time and space. He seems to be transported through space. He seems to have two existences, or to be conscious of two states, or to exist in two spheres. Delusions. Incoherent speech. Laughs at serious remarks. Laughs and weeps. Spasmodic laughter. Jesting. Moaning and weeping. Fear of death; of insanity; of the dark. Anguish and sadness. Mental symptoms ameliorated by walking in the open air. An opposite phase prevails with his weakness. He loses his sense and falls. Passes from the rational to the irrational in rapid succession, back and forth. Forgets words and ideas. Unable to finish his sentences. Thoughts crowding upon each other in such confusion prevent rational speech. His mind is full of unfinished ideas, and phantoms. Wonderful theories constantly form in -the mind. Loquacity He cannot control the mind to reason rationally upon any subject. Any effort to reason is interrupted by flights of wild imagination and theory. Vision upon vision passes before the perception. Hears voices, bells, music, in ecstatic confusion.

Feels as if the calvarium were opening and shutting, or being lifted and lowered into place. Pulsating pain through the head. Weight in occiput, with pulsation. Shocks in the brain on regaining consciousness, and on waking from sleep. Stitching pains in temples. Tension of scalp. Tenderness of scalp. Dimness of vision. Visual clairvoyance. Letters run together. Hearing acute. Singing and buzzing in ears; pulsating. Face pale and sunken. Insane look. Stupid look. Sickly, expressionless look. Grinding teeth during sleep. Stammering. Metallic taste. Desire for, and dread of water.

Flatulence, distending abdomen, ameliorated by eructations.

The urinary symptoms are numerous. Inflammation in the kidneys, with burning pain. Soreness in the kidneys, and dull aching. Stitching pains in the kidneys. Constant or frequent urination. Urine burns on passing. Burning, stinging in urethra, before, during and after urination. This remedy has cured many cases of gonorrhœa. It is useful in the first stage, and cures the symptoms set for *Cannabis. sativa.* Must wait for urine to start. Urine dribbles after urination. Much mucus in the urine. It is useful in chordee during gonorrhœa. The discharge in gonorrhœa is yellow.

Sexual desire increased in both sexes. Erections mechanical and painful. Menstruation profuse and fluid; painful; paroxysmal pains, like labor pains. Uterine spasms. Threatened abortion, threatened with gonorrhœa. Menses come every two weeks.

Spasmodic oppression of the chest with suffocation.

Palpitation during sleep. Pressing pain in the heart with suffocation during the whole night. Stitching pains in the heart. Pulse, slow or rapid and irregular; fluttering; a nervous pulse.

Pain in the back at the menstrual period. Pain across the dorsal region preventing walking erect.

Paralytic weakness of the limbs with trembling and thrilling. Numbness of limbs and soles. Pricking of soles. Rest ameliorates, and motion aggravates. Violent pains through the lower limbs on walking.

Sleepy, but cannot sleep. Starting of limbs during sleep. Dreams of dead bodies. Dreams prophetic. Nightmare.

Prickling of the skin. Formication and itching all over. The skin feels drawn tight over the body. Anæsthesia.

CANNABIS SATIVA

The resemblance of this remedy to *Cannabis Indica* is remarkable and has led to a belief that they are identical. The one has often been substituted for the other, and has cured symptoms produced by the other. Their mental and urinary symptoms are very similar. The sensation of opening and shutting has been cured by both remedies.

Things seem strange and unreal. He seems as though in a dream. Confusion as to his personal identity. Makes mistakes in writing and speaking, and misunderstands what he reads and hears said. Sounds in the room seem to come from a distance. When he speaks it seems as though some one else were speaking (*Alum*). Seems as though her senses would vanish. Despondent in forenoon, lively in the afternoon. Fear of going to bed. Hysterical feeling in the throat. Anxiety in the stomach. Confusion of mind and vertigo.

Rush of blood to the head, as though it came from the stomach. Opening and shutting of the vertex, begins on waking, lasts all day, and is worse from noise. Sensation of drops of cold water on scalp. Formication.

Inflammation of the conjunctiva and varicose veins. Sensation of sand in the eyes.

Noises in the ears.

Sensation of enlargement of the nose. Epistaxis. Pressure on the root of the nose. Dryness in the nose. One check red, the other pale. Nasty taste. Difficult speech. Dry mouth and throat. Aversion to meat. Eructations, bitter, sour, empty.

Inflammation of the kidneys. Ulcerative pains in the kidneys. Œdema of the prepuce with gonorrhœa. Thick yellow gonorrhœal discharge. Burning in the urethra during and after urination. Stitching in the urethra while the urine flows. Urethra sensitive, swollen. Chordee. Burning at starting and closing of urination. Stitching in urethra when not urinating. Most difficult and painful urination. Pain that extends from meatus back along the urethra while urine flows. Pressing out feeling at the orifice of the urethra after urination in a woman. Violent urging to urinate. Constant or frequent urging to urinate. Involuntary urination. Violent pain at the close of urination. Bloody urine.

Spasmodic closure of the neck of the bladder at the close of urination. Inflammation of the urethra. Inflammation and much swelling of the orifice of the urethra with burning pain during urination in the female.

Intense sexual excitement in both sexes. Much dropsical swelling of the prepuce. To the female it has a reputation for sterility. Menses profuse. Leucorrhœa in little girls (*Sepia*). Gonorrhœa. Uterine hæmorrhage after labor. Threatened abortion.

Catarrh of the chest. Bronchitis with wheezing. Asthma; must have window open. Green viscid expectoration. Salty sputum. Cough, with blood spitting. Stitching pains in the pleura. Asthma with bladder troubles. Palpitation.

Pressure as with a sharp point in the coccyx. Drawing pains in tendo-Achillis. Stitching in the skin all over while perspiring. Numbness of finger tips.

CANTHARIS

The most important feature of this medicine is the inflammatory condition, and the most important characteristic in the inflammation is the rapidity with which it develops into a gangrenous state. Inflammatory conditions usually follow a definite course for days, but when this medicine is put upon a part or taken internally the inflammatory state terminates in death of the part with great rapidity. When taken internally it proceeds almost immediately to attack the urinary tract and establish a uræmic state which brings about the mental symptoms; the local inflammatory condition comes on with great rapidity, and this brings the patient down violently sick in a great hurry. From strong doses in the poisonous effect we get startling and alarming symptoms; the whole economy is in disorder; grievous symptoms commonly of the urinary tract. The parts become gangrenous at an early stage.

The mental symptoms are striking. Among those that are guiding are *sudden* loss of consciousness with red face. Suddenly goes into stupor. Confusion of mind. Overwhelmed with strange ideas. Thoughts run riot, and go whatever way they will, as if possessed by outside influence.

Head hot, frenzy, delirium, with *great excitement and rage,* paroxysms renewed by dazzling or bright objects, by touching the larynx or by trying to drink water as in rabies. Fear and confusion of ideas. The mind often runs towards subjects that the inflamed parts would suggest. The bladder and

genitals are inflamed and the excitement and congestion of the parts often
arouse the sexual instinct, so that there are sexual thoughts and sexual frenzy.
Violent amorous frenzy, an excitement such as accompanies inflammation
attended with thoughts that correspond. The sexual instinct has gone mad.
The erections in the male are painful and violent. The penis is inflamed and
sore and it would be painful to have coitus, yet there is this frenzy. Insolence.
Blasphemy. Restlessness ending in rage. Restlessness causing him to move
constantly, a rage and delirium intermingled with amorous frenzy. This kind
of mental conduct in Cantharis is similar to what will take place in *Hyos.*,
Phos., and *Secale*, a violent delirious state intermingled with sexual ideas
and talk. In some instances he deliriously sings lewd songs and prattles on
the subject of human genitals, urine and fæces, a wild raving on subjects not
talked about in health except among the depraved. But in disease, chaste and
modest persons, virgins, will speak so that it is surprising where they have
picked up such language. In such cases it is well to exclude everybody from
the room except the nurse and doctor. I have seen a dear old mother weep and
wring her hands and say: "Where did my daughter learn such language?"
The daughter is not to blame. It is simply a condition of the urinary tract or
the menstrual function, brought on from cold or exposure, or through the
mother's neglect to tell her daughter what she should know in regard to her
menstrual function, and how there is inflammation of the ovaries or uterus, or
outside parts, and the urine burns and causes an inflammatory condition of
the outer parts, or the urine is retained and there is frenzy. Such is Cantharis.

Violent, bursting, lancinating headaches as if stabbed with a knife; an
inflammatory condition that takes hold of the mind violently.

Running all through the remedy there is *burning*. In the head burning,
throbbing and stabbing. Unconsciousness and delirium in the mental state.
Burning in the side of the head. Stitches in the side of the head and occiput.
Lancinating pains deep in the brain. Hair falls out.

It is seldom indicated in eye troubles alone, except such as come with
head and mind symptoms. Erysipelas of the face with large blisters. Burning
in the eyes and the whole atmosphere *looks yellow*. Burning and smarting in
the eyes. Erysipelas of the eyes, with gangrenous tendency. Eyes hot,
scalding tears. Erysipelas of the face, dorsum of the nose, involving the lids.
Rhus is more commonly used in this condition, but when it is violent, Canth.
will often be indicated and preferable to *Rhus*. *Rhus* has the blisters and the
burning, but in Canth. between your two visits the erysipelas has grown
black, it is dusky, a rapid change has taken place, and it looks as if gangrene
would set in. Burning in the erysipelatous area and the skin around burns
from the touch. In *Rhus* this is not so. In Cantharis the little blisters even if
touched burn like fire. *Eruptions burn when touched*, ever so lightly, *i.e.*,

those eruptions such as the remedy could produce.

This patient enters into a state of prostration, is pallid, has hippocratic countenance and dies. It corresponds to the lowest forms of disease, even gangrene and violent inflammation of the bowels, bladder, brain, spine and lungs; sinking and hippocratic countenance. Inflammation of the lungs, gangrenous type, prostration and the lung that is affected burns like fire, and immediately he expectorates cadaverous smelling expectoration, thin; bloody, watery; it has come on in an astonishingly rapid manner, and in a little while he will die; the nose is contracted, there is the hippocratic countenance, and the urine is suppressed. I remember one patient who had just come out of a prolonged drunk. I left the patient in the evening in just such a state as I have described. He was drooling a bloody saliva from his mouth and he was dying. He had had this condition come on in one night from being nearly frozen in a drunk. It would be Cantharis or death before morning, but by morning he was expectorating a rusty sputum and went on to a good recovery. *Arsenic* has the burning in the lungs and he spits up black sputum, pneumonia signs are present, with the restlessness and anxiety, and other symptoms of *Arsenic,* and *Arsenic* will stop it at once. These violent remedies are needed in those cases that will die.

Burning in the throat. Great thirst, with burning in the throat and stomach. Thirst, with aversion to all fluids, that is, the craving of the mouth and throat are antagonized by the mental state. Thirst in the throat and an aversion to water in the mind. Violent burning in the stomach, pylorus, abdomen. The abdomen is swollen and tympanitic; lancinating pains cutting and stabbing. Wherever there is a rapid inflammation in the bowels there is diarrhœa of bloody mucus or serum, watery, bloody fluids from the bowels and stomach. The same watery bloody fluid from the eyes. And wherever this watery fluid comes in contact with the skin it burns and excoriates. Bloody urine.

Desire for stool while urinating. The patient will sit on the commode with violent tenesmus to pass urine and stool, feels that if he could only pass a few more drops of urine or a little more bloody stool he would get relief, but no relief comes. All the parts are inflamed and on fire. Tenesmus and urging not only when the bladder is empty, but often when the bladder is full. Retention of urine. Passes none or only a drop or two. Violent tenesmus of the bladder: Cutting pains with tenesmus. Lancinating, stabbing like knives, in neck of bladder. Pains shoot off in different directions. Violent pains with frequent urging. Constant tenesmus. An anxious state and frenzy come on; most violent suffering and he has urging to pass urine and stool with sexual erethism tantalizing in the extreme. The whole urinary organs and genitalia are in a state of inflammation and gangrene. Burning when urinating. This bloody urine burns like fire in the bladder and about the genitals. Retention or suppression of urine. It is rare that one suffering from gonorrhœa has this violent inflammation, with burning and tenesmus of the bladder and rectum, but in such a case this remedy is indicated. The intensity and rapidity are the features of this remedy. It brings on pain and excitement found in no other remedy. Next to it comes *Merc. cor.*

In the female there is oversensitiveness of all parts. Inflammation of the ovaries and uterus. Burning in the vagina. Membranous dysmenorrhœa. Menses too early, profuse, black.

Puerperal convulsions. Retained placenta. Burning pains. When there have been no expulsive pains present to expel the afterbirth, with the symptoms running all through this remedy, after it has been given, normal contractions of the uterus have come on with expulsion of the membranes.

Violent lancinating pains through the kidneys and back. Pains in the loins, kidneys and abdomen. Pain on urinating, so that he moaned and screamed on passing a drop.

CAPSICUM

Most of the substances that are used on the table as seasoning in foods will in the course of a generation or two be very useful medicines, because people poison themselves with these substances, tea, coffee, pepper, and these poisonous effects in the parents cause in the children a predisposition to disease, which is similar to the disease produced by these substances.

In the fat, flabby red-faced, children of beer drinkers and pepper eaters, with poor reaction, a relaxed and flabby constitution, red face and varicose condition, those that have been overstimulated, children of overstimulated men, we find the sphere of Capsicum very often. In those constitutions in which the face looks rosy, but it is cold or not warm, and upon close examination the face is seen to be studded with a fine system of capillaries. Plump and round, with no endurance, a false plethora like *Cal.* The end of the nose is red, the cheeks are red, redness over the cheeks, red eyes, easily relaxed individuals. These constitutions react slowly after diseases and do not respond to remedies, a sluggish state, a tired, lazy constitution. In school girls who cannot study or work, who get home-sick and want to go home. In gouty constitutions, with cracking of the joints and gouty deposits in the joints, stiff joints, clumsy, weak, give out soon. There is sluggishness of the whole economy. They are chilly patients, are sensitive to air, and want to be in a warm room. Even in the ordinary weather the open air causes chilliness. They are sensitive to cold and to bathing.

In the mental state there is a no more striking thing than this symptom —*homesickness.* A sickness like homesickness runs through the remedy and is accompanied by red cheeks and sleeplessness, hot feeling in the fauces, fearfulness. They are oversensitive to impressions, are always looking for an offence or slight; always suspicious and looking for an insult. Obstinate to the extreme; it is a devilishness. Even if she wants a certain thing she will oppose it if it is proposed by some one else. After emotions red cheeks, yet with the red cheeks lack of heat, even with increased temperature; or one cheek pale and the other red, or the cheeks alternately red and pale. Children are clumsy and awkward.

The Capsicum mind is almost overwhelmed by persistent thoughts of suicide. He does not want to kill himself, he resists the thoughts and yet they persist, and he is tormented by these thoughts. There are persistent thoughts in many remedies, and it is necessary to distinguish between impulses and desires. If he desires to have a rope or a knife to commit suicide, that is altogether different from an impulse to commit suicide. An impulse is sometimes overwhelming and overbalances the mind, and he commits suicide. You should always find out from a patient whether he loathes life and wants to die, or if he has impulses which he wishes to put aside. Some persons lie awake at night and long for death, and there is no reason for it. That is a state of the will, insanity of the will. In another patient the thoughts jump into his mind and he cannot put them aside, and the thoughts are tormenting. The distinguishing feature of the remedy is often found by differentiating between the two. Desires are of the will; impulses come into the thoughts.

Headaches as if the skull would split when moving the head, when walking or coughing. Feeling as if the head would fly to pieces; holds the head with the hand. Feeling as if the head were large, aggravated by coughing and stepping, ameliorated by lying with the head high. Bursting pain and throbbing. Headache with pulsation in the forehead and temples. Headache as if the brain would be pressed through the forehead. On stooping, feeling as if the brain would be pressed out, as if the red eyes would be pressed out on stooping.

The senses are disturbed and are overacute; oversensitiveness to noise, smells, taste and touch, to impressions, to insults. The patient is excited.

Pains in the ears; itching pain; aching, pressing pain with cough, as if an abscess would burst. It has a peculiar action on the bones of the internal ear and mastoid process. Abscesses round about and below the ear and caries; petrous portion of temporal bone necrosed. It has been a frequently indicated remedy in mastoid abscess,

Old catarrhs. The patient takes cold in the nose and throat and this is followed by a collection of mucus. Very often in stupid patients it is difficult to get symptoms, and you must depend on what you see, the character of the discharge and a few other things, and you will find that some of these cases will be cured and all the other symptoms will go away; but in some of these old catarrhs no reaction seems to come after the most carefully chosen remedies, and all at once the doctor observes that the patient has a red face and it is cold and the end of the nose is red and cold, and the patient is fat and flabby and yet has not much endurance, never could learn at school, and if she exerts breaks out into a sweat and freezes in the cold air. He has a key to the patient and examines the patient by the key, that is, by the drug, a bad practice and never to be resorted to except as a *dernier resort* and in stupid patients. When he gives Capsicum to that patient it arouses her, it may not cure; but after it the *Silicea* or *Kali bich.* or other remedy which was perhaps given before and did not act takes hold and cures.

In the text it says, "Nose red and hot." The skin all over is red and burning, a capillary congestion. The cheeks are red and hot, and this alternates with paleness. Red dots on the face. Pains in the face like bone pains, from external touch. Pains are worse from touch. Pain in the zygoma, or the zygoma is sensitive. Sensitive to pressure over the mastoid. Swelling in the region of the mastoid.

Taste foul like putrid water. When coughing the air from the lungs causes a pungent offensive taste in the mouth. *A hot pungent air comes up from the throat,* tasting foul when coughing.

On the tongue and lips, flat; sensitive, spreading ulcers with lardaceous base. The mucous membrane of the lips and various parts of the body if pinched up with the fingers remain in the raised position, showing a sluggish circulation. This is the flabbiness of Capsicum. It wrinkles on pressure. It is a feeble circulation. The parts you touch are loose and flabby, red, fat and cold. That child will not react well if it has measles, until it gets Capsicum. The skin is moist and cold, and there is a fine measly condition of the skin due to capillary congestion. If the child is old enough it will complain of feeling cold. There is slow reaction after eruptive diseases, after glandular diseases, after bowel complaints. The child was fat and flabby, but now does not take on flesh.

He takes cold in the throat and nose, and the throat looks as if it would bleed, it is so red, a fine rash-like appearance—it is puffed, discolored, purple, mottled, flabby and spongy-looking; dark red. Burning soreness with ulceration in the fauces. Uvula elongated. Stitching in throat. Enlarged tonsils, inflamed, large and spongy. The throat remains sore a long time after a cold or sore throat. Burning, pressing pain in the throat, the throat dark red; relaxed sore throat; pain on swallowing, dysphagia. Throat sluggish for weeks, a do-nothing state, does not get very bad, but gets no better, a lack of reaction.

When the chill begins there is thirst. Thirst after every dysenteric stool, a sudden craving for ice-cold water, which causes chilliness. Craving for water before the chill and when taken it hastens the chill; it feels cold in the

---

stomach. He desires something warm, something stimulating, craves pungent things. This is seen in whisky drinkers; they crave pepper, and the pepper, on the other hand, turns round and craves whisky. These diffusable stimulants crave some stimulating thing, crave support. Dipsomania.

Let me give you a hint in *Arsenic.* In dipsomania the sinners who have been drinking a great many drinks in a day sometimes get to that state in which they must get up during the night for a drink or they will not be able to get up in the morning. In the morning the first three or four drinks will be thrown up, but the next one will stay down; they must take a number until one sticks. They have got to that state in which they must keep on taking it. If they sleep too long the first few drinks will come up, and so they must get up in the night or the whisky will not stay down in the morning until they have taken a number of drinks. You will see this in lawyers who do a great amount of work on stimulants. *Nux, Ars.,* and Caps. will do something for them if they will co-operate with you. I remember saying to one old toper, who had kept up altogether on champagne, that he would have to stop it. He whined, "I don't think it is worth while." If he could not get his champagne he didn't think life worth living. If these people want to get benefit they must co-operate.

Dysentery. After stool, tenesmus and thirst, and drinking causes shuddering. Smarting and burning in anus and rectum. Violent tenesmus in rectum and bladder at the same time. Hæmorrhoids; protruding, smarting, burning; smarting like pepper; they sting and burn as if pepper had been sprinkled on them. Tenesmus of the bladder; strangury. Burning, biting pain after urination. In old cases of gonorrhœa in which there is no reaction. *The discharge is creamy.* You take a picture of his face, you notice the plethora, but also that he has no endurance, plump, flabby, sensitive to cold, red face. He does not react after cold. He has the last drop or a creamy discharge with burning on urination. Capsicum will sometimes stop it suddenly. Coldness of scrotum. Prepuce swollen, œdematous. Pain in the prostate gland after gonorrhœa.

Coldness of the affected part. Coldness in patches. Coldness of the whole body.

It is useful in perplexing and troublesome chronic hoarseness. He has had a cold and remedies for the acute condition have been given, perhaps two or three remedies, *Acon., Bry., Hep., Phos.,* but all at once you wake up to the fact of his chronic constitutional state of hoarseness. He is rotund, chilly, red faced, and the hoarseness disappears under Capsicum. It is the same with the cough. After making several blunders you wake up and see it is a Capsicum case and that you have never yet gotten at the root of the trouble. This shows the importance of getting at the things general first. If there is much acute suffering of course you must give an acute remedy, but if the patient has delayed recovery and convalescence is slow the next remedy should be the remedy for the patient. Sometimes it is *Sulph., Phos., Lyc.,* and sometimes it is Caps. If the patient has a good constitutional state he will get over the cold on the acute remedy, but the old gouty, rheumatic, flabby patients need a constitutional remedy.

Cough in sudden paroxysms, convulsing the whole body. Cries after the cough from the headache. Stitches in the suffering part with the cough. Every cough jars the affected joint. The constitutional state comes first and the particulars must agree *i.e.,* prescribe according to the totality.

CARBO ANIMALIS

Carbo animalis is one of the deep-acting, long-acting medicines. Suitable in complaints that come on insidiously, that develop slowly, that become chronic and often malignant in character. Complaints in anæmic, broken down constitutions. Vascular conditions. The *Carbons* affect the veins more or less, relaxing, paralyzing. This one has its own peculiar feature of infiltrating little veins. Just as sure as an organ in the Carbo animalis patient becomes congested it becomes hard and purple from infiltration, and has a tendency to remain so. In an inflammation of a gland the veins become weak and infiltrated, the gland itself becomes hard and sore, the tissues around it indurate, and the skin over it becomes purple. The glands of the throat and axillæ grow purple and indurated with no tendency to soften. Some of these medicines, after infiltrating a gland, will hurry up the inflammatory action, produce sloughing, rapid breaking down, with pus—like *Hepar, Mercurius* and *Sulphur.* But this medicine paralyzes and infiltrates the little veins in the inflamed part, and there seems to be no tendency to suppuration.

We see that the economy of this patient is in a sluggish state; there are no rapid changes; but everything is slowed down. Even the inflammatory process is a passive one. Very often a slow quasi-erysipelatous inflammation comes on, the part becomes purple and will pit upon pressure. Just think what a contrast this is to *Belladonna. Belladonna* will inflame all the glands, they will swell, become hot and so sensitive that they can hardly be touched; at first bright red, then purple, with a tendency to resolution if let alone. But the Carbo animalis inflammation comes on slowly, its progress is slow, and there is no tendency to repair. Enlargement of veins here and there over the body, varicose veins. There is intense burning in the part inflamed, which is indurated and purple. The glands of the throat burn. Sluggish buboes in old broken down constitutions, in early stages of syphilis, inflame, become enlarged, purple, hard and burn. Lumps in the mammary glands. A purple lump the size of a hen's egg will form in the mammary gland. It does not go on to suppuration, as you would expect it to, it just stays there. It does not enlarge much, but it is hard

The woman has so much burning in the vagina that she persuades the physician to make a more careful examination than he has done. He will probably find the whole cervix inflamed, purple and somewhat enlarged. She says it burns like coals of fire.

Carbo animalis eventually produces ulceration of the tissues in various parts, especially in glands. After a while—but not early in the case—an ulcer forms, and perhaps after ulcerating for a time it comes to a stand-still; it has become a sluggish ulcer. Indurated ulcers. A bubo breaks down and forms an ulcer. All at once it stops suppurating and around about the tissues become hard and purple. The laudable discharge ceases, a bloody, ichorous discharge takes its place, and the surrounding parts burn. Now in ulcers and fistulous openings, where the walls become hard and burn, and the discharge becomes acrid, Carbo animalis is frequently the remedy.

It is not surprising that this remedy has been one of the most suitable for old, stubborn cancerous affections; for cancerous ulcers. They all burn. they are all surrounded by infiltrated, hardened, dark-colored tissue, and they all ooze an acrid inchorous fluid. It has cured these troubles in old feeble constitutions with night-sweats and much bleeding. It has relieved in incurable cases, and has apparently removed the cancerous condition for years, even though it comes back afterward and kills. This remedy is often a great palliative for the pains that occur in cancer, the indurations and the stinging, burning pains. Of course we do not want to teach, nor do we wish to have you infer, that a patient with a well-advanced cancerous affection, such as scirrhus, may be restored to perfect health and the cancerous affection removed. We may comfort that patient, and restore order at least temporarily, so that there is freedom from suffering in these malignant affections. Most patients that have cancer are really in such a state of disorder that only a temporary cessation of "hostilities" can be expected; and anyone who goes around boasting of the cancer cases he has cured ought to be regarded with suspicion. Do not dwell upon the cancer, for it is not the cancer but the patient that you are treating. It is the patient that is sick, and whenever a patient is sick enough to have a cancer his state of order is too much disturbed to be cured.

The proving of Carbo animalis presents the appearance of a broken down constitution. It brought out in the provers just such symptoms as occur in old, feeble constitutions, with poor repair and lack of reaction. Hence the medicine has been a great palliative for patients suffering frorn malignant infiltrations and indurations; suspicious indurations round about and under the bases of ulcers; suspicious indurations in glands. A gland becomes inflamed, hard and remains so. Carbo animalis stands at the head of the list of remedies that have that condition.

All through the remedy there is hypertrophy. Tissues pile up here and there into nodules; tissues pile up in glands and in organs. The economy has lost its balance, and the result is a disorderly distribution of material. Great prostration, want of energy, associated with palpitation, anxiety and disorders of the pulse. Weak pulse, rapid pulse, irregular pulse. Beating in blood vessels. There is turmoil in the economy, sometimes described as heat. A rushing of heat as though the body was full of steam. Awful sensation through the chest and in the head, like some great earthquake taking place. These are due to abnormal conditions of the venous side of the heart. Flushes of heat; pulsations here and there. Hæmorrhages. And of course the woman is more likely to bleed than the man; hence we have menses too early, too long, too copious. Prostration with every menstrual flow. The Carbo animalis woman sinks down at every menstrual period as if she would die. Such striking weakness is not at all accounted for by the quantity of the flow. Chronic induration, with enlargement of the uterus, which gradually grows from year to year (*Aur. m. n.*). Induration of the cervix and the whole uterus. Copious flow of the leucorrhœa. Offensive uterine discharges. Ulceration of the uterus, going gradually toward the malignant state. The menses are black and offensive. Finally this poor, feeble woman. who has been plodding along for years with this condition goes into malignant ulceration of the cervix, which burns, bleeds constantly and oozes a fœtid watery flow. The burning pains in the uterus extend down to the thighs.

Whenever this patient puts the child to the breast she has a sensation of emptiness in the stomach, sinking in the pit of the stomach, and she must take the child away.

There are many uterine troubles, with burning, stinging, smarting, a yellow brown saddle over the bridge of the nose, something like the mottled yellow saddle of *Sepia*. All sorts of disordered conditions of the uterus.

Surging of blood upward to the head, rousing up in sleep, with horrible dreams. This poor mortal is suffering from troubles in the base of the brain, has tearing pains in the head, and especially of the occiput, growing increasingly sensitive to cold, increasingly chilly, increasingly waxy, until we have phthisis or cancer, with varicose veins and all the conditions that I have described.

CARBO VEGETABILIS

We will take up the study of Vegetable Charcoal—Carbo veg. It is a comparatively inert substance made medicinal and powerful, and converted into a great healing agent, by grinding it fine enough. By dividing it sufficiently, it becomes similar to the nature of sickness and cures folks. The Old School use it in tablespoonful doses to correct acidity of the stomach. But it is a great monument to Hahnemann. It is quite inert in crude form and the true healing powers are not brought out until it is sufficiently potentized. It is one of those deep-acting, long-acting antipsoric medicines. It enters deeply into the life. In its proving it develops symptoms that last a long time, and it cures conditions that are of long standing —those that come on slowly and insidioasly. It affects the vascular system especially; more particularly the venous side of the economy—the heart, and the whole venous system. Sluggishness is a good word to think of when examining the pathogenesis of Carbo veg. Sluggishness, laziness, turgescence, these are words that will come into your mind frequently, because these states occur so frequently in the symptomatology. Everything about the economy is sluggish, turgid, distended and swollen. The hands are puffed; the veins are puffed; the body feels full and turgid; the head feels full, as if full of blood. The limbs feel dull, so that the patient wants to elevate the feet to let the blood run out. The veins are lazy, relaxed and paralyzed. Vaso-motor paralysis. The veins of the body are enlarged; the extremities have varicose veins.

The whole mental state, like the physical, is slow. The mental operations are slow. Slow to think; sluggish; stupid; lazy. Cannot whip himself into activity, or rouse a desire to do anything. Wants to lie down and doze. The limbs are clumsy; they feel enlarged. The skin is dusky. The capillary circulation is engorged The face is purple. Any little stimulating food or drink will bring a flush to that dusky face. When you see people gather round a table where wine is served you can pick out the Carbo veg. patients, because their faces will be flushed; in a little while it passes off and they get purple again: Dusky—almost a dirty duskiness. The skin is lazy; sluggish.

Running through the remedy there is *burning*. Burning in the veins, burning in the capillaries, burning in the head, itching and burning of the skin. Burning in inflamed parts. Internal burning and external coldness. Coldness, with feeble circulation, with feeble heart. Icy coldness. Hands and feet cold and dry, or cold and moist. *Knees cold; nose cold;* ears cold; tongue cold. Coldness in the stomach with burning. Fainting. Covered all over with cold sweat, as in collapse. *Collapse with cold breath, cold tongue, cold face.* Looks like a cadaver. In all these conditions of coldness the patient *wants to be fanned.*

Bleeding runs all through the remedy. Oozing of blood from inflamed surfaces. Black bleeding from ulcers. Bleeding from the lungs; from the uterus; from the bladder. Vomiting of blood. Passive hæmorrhage. On account of the feeble circulation a capillary oozing will start up and continue. The remedy hardly ever has what may be called an active gushing flow, such as belongs to *Belladonna, Ipecac, Aconite, Secale,* and such remedies, where the flow

comes with violence; but it is a passive capillary oozing. The women suffer
from this kind of bleeding; a little blood oozing all the time, so that the
menstrual period is prolonged. Oozing of blood after confinement, that ought
to be stopped immediately by contractions. There are no contractions of the
blood vessels; they are relaxed. Black venous oozing. After a surgical
operation there is no contraction and retraction of the blood vessels. An
injury to the skin bleeds easily. The arteries have all been tied and closed
but the little veins do not seem to have any contractility in their walls. An
inflamed part may bleed. Feeble heart; relaxed veins.

Again, ulceration. If you have a case, such as I have described, with
relaxation of the blood vessels and feebleness of the tissues, you need not
be surprised if there is no repair, no tissue making. So, when a part is injured
it will slough. If an ulcer is once established, it will not heal. The tissues are
indolent. Hence we have indolent ulcers; bloody, ichorous, acrid, thin
discharges from ulcers. The skin ulcerates; the mucous membranes ulcerate
Ulcers in the mouth and in the throat. Ulceration everywhere because of that
relaxed and feeble condition. Poor tissue making, or none at all. "The blood
stagnates in the capillaries," is the way it reads in the text.

You can see how easy it would be for these feeble parts to develop
gangrene. Any little inflammation or congestion becomes black or purple
and sloughs easily—that is all that is necessary to make gangrene. It is a
wonderful remedy in septic conditions—blood poisoning—especially after
surgical operations and after shock. It is a useful remedy in septic conditions; in scarlet fever; in any disease which takes on a sluggish form, with
purplish and mottled appearance of the skin. In Carbo veg. the sleep is so full
of anxiety that it may be said to be awful. On going to sleep there is anxiety
suffering, jerking, twitching, and he has the horrors. Everything is horrible
Horrible visions; sees ghosts. A peculiar sluggish, death-like sleep, with
visions. The Carbo veg. patient wakens in anxiety and covered with cold
sweat. Exhaustion. Unrefreshed after sleep. And thus the whole patient
prostrated by his sleep. So anxious that he does not want to go to sleep
Anxiety in the dark. Anxiety with dyspnœa as if he would suffocate. Anxiety
so great that he cannot lie down.

In Carbo veg. indifference is a very prominent symptom. Inability to
perceive or to feel the impressions that circumstances ought to arouse. His
affections are practically blotted out, so that nothing that is told him seems
to arouse or disturb him. "Heard everything without feeling pleasantly or
unpleasantly, and without thinking about it." Horrible things do not seem to
affect him much; pleasant things do not affect him. He does not quite know
whether he loves his wife and children or not. This is a part of the
sluggishness, the inability to think or meditate, all of which is due to the

turgescence. Sluggishness of the veins. Head feels full; distended. His mind is in confusion and he cannot think. He cannot bring himself to realize whether a thing be so or not, or whether he loves his family or not, or whether he hates his enemies or not. Benumbed; stupid. There is another state—anxiety and nightly fear of ghosts; anxiety as if possessed; anxiety on closing the eyes; anxiety lying down in the evening; anxiety again on waking. He is easily frightened. Starting and twitching on going to sleep.

The headaches are mostly occipital. His whole head is turgid, full, distended. He feels as if the scalp was too tight. Everything is bound up in the head. Awful occipital headaches. Cannot move, cannot turn over, cannot lie on the side, cannot be jarred, because it seems as if the head would burst, as if something was grasping the occiput. Dull headache in the occiput. Violent pressive pain in the lower portion of the occiput. Head feels heavy. When the pain is in the occiput the head feels drawn back to the pillow, or as if it could not be lifted from the pillow. Like *Opium;* he cannot lift the head from the pillow. Painful throbbing in the head during inspiration. The Carbo veg. patient takes short breaths, quietly, keeping just as still as possible, until finally he is compelled to take a deep breath, and it comes out with a sharp moan. Headache as from contraction of the scalp. Painful stitches through the whole head when coughing; the whole head burns. Intense heat of the head; burning pain. Rush of blood to the head followed by nose-bleed. Congestion to the head with spasmodic constriction, nausea, and pressure over the eyes. A feeling as of an oncoming coryza from an overheated room. Many of these headaches come on from taking cold, from coryza, from slacking up of an old catarrh. The Carbo veg. patient suffers from chronic catarrh. He is at his best when he has a free discharge from the nose, but if he takes cold and the discharge stops congestion to the head comes. He cannot stand suppression of discharges. Headaches come on every time he takes cold; from cold damp weather; from going into a cold damp place and becoming chilled. Awful occipital headache, or headache over the eyes, or headache involving the whole head, with pounding like hammers. These states are like *Kali bichromicum, Kali iodatum* and *Sepia.* Many of these headaches are due to stopped catarrhal conditions.

The hair falls out by the handful. Eruptions come out upon the head. School girls and boys, too, who are sluggish, slow to learn, and suffer from night terrors; they will not sleep alone, or go into a dark room without someone with them. They have headaches, worse from pressure of the hat. A long time after taking off the hat they still feel the pressure. Sweat, cold sweat; particularly sweat of the head and of the forehead. The Carbo veg. patient breaks out into a copious sweat, appearing first on the fore head, and the sweat is cold. The forehead feels cold to the hand, and any wind blowing upon it will produce pain; he wants it covered up. Head sensitive to cold. If

he becomes overheated and his head perspires, and then a draft strikes tha
sweating head, his catarrh will stop at once and headaches will come on. Hi
knees and hands and feet get cold, and he sweats without relief.

The eye symptoms are troublesome, and they often occur along with th
headache. Burning pain in the eyes. The eyes become lustreless, deep-set
and the pupils do not react to light. He feels sluggish mentally, and does no
want to think. He wants to sit or lie around, for every exertion gives him
headache. Whenever this state is present the eyes show it. You know he i
sick because the bright, sparkling look has gone out of his eyes. If he coul
only get somewhere by himself and lie down—provided it was not dark—h
would be comfortable. He wants to be let alone; he is tired; his day's worl
wears him out. He comes home with a purple face, lustreless eyes, sunke
countenance, tired head and mind. Any mental exertion causes fatigue. Weigh
in the head, distress and fulness in the head, with cold extremities. The bloo
mounts upward. Hæmorrhages from the eyes; burning, itching and pressin
in the eyes. The eyes become weak from overwork or from fine work.

Carbo veg. is one of the medicines for discharges from the ears. Offen
sive, watery, ichorous, acrid and excoriating discharges, especially thos
dating back to malaria, measles or scarlet fever—particularly to scarlet feve
A sluggish condition of the venous system. The veins seem to be mos
affected in all old complaints, especially whenever a patient says of himsel
or a mother says of her child, that he has never been quite well since an
attack of malarial fever. The daughter has never been quite well since she ha
the measles, or typhoid fever, or scarlet fever. Carbo veg. is one of th
medicines to be thought of when symptoms are in confusion, and the patien
has been so much doctored that there is no congruity left in the symptom
Old ear discharges, or old headaches, when all the symptoms have bee
suppressed. It is then Carbo veg. often becomes one of the routine remedie
to bring symptoms into order and to establish a more wholesome discharg
from that ear. It brings about reaction, establishes a better circulation an
partially cures the case, after which a better remedy may be selected.

Inflammation of the parotid glands, or mumps. When mumps change thei
abode, from being chilled, and go in the girl to the mammary glands, and i
the boy to the testes, Carbo veg. is one of the medicines to restore orde
very often it will bring the trouble back to its original place, and conduct it o
through in safety. Pains in the ear. Passive, badly-smelling discharges fror
the ear. Loss of hearing. Ulceration of the internal ear. Something heav
seems to lie before the ears; they seem stopped; the hearing is diminishec
especially in those cases that date back to some old trouble.

The Carbo veg. patient is always suffering from coryza. He goes into warm room, and, thinking he is going out in a minute, he keeps his overcoat on. Pretty soon he begins to get heated up; but he thinks he will go in a minute and he does not take off his coat. A procedure like that is sure to bring on a coryza. It will commence in the nose, with watery discharge, and he will sneeze, day and night. He suffers from the heat and is chilled by the cold; every draft chills him; and a warm room makes him sweat, and thus he suffers from both. He can find no comfortable place, and he goes on sneezing and blowing his nose. Perhaps he has bleeding from the nose. At night he is purplish. The coryza extends into the throat and brings on rawness and dryness in the mouth and throat. A copious watery discharge, filling the posterior nares and the throat. Then he begins to get hoarse, and in the evening he has a hoarse voice, with rawness in the larynx and throat. Rawness in the larynx on coughing; soreness to the touch. The more he coughs the worse the rawness becomes. This condition extends into the chest. Secretion of much thin mucus, finally becoming thick yellowish-green, and bad-tasting. Such is the coryza. Now, with it there comes a stomach disturbance that is commonly associated with Carbo veg. complaints. Great distension of the abdomen with gas. With this coryza he has belching, and sour, disordered stomach. Every time he disorders his stomach he is likely to get a coryza. Every time he goes into an overheated room he is likely to get a coryza, with sneezing, chest complaints, and catarrh.

This catarrhal state in the nose is only a fair example of what may occur anywhere where there is a mucous membrane. Catarrhal conditions with a flow of watery mucus and bleeding. Carbo veg. has catarrhs of the throat, nose, eyes, chest, and vagina. Old catarrhal conditions of the bladder; catarrh of the bowels and stomach. It is pre-eminently a catarrhal remedy. The woman feels best when she has more or less of a leucorrhœa—it seems a sort of protection. These discharges that we meet every day are dried up and controlled by local treatments, by washes, and by local applications of every kind—and the patient put into the hands of the undertaker, or made a miserable wreck. If these catarrhal patients are not healed from within out, the discharges had better be allowed to go on. While these discharges exist the patient is comfortable. It is quite common for the Carbo veg. patient to be feverish with the coryza, but with many other complaints he is cold; cold limbs; cold face; cold body; cold skin; cold sweat. It is not so common for the earlier stages of the coryza, and the catarrhal conditions to have these cold symptoms. He is feverish in the evening and at night. But after he passes into the second stage, when the mucus is more copious, then come the cold knees, cold nose, cold feet, and cold sweat.

The face of Carbo veg. is a great study. In the countenance and in the expression we see much that is general. The patient shows his general state in his expression, especially in the eyes. He tells you how sick he is; he tells you the threatening points. In Carbo veg. there is great pallor and coldness, with lips pinched and nose pointed and drawn in. Lips puckered, blue, livid, sickly, deathly. Face cold, pale, and covered with sweat. As the tongue is protruded for examination it is pale and cold, and the breath is cold, yet he wants to be fanned. This is true whether it be cholera, diarrhœa, exhaustive sweats, or complaints after fevers. Sometimes, after a coryza has run its course and ended in the chest, there is great dyspnœa, copious expectoration, exhaustive sweat, great coldness—and the patient must be fanned. Cough followed by dyspnœa, exhaustion, profuse sweats, with choking and rawness—and he wants to be fanned. Cold face; pinched face. So the sufferings are expressed in the face. The pains and aches, and anxiety and sorrow are all expressed in the face. The study of the face is a delightful and profitable one. The study of the faces of remedies is very profitable. It is profitable to study the faces of healthy people that you may be able to judge their intentions from their facial expressions. A man shows his business of life in his face; he shows his method of thinking, his hatreds, his longings, and his loves. How easy it is to pick out a man who has never loved to do anything but to eat—the Epicurean face. How easy it is to pick out a man who has never loved anything but money—the miserly face. You can see the love in many of the professional faces; you can single out the student's face. These are only manifestations of the love of the life which they live. Some manifest hatred; hatred of the life in which they have been forced to live; hatred of mankind; hatred of life. In those who have been disappointed in everything they have undertaken to do we see hatred stamped upon the face. We see these things in remedies just as we see them in people. The study of the face is a most delightful one. A busy, thoughtful and observing physician has a head full of things that he can never tell—things he knows about the face. So the face expresses the remedy. In Carbo veg. the face flushes to the roots of the hair after a little wine. This is a strong characteristic. All over the body the skin will become flushed. Sometimes a flush appears in islands which grow together and become one solid flush, creeping up into the hair. So great is the action of this remedy upon the capillary circulation that sometimes a tablespoonful of wine is sufficient to cause this flushing of the skin.

The old books talk about "scorbutic gums;" now we call it Rigg's disease—a separation of the gums from the teeth. Bleeding of the gums; sensitiveness of the gums. Separation of the gums from the teeth. The teeth get loose. We hear about "the teeth rattling in his mouth." The *Carbons* produce just such a state, a settling away and absorbing of the gums. They get spongy and bleed easily, and hence looseness of the teeth with bleeding of the gums.

which are very sensitive. Teeth decay rapidly. Bleeding of the gums when cleaning the teeth. Teeth and gum affections from abuse of *Mercury*. Teeth feel too long and are sore. Drawing and tearing in the teeth. Tearing in the teeth from hot, cold or salt food; pain from both heat and cold. This is in keeping with the general venous condition of the whole system.

Sensitiveness of the tongue. Inflammation of the tongue. In certain low forms of fever, like typhus and typhoid fevers, the gums turn black—that is, they throw out a blackish, bloody, offensive, putrid exudate. If disturbed or touched they bleed; and the tongue piles up that blackish exudate—that oozing of black blood from the veins. This is present in putrid forms of fevers like the typhoid—in zymotic states. This remedy is rich in those zymotic symptoms, such as are described in common speech as "blood poisoning." Carbo veg. is a sheet-anchor in low types of typhoid; in scarlet fever where a typhoid condition is coming upon the case, and in the last stages of collapse; in cholera, and in yellow fever at the time of collapse, where there is coldness, cold sweat, great prostration, dyspnœa—wants to be fanned. Great prostration with cold tongue.

The mouth and throat are filled with little purple aphthous ulcers, which were little white spots to begin with, but they have grown purplish and now ooze black blood. These aphthous patches bleed easily, burn and sting. Blisters form. Smarting, dryness of the mouth with bleeding aphthous ulcers. These are common features of Carbo veg. in any of the mouth and throat conditions. Tough mucus in the throat; bloody mucus in the throat. These little ulcers run together, spread, and become one solid mass. A large surface will become ulcerated, denuded of its mucous membrane, and then it will bleed. Little black spots come upon it. Food cannot be swallowed because the throat is so sore. Generally the throat feels puffed.

The Carbo veg. patient has a longing for coffee, acids, sweet and salt things. Aversion to the most digestible things and the best of food. For instance, aversion to meat, and to milk which causes flatulence. Now, if I were going to manufacture a Carbo veg. constitution I would commence with his stomach. If I wanted to produce these varicose veins and the weak venous side of the heart, this fulness and congestion, and flatulence, this disordered stomach and bowels, and head and mind troubles—sluggishness of the economy—I would begin and stuff him. I would feed him with fats, with sweets, puddings, pies and sauce, and all such undigestible trash, and give him plenty of wine—then I would have the Carbo veg. patient. Do we ever have any such people to treat? Just as soon as they tell their story, you will know enough about their lives to know that they are mince pie fiends; they have lived on it for years, and now they come saying, "Oh, doctor, my stomach; just my stomach; if you will simply fix up my stomach." But what are you going to do with him? He has made himself into a Carbo veg. patient for you and it may be quite a while before you can bring him down to a sensible diet Now he must begin at the foot of the ladder. I only brought this up to shov how a Carbo veg. patient is produced and what kind of a stomach he has, ane what he has been living on. He has burning in the stomach, distension of th stomach, constant eructations, flatulence, passing offensive flatus. In realit) he is in a fœtid condition, a putrid condition. His sweat is offensive. He ha heartburn; eructations; the stomach regurgitates the food that he takes.

Carbo veg. has much vomiting at the end of the chill. Vomiting and diarrhœa Vomiting and blood; with the vomiting of blood the body is icy cold; breatl cold. The pulse is thready and intermittent. Fainting; hippocratic face; oozin of thick black blood. Vomiting of sour, bloody, bilious masses.

There is an accumulation of flatus in the stomach, so that the stomacl feels distended. All food taken into the stomach seems to turn into flatus; h is always belching, and is slightly relieved for a while by belching. Carb veg. has cramps in the bowels and stomach; burning pain; anxiety; distension All these symptoms are ameliorated by belching, or passing flatus Amelioration from belching seems quite a natural event; but when we stud China, you will see that the patient appears to be aggravated from belching The idea is that the patient gets relief from belching, from eructation, bu under Lycopodium and China it seems that no relief comes. They belc copiously and yet seem just as full of wind as ever, and sometimes even seen to be worse. The Carbo veg. patient experiences a decided relief fron eructation. This is a particular symptom, but it becomes almost general, an sometimes quite general. Headaches are relieved by belching; rheumatic pain are relieved by belching; sufferings and distensions of various kinds ar relieved by eructations.

This abdominal fulness aggravates all the complaints of the body. Th fulness, which is described as if in the veins, is sometimes in the tissues under the skin, so that it will crepitate. This is a feature of Carbo veg., and, i rheumaitc conditions, part of the swelling is sometimes of this characte Food remains a long time in the stomach, becomes sour and putrid. It passe into the bowels and ferments further, finally passing off in the form of putri flatus. There is colic, burning pains, distension, fulness, constricting an cramping pains from this distension. The patient complains of feeling as i the stomach were raw. This is described as a smarting, sometimes from takin food; sometimes from taking cold water. Carbo veg. has cured ulceration o the stomach. It is a deep-acting medicine, and is capable of curing al disordered conditions of the stomach; such as disorders from eatin indigestible things, mince pie, too hearty food.

In Carbo veg. the liver, like all the other organs, takes on a state of torpidity and sluggishness. It becomes enlarged. The portal system is engorged, and hence hæmorrhoids develop. Pain and distension in the region of the liver; sensitiveness and burning in the liver, accompanied by a bloated condition of the stomach and bowels. A feeling of tension in the region of the liver; the part feels drawn, as if too tight. There are pressing pains in the liver, and it is sensitive to touch.

Much that I have said regarding the flatulence and fulness of the stomach applies also to the abdomen. Carbo veg. may be indicated in low forms of fever, as in septic fever, when there is a marked tympanitic condition, with diarrhœa, bloody discharges, distension and flatulence. Extremely putrid flatus escapes making the patient very offensive. A striking abdominal symptom of Carbo veg. is that the flatus collects here and there in the intestine as if it were in a lump; incarcerated flatus; a constriction of the intestine will hold it in one place so that it feels like a lump or tumor, that finally disappears. Colic here and there in the abdomen from flatus. There is burning in the abdomen. No matter what the trouble is, in Carbo veg. there is always burning. The part burns; it feels full; it becomes engorged and turgid with blood. Diarrhœa, dysentery, cholera, when there is a bloody, watery stool. Cholera infantum; stool mixed with mucus; watery mucus mixed with blood. The child sinks from exhaustion, with coldness, pallor and cold sweat. The nose, face and lips are pinched and hippocratic. With all diarrhœic troubles the prostration will indicate Carbo veg. as much as, if not more than, the stool. In the diarrhœa of Crabo veg. all the stools, no matter what kind, are putrid, with putrid flatulence. The more thin, dark bloody mucus there is, the better is the remedy indicated. Itching, burning and rawness of the anus and round about, are strong features of Carbo veg. Soreness—in all diarrhœic conditions— soreness to pressure over the abdomen. Round about the anus, in children, there is excoriation. The parts are red, raw and bleeding, and they itch. Itching of the anus in adults. Ulceration of the bowels. This tendency to ulceration of mucous membranes is in keeping with the character of the remedy. Whenever there are mucous membranes there may be ulceration. Aphthous appearance. Ulceration of Peyer's glands. The patient lies in bed and oozes involuntarily a thin bloody fluid, like bloody serum.

Old chronic catarrhal conditions of the bladder, when the urine contains mucus, especially in old people, with cold face, cold extremities and cold sweat. There is suppression of urine.

In both the male and the female organs there is a weakness and relaxation. The male organs hang down. Relaxation of the genitalia; cold and sweating genitals. The fluids escape involuntarily.

In the woman the relaxation is manifested by a dragging down sensation; dragging down of the uterus, as if the internal parts would escape. The uterus drags down so that she cannot stand on her feet. All the internal organs feel heavy and hang down.

Another strong feature of Carbo veg. is dark, oozing hæmorrhage from the uterus. It is not so often a copious, gushing hæmorrhage—the remedy has that also—but it is an oozing. The menstrual flow will ooze from one period almost to another. The blood is putrid and dark, even black, with small clots, and considerable serum escapes with it. It says in the text: 'Metrorrhagia from uterine agony." Atony is a good name for the condition; lack of tone; relaxation; weakness of the tissue. Atony is everywhere present in the Carbo veg. constitution. The muscles are tired, the limbs are tired, the whole being is tired and relaxed. This is in contradistinction to the gushing found in *Belladonna, Ipecac, Secale* and *Hamamelis,* where the blood escapes in great gushes, followed quite naturally by a contraction of the uterus, for there is more or less tonicity in connection with it. In Carbo veg., either in connection with confinement or menstruation, or in an incidental hæmorrhage, the uterus does not contract. Subinvolution from mere atony; no contraction; no tonicity; weakness and relaxation. After menstruation, confinement and the various complaints that woman is subject to, there is a period of weakness that Carbo veg. often fits. When there is a retained placenta, with scanty hæmorrhage—just an oozing, with no tendency to a gush of blood—the physician remembers that throughout the whole pregnancy and confinement there has been sluggishness and slowness of pains, and he says: "Why did I not think of Carbo veg. before?" The woman has needed Carbo veg. for a month. He administers a dose, and before he has time to think about it, the uterus will expel that placenta and fix up matters so nicely that he will not need the mechanical interference that might otherwise have been necessary.

Now-a-days we hear so much about this meddlesome midwifery, this curetting, and doing this and that and the other thing, that it makes a homœopathic physician disgusted. Just as if those parts were not made by Nature, and could not take care of themselves; as if they must be swabbed out and syringed out. These injections and bichlorides, etc., to keep the germs out of a woman are all nonsense. If a state of order is maintained there will be no germs. A homœopathic physician can manage hundreds of these cases, and have no trouble. If he sees clearly beforehand what remedy the woman needs there will be no bad cases; they will all take care of themselves. Irregular contractions that bring on abnormal conditions are all avoided if the woman is turned into order before she goes into confinement. Carbo veg is one of the medicines that prepares a woman well for confinement, that is the symptoms calling for Carbo veg. are often present in such conditions She is often run down, relaxed and tired. Pregnancy brings about a grea many unusual conditions. There is the nausea in pregnancy; the flatulence; the offensiveness; the weakness; the enlarged veins. They will tell you that the enlargement of the veins of the lower limbs is from pressure, but it is generally not from pressure, but from weakness of the veins themselves.

Suppression of milk; prostration or great debility from nursing. It is not natural for a woman in a healthy state to become prostrated when nursing her child. She becomes so because she is sick. She was in a state of debility before she began nursing, and the weakness should be corrected by an appropriate remedy. Then she can make milk and feed her child without feeling the loss of it. Such is the state of order. Carbo veg. is a friend to the woman, and a friend to her offsprings. You will be astonished, after ten years of real homœopathic practice, that you have so few deformed babies; that they have all grown up and prospered; that their little defects and deformities have been outgrown, and that they are more beautiful than most children, because they have been kept orderly. The doctor watches and studies him, and feeds him a little medicine now and then, that the mother suspects is sugar, to keep on the good side of the baby. She need not know that it is medicine, or that anything is the matter with the baby. So he watches the development of that little one, and grows him out of all his unhealthy tendencies. The children that grow up under the care of the homœopathic physician will never have consumption, or Bright's disease; they are all turned into order, and they will die of old age, or be worn out properly by business cares; they will not rust out. It is the duty of the physician to watch the little ones. To save them from their inheritances and their downward tendencies is the greatest work of his life. That is worth living for. When we see these tendencies cropping out in the little ones we should never intimate that they are due to the father or mother. It is only offensive and does no good. The physician's knowledge as to what he is doing is his own, and the greatest comfort he can get out of it is his own. He need never expect that anyone will appreciate what he has done, or what he has avoided. The physician who desires praise and sympathy for what he has done generally has no conscience. The noble, upright, truthful physician works in the night; he works in the dark; he works quietly; he is not seeking for praise. He does this when called to the house, and when members of the family bring little ones to the office. In this manner children can be studied and their symptoms observed and enquired into Whenever the mother brings the child, expecting medicine, she may know that he is receiving medicine, but when she does not ask for medicine let her suspect that Johnnie is getting sugar so the doctor can get on the good side of him. That is sufficient.

In Carbo veg. the voice manifests a great many symptoms. I described a part of them when going over the coryza. I explained how it began in the nose, and travelled to the throat, the larynx, and the chest. Now many of the complaints of the larynx begin with a cold in the nose, which finally locates permanently in the larynx—and in that way we bring out the Carbo veg. cases. It is only now and then that the Carbo veg. cold settles in the larynx first; it usually travels through the nose. Most remedies have a favorite place for beginning a cold. For instance, the majority of *Phosphorus* colds begin in the chest or larynx. Not so with Carbo veg.; its cold generally begins in the nose, with a coryza, and the larynx is simply one of the stopping places. If the Carbo veg. cold goes down into the chest it may have its ending in the bronchial tubes or the lungs. This is a favorite place for it to settle, and it seems as if it were going to remain there. Weakness in the larynx from talking. Tired larynx of speakers and singers, and feeble, relaxed persons. *The hoarseness comes on in the evening.* The larynx may be fairly well in the morning, but as soon as it becomes evening his voice becomes husky. In more serious forms he may be speechless in the morning, but hoarseness and huskiness in the evening are more characteristic. Huskiness and rawness in the evening. Rawness in the larynx when coughing. Some will say there is burning, some will say rawness. Rawness in the larynx and trachea when coughing. A continual formation of mucus in the larynx, which he has to scrape and cough out. We see the same tendency to weakness in the mucous membranes. No tendency to repair; no tendency to recover. He goes on from bad to worse, with a catarrhal condition of the larynx and trachea. Hoarseness and rawness from talking, worse afternoon and evening. He is obliged to clear his throat so many times in the evening that the larynx becomes raw and sore. Let me tell you another thing about the Materia Medica. Most of the provers were laymen, and hence there is some confusion of terms in the provings. This the physicians must see. Irritation in the throat from coughing nearly always means irritation in the larynx, though the prover said "throat." Now here is an expression, "obliged to clear his throat so often in the evening that the larynx becomes raw and sore." Clearing the throat would not make the larynx sore. Scraping the throat does not scrape the larynx; but he is obliged to clear his *larynx* so often that the part feels raw. Ulcerative pain, scraping and titillation in the larynx. Irritation in the larynx causing sneezing. Laryngeal phthisis. This catarrhal condition and lack of repair in the larynx goes on so long that tuberculosis begins.

Carbo veg. is one of the greatest medicines we have in the beginning of whooping cough. Its cough has all the gagging, vomiting and redness of the face found in whooping cough. It is one of our best medicines when the case is confused; when the cough indicates no remedy or when it remains in a partially developed state. A dose of Carbo veg. in such cases will improve matters very much, and minor cases of whooping cough may be wiped out in a few days. When the remedy does not cure permanently, it brings out more clearly the symptoms calling for another remedy. Most cases of whooping cough, in the care of a homœopathic physician, will get well in a week or ten days under a carefully selected remedy. When allowed to run, they continue a long time, gradually increasing for six weeks, and then declining according to the weather. If it is in the fall, the cough will sometimes keep up all winter; so whooping cough furnishes an opportunity for the homœopathic physician to demonstrate that there is something in Homœopathy.

The Carbo veg. patient suffers very much from difficulties of breathing. Suffocation; cannot lie down. A feeling of weakness in the chest, as if he could not get another breath. Sometimes it is due to cardiac weakness, and sometimes to stuffing up of the chest. The latter is most common. Sometimes the difficulty is asthmatic. The remedy cures asthma. We will see the patient propped up in a chair by an open window, or some members of the family may be fanning him as fast as possible. The face is cold, the nose pinched, the extremities cold and he is as pale as death. Put the hand in front of the mouth, and the breath feels cold. The breath is offensive; putrid. The extremities are cold clear to the body; not only the hands, but the whole upper extremities; and not only the feet, but the limbs clear to the body, are cold. The body only feels warm; even the skin is cold.

Carbo veg. has a rattling cough with retching and vomiting. A morning cough, with much rattling in the chest; the chest fills with mucus, and on endeavoring to expectorate he coughs and gags, or coughs and vomits. At any time during the day a peculiar choking, gagging, retching cough may develop from the mucus in the chest. He cannot get it up; it is tough, purulent, yellow and thick. Greatly reduced vitality; great relaxation; worn out persons, old people. Persons worn out from coughing or from prolonged exertion. Prostration. Catarrh of the chest, with copious expectoration.

At times there will be a hard, dry hacking cough, but finally, after prolonged coughing, it commences to loosen and he throws up great quantities of mucus. A dry, hacking cough, yet there is rattling in the chest, and the cough does not seem to do any good. He seems to cough and become exhausted, sweats and strangles. It seems as if he would suffocate with the cough. Finally he succeeds in getting up some mucus, and then follows mouthful after mouthful of thick purulent expectoration. Frequent attacks of spasmodic cough in violent paroxysms lasting for many minutes, sometimes an hour. Cold sweat, coldness and pinched appearance of the face. This increases as he goes into the paroxysm of coughing. His face looks haggard, so distressed does he become while in a paroxysm of coughing. This state is present in old phthisical cases, in the advanced stage, when they are incurable. Under such circumstances Carbo veg. furnishes an excellent palliative. It seems to strengthen the muscles of the chest so that the patient can expectorate better.

It mitigates the cough; the gagging and retching and dyspnœa are relieved, and he is temporarily improved. It is a wonderful palliative in. many incurable conditions with dyspnœa and weakness of the chest. In Bright's Disease, in phthisis, and in cancerous affections Carbo veg. stops the violent symptoms and mitigates greatly.

This remedy is one to begin whooping cough with. It simplifies the case greatly, and sometimes cures it in a few days. The patient coughs until the chest is sore, as if he had been beaten all over the chest. All night he has paroxysms of coughing. He sleeps into a paroxysm of coughing, like *Lachesis*. He rouses up from sleep with coughing, gagging, sweating and suffocation. He will go two or three hours without a paroxysm, and then on comes one that will last an hour. He has two or three hard paroxysms of coughing during the night. He commences to fill up, he hears the rattling breathing and he knows that before long he will have a hard time of it.

This goes on and on, to the end of his life in asthmatic cases—what is called "humid asthma." Real humid asthma comes on in persons who suffer from contractions of the small bronchial tubes, so that even at the best there are little whistlings in the chest. Every time such patients take cold their whistling increases. They expectorate mucus, at first copious, then tough and finally purulent. During all this there is great asthmatic dyspnœa. Carbo veg. is an excellent remedy in all those cases of asthma where the shortness of breath is so marked that there is only a partial oxidation, as a result of which he suffers much from occipital headache and wants to be fanned. Old cases of recurrent asthma. Every time there comes a warm wet spell his asthma comes on. It is common for Carbo veg. asthma to come on in the night. He goes to bed without warning of an oncoming attack, only he says, "I don't like the weather;" and he wakes up with asthma. He wakes up suffocating, springs out of bed and goes to the window or wants to be fanned.

Carbo veg. is required in old, badly-treated cases of pneumonia, with a remaining bronchitis; in cases where there has been hepatization that was not cleared up, and there are bad places in the lungs and bronchial tubes, with weakness of the chest. Weakness of the chest when coughing. He feels that there is not enough force in the muscles of the chest to get up a good cough, or to help him carry on the breathing. Pneumonia, third stage, with fœtid expectoration, cold breath, cold sweat, desire to be fanned. Threatened paralysis of the lungs. This is a combination of clinical states that the remedy covers well. Sometimes these asthmatic cases go on for a while, and then comes an infiltration of tubercle. If Carbo veg. can be given early it will prevent infiltration.

There is pain in the chest, and burning. Burning in the lungs; burning in the sides of the chest; burning with the cough; burning behind the sternum—

the whole length of the trachea; burning aggravated when coughing; a sense of rawness even when breathing. He feels a load upon the chest, an oppression, a great weight. These are the various words that he uses, all descriptive of the same thing.

The heart comes in for a great deal of trouble. It appears to be struggling. Of course it is the venous side of the heart that is in distress. The veins are engorged. It is a venous condition of the whole patient; the veins *are* performing their labor with great difficulty. A state of relaxation, struggling, and there are orgasms of blood—described by some of the authors as an orgasm, by others as a tumultuous action of the heart felt throughout the body. Pulsation felt all over the body. Flushes of heat mounting upwards, ending in a sweat. Suitable sometimes for women at the turn of life. Especially suitable to persons in advanced years.

Carbo veg. complaints come on in a weakly state in young people; as if it were a premature old age in the middle-aged people; or in the breaking down that naturally belongs to old age. It is a great comforter for aged people with enlarged veins, or fulness of the veins and coldness of the extremities. Oozing of blood, with palpitation—tumultuous action of the heart. The pounding goes on like a great machine, shaking the whole body.

The pulse is almost imperceptible. It seems as though the volume of blood ought to be tremendous, but it is not. Weakness of the whole vascular system. Pulse irregular, intermittent, frequent. Blood stagnates in the capillaries. Complete torpor; impending paralysis of the heart. Burning in the region of the heart. With this there is an awful feeling of anxiety in the chest—in the region of the heart—as if he were going to die, or as if something were going to happen. He feels that tumultuous action and tires out under it.

In going over the remedy I have said so much about the limbs, their coldness and the cold sweat, that I have practically covered most of the symptoms that belong to the extremities. Carbo veg. is an excellent remedy for the general constitutional disorder where there are indolent varicose ulcers upon the lower limbs—the legs above the ankles. There is no activity in these ulcers; thin watery discharge or it is thick, bloody and ichorous. Burning indolent ulcers; varicose ulcers; swelling of the limbs. A gangrenous state from the extremely feeble circulation. Gangrenous condition such as old people have, senile gangrene. The limbs wither; the toes and lower parts wither and look dusky. There are blisters upon them and they ooze a bloody, watery fluid. Burning like fire. Loss of sensation. Stiffness in the joints. Excoriating sweat between the toes, and numbness. Numbness in the limb lain on. If he lies on the right side, the right hand gets numb. It he turns over on the left side, the left arm gets numb. The circulation in the part is so feeble that if there is any pressure the part becomes numb. The surface is cold. The extremities are cold. He is indolent, weak and always tired, with an aversion to mental and physical work. Every little exertion brings on a feeling as if he would faint and collapse.

The sleep is full of dreams. He wakes up with dyspnœa, wakes with cold limbs, especially cold knees. Legs drawn up during sleep. Unrefreshed after sleep. The dreams he has are the kind that most of these patients have where the remedy acts so violently upon the veins, upon the basilar portion of the brain, and upon the voluntary system. They are awful. He dreams of fire, burglars, fearful and horrible things. Anxiety, restlessness and congestion of the head prevent his going to sleep. Rush of blood to the head. His head feels hot, but to the hand the skin feels cold. The inner chest feels as if burning, but the outer chest feels cold to the hand. So it is in the abdomen. The feeling of internal heat and burning, with external coldness, is a common feature of Carbo veg.

The fever is violent; it has a violent rigor or chill. Of course during the chill he is cold, but there is one strange feature, he wants cold water during the chill, and when the fever comes on he has no thirst. That is strange; it is uncommon. It is common for patients to be thirsty when they are hot with fever, and when cold not to ask for water. It is common not to ask for water during sweat. But in this patient you observe coldness, rigor, cold breath, and even in the chill sometimes a cold sweat, and you say that it is peculiar that he drinks so much cold water. It is strange; it is uncommon; rare. Hence it is one of the strong features of Carbo veg. febrile conditions.

With the chill of this remedy one side of the body frequently feels in its natural state of heat, that is, naturally warm, while the other side is cold. One-sided chill. Chill with icy coldness of the body. Chill with great thirst. Sweats easily, especially about the head and face. Exhausting night or morning sweats. Sweat profuse, putrid or sour.

Low forms of fever like yellow fever, and a very low type of typhus and typhoid fevers. After the fever has somewhat subsided he has prolonged cold spells with lack of reaction. He does not seem to rally, but he is cold, his knees are cold, his breath is cold, cold sweat, a sort of paralytic weakness. Cadaveric aspect of the face. Cyanotic face. Coldness of the limbs. Yellow fever in the last stage, the stage of hæmorrhage, with great paleness of the face. Violent headache, trembling of the body; collapse with cold breath, cold sweat, cold nose. Nose and face pinched. Vital powers very low, tells a great deal of the story of Carbo veg. Lack of reaction after some violent attack, some violent shock, some violent suffering. In weakly persons who give right out, with dyspnœa, coldness, copious sweat, exhaustion, collapse and cadaveric aspect, Carbo veg. must be given.

Carbo veg. is indicated after surgical shock, when the patient goes into collapse, and is in danger of dying from the shock of the operation. This is before inflammation sets in, for there is not vitality enough to arouse an inflammation. The heart is too weak to establish reaction enough for an inflammation. Inflammation comes after a reaction. But if reaction does not take place, Carbo veg. is one of our most important remedies.

CARBONEUM SULPHURATUM

The complaints and symptoms of Carbon bisulphide are worse in the MORNING, forenoon, afternoon, EVENING, NIGHT before midnight. It is a remedy of great depth of action, frequently indicated and long neglected. *Strong desire for open air and the open window;* better *in the open air* but worse from a draft. It is our most useful remedy in patients broken down from the long use of alcoholic stimulants. Weakness and suffocation from ascending stairs. Bathing brings on many symptoms. Many symptoms are worse after breakfast. It is a most useful remedy to restrain the growth of cancer (like *Graphites*) and it has cured lupus. He is extremely sensitive to every change of weather, especially to *warm damp weather.* A condition not unlike chlorosis is produced by this drug. It is very useful in chronic rheumatism, especially of the joints. Extremely sensitive to the clothing. He is sensitive to both cold and heat. Cold in general aggravates or brings on many symptoms. Worse from becoming cold; from cold air; after becoming cold; takes cold easily; takes cold from exposure to cold air when overheated. Like *Carbo veg.* it is a most useful remedy in *collapse.* Marked venous stasis in organs and parts. Constriction of any parts. Constriction like a band around parts. Constriction of the heart. It is suitable in clonic and epileptic spasms. Dwarfishness of body and mind. Distension of the blood vessels and varicose veins. Œdema of the extremities. It is both better and worse after eating. Gradual shrinking of all the muscles, even to marked emaciation. The lymphatic glands are enlarged. Fainting followed by stupefaction and loss of memory. Symptoms are worse from cold feet; fat food; milk; warm foods; warm drinks ameliorate. Full feeling internally and general venous engorgement. Gouty condition of joints. *Passive hæmorrhage.* Lack of vital heat. Internal and external heaviness Induration of glands. Marked lassitude and constant desire to lie down

Many conditions are worse from a jar and from stepping. Anæsthesia of the skin and mucous membranes.

Weakness follows straining of muscles. Lying ameliorates except respiration and head symptoms. Feels better while lying. Complaints worse before, DURING and *after* menses. Motion increases all symptoms and he dreads

motion. Mucous secretions *copious,* thick and viscid. Numbness of single
parts and parts lain on. Orgasm of blood in the body. Pain in bones and
glands. Pains of many kinds in all parts of the body. Short and quick attacks
and at regular intervals. Paroxysmal pains. Sore bruised pains in body and
limbs. Burning pains internal and external. Cutting, JERKING and shooting
pains. Pressing pains are very common in all parts. Stitching pains and itching
stitching pains in all parts. Violent tearing pains; extending downwards.
Wandering pains; wandering, jerking, stitching pains. Paralysis one-sided;
of organs; painless. Pressure helps most symptoms. Pulsation all over the
body. Pulse spasmodic and rapid; pulse slow; 52. Rheumatic conditions with
or without fever. Chronic rheumatic states. Extreme sensitiveness to pain. He
is worse after pain and from standing. Stiffness in body and limbs. Complaints
from summer heat. Dropsical swelling and swollen glands. Trembling all over;
tubercular tendency; lungs and bowels. Twitching of muscles. Wine increases
all his sufferings and brings on many complaints. Walking increases
sufferings; walking in open air aggravates many symptoms. He is worse from
the heat of summer and from the cold of winter. Worse from warm wraps,
warm room, warm bed and warmth in general, yet he is sensitive to cold.
EXTREME WEAKNESS in the morning; *in old drunkards;* in the heat of summer;
during menses; after stool. Painful weariness in the morning.

Very absent minded and so irascible that he breaks things that happen to
be in his hands; when spoken to. Anxiety in the *morning; evening in bed;
night;* before midnight; of conscience, with fear; about the future; before
menses. Biting things in delirium. Capricious at times. Cheerful in the morning
after passing much flatus. Aversion to company. Concentration difficult when
reading. Confusion of mind in the morning on waking; from mental exertion;
from pain in the head; as if intoxicated. Very conscientious about small matters.
Fantastic delirium at night, raving and tries to bite. Sees visions; excitement
at night. Illusions of fancy. There is despair, discontentment, discouragement
and DISTRACTION Dulness of mind, in the morning; thinking is very difficult.
Very excitable. Exhilaration—bordering on drunkenness. Fear; morning;
night; of death; of insanity; of misfortune; of people; of walking in the dark.
Forgetful; forgets what she was to do with the things and held them in her
hand. *Frightened easily.* Hilarity and extravagant gaiety. *Hurried feeling.
Hysterical conduct.* Irresolution, indifference and mental sluggishness. *Indolence.* Worse in the morning. *Imbecility* and insanity. Ideas abundant at first,
later confusion and stupefaction. Irritability in the morning. Weak memory;
cannot find the right word; misplaces words when writing. His mood is
constantly changing; morose; easily offended; rage; mental prostration.
Religious affections. Very restless during the night; worse before midnight.
Sadness in the evening; during chill; during fever; during perspiration. He

sings and whistles. Inclination to sit in silence. Averse to being spoken to. Maniacal conduct. Jumps out of the window. Stares at her hands with a vacant look. Starting during sleep. Suspicious. Talkative at first, later indisposed to talk. Talking in sleep. Persistent tormenting thoughts. Timidity. Unconscious. Violent actions. Weeping much; alternating with laughing; in sleep. *Vertigo,* in the morning on rising; afternoon; evening; better in open air; as if intoxicated; during menses; *while sitting;* when stooping; a tendency to fall forward; when walking; when walking in open air.

Coldness of the forehead. Constriction; like a band; of *forehead;* of the *occiput.* Dandruff on the scalp. A sensation, of emptiness in the head. ERUPTIONS; *crusts;* ECZEMA; *itching;* MOIST; scaly; pimples, sore and painful. Erysipelas of the scalp. The head falls forward when walking. A sensation of fluctuation in the head on moving the head: Fulness in the head; in the forehead. *The hair falls out. Heat* in the afternoon; in forehead; IN THE VERTEX. Heaviness in the head; after breakfast. Hyperæmia of the brain. The scalp itches violently. Movements felt in the head. Nodules in the scalp sore to touch. Numbness of the vertex. Pain in the head in the morning in bed; on waking; at 9 A.M.; in the afternoon; in the evening; at night; 10 P.M.; better in the open air; worse ascending steps, binding up the hair; after *breakfast;* after dinner; after eating; from becoming heated; from a jar; from heavy stepping; from mental exertion; from motion; from shaking the head; *after sleep; after stool;* in a warm room. Headache comes on from taking cold; during chill; during fever. Rheumatic headaches. Catarrhal headaches. Headache with pain in back of the neck. Pulsating pain on motion of the head and when thinking or reading. Violent headache, increased until the mind is affected. Pain in the forehead in the morning on waking, lasting all day, violent in the forenoon. Pain in OCCIPUT evening and night. Pain in sides of head. One-sided headache, worse left. Pain in temples in the afternoon, worse shaking head and on stooping. Pulsating pain in temples in the morning on waking 6 A.M. Pain in *vertex.* Boring pain in forehead and temples. Burning pain in *vertex.* Cutting in temples, worse after dinner. Drawing pain in forehead 10 P.M. in occiput; in temples. Dull pain in head toward evening. Jerking pain in forehead. Pressing pain in the head in forenoon. Pressing pain in forehead with sleepiness, worse reading and stooping; over eyes; extending to eyes and temples. PRESSING PAIN IN OCCIPUT; in temples, extending to vertex; in VERTEX ALL DAY. Sore bruised pain in head. Stitching pain in temples worse on left side, extending to occiput. Tearing pains better in open air and during rest; in *forehead;* occiput; sides; temples; worse on left side. Cold perspiration on forehead. The scalp is sensitive to the brush. Pulsation in occiput and temples. Electric shock in the head.

The eyelids stick together during the night. The discharges are acrid, bloody, purulent and yellow. Dulness of the eyes. Eruptions about the eyes;

on the lids, pustules on upper lids that itch and burn. Falling lids. Granular lids. The eyes feel hot. Heaviness of the lids and they are sore on moving them. Catarrhal inflammation of eyes and lids. Conjunctiva full of dark veins. Insensibility of the cornea. Itching of the eyes and *lids*. Lachrymation in the open air and when reading. Pain in eyes on moving them; aching; burning pain with headache, morning; when reading; evening; margin of lids when reading; in canthi. The pains are cutting, pressing; as from sand; sore, itching and tearing. Drawing backwards. Pressing in the evening with great heat in the eyes. Itching while reading and after stool. Pupils contracted, also dilated. *Photophobia*. Quivering in lids. Redness of eyes; of lids; edges of lids. Recurrent styes. Staring and sunken eyes. Swollen lids. Thick lids. Twitching lids. Ulceration of the cornea; of the lids. Weak eyes. Vision *dim;* objects seem too far off. *Diplopia. Flickering.* Loss of vision. Vanishing of sight. Myopia.

Discharge from ear; bloody, fœtid, *offensive,* purulent. Redness of the ears. Eruption behind ears. Sensation of flapping in ears. The ears are red and hot. Inflammation in middle ear and auditory canal. Itching in ears. Noises in ears; morning; evening; night; buzzing; cracking; chirping; fluttering; humming; reverberations; RINGING; ROARING; rushing sounds. Pain in ears afternoon and evening; when swallowing. Pressing, STITCHING and tearing pains. Stitching after stool worse in *right ear.* Pulsation in ear. Stopped sensation in ear. Hearing at first acute, later *impaired* and finally lost. It has cured ear cough.

It is a most useful remedy for chronic catarrh of the nose. The *nose* is cold. CORYZA in open air; with chill; constant; with cough; fluent; *dry in evening.* Discharges from nose of all kinds and consistency. Clear; copious; crusts and scabs; *excoriating;* greenish; hard chunks; offensive; *purulent;* thick; VISCID; water; thick yellow pus. Redness and burning of the tip of the nose. DRYNESS IN NOSE. Epistaxis morning and evening, dark blood; on blowing nose. Itching in nose. OBSTRUCTION OF NOSE. Fœtid odor from nose. *Ozæna.* Pain and soreness in nose. Burning in root of nose. It has cured polypus in nose. Smell acute for odors, later smell is *wanting. Frequent sneezing.* The nose is swollen. Ulcers high up in nose.

The face is bloated and chlorotic. Sensation of tension in the face. The face is cold and the lips are *cracked.* The face is discolored; *bluish; dark;* PALE; sickly; yellow. Dry burning lips. Eruptions on chin; lips; around mouth; on nose. Acne rosacea on face and forehead. Acne of drunkards. *Comedones.* Crusty eruptions on face and nose. Herpes on face with tearing pains in limbs. *Moist itching* eruptions. Pimples, pustules, rash. Red eruptions on *cheeks* and nose. Scurfy, scaly eruptions. Tetter on left cheek. Vesicles on face. Phlegmonous erysipelas. Expression is anxious; bewildered; sickly; suffering; vacant. Heat of face evening; during chill; FLASHES. Itching of face. Pain in face in *cold air;* while lying. Burning face and lips.

Drawing, sore, bruised, stitching and tearing pain in face. *Cold sweat on face.* Stiffness of jaw. Sunken look. Swelling of face; œdematous; glands; parotid; sub-maxillary. Tension in muscles of lower jaw. Ulceration of lips.

Anæsthesia of mouth and tongue. Aphthæ of mouth and tongue. Bleeding of mouth and gums. The tongue feels cold. The tongue is cracked. The gums are detached from the teeth. The tongue is coated white; dryness of mouth and tongue in the morning with unquenchable thirst. Odor from mouth offensive; putrid. Burning mouth and tongue. Saliva is bloody. Copious flow of saliva. Speech difficult and stammering. Gums swollen. Taste is bad; BITTER in the morning; foul, metallic; nauseous; pasty; saltish; sour; sweetish. Tickling of soft palate after lying down. Ulcers in the mouth. The teeth are on edge and loose. Pain in teeth evening and night; in cold air; from cold water; during and after eating; when masticating; from touch; from warm food and drink; from external warmth; from both warm and cold things. The pains arc drawing; jerking; jerking-stitching; pulsating; *stitching; tearing;* jerking-stitching at 9 A.M.; pulsating evening and night. Tearing in afternoon and in cold air.

Catarrh of the throat in cold weather with choking dryness, redness and sensation of fulness. Constant desire to hawk. Inflammation of the throat with gangrenous tendency. Sensation of a lump in throat. Mucus in throat in morning; viscid; tasting salty. Pain in throat on coughing; on swallowing; on empty swallowing. Burning in throat extending to stomach. Burning in œsophagus. Rawness and soreness. Stitching on swallowing; in œsophagus as if bone had lodged in throat. Scraping the throat; spasms of the œsophagus. Constant disposition to swallow. Difficult swallowing. Swelling of throat and tonsils. Ulceration of throat: Induration of glands of the external throat. The glands of neck are swollen. *Enlarged thyroid gland.*

Appetite diminished or wanting with easy satiety. Appetite is RAVENOUS without relish of food; with aversion to food. Aversion to fats; fish; food; MEAT; milk. Cold sensation in stomach. Sensation of *constriction.* Desire for beer. Cold drinks; sour things; distension after eating. Sensation of emptiness. Eructations empty; after eating; ineffectual; after milk; while walking. *Eructations ameliorate.* Eructations acrid; bitter, EMPTY; of food; foul; loud; nauseous; rancid, sour; waterbrash. Fulness in stomach after eating. Gnawing in stomach. Heartburn after eating. Flushes of heat in stomach. Heaviness. hiccough and loathing of food. Nausea in morning; afternoon; night; after eating; with fainting; better after eructations; during headache; on entering a room or going into open air. Pain in stomach in the morning; in night; after breakfast; after cold drinks; after eating; during menses. Burning after stool. Cramping and pinching. Pressing pain in stomach after eating and after stool. Soreness in stomach. Stabbing extending to back. Stitching pains. Pulsation. Retching with the cough. "A tied together feeling." Thirst in the morning;

burning thirst; during chill; extreme thirst; during heat; drinks large quantities of water. Vomiting in the morning; on coughing; after eating; with headache; during menses; vomiting bile; bitter water; blood; food; green mucus; sour; watery.

Sensation in abdomen as if diarrhœa would come on. Distension after eating; tympanitic. Abdominal effusion. Flatulence in abdomen; obstructed; in cæcal region. Fulness after breakfast. Heaviness and gurgling. Hardness of the abdomen; of the liver. *Liver affections* with dropsical swelling of feet. Pain morning; afternoon; evening; night; as if diarrhœa would set in; after eating; on inspiration; before and during menses; on motion; on *pressure;* in cæcal region; in hypochondria after sitting; in hypogastrium; in the inguinal region; in *the liver;* in the left lobe of liver; in umbilicus. Burning pain in abdomen; in hypochondria; in *liver.* Cramping in abdomen; in the morning; 10 A.M.; afternoon; night; before stool; after stool; in umbilicus; in ypogastrium. Cutting in abdomen; before stool; in hypogastrium. Drawing pain in abdomen; in navel. Dragging in abdomen, Jerking pain in abdomen; in left hypochondrium. Pressing pain in abdomen; in hypogastrium; in *liver.* Sore bruised pain in abdomen; in *liver.* Stitching pains in abdomen; in hypochondria; in hypogastrium; in inguinal region; sides of abdomen; liver. Tearing in abdomen; in umbilical region extending to bladder. Retraction of navel (*Plumbum*). Rumbling in abdomen; before stool. *Tension.* Trembling after stool. Weak feeling after stool. Constipation with much belching; *difficult* stool; ineffectual urging, insufficient stool. Diarrhœa in the morning; 5 A.M..; after breakfast; night; noon; after eating; after dinner; painless; with much rumbling; chronic; pain in region of umbilicus with thin, yellow, frothy stools; stool OFFENSIVE; sour; pasty; THIN; WATERY. Some workers in carbon bisulphide suffer from constipation and some from diarrhœa. Dysentery with bloody mucous stools. Eruptions about the anus. Excoriations at anus and between the nates. Fistula in ano. FLATUS COPIOUS OFFENSIVE; while walking; ameliorates. Fornication in the anus. Hæmorrhage of bright red blood. HÆMORRHOIDS; bluish; chronic; *external;* large; during menses; *very sore; inactivity of the rectum.* Involuntary stool during urination. *Moisture at the anus,* itching and burning. Itching in the morning. Pain in the rectum after stool; during stool. Burning and itching. Burning during stool; after stool. Cramping stitching in anus and neck of bladder during urination. Cutting and pressing outward. Soreness in anus; after stool. Stitching pain in anus; evening; during stool; stitching in anus and neck of bladder to urethra during urination. Tearing in anus. Tenesmus during stool. Constant prolapsus of rectum. Urging to stool in the morning; after breakfast; 8 A.M.; 10 A.M.; during stool. Worms. Ascarides; lumbricoides; tæniæ. The stool is acrid, black, *bloody,* brown, HARD, knotty, *lienteric,* light colored, like sheep dung.

Catarrh of the bladder with mucous sediment in the urine; pain in the bladder; aching; cramping in the neck of the bladder; pressing pain; stitching in the anus and neck of the bladder to the urethra during urination. Paralysis of the bladder. Retention of urine. Tenesmus of the bladder. Urging to urinate; at night; constant; ineffectual; painful. Urination; dribbling; dysuria; feeble stream; frequent, especially at night; involuntary at night, in sleep. Suppression of urine. Gleety discharge from urethra. Bleeding from urethra. Itching in the urethra with a sensation of drops of urine. Burning in the urethra during urination and during stool. Cutting during urination. Urine; acrid, albuminous; bloody; burning; cloudy on standing; dark; red; copious; offensive; SCANTY. Sediment purulent; mucous; white. Atrophy of testes. Erections violent. Erections absent. Complete impotency. *Hydrocele.* Inflammation of glans penis. Itching of the genitals; scrotum. Pain in testes; during rest. Burning in spermatic cords. Drawing in testes. Stitching pain in testes; in spermatic cords. Perspiration on genitals in evening; on scrotum. Relaxed genitals. Seminal discharge too soon during coition Seminal emissions at night; shrunken organs. Sexual desire wanting. Swelling of the prepuce; of testes; of epididymis. Tuberculosis of testes.

Atrophy of the ovaries. Cancer of the uterus. Aversion to coition. Eruption and excoriation. Inflammation of the uterus. Itching of the vulva. LEUCORRHŒA; ACRID; bloody; burning; copious; before and after menses; milky; thin; white; watery. Menses absent; excoriating; black; dark; delayed first menses; irregular; LATE or too soon; offensive; painless; copious at first, later SCANTY, short; suppressed; slow passive hæmorrhage from uterus. Pain in uterus; burning; soreness; weak labor pains. Women who work in carbon bisulphide are often sterile. Encysted tumor on vulva.

Catarrh of air passages. Constriction of larynx causing cough. Heat in larynx. Inflammation of larynx. Irritation of larynx and trachea. Mucus in larynx. Pain in larynx. Burning in larynx. Rawness in larynx and trachea. Soreness in larynx and trachea. Laryngeal phthisis. Rattling in the trachea. He constantly clears the larynx. The larynx very sensitive. Tickling in larynx and trachea. Hoarseness morning and evening; with coryza; in damp weather. Voice is lost.

Fast breathing. It has served well in asthma. Asphyxia from alcohol and from coal gas. *Difficult breathing; evening;* night ascending; in a close room; when coughing; after eating; after slight exertion; while lying; must have windows open, on falling asleep; on waking. Respiration rattling; short; sighing. Suffocation at night and in a warm room; wheezing; whistling.

Cough in morning; evening; NIGHT; before midnight; in cold air; asthmatic; on becoming cold; from constriction of larynx, dry; hacking hoarse, from irritation in larynx, bronchial tubes and trachea; loose morning cough; lying down in evening; paroxysmal; from rawness in larynx; from scraping larynx;

short; waking one from sleep; spasmodic; suffocative; from talking; from tickling in larynx and trachea; whooping cough. Expectoration: in daytime; *morning;* evening; night; bloody; copious; GREENISH; mucous; offensive; purulent; tasting putrid and salty; viscid; yellow. It has cured paroxysmal ear cough.

Anxiety in chest; *in the heart. It* has been of great service in cancer of mammæ. Very stubborn catarrh of chest. A sensation of coldness in chest. *Constriction of chest in evening;* pleural dropsy. Emphysema. Eruptions on the chest; vesicles. Erysipelas of the mammæ. Feeling of fulness in the chest. Heat in chest and bleeding from lungs. The mammæ are indurated. Inflammation of bronchial tubes; heart; lungs; pleuræ; mammæ. Itching all over chest but especially in axillæ and mammæ. VIOLENT OPPRESSION OF CHEST. Pain in chest on coughing; on motion; in sides of chest; in heart; aching; *burning;* burning in middle of chest and in left side. Cutting pain in chest; in left lower chest to back in breathing; *pressing pain* in chest; in mammæ; in left side. Rawness in chest with cough. Soreness in chest from coughing. Stitching pains on deep breathing, in left side of chest through to back; in the sternum extending upwards; in heart; flying burning stitches in chest. Tearing pains in chest. Palpitation of heart in evening; in anæmic patients; with anxiety; from slight exertion; from motion; visible; tumultuous. Perspiration in axilla. A very useful remedy in phthisis. A continuous sensation of weakness in chest.

Coldness of the back; lumbar region. Eruptions on the back. A heavy load between the scapulæ. Itching of the back. Pain in the back; night; on breathing; during chill; during menses; on motion, while sitting. Pain in cervical region; between scapulæ. Pain in lumbar region morning on waking; during menses; while sitting. Pain in lumbar sacral region in morning on waking. Pain in sacrum in morning on waking; during menses. Pain in coccyx. Aching in back; in lumbar region; in sacrum. Bruised feeling in lumbar region. Burning in back; between scapulæ. Drawing in the cervical region; in lumbar region. Pressing pains in the back; in lumbar region. Stitching pains in hack; in cervical region; in scapulæ; in lumbar region. Tearing pain in cervical region; in lumbar region. Stiffness in cervical region. Tension in back; in cervical region; in lumbar region on ascending; in sacrum worse on ascending. *Weakness in back;* in lumbar region.

Anæsthesia of arms and hands. Coldness of limbs; with headache. Upper arms; hands; fingers; lower limbs; knees; legs; FEET in evening in bed. Constriction of lower limbs. Contractions of muscles and tendons; upper limbs; hands; fingers. Cracked skin of hands. Cracking in the joints; in the right shoulder. Cramps in the limbs; upper limbs; *thighs; legs;* CALF IN BED; FOOT; SOLES; toes. Blueness of nails; during chill. Emaciation of limbs. Eruptions on limbs; herpes on back of hands; pimples; impetigo; vesicles between fingers. Excoriations between nates; between thighs. Formication of limbs; upper limbs;

forearms; hands; legs; feet. Heat of hands; palms; feet; soles. Heaviness of limbs; upper limbs; *lower limbs; legs; feet.* Hip joint disease. Itching of the limbs; upper limbs; upper arm; forearm; hands; lower limbs; thighs. Milk leg has been cured by this remedy. Convulsive motion of limbs like chorea. NUMBNESS OF UPPER LIMBS;lower limbs. Pain in limbs; during chill; PAROXYSMAL; *rheumatic;* in *joints; gouty.* Pain in upper limbs; *during the night;* paralytic in left arm; rheumatic in shoulder; in elbow on motion; rheumatism in elbow, in hand; gouty in hand. Pain in lower limbs; rheumatic; worse on motion; sciatica from taking cold; in thighs after dinner; neuralgia in thighs; in knees; in hips; in hollow of knee. Pain in leg; rheumatic; in ankles in morning; in os-calsis on ascending steps; in feet after dinner and while walking. Aching in forearm. Burning pain in limbs; in shoulder; upper arm; forearm; hand; palm; thighs; feet; soles; joints of feet. Drawing pains in limbs; shoulder; upper arm; elbow; forearm;. wrist; hands; fingers; lower limbs; hips; thighs while walking; hollow of knees; legs; calf; feet. Itching, stitching pains in deltoid muscle. Jerking pains in hip and ankles on ascending. Jerking-stitching in all the limbs; in biceps; in fingers; in thumb; in thighs; in legs; in toes. Pressing pains in left forearm, worse leaning on it; in left heel. SORE, BRUISED LIMBS; *joints;* upper limbs; lower limbs; thighs; legs; soles when walking. Stitching pains in limbs from every change of weather; in joints; in upper limbs; in *right shoulder;* in cold, damp weather, extending down arm; in upper arm; forearm; elbow; wrist; hand; fingers; lower limbs; hips; thighs; ankles; feet; toes while walking. Tearing in all the limbs, wandering about, sudden pains; in joints; upper limbs; shoulder; upper arm; elbow; *forearm;* wrist; hands; finger joints; lower limbs; knee; calf; ankles; feet; toes; first toe. Paralysis of extensors of wrist; of lower limbs. Perspiration of hands; of FEET; COLD; offensive; profuse. Restless legs and feet. Stiffness of limbs; fingers; of lower limbs, of knees. Swelling of hands; lower limbs; legs; ankles; feet. Dropsical swelling of limbs with liver affections. Tension in hollow of knee and legs. Tingling of limbs; uipper and lower hands and feet. Trembling of limbs; upper limbs; forearm; hands; lower limbs. Twitching of the limbs; upper limbs; hands; lower limbs; thighs; legs; feet. Ulcers on lower. limbs; LEGS; feet; ABOUT THE NAILS. Varicose veins, *lower limbs;* LEGS. Weakness of all the limbs; joints; *upper limbs; lower limbs;* thighs; knees; legs.

Deep morning sleep. Dreams; amorous; ANXIOUS; of danger; of death; distressing; of previous events; fantastic; frightful; of ghosts; horrible; unpleasant; VEXATIOUS; vivid. Late falling asleep. Restless all night. SLEEPINESS IN MORNING; afternoon; after 3 P.M.; evening; after dinner; after eating; while reading; sleepless before midnight; with sleepiness; from thinking; after waking. He is not refreshed after sleep. Waking difficult; early or late; frequent.

Coldness in morning in bed; in afternoon; *evening;* 7 P.M.; 8 P.M. Icy coldness. Chilliness during menses. Chill after eating; in evening; then sweat; during sleep. Fever in the evening and during the *night*. NIGHTLY FEVER; with chilliness; burning heat at night. Fever without chill. Dry heat at *night*. Extreme heat. Flashes of heat. Fever without perspiration. Septic FEVERS. Fever with shivering. Perspiration in daytime; morning; evening; *night;* during anxiety. Cold, on coughing; WHILE EATING; AFTER EATING; on slight exertion or motion. Profuse sweat during the night. Sweat during and after sleep; offensive; sour at night. *Complaints come on* if exposed while sweating.

Anæsthesia of the skin. Biting after, scratching. Burning of the skin after scratching. Coldness of skin. Chapping and *cracks in winter*. Discoloration. Blueness, liver spots; red spots; yellow. Dryness with burning. *Eruptions*. Biting; blisters; boils; *burning;* discharges, corrosive, glutinous, yellow fluid; dry; eczema. Herpetic eruptions; scabby; scaly; tearing pain; zoster. Eruptions; itching; like measles; phagedenic; pimples; pustules; rash after scratching. Scabby eruptions, moist, worse after scratching. SCABIES. Smarting eruptions. Eruptions worse after scratching. Suppurative eruptions; tubercles; urticaria, nodular worse after scratching. Vesicles filled with yellow fluid. *Erysipelas with much swelling* and *covered with vesicles*. EXCORIATION; after scratching. Excrescences. Formication all over body. *Induration* in skin. Itching-jerking all over body. ITCHING at NIGHT; in a warm bed. Itching-pricking here and there, all over. Sticking in the skin; after scratching. Ulcerative pains in skin. ULCERS: black; bleeding; burning; *cancerous;* deep; discharging; bloody; copious; ichorous; OFFENSIVE, yellow pus; fistulous; indolent; indurated; painful; phagedenic; fungous; sensitive; SPONGY; stinging; suppurating. Unhealthy skin; *small wounds fester*.

CARDUUS MARIANUS

This is one of the most important liver remedies, if a homœopathic author can be excused for the expression. There are many pains, pressing, dragging, drawing, burning; worse from motion. The patient is very sensitive to cold, and is subject to attacks of bilious vomiting at regular or irregular intervals. The author has cured many violent sick headaches ending in vomiting bile, and cases in the habit of taking calomel, with this remedy (*Sang.*). Dropsical effusions with liver diseases. It is useful in hæmorrhages and jaundice, when symptoms agree.

Sadness, irritability and weeping. Congestive headaches; pressing pains coming periodically Fulness and heaviness in the head. Sensitiveness of the scalp to cold air. Pressing outward of the eyeballs. Yellow sclerotics. Burning in margins of lids. Burning inside of the nose. Epistaxis.

Taste bitter, insipid, or wanting. Foul tongue. No desire for food. Nausea, and vomiting mucus, then bile. Painful retching. and then vomiting sour greenish fluid. Drawing pains from left to right in the stomach. Burning in the stomach. Vomiting blood, very black.

The most important of all the liver symptoms. Dragging pain in right hypochondrium when lying on left side; like *Arn., Mag. m., Nat. s.* and *ptel.* Pressing, drawing, stitching in right lobe of liver. This remedy establishes a healthy flow of bile, and thereby cures the condition that favors the formation of gall-stones. It has many times broken up the tendency to gall-stone colic. Portal congestion and hæmorrhoids. Sore, bruised, hard liver; sometimes the left lobe, but oftener the right. When complicated with lung and heart symptoms; with expectoration of blood.

Drawing, stitching or burning pains in the abdomen. Distended abdomen. Cutting pains.

The stool is black. Stool hard and knotty. Clay-like, bileless stool. Burning in rectum and anus. Itching piles. Bleeding piles. Inveterate constipation.

Burning in the urethra. Copious high-colored urine, with copious sediment. Turbid urine. Retention of urine.

Menses copious. Menses suppressed. Uterine hæmorrhage with portal congestion. Drawing in vagina, and leucorrhœa.

Liver cough, when lower portion of right lung is affected, with chronic congestion of the liver.

Pains in the chest with liver pains. Stitching pains. Drawing pains. aggravated by motion.

Pain in the back under the right scapula (much like *Chel.* and *Æsc.*). Drawing pains in the back. Sensitive spine.

Cramping, drawing, pressing, rheumatic pains in the limbs. Violent pain in the right deltoid. Pain in the hip joints, aggravated from rising, stooping, and motion. Neuralgic pains in the lower limbs, worse from motion. Œdema of the feet. Varicose veins. Ulcers. Rheumatism, and jerking of the muscles. Cramps in the calves and feet. Walking almost impossible.

Gastric and bilious fevers.

CAULOPHYLLUM

Weakness in the reproductive system of the woman. From weakness she is sterile, or she aborts in the early months of gestation. During parturition the contractions of the uterus are too feeble to expel the contents, and they are only tormenting. Labor-like pains during menstruation with drawing pains in the thighs and legs, and even the feet and toes. Uterine hemorrhage from inertia of the uterus. Relaxation of muscles and ligaments. Heaviness, and even prolapsus.

Subinvolution. Excoriating leucorrhœa. Menses too soon, or too late. She is sensitive to cold and wants warm clothing, quite unlike Pulsatilla. She is hysterical, like Ignatia. She is fretful and apprehensive. She is rheumatic, Like Cimicifuga, only the small joints are likely to be affected. Later she suffers from after pains, and they are felt in the inguinal region. Rheumatic stiffness of the back, and very sensitive spine. She is sleepless, restless, and withal very excitable. This remedy has cured chorea at puberty when menstruation was late.

CAUSTICUM

Causticum is a very searching medicine, suitable in old, broken down constitutions, suffering from chronic diseases. Only occasionally is it indicated in acute diseases. Its complaints are such as are progressive, slow, and accompanying a declining state of the economy. Gradual decrease of muscular power, a paralysis. Paralysis of the œsophagus, paralysis of the throat, such as occurs after diphtheria; paralysis of the upper eyelids; paralysis of the bladder paralysis of the limbs, of the lower limbs; great lassitude, muscular relaxation indescribable fatigue and heaviness of the body. And there is a tremulousness a quivering, jerking, twitching of the muscles, twitching in sleep.

The next most striking feature is found in the tendons, which become shortened, resulting in a temporary or permanent contracture, and the limb i drawn up. Tendons of the forearms contract and there is gradually increasing flexion. Sometimes a whole muscle will harden and shorten, so that it can be felt by the hand as a hard ridge. *Contractures of muscles and tendons.*

Closely related to this is a rheumatic state of the tendons and ligament about the joints, sometimes with swelling, but always with pain and ending in a shrivelling of the joint, a tightening up of the joint so that it become ankylosed. Great stiffness of the joints, and while this is going on the patient is growing weaker, is running into a state of melancholy, of hopelessness anxiety and fear. Constantly present in his mind is the hopelessness, and feeling that something is hanging over him, that something is going to happen These are general features of Causticum. They all go to make up one picture they are inseparable.

Another kind of progressive trouble in Causticum is hysteria. Gradually increasing hysteria. Hysterical cramping. The woman loses all control of herself and says foolish things. Her nervous system becomes extremely sensitive to noise, touch, excitement or anything unusual. Starting from the slightest noise; starting in sleep; twitching and jerking; the child is easily startled, or acts as if startled without cause.

The paralytic weakness is associated with the rheumatic diathesis. The rheumatic states are peculiar. The patient himself can endure neither heat nor cold. They both aggravate his rheumatic conditions, his nervous conditions and himself in general. His pains are ameliorated by heat, but they are aggravated in dry weather. Great deformity of the joints; they are enlarged, soft and infiltrated, always worse in dry weather; more pains and aches during dry weather. Rheumatism that affects both the muscles and the joints. This patient is also aggravated by exposure to cold, dry winds. Many an individual who has gone from the low lands of the East up into Colorado will come down with rheumatism from the cold, dry winds. Let such a patient as I have described take a ride in the cold lake wind and he will have paralysis of the side of the face exposed to the wind. A long drive with the east wind coming against the face. The next day that side of the face will be paralyzed. Such a paralysis will almost always recover under Causticum.

Rending; tearing, paralytic pains; pains that benumb; pains that fairly take the life out of him, they are so severe. And they are likely to remain in one place for a long time. Causticum has often greatly mitigated the lightning-like pains of locomotor ataxia.

Now, with all these sufferings the patient is slowly growing weaker, till at length he can no longer walk, he can no longer sit up, he is so tired and weak that he must lie down. He is tired in body and mind. It is a paralytic fatigue.

Convulsive symptoms. Cramps, now here, now there. If frightened he is almost sure to have some form of convulsive condition. The woman with tendency to hysteria will have hysterics from fright; nervous girls that are more inclined to chorea, will start with jerking of muscles and will keep it up day and night. Chorea even at night. Localized chorea, jerking of single parts, chorea of the tongue or of one side of the face.

Epilepsy in young persons at the age of puberty, from fright, from being chilled or exposed to some great change in the weather. Epilepsy, chorea, paralysis, hysteria worse during menses. We see that Causticum is a deep medicine. Worse from exposure to cold, dry wind. It also has rheumatic complaints aggravated in the warm, damp days, in wet weather, but this is not so striking.

Any one of the complaints that I have mentioned may be brought on by bathing in cold water. A long, dry, cold spell will aggravate the rheumatic troubles, getting wet or becoming chilled by bathing will start them.

Causticum has cured insanity; not acute mania with violent delirium, but mental aberration of the passive kind, where the brain has become tired. The constitution has been broken down with long suffering and much trouble, and finally the mind is in confusion. At first the patient recognizes his inability to do anything and then comes this foreboding that something is going to happen. He is unable to think, and consequently unable to carry on his business. He is going into imbecility. Full of timorous fancies. "Timorous anxiety," overwhelmed with fearful fancies. At every turn there is fear that something is going to happen. Fear of death, fear that something will happen to his family. Always anticipating some dreadful event. That is a striking feature of the Causticum mental state. It is found in old, broken down mental cases, after prolonged anxiety; after a prolonged struggle of some sort. Anxiety before falling asleep. In addition to this, the Causticum patient lacks balance. Everything excites him. The more he thinks about his complaints the worse they become. Mental and other ailments from long-lasting grief and sorrow. The injurious effects of fear and prolonged vexation. Tired from vexations of business.

The suppression of eruptions is apt to bring out mental symptoms. Mental exhaustion, hopelessness, despair, appearing after the suppression of an eruption with zinc ointment. He was fairly well while he had the eruption, but when it disappeared his mind gave out. Eruptions on the side of the head and face, and extending over the whole head. Thick, crusty eruptions covering the whole occiput. When these eruptions are suppressed in children, chorea is apt to follow. In the adult there will be trembling, paralytic weakness and the mental state, sometimes pains in the nerves. The driving in of a facial eruption will frequently result in facial paralysis. The healing of an old ulcer with stimulating lotions and ointments will have a similar result. Then he also suffers from violent headaches, congestive, pulsating headaches; violent stitches in the head, worse in the evening. But the headaches are, as a rule, nondescript; only occasionally do we find a Causticum headache standing out by itself. It will usually be associated with rheumatic and gouty conditions which also affect the scalp. The scalp contracts and tightens up in places like the contractures in other parts. Rheumatic headaches; sometimes the pain is so severe as to cause nausea, and vomiting. Blinding headaches followed by paralysis.

Torticollis. The head is sometimes drawn to one side by the shortening of the muscles of the neck. Causticum is a curative remedy in this shortening of the tendons and muscles.

Causticum is rich in eye symptoms. Very often the patient says that the eyelids feel so heavy that he can hardly hold them up. This gradually increases until it becomes an actual paralysis. Sometimes there is the appearance of a veil before the eyes; foggy vision. Flickering before the eyes. Air seems full of little black insects. Then, again, large black or green spots are seen. After looking at the light a green spot appears and remains in the field of vision for a long time. Diplopia. And the vision gradually grows weaker until it is lost. Paralysis of the optic nerve. Lachrymation, tears acrid, burning; ulceration, copious discharges from the eyes, agglutination of the lids, paralysis of the eye muscles. Causticum cures scrofulous ophthalmia with ulceration of the cornea; chronic, purulent ophthalmia of psoric origin. The cornea is covered with little veins.

Another very strong feature of this medicine is its tendency to grow warts. Warts on the face, on the tip of the nose, on the ends of the fingers, on the hands. Hard, dry. horny warts come out on various parts of the body.

It is a natural feature of this remedy to produce copious, thick, tough, gluey discharges from mucous membranes. The catarrhal troubles creep up the Eustachian tube, from the nose and throat into the ear, resulting in roarings, cracking noises and reverberations in the ear. There is great accumulation of ear wax; deafness of catarrhal origin and deafness from paralysis of the auditory nerve. Severe, dragging pains in the ear.

The nasal catarrh is very troublesome. Old, atrophic catarrh with accumulation of crusts throughout the whole nasal cavity; post-nasal catarrh with ulcerations, granulations and copious, thick, yellow or yellowish-green discharge; nose-bleed; frequent attacks of acrid, watery coryza. Much itching of the nose. A wart grows upon the tip of the nose.

The pains in the face are violent. Neuralgic pains from exposure to cold. These pains often accompany the facial paralysis. Tearing pains in the face, stitching pains, pains of a rheumatic character.

Ulcerations about the mouth and nose. Fissures about the lips, the wings of the nose and the corners of the eyes. Fissures seem to form upon the least provocation. Fissures of the anus, of the skin about the joints. Old cases of salt rheum with fissures in the bends of the joints. Fistulous openings with indurated walls.

The gums become scorbutic and settle away from the teeth; bleeding and ulceration of the gums. Violent, tearing pains in the roots of the teeth from riding in the wind. Old rheumatic subjects suffer all through every dry spell with toothache. Stitching, tearing, pulsating pains in the teeth; even in the sound teeth on drawing in cold air. Frequently recurring abscesses of the gums. Putrid sour or bitter taste in the mouth.

When the paralytic condition affects the tongue then we have stammering. There is also the condition of complete paralysis of both the pharynx and œsophagus. Hence Causticum is useful in the results of diphtheria when it has been maltreated or when the remedy has not been sufficient to cure the disease. The food goes down the wrong way or enters the larynx or the post-nares. Paralysis of the organs of speech, paralysis of the tongue, awkward at talking, awkward at chewing; bites the tongue and cheeks while chewing. Post-diphtheritic paralysis is a serious condition and only a few remedies can cure it. Causticum is one of them. *Lachesis* and *Cocculus* are also important. Dryness of the mouth and throat; rawness of the throat; must swallow constantly on account of a sensation of fulness in the throat, a nervous feeling in the throat. This is often a forerunner of paralysis. The *Staphysagria* patient when excited will keep up a constant swallowing and this goes on until it becomes a source of great annoyance. Burning in the throat; jerking in the throat; constantly scraping thick, tough mucus from the larynx. Study the sounds that patients make in order to ascertain where the mucus comes from. The presence of hoarseness shows that the trouble is in the larynx.

The Causticum patient sits down to the table hungry, but on seeing the food his appetite vanishes. The thought, sight or smell of food takes away the appetite. This is a common symptom in the pregnant woman. Although hungry, on sitting down at the table, she cannot eat. *Kali carbonicum* has an empty, all-gone feeling in the stomach, with aversion to food. *China* has canine hunger, but loathes the sight of food.

Thirst after eating; thirst for cool drinks with aversion to water; desire for beer, smoked meats, pungent things, aversion to sweet things our delicacies. Most remedies that have loss of appetite have desire for sweet things, pastry, etc. The symptoms of thirst with aversion to drinking is very much like *Lachesis*. The two run very closely together in the paralytic condition of the throat.

There is a queer sensation in the stomach as if lime were slaking there. Trembling in the stomach; burning. Bread causes a sensation of heaviness and pressure; coffee seems to aggravate all the symptoms of the stomach, but a swallow of cold water relieves. Many symptoms in this remedy are made better by a swallow of cold water. The violent, spasmodic cough may be stopped at once by a drink of cold water. Cold water seems to tone up the paralytic condition. Warm water applied to the hands brings on pains in these old sensitive spinal conditions. Cold washing is their only relief.

Causticum has belching, nausea, vomiting, distension and violent pains in the stomach. Pinching colic. In the rectum there is the same tendency to paralytic weakness that is found in other parts of the body. It is inactive and fills up with hard fæces, which pass involuntarily and unnoticed. *Aloe* has involuntary dropping of little, hard balls, especially in children. Even when old enough to understand about such things, they will pass little balls unnoticed.

On account of the paralytic condition the stool passes with less straining while the patient is standing. Retention of urine except when standing; unable to pass it in any other position is *Sarsaparilla.*. Constipation, frequent, unsuccessful urging to stool. The stool is tough and shining, and is passed with great difficulty and exertion.

Fissures in the anus; itching and stitching in the rectum, excessive itching day and night; hemorrhoids; pulsating in the perineum; fissures and hæmorrhoids pulsate and burn like fire. The hæmorrhoids become infiltrated and hardened.

This remedy has two kinds of paralysis of the bladder, one affecting the muscles of expulsion and the urine is retained, and the other centering upon the sphincter vesicæ, and then the urine is passed involuntarily. "He urinates so easily that he is not sensible of the stream and scarcely believes, in the dark, that he is urinating, until he makes sure by sense of touch." Causticum is unconscious of the stream as it passes. It is a very useful remedy in children that wet the bed. Especially is it a wonderful remedy in the woman. *The urine escapes involuntarily when coughing.* Retention of urine in the woman. Retention after labor. Paralysis of the bladder. A woman who is too greatly embarrassed to pass through a crowd of observing men to the closet at the end of a railroad car, at the end of the journey finds that she is unable to pass the urine. Retention of urine from straining the muscles of the bladder. If the patient is chilled at the time the remedy may he *Rhus. Rhus* and Causticum are the two great remedies for paralytic weakness of muscles from being overstrained, or from being overstrained and chilled.

Great weakness at the time of the menses. Anxious dreams before menstruation; melancholy; cramp-like spasms; pains in the back. The woman suffers from many annoyances during menstruation. Just about the time for the flow to start violent cramp-like pains come on. In a woman who is nursing a child the milk almost disappears in consequence of fatigue, night watching and anxiety. The nipples get sore and crack, another instance of the tendency to form fissures.

The Causticum patient has trouble with the voice. You remember, when we were going over the symptoms of *Carbo vegetabilis,* I told you that the hoarseness was worse in the evening. Now observe that the hoarseness of Causticum is worse in the morning. He gets up in the morning with a hoarse voice; if it is an ordinary case, after moving about and expectorating a little mucus, it is better. Sudden loss of voice from paralysis of the vocal cord. It sometimes begins with the morning aggravation, gradually increasing until it lasts all day and all night.

The Causticum cough is a hard cough and racks the whole body. The chest seems full of mucus and he feels if only he could *cough a little deeper* he could get it up, and he struggles and coughs until exhausted or until he finds out that a drink of *cold water will relieve.* But it must be ice cold. The cough is hollow, it sounds as if he were coughing into a barrel. It is relieved by expectoration if it can only get deep enough to reach the mucus. Sometimes such a cough precedes quick consumption. It is a deep-acting medicine; it cures phthisis, especially mucous phthisis or quick consumption. "Cough with a sensation as if the patient could not cough deep enough to start the mucus; produced by tickling, accompanied by rawness. Cough wakens her from sleep in the evening and morning. Cough relieved by a swallow of cold water. Cough worse by bending forward. Continual, annoying cough; with each cough escape of urine." Influenza with tired aching of the limbs as if they had been beaten. "Whooping cough in the catarrhal stage."

Great soreness and tightness of the chest, oppression of the chest; it feels as if a load were upon it. It seems to be filling up with mucus, and the patient coughs until he raises a mouthful and then he feels a little better for a time. Pale as death, covered with sweat.

There are many symptoms in the back. Pain and stiffness; stiffness on rising from a seat. Stiffness in the limbs, through the hips and in the back, so that he rises up from sitting or the recumbent posture with great difficulty. In most cases the pains and aches are ameliorated by the warmth of the bed and by applied heat. Only the pains in the fingers are sometimes brought on by heat.

CENCHRIS-CONTORTRIX PROVING
(Copperhead)

Bulletin No. 24 of National Museum gives check list of North American reptilia Ancistrodon Contortrix. Dr. Albert Gunther, who furnished the article for The Encyclopedia Britannica, calls the "Copperhead" Cenchris-Contortrix, and considers it very similar to the Trigonocephalus family, but smaller in size, generally found near the water-courses, closely related to the Chenchris Piscivarus, which is the water-snake or crater-moccasin.

The Cenchris family belongs to the temperate parts of North America, and its venom is of a deadly nature.

PROVERS

No. 1   Mrs. K., 6th potency, one dose only.
No. 2. Dr. Mary S., 6th potency, one dose only.
No. 3. Dr. Eliza M., 6th potency, one dose only.
No. 4. J. A. T., 6th potency, one dose only.
No. 5. Dr. Mary S., 2nd proving, 10m.
No. 6. Dr. Eliza M., 2nd proving, 10m, one dose.
No. 7. Geo W. S., 6th and 30th potencies.

MIND—Loss of memory. Feeling of intoxication. Anxiety, with a feeling that she will die *suddenly*[1] (8th day, lasting many days). The horrors of the dreams of the previous night seemed to follow her[1] (8th day). She could not banish the horrors of her dreams[1] (9th day). Instantly after lying down at night she was seized with a horrible, sickening anxiety, all over the body, but most at the heart and through the chest, exclaiming, "I shall die! I shall die!" This soon passed into profound sleep, which was not interrupted until morning, but full of horrible dreams. Afternoon and evening thinks her family plotting to place her in an insane asylum (this lasted four afternoons and ended fourteenth day of proving). Suspicious of everybody. Melancholy (old symptoms worse). No inclination to attend to her usual duties which are pleasant.[3] Angry when disturbed.[3] Not able to rest in bed, must walk the floor to ease mind.[3] Wants to be alone[3] (4th day). Nervous and irritable[3] (14th day). Catch myself staring into space and forget what people are saying to me, or that there is any one in the room[2] (4th day). Inability to concentrate mind[2] (4th day, 6th and 10m.). Absent-minded[2] (two provers, 5th, 6th and 10m.). *Dreamy, absent-minded, took wrong car without realizing where was going.* Misdirected letters[2] (13th day, 6th and 10m.). Very gloomy and discouraged[3] (7th day). So absent-minded and stupid that I tremble and shiver, and my teeth chatter for some time before I begin to realize that I feel cold[5] (3rd day). Foreboding, gloomy without cause, frequent sighing[2] (21st day, 6th and 10M.). Crying and very frequent sighing, as if very sad[2] (Many days, 6th and 10m.). Lack of determination and snap, have to use all my reserve mental force to make myself get up and go out[5] (many days). Painful procrastination, indecision.[5] Times passes too slowly, seems to drag along. I am longing to go, yet I cannot tear myself out of my chair and move along. When at last I do pick up enough determination to go, I go very suddenly.[5] Feel hard and uncharitable[5] (8th day). Selfish, envious, easily slighted. Transient attacks of anger 6 P.M.[5] (9th day, 6 P.M. and 8-30 P.M. 14th day, and 6-30 P.M. 17th day). Longing for the woods so intense I wandered out to the park alone[5] (2nd day). Great depression and gloomy foreboding followed by great hilarity[5] (9th day). Alternation of opposite moods and desires[5] (9th day).

SENSORIUM—Sensation of intoxication in evening[3] (2nd day). Sensation of intoxication came on at 4 P.M., lasting 3 hours, feeling as if I would fall; unable to walk in a direct line; go from side to side of pavement[3] (2nd day). Same symptoms 4 P.M. (3rd day). (Same symptom 4 P.M. to 7 P.M. 4th day, and came every day for 4 weeks). Vertigo, coming and going, with no inclination to attend to her usual duties that are very pleasant; nervous and tired all the time[3] (6th day). Vertigo. Angry when disturbed[3] (6th day). Compelled to lie all afternoon. So dizzy[3] (9th day). Vertigo very bad from 4 P.M. to 7 P.M.[3] (2nd to 10th and 11th days). When riding in the car, she rode by the place she intended to get off at.[3] Her mind is all a blank for ten minutes, but people did not observe anything wrong with her appearance. Dreamy feeling[2] (6th day). *Fainting spells.*

INNER HEAD—Sensation of fulness about the head[1] (18th day). Dull, aching pain in the forehead, which finally extended to the occiput, leaving forehead[1] (1st day). Feeling as if all the blood in the body rushed to head[1] (8th day). Violent headache in both temples in forenoon; could not stand any warmth in the room; lips dry and parched[1] (13th day). Headache in both temples on rising, passing off after breakfast[3] (4th day). Headache in temples; passes off after eating.[3] Headache, not defined, with disgust for food[3] Aching in the frontal sinuses, nose, and throat, as though she had taken a severe cold, but no discharge of mucus[2] (4th day). Dull ache in the occiput[2] (4th day). Dull aching in the frontal eminence[2] (4th and 8th days). Dull ache in left frontal eminence[5] (7th day). Hard, aching pain commenced in left frontal eminence and spread down left side to teeth, then spread to right frontal eminence then to teeth on right side[5] (16th day). Hard pain over left eye[5] (9th day). Dull frontal headache during menstruation[2] (23rd day). Dull throbbing in vertex (18th, 19th and 20th days).

OUTER HEAD—Sore feeling in the scalp after the headache passed away (2nd day). Itching of scalp, better by scratching[2] (1st and 6th days—6th and 10m.). Transient sensation of prickling in the scalp, like a gentle current of electricity[5] (4th day). One large, dry, scabby pimple on scalp, long and narrow oval shaped[5] (12th day).

SIGHT AND EYES—Eyes ache, and there is dimness of vision.[3] Lachrymation from left eye; left eyelid red on edges[2] (7th day). Twitching in left eyelid (17th day). Dull ache in eyes, with sense of weakness[5] (16th day). Itching of eyes; begins in left eye and extends to right[1] (17th day). Margins of eyelid red, especially at night[5] (many days).

HEARING AND EARS—Itching of ears at night[3] (an old symptom not had for a year; 5th day). Itching of ears during the day[3] (7th day). Dull pain in and around the left ear[5] (6th day).

SMELL AND NOSE—Sickening odor in the nose (1st day). Copious flow of mucus, thin and watery.[2] Copious flow of mucus. Coryza. Cold nose[2] (several days). Cold nose[2] (6th day, evening 7 P.M.). Aching in throat and nose, tickling sensation in nose, as though discharge would flow, but very little discharge when blowing it[2] (5th and 6th days). Aching in left side of nose as though in the bones, with dull headache[2] (7th day). Sneezing occasionally and eye filled with water[2] (6th and 8th days). Sneezing in morning when waking[2] (7th day—6th and 10m.; many days). Sneezing violently on awaking in the morning[2] (6th and 8th days). Tingling from left nostril to left eye (lachrymal canal). Slight discharge of water from left eye, sensation of weakness in the eye[2] (6th day). Nose burning sensation inside as though full of pepper[2] (7th day). Nostrils sore, worse left side[2] (7th day). Discharge of yellow mucus sometimes tinged with blood[2] (7th and 9th days). Discharge of mucus from nose, varying from cream to amber color, specked with blood[2] (8th day). Cannot breathe through the nose[2] (8th day—6th and 10m.; many days). Impossible to breathe through the nose[2] (9th, 10th, 11th days). Scabs in the nose, lasting many days[2] (10th day—6th and 10m.). Dry mucus in nose, cannot breathe through it[2] (13th day). Slight tingling in left nostril[5] (4th day).

FACE—Flushes of heat about the face and head[1] (1st day). Bloating of face, as if intoxicated[1] (9th day). Bloating above and below eyes[1] (9th day). *Besotted countenance.* Mottled skin; purple, deep, dark red face. Dry parched lips in evening, with fever that began at 3 P.M.[1] (10th day). Swelling above eyes, below brow[1] (like Kali c.—12th day). She can see the water bag that fills the upper lid[1] (12th day). Baggy swelling under eyes[5] (many days). Face pale all through the proving.[3] Flushing and burning of face[2] (1st day). Great burning of the face, worse at night[2] (6th and 7th days). Cheeks began to get red and hot about 2 P.M.; keep growing hotter and redder until she goes to sleep at 10 P.M.; became dark red like erysipelas[2] (9th day). Woe-begone expression of face[2] (12th day). Burning face, 2 P.M.[2] (16th day). Burning begins in left cheek and ear, spreads to right cheek 6-30 P.M.[5] (2nd day). Blue circles under eyes[5] (all through the proving). Face sallow.[5] Very small red pimples in little clusters, between the eyes and on the upper lip[5] (15th day). Same tiny pimples on end of nose[5] (16th day). Formication on left cheek. like crawling of a fly, also on septum of nose[7] (8th day).

LONG FACE—Lips cracked and hot. Face chapped, dreads washing it[2] (18th day—6th and 10m.).

TEETH AND GUMS—Aching through jaws after lying down at night, lasting until after midnight[1] (12th day). Teeth ache from hot or cold drinks[5] (12th day). Teeth feel edgy, can feel that I have teeth[5] (12th pay). Dull ache in right upper teeth when eating [5] (19th day).

TASTE, SPEECH AND TONGUE —Dry tongue. Bitter taste in mouth on waking in the morning. Taste of copper in the mouth[2] (14th day). Dry tongue[7] (4th day—30th potency).

MOUTH—Dry mouth in evening.[1] Increase of saliva[2] (7th and 8th days). Profuse saliva[2] (8th day). Profuse saliva, running out of mouth on pillow in sleep[7] (4th day—30th potency).

PALATE AND THROAT—Constantly hawking up thick, tough, stringy mucus, difficult to raise[1],[5] (1st day). Throat full of mucus, thick and yellow, slightly tinged with blood from posterior nares, in the morning on waking[2] (6th day). During morning, twice discharged glossy, thick mucus from throat, looking like gelatine with bluish tinge, not tough, easily broken up[2] (6th day). Sore throat; painful, empty swallowing, but water swallowed without pain. Sore all over throat, after an hour it located on left side in tonsil, and muscles of left side of neck, was gone next morning[1] (11th day). Throat feels scraped, warm drinks are grateful[2] (4th, 22nd, 26th days—6th and 10m.). Right side of throat red and swollen[2] (6th and 7th days). Throat full of mucus, yellow with specks of blood in it[2] (8th day). Throat feels strained from the exertion of hawking[2] (6th day). Slight pricking in the throat on empty swallowing, but no pain on swallowing liquid or solid food[2] (6th day). Rawness of the throat with increase of saliva, which she swallows[2] (7th day). Throat full of mucus, yellow, with blood vessels plainly outlined on uvula, fauces and pharynx[2] (7th day). Right side of throat (pharynx), behind the posterior pillars of fauces, swollen and dark red, with sticking pains[2] (7th day). Throat feels sore and full, have to swallow often in order to breathe[2] (8th day). Aching in right side of throat[2] (8th day). Constantly swallowing[2] (9th day). The mucus is difficult to raise, loses her breath, and strangles in trying to raise it[2] (9th day). Eustachian tubes filled with mucus[2] (9th day). Had to hawk a half hour before I could get the mucus out of the throat so I could go to sleep; *mucus thick, tough* and yellow[2] (9th day). Throat painful on empty swallowing, but not when swallowing solids or liquids[2] (11th day).

APPETITE, THIRST, DESIRES AND AVERSIONS—Intense thirst for cold water in the evening. Every evening during proving.[1] Intense thirst in evening, with dry mouth.[1] Dislike for everything put before her to eat, and finds fault with everything[3] (5th day). No appetite for anything at breakfast[3] (7th day). Craves salt bacon (7th day). Disgust for food at breakfast[3] (9th day). No appetite.[7]

HICCOUGH, BELCHING, NAUSEA AND VOMITING—Eructations of tasteles gas a short time after eating[2] (3rd and 6th days). Vomiting of white gruel-like substance, with mucus and undigested food[5] (2nd day). Nausea > by ice; water makes sick[6] (2nd day).

STOMACH—Transient throbbing in the stomach[5] (6th day). Acute cramping sensation in stomach, > by belching.

HYPOCHONDRIA—Pain in the attachment of the diaphragm, right side[2] (3rd day). Cough felt at the attachments of the diaphragm .[3] Aching all round the waist, at the attachments of the diaphragm.[2] Felt as though a cord were tied around the hip.[2] Pain in the attachment of diaphragm when laughing[5] (9th day). Hard ache in the attachment of diaphragm, both sides, < by breathing deeply[5] (11th day). Feeling of a bottle of water in left hypochondrium, shaking up and down with motion of carriage[7] (11th day).

ABDOMEN—Dull pain in two spots directly ove. pubic arch. 10 A.M., passing off after two hours[3] (2nd and 3rd days). Feeling as though that part of abdomen below umbilicus was not sufficiently expanded, on waking in the morning (2nd day). *Bands around the waist unbearable most of the time during the three weeks of proving.*[2] Dull pains in lower abdomen[2] (2nd day, 12th day—6th and 10m.). Dull pain in abdomen when coughing[2] (14th day). Transient aching in a spot just above the umbilicus[2] (11th day). Sensation of a hard lump in left side of abdomen. Bloating of abdo-men after small amount of food, with diarrhœa[7] Great deal of rumbling in the bowels, left side[7] (11th day). During breakfast, sharp, cutting pain in the left hypochondrium, from above downward; pain deep, took breath away, lasting but short time[7] (2nd day—30th potency).

STOOL, ANUS AND RECTUM—Itching and soreness of the anus[1] (13th day). Soreness of anus[5] (20th day). Hemorrhoids that itch and are sore[1] (13th day). Urging to stool, which passes away before the closet can be reached[2] (3rd day). Unsuccessful urging to stool strain until rectum feels as though prolapsed, but have no stool[5] (3rd day). Waked in morning with itching of anus[5] (13th day). Diarrhœa with tenesmus[5] (35th day). On waking in the morning, had to hasten to the closet; stool watery, dark with a black sediment like coffee grounds; stool intermits, have to sit a long time, passing small quantities every minute or two[6] (2nd and 40th days). Stool looks like bran porridge and of some consistency[7] (10th day). Stool gushing and frequent, watery, with a dark sediment at first without pain; after several hours great pain before stool[6] (20th, 21st. and 22nd days). Flatus at termination of stool. Painless and involuntary stool when passing flatus. Soiled the bed twice in sleep[7] (10th day). Had several diarrhœic stools at night, copious, gray in colour, not debilitating. Several copious stools during the day with spluttering flatus, with bloating of abdomen after the smallest amount of food. Desire to be in a warm room, with above symptom[7] (14th day). Several stools, not so frequent; weak today, good deal of rumbling in left side of abdomen. Stools profuse, each seems as if it would empty the bowel, but soon full again. Sensation of intestines filled with water (Crot. tig.). Stool frothy, foamy, air bubbles like yeast[7] (16th day).

URINARY ORGANS—Loses her urine when coughing.[3] Desire to urinate at night, just after getting in bed; must get up and press a long time before a few drops pass[5] (many days). When doing mental work, frequent desire to urinate, pass large quantities of colorless urine[6] (several days).

MALE SEXUAL ORGANS—Violent sexual desire.[4] No sexual desire (unusual) since began the proving[7] (10th day)

FEMALE SEXUAL ORGANS—Yellow leucorrhœa; never had any leucorrhœa before[1] (11th day). White leucorrhœa, only while at stool, during the whole proving.[6] Sexual desire strong, in a widow who had long been free from such sensations. Pain in right ovary[3]. Herpetic eruption on labia majora.[3] Dull aching in the small of the back and sacral region, at night during menses[2] (23rd day). Soreness in coccyx and gluteal muscles, and aching in abdomen at night, during menses[2] (23rd day). Menstrual flow very profuse, bright red, with dark clots (23rd day). Menses two weeks late[5] (old symptom, 13th day). During menses, aching in small of back, when sitting up, must lie down. Easily moved to tears. Throbbing about umbilicus[5] (13th day). Sharp shooting pain in left ovary, upon motion[5] (3rd day). Pain in left ovary during menses (10th and 38th days). Cramping pains in uterus at each menstrual period, for four months.[6] Labor-like pains in uterus during menses.

VOICE AND LARYNX—Slight hoarseness, worse at night[2] (26th to 30th days—6th and 10m.). Hoarseness[2] (8th day).

RESPIRATION—Suffocating feeling after lying down in the evening[1] (7th day). Dyspnœa as if dying from anxiety[1] (7th day). Stops breathing on going to sleep[1] (8th day). She was prevented from sleeping by thinking of dreams of the previous night[1] (8th day). After lying down, a suffocating feeling came over her, with anxiety[2] in the chest as if she would die, worse on first lying down, She must lie with head drawn back, as she chokes so[1] (9th day). Dyspnœa on lying down. and the thought of sleep brings on great anxiety[1] (12th day). She says: "There is no use lying down, that suffocation will come[1]" (12th day). *Frequent sighing*[2] (8th day). Impossible to breathe through the nose and very hard to breathe through the mouth, because of mucus in the throat[2] (9th day). Can hardly find breath enough to talk, have to stop and gasp in the midst of a word or short sentence[2] (9th day). Great difficulty of breathing at night, she had to gasp and struggle for breathe[2] (9th day).

COUGH AND EXPECTORATION—Dry, hacking cough, coming on at 3 P.M., continuing through the evening.[3] Irritation to cough, felt in pit of stomachs.[3] Soreness in abdomen when coughing.[3] Cough comes on when walking fast or walking upstairs.[3] Coughs only when in the house.[3] Cough at night after retiring[2] (7th day). Cough caused a feeling of hclplessness[2] (7th day). Concussive cough, causing watering on left eye[2] (7th day). Only cough twice, but felt quite concerned about it; a hopeless feeling comes over her at each cough[2] (7th day). Dark, bloody expectoration; also bright red blood seems to come from throat[2] (12th day). Cough seems to come from the diaphragm, causing violent contraction there. At other times it causes contraction of the umbilicus[2]. Expectoration frothy white, all shades of yellow in morning[2] (14th day). Loose cough in morning, with frothy sputa.[2] Concussive cough at night[2] (18th and 19th days). Dry, short cough at 4 P.M., with constant irritation to cough, lasting until 10 P.M. Cough very hard, dry, frequent[2] (14th day). Concussive, forcible, dry cough, shaking chest walls, cannot be repressed, lasting many days[2] (16th day). Expectoration of white mucus of a metallic taste[2] (18th day). Cough only in evening[2] (20th day). Hoarse, paroxysmal cough, with whitish expectoration[2] (21st day).

LUNGS—Transient hard ache in lower lobes of lungs; and afraid to draw a long breath on account of the pain[5] (9th day).

HEART AND CHEST—Anxiety about the heart in evening after lying down[1] (7th day). Anxiety about the heart with palpitation[1] (8th day).

Anxiety in the chest, as if she would die, worse on lying down; must lie with head drawn back, as she chokes so[1] (9th day). Feeling as though the whole chest was distended and the heart very sore[1] (9th day). Feeling as if the heart was distended, or swelled to fill the chest[1] (many days). Anxiety in the region of the heart all night[1] (9th day). Extreme realization of the heart[1] (strongest 12th day, lasting many days). Pulse 120 in the morning[1]. Pulse 105 in the evening[1]. At 3 P.M. sensation of fluttering of heart followed by feeling that heart fell down into abdomen; then pulse became feeble, with heat lasting until after midnight[1] (10th day). At 11 P.M. sudden, sharp stitching pain in the heart, followed by dull pain, which gradually subsided[2] (1st day). Throbbing or fluttering under left scapula[2] (2nd day). Sudden, sharp stitches in apex of heart, worse evening[2] (3rd day). Pain through the attachments of the diaphragm, just below apex of heart. Pain in same region on right side of chest; hard aching, worse from deep inspiration[2] (3rd day). Sharp stitches in the heart[2] (4th day, lasting through the proving—four weeks). Dull pain in region of heart at 10 P.M. (7th day). Drawing pain in right side of chest, below mammary gland, on lying down at night (three nights); makes him put the hand on the pain; > by lying on that side and < lying on left side.[4] Sharp stitches in right side of chest[2] (7th day). Dull pain in apex of heart. transient[5] (2nd, 4th, 9th and 17th days). Hard ache in heart at 10-30 P.M.[5] (10th day). Sharp, darting pain under right breast[5] (13th and 16th days).

OUTER CHEST—Hard dull aching across the chest, extending to axilla on both sides, < on pressure; moving the hand to opposite shoulder causes pain in muscles of chest[2] (6th day). Transient sense of pressure over the lower sternum[5] (12th day).

NECK AND BACK—During the day, constriction about the neck, clothing disturbed her, choking feeling[1] (8th day). Sore aching feeling below the left scapula, rubbing >[1] (lasting many days). Transient lame stitch in back of neck[2] (4th day). Transient aching feeling in sacrum[2] (5th day). Throb-bing under the scapulæ, dull aching in small of back[2] (13th day). Transient dull aching in back of neck[2] (18th day). Dull aching in small of back[2] (21st day). Throbbing in buttocks[2] (21st day). Soreness in coccyx and gluteal muscles when sitting[2] (21st day). Awoke with throbbing in vulva and in anus, followed by a dull aching in sacral region, relieved by walking about (12th day). Throbbing carotids when lying down[5] (12th day). Awoke at night with pain in region of left kidney, worse lying on left side, better by turning on right side and drawing up limbs[7] (3rd day).

UPPER LIMBS—Transient aching in middle of right forearm, on the radius[2] (3rd day). Heat in palms in evening[2] (3rd day). Hands get chapped easily.[2] Hands vary, one minute hot and dry, then cold, then sweating in palms[5] (3rd day). Dull ache in metacarpal bone of thumb[5] (4th day). Dull ache in cushion of right and left thumbs[5] (12th day). Dull ache in left palm[5] (21st day). Itching of left palm[5] (17th day). Cold air makes the hands look red and as though the little red points of blood would ooze out. In the house hands merely look rough[5] (20th day).

LOWER LIMBS—Feet painful in morning[3] (7th day). Sharp itching in 3rd toe[3] (old symptom, 5th day). Awoke with dull aching in four lesser toes of right foot, acute pain when stepping or moving foot, gradually subsided after bathing in hot water[2] (19th day). Want to put feet up; unconsciously cross the limbs[5] (throughout proving). Profuse foot-sweat, can almost wring the stockings, not acrid nor offensive[5] (12th day). Corn burns and twinges, cannot bear her usual shoes: < in wet weather[5] (21st and several days following).

LIMBS IN GENERAL—Hands and feet get numb early during proving.[2]. Small varicose veins.[5]

NERVES—Extremely restless during night, compelled to move constantly[1] (Rhus—11th day). Not able to rest in bed, must walk the floor to ease mind and yet has no mental trouble[3] (6th day). Restless after stools[7] (11th day). Hysterical fainting at 7-30P.M.[3] (an old symptom—11th day). Fainting from nervousness[6] (30th day).

SLEEP AND DREAMS—Unusually sound sleep during entire night[1] (7th day). The night was full of horrible dreams of drunken people, dead people, naked people, robbers, indecent conduct of men and women[1] (7th day). While sleeping in afternoon the breathing ceased and she awoke suffocating[1] (8th day). Sleepless until 3A.M.[1] (9th day) Wakeful with horrible anxiety and feeling that she must die[1] (many nights). Wakeful until 3 A.M.[1] with anxiety. Sleepless until 1 A.M. (10th day). Sleepless before midnight[1] (11th day). Restless all night, could not lie in one place long enough to go to sleep[1] (12th day). Dreams of wandering in the field with cattle, with fear of being hurt[3] (3rd day). Dreams of male animals following her in the field to injure her[3] (6th day). Wakeful until midnights[3] Dreams of seeing animals copulating (two provers). *Dreams of rape* (confirmed). Late falling to sleep; voluptuous dreams[3] (8th day). Wakeful night with dreams of animals; voluptuous dreams[3] (9th day). Dreams of male and female terrapin. Wakeful, after these dreams of animals[3] (13th day). Dreams of wandering; of naked people; of wild animals pursuing her[3] (14th day). Vivid dreams first night.[2] Vivid, horrible dreams; of dissecting living and dead people; of going up and down ditches; being in peril of engines; woke feeling as though that part of abdomen, the umbilicus, was not sufficiently expanded (constriction)[2] (2nd day). Dreams confused[3] (3rd day). Sleepy at dark[2] (4th day). Dreams, horrible; of the dead; seeing dead infants[2] (5th day). Very sleepy at 9 A.M., can hardly hold eyes open while people are talking to her[2] (6th and 7th days). Dreams vivid and pleasant[2] (13th day). Dreams vivid and fantastic

(6th day). Dreams vivid[5] (6th, 7th, 8th days). Dreames had all the upper incisiors pulled out[7] (8th day). Dreamed all night of snakes, they were coiled ready to strike, was bitten on left hand by one and hand swelled and pulse went upto 160 per minute[7] (9th day). Cold when in bed; not when had my clothes on[7] (10th day). Coldness of body, especially nates, early in bed, 8-30[7] (10th day). Sleepy at 11 A.M., took nap. Biting sensation in left temple on waking[7] (3rd day—30th potency). Sleep all night on left side without moving. Dreams of plotting to fire the town or any building[7] (4th day—30th potency). Tongue dry; saliva running upon the pillow during sleep (unusual). Body always cold in bed since began the proving[7] (5th day—30th potency).

TIME—Suffocating feeling after lying down in the evening[1] (7th day). At 3 P.M., most symptoms; chill, fever, thirst, dry mouth, constriction of neck. Most symptoms better in the morning. Tired at 10 A.M., wants to lie down. During breakfast, cutting pain in left hypochondrium. At 11 A.M. sleepy, took a nap.

CHILL FEVER AND PERSPIRATION—Chill at 3 P.M., icy cold hands and feet.[1] flushes of heat to face and head (1st day). Fever at 3 P.M., lasting until midnight.[1] Fever, afternoon and evening. At 3 P.M., dry mouth and lips, mouth feels parched, intense thirst, pulse 105, choking and sensation as if chest was filling up, causing constriction and difficult breathing[1] (10th day). Considerable chilliness[3] (10th day). Chilly all morning[3] (12th day). Very chilly, shiverings pass over body every few minutes, absent 9 to 10 P.M.[2] (5th day). The body feels flushed, but the contact of cold things is disagreeable, causing chills[2] (7th day). Chilly at night[2] (8th day). Feels flushed all over the body[2] (9th day). Face and hands feverish in afternoon[2] (12th day). At 10 P.M., cold chills in the back and chest, face and hands still burning[2] (12th day). Felt very cold for about a half hour, could not get warm even when wrapped up warinly[2] (12th day). Went to bed at 11 P.M., still feeling feverish[2] (12th day). Awoke at 5 A.M., still feeling flushed with fever[2] (13th day). At 10 P.M., hands hot and dry, nose cold[2] (14th day). Inclined to be chilly all day and more so at night, must keep wrapped warmly, even when feeling feverish[2] (14th day). Chilly at 11 A.M.[2] (16th day). Chilly, shaking and trembling with cold at night in bed[2] (16th day). Shivering in bed, during evening and night, though (10 A.M.) loaded with blankets[2] (17th day). Sensitive to draft of air.[2] Heat and chilly sensations alternate from 6 to 10 P.M.[5] (8th and 9th days). Chilly, yet face is burning[5] (10th day). Chilly, yet heat gives her a dull headache and makes her feel smothered[5] (12th day). Fever, beginning left side of face and spreading over body about 4 P.M.[6] (2nd, 3rd, 4th, 16th, 17th days). Chill from 9 to 11 A.M., worse from least motion, even moving finger[6] (2nd, 3rd, 4th, 16th, 17th days).

SENSATIONS—Sensation of warmth over region of liver[5] (many days). Sense of fluttering and beating, or throbbing in a small spot on the outer side of right thigh, near its middle, commenced at 5 P.M. At 6 and 7 P.M., same sensation under right breast, alternates with that sensation in the thigh. This beating sensation is next felt in left hypochondrium, then in stomach pit, then in right ankle[5] (18th day). Throbbing in left calf[5] (9th day). Throbbing under right breast[5] (21st day). Heat over region of liver extends to heart region[5] (19th day). Cramping sensation[7] (1st day—30th potency). Sensation as though hack were going to have a crick, while sitting on feet, < on left side, had to hold back with hands, soon passed off[7] (3rd day—30th potency). Biting sensation, as of a fly[7] (3rd day—30th potency).

TISSUES—*Abscesses.* Hard pain in left iliac bone[5] (1st day).

TOUGH MOTION AND MODALITIES—Immediately after lying down: suffocation; anxiety; palpitation; sinking; sensation of dying. Horrible anxiety comes over her on lying down at night, also on lying down in afternoon. Must lie with head drawn back, she chokes so. Compelled to move constantly, which seems to quiet for a moment; compelled to change position from restlessness. Sensitive to clothing about the body and neck. Symptoms > from heat, < evening and night. *Restless.* Stomach symptoms > by belching. Catching sensation in back, < by holding with hands.

SKIN—Spot on the right calf became red, then copper-colored; it seemed deep in the skin.[3] Some old scars from a burn, which became blue and deep red during the proving, have again become white.[2] Itching all over the body; flying over the body[2] (10th, 13th days).

GENERALITIES—Feeling of general anxiety throughout the body[1]. Feeling as if the entire body was enlarged to bursting[1]. All symptoms come on when lying down at night[1]. Tired at 10 A.M., wants to lie down. Weak, sick feeling all day[3] (11th day). He lost much flesh, emaciation spreading from above downward, about the neck and face, then mammæ, then thighs and legs. Most of symptoms come after 3 P.M.[1] Weary[2] (4th day). A dog was bitten and an abscess forms upon his neck, which has reopened three times; when it is about to open, he scratches it violently until it opens and discharges a yellow watery fluid. Tight clothing unbearable[2] (throughout the proving). Throbbing in entire body[2] (21st day). So tired, the weight of her clothing is burdensome[5] (4th, 5th, 6th days). Bloated feeling, lasting all day[7] (13th day). Lost from 10 to 20 lbs. during proving[7].

RELATIONSHIP—Chamomilla antidoted its uterine hæmorrhage. Cenchris antidotes Pulsatilla. Amin. c. > general symptoms.

CHAMOMILLA

The general constitutional state of Chamomilla is *great sensitiveness*, sensitive to every impression; sensitive to surroundings; sensitive to persons and, above all, *sensitive to pain*. The constitutional irritability is so great that a little pain brings forth manifestations as if the patient were in very great suffering. It naturally belongs to the woman's nervous system, when she is wrought up and extremely sensitive and in pain.

The mental state goes along with this. Sensitiveness of the mind. Great irritability. These two run through Chamomilla so closely that they are inseparable. *Sensitiveness to pain. Easily affected* by mortification, by chagrin, so that the nerves become extremely sensitive from these causes, and pains, convulsions, colic, headaches and other kinds of nervous symptoms set in. The nervous child when punished will go into convulsions. The oversensitive nervous woman will suffer from chagrin. Jerking and twitching of muscles from mortification and excitement. Excessive sensibility of the nerves, so excessive that only a few remedies equal it, such as *Coffea, Nux vom.* and *Opium*. Of course, without hearing a lecture on *Opium* you naturally think of *Opium* as capable of producing stupor: Those of you who have seen the awful state of mind and distress that follow the administration of the crude *Opium* will understand what I mean by the Chamomilla sensitivity. Convulsions of children. It is not an uncommon thing, even now-a-days, and especially when practicing in the country, for the young mothers and the nurses to give the baby Camomile tea for colic, and the baby goes into convulsions. No one attributes it to Camomile tea, but the doctor will see at once, if he knows Chamomilla, that these convulsions are due to Camomile. Then you see the jerkings. the convulsions are the hot head, the great sensitivity; sensitiveness to noise, and to persons, and the great irritability between the convulsions. Convulsions of children; they become stiff; roll the eyes; distort the face; twitchings of muscles; throw the limbs about; clinch the thumbs; bend the body backwards. Such is the natural appearance of the Chamomilla convulsions; those convulsions that come on in oversensitive children, when they have suffered a good deal of pain from teething. Teething ought to be a perfectly healthy process, but it is really looked upon as a disease, and many doctors carry medicines for "teething children," and administer them; first one and then another. Chamomilla has fallen into that bad use of being given "for teething". It is true that many children suffer from irritability of the brain, convulsions, stomach disorders and vomiting about the time of dentition, but I say dentition should not be a diseased state, it should be normal. If they were in health they would cut teeth without sufferings. But slow teething we have to contend with, and that irritable state, that oversensitiveness, so that the child does not sleep. Wakes up as if it had awful dreams. Wakes up in excitement, vomits, has diarrhœa green, slimy diarrhœa, like chopped grass. Offensive diarrhœa with teething. These symptoms come at this time when the child has not been properly looked after. Or perhaps the mother has not been properly qualified for parturition. "Tetanic convulsions.

Twitching in the eyelids. Pain in the limbs. General prostration, faintness."
Neuralgic pains all over the body with numbness. Twitching, darting, tingling
pains. The pains are mostly ameliorated by heat, with the exception of the teeth
and jaws. Toothache, pain in the teeth ameliorated by cold, and made worse by
heat. But the earaches and pains in the extremities are made better by heat.

You will see in the text under "Temperature and Weather" the symptom
"Pains are worse from heat," with two black bars as if it were the most important
symptom in it, and then below, without any bar, "Sensitive to cold. Chilly." and
"Better from heat;" but the fact is the pains that are worse from heat are about
the teeth and jaws, and it is decidedly a particular symptom relating only to a
part; whereas it is true that the patient in the general state, entirely contrary to
what this says, is better by heat. The pains in general are better by heat. The
patient himself is better by heat. Consequently, this being a particular, it should
state that the pains that are so commonly worse by heat are of the teeth.

The most important part of Chamomilla is the mental state. It pervades the
whole economy and you will see that every region that is taken up, every part
that is studied, brings into it the mental state of the patient. This remedy has
more mental symptoms than symptoms in any other part. Crying. "Piteous
moaning. Irritable." The irritability is so great that it manifests itself sometimes
in a very singular way. The patient seems to be driven to frenzy by the pains,
and she forgets all about her prudence and her diplomacy. Loss of generosity;
she has no consideration for the feelings of others. She will simply enter into
a quarrel or dispute regardless of the feelings of anybody. So, when you go
into practice, do not be surprised when you go to the bedside of a patient in
labor, who is full of pains and sufferings, if she says: "Doctor, I don't want
you, get out." Just such a one will pass under other circumstances as a lady.
The awful pains that she is having drive her to frenzy, and this frenzy, this
oversensitiveness to pain, is coupled with the mental state. Inability to control
her temper, and the temper is aroused to white heat. Now, in the child, the
child whines and cries and sputters about everything. It wants something
new every minute. It refuses everything that it has asked for. If it is for
something to eat, for something to play with, for its toys, when these are
handed to the child it throws them away; slings them clear across the room.
Strikes the nurse in the face for presuming to get something or other that the
little one did not want, yet had asked for. *Capriciousness.* It seems that the
pains and sufferings are sometimes ameliorated by passive motion, this very
particularly in children. The pains seem to be better when the child is carried,
so the child wants to be carried all the time. This is true in the colic and in the
bowel troubles. It is true with earache; it is true with the evening fevers, and
the general sufferings from cold and conditions while teething. *Children must
be carried.* The nurse is compelled to carry the child all the time. And then

there is the restlessness and capriciousness about the members of the family. The child goes two or three times up and down the room with the nurse, and then reaches our for its mother; goes two or three times up and down the room with her and then wants to go to its father. And so it is changing about. Never satisfied. It seems to have no peace. When it has earache the sharp shooting pains cause the child to screech out. Carries the hand to the ear. The pains often cause that sharp, piercing tone of the voice. Adults in pain cannot keep still, the pains are so severe; it is not always that they are decidedly ameliorated by moving, but they seem to be. But they move because they cannot keep still. So the Chamomilla patient is tossing in bed, if in bed; not an instant quiet. And along with all of these the same irritability; becomes violently excited at the pain; angry at the pain; irritable about the pain; will scold about the pain; the pain is so torturesome. Aversion to talk, and snappish. The patient is constantly sitting and looking within herself when pains are absent.

Chamomilla has melancholy, and has suffering of the mind, without pain. Then the Chamomilla patient sits and thinks within herself—a sort of introspection. Cannot be induced to say a word. Sadness. The Chamomilla child cannot be touched. Wants to do as he pleases. Wants to change; wants to do something new. The answer from both the adult and the child are snappish. Complaints come on from contradiction; from anger. Convulsions come on from anger. If the child is suffering from whooping cough it will have a coughing spell, a spasmodic cough from being irritated. Goes into a spunky state, gets red in the face, and then gets to coughing. Peevishness. "Quarrelsome. Easily chagrined or excited to anger. Bad effects of having the feelings wounded." Such is the mental state, and, as I have remarked, that mental state will be found wherever there is an inflammatory condition that Chamomilla fits. In pneumonia, in bronchitis, laryngitis, inflammations of the ear, erysipelas, headaches, fevers, Chamomilla is capable of curing when the mental state is present, and the symptoms, in particular, are present.

The headaches of Chamomilla are found in sensitive people, sensitive women. Nervous; overstrained; overtired. Fidgety. Excitable women that suffer from pain. A little headache seems an enormous thing. Throbbing, tearing, bursting pains. Congestive headaches. Worse when thinking of the pain, or when thinking about the sufferings. The headaches are worse evenings. A particular time in the evening for many complaints to be worse is 9 o'clock. Sometimes 9 o'clock in the morning, and sometimes 9 in the evening. Fever conditions .worse 9 o'clock in the morning. Pains worse in the evening, and especially worse about 9 o'clock. Stitching, tearing pains in the temples and head. Wandering pains in the temples. Pressing pain in the head as soon as attention was directed to it, better by busying the mind at something else, or by occupation; forcing one's self to do something, and to think of something

CHAMOMILLA

else. Congestion to the head. Violent neuralgia of the face, teeth, ear, sides of the head. Pains inside of the mouth are ameliorated by cold. Pains of the ear and sides of the head are ameliorated by heat; earache ameliorated by heat.

There are pains in the eyes. Inflammation of the eyes with bleeding. Oozing of a bloody water from the eyes of the new born infant. Chamomilla will cure if there is irritability of the temper. Profuse acrid discharges; yellow discharges; discharges of purulent matter from the eyes. Violent pressure in the orbit. Lachrymation accompanying coryza with sneezing. Stuffing up of the nose. Headaches, irritability. Associated with the above is a symptom: "Face red and hot on one side, the other side pale." Like the whole constitution of the remedy there is a great sensitiveness of hearing. Roaring, ringing and singing in the ears. Stitching pains in the ears, ameliorated by heat. Pressing earache. You will see the little one when the pain comes on put its hands up to its ears, and spitefully moaning, yelling and screaming. Violent pains in the ear. When old enough to talk about it will complain of heat in the ear, and a feeling of fulness as if the ear were obstructed or stuffed up. In adults, nervous, sensitive women who cannot ride in the wind without covering up their ears. The ears are so sensitive to air when other parts of the face and head are not sensitive to air. You will find some patients that cannot have air touch the neck. Others have extra covering between the shoulders. Chamomilla singles out the ears. The whole body is sensitive to air and to cold, and he wants to dress with plenty of covering.

Sneezing, watery coryza. Hot face on one side, and often with pains in the head and jaws. Fluent coryza, viscid, acrid, with loss of smell. Loss of smell lasting while the cold lasts.

Rending pains in the face, sometimes involving the teeth and the outer face at the same time. It is not an uncommon thing to have a very sensitive woman if she is disturbed by chagrin, if she has been vexed by her servant, to go to her room and suffer tortures from pain in the face from that excitement, from anger. If it is the outer nerves in the face the pains will be ameliorated by heat; but when it affects the teeth the pains will he ameliorated by cold. Heat of the face, while the rest of the body is cold. "The face sweats after eating or drinking." It is common feature of this remedy to sweat only about the head, the hairy scalp. Sometimes during measles or scarlet fever we will have Chamomilla manifestations. Sweating about the head, face red on one side. "One-sided swelling of the cheek;" that is, an inflammatory attack, gets redder and redder, and finally purple, going into erysipelas, with the mental symptoms. Hot face, redness of one side. Burning in the face. Neuralgia of the face. If anything warm is taken into the mouth it will bring on aching in the teeth, and sometimes burning and throbbing in the roots of the teeth; tearing, stitching, stinging pains, aggravated by talking; aggravated in the open air; aggravated in a warm room, or getting warm in bed, anything that heats up the body will aggravate this toothache; ameliorated by holding cold drinks in the mouth. Toothache that is entirely absent in the daytime; as soon as it comes night, and the patient gets into the warm bed, then these shooting, tearing pains begin; with the irritability, oversensitiveness to pain, the mental, state, hot head, you have the Chamomilla toothache. "Swelling and inflammation of the gums. Threatened abscess of the gums. Toothache when coming into a warm room," when it has been better in the cold air. This toothache is one that may be brought on by taking cold, by exposing one's self to cold air when sweating; and yet the toothache itself when present is ameliorated by cold. "Toothache from a draft of air." "Ameliorated from eating cold things. Worse before midnight." The most of the troubles of Chamomilla that come on in the evening and night subside about or sometimes before midnight. From midnight to morning almost all of the complaints of Chamomilla are absent. Many of them are absent during the day. It has aggravation in the *fore-part of the night.* "Teeth feel too long. Swollen gums." The Chamomilla infant will often hold a glass of cold water against the gums. The little one has inflamed gums, painful gums, the coming forth of the teeth is painful, and it seems to want to prolong the cold in the mouth; when it is so young you would not think it would realize the good of making use of the cold edge of the glass. Offensive fœtid smell from the mouth.

The spasms that affect the child all over are likely to affect the larynx, and sometimes affect the larynx without affecting the child anywhere else. "Spasms of the larynx during cough, or without cough. Spasmodic constriction of the larynx. Choking. Spasms of the throat. Sore and inflamed." Chamomilla cures sore throat when the throat is of a uniform redness, spreading pretty evenly over the whole throat, with considerable swelling. Inflammation of tonsils. Much redness; when the mental state is present. It will never cure a sore throat except in these irritable constitutions, such as suffer from pain, such as are easily angered in a constant fret. The Chamomilla mental state determines when you are to give Chamomilla in sore throat.

"Want of appetite. Great thirst for cold water and desire for acid drinks. Unquenchable thirst." Aversion to coffee, warm drinks, to soups and liquid foods. The aversion to coffee is a strange thing. Chamomilla and coffee are very much alike in the general sensitivity of the economy. They antidote each other. When persons have been overdrinking coffee, nurses drinking coffee to keep up at night to take care of the patient; persons overdrinking coffee when tired and overworked, Chamomilla is its antidote. "Thirsty, and hot with the pains." When the Pains come, no matter where. she heats up, and sometimes becomes really feverish. Face red, especially on one side. Head hot; extreme irritability.

Chamomilla has much vomiting. Eructations of gas which smells like sulphuretted hydrogen. The Chamomilla patient has violent retching. Making violent efforts to vomit. Seems that it will tear the stomach. Covered with cold sweat. Exhausted. That is just what *Morphine* does. If you have ever seen a patient who has been overdosed by a doctor—I hope that you will never see one that has been overdosed by yourself. Do not make a case, you will have one soon enough—but if you get into a town where there is an allopathic physician, and he happens to give *Morphine* to one of these oversensitive patients; it may relieve her pain for a little while, but on will come the awful eructations, and she will retch and vomit, and continue to retch when there is nothing to vomit. Chamomilla will stop that, the first dose, in a few minutes, and it is the only remedy you will need. It will always stop the vomiting from *Morphine after the* crude effect of *Morphine* has passed away and the vomiting comes.

Colic, especially in the little ones, in the infants. Pain in the stomach and abdomen. The child doubles up, and screams, and kicks; wants to be carried; is extremely irritable; attack comes on in the evening; one side of the face red, the other side pale; wants things, and when they are given does not want them; and you have a Chamomilla colic. It is a wind colic. It lasts a fraction of a minute, and then it straightens out again. It shows, that it is a cramp, a wind cramp. In adults, who have felt these symptoms, they are said to be cutting, burning, griping. Griping pains. Of course, such are the pains that are called colicky. Cramps in the bowels. Griping pains. Sometimes griping as if must go to stool. The abdomen distended like a drum. Sometimes ameliorated by warm applications. "Colic while urinating;" that is an uncommon symptom. "Colic in the morning. Tympanitic abdomen."

The most striking Chamomilla stool is *grass green, or* like chopped eggs, or like these two chopped up; yellow and white, intermingled with mucus that is grass green, like chopped grass; chopped spinach. Greenish, slimy discharges, greenish water. Those old enough to express themselves in the proving said that the stool felt hot while it passed. It smells like sulphuretted hydrogen. Copious stool; scanty stool, with dysenteric straining. Watery diarrhœa, six or eight passages daily. Mucous diarrhœa. Green, watery stool, fæces and mucus. "Yellowish brown stool." Also constipation, with no ability to strain. A paralytic weakness of the rectum; inactivity of the rectum. Much itching and rawness about the parts, especially in the evening. Anus is "pouting," with swollen appearance and redness.

The woman, such as I have described, oversensitive to pain, snappish, suffering intensely from a little pain, takes on many symptoms at the menstrual period. The menstrual flow is black, clotted, offensive. Cramping pains in the uterus, clutching and griping, ameliorated by heat. "Oversensitive to pain," with all the pains and complaints, and the mental state, the irritability, the snappish mental state at a menstrual period. Whether it be a menorrhagia, or a metrorrhagia, there are copious black clots. "Menstrual colic following anger," which means violent cramping pains in the uterus during menstruation if she has had any great excitement to anger her. Sexual irritability, emotions, disturbance of mind, will bring on cramps at the menstrual period in a woman who is not subject to cramps, affecting her as if she had taken cold. It is a very useful remedy in membranous dysmenorrhœa. It, perhaps, has existed from the first menstrual period. Every month the woman throws off a little membranous formation. This is thrown off with violent labor-like pains, and often with clots. Chamomilla may be a palliative. It is not the constitutional remedy that clears away, and prevents the future formation of this membrane, like the deeper anti-psorics, but it is often palliative in the more severe attacks, with the irritable condition of the mind; feverish condition ameliorated by heat; cramping, and clutching like labor pains. "Yellow, smarting leucorrhœa. Excessive menstruation; blood dark, nearly black, clotted, with pain through from back to front, attacks of syncope, coldness of limbs, much thirst."

In pregnancy the woman has also Chamomilla conditions. Irregular contractions; false labor pains. Labor pains that are felt in wrong places. Labor pains that are felt too much in the back. Contractions that are most painful, cutting, tearing, bringing out screams. So irritable; she scolds the pains; she scolds the doctor; she scolds everybody; drives the doctor out of the room; drives the nurse off, and then calls for her again; refuses things that are offered. Labor pains that are clutching here, and clutching there, and cramping, showing that certain fibres of the uterus are contracting in one direction, and certain other fibres in another. There is not that uniform, regular contraction that should take place in the expulsion of the contents of the uterus; expulsion of a mole or expulsion of a child. If the physician can have the pregnant woman under his care during the period of gestation he ought to be able to select remedies to remove these irregular contractions of the uterus, or to prevent them when it comes time for labor. The pains are then not so violent. She feels the contractions, but in many instances they are painless. You will not always be able to prepare women, they will not always permit it. Women are more inclined to be notional and whimsical and to have their own way a short time before confinement than at any other time. A woman ought to be under treatment all through gestation, and sometimes it takes longer. Gestation is a fortuitous time for the woman to take treatment. Symptoms representative of her disordered state come out then that do not appear at any other time. If she has a psoric condition it may remain dormant until pregnancy comes on, which may act as an exciting cause to bring out the conditions that are in the constitution. It furnishes, therefore, a good time for the homœopathic physician to study the case and give that woman a constitutional remedy based upon those symptoms that will not only remove those symptoms and prepare her for confinement, but will remove very much of the disorder in her economy, and she will go on through life liberated from much distress, cured from many conditions that perhaps would not have come out until some other occasion brought them out. A woman that knows much about Homœopathy would submit herself regularly to constitutional treatment during gestation, that is, would be particular to give the physician everything, all the details, all the sufferings, all the trouble, that he may study that case. The things that are to be observed during gestation are to be added to the constitutional symptoms found when gestation is not present, because they are all evidence of a disturbance in that one patient. And it is the *patient* that is to he treated, not a disease. It is simply another form of disturbance, of disorder of the economy. The things that Chamomilla reaches during confinement, and during its course, and at the close of it, are irregular contractions, like hour-glass contractions. "Rigidity of the os." After confinement, after-pains. With all these the same mental condition, the same oversensitiveness to pain. "Post-partum hæmorrhage." Every time the child is put to the breast, cramping of the uterus; cramp in the back. Either of these, or both, Chamomilla cures. The two principal remedies you will have to rely on for these conditions, cramping in the back and cramping in the abdomen every time the child is put to the breast, are Chamomilla and *Pulsatilla.* They are two decidedly different remedies in the mental sphere. One is mild and gentle, though whimsical; and the other is snappish and irritable. Both are sensitive to pain, but Chamomilla is far more sensitive to pain than *Pulsatilla.*

Chamomilla has inflammation of the mammary glands. You cannot prescribe for that unless you have something along with it, and I am sure you will recognize a Chamomilla *patient.* The woman goes into convulsions. At the beginning of the confinement the husband comes into the room in some snappish way, "to make his wife behave herself; it makes her mad, and she goes into convulsions. The doctor, perhaps, has just turned his back upon it, but now he says, "Well, why did I not think to give this woman a dose of Chamomilla? If I had done that I would have prevented these convulsions." She becomes very philosophical after a dose of Chamomilla, and often goes to sleep.

There are many suffocative attacks and difficulties of breathing, inflammation of the larynx, etc., that you can read up easily. The cough of Chamomilla has some striking things in it. It is a hard cough, a dry, hacking cough. The child goes to sleep at night and coughs and does not wake up. Coughs in its sleep. It is a little feverish, has taken cold, and one side of the face is flushed. It is crabbed when it is awake. The child becomes angry when it has a cold and a little cough, and a little disturbance of the larynx and bronchial tubes has been noticed coming on, and all at once it becomes more excitable, wants to be carried, and if not pleased, or is angered, it will go into a hard coughing spell, and cough and vomit. "Coughing spells from anger." That is, he coughs when there is already a cold or a cough, and if the patient becomes angry he has a fit of coughing. The coughing complaints, and chest complaints, and laryngeal complaints are generally worse at night. The feverish condition comes on at night with the Chamomilla colds, with the Chamomilla whooping cough, with the Chamomilla chest complaints. Most of the complaints of Chamomilla are better after midnight. From 9 o'clock to midnight they are worse. "Dry cough worse at night and during sleep." Dry cough from catching cold. Rough, scraping cough of children in winter, with tickling in suprasternal fossa, worse at night. Dry cough, continuing during sleep. Amelioration of cough when getting warm in bed. Chamomilla is a very common remedy in whooping cough, where the child wants to be carried; keeps the nurse busy all the time. Coughs and gags and vomits, and it is very irritable and capricious in all of its wants and coughs during sleep.

You can now easily detect the chest symptoms. They go with the mental symptoms and the irritability and cough. The cough in the chest is scarcely different from the cough in the larynx and the cough from cold. It is the same Chamomilla cough. *Cough during sleep.* During most of the complaints, fevers, colds, acute complaints and little attacks, burning of the extremities. Stitching pains in the limbs. Cramping in the muscles. Limbs go to sleep. With the pains in the limbs, and sometimes in other parts, but particularly in the limbs, *a benumbed feeling,* or pains with the feeling of deadness, pains accompanied by a benumbed feeling, sometimes almost complete loss of sensation of the skin, yet the pains in the long nerves, in the extremities are very violent, and the patient seems just as sensitive to pain as at other times. Extremely sensitive to pain, but the pains themselves cause a *benumbing feeling to follow them.* It has been called in older books a paralyzing pain. Convulsions of the extremities. Convulsions of the whole body. "Cramps in the legs and calves. Tearing pains in the feet following a severe chill. Burning of the soles at night; puts the feet out of bed." All the routine prescribers whenever the patient is known to put the feet out of bed *give Sulphur,* yet there is a large list of remedies with hot feet, burning soles, and all of them will put the feet out of bed, of course, to cool them off. There is no reason why they should all get *Sulphur.*

Another feature of the pains that come on at night, sometimes before midnight is, they are so violent that he cannot keep still. When the child has pains he wants to be carried, that seems to do him good. When the adult has pains at night in bed he gets up and walks the floor. Benumbing pains, pains ameliorated by heat, pains that drive him out of bed at night, with twitchings of the limbs. Oversensitiveness to pain. Great irritability. The Chamomilla patient cannot go to sleep at night. He is sleepy, like *Bell., but* he cannot sleep. If he quiets down during the day he wants to go to sleep. But as soon as the time comes to go to bed he is wide awake, he is sleepless and restless at night, especially the fore part. At times the Chamornilla patient becomes so full of visions and so much excited during the fore part of the night in his efforts to go to sleep that when he does go to sleep he jerks and twitches and has horrid dreams, and is full of sufferings. "Anxious dreams. Sees horrible apparitions and starts: dreams about fatal accidents." Worn out mentally from trying to go to sleep, and he is tired out.

CHELIDONIUM

Chelidonium is a remedy more suitable for acute diseases, though it cures certain chronic conditions. It is not a very deep acting remedy. It is about like *Brvonia* in its general plane, length and depth of action. It has been used principally in gastric and intestinal catarrhs, in acute and semichronic liver troubles, and in right-sided pneumonia. The skin is likely to be sallow, and gradually increases to a marked jaundice in connection with these complaints. Semi-chronic gastritis, with jaundice. "Gastro-duo-denal catarrh. Congestion and soreness in the liver, with jaundice. Right-sided pneumonia, complicated with liver troubles, or jaundice." This remedy seems to act throughout the system, but almost always along with it the liver is involved, and it is suitable for what the old people and the doctors called "biliousness". The patient is generally bilious, has nausea and vomiting. Distension of the veins. Yellowish grey color of the skin.

Very few mental symptoms have been brought out in its proving, not enough to give us a good idea of the desires and aversions. We do not get a clear idea of the intellectual faculties. It needs further proving, yet in many regions it has had superabundance of proving. "Sadness and anxiety." Brooding over some sort of trouble generally runs through the mental state. "Anxiety, allowing no rest," keeping the patient uneasy day and night. Sadness, as if she had committed a crime; as if some dreadful thing was going to happen. So sad that she thinks she must die. Weeping despondency. Distaste for mental exertion and conversation. If you examine those medicines that act primarily upon the liver, that slow down the action of the liver, you will find the word "melancholia". With heart troubles, great excitement. With liver troubles, slowing down of the mental state, inability of the mind to work, sluggishness of the mind, inability to think, inability to meditate, slow pulse. Sluggishness of the whole economy. The sensorium is very commonly disturbed, and the patient is dizzy. "Things go round in a circle." Dizziness comes, and it does not let up until nausea, and sometimes vomiting, follows. "So much turning in the head that he vomits. Confusion of mind. Loss of consciousness and fainting." These are also common features with liver troubles.

The mind symptoms are present more or less with the following liver symptoms: There are pains of a dull aching character, "soreness". Bruised pains. Tenderness of the liver to touch. Aching pains, that seem to involve the whole right lobe of the liver; creating a sensation of fulness. Pressure upwards, with difficulty of breathing. Pressure downwards, sympathetic with the stomach, with the nausea and vomiting. And then more intense pain felt *under the right scapula.* "Dull aching pains under the right scapula; sharp, shooting pains under the right scapula;" these complicate themselves again with pneumonia, with pleurisy. It cures pneumonia and pleurisy; it cures various forms of congestion in the liver, when these pains go from before backward, and seem to be felt through the back. "Stitching in the region of the liver, extending through to back. Hard pains felt through the back." Some patients will describe these pains as shooting pains; some as tearing pains, and others as sharp pains, going through the right hypochondrium or through the right lobe of the liver to the back. "Pains from the region of the liver, shooting towards the back and shoulders. Spasmodic pain in the region of the liver. Pressing pain in the region of the liver." In congestion or inflammation, fulness and enlargement, semi-chronic cases, or even acute, this medicine proves suitable for such conditions. The right hypochondrium is tense and painful to pressure.

This remedy has cured gall-stone colic. Practitioners, who know how to direct a remedy, relieve gall-stone colic in a few minutes. We have remedies that act on the circular fibers of these little tubes, causing them to relax and allow the stone to pass painlessly. In a perfect state of health, of course, there are no stones in the bile that is held in the gall-bladder, but this little cystic duct opens its mouth and a little gall-stone engages in it, and it creates an irritation by scratching along the mucous membrane of that little tube. When this pain is a shooting, stabbing, tearing, lancinating pain, extending through to the back, Chelidonium will cure it. The instant it relieves the patient says: "Why, what a relief; the pain has gone." The remedy has relieved that spasm, the little duct opens up and the stone passes out through the ductus communis choledochus. Every remedy that is indicated by the symptoms will cure gall-stone colic.

A patient lying in bed, with great heat, extreme sensitiveness, cannot have the body touched, screaming with pain, red face and hot head, with gall-stone colic, will be relieved in three minutes by *Bell.,* but that is not at all like this remedy. *Natrum sulph.* and many other remedies have cured gall-stone colic in a few minutes, when the symptoms agree.

Now as to the pneumonia, it is generally of the right side, or right-sided spreading to the left. The right-sidedness is marked, and but small portions of the left lung are involved. The pleura is generally involved, and so there are stitching, tearing pains. One may not practice long before he will find a Chelidonium patient, sitting up in bed with high fever, bending forward upon his elbows, holding himself perfectly still, for this medicine has as much aggravation from motion as *Bry.* All of the pains are extremely aggravated from motion. This patient is sitting with a pain that transfixes him; he cannot stir, he cannot move without the pain shooting through him like a knife. The next day you will see that his skin is growing yellow. If you see him in the beginning Chelidonium will relieve him and you will prevent that pneumonia. It is not uncommon in children, and it is extremely common in adults.

Do not get confused with *Bryonia.* Both are violently worse from motion. *Bryonia* wants to lie on the painful side, or wants to lie on the back if the pneumonia is mostly in the posterior part of the right lung. In Chelidonium he is worse from touch and motion.

Bell. has that extremely painful, tearing, rending of the right lung with pleurisy, but in *Bell.,* one cannot touch that right side, cannot press it, but must lie on the other side and he cannot move. Cannot stand a jar of the bed, because of the extreme sensitiveness to motion. I mention all three in this particular way because they have some things in common, but the remedies are different.

Chelidonium has cough with chest symptoms *of the right side,* liver affections, and the mental affections that commonly belong to these, violent aggravation from motion. The pains are ameliorated by heat. Pain that extends to the stomach, ameliorated by heat. Mental symptoms ameliorated by eating. Craves hot milk; hot fluids. Eating warm food ameliorates the liver, the chest and stomach symptoms.

"Bilious vomiting. Retching; bilious eructations. Nausea and retching during an attack of anxiety." These are all commonly present during the complaints described. The pains, when they become severe, seem to strike the stomach and cause vomiting. Ameliorated by something hot. "A feeling of anguish in the pit of the stomach. Persistent pain in the stomach; aggravated by motion and ameliorated by eructations. Constriction and sensitiveness in the pit of the stomach." These are all aggravated by touch and ameliorated by eating. "Constant aching pain in the stomach, ameliorated by food. Constrictive, pinching pain in the stomach better from drawing up the limbs and lying on the left side, ameliorated by eating."

It has many eye symptoms. Stitching pains. "Opacity of the cornea." Inflammations. "Bruised pain in the eyes. Right supra-orbital neuralgia. In many instances it prefers the right side.

In the face the jaundice is the most marked thing that is expressed; and, then, we have the dirty gray complexion. "Pale, dirty-yellow face."

The headaches are brought on from heat, unlike the stomach and the liver, and the lungs, etc. The head is aggravated from motion, aggravated from heat, aggravated from a warm room, aggravated from warm applications. There is where it differs from the internal or general state. There are numerous headaches. Periodical bilious sick headaches, with vomiting of bile, brought on from exposure to heat, from being overheated, aggravated from motion, wants to lie perfectly quiet in a dark room, and better from vomiting bile. Old-fashioned bilious sick headaches.

Bilious diarrhœa. Along with jaundice, clay-like, pale, fæcal, putty-like stool. Bileless stool. Stool too light colored. Stool quite white in children. Diarrhœa and constipation alternate. Stool brown, white, watery, green mucus, thin, pasty, bright yellow, or gray tinged with yellow.

Hoarseness. "While coughing, pain in the larynx, and pressure in the larynx."

The difficult breathing comes on with liver symptoms and pneumonia and chest troubles in general. "Difficult respiration, with short fits of coughing. Short, quick breathing. Anxiety as if he must choke. Difficult breathing; tightness over the chest as if breathing would be hindered." It has also nightly attacks of humid asthma. This is brought on from every change of the weather. All its complaints are brought on from changes in the weather. He cannot stand weather changes, either too cold or too warm. Rheumatic complaints in the shoulders, hips and limbs, from changes in the weather.

With complaints of the liver, lungs and chest, there are coughs. They are spasmodic. The chronic cough is violent, spasmodic, dry, coming in paroxysms. "Spasmodic cough, without expectoration." After it has existed a while there will be some expectoration. "Repeated attacks of short cough. Short cough, with little grayish phlegm. Rattling, fatiguing cough."

In the limbs there are rheumatic and neuralgic pains. Neuralgia of the limbs in general, most violent. Limbs feel heavy and stiff. Limbs flabby. Later the patient runs down somewhat, weak heart, weak circulation; dropsical conditions of the limbs. Great restlessness. "Trembling and twitching of the limbs. Weariness. Indolence. Indisposition to work."

The neuralgias are more common in the head and face than in the lower parts of the body, in the limbs and in extremities.

It has sharp, febrile attacks, such as found in pneumonia with chill; and in inflammation of the liver. It has cured intermittent fever, coming in the afternoon and evening.

Itching of the skin. Jaundice. It has cured old putrid ulcers.

CHINIUM ARSENISOCUM

Complaints come on at night. Open air aggravates most complaints. General increasing anaemia. Inflamed parts turn black. *Chlorosis. Sensitive to cold,* and complaints are worse from cold and from becoming cold. Tendency to take cold.

This is a useful remedy in weakly constitutions. Cold, pale, emaciated people. In prolonged suppuration; after hæmorrhages. Chronic diarrhœa, when the weakness is the most prominent feature. Fulness of blood vessels. Dropsy in sacs, or *œdema*. Emaciation. Cannot sustain a physical exertion. Faints on slight provocation. Wants to be warm; wants warm drinks and warm food. Warm room ameliorates. Wants to lie down. Aversion to motion. Stitching and tearing pains. Periodicity is most marked. Pulsation all over the body. Pulse fast, *feeble and irregular.* Relaxed and flabby (*Calc.*). Sensitive to pain. Many symptoms come during sleep. Standing increases many symptoms. *Sensitive to touch. Trembling.* Walking in the open air aggravates. Weakness from walking. Complaints come on in windy, stormy weather.

Easily angered, and refuses to talk or to answer questions. Anxiety day and night, but worse in the evening, worse during chill; anxiety with fear. Anxiety during fever, even becomes wild. Anxiety on waking. Desires things which he cares nothing for after he gets them. Becomes critical with his most intimate friends. Complaining. Confusion of mind in the morning on waking. Over-conscientious about trifles (*Silicea, Thuja*). Delirious at night; after haemorrhage. Many imaginations, illusions of fancy: sees images, frightful images. Despair during chill, heat and,suffering. Discontented with everything. Discouraged easily, and faint-hearted. Dulness of mind. Becomes excited over small matters. Exaltation of fancy. Fear at night that evil will come to him; fear of ghosts. Forgetful. Mind overwhelmed with ideas at night. Impatience in intermittent fever. Becomes indifferent ro all enjoyment. Aversion to work. *Irritable* during chill, and on waking. Jumps out of bed during the fever. Moaning during the chill and the fever. Loathing of life. Weakness of memory. He is easily offended, and looks for insults. Great restlessness at night, and during fever. Anxious restlessness, driving him out of bed; driving to despair. Extreme sadness, especially during chill and fever, and sometimes during the sweat. Over-sensitiveness to noise, and in general. Sentimental. Mental symptoms from sexual excesses, and loss of vital fluids. Refuses to talk, and remains silent. Sits by the hour in silence without moving. Wandering speech. Starting on falling asleep, and waking as from fright. Lies in bed in a state of stupefaction in low forms of fever. Suicidal disposition. Suspicious. Persistent thoughts. Timid. Weary of life. Weeping. The chilliness is brought on by thinking of it. The headache is worse by mental exertion.

Vertigo comes in the evening, with nausea; while walking in the open air. Cerebral congestion with great heat of the head. The forehead becomes cold and covered with sweat. Constriction of the head. Great heat in the forehead. Heaviness in the head in the morning. Motion is felt in the brain on moving the head. Sensation of rushing in the brain, down right side of the neck and arm becoming convulsive, and ending in real convulsion. Violent darting pains in the head preventing sleep. Pain in the whole head. Pain; in the morning on waking, in the afternoon, but most severe at night. Night headaches. Cold air brings on the head pains. The scalp is sensitive to touch, to combing the hair, and to binding up the hair during the suffering. Catarrhal headache. Pain very severe during the chill and heat, but ameliorated as the sweat becomes free. Pains worse or brought on from becoming cold. With coryza the pain is violent; worse coughing or jarring, after eating. Hammering headaches. Headaches during menses. Mental exertion aggravates the headache. Nervous headache, and headache from *excitement or noise.* Paroxysmal pains. *Periodical* headaches; headache every two weeks. Pulsating pains. Pains worse walking. Neuralgic pains, worse in left side, ameliorated by rubbing. Aching felt deep in the head. Pains in the forehead, mostly on the right side; in *occiput* after sleep; in sides of head in the evening; in temples and forehead; in vertex. Bruised pain all over the head after fever, and after sleep. Burning pain in left occipital region extending down the neck in the morning. Bursting pain. Press-ing pain. Pressing in the forehead; over the eyes. Pressing in the occiput and temples. Stitching and tearing pains in the head. Perspiration on the forehead. Complaints come on from uncovering the head in cold air.

Inflamed eyes. Lachrymation. Intense photophobia and spasms of orhicularis muscles. Gushing hot tears. Large ulcers on each eye, worst from midnight until 3 A.M. Scrofulous ophthalmia, worse after I A.M. Flickering before the left eye. Pain in the eyes at night. *Burning pains.* Pressing. Sunken eyes. Dim vision. Sparks before the eyes. *Weak vision.*

Noises in the ears; buzzing, humming, ringing, *roaring, singing.* Stitching in the ears. Earache. Pain burning, *stitching, tearing.* Hearing acute. Hearing impaired.

Coryza with discharge. *Dry coryza.* Nasal catarrh with bloody discharge, or *purulent* discharge. Dryness in the nose. Epistaxis. Nose obstructed. Sneezing. Excoriation of the corners of the nose. Especially useful for periodical coryza and frequent taking cold in the nose which keeps a catarrh in constant activity.

Chlorotic face. Cracked lips. Bluish lips. Pale earthy face. Circumscribed red cheeks with pale face. Sickly color of face. Jaundiced face. Expression anxious. The pains of the face are worse in the open air; burning, tearing.

Periodical pains. Swelling of sub-maxillary and parotid glands. Perspiration cold. Œdema of face. Ulceration of the lips.

Burning canker sores in the mouth. Bleeding from mucous membranes of the mouth. Cracked tongue. *Tongue black,* brown, white or yellow. Dry mouth and tongue. Hot mouth. Burning rawness of the tongue. *Sore tongue.* Salivation. *Swollen gums* and *tongue.* Taste bad, *bitter* while eating; insipid, metallic, saltish, *sour,* sweetish. Vesicles on the tongue. Pain in the teeth at night, < by biting the teeth together, from touch; cold drinks. Pains come on periodically, are jerking, *pulsating.* tearing, and date back to malarial fever.

Contraction in the throat. Dryness in the throat. Gangrenous inflammation of the throat with putrid odor, in malignant scarlet fever. The throat feels hot. This remedy has been used in diphtheria when the exudation was blackish, and putrid odor from the mouth. *Great pain on swallowing.* Burning in the throat. Stitching in the throat on swallowing. Difficult swallowing. Swollen throat. Constant clearing of the throat.

Appetite diminished, or *ravenous.* No appetite for breakfast. Strong appetite without relish of food. Aversion to rich food and fats; *aversion to food, to meat.* Desires wine; *cold drinks,* sour things, sweet things. Sensation of coldness in the stomach. Emptiness, better by eating. Eructations after eating, *bitter,* empty, of food, *sour.* Waterbrash. Sensation of fulness after eating. Heartburn. Great weight in the stomach after eating. Hiccough. Stomach easily disordered. Cannot digest eggs or fish. Water tastes bitter. Nausea after eating, during headache. Pain in the stomach from coughing; *after eating.* Burning; cramping; *pressing, soreness;* stitching, tearing. Pulsating. Retching with cough. Strong *thirst,* in the evening, during *perspiration;* for small drinks during heat. Vomiting at night, on coughing, *after drinking, after eating,* with headache; of *bile, black, blood, food,* mucus; *sour;* water. Nausea and vomiting followed by sleep. Sudden inclination to vomit at 2 P.M.

Sensation of coldness in the abdomen during chill. *Distension* morning, after eating, *tympanitis, ascites;* enlarged liver and spleen from malarial influences. *Flatulence* in intermittent fever. Fulness in the abdomen. *Hardness of the liver.* Heaviness as from a load in the abdomen after eating. Great pain in the abdomen during chill, like colic; during diarrhœa; after eating; before stool; ameliorated by lying on the abdomen. Great pain in the region of the liver, in the hypogastrium, in the region of the umbilicus. The kinds of pain in the abdomen are burning, cramping, cutting, dragging; *soreness;* stitching. *Much rumbling* and tension.

Constipation, with hard, knotty stools. *Diarrhœa,* morning, *afternoon,* NIGHT, *after midnight;* after cold drinks; from taking cold; AFTER EATING; *after fruit;* in hot weather. Dysentery. *Much flatus,* offensive. Bleeding from anus. Hæmorrhoids. Involuntary stool and urine. Itching of the anus. Moisture about the anus. Pain in the anus during stool. Burning in the anus during diarrhœa, during stool. Pressing pain. Stitching. Paralytic weakness of the rectum. Ineffectual urging to stool. Stool bilious, *black,* bloody, clay colored, copious, *fi .quent,* LIENTERIC, offensive, *liquid, watery.* Diarrhœa with intermittent fever.

Spasmodic retention of urine. Urging to urinate, frequent, ineffectual. Involuntary urination at night; after stool. *Urine albuminous, bloody,* burning; cloudy on standing; *dark, greenish,* pale, copious at night, offensive, *scanty.* Sediment is red and sandy. Sugar. Clear watery urine.

Erections feeble. Seminal emissions.

Itching of vulva. Leucorrhœa, excoriating, bloody, copious, after menses, offensive, thin. Menses absent; *copious, dark,* too frequent, offensive, painful, pale, protracted; suppressed. Uterine hæmorrhage. Prolapsus.

Catarrh of larynx and trachea. Rawness in larynx. Soreness in larynx. Hoarseness; rough voice.

Respiration quick, *asthmatic,* deep, *difficult in* evening and *night;* difficult with cough; difficult while lying; *rattling; short. Suffocation. Wheezing.* Whistling. Suffocation in the forenoon during phthisis. Must sit bent forward by an open window in the attack of suffocation, worse in any other position. Every day at 9 A.M. Suffocation.

Cough, *morning,* afternoon, *evening, night; after* midnight; asthmatic, from deep breathing; from full feeling in chest; *during chill.* Dry cough, at night, during fever. Cough exhausting. *Cough during fever.* Hacking cough. Irritation in larynx and trachea. Loose cough. Motion aggravates the cough. Short cough. Spasmodic cough. *Suffocative cough.* Talking aggravates the cough. Tickling in air passages causes cough. Expectoration bloody, copious; difficult; MUCUS, offensive, *purulent;* tastes bitter, flat, salty. Expectoration is viscid, white.

Anxiety in chest, region of heart. Constriction. Hæmorrhage of lungs. *Oppression* of chest. *Angina pectoris* with dropsical symptoms. Pain in the chest, during cough. Pains in the sides of the chest. *Rawness in the chest.* Stitching in the chest on coughing. Stitching in the heart. *Palpitation of the heart,* anxious, aggravated on slight exertion, leaning back against chair *violent.* Sensation as if heart ceased to beat. Full pulse. Weakness in chest. Weakness of respiratory muscles. Violent pain in left mammary region, as though part were torn with red hot tongs. Aching in region of seventh rib on inspiration.

Coldness of the back at night. Eruptions on the back. Pain in the back, during chill. Pain in the cervical region, in scapula, between scapulæ, in lumbar region; in sacral region; in spine. Aching; bruised; drawing; soreness in spine; tearing. Stiffness in cervical region. Weak feeling in back.

Limbs icy cold. Upper limbs cold. *Cold hands and feet. Cold knees. Cold legs.* Cramps in calves. Blueness of finger nails. Eruption on limbs. Excoriation between thighs. Heaviness of limbs, of lower limbs. After prolonged suppuration in hip joint disease. Stitching in limbs, in lower limbs. *Weakness of limbs,* forearms, lower limbs, legs. Gooseflesh on lower limbs with chilliness. Palm, hot and dry. Pain in limbs, *rheumatic,* in the joints; *gouty joints, Pain in* the upper limbs, shoulders. Pain in the knees. Aching pains in all the limbs. Wandering aching pains. Aching of the biceps of left arm. Pain in flexors of left forearm, in radial side near elbow. Burning in the limbs, in the feet. Drawing pain in the limbs, upper limbs; *thighs, knees,* feet. Stitching in shoulders; upper arms, *hips,* thighs, knees, feet. *Tearing pain in the limbs;* upper limbs, shoulders, *elbows,* wrist, hand, *fingers; lower limbs, thighs, legs,* ankles, feet. *Restlessness of the limbs; lower limbs, legs, feet.* Stiffness of the limbs, hands, fingers; lower limbs. Dropsical swelling of the hands and feet. Trembling of the limbs; hands; lower limbs. Weakness of the lower limbs. Weakness of the limbs, joints, upper limbs; *lower limbs, knees, thighs.*

Sleep deep. Sleep during fever. Dreams anxious, of death, frightful, misfortune, vexatious, vivid. Falling asleep late, restless until 3 A.M. *Restless sleep. Sleepiness* afternoon, evening. *Sleeplessness,* before midnight. Sleep is unrefreshing. Wakens too early, frequently. Yawns much.

Intermittent fever. CHILL, morning, *forenoon,* noon, AFTERNOON, evening, night, midnight; *open air;* walking in the open air; anticipating; in bed. *Drinking aggravates chill.* Quotidian chill; quotidian or *tertian.* Hard, *shaking chill.* Chill like cold waves with goose-flesh all over body. Warm room ameliorates. *External* warmth ameliorates. High fever follows chill. Fever without chill afternoon and evening. Fever and chill alternate. Burning fever. Feverish all the time, but more so at night. Dry heat at night. *Hectic fever.* Heat during sleep. Chill, heat, then sweat. During the heat he desires to uncover. *Perspiration, morning, night;* during anxiety, COLD; from coughing; *with weakness; during slight exertion; following fever;* from motion; PROFUSE; *during sleep; after waking;* staining linen yellow. Fevers from living in damp rooms. Malarial fevers. Symptoms increase while perspiring. *Fevers with extreme prostration.*

Anæsthesia of the skin. Burning. *Cold skin.* Bluish discoloration; *pale; yellow;* jaundice every summer *Dryness.* Burning eruptions, boils, pimples. Urticaria after scratching. Vesicles. *Formication.* Gooseflesh. *Itching,* burning, *Skin very sensitive,* a feeling of soreness. Sticking. Dropsical swelling of skin. Ulcers, burning, sensitive, stinging.

CICUTA VIROSA

This remedy is of interest because of its convulsive tendency. It puts the whole nervous system in such a state of increased irritability that pressure on a part causes convulsions. The convulsions extend from center to circumference; the head, face and eyes are first affected. An aura in the st⁻mach gives warning of the convulsion. Some complaints spread from the chest, especially from the heart; the rigors and chills begin in the chest; and there is a sensation of coldness about the heart, and from there it extends to other parts. Convulsions often begin about the head and throat and extend downward. The whole body is in such a state of tension that, after excitement, a fire rages throughout the economy and causes convulsions. Any irritation in the throat or œsophagus will cause violent convulsions in this region. On swallowing a fish bone, instead of only a pricking sensation as would occur in phlegmatic individuals, the irritation is so great that a spasm commences and spreads to other parts. It was the old remedy for tetanus and spasms caused by splinters in the skin or under the nails, competing with *Bell.* At the present day we find the most frequently indicated remedies for injuries to nerves are *Led.* and *Hyper.*

A peculiar feature about some of the symptoms is that they resemble catalepsy. The cataleptic condition may be present or a condition very similar to it. He recollects nothing that took place or that he said during a certain period. He knows nobody, and lies without recognizing anyone, but when asked questions he answers correctly, and subsequently he has no recollection of what took place.

It is a cerebro-spinal irritant; the head is drawn back, opisthotonos; all the limbs are convulsed and rigid. It has cured traumatic tetanus lockjaw. epilepsy, epileptiform convulsions.

With severe pains in the bowels come convulsive movements and convulsions. If the stomach is disordered or chilled, or if he has fear or other mental conditions, convulsions come on. He is extremely sensitive to touch, and touch and drafts bring on convulsions. The convulsions spread from above downwards, and thus it is the opposite of *Cupr.* The convulsions of *Cupr.* spread from the extremities to the centre; *i.e.*, the little convulsions, merely cramps, are first felt in the fingers and then in the hands and later in the chest and whole body. In Cicuta the little convulsions of the head, eyes and throat spread down the back to the extremities with violent contortions. The convulsions of *Secale* sometimes begin in the face.

At times he knows no one, but when touched and spoken to he answers correctly. Suddenly consciousness returns and he remembers nothing of what has occurred. He confuses the present with the past. He imagines himself a young child. Everything is confused and strange. He does not know where he is. The faces of old friends look strange; he looks at them and wonders if they are the same persons he used to know. His house and familiar places look strange. Voices sound strange. The senses of sight and smell and all the other special senses are disturbed and confused. He is confused as to himself, his age and circumstances. A woman on coming out of the cataleptic attacks often takes on childish behaviour. A man thinks that he is a child and acts like one; silly laughter, playing with toys, and other acts of childish behaviour. He feels as if he were in a strange place. and this causes fear. Thinks of the future with anxiety. Mental torpor; loss of ideas and sensation extending over a certain period. Memory a blank for hours or days with or without convulsions. Convulsions generally take the place of the ecstatic or cataleptic condition. *Natr. m.* is somewhat similar to the mental condition of this remedy, as the *Natr. m. patient* goes about doing all her household work and other functions and next day knows nothing about it. *Nux mos.* is another remedy that has such a complete blank when going about doing things, a complete abstraction of mind.

This patient has strange desires; desires to eat coal and many other strange articles, because he is unable to distinguish between things edible and things unfit to be eaten; eats coal and raw potatoes. Wants to be alone; dislike to society. Singing, shouting, dancing; likes toys, jumps about like a child. Lies in bed lamenting and wailing. Great agitation; child grasps at one's clothing in a frightened manner. This is likely to occur before the convulsion, great horror in the countenance, yet he has no recollection of the horror when he comes out of the convulsion. That state of anxiety and fear comes after the attack has begun, though the convulsions have not yet come on. Between the convulsions the patient is mild, gentle, placid and yielding, which distinguishes it from *Strych.* And *Nux v.* convulsions. The *Nux* convulsions are all over the body and are worse from touch and draft, blueness and purple color of the body, but between the convulsions the patient is very irritable. Of course, when they go out of one convulsion into another you cannot see this, but when out of the convulsion, the *Nux* patient is very irritable. The Cicuta patient, out of the convulsion, is full of sadness, anxiety, and darkness, borrows trouble from the future, is affected by sad stories, is pessimistic. He is afraid of society, afraid of company, and wants to he alone. He is suspicious and shuns people; des-pises others; over-estimation of himself. In this it approximates *Plat.,* but there is no further resemblance between the two remedies. Full of fear; fright will bring on convulsions, like *Op., Ign.,* and *Acon.*

Full of vertigo. The whole sensorium is violently excited. Things turn around in a circle. Vertigo on walking, glassy eyes, etc. Complaints brought on from injuries to the skull, from blows on the head. Many times there is no trouble in the region of the injury; there may be compression and yet all the pains be in distant parts; drawing of the muscles and cramps. Concussion of the brain and chronic injuries therefrom, especially spasms. Semi-lateral headaches forcing the patient to sit erect. Headache as if the brain were loose on walking. When thinking of the exact nature of the pain it ceased. It has cured cerebro-spinal meningitis when there were convulsions and the convulsions were aggravated from touch, with fever and even spotted mottled skin. Mind and head symptoms after injuries. On going into a cerebro-spinal meningitis the patient sits in a chair talking as if nothing were wrong, when, quick as a flash, he passes into another state in which he knows no one; he falls over limp, he is put to bed, and though he answers questions he remains in a semi-conscious state, knowing no one. This may change into a spasm. The head is bent back in spasms; jerking back of the head; spasms begin in the head and go downward. Violent shocks in the head, arms and legs. Head hot and extremities cold, like *Bell.* in its convulsions. Sweat on the scalp when sleeping. Child rolls head from side to side. Hot head.

Convulsive action about the eyes; pupils dilated and insensible; patient lies fixed in one place, with staring, fixed, glassy, upturned eyes, like *Cupr.* Strabismus may be the only spasm the child is subject to from cerebral irritation. Every time the child is frightened it has strabismus; when touched or when it has cold, or after a fall hitting the head, or coming periodically, it has strabismus.

The nose is sensitive to touch. Touch and jarring bring on complaints, and hence it was so useful in, and was the first remedy for, the result of injuries and irritability and over-sensibility.

It has troubles from shaving; it is useful in such eruptions as come in the whiskers; barber's itch; a solid crop of eruptions all over the face wherever the whiskers grow. Eruptions on the cheek like eczema. Swelling of the submaxillary glands. Erysipelatous eruptions. It is closely related to *Conium* about the lips and lids, in that a small amount of pressure causes induration. It has cured epithelioma of the lips.

The throat troubles are mostly spasmodic. After swallowing a fish bone or stick which lodges in the throat a spasm comes on. After Cicuta the spasms will cease and it can be taken out. It is useful in cases of injury, accompanied with violent choking, so that he cannot allow an examination to be made.

Cold sensation in the chest. Spasms of the chest. Feels as if the heart stopped beating. Spasmodic symptoms of the back. Opisthotonos. All conditions of the limbs are of a spasmodic character.

CINA

Cina is pre-eminently a child's remedy, but it is suitable for conditions in adults that are seldom thought of. A marked feature running through is *touchiness,* mental and physical. The child wants something, but does not know what. The child is aggravated by touch and even by being looked at, and is worse from seeing strangers. The skin is sensitive to touch. The scalp and back of the neck, the shoulders and arms are so sensitive, that it is almost a soreness as if bruised. The hyperæsthesia is both mental and physical. The old routine of giving Cina for worms need not go into your notes, for if you are guided by symptoms the patient will be cured and the worms will go.

This patient is disturbed by everything, worse after eating even a moderate meal. The child takes a moderate supper and dreams all night, jerks and twitches in sleep, rouses up in a fright, talks excitedly about what he has dreamed, thinks it is real, and sees dogs; phantoms, and frightful things he has dreamed about. The dream is prolonged into the wakeful hours. Screams and trembles, with much anxiety on waking; whines and complains. While this little patient is aggravated by being handled yet he wants to be carried and kept busy, like *Chamomilla;* although not so intensely irritable as that remedy, yet he must be carried. At first on taking him out of the crib he screams when taken hold of; the first touch aggravates. This aggravation from touch and sensitiveness runs through the convulsions and fevers, with delirium, glassy eyes, drawn mouth and white ring around the nose and mouth. With a disordered stomach he has convulsions after eating, with the head drawn back and glassy eyes. The stomach is sour and the child is always spitting up sour milk and belching sour wind. The child smells sour. The mother says that "Baby has a worm breath," but the same odor is present when there are no worms. In the convulsions there are loss of consciousness and frothing at the mouth.

Hallucinations of smell, sight and taste, in the delirious state, after taking cold, or on waking from sleep; wakes up with the delusion. Things taste and smell differently. The senses of taste and touch are exaggerated or perverted.

In some cases of internal hydrocephalus, not with enlarged skull, but with increase of the fluid in the ventricles and central canal of the spinal cord, the patients take on Cina symptoms. Rolling of the head; frequent headaches; sensitiveness to jar; cannot be touched or tapped along the spinal cord without headache; always worse in the sun; the head is hot and the feet are cold in the sun. Cina will cure some of these cases. They cannot stand any kind of disturbance; it produces a convulsion. They cannot be punished because they go into convulsions. If the *iter a tertio ad quartum ventriculum* is closed they will be incurable, the internal pressure will go on and they will die from it. Such congenital states are incurable.

Dull headache with sensitiveness of the eyes,, Headache before and after epileptic attacks and after intermittents. Before and during the headache sensitiveness of the skull. Cina children cannot have the hair combed, and the Cina woman must have her hair down in head and nerve complaints.

There is coldness of the extremities and also some itching of the skin, but the head symptoms are predominant. From slight disturbances of the mind he cannot digest, and he has diarrhœa. The complaints are aggravated in summer; the heat affects the brain, arrests his functions, and on comes diarrhœa with green, slimy stools or white stools, and the child vomits. It is pre-eminently *brain* in Cina; the orders are not received from the brain and so stomach symptoms develop, and worms hatch out. If he is cured, the healthy gastric juice will chase the worms out.

The child turns his head from side to side. The pains are sometimes better from turning the head from side to side. You will see this in sensitive women, who must have their hair down; *rolling* the head relieves, not *shaking* as *in* the text, that is too violent.

All sorts of colors before the eyes. Objects look yellow. It is useful in sensitive women, sensitive nervous women, who are always worse from using the eyes, and get pain in the head and eyes from sewing. It is like *Ruta* in that respect, symptoms of eye-strain. It is not so much indicated in young people but more when presbyopia is beginning in middle-aged women, and there is the effort to strain the eyes on fine work or print. Rubs the eyes and can then see more clearly. On rising from the bed blackness before the eyes; different colors, especially yellow. Strabismus when worms are present, depending really on brain trouble because the worms are dependent upon that.

Face sunken, pallid, wings of nose drawn in. Blue ring or gray streak around the mouth. "A sure sign of worms," the mother says. Child rubs its nose with the hands or on the pillow or on the nurse's shoulder. Child bores into the nose until the blood comes. The sickly aspect is striking, but it is representative of brain trouble, central trouble. The brain symptoms are the highest and most important. If frightened, whipped, or scolded, the brain is disturbed and the stomach disordered. They get indigestion and breed worms; white or blue appearance about the mouth, grinding of the teeth during sleep. Before the child has teeth it has a chewing motion, a side to side movement. Sensitiveness of the teeth to the cold air and cold water. Bleeding from the mouth and nose. Inability to swallow liquids; they gurgle down the œsophagus—before and after convulsions. When the head symptoms are present, the milk or water gurgles down the œsophagus with a gurgling cluck. This is present in diarrhœa and vomiting with brain symptoms. *Ars.* and *Cupr.* are also prominent in gurgling down the œsophagus when swallowing. Choreic movements extend to the tongue.

The child or adult is not relieved by eating, is still hungry. The stomach is loaded and yet he is hungry. After vomiting you would expect there would be an aversion to food, but there is in Cina the same empty, hungry feeling. When there is gnawing in the stomach after eating, or when the child has taken all it can hold yet cries for the bottle, or empties its stomach by spitting up and vomiting the food and then reaches out whining and crying for more, think of Cina. Shuddering when drinking wine as if it were vinegar.

438 CINCHONA

Abdomen hard and bloated. Very often the Cina child will flop over on its belly and get to sleep in that way. If it is turned on the side it wakes up again. While in the mother's arms it will go to sleep with the abdomen resting on the mother's shoulder, but when she puts it on the side in bed it wakens. If you had a child with copious, gushing, violently fœtid stool, ameliorated by lying on the abdomen, and it would have another stool if lying any other way, *Podoph.* would be the remedy. That would not be Cina. The Cina stool is not very copious, and often white.

Gagging cough in the morning. Short, hacking cough at night. Spasmodic cough. Whooping cough.

Oversensitiveness to touch; trembling, spasms, chorea. Spasmodic yawning. Child cannot sleep unless on the belly or in constant motion.

CINCHONA

Now we shall take up the study of Cinchona, or China. Persons who have suffered much from neuralgias due to malarial influences, who have become anæmic and sickly from repeated hæmorrhages, are likely to develop symptoms calling for China. China produces a gradually increasing anæmia, with great pallor and weakness. It is sometimes indicated in plethoric individuals, but this is the exception, and even in this class we find that the symptoms are tending towards the cachectic state, which is avoided by the prompt action of the remedy.

Throughout the body there is a gradually increasing sensitivity, a gradually increasing irritability of the nerves; the nerves are always in a fret, so that these people will say:" "Doctor, what is the matter with me, I am so nervous?" Everywhere there are twining, tearing, cutting pains—in the limbs and over the body. And so great is the sensitiveness to touch that the nerves can many times be outlined; as, for instance, the little nerves in the fingers, because of their extreme sensitiveness. The China patient grows increasingly sensitive to touch, to motion, to cold air, so that he is chilled from exposure. The pains are brought on by exposure to the wind, by cold air, and are increased by motion and touch. Old malarial conditions that have been suppressed with quinine; gradually increasing pallor, bloodlessness, cachexia, until the patient is always catching cold, has liver troubles, bowel troubles, disordered stomach, is made miserable and sick by nearly everything he does. He cannot eat fruit without having indigestion; he cannot eat sour things. He is debilitated, pale, waxy, suffers from pains, such as are found in quinine subjects, and breaks out into a perspiration upon the least exertion.

This patient bleeds easily; bleeds from any orifice of the body—from the nose, from the throat, from the uterus. And after hæmorrhage complaints come on. Running through the remedy as a general constitutional state is a tendency to congestion and often inflammation in connection with hæmorrhages. Inflammation of the part that bleeds or of distant parts. For instance, a woman aborts, has a hæmorrhage, but with apparently no provocation, inflammation of the uterus or of the lungs, sets in. With these inflammations there is also great irritability of the tissues, tearing pains, cramping in the muscles and actual convulsions. When a China patient bleeds a little, for instance, in confinement, right in the midst of the bleeding convulsions come on. You would scarcely need to think of any other remedy. *Secale* is the one other medicine that has this, but the two do not look alike. *Secale* wants the covers all off and the windows open, even in cold weather. If a draft of air blows on a China patient, while in labor, she may go into convulsions. In the midst of labor the pains cease and convulsions come on. Another feature about this inflammation is its rapid progress and intensity, quickly going into gangrene. Inflammation after hæmorrhage and the parts rapidly turn black.

China has a fulness of the veins. Not exactly a varicose condition, but a sort of paralysis of the coatings of the veins. The veins become full during fever.

All of these complaints are such as we find in broken down constitutions, in feeble, sensitive patients, especially in sensitive women. Sensitive to the odors of flowers, of cooking, of tobacco. Weak, relaxed, emaciated, pale, with feeble heart, feeble circulation and tendency to dropsy. Dropsy runs through the remedy; anasarca and also dropsy of shut sacs. A peculiar thing about this dropsy is that it comes after hæmorrhage. In the anæmic condition, directly following the loss of blood, dropsy appears. This is the typical China patient.

Catarrhal condition of all mucous membranes. Gastro-duodenal catarrh, ending in jaundice. Old liver subjects with jaundice. They have lived for a long time under the influence of the malarial miasm. Feeble, sensitive, anæmic. We see such cases in the South and South-west, and along the Mississippi Valley.

Periodicity is regarded as the most important indication for China, but it is a mistake. Periodicity is the symptom upon which *Quinine* is given. China has periodicity, but in no greater degree than many other remedies and is not so frequently indicated as routine prescribers suppose. Allopaths give *Quinine* whenever there is any periodicity in complaints. Still periodicity is a strong feature in this remedy. Pains come on with regularity at a given time each day. Intermittent fevers appear with regularity and run a regular course.

A part of this periodicity is an aggravation at night, and sometimes sharply at midnight. In colic that comes on regularly every night at 12 o'clock, and it may be, perhaps, a week before you suspect it to be a China colic. A lady had colic and bloating of the abdomen every night at 12 o'clock. After suffering many nights a single dose of China prevented any further trouble. Hæmorrhage from the nose coming on with regularity. Diarrhœa at night. Several gushing, black, watery stools during the night; in the daytime, *only after eating*. There is a general aggravation after eating.

Remember that this is a chilly patient, sensitive to drafts, sensitive to cold, whose complaints are brought on by being exposed to cold air; sensitive to touch, sensitive to motion. Extreme irritability of the tissues.

China is indicated in conditions following the loss of blood and other animal fluids; as, for instance, in those who are suffering from sexual excesses, from secret vice. They have become feeble, sleepless and irritable. There is weakness and general coldness of the skin; twitching and jerking of the limbs; drawing and cramping in the muscles; chronic jerking; epileptiform convulsion; paralytic weakness; rush of blood to the head; ringing in the ears; darkness before the eyes; fainting on the slightest provocation. Such is the China cachexia, and with this in view, the mental stare will scarcely be a surprise to you. It is just such as you would expect in this nervous, sensitive patient. Weakness of mind. Inability to think or remember. Full of fear at night. Fear of animals, dogs, of creeping things. Wants to commit suicide, but lacks courage. Gradually the mind grows weaker; he uses wrong expressions or misplaces words. Lies awake at night making plans; theorizing, building air castles, thinking of the wonderful things he is going to do some day. In the morning he wonders how he could have thought such foolish things. After sleep his mind is clear and he looks more philosophically on the affairs of life. Unable to entertain any mental proposition that means work. He dreads work. He is apathetic, indifferent, low spirited, silent, disinclined to think. He is unable to control the mind, to make it do what he wants it to do. You see it is not as yet a real insanity.

This state of mind comes on after hæmorrhage. Insomnia after hæmorrhage. A woman, after having suffered great loss of blood, will be sleepless night after night.

After hæmorrhage we may have dizziness. It is a natural consequence; dizziness and fainting. But ordinarily, after the proper diet for a few days, these symptoms will have disappeared. With the China patient they go from bad to worse. The woman after severe hæmorrhage does not make blood. There is malassimilation, and the vertigo persists for days and weeks. China will restore order.

The remedy is full of headaches. Congestive headaches in broken down constitutions. Extremities cold and body covered with a cold sweat. Rending, tearing pains. Pressing and throbbing. As soon as the air strikes the head those pains come on. Headache better in a warm room; worse from touch; worse from motion; worse from cold. These are the principal features. A slight touch will aggravate the disturbance. But notice the exception. *Hard pressure* ameliorates the China pains, as light pressure aggravates. Sensitiveness of the tissues; sensitiveness along the course of the nerves; the pains are brought on by touch, by cold air. Stitches in the head with pulsation in temples, which can be felt with the fingers; ameliorated by hard pressure, but aggravated by touch. The jar and motion of walking hurt the head. Even turning over in bed aggravates. Cannot ride in a carriage or anything that jolts. Ameliorated by hard pressure. Throbbing headaches, aggravated by a draft of air, in the open air, from the slightest touch; ameliorated by hard pressure. The scalp feels as if the hair was grasped roughly. It is sensitive to touch. Profuse sweating of the scalp. Headaches aggravated at night. Headaches from sexual excesses; loss of animal fluids.

Now we come to the eye. Photophobia. Yellowness of the sclera. Exposure to cold wind will bring on neuralgia; ameliorated from keeping quiet and from keeping warm. "Nocturnal blindness, dimness of vision. Feeling as if sand were in the eyes. Pains worse from light. Better in the dark."

In the ear and the nose you find the same sensitiveness as in eyes; every little noise is painful. Ringing, roaring, buzzing, and singing, chirping like crickets in the ears. Dry catarrh of the middle ear. Hardness of hearing is not infrequently the result of this condition. It gradually increases until there is total deafness, and the noises in the ear continue long after the patient has lost the ability to distinguish articulate sounds. Hæmorrhage from the ear. Offensive, bloody, purulent discharges.

Frequent nosebleed in anæmic patients. Here, again, the dryness and catarrhal conditions. Dry coryza; or fluent coryza, suppressed and causing violent head pains. Odors nauseate. Sensitiveness to the odors of flowers, cooking, tobacco.

The face is withered, shrunken, sallow, anæmic, sickly Red when the fever is on and sometimes when the chill is on, but in the apyrexia pale, sickly and sallow. Neuralgia of the face; tearing, rending, knife-like pains with the usual modalities. The veins of the face are distended. This is frequently observed during the fever and sweat of the China intermittents.

The teeth get loose, the gums swell. The teeth are painful while chewing; they feel too long. Toothache with every little cold. Rending as if teeth were being pulled out, every time the child nurses at the breast. Exudations about the teeth and gums. Black, and fœtid; great putridity in the lower forms of fever.

The taste is extremely acute. Exaggerated so that nothing tastes natural. "Bitter taste in the mouth. Food tastes bitter or too salty. Burning as from pepper on tip of the tongue. Dryness in the mouth and throat. Difficult swallowing." Sometimes there is canine hunger, but one of the most common features is loathing of everything; aversion to all food. The China patient is often passive in regard to eating. Sits down to eat and the food tastes fairly good and he fills up. But it does not matter much whether he eats or not. "Loathing and violent hunger." "Hunger and yet want of appetite. Indifference to eating and drinking. Only while eating some appetite and natural taste for food return. Loss of appetite. Aversion to all food. Aversion to bread." His appetite varies. Thirst is peculiar. The patient will say: "I know my chill is coming on now because I have thirst." Thirst before the chill, but as soon as the chill comes on there is no thirst. But when he begins to warm up he begins to get thirsty; that is, during the period in which the two lap he is thirsty, but when the chill has fairly subsided and the heat is upon him his thirst subsides also and he only wants to wet his mouth. But as the hot spell begins to subside he increases the amount taken, and all through the sweat he can *hardly get water enough.* Thirst before and after the chill and thirst *during the sweat.* No thirst during the chill. No thirst during the hot spell. You will cure more cases of intermittent fever with *Ipecac* and *Nux vomica,* than with China. China has well-defined chill, fever and sweat.

Gastric symptoms from eating fish, fruit, and from drinking wine. Flatulent distension almost to bursting. There are constant eructations, loud and strong, and yet no relief, so extensive, is the flatulence. In *Carbo veg.* after belching a little, there is relief. *Lyc.* has both. Tympanitic distension of the abdomen and stomach in low forms of fever. Cannot move on account of soreness in the bowels. Vomiting of blood. Sometimes followed by dropsy of the extremities. "Hiccough. Nausea. Vomiting. Eructations, tasting of food, or they are bitter, sour. Frequent vomiting. Vomiting of sour mucus, bile, blood." Likely to occur at night. Pulsation in the stomach and rumbling. Cold feeling in the stomach. Fermentation after eating fruit. Acidity. Disorders of the stomach after milk.

Diarrhœa. Copious, watery black discharges from the bowels. Gurgling and rumbling in the abdomen. Stool immediately after eating and at night. Great quantities of flatus expelled from the bowels. Diarthœa comes on gradually. Stools more and more watery. Chronic diarrhœa, with emaciation and aggravation at night. *Petroleum* has a chronic diarrhœa, but only in the daytime.

Of the male genital organs the most striking feature is weakness. Of the female genital organs there is a different class of conditions. In the woman who has been subject to uterine hæmorrhages you may look out at any moment for a sudden, sharp attack of inflammation of the ovaries. Hæmorrhage from the uterus. Prolapse. Menses too early and too profuse; black, clotted blood; menstrual colic; metrorrhagia. Pains and convulsions; convulsions come on in the midst of the hæmorrhage; cramps in the uterus along with hæmorrhage; labor-like pains; ringing in the ears; loss of sight; sliding down in bed. In confinement the lochia is profuse and lasts too long. Deterioration of health from prolonged lactation; toothache; neuralgia of the face.

Difficult respiration, rattling and filling up of the chest with mucus; asthma. "Pressure in the chest, as from violent rush of blood; violent palpitation, bloody sputa, sudden prostration." Dry, suffocative cough at night; profuse night sweats. Pains in the chest, increasing sensitiveness to cold, heat and redness of the face with cold hands.

Along the spine there are sore spots. Tearing. darting pains in the limbs, ameliorated by heat and hard pressure, brought on by touch, by becoming chilled. Worse at night. "Knees weak, especially when walking."

China cures low forms of fever, remittent or intermittent, typhoid or malarial.

CISTUS CANADENSIS

This remedy is an antipsoric, a deep-acting remedy. It runs very close to *Calcarea*. but is milder in its action. It has the same exhaustion from exertion, dyspnœa, sweating and coldness that we find in *Calcarea.*

What will forcibly call your attention to a remedy will be the curing of a bad and typical case. I remember the first time my attention was decidedly called to Cistus. I had put it on my list to study from time to time and had come to the conclusion that it was only a side issue, until a young lady, nineteen years of age, fell under my observation. The glands of the neck were large and hard, the parotids especially; she had fœtid otorrhœa; her eyes were inflamed and suppurating; there were fissures at the corners of the eyes; her lips were cracked and bleeding, and she had salt rheum at the ends of the fingers. I could not make *Calcarea* fit the patient, but after much study this little remedy seemed to be just what I needed; and although she had had an immense amount of Homœopathy, good and bad, this remedy cured.

The glands inflame, become swollen and suppurate. It causes caries and cures old ulcers. It has a scrofulous constitution. It is useful in chronic diarrhœa, with enlarged glands, even in those who are flabby, sickly and pallid and who cannot go upstairs without losing their breath. All the mucous membranes throw out a thick, yellowish, offensive mucus and hence it is suitable in old and troublesome catarrh. The chest fills up with mucus and he feels relieved after expectoration, but after he empties the chest it feels raw. It has eruptions, herpes, tetter, scaly eruptions, salt rheum on the hands and ends of the fingers, with cracking and bleeding of the fingers in winter and from washing in cold water.

All its complaints are worse from mental exertion. He is excitable. His cough. headache and pains are worse from mental exertion. Pains shoot from the head to the ear. Shooting, stitching, tearing pains in inflamed parts. Old discharges from the ear date back to eruptive diseases. He feels as if paralyzed after mental exertion, and mental excitement increases his sufferings, like *Calcarea* and *Borax*. If he is compelled to fast headache comes on, and like *Lyc.,* the headache will be relieved after eating. Frontal headache with coldness. In a warm room the perspiration comes out, and it is cold, and the more he sweats the colder he gets. Pain in the forehead with cold sweat, and the colder he gets the worse the pain becomes. Sick headaches and great prostration with the headache. Sensation of internal coldness of the forehead, especially in warm room. Pressing pain at the root of the nose with headache. The parotid gland is so much enlarged that it pushes the head to one side. The glands of the abdomen swell with chronic diarrhœa, and the swelling may be tuberculous. Enlarged glands, with or without eruptions.

All over the body there is a sensation of crawling; formication; tingling and creeping like ants, and no eruption. He scratches till the skin is raw trying to get relieved of the itching and prickling. Eruption upon the face; eczema. Eruptions about the ear.

Cold feeling or burning in the nose. This is difficult to distinguish. In acute coryza the nose fills up with thick, yellow mucus, and when this is blown out it leaves the nasal cavity empty, and there is irritation; one will say it is a rawness, another will say a coldness, and another will describe it as a burning. There is relief when the nose fills up again with mucus. In *Ars.* the mucus in the nose is so acrid that it burns, but in *Ant. c., Æsculus,* and in this remedy when the nose is empty there is a burning or rawness. The sensation of rawness, coldness or burning is caused by the inhalation of air. An epidemic of coryza was prevalent, and this was the strongest symptom—the pain caused by inhaling air, great burning from inhaled air. But it is not in the acute coryza that we see the value of this remedy, it is in the old, chronic case, with thick discharge, and a cold feeling or burning in the nose when inhaling air.

"Sharp shooting, intolerable itching and thick crusts, with burning on right zygoma." This remedy has cured lupus on the face. Caries of the lower jaw. Open, bleeding cancer on the lower lip. Lupus exedens. Pain in all the joints of the face. It cures old, deep-seated, eating ulcers about the ankle and shin, with copious acrid discharge, formication and swollen glands, aggravation from bathing, extreme sensitiveness to the open air, only comfortable when very warm.

The teeth have all sorts of disturbances; the gums settle away, the teeth become loose; scorbutic gums. The same cold feeling is described in the throat as in the nose—smarting and coldness. Mouth and throat full of mucus. The throat feels rough, as if full of sand. Dry spots in the throat The throat looks glossy, shining as if varnished, in old atrophic catarrhs.

Every cold settles in the throat. Hot air feels good everywhere. In old cases there is trouble with scrofulous glands, which are enlarged, and the patient wants the heat; goes to the register and turns the heat on, wants to feel the heat in the nose, throat and lungs. Patients going into tuberculosis have that desire for heat; chilly persons. They do not feel cold to touch, but they are cold subjectively, chilly. Hawking of gum-like mucus, especially in the morning, fauces inflamed and dry. Suppuration of the glands of the throat.

These patients crave pungent things, and especially want something to warm them up, something to build them up, something stimulating; herring, cheese; something "strong".

"Chronic induration and inflammation of the mammæ. Left mamma inflamed, suppurating, with a feeling of fulness in the chest. Sensibility to cold air," with the inflamed glands. We see its tendency to produce enlargement of the glands, and this would make us think of it in growths with involvement of the glands all around. The glands of the neck are enlarged in lines, like knotted rope, as in Hodgkin's disease. Only a limited number of remedies have this knotting.

Itching of the skin and mucous membrane. The itching in the ear is not relieved by scratching, and the part is raw from the constant rubbing and scratching. The eyes constantly itch. In the throat there is continuous itching. In the chest there is a constant tickling, causing cough. At the anus and all other orifices there is itching, and the itching parts are rubbed until raw and bleeding.

Scrofula; swelling and suppuration of the glands of the neck. Eruption on the back like shingles. Scrofulous ulcer on the back. Burning, bruised pain in the coccyx, worse from touch. That is like *Carbo an.*, in which the coccyx burns when pressed on, especially after a slight injury in a nervous woman.

Tetter on the hands; blisters oozing after scratching. Diseases of the nails. Hard, thickened places on the hands of workmen, with deep cracks.

The febrile symptoms have not been sufficiently brought out. In chronic cases there is copious sweat with exhaustion. Night-sweats.

CLEMATIS ERECTA

Clematis has only been partially proved, and consequently it applies only to a few conditions, but these are very important, so that it cannot be passed over. It has vesicular eruptions almost erysipelatous in character. One almost constant mental state is that he fears to be alone, yet dreads company. He dreads the necessity of having company, and it seems that the atmosphere is full of frightful and distressing things to worry him.

This makes him low-spirited. The remedy seems to fit the sycotic constitution in its mental state and its generals. It seems to be fitted to those who
had gonorrhœa recently suppressed, because after that suppression will come
on this mental state with inflammation of glands.

It is rather singular about the eruptions. One would not think that from so
harmless a little shrub so much trouble would come; but there are persons who
are just as sensitive to this vine as to *Rhus,* and it resembles *Rhus* to a great
extent in its manifestations. It produces just as poisonous a condition as
Rhus. Here I might speak of several remedies which relate to the *Rhus* poison.
There are many vesicular remedies that look like *Rhus,* and all of them you will
have to use more or less in their antidotal relation, to each other, but it is well
to be sure in a given case which one of them produced the poison. *Croton tig.,
Rhus, Ranunculus, Anacardium* and Clematis at times look so much alike that
I am unable to tell them apart by their eruptions. They are all similar enough to
each other to become universal antidotes. The others are all deeper acting
than *Rhus.* The *Ranunculus,* the little buttercup, has cured epithelioma of the
lids. It has cured cancerous affections, so we say it goes deep into the tissues.

On the outer head we have a part of the manifestations of Clematis;
vesicular eruptions with great itching, stinging and crawling. Now what is
true of the eruption here will be true of the Clematis eruption everywhere. It
is aggravated from washing. It will smart and burn, and a quasi-inflammation
will set in from washing. Contrast this with the internal features of the remedy.
In the teeth and jaws the pain is violent, but while the eruption is made worse
from cold applications, the pain inside the jaw and the teeth is relieved by
cold water held in the mouth, and aggravated violently from heat, and from
the warmth of the bed. The eruption is aggravated from the warmth of the
bed, and also from cold washing. We have to go into the details a little to see
whether an eruption is *Rhus* or whether it is Clematis, or something else.
Vesicular eruptions filling with yellow fluid and with induration under the
vesicles. It produces eruptions very closely related to herpes and eczema,
and they spread. About the eyes we have vesicular eruptions. If seen in one
stage it will be vesicular, and if later, it will be seen as an ulceration. Simple
and graver forms of herpes. Herpes zoster about the body. "Burning and
smarting of the eyes; worse from closing them. Inflammation of the iris. Eyes
inflamed, protruded, dim. Chronic irritation of the lids."

The pains in connection with the teeth are aggravated from the warmth of
the bed, which is general; they come at night, are aggravated from warm
things held in the mouth and ameliorated from holding cold water in the
mouth. Stitching and drawing pains in the teeth; worse at night; better for a
short time from holding cold water in the mouth; better from drawing in cold
air; worse from the warmth of the bed. The toothache is tolerable during the

day, but as soon as he lies down in bed and assumes a horizontal position it increases to an intolerable degree. Pain in hollow tooth, better by cold water or drawing in cold air.

Swelling of the glands of the groin is a striking feature even when connected with scirrhus. It is connected also with suppressed gonorrhoea, and with rheumatism of the joints. Pain and swelling of the right spermatic cord; this is worse at night, worse from walking and from the warmth of the bed. While it has both sides, strange to say there is more trouble in the glands that are on the right side of the body than on the left. It has produced much trouble in the bladder. Constant urging to urinate, most painful tenesmus. Flow stopping and starting. The urethra is painful to pressure. Micturition is remarkably slow, only a feeble stream because of the smallness of the urethra.

It is the nature of this remedy to infiltrate and inflame tissues, and hence it is useful in those cases of gonorrhœa where they have been slow in passing away, where they have been treated by injection. That slow inflammation of the urethra will infiltrate and the urethra feels like a large whipcord, painful upon pressure, and this goes on until the canal is almost closed. You will be surprised to find, when Clematis is indicated, that after giving that remedy the discharge is re-established, and soon the old stricture goes away. At the end of two or three months he feels nothing of it.

A striking feature in connection with the urine, bladder, etc., is that the patient cannot quite empty the bladder. He always feels as if there was a little more, and when he appears to have finished it will keep dribbling away. This is a common feature of stricture. "Inability to evacuate all the urine at once. When beginning to urinate it burns the worst, while urinating it sticks in urethra, and after urinating it still continues to burn. Discharge from the urethra of thick pus." It is seldom indicated in the very first stage of gonorrhœa during the highest inflammation, but in those cases that are inclined to hang on. Then come the sequelæ if gonorrhœa be suppressed. Inflammation of the testes is common, and this is one of the medicines suitable. Strange to say, the right side of the body is more commonly affected than the left. Intermittent flow of the urine. Urine stops and starts with the chordee still present. The right spermatic cord is very sensitive. Pain in the testes, drawing. Painful, inflamed and swollen testes. Orchitis with much painful swelling and hardness. Now when the swelling has gone down—perhaps you gave *Puls.*, which was the remedy for the time, but it did not finish the case—there is induration of this portion. Swelling of the right half of the scrotum with thickening and hanging low down.

Provings have not been made very much in women, which is to be regretted, because it would be well to know if this remedy affects the ovaries as it does the testes. It has been clinically used, and has cured many troubles in women, especially inflammation in the mammary gland. "Ulceration and hardness of glands. Scirrhus of the breast with induration and ulceration. Scirrhus of the left mamma with stitches in the shoulder;" this is a clinical symptom, "worse in the night". She canot bear to be uncovered.

It has rheumatic conditions of the limbs from suppressed gonorrhœa. Great nervous weakness and twitchings of the muscles. It has pain on lying down and preparatory to going to sleep. An electric shock; twitching, jerking, as if a faradic battery had been turned on. It has also a general febrile condition, but nothing very striking.

Vesicular eruptions on the body. Herpetic eruptions here and there; it has a herpetic constitution. "Eruption of vesicles and pustules; from the former exuded a clear, watery secretion, from the latter a purulent fluid." Yellow vesicles and yellow pustules. Both are common to this remedy. "Dark, burning eruptions with violent itching." Herpes that ulcerate. Ichorous, spreading ulcers.

COCCULUS INDICUS

We will study the general system and the mind as usual. Cocculus slows down all the activities of the body and mind, producing a sort of paralytic weakness. Behind time in all its actions. All the nervous impressions are slow in reaching the centres. If you pinch this patient on the great toe he waits a minute and then says "oh," instead of doing it at once. In response to questions he answers slowly, after apparent meditation. but it is an effort to meditate. And so with all nervous manifestations, thought, muscular activity, etc. He cannot endure any muscular exertion, because he is weak; he is tired. First comes this slowness, then a sort of visible paralytic condition, and then complete paralysis. This may be local or general. There are certain causes which produce these effects. A wife nursing her husband, a daughter nursing her father, becomes worn out by the anxiety, worry and loss of sleep. She is exhausted; unable to sustain any mental or physical effort; weak in the knees, weak in the back, and when the time comes for her to sleep she cannot sleep. Sickness brought about in this manner is analogous to that caused by the Cocculus poison, and hence Cocculus from the time of Hahnemann to the present time has been a remedy for complaints from nursing. not exactly complaints that come on in the professional nurse, for Cocculus needs the combination of vexation, anxiety and prolonged loss of sleep, such as you have in the mother or daughter who is nursing, or the nurse when she takes on the anxiety felt by a member of the family; a wife nursing her husband through typhoid, or other long spell of sickness. At the end of it she is prostrated in body and mind, she cannot sleep, she has congestive headaches, nausea, vomiting and vertigo. That shows how a Cocculus case begins. One who is thus exhausted in body and mind goes out for a ride. She gets sick headache, pain in the back, dizziness, nausea and vomiting. She gets into the car to take a journey. Sick headache comes on. She goes on a mile or two and will have nausea: vomiting and sick headache. She feels weak atl over, feels as if she would sink away.

The Cocculus patient gets into a wagon to ride, sick headache, nausea, vertigo come on. The Cocculus patient cannot endure motion. Aggravated by talking, by motion, by the motion of the eyes, by riding. Wants plenty of time to turn the head cautiously to see things. Wants plenty of time to move, to think, to do everything. The whole economy is slowed down, inactive.

Tremulous, tired, excitable. The hands tremble when taking hold of anything, or he takes hold of it awkwardly and drops it. Incoordination runs through this remedy, and hence it has been used with good effect in loco-motor ataxia. It has staggering and numbness. Numbness is quite a feature of this remedy. Numbness of the lower extremities, in the fingers, in the shoulder, of the side of the face. Complaints from anxiety.

Extreme irritability of the nervous system. The least noise or jar is unbearable. You have heard that *Bell.* is worse from a jar. So is Cocculus, and quite like *Bell.* Cocculus is also like *Belladonna* in its sleeplessness, and other general conditions. This sensation of sea-sickness and dizziness is sometimes felt all over the body; a sort of faint feeling which is followed sometimes by loss of consciousness, or a paralytic rigidity. Stiffness of the joints is a common feature in Cocculus. It belongs to the limbs in general. But it is such a strong symptom I will mention it here. Limbs straightened out and held there for a while are painful when flexed. Persons who have been suffering from anxiety, prostrated, will lie on the back, straighten out the limbs, and get up only with great difficulty. The doctor comes and he discovers what is the matter. He bends the limbs and she screams, but she is relieved after the bending, and then she can get up and move about. You cannot find that anywhere else. It is entirely without inflammation. It is a sort of a paralytic stiffness, a paralysis of the tired body and mind. The Cocculus headaches and backaches, pains and distress are present. A man will stretch out his leg on a chair and he cannot flex it until he reaches down with his hands to assist. Such things are strange. Faintness on moving the body, fainting from pain in the bowels, from colic. With all this slowing down of the thoughts and activities the patient remains extremely sensitive to suffering, sensitive to pain.

Spasms through the body like electric shocks, convulsions after loss of sleep. This patient goes on with nervousness and excitement, anxiety and loss of sleep until convulsions supervene. Tetanus. Cholera, attacks of paralytic weakness with pain, paralysis of the face, of the eyes, paralysis of the muscles everywhere, paralysis of the limbs. Even diphtheria has been known to induce a state very much like I have described as due to loss of sleep and anxiety. I remember a case of paralysis of the lower extremities that was prescribed for by a very careful homœopathic physician many years ago. It was one of the things that surprised me in the early days of my prescribing and observation. It was the case of a little girl with paralysis of lower extremities after diphtheria and no hope was given. But Doctor Moore (he was then an Octogenarian) looked over the case. I was acquainted with the family and with the doctor. He studied the case carefully and gave Cocculus c.m. It was not many days before the child began to move the legs, and the condition was perfectly cleared up, and I have never ceased to wonder at it. It was a good prescription, perfectly in accord with all the elements of the case. Doctor Moore was one of the pupils of Lippe and Hering.

You can readily see what is coming when the mental activities are slowed down, from anxiety, and loss of sleep, such as we have in nursing. The mind appears like approaching imbecility, and as you look upon the true Cocculus case you wonder if that patient has not been growing insane for a year or two, because the mind seems almost a blank. He looks into space and slowly turning the eyes toward the questioner answers with difficulty. It occurs in nervous prostration, in typhoid fever. It is so nearly like *Phos. acid* that the two remedies must be carefully individualized. Time passes quickly. He cannot realize that it has been a whole night. A week has gone by, and it seems but a moment, he is so dazed. Slowness of comprehension; cannot find the right word to express his thoughts, so slowly does his mind work; what has passed he cannot remember; forgets what he has just read; cannot talk; cannot bear the least noise; cannot bear the least contradiction. The tongue will not respond. There is confusion of mind and difficulty of articulation. An idea comes into his mind and becomes fixed. He cannot convert it or move it, but it just stays there, and if he speaks he will say something that will cause you to realize that that same idea is holding on to him. So he appears to he in a state of imbecility. Mental derangement with vertigo. With most all the mental symptoms there is vertigo. He lies in a state of apparent unconsciousness, yet knows all that is going on and at times is even able to remember and describe what was going on, but does not even wink; does not move a muscle. There is an appearance of ecstasy, a smile upon the face. Knows what is going on, yet with complete relaxation of the muscles without speech or apparent recognition of anyone. Perfectly relaxed, and yet knowing what is going on. That resembles catatonia. Unable to think. Fears death. Feels as if some awful thing was about to happen. All this is the result of grief, anxiety, vexation, prolonged loss of sleep. The vertigo is usually attended with nausea.

A Cocculus case cannot look out of the car window, cannot look down from the boat and see water moving, without nausea immediately.

Perhaps you can even now surmise what the head symptoms are to be With the headaches come dizziness, extreme nausea and gastric symptoms. Headaches brought on from riding in a wagon or riding in the cars or on shipboard; headache from motion. Cannot accommodate the eyes to moving objects; dizziness and whirling and headache. Congestion of the head, pressing, throbbing headache. Headache as if the skull would burst, or like a great valve opening and shutting. Sick headache with vertigo. Headache again from working in the sun. Sick headache from riding in a carriage.

Dim sightedness and disturbance of vision. Paralytic weakness of the muscles of the eyes, as well as the muscles of accommodation. The face becomes pale and sickly. Pale as death, with pains in the face, vertigo and nausea. Tearing pains in the face. Neuralgia of the face. Face bloated. Quivering and twitching of the muscles of the face. Paralysis of the muscles of the face. Numbness of the face. Twitching, jerking, numbness, paralysis. tearing pains.

Prostration and nervous exhaustion accompany most of the complaints of Cocculus.

Stomach symptoms. Loathing of food. Metallic taste in the mouth. Bitter taste in the mouth. Sour, nauseous taste in the mouth, and no food tempts him. He lies there sick with a little fever or a "cold". Headache, vertigo, nausea, loathing. Intermittent fevers with pains in the limbs, especially in the knees and bones of the legs, with that peculiar stiffness, nausea, and loathing of food. In intermittent fever or perhaps a low typhoid state, we have this loathing of food with nausea. You go to the bedside and you ask the nurse, "What have you been feeding the patient?" and the patient gags. The thought of food makes the patient gag. The nurse will say that every time she mentions food the patient gags. That thought of food or the smell of food in the other room, or in the kitchen, will nauseate the patient. Two medicines have this Cocculus and *Colchicum*.

Paralytic conditions. Paralysis of the œsophagus. Cannot swallow. "Paralytic condition of the throat after diphtheria." Sore throat with low forms of fever. The fever is gone but the patient does not rally, there is much nervous trembling,, numbness, twitching of muscles and great weakness. Sensation as though a worm were crawling in the stomach. Spasms of the stomach. Violent attacks of gastralgia, violent cramp of the stomach. Griping, pinching, constrictive pain. The pain in the bowels feels as if the intestines were, *pinched between sharp stones*. This causes fainting and vomiting. Colicky pains in the bowels; great distension of the abdomen, such as is found in typhoid fever; tension of the abdomen after drinking; flatulent colic. Tearing, cutting, spasmodic pains in the bowels. Radiating pains in the bowels accompanying diarrhœa. A paralytic condition of the rectum. Inability to press at stool. Urging to stool and burning in rectum. Disposition to stool, but peristaltic motion in upper intestines is wanting.

Copious menstrual flow, menses too soon; last too long. Catamenia two weeks before the time. In women prostrated from grief and from anxiety, and from prolonged loss of sleep, menses come too soon, are copious and prolonged. Headache, vertigo, nausea. Violent, cramping pains in the bowels, clutching pains in the uterus during menstruation. Again, just such a patient as described will have a suppression of the menstrual flow, or for weeks and months will have no menstrual flow; or just at the time the menstrual period should come on there is a copius *leucorrhœa that takes the place of the menses*. The woman is emaciated, and grows more and more sickly and chlorotic. The face is of greenish, yellow, sallow hue. "Leucorrhœa in place of the menses", or "copious leucorrhœa between the menstrual periods".

The heart is weak, pulse feeble. Paralytic weakness in the limbs, numbness, jerking of the muscles, twitching, quivering, loss of sensation, loss of power, muscular weakness in all the limbs. Numbness and paralytic feeling in the limbs. Awkwardness of the fingers and hands. On attempting to grasp the one hand with the other there is migratory numbness, or a more permanent numbness associated with paralytic weakness, sometimes changeable; sometimes one side is numb and the other paralyzed. The soles of the feet go to sleep. Numbness of the soles of the feet, such as we have in locomotor ataxia; cold feet. The knees give way from weakness. Totters while walking and threatens to fall to one side. Knees stiff. Paralysis of the lower extremities, proceeding from the small of the back. Arising from cold, from the abuse of *Mercury*. Paralysis of the lower limbs, with stiffness, numbness and bruised feeling.

Sleeplessness from long nursing and from night watching; that is a symptom that I have called your attention to so often. Anxious, frightful dreams; ill effects from loss of sleep and night watching. "Slightest loss of sleep tells on him."

COCCUS CACTI

There is a little remedy and wilt be a relief after the study of so many difficult ones. With fuller proving it will doubtless show itself a deep-acting constitutional remedy. Although it has cured some deep-seated chronic troubles, it has been used chiefly in acute affections. This is only because of the scantiness of its provings and our lack of knowledge concerning it in a general way. Very few mental symptoms have been brought out. Its use, so far as demonstrated, is mostly in catarrhal conditions of the air passages, and whooping cough, with copious, ropy, jelly-like mucus. Great quantities of this mucus form in the nose, in the throat, in the air passages generally, and in the vagina. The routine practitioner, whenever he sees thick, ropy, gelatinous mucus, thinks only of *Kali bi*. That comes from the study of key-notes. But it must be remembered that other remedies besides *Kali bi.* have this.

Spasmodic cough; whooping cough; the cough of drunkards. The chronic catarrhal state of the Coccus cacti patient comes on especially in the winter. It comes on when the cold weather begins and lasts till the warm weather comes. The patient is cold, and his complaints come on in cold weather. He is sensitive to cold, easily takes cold. But you must distinguish between the patient himself and his complaints, because they are entirely opposite to each other. When he once becomes sick from exposure to cold, he is always worse in a warm room and better in the cold air. His cough is brought on in a warm room; from being too warm in bed; from. drinking warm things. It is better from drinking cold things in a cold room; worse from exertion; from getting heated up; from becoming warm; that is, after the complaint has once set in, it reverses itself.

This is not unlike many other remedies. I have received many letters from doctors, saying: "Why is it that in your repertory and in Bœnning-hausen's, certain remedies are put down as better from cold and worse from cold? They certainly cannot have both." But they do have both, sometimes under different conditions and sometimes under the same conditions. Sometimes these are primary, sometimes they are secondary symptoms. A remedy must be examined to ascertain how it is that these circumstances can be the very opposite of each other. But commonly Bœnning-hausen registers both those things that belong to particulars and those things that belong to generals, and if the symptom, in his judgment, is strikingly worse by a certain circumstance, even if it is the very opposite of the general, he has that symptom in boldfaced type. *Phos.* is a good illustration of what we have been talking about. If you make a careful study of *Phos.* you will see that the complaints of the chest are all worse from cold, from cold air and from being cold. He catches cold and it settles in the chest, and the cough and irritation in the chest are worse from cold and being exposed to cold air. But he wants cold things in the stomach. His stomach feels better from cold things. Let him have head trouble and his head is better from cold, he wants cold things in his stomach. If he has stomach trouble, it is made worse by anything hot; he wants cold water to drink, and as soon as it gets warm, he vomits it up. You see *Phos.* is worse from cold and worse from heat. The pains in the extremities are better from heat.

The chronic cough, as has been said, is likely to begin with cold weather and last all winter, with a copious formation of mucus in the chest. It is a spasmodic cough, forcing the patient into the most violent efforts. The face becomes purple. Finally he retches and vomits long strings of tough, ropy mucus, filling the mouth and throat and causing him to choke. This is due to the fact that the mucus is so tenacious that it cannot be ejected from the pharynx in the usual way, therefore he must vomit. Now, there is a striking feature of this remedy. Anything coming in contact with the pharynx, the inside of the mouth, or even the gums, produces gagging and retching and will bring on the cough. We find this in the chronic states of sensitive persons, who are unable to brush the teeth or rinse the mouth without gagging and sometimes vomiting.

There is a general hyperæsthesia of the skin and mucous membranes Sensitive to the pressure of the clothing.

With the chest troubles there is much dyspnœa. He cannot walk without bringing on difficult breathing. He cannot ascend a height without suffocation. After the quantities of mucus are cleared out the cough is better and he goes on for two, three or four hours, when another one of these awful attacks comes on. They are apt to be worse at night when he becomes warm in bed. If he can lie in a cool room without much covering he will go longer without coughing.

The whooping cough is of a similar character. You will see the child lying in bed with the covers off. It wants the room cold, and the mother will tell you that if she can get to it quickly enough with a drink of cold water she can ward off the paroxysm. The chest fills up with mucus until respiration cannot be carried on any longer and it must he cleared out, yet the chill will resist and hold its breath to prevent coughing. You will be astonished to see how speedily Coccus cacti will change the character of that cough. One of the earliest signs of improvement will be observed in the easier respiration. The cough becomes less violent, the retching passes away, and in a week or ten days the cough will go, too. Cough worse after eating, worse on waking, worse in a warm room.

In the early stages of whooping cough Carbo veg. will develop and bring out the symptoms and furnish a good picture for a second Prescription, even if it does not cure.

Discharge of thick yellow mucus from the nose; nose stopped up. with inclination to sneeze. Great dryness of the nose. The air passages burn after the mucus has been cleared away. The chest burns from the mere exhaling of air. Sore throat with redness. Tickling in the throat. Sensation of a hair or crumb lodged in the throat behind the larynx. Fauces very sensitive. Arch of palate and fauces, as far as visible, very red. Burning in the throat < in the warmth, especially when warmed up in bed, < from warm drinks, though hot drinks are not so bad. Better from cold drinks. If the patient gets warm in bed or the room gets .warm he commences to clutch the larynx and cough. The slightest touch on the palate. or even the gums in examination of the throat will cause gagging sometimes when the parts look normal. He cannot hawk without gagging.

On swallowing food sometimes it will come right back again and cause gagging and retching.

Great thirst; wants water often and in large quantities. Nauseous taste in the mouth; never rid of it. Nausea in the throat Vomiting of white, bitter tasting froth. Toothache; sudden drawing pains in the teeth, worse from cold and from touch.

The mental symptoms are chiefly depression and anxiety. Great sadness; a cloud seems to hang over everything. Apprehensiveness. especially at 2 to 4 A.M. This state may alternate with loquacity and liveliness, like *Lachesis*. There are other symptoms worse after sleep; wakes in the morning with basilar headache, or with headache in the forehead; < mental exertion; after lying down; sometimes > from slow motion; < on coughing and from exertion; < after sleep.

A strong feature is its action on the kidneys, resembling acute parenchymatous nephritis. Albumen in the urine. Dark red sediment in the urine. Pain shooting from the kidney to the bladder and down the legs; < from motion. Renal colic. Urging to urinate, but inability to pass urine until a large clot of blood has been passed. In Coccus cacti the right side of the heart affected, the vessels become friable and there is hæmorrhage, oozing of blood, forming great black clots. The above symptom suggests a woman with uterine hæmmorrhage. There are haemorrhages of the uterus where the blood flows freely, coagulates slowly and does not form much of any clot in the vagina. But in this remedy the clots form very rapidly and the vagina becomes packed, and the bladder cannot be emptied until the clot is expelled. Uterine hæmorrhage is a strong feature of this remedy. Copious, frequent, prolonged menstrual flow. Large, hard, black clots fill the uterus, are expelled by labor-like pains, and form again. Inflammation of uterus and vagina, with copious, thick, white, jelly-like, ropy mucus. Soreness of the vulva; cannot bear the pressure of the clothing.

Hæmoptysis, dark, clotted; .< from exertion.

In the male there is impotence with dull pain in the loins. Dull pains in the region of the kidneys, with albuminuria; heavy sediment in the urine, etc., just such a state as you would find in a child that had taken cold after scarlet fever.

COFFEA

This drug is characterized by a general sensitivity. Sensitiveness of vision, of hearing, of smell, of touch; sensitiveness to pain. It is most astonishing sometimes about this great sensitiveness. *Pains are increased by noise.* Sensitiveness of hearing is so great that sounds are painful. Pains in the face, toothache, headache; pains in the lower limbs; everywhere *aggravated* by noise. All the nervous disturbances possible are found in this medicine, and they are all aggravated by noise. Even the opening of the door and the ringing of the door-bell produces great suffering. Such patients are so sensitive that they hear sounds which those in a state of health cannot hear. Perhaps no medicine in the Materia Medica approximates this sensitiveness of hearing where it is accompanied with pain, unless it be *Nux vom.* Those practitioners who do not know this generally resort to *Nut vom.* for pains aggravated from voices in another room, or from noise or the sound of children. Many remedies have increase of nervousness from noise; noise aggravates headache, and aggravates suffering about the head, and makes some persons nervous. But pain in the extremities aggravated by noise is peculiar. It seems that the noise disturbs him so that he cannot bear pain.

The Coffea state is brought on by emotions or Violent excitement of the mind, but especially by joy or "pleasant surprise". The result is sleeplessness, nervous excitement, neuralgia, twitching of muscles, toothache, faceache, red face and hot head.

You may be called to the bedside of a woman who has been laboring for some great cause. She works persistently, is successful, but goes to bed with weeping, delirium, neuralgia, sleeplessness. Her heart palpitates, her pulse flickers, she has fainting spells, and without Coffea she may die. Coffee drinkers who kept up through some ordeal and then break down are similarly affected.

The Coffea patient is sensitive to wine. A small amount of wine intensifies the nervousness, produces sleeplessness, flushed face, feverishness, great excitement. Not necessarily intoxication, but nervous excitement. Coffea has a painful sensitiveness of the skin beyond comprehension. I remember one particular case. A woman had her lower limb out of bed and it was as red as fire down one side. I walked toward it to put my hand on it But she said, "Oh, don't touch it, I can't bear to have it touched; I can't touch it myself." I asked how long this had been coming on. She said, "Oh, it all came on within an hour." Such a symptom is common in coffee drinkers. There was no fever. Intense stinging, burning pains in the skin with the redness and heat with coarse rash coming on suddenly, leaving just as suddenly. The sensitive part is aggravated by cold air, aggravated by any wind or from fanning, from motion, yet aggravated by warmth. Aggravated from anyone walking across the floor. The woman I referred to scowled when I was walking toward the bed. A number of times I have seen such things relieved within a few minutes by Coffea.

Fainting from sudden emotions. Hysteria, nervousness, weeping. Pitiful weeping from pain; trembling and weeping from hurt feelings; the slightest neglect. The greatest mental and physical exhaustion; great restlessness; lying awake most of the night. The wakefulness produced by Coffea is well known, even to the laity. It is taken by nurses to keep them awake nights with their patients. The Coffea patient is quick to act and to think. So full of ideas that she lies awake nights making plans, thinking of a thousand things; utterly unable to banish the thoughts that flood the mind; hears the clocks on the distant steeples, as do *Opium, China* and *Nux vam.* Hears the dogs barking. So great is the brain activity, the mental excitement, that she hears noises that are purely imaginary. Memory active, easy comprehension; full of ideas; increased power to think and to debate. Coffea increases the mental capacity. But after a while reaction follows; she becomes stupid and sleepy. There is no end to the fancies, to the visions. Fanciful visions come before the mind. Recalls things not thought of for years; recalls poetry that was recited in childhood. Eyes brilliant; pupils dilated; face flushed; head hot.

With all these nervous states the patient dreads the fresh air. He is extremely sensitive to cold, sensitive to the wind and cold weather. Complaints come on in the cold weather, from the cold air. Pain in the mouth and jaws, *better from holding ice-cold water in the mouth.* This applies to toothache and faceache where it is deep in the jaws. Hot head; inflamed condition of the gums. Pain in the teeth; rending, tearing pain in the teeth, brought on from exposure to cold, from emotions, from excite ment, from joy; aggravated from motion; ameliorated by ice or ice-cold things; aggravated by warm food. Cannot drink warm tea, it so intensifies the pain. That is a particular. The particulars contrast with the generals. In one place you may see "better from cold" in black-faced type, put it relates to the face and jaws. Worse from cold is a general. Aversion to cold air, aversion to the open air unless it is very warm and still. Aversion to wind. "Neuralgic toothache entirely relieved by holding cold water in the mouth, returning as it becomes warm. Toothache during the menstrual period. Complaints of anæmic children during dentition." Those nervous, excitable children that talk to the nurse and the mother very rapidly with brilliant eyes, red face, cannot go to sleep. It will quiet the patient and actually favor the growth of the tooth in a painless manner. That is the description of a nervous child with many nervous brain and mental troubles. This child is extremely sensitive; it takes cold. The routine prescriber gives *Belladonna* to a child who has hot head, hot face and throbbing carotids, and when it does not help he gives more *Belladonna,* and increases the size of his dose until the child has a proving. He makes a *Belladonna* child out of it when Coffea would have cured it. In most instances where *Belladonna* is indicated the child is sluggish and stupid, and would like to sleep. With Coffea there is excitement. The child hears things its mother cannot hear; sees things; imagines things. Wakes up in fright. Sees this, that and the other thing in the room. Wakes up excited as if it had visions. Looks for things, and finally sees they are not there. Such things are strong features of Coffea.

At times the head is hot, the face is flushed and the eyes so brilliant that one fears apoplexy. Patients will often tell yon that they hear a "noise" in the head, a ringing and roaring in the occiput. The ear is the one organ capable of registering sounds. But strange to say, the ears are sometimes very deceiving. Roaring in the ears sometimes seems as if it were in the occiput. ,Sometimes it is accompanied with a sensation of tingling or bubling in the head. When patients say, "I have a roaring in the head," you know that means in the ear; many times accompanying roaring, ringing in the ears, buzzing in the ears, is a peculiar sensation of vibration in the head that is mistaken by the patient for a sound. I mention that because the Coffea patient feels a crackling or a bubbling in the occiput. The head feels badly; it feels too small. Headache, as of something pressing hard upon the surface of the brain. You would naturally suppose there was a pressing because of the congestive state heretofore described. "Headache as if the whole brain were torn and bruised, or dashed to pieces. Worse from motion, noise or light." The eye and the head symptoms are worse from noise and light. "Headache intolerable. Head feels small, and as if filled with fluid. Nervous hysterical headache. One-sided headache." There is another head symptom which is quite common. A feeling as if a nail were driven into the head Coffea headaches are worse from walking, from motion; from the mere moving across the floor, he says he feels a draft of air on his head. And that is true of the pain in any part of the body. If a Coffea patient should have a pain in the hand, swinging of the hand through the air will aggravate. It is worse both from the motion and from the air. I want to illustrate that in this way in order to show how sensitive he is to air, and especially the painful part to cold air; when he moves against the air, against even still air he feels it. But the amelioration of the toothache from cold is an exception, is a particular.

The neuralgia of the face is a common feature of old coffee drinkers. Sensitive persons take coffee and finally become habituated to it. They say they cannot get along without it. They must have coffee. Such individuals should stop coffee. When coffee furnishes a crutch it is a sure indication that drinking it must be stopped. So it is with tea or any beverage. Such persons sometimes become sensitive to coffee, and they drink it in great quantities; the face becomes red; headaches come on, and other symptoms of Coffea. Stopping coffee brings out quite a proving, and you have to study *Chain.* and *Nux* for an antidote. In all these remedies you get opposite effects. Now *Opium* will illustrate that. The first effect of *Opium* is to constipate. Let several doses be given, and as the effects of the Opium wear off he may have diarrhœa. *Opium* eaters can seldom stop because a diarrhœa comes on. If you should ever have an *Opium* case and diarrhœa comes on *Puls.* will nearly always control it. But there are individuals who reverse that. Often small doses of *Opium* will bring on dysentery, and if it is increased, bloody dysentery and inflammation of the bowels come on. Of course, one is action and the other the reaction.

A woman who is a confirmed coffee drinker will have menses too soon and lasting too long. Uterine hæmorrhage is not uncommon. Another feature of Coffea is that the woman can scarcely wear the napkin during menstruation (*Platinum*). The parts are in a state of hyperæsthesia. The vagina is hot and sensitive, often preventing coition. In the text it reads "Great sensitiveness of female genital organs, with general excitability. She is in a state of ecstasy. Uterine hæmorrhage with excessive sensitiveness of organs and voluptuous itching. Metrorrhagia; large black lumps," Sometimes large bright red lumps. "Worse from every motion, with violent pain in the groins, and fear of death." Excessive sensitiveness about the vulva with voluptuous itching, is a strong feature of Coffea, and you will often find such symptoms in coffee drinkers.

During and after labor we also see this great excitement, all these nervous manifestations The nervous system is in a fret, and such a mental state as described comes on with after-pains; extremely sensitive to pain, cries out; sees visions; hears all sorts of noises. Pains aggravated from motion; aggravated from noise. Wants everybody to keep still in the house.

Convulsions of children. "Puerperal convulsions. Extreme excitability." "Palpitation of the heart, pulse fluttering." "Strong, quick palpitation of the heart with extreme nervousness, sleeplessness and cerebral erethism caused by unexpected news of great good fortune." Let a woman about to go into confinement hear suddenly some unusually good news and she becomes almost ecstatic; carries the symptom all through confinement. The child is affected, the milk is affected. The milk flows away. Hæmorrhage is likely to come on. Great nervousness, excitability, fear.

COLCHICUM

It is rather singular that traditional medicine used Colchicum so much for gout. In all the old books it was recommended for this malady. The provings corroborate the fact that Colchicum fits into many conditions of gout. Acute rheumatism and uric acid diathesis; rheumatic complaints in general, with swelling and without swelling. But traditional medicine does not tell us what kind of gout to give it in or what kind of rheumatism. It was really the medicine of experience. "If it is gout, try Colchicum." The question of what was to be done with the *patient* when the remedy failed never came up. It was "Give the prescription and keep at it," and drugs were administered until the patient, steadily growing worse, passed from one doctor's hands to another's. It is true that Colchicum fits into the gouty state. Spells of cold, wet weather will slack up the flow of urine. make it scanty, or decrease the quantity of solids in the urine. This takes place in the provings of Colchicum and has been verified many times. It is well known that such a condition will bring about or intensify the gouty state. If the solids in the urine are deficient, if they are not carried off in the urine, something must happen, and the gouty state comes on.

Colchicum is aggravated by cold, damp weather; by the cold rains in the Fall. It is aggravated by anything that will debilitate. It is aggravated in the extreme heat of summer; it has a summer rheumatism; the heat will slack up the flow of urine or the quantity of solids in the urine.

A striking feature running through the remedy is its tendency to move from one joint to another, from one side to another, from below upwards, or from above downwards. Rheumatic conditions with swelling or without swelling; first here, next there, changing about from place to place. Another striking feature is the general dropsical condition. When the hands and feet swell, and there is pitting on pressure. Dropsy of the abdominal cavity; of the pericardium; of the pleuræ and dropsy of serous sacs. Swellings that are inflammatory and rheumatic; swellings that are dropsical, with pale urine. Whether copious or scanty, still it is pale.

Muscular rheumatism and rheumatism of the white fibrous tissues of the joints. Rheumatic troubles that have been going on for some time will end in cardiac troubles. When cardiac troubles with valvular defects are present, almost the first thing the busy doctor, thinks of is a history of rheumatism. Let me say that a part of the study of Materia Medica consists in the observation of sick people. A busy physician learns without books, though of course he should familiarize himself with the literature, so that from reading, as well as observation, he may acquire a knowledge of the general nature of sickness. When he listens to the patient's story or makes a physical examination, he knows how such cases usually conduct themselves. He knows what to expect. He knows the natural trend of sickness and instantly recognizes what is strange and unusual. He will not recognize what is strange and unusual unless he knows what is natural. So your books on symptomatology and pathology, diagnosis, etc., will tell you much of this, but as you gain experience in homœopathic practice you will get a much finer idea of this because your Materia Medica teaches you to observe more closely. The Materia Medica man learns to single out and trace every little thing in order to individualize. So it may be said that years of observation in studying disease, studying the sick man along with the Materia Medica, will open to the mind a much grander knowledge of the sicknesses of humanity than can he had by practicing traditional medicine. Traditional medicine benumbs the ability to observe.

All the complaints of this remedy are aggravated from motion. The painful complaints, the head complaints, the bowel complaints, the liver complaints, the stomach complaints, are all worse from motion. Such an aggravation from motion that he dreads to move. About as marked as we find in *Bryonia*. Aversion to motion, and aggravation from motion. Aggravation from becoming cold and in cold, damp weather. He is a chilly patient, sensitive to cold. Most rheumatic patients are sensitive to cold, but there are a few exceptions. There is no greater rheumatic patient than the *Ledum* patient. He presents both sides. Though he is cold, his pains are ameliorated by cold. In Colchicum the pains are ameliorated by heat, by wrapping up, by being warm. If he moves, any suffering that he may have will be intensified. Great prostration accompanies the complaints of this remedy. Weakness of the limbs, great exhaustion, nervous exhaustion of a typhoid character. He gradually grows weaker like one going into Bright's disease. He has grown weak for some time, and he is pallid and waxy. His hands and feet pit upon pressure. Examine the urine and you will find albumen in it. The urine becomes black like ink with albumen. There is an unusual degree of irritability of the tissues, soreness, sensitiveness to touch, sensitiveness to motion; bruised feeling of the joints and of the whole body. Touch and motion bring on a painful sensation in the body as of electric vibrations. Great weakness and exhaustion. He cannot exert himself in the least without causing dyspnœa. Must lie down; does not want to move; sinking of strength; seems as if his life will flow our of him from motion and from exertion; so tired and exhausted. This naturally occurs when going towards Bright's disease, when going towards a continued fever. Kidney affections and liver affections. Lassitude, prostration, anxiety. The muscles twitch and electric shocks pass through the body. A paralytic weakness was observed in the poisonous effects and too prolonged provings. The jaw hangs down, the muscles are flabby, relaxed. He lies on the hack as if sinking; slides down in bed like one in typhoid, in low forms of rheumatic and in continued fevers, so great is the exhanstion. Paralysis of the limbs or of one limb, or of any part.

The Colchicum patient is almost constantly sweating, even with fever, and sometimes the sweat is cold. A draft blows upon him, suppresses that sweat and the paralytic condition of the limbs comes on; suppression of urine and retention of urine. This describes the profound character and type of sickness. Low forms of sickness; prostrating sickness; sickness with nervous trembling; with great exhaustion. After acute disease has passed away, great weakness and dropsy follows. Dropsy after scarlet fever.

With all these troubles, the stomach and the bowel symptoms are very decided. This is like *Cocculus*. Absolutely unable to touch food. Nausea, gagging, retching at the bare mention of food in his presence. The thought and smell of food bring on nausea and vomiting. With all these low forms of disease, these states described, we can see that this kind of weakness is little different from the *Cocculus* weakness. Colchicum has delirium, prostration, depression of mind, great sensitiveness to pain, which he seems to feel in his mind, and it brings out mental symptoms. Very sensitive to pain; confusion of the mind; disorders of comprehension. Cannot understand what he reads. The headaches are all of a rheumatic character. Very often the 'whole skull,' the pericranium, is sore as if bruised. The scalp is sensitive. Pressure in the head—constriction; pressing, bursting headaches. Heat in the head. Tearing in the scalp. Headaches are all aggravated by motion.

The eye symptoms are of a rheumatic character, are connected with rheumatism, rheumatic fever. It is not very uncommon to have iritis in connection with rheumatic fever and it is a strong feature of Colchicum. Ulcers of the lids, styes, much lachrymation in the open air. The tears excoriate and cause redness of the lids.

He takes cold easily. Sneezing, stuffing up of the nostrils. Nosebleed in rheumatic and gouty constitutions. But there is one feature that is more marked in Colchicum than all others. He is so sensitive to odors that he smells things which others do not smell. He smells odors from which he is nauseated. "Strong odors make him quite beside himself." You say "soup" or "broth," or something to eat, and he gets sick. He can smell the things in the kitchen, in spite of much precaution, and this runs through the remedy. In typhoid fever, prostrated beyond the usual—and typhoid is always prostrated enough—he is unusually prostrated. He cannot take milk, cannot take raw eggs, cannot take soup, because he gags at the mere thought of them. He has gone on for days, and his family are afraid that he is going to starve to death. That aggravation from odors is so strong with him that it seems to take possession of him. It involves his appetite, his weakness, his stomach. So it does seem that it is a strong feature. Notice that this is one of his loves; it is a perverted love, and the loves are general whether they are manifested through the eyes, nose or touch. It enters into his very life because it involves hatred to odor, and when it stands out in low forms of disease like the continued fevers, the exhaustive fevers and rheumatic complaints it becomes a general. It would be a particular if it were something that applied to the things alone, but you see it enters into the very innermost. Involves a hatred, becomes mental, becomes a part of the man. He himself may be said to hate odors, hate the smell of food and the thought of it. Do not say "food" in the presence of a Colchicum patient, but give him Colchicum first, and pretty soon he will want something to eat. It removes that hatred for food. What a vital thing it must be when a man hates that which will keep him alive.

The teeth are very sensitive. "Rheumatic teeth." The gums settle away; after a while the teeth become loose. Pain in the teeth; rheumatic condition of the jaws and the teeth. "Grinding of the teeth, teeth sensitive when pressed together."

"Aversion to food; loathing the sight and smell," more the smell of it. "The smell of fish, eggs, fat meats or broths causes nausea even unto faintness." The Colchicum patient may have much thirst or no thirst, or these may alternate, Nausea and vomiting are very strong features. "Nausea and inclination to vomit, caused by swallowing saliva. Nausea, eructations and copious vomiting of mucus and bile. Violent retching followed by copious and forcible vomiting of food, and then of bile."

In the stomach there is sometimes coldness and sometimes burning. Now it may be that the Colchicum patient has both coldness and burning. They are both recorded in the Repertory and in the provings, but it is sometimes difficult to tell which is which, more difficult than you will imagine unless you try a piece of ice somewhere and something very hot.

"Burning in the pit of the stomach." Coldness in the stomach. Now the abdomen furnishes us still more to observe. The abdomen is distended with flatus, tympanitic. Great soreness in the whole abdomen. Just such a tympanitic condition as we have in typhoid. If you ever happen to be in the country practicing medicine, and the farmer's cows get into a fresh clover patch and eat themselves full and become distended so that you are afraid they are going to explode offer your services and give each one of those cows a few pellets of Colchicum. It will be but a few minutes before the wind will get out of there to your surprise and the farmer's, too; and you may convert him to Homœpathy. Farmers have been known to put a butcher's knife into the pouch of the cow between the last short ribs to let the wind out. The cow will get well, but Colchicum is better than the butcher's knife. The same is true of the horse; in fact, of man or beast. When the abdomen is violently distended and tympanitic, Colchicum is often a suitable remedy.

Spasmodic pains, colic, tearing pains, burning, griping pains, forcing the patient to bend double. Aggravated from motion. Great tenderness and soreness with the colic. Aggravated from eating; ameliorated from bending double. And then comes the diarrhœa. It has just such a diarrhœa as is found in low forms of fever. Dysenteric or diarrhœic stools that are jelly-like. They form in the pan a solid mass of jelly-like, coagulated mucus. Very painful, extremely painful is the Colchicum stool. Great soreness in the abdomen. Great relaxation of the parts. Prostrusion of the rectum. Putrid, dark, bloody mucus. "Bloody discharges from the bowels with deathly nausea." Fell dysentery, with discharges of white mucus and violent tenesmus. Putrid, dark, clotted blood and mucus pass from the bowels. Diarrhœa with violent, colicky pains. Bloody stools with scrapings from the intestines and protrusion of anus. Profuse, watery stools in hot, damp weather or in the Autumn. Watery, jelly-like mucus passes from anus with violent spasm in sphincter. It passes as a thin, watery flow; but as soon as it cools, it forms a jelly.

The urine burns when it passes. It is attended with much pain. inflammation of the kidneys, inflammation of the bladder; tenesmus; retention of urine. The kidneys manufacture no urine; scanty urine with dropsy. The urine is inky, that is, very dark brown and sometimes almost black, loaded with albumen. This remedy conforms principally to the acute form of Bright's disease.

Great dyspnœa, rapid, short breathing; the heart's impulse strong. Respiration accelerated. The heart's impulse can be heard all over the room. Palpitation; oppression of the chest. Feels as if he had a great weight on the chest; cannot breathe. Hydrothorax; the pleural cavities distended with serum, causing the dyspnœa. "Heart's action muffled, indistinct, very weak." Stinging, tearing pains in the muscles of the chest.

Paralytic pains in the arms; enlarged finger joints. This also tells what a low form of sickness, what a feeble circulation the medicine brings about. "Weakness so that he strikes the knees together when walking; pain all over as if bruised. Swelling of the joints." The joints are most affected. Muscular rheumatism. Numbness, œdema, swelling of the limbs.

COLOCYNTH

The principal feature of Colocynth is its severe, tearing, neuralgic pains; so severe that the patient is unable to keep still. Sometimes they are > by motion—at least it appears that they are worse during rest— > by pressure and sometimes > by heat. Pains occur in the face, abdomen, along the course of the nerves.

These pains are often due to a very singular cause, namely, anger with indignation. Hence persons who are haughty and easily offended or chagrined have Colocynth complaints. Anger will be followed by violent neuralgia in the head, eyes, down the spine and in the intestines.

In spite of extreme restlessness there is great weakness with the pains. A patient suffering with chronic diarrhœa, with severe colic, will sometimes become so weak that he can hardly speak. A feeling of faintness, or even fainting, is by no means an unusual concomitant of the pains. Griping occurs along the course of nerves, and in some cases numbness, pricking and tingling, like the crawling of ants in the part affected.

With many doctors Colocynth is a routine remedy for sciatica; and only when it fails to do they take the symptoms of the case in order to find the remedy that is indicated. There is no excuse for such practice. Where the pain is better from hard pressure and from heat, where it is worse during repose and drives the patient to despair, Colocynth will generally cure. But it is not indicated in all cases. Some remedies select the muscles and tendons, some the bones and periosteum, while others select the great nerve trunks in which to manifest their symptoms. The pains of Colocynth appear, as a rule, in the larger nerves.

The mental symptoms are not very striking. As soon as the prover of Colocynth begins to have pains along the course of nerves he becomes irritable; everything vexes him; he is worse from vexation.

Screams with the pains. Walks about the room and becomes increasingly anxious as the pain goes on. Disinclined to talk or to answer, or to see friends.

His friends irritate him and he wants to be alone.

He has all he can do to stand those terrible pains.

Vomiting and diarrhœa frequently come with the pains, especially if they are in the abdomen.

Colic comes on in paroxysms that grow in intensity.

The patient becomes increasingly nauseated until finally he vomits and he continues to retch after the stomach is empty.

Colocynth produces a state in the nervous system like that found in individuals who have for years been laboring under annoyances and vexations. A man whose business affairs have been going wrong becomes irritable and nervous exhaustion follows. A woman who must watch her unfaithful husband night and day to keep him away from other women gradually assumes a sensitive irritable state of mind, and is upset by the least provocation. This is the state of the Colocynth prover.

You will seldom find this medicine indicated in strong. vigorous, healthy people who have suddenly become sick. It is more likely to be in the constitution just described, and those who are in the habit of overeating.

We find tearing pains in the scalp, brought on by anger; exhaustion; pains that are better from pressure and heat, and worse when not in motion.

Constant, gnawing pains in the head.

Painful, tearing, digging through the whole brain, becoming unbearable when moving the eyelids.

Intense pain through the whole head; worse from moving the eyes. Severe, pressing, tearing headache, causing her to cry out.

Intermittent headache in those of a rheumatic, gouty or nervous diathesis.

Pain tearing and screwing together.

Violent periodical or intermittent headache.

Such are some of the expressions in the text. But the particular character of the pain is not as important as the circumstances that are likely to cause it and the conditions in which the patient has been living. Knowing the life of a patient affords much knowledge of the patient himself.

The same violent neuralgic pains are found in the eye.

Rheumatic iritis, worse in the evening and night.

Severe, burning, cutting and sticking pains in the eye.

Burning is more characteristic of the pains of the eyes than of other parts of the head and face.

Sharp. cutting stabs; pressing pains.

The faceache is especially important, because Colocynth is one of the most frequently indicated remedies for neuralgia of this region. There are three remedies which are indicated in faceache more often than any others, *Belladonna, Magnesia phosphorica* and Colocynth.

The *Belladonna* pains are as violent as any, and are accompanied by red face, flashing eyes, hot head, and great sensitiveness of the part to touch.

In Colocynth the pains come in waves, are better from heat, from pressure, worse if anything during rest, and are brought on by excitement or vexation. They are generally on the left side; while those of *Belladonna* are on the right, and are caused by cold.

Magnesia phosphorica has tearing pains that shoot like lightning along the nerves and are relieved by heat and pressure.

The expression of the Colocynth face is one of anxiety from the severity of the suffering. No matter where the pain is the face is distorted. Finally, it becomes pale and the checks become blue.

Tearing pains in the check-bones, or more correctly, in the infraorbital nerve where it emerges from the foramen. Sometimes this pain feels like a hot wire, sometimes like a cold nail, and sometimes it is tearing, burning or stinging. Frequently it spreads over the face, following the ramifications of the small branches of the nerve, usually on the left side. The patient cries out and is very restless.

Tearing or burning pain extending to the ear and head.

All pains are better from pressure, but this is in the beginning. After the pain has been going for several days with increasing severity, the part becomes very sensitive and pressure cannot he endured.

Aversion to food.

Violent thirst.

Colic brought on from drinking while overheated; from eating indigestible things, from high living; colic from eating potatoes.

Potatoes and starchy foods disagree with the Colocynth patient like *Alumina.*

The vomiting of Colocynth is different from that of most other remedies. Nausea does not appear at first, but when the pain becomes sufficiently intense nausea and vomiting begin, the contents of the stomach are ejected, and the patient continues to retch until the severity of the suffering decreases.

The stomach pains are clutching, cramping and digging, as if grasped by the fingers.

Similar pains occur lower down in the abdomen, but they are still better from hard pressure, and from doubling up—which amounts to pressure—come on in paroxysms of increasing severity, until the patient is nauseated and vomits, and are associated with great restlessness and faint, sinking feeling at the pit of the stomach. The victim bends down over the back of a chair, or ever the foot-board if unable to get out of bed.

In the Guiding Symptoms we find several pages of repetitions, showing how extensively this medicine is applicable in abdominal complaints where these symptoms are present. It would be well to read them.

The pains in the lower part of the abdomen are relieved by drawing up the limbs and pressing with the fists. In the violent ovarian neuralgias of Colocynth, the woman will flex the limb of the painful side hard against the abdomen and hold it there.

The physician asks: "What has happened to give you these pains?" Her answer is likely to be: "My servant spilled some dirty water on a handsome rug, we had some words over it, and this is the result."

Colic from anger with indignation; better from bending double and worse in the upright position, while standing or bending backwards.

Colic of infants when they are relieved by lying on the stomach; as soon as the position is changed they begin to scream again.

The same symptoms accompany the diarrhœa and dysentery. The stools consist of white mucus, are thick, ropy and jelly-like; at times bloody. At first they may he copious, strong smelling, pappy, and later watery, yellow, scanty and almost inodorous.

Diarrhœa and dysentery from anger with. indignation; the most awful tenesmus during stool; urging to stool with colic.

Eating ever so little, brings on the colic, urging and stool.

Watery stools after eating.

Many of these cases find relief from heat and the warmth of the bed.

CONIUM MACULATUM

This medicine is a deep, long acting antipsoric, establishing a state of disorder in the economy that is so far reaching and so long lasting that it disturbs almost all the tissues of the body. The complaints are brought on from aking cold, and the glands become affected all over the body. From every little cold the glands become hard and sore. Infiltration in deep-seated diseases in he region of ulcers and in the region of inflamed parts; in the glands along the course of the lymphatics, so we get a chain like knots. The glands under the arm inflame and ulcerate. The glands in the neck, in the groin and abdomen become enlarged. Ulcerated parts indurate. An abscess of the breast becomes surrounded by lumps and nodules. Nodules in the breast even where milk has not yet formed; lumps and nodules, indurations and enlarged glands form under the skin all over the body. Conium has been used extensively for malignant affections of glands, because it takes hold of glands from the beginning and infiltrates, and they gradually grow to a stony hardness, like scirrhus. Now, another grand feature running through this remedy is the action upon the nerves. The nerves are in a state of great debility. Trembling, jerking of the muscles and twitching from the weakness of the nerves. Inability to stand any physical effort without great exhaustion. Gradually growing paralytic weakness, somewhat as was described in *Cocculus*. Exhaustion of body and mind, that is, a general slowing down of all the activities of the body. The liver becomes indurated, sluggish, enlarged. The bladder is weak, can expel only a part of the urine. Or sometimes there is a paralytic condition and no expulsive power. This shows that the remedy increases toward a paralytic weakness.

Hysteria. Hypochondriacal state of mind, with the nervousness, trembling and weakness of the muscles. He gets tired in the earlier stages, but finally this goes on until the limbs are paralytic.

A great many of the complaints are painless. The ulcers and the paralytic conditions are painless. Great physical and mental debility; great prostration of the muscular system; exhaustion, tremulous weakness. Paralysis of the legs and hip. Mental symptoms, nervous symptoms, trembling, in widows and widowers who have suddenly been deprived of their sexual relations. When in a state of considerable vigor, if suddenly deprived, the woman or the man takes on a state of trembling weakness, inability to stand any mental effort, and inability to put the attention upon things said by others. Not so marked or not so common in the woman as in the man. When this state comes on in a woman who is of unusual sexual vigor there may be severe congestion of the uterus and ovaries, *Apes* is more likely to fit her symptoms than Conium. But with hysteria and excitability Conium is often the remedy. Many of its symptoms come about from such a cause.

Conium has such a deep action that it gradually brings about a state of imbecility. The mind gives out. The mind at first becomes tired like the muscles of the body. Unable to sustain any mental effort. The memory is weak. The mind will not concentrate, it will not force itself to attention; it cannot meditate, and then comes imbecility. Inability to stand any mental effort or to rivet the attention upon anything are some of the most important symptoms in this medicine. Insanity of a periodical type. Imbecility, though, is far more frequent than insanity. When you come to examine the mental states you will see symptoms that will make you think the patient is delirious, but that is not quite it. It is a slow-forming weakness of mind; not that rapid, active state, such as accompanies a fever; it is a delirium without a fever, so to speak, which is not constant. Forms of insanity that are passive. He thinks slowly, and he continues in this stage for weeks and months, if he recovers at all. Those excitable cases that have more or less violence and activity in mental states are such as will correspond to *Bell., Hyos., Stram.* and *Ars.* You see nothing of that in this medicine. This state of the mind has come on so gradually that the family has not observed it. The mind is full of strange things that have come little by little, and when the family look over the many things that he has done and said they begin to wonder if he is not becoming insane, but he is travelling toward a state of imbecility. Conium is of a slow, passive character. Complete indifference; takes no interest in anything, particularly when walking in the open air. "He is averse to being near people and to talking of those passing him; is inclined to seize hold of and abuse them." That, of course, is an insane act. "Sad and gloomy. Great unhappiness of mind, recurring every fourteen days," showing a two weeks periodicity. The Conium patient will sit and mope in the corner in a state of sadness and depression, giving no reason only that he is so sad. A hypochondriacal subject going around with whims and notions that people attempt to reason him out of, and the more they attempt to reason with him the more sad he is. Morose, peevish, vexed. Everything vexes and disturbs him. Cannot endure any kind of excitement, it brings on physical and mental distress, brings on weakness and sadness. Sometimes Conium symptoms will be found in persons who have suffered from grief; they become broken in memory. This is likely to come first. They forget, never can recall things just as they want them. And so they grow weaker and weaker until they become imbeciles. If it is decidedly mental, imbecility results; if it is taking a physical course the ending is paralysis, and it is not uncommon for a general paralytic weakness to come on, so that body and mind progress toward weakness together until some decided manifestation is made, and then it will be seen to be going toward paralysis, or some decided manifestation is made which will send it toward imbecility, and then the body will seem to remain stationary. There comes a time in these cases where there is a sort of division between the body and the mind. Whenever under homœopathic treatment the physical improves and the mental grows worse, that patient will never be cured. There are such cases. I never like to see the physical grow better and the mental grow worse in any degree. That does not mean the aggravation caused by the remedy. If the mental does not improve it means that the patient is growing worse. There is no better evidence of the good action of a remedy than mental improvement.

Conium patients cannot endure even the slightest alcoholic drink. Any wine or stimulating beverage will bring on trembling, excitement, weakness of

mind and prostration. There are many headaches in these patients. Patients
going into decline will manifest headaches. Stitching, tearing pains in the head;
throbbing in the head. Signs precursory to a giving out of the brain. Neuralgia.

Weakness of muscles. Weakness of muscles on one side of the face.
Paralysis of the upper lids. Tingling pains. These are only in keeping with the
signs of a general breakdown. We would not think of giving Conium for those
sudden, violent congestions of the brain, or sudden, violent attacks of pain
in the head, face or eyes, but those that accompany a general progressive
disease. There are stitching, lancinating, knife-like pains along the course of
nerves about face and eyes and head. Stitching in the top of the head. Burning
on top of the head. Often the symptoms will lead the homœopathic physician
to make a physical examination. A great deal more important than the physical
examination are the symptoms that point out a remedy.

Excitement will bring on headaches. Numbness of the scalp is one of the
common symtpoms of Conium. It is a general; wherever there is trouble there
will be numbness, numbness with pains, very often numbness with the
weakness. Paralytic conditions are attended with numbness. Sick headache
with inability to urinate. Great giddiness. Everything in the room seems to go
around. Confused feeling in the head. Often sits lost in thought. Vertigo and
pressure in the head with unaltered pulse. Vertigo worse from stooping. The
slightest spiritous drink intoxicates him. Vertigo when turning the head, like
turning in a circle, when rising from a seat; worse when lying down, *as though
the bed were turning in a circle; when turning in bed* or when looking
around. The vertigo most common in Conium is that which comes on while
lying in bed rolling the eyes or *turning the eyes.* This is somewhat as it is in
Cocculus, not as to vertigo alone, but the general slowed down condition of
the muscles. The paresis, or weakness of the muscles all over the body is
also present in the eyes. There is a muscular weakness of all the muscles of
the eye, so that the Conium patient is unable to watch moving objects without
getting sick headaches, visual and mental disturbances. Riding on the cars,
watching things in rapid motion, and inability to focus rapidly—slowness of
the accommodation is what we must call it—is the cause for many sicknesses.
Inability to follow moving objects with sufficient rapidity and a headache
comes on. "Objects look red, rainbow-colored, striped; confused spots;
double vision; weakness of sight. Short-sighted; cannot read long without
letters running together." All this is due to defective accommodation.
"Sluggish adaptation of the eye to varied range of vision. Vision becomes
blurred when he is irritable. Weakness and dazzling of the eyes, together
with dizziness. *Aversion to light without inflammation of the eyes.*" The
pupil will not accommodate itself to the changes between strong light and
dim light, and he suffers from it. Severe photophobia and lachrymation

Photophobia without congestion of any tissue without or within the globe of the eye. Sometimes the pupils are contracted and sometimes dilated. Conium has cured ulcer of the cornea. "Burning in the eyes when reading." Shooting, smarting, cutting, burning pain in the eyes. The lids indurate, thicken and are heavy and fall. It is with difficulty that he can lift them up. So this paralysis extends all through the muscles of the body and affects the mind similarly. "Could scarcely raise the eyelids, they seemed pressed down by a heavy weight. Burning on entire surface of lids; hordeola; paralysis of muscles of the eyes." A marked condition is that of swelling of the glands about the face, ear and under the jaws. The parotids are swollen and hard. The same gradually increasing hardness in the submaxillary and sublingual glands. Enlargement of the glands of the side of the neck in cancerous affections. It has cured epithelioma of the lid, and of the nose and of the cheek. Ulcers about the lip with induration. Deep under the ulcer there will be hardness, and along all the vessels that send lymph towards that ulcer there will be a chain of knots.

Paresis extending to paralysis of the œsophagus; difficulty in swallowing; food goes down part way and stops. As food is about to pass the cardiac orifice it stops and enters with a great effort. "Strange rising in the throat, with sense of stuffing, as if something were lodged there. Sense of fulness in the throat as of a lump, with involuntary attempts at swallowing. Fulness in throat with suppressed eructations. Pressure in œsophagus as if a round body were ascending from stomach." That is a nervous affection found in nervous women and has been called globus hystericus. When a woman feels as if she wanted to cry, and she swallows and chokes, she will have a similar lump in the throat. Nervous, broken-down constitutions; tired of life; sees nothing in the future but sickness and sorrow and paralysis or imbecility. When they have their lucid moments they weep, become sad over their enlarged glands and weakness, and have a lump in the throat.

There are many stomach troubles; ulceration of the stomach; cancer of the stomach. Conium is one of the greatest palliatives in symptoms of the stomach when all the symptoms agree. It will palliate cancerous conditions for a while, then on comes the difficulty again, because when the symptoms have advanced sufficiently to indicate Conium many times there is no hope of cure.

Hardness of the abdomen, great sensitiveness of the abdomen. Pinching pains, stitching pains, colicky, cutting pains, cramping pains. Bearing down in the abdomen—in the woman—as if the uterus would escape. Often more common than diarrhœa is constipation with ineffectual urging, hard stool, paralysis of the rectum. Inability to strain at stool, inability to expel contents because of the paralytic weakness of all the muscles that take part in expulsion.

Pulsation and emptiness in the abdomen after a normal stool. The woman strains so much at stool that the uterus protrudes from the vagina. After every stool tremulous weakness and palpitation. The urine will stop and start. He strains to expel the urine and gets tired and stops. The stream of urine stops and without any pressure whatever it starts again, and it does that two or three times during urination. Irregular muscular actions while passing urine. "Intermittent flow of urine, with cutting after micturition. Urine turbid after standing."

Weakness of the sexual powers of the male; impotency. He may have most violent sexual desire yet he is impotent. "Great sexual desire with partial or complete incapacity. Emissions without dreams. Painful emissions and painful ejaculations." There is a catarrhal state of the seminal vesicles attended with much soreness, so that when ejaculation takes place there is cutting like a knife, as if the semen were acrid. Bad effects from suppressed sexual desire in widowers and those who have been accustomed to coition. "Sexual weakness. Insufficient erection, lasting only a short time; weakness after embrace. Swelling and induration of testicles." Hardness and swelling of the testicles gradually comes on. 'Discharge of prostatic fluid on every change of emotion, without voluptuous thoughts, or while expelling fæces; with itching of the prepuce." Hence we have a strange intermingling of increased irritability of the parts, the neck of the bladder, sexual organs, prostate gland, with weakness, with impotency. In the male, remember, there is induration and enlargement of the testicles; in the woman induration and enlargement of the ovaries and uterus. "Uterine spasms during too early and scanty menses." Soreness in the abdomen in the early stages of gestation, motions of the child are painful. Burning, stinging, tearing pains in the neck of the uterus. Great soreness of the breasts. This medicine has dwindling of the mammary glands as well as enlargement and induration. Suppressed menstruation, painful menstruation, throbbing, tearing, burning pains in the uterus and in the ovaries, in the pelvis. It has cured fibroid tumors of the uterus. It has restrained cancerous growth of the cervix. One of the most distressing growths known to women is a cancerous growth of the cervix. It is the most difficult to check of all the cancerous affections known. It will progress most rapidly, but Conium is one of those remedies that will slow down that inflammation and restrain somewhat the hæmorrhages. Conium has produced induration and infiltration of the cervix.

Difficult breathing. Dry cough almost constantly, worse lying in bed. Cough when first lying down. Is obliged to sit up and cough it out. Taking a deep breath causes cough. Such are the striking features of a Conium cough. In the chest, violent stitches. Painful swelling of the breasts. Rending, tearing pains in the chest.

In the back, weakness is a most striking thing, with some dorsal pains. Lancinating pains are spoken of. "Ill effects of bruises and shocks to the spine." After injuries, especially in the lumbar region, pains and filling up of the veins of the lower limbs. Rheumatic pains; paralysis of the lower limbs; ulceration. And the sufferings and conditions are *better by letting the limbs hang down.* Conium differs from a great many medicines. It is common for pains and aches to be relieved by putting the feet up on a chair; by putting them up in bed. But the patient with the rheumatism, with the ulceration of the legs and the other strange sufferings of the legs, will lie down and permit his legs to hang over the bed up as far as the knee. That is something that somebody ought to undertake to account for, so we could have at least one thing we could prescribe for under pathology. But up to date we have no explanation. Tottering gait in middle-aged men.

Another grand feature of the remedy; he sweats copiously during sleep. Sometimes the patient will say that if he merely closes the eyes he will sweat. It is certainly true on closing the eyes preparatory to going to sleep he will break out in a sweat. Owing to the fact that Conium produces such a marked induration and infiltration of tissues that have been inflamed, stenoses are apt to form where inflammation has been present. Stricture of the urethra and stenosis of the os uteri have been cured by Couium.

CROTALUS HORRIDUS (RATTLESNAKE)

The first impression would be to rebel against the use of such substances as Crotalus, *Lachesis, Apis* and other animal poisons, and it is true that the lay mind must look with something like horror upon their administration; but when they are properly used and when we consider the dreadfulness of the necessity demanding them, and also when we have ascertained that there can be no substitute when demanded, and again that they are potentized and changed until they are perfectly pure, because reduced to a state of simple substance, the horror passes away from the mind. It is true that the diseases that call for the use of such substances as Crotalus are very grave. When at the bedside of a Crotalus patient one feels that death is very near, the subject is horrible to look upon, and the mother in regard to her child, or the husband, would immediately say, "Doctor, use anything in order to save the life, resort to anything in order to heal this sick one."

The symptoms are peculiar in Crotalus. The remedy stands out by. itself. There can be no substitute for it, as there is no other remedy, taken as a whole, that looks like it. The other snake poisons form the nearest resemblance, but this one is the most dreadful of all, excepting, perhaps, the *Ancistrodon contortrix* (*Copperhead*). In the case of snake bites we get the most dire effects; we see death itself, we see the ending after a very rapid course, the very highest type of zymosis. These snake poisons are supposed to be cyanhydrates of soda and other salts. It is known that alcohol is the natural solvent of the cyanhydrates, and because of this alcohol has been used in great quantities in snake bites, and it has frequently prolonged and even saved life. If he lives through the violent attack he goes on forever manifesting the chronic effects, and from these we have collected symptoms. Dogs that have been bitten manifested the chronic effects of rattlesnake bite, and in them a peculiar periodicity has been manifested, viz., *every spring* as the cold weather subsides and the warm days begin. I once had the privilege of tracing up a dog that had been bitten by the *Cenchris* and had survived. It was bitten in the region of the neck, and in that region a large abscess formed every spring as long as that dog lived, until old age, when he died from that disease. The periodicity in the snake poisons is related to the spring, to the coming on of the warm weather.

Another marked general feature in Crotalus, as in most of the other Ophidians, is that the patient *sleeps into the aggravation*.

The poison of' the Crotalus horridus, in its earliest manifestations, is like unto the zymotic changes that we find in scarlet fever, in diphtheria, in typhoid and low forms of blood poisoning, those cases that come on with great rapidity, breaking down of the blood, relaxation of the blood vessels, bleeding from all of the orifices of the body, rapidly increasing unconsciousness like one intoxicated and besotted in appearance. A mental and physical prostration that is almost paralytic in character. Scarlet fever when it becomes putrid; typhoid when it becomes putrid, diphtheria with much bleeding and putridity. The body appears mottled, blue intermingled with yellow. Jaundice comes on with astonishing quickness, and the eyes become yellow, and the skin becomes yellow and mottled. Blue in spots. Black and blue spots as if bruised, intermingled with yellow. After hæmorrhages the skin becomes extremely anæmic. It is yellow, pale, bloodless. The body looks like wax. Hæmorrhage from the ears, eyes, nose, lungs, from the muzous membranes everywhere, from the bowels, from the uterus. A hæmorrhagic constitution. Crotalus is indicated in disease of the very lowest, the most putrid type, coming on with unusual rapidity, reaching that putrid state in an unusually short time. One who has been poisoned rapidly sinks into this besotted, benumbed, putrid, semi-conscious state. There is a feeling as if death were coming over him. As the blood oozes out it becomes black. It is sometimes fluid.

An awful state of nervousness prevails. Trembling of the limbs, tremulous weakness. On protruding the tongue it comes out quivering. Tired by the slightest exertion. Sudden prostration of the vital powers. A paralytic weakness prevails throughout. Twitching of the muscles, trembling of the limbs. Sliding down in bed occurs in the typhoid conditions where this remedy has proved of benefit, the forms of yellow fever with great prostration. This species of yellow fever has been cured by this remedy. Convulsions and paralysis. It has twitching of muscles something like chorea, trembling, localized spasms, hysterical manifestations.

The mental symptoms are well worth examining. The low form of delirium, muttering, talking to himself is a peculiar form of loquacity. It differs somewhat from *Lachesis*. Both have loquacity. The *Lach.* loquacity is so rapid that if anyone in the room commences to tell something the patient will take it up and finish the story, although he has never heard anything about it, so active is his mind. No one is permitted to finish a story in the presence of a *Lach.* patient. One will commence to tell something. He will say, "Oh, yes; I understand it," and he will go off on another line and finish up with something entirely different. Crotalus does that, too, but Crotalus will take it up and mumble and stumble over his words in a clumsy manner. It is a low passive state like intoxication; in *Lach.* it is wild excitement. "Delirium with languor, drowsiness, stupor." That tells it. "Loquacious delirium with desire to escape from bed." It is passive, however. His motions are slow. "Muttering delirium of typhus. Sadness." His thoughts dwell on death continually.' "Excessive sensitiveness. Moved to tears by reading. Melancholy with timidity, fear. Anxious and pale, with cold sweat. Irritable, cross, infuriated by least annoyance." On motion there is vertigo, dizziness. On keeping still there is pain. On going to sleep there is pain, and he is roused by violent pain. The longer he sleeps the more severe that pain in the head.

He sleeps into his symptoms. All the snake poisons more or less sleep into troubles. The head troubles come on after sleep. He sleeps into headache. The longer he sleeps the harder are the headaches. The headache is so hard in the back of the head that it is almost impossible to raise it from the pillow. The muscles become so tired he has to take hold of it with his hands. This belongs also to *Lach.* A congestive headache with waxy face, yellow, purple, mottled face, as if there had been bruises. "Headache extending into the eyes. Bilious headache every few days." Severe sick headache, together with dizziness, throbbing in the top of the head. Dull, pulsating headaches. *"Dull, heavy, throbbing, occipital headaches,"* or the whole head is in a state of congestion. He is confused and dazed. Head feels too large. Head feels full, feels as if it would burst. Headaches that come on in waves as if they came up the back, a surging of blood upwards, an orgasm described as if the blood rushed upwards. Headache with surging in waves and excited by motion or jar, by turning over in bed, by rising up in bed, or by lying down. Change of position will cause this surging. In *Lach.* it is described, and I have seen it verified, as beginning away down in the spine and surging upward coincident with the pulse.

Hæmorrhage from the eyes. Yellow appearance of the eyes. "Blood exudes from the eye, burning in eyes; redness with lachrymation." Pressure in the eyes as if the eyes would be pushed out from the head. Paralysis of the upper lids. Inflammation of the mucous membrane of the lids.

Surging in the ears. "Sensitive to noises." Dull aching and throbbing in the ears. Fœtid, copious, yellow, offensive, bloody discharges from the ears. Blood oozing from the ears in drops in zymotic diseases, low forms of scarlet fever, or of diptheria where there is oozing from the eyes and ears, and copious bleeding from the nose. The nose is the most common organ to bleed in zymotic diseases. The rush of blood seems to get relief from bleeding from the nose. In this medicine the congestion to the head is violent with bleeding from the nose. It has cured all forms of fœtid discharge. Horrible, fœtid, putrid discharges from the nose. Ozæna.

Inflammation of the parotid gland. Blueness and discoloration of the face. Yellow appearance of the face, a marked condition of jaundice. In girls who appear waxy or anæmic, yellowish green, have for a long time missed the menstrual period and break out in pustules and pimples.

The patient often wakes up during the night grinding the teeth. The taste is bad, putrid. Inflammation of the gums. Bleeding from the mouth. Inflammation of the throat with bleeding of the throat. Burning in the throat and mouth. Trembling, quivering and swollen tongue. Trembling of the tongue when it is put out. Trembling of the hands when they are moved. Those cases of diphtheria that ooze blood from the nose and mouth are very low types, and are sure to die without a well-selected remedy. The throat will be filled up under such circumstances with a diphtheritic membrane that looks dark. There is bleeding all around it. Sore mouth with bleeding. Ulcers in the mouth. Ulcers after *Merc.* in those who. are pouring forth saliva on the pillow at night. Bleeding ulcers in the mouth. Difficult swallowing. Malignant diphtheria. Cannot lie on the right side or back without instantly producing black, bilious vomiting. This is a wonderfully bilious remedy, sick headaches, vomiting of bile in great quantities. The various low forms of disease calling for Crotalus often begin with vomiting great quantities of bile, sometimes bile mixed with blood.

Pain in the stomach, coldness as if a piece of ice were in the stomach or the abdomen. Stomach irritable, unable to retain anything, constantly throwing up blood. Crotalus has cured ulceration of the stomach. It has greatly restrained the growth of carcinoma when there is much vomiting of bile and blood. Vomiting in many instances where the blood has no tendency to coagulate. Now, with these ulcerations of the stomach, cancerous affections, low zymotic disease, jaundice is nearly always present; jaundice and more or less of bleeding; fever seldom runs high; sometimes the temperature is subnormal, but with oozing and bleedings, with dark hæmorrhage from the nose and mouth and dark, scanty, bloody urine containing albumen. The abdomen is greatly distended like the tympanitic abdomen of typhoid and the low zymotic diseases. Ulceration of the bowels, hæmorrhage from the bowels. Much pain and soreness in the abdomen with numbness. Feeling in it as if it were made of wood. "Stool black, thin, like coffee grounds. Dysentery of septic origin from foul water, food, etc. Diarrhœa from noxious effluvia." Inflammation of the ovaries and of the uterus. Low form of putrid fever. Hæmorrhages. Either dark clots or blood that has no tendency to coagulate and keeps on flowing. There is great trouble at the climacteric period. Hot flashes. Jaundice. Hæmorrhage from the uterus or from other parts. Cancer of the uterus with much bleeding. Great offensiveness. Patient becomes yellow, jaundiced, great exhaustion, mottled appearance of the skin, swelling of the face, of the leg, especially along the course of the veins. Phlegmasia alba dolens. Worse from the slightest touch. Worse from jar, from motion.

There is some reason to think that this will be more or less a heart remedy from the great cardiac weakness it produces. But the other snake poisons like *Naja, Lach.* and *Elaps* have had more clinical application than this one. This one seems to prostrate the heart, but also to prostrate the whole body, and its complaints are more general. Mottled appearance of the limbs. Gangrenous appearance of the extremities.

Boils, carbuncles and *eruptions are* surrounded by a purplish condition of the skin, a mottled, blue, splotched or marbled state. It produces boils, abscesses and a condition somewhat resembling a carbuncle, with burning and violent pains, but the peculiar feature is the doughy centre. Around the boil or carbuncle for many inches there is œdema, with pitting upon pressure. The boil, or abscess, or carbuncle will bleed a thick, black blood that will not coagulate. Carbuncles that come upon the neck and upon the back begin with a pustule, and then several come and they are surrounded by little pustules and papules and there is pitting upon pressure. For these carbuncles you will need to study particularly *Arsenicum, Anthracinum, Lachesis, Secale* and Crotalus. They are the medicines that have in their nature malignancy and manifestation.

In *puerperal fever* there is a continued oozing of black offensive blood that will not coagulate; bleeding from every orifice of the body as well as from the uterus. Imagine a woman who is pregnant suffering from typhoid fever. She aborts and a low zymotic state comes on with the symptoms that I have described and with all the appearances as if she would bleed to death after the abortion. The blood will not coagulate and the flow continues. Or in a woman during a typhoid fever menstruation comes on. It is not a true menstrual flow, that is, it does not resemble the ordinary flow, because it is copious, dark and liquid, a continuous oozing with all the grave symptoms described, and especially the besotted countenance, the comatose state, the appearance as if she were intoxicated, lying as one dead. When aroused every muscle trembles; if the tongue is protruded it trembles, and there is inability to articulate. Crotalus may save her life. Would it be possible to think of graver states of sickness than such as are produced by the ophidia? When a physician sees these symptoms coming on he immediately thinks of a class of remedies that can cover such a state, remedies like *Baptisia, Arsenicum, Secale* and the *Ophidia,* and sometimes *Arnica, Phosphorus* and *Pyrogen.*

In the more chronic conditions the individual manifests a terrible state as *to* his sleep. He rises from sleep as in a fright; has horrible dreams of murder, of death, of dead bodies and dead people, of associating with the dead and with corpses, of being in graveyards; even the smell of the cadaver is dreamed of. While he is awake he is tired, he is stupid, he cannot add figures, he makes mistakes in writing, he transposes sentences, and in words he makes mistakes in writing, he transposes sentences, and in words he transposes letters. He is unable to take care of his own accounts, for he cannot add up things that are at all particular. Sleep alternates with long and tedious periods of wakefulness. He is disturbed by any change to warm weather. Great irritability, sensitive to spheres, easily disturbed by his surroundings, and easily wrought up into a pitch of excitement are also features of this remedy. Following this up he is suspicious of his friends and is unable to reason upon a rational basis. He craves intoxicating drinks and is unable to resist the craving. This wonderful resemblance to old inebriates has led to the use of Crotalus in delirium tremens; it has the besotted countenance, the purple aspect of the face, the peculiar kind of hunger in the drunkard, the craving by spells for stimulants. There is every reason to believe that in fat, robust, besotted drunkards it may, if properly used, be a remedy deep enough to remove the appetite for strong drink.

CROTON TIGLIUM

Croton oil when applied to the skin, produces both vesicles and pustules upon an inflamed base, and the part becomes very red and sore. The inflammation often increases until it resembles erysipelas, but more commonly the eruption produced resembles a vesicular eczema. This eruption will come on for a few days and will then desiccate, and in a few days longer it will desquamate.

When one has been overdosed, as is done in a too prolonged proving, or by the crude drug, or when the prover has been markedly sensitive, we get an alternation of states, the internal alternating with the external. After the eruption is out the internal manifestations are not present, as is seen in the rheumatic state, the cough and the bowel symptoms. If we study these groups separately we will find they are all interesting. First, its cough. It has an asthmatic cough, coming on in the middle of the night, often arousing the patient from a sound sleep. Attacks of violent coughing, with dyspnoea and choking, worse at night and worse on lying down, compelling him to sit up, to be bolstered up in bed, or to sit up in a reclining chair. His friends wonder if he is not going into consumption. If it is a child they wonder whether it is not whooping cough. There is extreme irritation of the air passages, so that the inhalation of air brings on the cough. Sensitive to deep breathing. Now, this will go on for a while and finally he will break out with an eruption somewhere upon the body, vesicles and pustules, in clusters and patches, that become inflamed and red and finally dry up and desquamate and disappear, and then back comes his cough. This may go on as a chronic state, and when such is the case it will be very well to know this remedy.

The next most important symptoms are the bowel symptoms, and perhaps they are the best known of any of its symptoms outside of the eruption. It is suitable in both acute and chronic diarrhœa. It is suitable in cholera infantum. The marked feature is the extreme suddenness with which the stool is ejected. It seems to come out in *one gush of yellow. watery* or pappy stool; soft, thin fæces, coming out *with one gush.* So marked is this that it is not an uncommon thing for a rural patient to describe it as "like that of a goose". It all gushes out in one squirt. The mother says of the little patient: "You would be astonished, doctor, at the violent rush, for it all comes out with one squirt." That is descriptive. Many remedies have a holding on and a prolonged effort at stool, until it takes quite a long time. Many of the diarrhœas are prolonged with numerous little gushes of thin fæces or water, but this particular feature is striking. It may not always be so, but this violent gush of thin, yellow fæces or yellow water is a striking feature of the remedy. With this the abdomen is very sensitive, and is greatly distended; there is much gurgling in the bowel, and when the physician puts his hand upon it the patient will say he feels the gurgling, as if he were full of water, and it probably is so, for the expulsion of the stool would not occur in one strong gush were it not for the fact that the colon and rectum were full of fluid. Another peculiar thing commonly attending Croton tig. diarrhœas is that pressure over the abdomen or pressure about the umbilicus causes a pain in the rectum and urging to stool, and a feeling, with the expulsion of the stool, as if the rectum would protrude. Clinically it has been described as if the pain followed the intestines all the .way down to the anus. The taking of a little water, or of a little milk, what would ordinarily be suitable food for such a diarrhœa, will at times cause an instant urging to stool; he must go to stool immediately after eating. This gives the general features of the Croton tig. diarrhœa. If it is in an infant there is great exhaustion, tympanitic abdomen, much rumbling of the bowels, great sinking, and as soon as the infant takes one mouthful of milk or draws from the mother's breast it expels a gush of liquid or pappy stool.

Another most important group of symptoms is its eye symptoms. It has eye symptorns of an inflammatory character, and around the eyes and upon the lids are vesicles and pustules. Pustules upon the cornea, granular lids. Inflammation of all the tissues of the eye. It has an inflammation of the iris and conjunctiva. The bloodvessels of the eyes are distended, the eye looks red and raw. The eyelids when turned out are seen to be greatly inflamed and granular, covered with vesicles and pustules. With this inflammatory condition there is a sensation very commonly present in the Croton tig. eye cases, as if the eye were drawn backwards by a string, or as if the optic nerves were dragging the eyes backwards into the head. This drawing in the back of the eyes as with a string is also peculiar to *Paris quadrifolia,* but the condtions are different in *Paris quad.* In headaches from overuse of the eyes in engravers or those doing fine needle work, with much neuralgia in the head, due probably to the overuse of the eyes, when the pains in the eyes are not attended with inflammation but are more of the type of dull aches and pains that you might call only rheumatic or neuralgic. with this sensation as if the eyes were drawn back into the brain; in these neuralgic cases use *Paris quad.* But in the inflammatory conditions such as I have described, with the same drawing back as with a string, Croton tig. is the remedy.

Troublesome eczema of the scalp in infants, either purely vesicular or intermingled more or less with pustules. The vesicles dry up and then desquomate, and now there is a red, raw, inflamed surface, sensitive to touch. After desquamation has pretty nearly finished, a new crop of pustules and vesicles comes out, and while one place is clearing off another is vesicular. This is how it goes on with a chronic eczema. The eruptions are often about the eyes, on the temples, over the face and on top of the head. The appearance is so nearly like *Sepia* that the two very often cannot be distinguished. *Sepia* has the same vesiculation intermingled with pustules, the bleeding and rawness of the surface and the eruption of new crops. *Sepia* is more frequently indicated in this raw and bleeding state of the scalp, in crusta lactea, or the eruption of children than Crot. tig. Under Croton tig. infants in this state very often have attacks of gushing diarrhœa, coming on from the slightest disturbance or indigestion; this is a grcat help in guiding to the remedy. When the two groups of symptoms are combined, the scalp symptoms and the diarrhœa, you can hardly make a mistake. You will see this also, that if the diarrhœa is at all prolonged, the head will steadily improve and you will think your patient is getting well of the scalp trouble, but when the diarrhœa slackens up a little out will come a fresh crop. If the diarrhœa becomes chronic the external eruption will disappear, and if the diarrhoea improves the exrnal eruption gets worse. It seems necessary in such a constitution to have a vent. The mucous membrane is but the internal skin, and the integument of the body the external skin, and this remedy especially manifests itself upon one or the other of these, the mucous membrane or the integument.

It has another manifestation that you want to carry in mind, a group of symptoms in relation to lactation. After confinement the mother may go on a little while with all things following normally, but all at once she commences to have pains in one or the other mammary gland, and the drawing as with a string comes up again. It feels to her as if a string were attached behind the nipple pulling backward, a sharp, drawing, stinging pain that will in some instances keep her walking the floor night and day. Though it is but a little thing it is a very important symptom to know with Croton tig. We see this drawing, as with a string, in the eye and in the breast, and also the symptom, very like the *Plumbum* symptom, drawing in the navel upon pressure, somewhat like a string. Associating such things together will enable you to understand them as a part of the nature of the remedy and to keep them in mind. I once cured a woman of this painful drawing from the nipple as with a string. I watched her walk the floor and saw that the suffering must be very intense, for at times it brought tears to her eyes. She had borne it several nights, which shows that Croton tig. is capable of curing a pain that is very prolonged or tedious. The breast had been poulticed, hot applications had been put upon it, and they did not give relief, a point which is worth remembering.

In cholera infantum we will naturally have the symptoms of vomiting, which, however, are not so common to Croton tig., although it has some vomiting. So in cases of cholera infantum, in which the vomiting is not so important a feature as the loose bowels, the remedy may be Crot. tig. A symptom is reported that is of great value. Excessive nausea with vanishing of sight, vertigo, worse, after drinking, with frequent discharges of yellowish-green water from the bowels; excessive nausea, much water in the mouth. So we note the excessive nausea and not so great vomiting. The nausea is more like that of *Ipecac.*, but in *Ipecac.* we have nothing like the stools of Crot. tig., we have only scanty little gushes, every minute a little gush with tenesmus. Vomiting is the all important symptom in the cholera infantum of *Ipecac.*, and when the stomach is emptied there is overwhelming retching and exhaustion from it, and the stools are scanty; but in Croton tig. the stools are copious, and while there is nausea the vomiting is seldom and scanty.

Another feature to be considered in this remedy is its relation to *Rhus.* It is an antidote to *Rhus.* Croton tig. is closely related in its vesicular eruption to the *Rhus* family (particularly *Rhus tox.*). *Anacardium, Sepia* and *Anagallis.* The eruptions of Croton tig. very often select as a location the genital organs. *Rhus* does the same, and when the genital organs are the principal seat of the eruptions in *Rhus* poisoning Croton tig. will commonly be its antidote; also when the eruptions are most about the eyes and scalp Croton tig. will often furnish an antidote. When the symptoms, however, confine themselves to the palms of the hands Croton tig. is not the remedy, but it is *Anagallis. Anagallis* does upon the palms of the hands just what Croton tig. does upon the genitals. If you examine *Anagallis* you will find that the eruptions will come out and desquamate, and no sooner does the surface look as if it would heal than a new crop comes out. *Rhus* is similar in that ,it locates upon the palms of the hands. but *Rhus* does not repeat itself upon inflamed surfaces. In the Croton tig. eruption there is some burning, but nothing like that of *Rhus.* The *Rhus* burning pain in eruptions that are marked is almost like fire. It is worse from the air, and it is better from dipping the part in water as hot as it is possible to endure it. Persons who have these *Rhus* eruptions talk about scalding their hands to relieve the itching and burning. So it is with Croton tig., but it is usually so sore he cannot touch it; when the eruption is so mild that he can handle it, we find that the slightest rubbing relieves the itching. In *Rhus* touch aggravates the itching. In bad cases of *Rhus* poisoning he will hold his fingers far apart if they have very large blisters upon them, and he will not touch the place because it establishes a voluptuous itching that nearly drives him wild. Although this is not so with Croton tig., still they are similar enough to each other to be antidotal; they do not have to be exactly alike, but they need to be similar. It is true that remedies that are relieved by scratching are more nearly antidotal to such remedies as are relieved by scratching. The more similar the better; but medicines will antidote each other when they are similar only in general character; and they will cure disease when they are similar in general character. It is also true that medicines while they are not similar in general character may be similar enough in special localities to remove the symptoms in these localities, while the disease will go on. The remedy in this case is not similar enough to cure the disease, but it has removed some of the symptoms. That is the most miserable kind of a prescription, as it changes the manifestations of the disease without changing its nature. In that way a very poor prescriber may hunt around and get one remedy for one group of symptoms and another remedy for another group, and the patient be worse off than before. If the remedies are similar as to their general nature, then the little superficial symptoms are not so extremely important.

"Frequent, corrosive itching on glands and scrotum." "Vesicular eruption on scrotum and penis." It is a remedy for vesicular and pustular eruptions upon the genital organs. It is closely related to *Petroleum,* which has fine red vesicular and granular elevations, intermingled with fine red rash upon the genitals, itching intensely, worse at times by scratching until burning comes on and then bleeding which relieves.

CULEX MUSCA

When this remedy is needed your patient will present to you a picture of something on fire; he burns like something he would like to mention, and perhaps does mention the place; the itching and burning are present everywhere in this remedy; he rubs and scratches wherever the eruptions appears.

The mental symptoms are just what you would expect would follow the physical symptoms of Culex; impatience, a willingness to quarrel, anxiety and fear or death; poor memory and a disinclination for all work; he is so busy scratching to relieve the itching and so busy walking to relieve the restlessness, that any interruption makes him impatient and ready to quarrel.

The dull frontal headache begins on waking at five a.m. and passes away after lying awake for a while; during the forenoon there is pain, fulness and pressure in the forehead with heat of the face, getting worse by spells until afternoon when it extends to the outer part of the right orbital ridge and extending through to the occiput is accompanied by nausea which lasts until evening. Some of the head pains go from the cerebellum to the forehead or right temple; the boring pains in the temples come on several times a day; the pain comes and goes across the forehead just above the eyes; a rending pain back of the eyeballs. The headache is made worst by the least motion followed by intense vertigo which comes on in the afternoon and is located in a spot over the right eye. Itching and stinging of the scalp.

In the right eye there is a feeling of fulness extending to the parotid gland, from there to the sub-lingual and finally involves the right side of the face and head. The margins of the lids are sore and crusted over; the inflammation of the lids is worse in the morning with a discharge of sticky fluid; the eyeballs are inflamed and there is stye-like ulceration. Rending pains in the eyeballs; he could not keep his eyes open yet it pained to keep them shut; the eyes feel tired.

The ears come in for their share of trouble with swelling of the parotid glands and soreness on pressure; pain as if he were going to have mumps; sharp pains in both ears followed by watery discharge of the same sticky character that is present in the saliva.

From the nose there is a watery discharge with bloody scabs on the inside; small scabs come from the nose which may be dry or moist and bloody; usually mixed with a copious discharge which may be greenish or light-colored and the head feels stuffed; the itching, stinging and tickling are always present; he rubs and scratches because his nose itches inside and outside and the more he rubs it the more it burns so he stops for a while until he is driven to rub and scratch again only to be compelled to stop while there is a little skin left on his nose. On top of his nose is a shining redness like a rum blossom; the nose is swollen and the eruption on it contains a clear colorless fluid; as the swelling goes down it is followed by itching and to rub it only increases the desire for more rubbing.

There is pain in the posterior nares with green scabs with bleeding after removal of the scabs. Epistaxis morning and night on blowing the nose. The redness is like erysipelas; shining, red, and sore to touch; it is more marked on the right side in the beginning and then extends to both sides of the nose and to the face. An ineffectual desire to sneeze.

Pain over the right malar bone going to the left the next day and here you will see one of the characteristic red spots the size of a twenty-five cent piece feeling as if red pepper had been rubbed in; from the malar bone will be shooting pains to the temple and forehead in the evening, made worse by setting the jaws together. The submaxillary gland is swollen and tender on pressure. The eruption on the face and between the eyes contains a colorless fluid; there will also be swelling and puffiness under the eyes; in keeping with this remedy we find the heat and redness of the whole right side of the face with a sore bruised feeling.

Constant wetting of the lips; a symptom common to many remedies perhaps from nervousness but in this patient it ameliorated the dryness and the ever present burning; the saliva is of such a character that it leaves the lips sticky; this bad tasting whitish saliva leaves a bad taste in the mouth in the morning on waking; a sickish taste as if he had been drinking warm mineral water. The tongue is coated white and is dry, swollen, thick on waking; there is also numbness of the tongue. Periodical attacks of salivation for months; at night the pillow is wet and the daytime the saliva accumulates and causes continued swallowing. If you prescribe a remedy on, one symptom this patient would probably be given Merc. The entire edge of the tongue is covered with a double row of small painful vesicles. This remedy cured a case of numbness of the tongue with ulceration at the tip following scarlet fever.

On rising in the morning in addition to the other troubles, he must spend much time hawking up from the pharynx dark green scabs and strings of tough mucus tinged with dark blood and coughing from the trachea green scabs corresponding to the green discharge from the nose.

There is burning and dryness of the throat with soreness in throat and in the posterior nares on swallowing solids or fluids. The right side of the throat is always sore.

The appetite is increased but the food does not digest; it sours in the stomach; his appetite is quite likely to be ravenous and he must have his dinner on the minute or he feels faint; he is especially hungry and faint in the morning and cannot wait for the breakfast to be prepared; with this sour condition of the stomach you would expect nausea and it is often present day and night; sometimes even the thought of food will bring on nausea with gagging and retching and inability to vomit; with the disordered stomach are sickening pains and eructation of much offensive gas.

Thirst for cold water which causes burning in the stomach with urging to stool, followed by loose and dark brown offensive stool, much tenesmus lasting several days and gradually subsiding into painless diarrhœa.

On the abdomen are blotches the size of a twenty-five cent piece, itching burning, with little pimples on the blotches; this is the form of the eruption wherever it is present.

A dull pain in the right side in the region of the kidney extending up the back to the occiput.

Cramps in the abdomen during stool with rumbling and the passing of much offensive flatus; these colicky pains come on about ten a.m. and last from one to three hours. The usual desire for morning stool is absent; the stool is scanty, lumpy, and expelled with effort; the first part of the stool is hard and scratches the anus; it is followed by a soft stool; after stool he has the sensation that he has not finished so he sits and strains until blood comes (Merc.).

Itching and burning of the anus; it is scalding hot and raw as from a bite; burning of the glans penis and there is a strong smelling discharge from the glans; the itching of the scrotum comes from spots like bee stings; these spots are of the usual circumscribed character that swell and burn and itch; rubbing only aggravates the itching, stinging, burning.

The majora has the same itching, burning that runs all through the remedy. The itching of the vulva is so intense that she feels as if she could tear it to pieces; this symptom returned at intervals for years and was cured by Culex.

Menses come too soon with a profuse dark clotted flow; violent pains in the uterus compelling her to go to bed.

Hoarseness so that he could scarcely speak a word; usually there is great hoarseness in the morning.

Deep sighing breathing with constant desire for a deep breath; the breath is foul and it seemed as if he could smell it himself.

A distressing cough caused by burning in the chest; a whistling strangling choking cough with red face and water running from the eyes or it may be a dry hacking cough, present day and night; the cough is mostly in the morning with the feeling as if he would vomit; with the cough there is pain low down in the back; there is coughed up a small amount of yellowish white expectoration; sometimes there is one constant racking cough lasting fifteen minutes ending in a long loud inspiration with blue face and protruding eyes followed by great languor and sweat. There is constant desire to sneeze and cough alternately with a discharge of quantities of mucus from the throat which does not relieve the inclination to cough.

In the apex of the right lung there is soreness which is aggravated by deep breathing or raising the right arm, and occasional dull pain in the lower part of the right lung; a painful condition when you consider the desire for deep breathing which is present with oppression and anxiety in the chest; other symptoms give him much trouble; a sensation of fulness in the right lung, soreness on stooping, leaning forward, raising the right shoulder, and with it all there is the sensation of a rubber band around the right lung; not all the pains are dull, there are sudden cutting pains running up and down lasting a minute; there is rawness, a bruised feeling in the right chest; drawing, clawing pains in the right lung going to the left lung and staying there; these pains lasting several hours each day; with these conditions you would expect soreness on stooping, leaning forward, or raising the right shoulder.

Culex Musca has very few heart symptoms which is fortunate considering the many lung symptoms; there are occasional cutting pains that are neither severe nor long lasting; there are pains in the right pectoral muscles and the right side of the neck is swollen.

The hands and fingers are hot and burning, as if frozen, with severe pain; the burning of the palms and on the thumb is as if the hand had been rubbed against nettles; itching, burning, as if he must tear the flesh for relief while the back of the hands felt cold and benumbed.

Rose red, colored, burning eruption on the arm aggravated by heat; the arms and hands are numb and prickling; there is the everlasting itching that is present all through this remedy; the eruption with its colourful fluid, burning after scratching and with it the desire to tear the skin off. There is coldness of the right hand while the left hand is warm.

The lower limbs feel heavy with an uneasy restlessness that is made better by the open air; his feet are tired all day long yet he must drag himself into the open air for relief; he wishes that he knew some place where he could put his poor, tired, heavy limbs that would give him rest. On the thigh there is the blotch the size of a twenty-five cent piece, with little pimples on it, that itches and burns like a flea bite. There is aching of the legs from the knee down; there is no position that will make the pain less so he must get up out of his chair and take a walk in the open air; there is little comfort to his feet while walking as the soles are tender and there is intense itching on the tops of the feet.

Of course his sleep is restless with much tossing about in sleep; the heat of the bed causes him to waken frequently; he must rise early in the morning to move around for relief; he is unrefreshed by sleep which has been restless, and full of dreams of quarrels, fights, and of the dead.

There are hot flushes as if a chill would follow, followed by warm perspiration which is strong smelling and sticky, this stickiness is also noticed in the saliva.

His skin torments him almost beyond endurance, itching, burning, heat, all combine to make him miserable; the skin feels better while scratching but worse after scratching; there is no comfort at home or abroad, in bed or out of it and a place of amusement is not to be thought of; he scratches which makes more trouble yet he must scratch to relieve that terrible, constant itching; you may truthfully say that this remedy has many out-ward manifestations.

This may be summed up as a right-sided remedy with the strange feeling of having been poisoned; there are sharp stinging pains all over the body like needles; lightning-like; darting here and there, aggravated by light pressure and ameliorated by hard pressure.

Head, nose and limb symptoms seem to grow worse until seven p.m. and are ameliorated' about eight P.M.; in an hour or two they are gone; the symptoms seem most severe from six to seven p.m.

All symptoms, pain, itching, burning, are worse in a warm room and better in the open air, although he is so tired and weak that he can scarcely move, cannot walk straight, with soreness and aching all over the body, yet he is so nervous that he finds it impossible to keep still; there is almost constant motion of the hands and feet.

CUPRUM METALLICUM

Cuprum is pre-eminently a *convulsive* medicine. The convulsive tendency associates itself with almost every complaint that Cuprum creates and cures. It has convulsions in every degree of violence, from the mere twitching of little muscles and of single muscles to convulsions of all the muscles of the body. When these are coming on the earliest threatenings are drawings in the fingers, clenching of the thumbs or twitching of the muscles. It has twitching, quivering, trembling, and it has also tonic contractions, so that the hands are closed violently. In this condition the thumbs are first affected; they are drawn into the palms and then the fingers close down over them with great violence. In the fingers and toes and in the extremities the spasmodic condition increases and extends until the limbs are in a state of great exhaustion. Tonic contractions, the limbs being drawn up with great violence and it seems as if the frame would be torn to pieces by the violent contractions of the muscles everywhere. Often the' contractions assume a clonic form, with jerking and twitching.

Cuprum has many *mental symptoms*. It has a great variety in its delirium,

incoherent prattling, talking of all sorts of subjects incoherently. It has produced
a variety of mental symptoms: delirium, incoherency of speech, loss of memory.
During its different complaints, such as cholera, some forms of fever, the
puerperal state, dysmenorrhœa, congestion of the brain, etc., there is delirium,
unconsciousness and jerking and twitching of the muscles. The eyes roll in
various directions, but commonly upwards and outwards or upwards and
inwards. There is bleeding from the nose and the vision is disturbed. Between
the convulsive attacks there is incoherent talk, delirium, during which the
patient is spiteful, violent, weeping or shrieking. They go into convulsions
with a shriek. In one place it is spoken of as bellowing like a calf.

This drug has the ability to produce a group of spasms followed by the
appearance as if the patient were dead, or in a state of ecstacy. Convulsive
conditions sometimes terminate in a state of stasis during which the mind
ceases to act and the muscles remain quiet or only quiver. This is often one of
the leading features in *whooping-cough* when Cuprum is indicated. To bring
it down to the language of the mother, the description which she gives of the
little one, which will probably make you remember it better than if I use the
text, she says that when the child is seized with a spell of this violent whooping-
cough, the face becomes livid or blue, the finger nails become discolored, the
eyes are turned up, the child coughs until it loses its breath, and then lies in
a state of insensibility for a long time until she fears the child will never
breathe again, but with violent spasmodic action in its breathing, the child
from shortest breaths comes to itself again just as if brought back to life. You
have here all the violent features of a convulsive whooping-cough. In addition
to what the mother says you may also observe a few things, but the whole
make-up of such a case, its whole nature, shows that it is a Cuprum whooping-
cough. If the mother can get there quickly enough with a little cold water she
will stop the cough. Cold water especially will relieve the spasm, and so the
mother soon gets into the habit of hurrying for a glass of cold water, and the
child also knows, if it has tried it once, that a glass of cold water will relieve it.
Whenever the respiratoury organs are affected there is *spasmodic breathing,*
dyspnœa. There is also rattling in the chest. The more dyspnœa there is the
more likely his thumbs will be clenched and the fingers cramped.

In the lower part of the chest, in the region of the xiphoid appendix, there
is a spasmodic condition that is very troublesome. It seems to be at times a
constriction so severe that he thinks he will die, and at others a feeling as if
he were *transfixed* with a knife from the xiphoid appendix to the back. Some
say it feels as if a lump were in that region and others as if much wind were
collected in the stomach. It destroys the fulness of the voice, and it seems as
if his life would be squeezed out. Sometimes then it takes the form of colic
and sometimes of neuralgia. If you examine the sensation of tightness in the

region of the stomach you will see at once how the voice is affected. You will find the patient sitting up in bed; he tells you in a cracked and squeaking voice that he will soon die if he is not relieved; his face is a picture of fear and anguish; he really looks as if he were going to die; the sensation is dreadful. Cuprum speedily cures this complaint. This constriction and dyspnœa occur sometimes in cholera morbus and in painful menstruation. Spasms of the chest are also accompanied by this constriction and a nervous spasmodic breathing. He is not able to take a full breath.

The Cuprum patient is full of *cramps*. There are cramps in the limbs and in the muscles of the chest, with trembling and weakness. In old age, and in premature old age, it is useful for those cramps that come in the calves, the soles of the feet, and the toes and fingers at night in bed. In debilitated, nervous, tremulous old people, Cuprum serves a peculiar purpose. When an old man, who has been single a long time, marries, his cramps will sometimes prevent him performing the act of coition. He has cramps in the calves and soles as soon as he begins the act. It is especially suitable to young men who have become *prematurely old from* vices, from strong drink, from late nights and various abuses, and these cramps are not unlikely to occur in such subjects. Cuprum and *Graphites are* the two remedies for cramps coming under these circumstances, but whereas Cuprum is said to produce cramps that prevent the act, *Graphites* is said to bring on the cramps during the act. The two remedies however compete closely with each other, and hence if *Graphites* corresponds to the constitution of the patient, it should be given, and the same in regard to Cuprum. *Sulphur* also has cured this state.

In spasmodic conditions that come on during menstruation Cuprum is also useful. *Painful menstruation with spasms* commencing in the fingers and extending over the body. Tonic contractions that look like hysterical manifestations. They may be hysterical, but that does not interfere with Cuprum curing, if they are only spasmodic or convulsive. Violent dysmenorrhœa with delirium, turning up of eyes, contortions of the face and epileptiform manifestations.

In *epilepsy* calling for Cuprum we have the contractions and jerkings of the fingers and toes. He falls with a shriek and during the attack passes urine and fæces. It is indicated in epilepsy that begins with a violent constriction in the lower part of the chest as I have described, or with the contractions in the fingers that spread all over the body, to all the muscles.

Again, it is a remedy sometimes needed in the *puerperal state* before or after delivery. The case may be of uræmic character, but no matter; the urine is scanty and albuminous. During the progress of the labor the patient suddenly becomes blind. All light seems to her to disappear from the room, the labor pains cease, and convulsions come on, commencing in the fingers and toes. When you meet these cases do not forget Cuprum. You will look a long time before you can cure a case of this kind without Cuprum.

In *cholera morbus* with gushing, watery stools and copious vomiting, the stomach and bowels are emptied of their contents. The patient is fairly emptied out, becomes blue all over, the extremities are cold, there is jerking of the muscles, cramping of the extremities and of the fingers and toes, spasms of the chest; he is cold, mottled, blue in blotches, going into collapse; the finger nails and toe nails and the hands and feet are blue. There are several remedies that look like Cuprum in such a condition. In cholera we would naturally hunt for such remedies as produce cholera-like discharges, more or less spasmodic conditions, the great blueness, coldness, sinking and. collapse. We would here refer to Hahnemann's observation. Hahnemann had not seen a case of cholera, but he perceived that the disease produced appearances resembling the symptoms of Cuprum, *Camphor* and *Veratrum*. He saw from the description of the disease that the general aspect of cholera was like the general aspect of Cuprum, *Camphor* and *Veratrum;* and these three remedies are the typical cholera remedies. They all have the general feature of cholera, its nature and. general aspect. They all have the exhaustive vomiting and diarrhœa, the coldness, the tendency to collapse, the sinking from the emptying out of the fluids of the body.

From what I have said you will see that the Cuprum case is, above all others, the *spasmodic case.* It has the most intense spasms, and the spasms being the leading feature, they overshadow all the other symptoms of the case. He is full of cramps and is compelled to cry out with the pain from the contractions of the muscles. *Camphor* is the *coldest* of all the three remedies; the *Camphor* patient is cold as death. *Camphor* has the blueness, the exhaustive discharge, though less than Cuprum and *Veratrum;* but whereas in the two latter remedies the patient is willing to be covered up, in *Camphor* he wants the windows open and wants to be cool. Though he is cold he wants to be uncovered and to have the windows open. But just here let me mention another feature in. *Camphor.* It has also some convulsions which are painful, and *when the pain is on* he wants to be covered up and wants the windows shut. If there are cramps in the bowels with the pain, he wants to he covered up. So that in *Camphor,* during ill of its complaints in febrile conditions (and fever is very rare in *Camphor*), and during the pains he wants to be covered up and warm, but *during the coldness* he wants to be uncovered and have the air. In cholera, then, the extreme coldness and blueness point to *Camphor.* Again, with *Camphor* there are often scanty as well as copious discharges, so that the cholera patient is often taken so suddenly that he has the coldness, blueness and exhaustion and almost no vomiting or diarrhœa, a condition called *dry cholera.* It simply means an uncommonly small amount of vomiting and diarrhœa. This is *Camphor.* Another prominent feature is the great coldness of the body without the usual sweat that belongs to the disease. Cuprum and *Veratrum* have the cold clammy sweat, and *Camphor* also has sweat, but more commonly the patient needing *Camphor* is very cold, blue and *dry* and wants to be uncovered. That is striking. Now we go to *Veratrum* and see that we can have three remedies very much alike, and so perfectly adapted to cholera and yet so different. *Veratrum* is peculiar because of its *copious exhaustive discharges,* copious sweat, copious discharges from the bowels, copious vomiting, and great coldness of the sweat. There is some cramping and he wants to be warm; he is ameliorated by hot drinks, and by the application of hot bottles which relieve pain and suffering.

These three remedies tend downward into collapse and death. Now to repeat: Cuprum for the cases of a *convulsive* character, *Camphor* in cases characterized by *extreme coldness* and more or less dryness, and *Veratrum* when the *copious* sweat, vomiting and purging are the features. That is little to remember, but with that you can enter an epidemic of cholera with confidence.

In cholera-like states there are other remedies which relate to Cuprum and which ought to be considered. *Podophyllum* has cramps, mainly in the bowels. It has a painless, gushing diarrhœa with vomiting as well, and hence is useful in cholera morbus.

The cramps in *Podophyllum* are violent, they feel to him as if the intestines were being tied in knots. The watery stool is yellow, and, if examined a little while after, it looks as if corn meal had been stirred into it. The odor is dreadful, smelling like a *Podophyllum* stool. If you say it smells like stinking meat that only partly describes it; it is not quite cadaveric but it is horribly offensive and penetrating. The stool is gushing, copious, and is accompanied by dreadful exhaustion. "It is a wonder where it can all come from," says the mother, speaking of the exhausting diarrhœa in an infant or in a child. The stool runs away gushingly, in prolonged squirts, with a sensation of emptiness, sinking, deathly goneness in the whole abdomen. *Phosphorus* also ought to be thought of in relation to Cuprum. It also has cramps in the bowels, exhaustive diarrhœa, sinking as if dying, but commonly with heat of the skin, with burning internally, with gurgling of all the fluids taken into the stomach; as soon as they come to the stomach they commence to gurgle, and gurgle all the way through the bowel. A drink of water seems to flow through the bowel with a gurgle. Now this gurgling in Cuprum commences at the throat; he swallows with a gurgle; gurgling in the œsophagus when swallowing.

Convulsive cramps all over the body with twitching, jerking, trembling and blueness of the skin. Everything he does, all his actions are spasmodic, are convulsive. All the sphincters are convulsive. All the activities are irregular, disorderly and convulsive when poisoned with copper. Bear these things in

mind as we study every region in Cuprum. Repression or driving in of
eruptions, attended with diarrhœa and convulsions, sometimes only
convulsions. We note a case of measles or scarlet fever with a rash that has
been suppressed by a chill or exposure to wind and convulsions have come
on. That belongs to *Zincum* and Cuprum, sometimes to *Bryonia,* but to *Zincum*
and Cuprum particularly. Twitching of the limbs from a sudden suppression
of a scarlet fever, with suppression of urine, chorea, etc. Cramping of the
muscles of the chest; cramping of the calves; cramping all over. Suppressed
eruptions. Discharges that have been in existence quite a long time. The
individual has become debilitated and worn out with excitement, but this
discharge barely kept him alive. He has gradually grown weaker, but he has
kept about because he had a discharge. It has furnished him a safety-valve. If
stopped suddenly convulsions will come on. That is like Cuprum. A woman
has suffered a long time with a copious, leucorrhœa and some unwise doctor
tells her she must take injections and she checks it up for a few days, hysterical
convulsions, crampings and tearing of the muscles come on; contractions of
the fingers and toes. Discharges from old ulcers, fistulæ suppressed.

Cuprum will re-establish a discharge that has been suddenly suppressed
and convulsions followed. It stops the convulsions and re-establishes the
discharge. It has caries, it has senile gangrene, or the gangrene that belongs
to old age: old shrivelled up octogenarians, whose toes and fingers dark in
spots; feeble circulation.

In the Cuprum patient the nerves are all the time wrought up to the highest
tension; wants to fly, wants to do something dreadful. Impulsiveness.
Compelled to do something; restless and tossing about—a constant
uneasiness; nervous trembling; always tired. Great weakness of the muscles,
and relaxation of the body when the convulsions are not on. Twitching and
jerking and starting during sleep. Grinding of the teeth with brain affections.
Inflammations cease suddenly and you wonder what has happened. All at
once comes on insanity, delirium, convulsions, blindness; evidence of cerebral
congestions and inflammation appearing with wonderful suddenness.
Metastasis. A perfect change from one part of the body to another. The same
thing may occur from a suppressed eruption, or suppressed discharge, or, a
suppressed diarrhœa, and it goes to the brain, affects the mind and brings on
insanity; a wild, active, maniacal delirium. Cuprum is not passive in its
business. Violence is manifested everywhere. Violence in its diarrhœa, violence
in its vomiting, volence in its spasmodic action; strange and violent things in
its mania and delirium. Hysterical cramps and hysterical attitudes may change
in a night or in a day to St. Vitus' dance, and go on with it as if nothing had
happened. Such is the suddenness with which it changes its character. This
is not generally known of Cuprum, this constant changing about. Spasmodic

affections in general. Spasmodic coughs, spasms all over the body. The face becomes purple. He loses his breath; suffocates. The mother thinks the child will never come to life again. Spasms of the chest; spasms of the larynx; spasms of the whole respiratory system of such a character that the child seems to be choking to death.

Whooping cough. With every spell of whooping cough comes this awful spasmodic state, this spasmodic coughing. Jerking of the muscles. Cuprum has spasms of the limbs with all sorts of contractions such as are found in hysterical constitutions. Puerperal convulsions. Convulsions where a limb will first flex and then extend—an alternation of flexion and extension. In a child you will see the leg all at once shoot out with great violence, then up against the abdomen again with great violence, and then again shoot out. It is hard work to find another remedy that has that. *Tabacum* has it, but not many others. Convulsions with flexion and extension are common to Cuprum. Convulsions of the limbs, twitching and jerking of the muscles. We get a part of the symptom picture in one and part in another.

Violent congestion in the head, violent pains in the head. Tingling pain in the vertex, severe pain in the vertex, bruised pain. Crawling sensation in vertex, stitches in the temples. Congestion of the brain. Meningitis. Headache after epileptic attacks. Paralysis of the brain with symptoms of collapse. Metastasis to the brain from other organs.

About the face; convulsions, jerking of the eyes; twitching of the lids. Bruised pain in the eyes. Spasms of the muscles of the eye so that the eyes jerk and twitch, first from one side and then the other. Rolling of the eyes. "Quick rotation of the balls with the lids closed. Lids spasmodically closed." Closed so that they seem to snap. "Inflammation of the periosteum about the eyes and cellular tissue of the lachrymal glands." Spots of ulceration on the cornea. Face and lips blue. The face is purple in convulsions and whooping cough; lips blue.

Inflammation of the tongue. Paralysis of the tongue. It is not an uncommon thing to find paralysis in Cuprum after convulsions. The violence of the convulsions seems to have brought about a reaction and paralytic weakness, a numbness and tingling, a loss of motility. "Spasms of the throat, preventing speech. Sensation as if constricted on swallowing. Great thirst for cold drinks." Many complaints are ameliorated by drinking cold water. The spasms are sometimec mitigated by drinking cold water. The cough is brought on sometimes by inhaling cold air, but stopped by drinking cold water, like *Coccus cacti.* "Desire for warm food and drinks. Eats hastily." Indigestion from milk.

Then there is nausea, vomiting and diarrhœa connected more or less with spasms. Spasms of the stomach. Spasms of the chest with diarrhœa and vomiting. Cramps of the calves and the fingers and toes. "Pressure in the stomach." In the stomach and bowels periodical cramps. Cramps coming periodically. It has cured colic in the form of violent cramps coming every two weeks with perfect regularity. It has pain in the stomach, and a pain under the xiphoid appendix that seems as if it would take his life. If it is not removed he will certainly die in a little while. Constriction across the chest, suffocation, cramps of the legs. Cuprum goes deep into the life, and it has many a time taken such a grand hold of an old hysterical subject that it has completely eradicated in a short time the hysterical tendency to cramps. In Cuprum particularly, early in the cramps the thumbs commence to draw down. It is with difficulty that they can be lifted up. They will draw back again, and then the fingers will clinch over them and draw so tightly that it is painful. In children with such convulsions, and in hysterics with such convulsions, Cuprum goes deep into the life and eradicates this tendency to convulsions and cramps. Uræmic convulsions. Convulsions with suppressed or scanty urine. No urine in the bladder. In young girls beginning to menstruate, violent cramps in the limbs, cramps in the abdomen, diarrhœa, cramps in the uterus. Epileptic spasms coming at every menstrual period. Before or during menses, or after suppression, violent, unbearable cramps in the abdomen. A case something like this is not so very uncommon. Girls, at about the time of puberty, go in bathing, when their mothers have been a little too prudish, a little too sensitive, and have not told their daughters what they might expect, and to look out for bathing in cold water at certain times. The menstrual flow starts. From a cold bath she suppresses that flow and on come convulsions. That is in keeping with Cuprum. Hysterical convulsions they may be called. They will take the form, quite likely, of hysterical convulsions; they may take the form of chorea. Instead of convulsions it may take the form of congestion of the brain with violent delirium. Again, the menses not appearing after suppression, after sweat, and convulsions come on; frequent spasms during menses, Cuprum is not generally known to be such a wonderful medicine where there is anæmia; but it has chlorosis. It is a deep acting medicine. It affects with great power the whole voluntary system, the desires and aversions. It is suitable in those girls who have always had their own way, have never been crossed, and when they grow older, and reach puberty, and have got to submit to some sort of discipline or never become women, they have mad fits, have cramps. Cuprum will sometimes make them sensible, so in that way it fits into the loves and hates. It belongs to the voluntary system most prominently

Spasmodic respiration; great dyspnœa, asthmatic breathing. Attacks of spasmodic asthma and most violent spasmodic coughs. "Dry, hard, difficul cough, rattling in the chest, spasms. Dry spasmodic cough until he suffo cates. Face is red or purple."

CYCLAMEN

Aversion to motion, yet *motion ameliorates* her pain and uneasiness.

Aversion to the open air, yet open air ameliorates some symptoms, especially the coryza and cough.

The marked dulness of the senses and special senses is a striking part of this picture.

Chlorosis; irregular menses; and palpitation.

Stitching pains.

Weakness and aggravation from exertion.

Flabby muscles.

Most symptoms ameliorated by walking.

Very restless at night.

Great lassitude.

Weakness in the evening, ameliorated by moving about.

Sensitive to cold, and cold air.

Complaints from being overheated.

Alternation of moods is a striking feature of the mental state.

Great flow of ideas alternates with weak memory.

Joyous feeling alternating with irritability.

Serene humor changes suddenly into seriousness or peevishness.

Grief and fear keep her in continuous mental agitation.

Dulness of mind prevents mental labor.

Absorbed in thought; seeks solitude; thinks about the future.

Answers incoherently; confusion of mind.

Aversion to work, and dread of open air.

Wants to remain in a warm room, and in solitude.

Remains a long time silent. Excitement with trembling.

Sadness, as if she had wronged somebody (*Aur.*).

Tearful and meditates upon her grief, which is only imaginary.

Thinks she is alone in the world and persecuted by *every* one (*China*).

Obstinate and censorious. She grows steadily weaker; fainting spells come on; she becomes pale and anæmic.

These symptoms are important if associated with scanty menses or amenorrhœa.

Vertigo when walking in the open air; objects turn in a circle; ameliorated in a room, and when sitting. Everything turns dark before the eyes, and she falls as if fainting.

The pain in the head is stunning, and makes her fear she will lose her senses. Boring, darting, pressing in forehead and temples. Violent pains in the forehead. Pains worse lying on painful side or back. Pains one-sided.

Pain morning and evening, ameliorated by vomiting; worse by motion and in open air. Obscure vision with the pains. Pressure in vertex, as if brain were enveloped in a cloth, which would deprive him of his senses. Headache with flickering before the eyes on rising in the morning. Pulsating in the head. Rush of blood to the head; anxiety and confusion of mind; obscuration of vision; vertigo; general coldness, after dinner. Headache ameliorated by cold applications. Headaches from disordered stomach. Head feels as if he had on a skull cap. Tearing pains in the scalp.

In the field of vision there are spots, fog, bluish colors, flickerings, glittering objects; various colors—now yellow, and again green; fiery sparks, smoke; halo around the light, black specks or flies. Dimness of vision. Diplopia. *Convergent strabismus.* Dilated pupils. Hemiopia. Heat and burning. Lids œdematous. Swelling of upper lids. Dryness and itching of lids. Dim vision during headache. Impaired vision, smell, hearing and taste.

Dulness of hearing. Humming, ringing and roaring in the ears. Drawing pains.

Sense of smell diminished. Dryness in the nose. Dry, or fluent coryza, worse in a warm room, better in the open air or cool room. Sneezing and watery discharge in a warm room, entirely relieved in the open air. Walking in the cold open air is his most comfortable pastime. Pressing pain over nasal bone during coryza. Takes cold from being overheated and from overheated rooms.

Pale, sickly face; dark under the eyes in woman. Contracted forehead— a frown.

Dry lips. Numbness of upper lip.

Boring, stitching, tearing in the teeth. Jerking in the teeth at night. Taste is lost, or perverted; flat; bad; putrid; rancid; *all food tastes too salty.* Tongue white, or yellowish. Burning blisters on tongue. *Saliva increased.* Burning, tip of tongue. *Saliva tastes salty.* Viscid mucus in the mouth.

Burning, dryness and scraping in the throat.

Loss of appetite and even aversion to food. Thirstless, except in the evening during fever. Desires lemonade (*Nit. ac., Bell., Sab.*). Aversion to bread and butter, and fatty things; but desires inedible things. Disgust for meat; craves sardines. Satiety after the first mouthful (*Lye.*) and then he loathes food. Stomach weak. Nausea after eating. Pork disagrees. The stomach symptoms are much like *Pulsatilla.* Symptoms worse after coffee. Vomiting after eating. Vomiting in the morning. Vomiting watery mucus. Eructations. Aching in the stomach and burning in œsophagus, better by walking about. Fulness, as if he had eaten too much. Weight in the stomach after eating. Stitching pains in the stomach.

Colicky pains in the abdomen, ameliorated by walking about. Tenderness all over the abdomen, even hypogastrium. Gnawing pains in the evening.

Gnawing pains after food. Rumbling and gurgling in the abdomen. Paroxysmal cramps during the night, ameliorated by walking about.

Stitching pains in the abdomen and liver.

Diarrhœa after coffee. Diarrhœa in chlorotic women subject to sick headaches and menstrual irregularities. Watery, forcible stool, odorless, brownish, yellow. Diarrhœa in the evening. Constipation; stool hard. Nausea. Colic before stool. Colic and urging after stool. Hæmorrhoids that bleed. Drawing, pressing pain about the anus, as if a spot would suppurate.

Frequent urging to urinate. Ineffectual urging to urinate. Urine profuse, watery. Flocculent sediment; iridescent cuticle. Stitching in the urethra with desire to urinate.

In the male the sexual desire is diminished. Irritable prostate gland, with stitching pains; urging to stool and urine (*Nux*).

Menses too soon, or too late; irregular, or suppressed; copious, prolonged, or scanty. When profuse, the mental symptoms are better. Flow black and clotted. Labor-like pains at the menstrual period, commencing in small of back and running down each side of the pubes. Uterine hæmorrhage. Dread of open air. Menses suppressed, palpitation of the heart, weeping, aversion to company and dread of open air. Rush of blood to the head, and scanty flow. Suppressed menses from overexertion, or being overheated. Fainting at the menstrual period. After menses, milk in mammæ. Complaints after weaning (*China*).

Much scraping in the larynx at night, thick, white mucus. Tickling in the larynx and trachea. Oppression of chest. Suffocative cough. caused by scraping and dryness in the trachea. Cough comes on during sleep, from dryness and constriction of larynx. Cough ameliorated in the open air, even in a cold wind.

Pressure in the middle of the sternum. Weakness in the chest. Stitching in the chest and heart. Tearing, stitching, and shortness of breath during motion and rest.

Palpitation and anæmic murmurs. Tumultuous action of the heart; great lassitude. Weak pulse. Sensation as if air streamed from nipples. Mammæ swollen, containing milk in non-pregnant women. Mammæ swollen and very hard after menses.

Drawing pains in the neck, with stiffness. Twinges up the back, ameliorated by drawing the shoulders back. Stitching in the region of the right kidney, worse during inhalation. Pain in the small of the back while sitting. ceases on rising.

Tearing, drawing pains in the limbs. Hyperæsthesia of the skin. Flabby muscles. Tearing, drawing in the upper limbs. Sensation of weakness of the hands, as if she must let fall what she holds in her hands. Writer's cramp. Drawing pains in flexors of the leg. Burning sore pain in heels. Toes feel dead after walking. Weakness in the limbs.

Sleep not restful, disturbed by anxious dreams; frightful, vivid dreams. Restless sleep. Late falling asleep. Wakens early, but wants to sleep late. Nightmare. Wakens early, but too tired and sleepy, cannot rise. Pollutions in dreams.

Chill, fever and sweat. Chill not ameliorated by warm clothing. Chilliness during menses. Chill forenoon or evening. Chill predominates in the evening. Heat of face follows chill. Chill and heat alternate. Sensation of heat through whole body, particularly in face and hands. Heat, with swelling of the veins (*China*). General heat after eating. Sweat at night during sleep, offensive. Sweat sometimes on lower part of body.

Itching at night in bed. Numbness after scratching, or changing places by scratching.

DIGITALIS

This drug as used by the Old School has done more mischief than any one drug in their Materia Medica. Every patient who had a fast heart, or anything the matter with the heart, was given Digitalis. It has caused more deaths. than any drug. If administered when the heart is going fast it will soon produce a peculiar kind of paralysis; the heart then having lost its balance-wheel, compensation gives out, the patient sinks and finally dies. They do not know that many patients would have lived through fevers, pneumonia and other acute diseases if it had not been for this medicine, used as they have used it in the tincture, in many-drop doses, until the heart was slowed down. They call it sedative; yes, it is a sedative. It makes the patient very sedate. You have seen how very sedate a patient looks after he has been in the hands of an undertaker and has on his best garments. That is what Digitalis does. In that way it is a sedative in the hands of the allopath. A homœopathic physician never prescribes to bring down the pulse. He prescribes for the patient and the heart's action takes care of itself.

Digitalis is a very poor fever medicine. Instead of being indicated when the pulse is fast, the proving says it is indicated when the pulse is *slow*.

It produces a great disturbance of the liver. "Congestion and enlargement of the liver. Soreness of the liver." Tenderness about the liver—but during that time the pulse is slow. It makes the bowels very sluggish, produces inactivity of the liver, and stools are bileless, light colored, putty-like—and the pulse is slow. Add to that jaundice and you have a grand picture of Digitalis. Jaundice, with slow pulse, with uneasiness in the liver, pale stool, and even if you have never seen or heard of Digitalis before you will scarcely miss it. Now, you might add a myriad of little symptoms, but it does not change the aspect of things. It is Digitalis.

Another group of symptoms that belongs with the Digitalis heart, the Digitalis liver and the Digitalis bowels, is a gone, sinking feeling in the stomach. It seems as if he would die, and he does not get better from eating. It is a nervous, deathly sinking that comes with many heart troubles. You would not be surprised to find in Digitalis much nervous prostration. Restlessness and great nervous weakness. "Feels as if he would fly to pieces. Anxiety. Feels that something is going to happen." Seems as if his whole economy were full of anxious feelings and restlessness. Lassitude, faintness, exhaustion and extreme prostration. Faints on the slightest provocation. It begins in the stomach; an awful sensation of weakness in the stomach and bowels.

His sleep is full of horrible dreams, nightmare, fright. Dreams of falling — that is very common with cardiac affections. When the pulse is too slow, when it is irregular, the 'brain is irregularly supplied with blood during sleep, and there is a turbulent state. A shock goes through the body like an electric shock, like internal jerkings, twitchings. Sudden muscular movements, as if a current of electricity passed through the body. This, with slow pulse, with a sense of faintness, and great weakness. Bluish paleness of the lips in persons who suffer at times with cardiac spells—it seems at times as if the pulse would cease. Face becomes blue, the fingers become blue. Wants to lie on the back. Frequently startled in sleep; jerking at night.

The heart symptoms are numerous, but none is so important as the slow pulse. The pulse is slow in the beginning of the case. It may now he flying like lightning. He is anxious, restless, has horrible dreams and sinking in the stomach—that sounds like the advanced stage of Digitalis—but I want to know if in the beginning, the pulse was slow. The patient himself seldom knows, but someone says that in the beginning the pulse was 48; that is Digitalis. If the pulse in the beginning was rapid do not think of Digitalis, for it will not do any good. The Digitalis pulse is at first slow and perhaps remains so for many days, until finally the heart commences to go with a quiver, with an irregular beat, intermits, feels as if it would cease to beat, and then we have all these strange manifestations. Weakness is the very character of the Digitalis pulse, and all these characteristics go along with it. First it is slow, and sometimes strong. Slow, strong pulse when rheumatism is threatening the heart. "Violent, but not very rapid pulse. Sudden violent beating of the heart, with disturbed rhythm." The slightest motion increases anxiety and palpitation. When the pulse is going very slow, sometimes down to 40, the patient turns the head and the pulse flutters and increases in its action. If he turns over in bed it seems as if the heart would stop. If he moves he feels it fluttering all over him, and it settles back and is slow again; but, finally, it changes and flutters all the time.

Palpitation of the heart originating in grief. Sudden sensation as though the heart stood still. Fluttering of the heart. The least muscular exertion renders the heart's action labored and intermittent—in a feeble heart. A person with an enlarged liver, with a slow pulse. with jaundice and pale stool. With that he will have a troublesome cough. Digitalis is not much of a remedy for a cough unless it is a cardiac cough. Cough at midnight. Cough, with expectoration of "boiled starch". Cough, with expectoration of bloody mucus in hypostatic congestion of the lungs. Cough, brought on by talking, walking, drinking anything cold, bending the body. These are coughs associated with other troubles.

The same thing is to be said of the respiration. There are difficulties of respiration, along with cardiac troubles and liver troubles. "Respiration irregular and performed with great difficulty. Constant desire to take a deep breath. When he goes to sleep the breath seems to fade away, then he wakes up with a gasp. *Lachesis, Phosphorus, Carbo veg.* and some other remedies have that; remedies that affect the cerebellum particularly, producing a congestion of the cerebellum. When a patient goes to sleep the cerebrum says to the cerebellum: "Now you carry on this breathing a little while, I am getting tired." But the cerebellum is not equal to the occasion. It is congested, and just as soon as the cerebrum begins to rest the cerebellum goes to sleep, too, and lets the patient suffer; and in that way we get suffocation. The cerebellum presides over respiration during sleep and the cerebrum presides over respiration when the patient is awake. We might learn that from the provings of medicines if we never found it before.

"Fear of suffocation at night." Now, to analyze that. He knows from experience that every time he drops into a sleep he suffocates, and hence he fears to go to sleep for fear he will suffocate. The fear of suffocation at night is from this origin. It is the same if he falls asleep in the day time. "Can only breathe in gasps." Digitalis is a useful medicine when there is a filling up of the lower part of the lungs. The patient is sitting up in bed, and there is dulness in the lower part of each lung and plenty of resonance in the upper portion. Then it is, if he Lies down, he will suffocate. Digitalis likes mostly to lie flat on the back with no pillow, when there is no filling up of the lungs. But when there is hypostatic congestion he suffocates. If early in the case the pulse was slow and it has become fast, Digitalis may be of some benefit.

Now, a feature in connection with the genito-urinary organs. In old cases of enlarged prostate gland I do not know what I would do without Digitalis. Where there is a constant teasing to pass urine. In many instances where the catheter has been used for months or years because he is unable to pass urine in a natural way, and where there is a residuary urine in old bachelors and old men, Digitalis is a good remedy. It diminishes the size of the prostate gland and has many times cured. "Dropsy with suppression of urine." In uræmic poisoning and in various phases of Bright's disease of the kidneys we have symptoms indicating Digitalis. Retention of urine; dribbling of urine. Spermatorrhœa. Nightly emission. In persons addicted for years to secret vices. Enlarged prostate gland.

It is capable of curing chronic gonorrhœa. It has cured acute gonorrhœa. It has cured inflammation of that thin, delicate membrane covering the glands penis. Dropsical swelling of the genitals.

"Loss of appetite and violent thirst." Most doctors give *Sulphur* when the patient drinks much and eats little. The nausea of Digitalis is not like that of *Ipecac.* and *Bryonia.* It is a singular nausea. The smell of food excites a deathly nausea, a sinking, a goneness, associated with cardiac troubles, with jaundice and liver troubles. The nausea is accompanied by a deathly feeling, as if he is sinking away. Sometimes the nausea is relieved by eating, but the sinking remains after eating, showing that it is something besides hunger. "Persistent nausea. Extreme sensitiveness in the pit of the stomach. Faintness and sinking in the pit of the stomach as if he would die. No appetite, but great thirst. Soreness and hardness in the region of the liver. Sensitiveness to pressure in the region of the liver." Now remember the liver and the heart symptoms, the jaundice, the slow pulse, the awful sinking in the stomach, the enlargement of the prostate gland, the gray stool, and you have the principal symptoms of Digitalis.

After all that I have said you are not surprised at the horrible anxiety that the Digitalis patient carries with him all the time. He wants to be alone; sadness, melancholy, despondency and restlessness. He can't decide upon anything that he ought to do; tremulousness. The stomach, bowel and liver troubles are just what you see sometimes in a hard drinker after trying to break off. He is prostrated; his heart gives out, is irregular, weak, slow; and he has sadness and melancholy; inability to apply himself. Digitalis will help him straighten out.

DROSERA ROTUNDIFOLIA

The use of this medicine has been mostly limited to whooping cough, but it has a more extensive use. When we examine its spasmodic nature, its exhaustion, its cramps, which extend through a large number of complaints, we must realize that it is a more extensive remedy. Epileptiform spasms, prolonged sleeplessness, copious sweat on waking from sleep, restlessness and anxiety. Imagines that he is constantly persecuted. Flashes of heat, dread of the night. Many complaints come on in the night. Anxiety, sleeplessness,

and fear of ghosts. Spasmodic cough. Fear of being alone and suspicious o
his most intimate friends. Confusion of mind and much dizziness. Lancinating
pains in various parts of the body, especially in the head, and must suppor
the head with the hands. Must support the chest when coughing. Mus
press upon the abdomen. Pressive, congestive headaches. Corrosive itching
in various parts of the body with measle-like eruptions. The eyeballs become
prominent and congested from coughing during measles and in convulsions
Stitching pain in the eyes. Noises in the ears, roaring, humming and drumming
Earache in children. Stitching in the ears. Bleeding from various orifices
especially from the nose, throat, larynx, and chest when coughing, i
connection with the spasmodic coughs. Ordinarily the face is pale and sunke
with heat of the face and he has cold extremities, except when coughing, a
which time the face becomes red, congested, and purple like *Bell.* and *Cupr*
Stitching pains will be found in many complaints. Putrid taste in the mouth i
a common symptom when it is found in phthisical conditions of the lungs
larynx, and also in whooping cough. Bloody saliva and hæmorrhage from th
mouth. Difficulty in swallowing solid foods. Constriction of the throat and o
the larynx and constriction of the œsophagus preventing swallowing
Cramping constriction runs all through the remedy. Cramping of the hand
upon undertaking to hold on to something. When grasping the broom handle
In the throat there is burning and scraping. Stitching pains in the throat. Th
throat is dark red or purple. I believe that Drosera has a clinical symptom o
great value. Scraping in the larynx and cough after eating. In its proving
has cough after drinking. It has especially cough after eating and drinkin
cold things. This cough comes from tickling in the larynx and constriction
in the larynx. Nausea and vomiting. Vomiting of blood and bile in the mornin
and vomiting of mucus and food when coughing. Coughing until he retche
and vomits. Constricting pains in the pit of the stomach. Constricting pain
in the sides of the abdomen. Colic after sour food. Perhaps the mos
troublesome irritation found in this remedy is in the larynx, where there wi
be found clutching, cramping, constricting, and burning. Hoarseness an
continued irritation causing coughing and continued irritation and scrapin
of the larynx. Accumulation of mucus in the larynx, dryness in the laryn
spasms of the epiglottis. Violent spasmodic cough from tickling in the laryn
Violent tickling in the larynx brings on cough, rousing him from sleep, comin
on every few hours with increasing intensity making the remedy resembl
Whooping cough, in which it has been very useful. Sensation in the laryn
like a feather. Spasms of the larynx. Spasms of the extremities when coughin
The cough is brought on from tickling, from accumulation of mucus in th
larynx. These conditions are found in phthisis of the larynx, in whoopin
cough, in laryngitis, and in catarrh of the larynx.

Spasmodic difficulties of the chest and larynx cause difficult breathing and suffocation. Sensation as if something in the chest preventing breathing when talking or coughing. Difficult breathing and cough coming after midnight. Difficult breathing especially on waking. Not able to utter a sound. Difficult breathing and suffocating sensation. The face becomes purple from spasms in the larynx. Compression of the chest. These attacks of suffocation come on with the cough or come upon lying down. Asthmatic breathing from talking and constriction in the larynx Deep sounding, hoarse cough, rough scraping cough, loud whooping cough, spasmodic whooping cough. Violent constriction of the chest and muscles of the throat and larynx with whooping cough. Whooping cough coming in paroxysms of two or three hours, but violently worse after lying down at night and toward 3 o'clock in the morning. Most tormenting tickling in the larynx urging to cough. Paroxysmal dry cough from tickling in the larynx. Spasmodic cough, sympathetic cough from spinal irritation. Violent spasmodic cough in young girls going into consumption. Cough with expectoration of bright red or black clotted blood. Bloody expectoration. These spasmodic coughs come often during measles or after an attack of measles. An irritation in the larynx remains. It is one of the most frequently indicated remedies for measles. Like *Carbo veg.* Severe attacks of stitching in the chest when sneezing or coughing. He must press on the chest with the hand for relief. Makes an effort to hold chest with the hand when coughing, the cough is so violent. Compression of the chest, burning sensa-tion in the chest, stitching pains in the chest. It is a very useful remedy in chronic bronchitis with spasmodic cough. It is a great palliative for the spasmodic cough that occurs in consumption and all along the course of tuberculosis of the lungs. In these chest complaints, pains between the shoulders, pains in the back as if bruised from coughing. Coldness in the hands and feet and blueness of the extremities. Cramps in the extremities with the cough. The cough becomes so violent that the patient goes into convulsions. Along with these spasmodic coughs especially in phthisical conditions there are febrile attacks. Chill and chilliness and one-sided chill. Chill and fever with whooping cough. Chill and fever with inflammation of the larynx The heat as well as the cough is worse after midnight. Cold sweat on the forehead and on the extremities. Sweat over the whole body following the fever. Copious sweat all over the whole body with the cough. The cough ends in great exhaustion. Whooping cough with fever.

DULCAMARA—BITTER SWEET

This medicine seems especially to affect the mucous membranes. It appears to have a tendency to establish or ultimate discharges, both acute and chronic.

The Dulcamara patient is disturbed by every change in the weather, from warm to cold, from dry to moist, and from suddenly cooling the body while perspiring. He is ameliorated in dry, even weather; cold and damp aggravate all the conditions. He is worse evening and night and during rest.

Dulcamara produces catarrh of the stomach, intestines, nose, eyes, ears, and inflammatory conditions of the skin with eruptions. If you go through any of these in detail, you will be astonished to find how disturbed is the constitutional state of this patient by weather changes.

It is a medicine wonderfully useful in diarrhœa, at the close of the summer, hot days and cold nights, with changeable stool; diarrhœa of infants. There seems to be no digestion; yellow, slimy stool; yellow-green stool, with undigested stool; frequent stool, blood in the stool and quite a mass of slime, showing a marked catarrhal state. This gets better and worse; this gets better under ordinary remedies; it will often get better from *Pulsatilla,* because *Pulsatilla* symptoms seem to predominate, and sometimes it is relieved by *Arnica;* but every time the child takes cold, it comes back again, and soon the physician will realize that he has not struck the remedy belonging to all the symptoms. It is very often an annoying condition, because the symptoms are not recognized until two or three attacks have come. It is not easy to discover that the attacks come on from cold.

Every year women bring their babies back from the mountains, at the end of the season, and then we get some Dulcamara cases. One needs to be in the mountains at the close of the summer season to know what the condition is. If you go into the mountains at such a time, either in the North or West, you will notice that the sun's rays beat down during the day with great force, but along towards sunset if you walk out a draft of cold air comes down that will chill you to the bone. This will make the baby sick; it is too warm to take the child out in the middle of the day, and so he is taken out in his carriage in the evening; he has been overheated in the house during the day, and then catches this draft in the evening. Dulcamara is suitable for conditions that would arise from just such a state. So with an adult who has been out in the heat of the sun and catches the cold draft by night, which means hot days and cold nights, such as occur in the fall of the year, at the close of the summer and coming in of the winter; this intermingling of hot air and cold drafts. You go up towards the foot of the hills after a hot day, you will walk through a stratum of air that will make you perspire and the next minute a cold air that will make you want your overcoat on, and then again a stratum of hot air and so on. Such a state will bring out a sweat and then suppress it. The symptoms that come from Dulcamara seem to be like symptoms that arise from just such causes. And we are free, then, to infer from such an experience that Dulcamara cures these cases. I have been puzzled in times past over these babies that have brought home from the mountains, and have prescribed upon the visible symptoms, until I thought about the matter carefully and figured it out that they had come from these hot and cold regions. Babies have to be hurried home at times, because of the diarrhœas that cannot be cured in the mountains. but a dose of Dulcamara will enable them to stay there and live right in that same climate. Chronic recurrent dysentery from cold. If they have a dose of Dulcamara it fortifies them against the continual taking of cold.

There are people in a certain kind of business that really constitute a Dulcamara state. Suppose we look at our ice-cream men and our ice handlers and cold storage men; in a cold room they are handling ice; the summer weather is hot, they must go out and take some of the heat, and then they go back into their cold rooms and handle the ice, I have seen these things and have had occasion to follow them out. These men are subject at times to bowel troubles, and other catarrhal affections, but generally to diarrhœic affections. Their business cannot stop because it is their means of living. Dulcamara cures such chronic diarrhœas when the symptoms agree. *Arsenicum* is a medicine that would be suitable for such patients if the symptoms agreed, but the symptoms at times agree with Dulcamara, for that is the nature of the remedy, to take cold from cold, damp places, from suppressing a sweat, from going out of a hot atmosphere into an ice house, into icy rooms; into cold rooms; in this climate such complaints as come on from overexertion, overheating; and then throwing off the clothing and becoming chilled, suppressing the sweat; fevers may come on, aching in the bones, trembling with the aching, trembling in the muscles, and as the fever goes on, he is in a distressed state, cannot remem-ber, forgets what he was about to speak of, forgets the word that would naturally express his idea, and he enters into a dazed state, a state of confu-sion. It suits these colds that have this sluggish circulation of the brain, with trembling and chilliness, coldness as if in the bones.

Dulcamara is full of rheumatism, full of rheumatic pains and aches, sore and bruised all over, the joints are inflamed, become red, sensitive to touch and are swollen. It is suitable in cases of inflammatory rheumatism, due to *suppressed perspiration,* induced by changing from a high to low temperature, or from cold, wet weather. Worse evening and night and during rest.

Now, it has many chronic complaints. A catarrhal condition of the eyes, purulent discharges, thick, yellow discharges, granular lids; eyes become red every time he takes cold; "every time he takes cold it settles in the eyes," is a common expression of the patient. The patient will often ask the question, "Why is it, doctor, that every time I take cold it settles in my eyes? If I get into a cold atmosphere, or take off my coat after being heated, I have to look out."

If it becomes cold in the night and he has thrown the clothes off, he takes cold, or, if a cold rain comes on, he takes cold and then has sore eyes. Such eyes are very often effectually cured by Dulcamara. As to the eye itself, it is only an ordinary catarrhal state, but the manner in which it comes on is the important thing. That is the nature of the patient to have sore eyes whenever he takes cold; it belongs to some other remedies as well, but this one particularly.

Dulcamara has also catarrhal discharges from the nose, with bloody crusts blowing out thick, yellow mucus all the time. In infants and children who have sniffles, they are always worse in cold, damp weather. When the patient says "Doctor, in cold, damp weather I cannot breathe through my nose; my nose stuffs up;" or, "I must sleep with my mouth open." Dulcamara is a very useful remedy to know in caarrhal cases that always stuff up when there is a cold rain.

It is markedly an autumnal remedy. The Dulcamara patients go through the summer very comfortably; their catarrhal conditions to a great extent pass away; the warm days and warm nights, because of the even temperature, seem to agree with them, but as soon as the cold nights come on and the cold rains come, all their difficulties return; there is an increase of the rheumatism and of the catarrhal discharges. This medicine has been used a long time by our mothers. They used to make ointments out of Dulcamara. You will find that the old ladies, in almost any rural district in which Dulcamara grows, gather it and make it into a salve for ulcers. Well, it is astonishing how soothing it is when applied externally to smarting wounds, whether in solution or salve or any other way. But it is a better medicine, of course, when indicated by symptoms of the constitutional state; it is a better medicine if used internally. It produces ulcers and a tendency to ulceration of the mucous membranes and this condition will become phagedenic. Sometimes it starts as nothing more than an herpetic eruption, but it spreads and finally yellow pus forms and then the granulations that should come, do not come; an eating condition appears and the surface does not heal. Especially along the shin bone there will be raw places, which even extend to the periosteum, to the bone, producing necrosis and caries; so we have affections of the mucous membranes or skin, first becoming vesiculated and then breaking open and eating. It is especially related to very sensitive, bleeding ulcers with false granulations, phagedenic ulcers. This is not generally known; it is a matter of experience with those that have watched this medicine; and again, strange to say, *Arsenicum,* which I have already mentioned once or twice, has this state. *Arsenicum* leads all other medicines for ulcers that eat, phagedenic ulcers. *Arsenicum* is a typical remedy for spreading sores, for spreading ulcers, and especially those that come from a bubo that has opened and will not heal.

Another feature of this medicine is its tendency to throw out eruption.

over the body. It is a wonderfully eruptive medicine, producing vesicles, crusts, dry, brown crusts, humid crusts, herpes. Dulcamara produces eruptions so nearly like impetigo that it has been found a useful remedy in that condition. *i.e.*, multiple little boil-like eruptions; it produces little boils, and the boils spread. Enlargement and hardness of the glands. Eruptions upon the scalp that look so much like crusta lactea that Dulcamara has been found a very useful medicine. Extreme soreness, itching; and the itching is not relieved by scratching, and the scratching goes on until bleeding and rawness take place. Eruptions that come out upon the face, upon the forehead, all over the nose, but especially on the cheeks, which become completely covered with these crusts; eczema of infants. Children only a few weeks old break out with these scalp eruptions, and Dulcamara is one of the medicines that you will need to know. It is about as frequently indicated as any of the medicines. *Sepia, Arsenicum, Graphite's*, Dulcamara, *Petroleum, Sulphur* and *Calcarea* are about equally indicated, but of these, in this climate at least, I think *Sepia* is probably more frequently indicated.

All of these catarrhal symptoms, the rheumatic symptoms, the eruptions upon the skin, are subject to the peculiar aggravations of the constitutional state. No matter what the symptoms are, the constitutional state is worse in cold, damp weather.

"Catarrhal and rheumatic headaches in cold, damp weather." When the headache is the main trouble, the catarrh takes a different course from what it does when the catarrh is the principal ailment. There are two ways in which that conducts itself. In some Dulcamara patients, whenever he takes cold from the cold, damp weather, he commences to sneeze, and to get a coryza, and soon comes a copious, thick, yellow flow from the nose. On the other hand, Dulcamara has a dry catarrh in its first stage, and a fluid catarrh only in the second stage. One who is subject to Dulcamara headaches, has the dry catarrh; whenever he takes cold instead of the usual catarrhal flow with it, he at first sneezes and then feels a dryness in the air passages, a slacking up of the usual discharge, which would give him relief, and then he knows that he must look out, for along will come the neuralgic pains, pains in the occiput, and finally over the whole head. Congestive headaches, with neuralgic pains and dry nose. Every spell of cold, damp weather will bring on that headache. The catarrh is not always acute enough for him to pay attention to it. He does not say very much about it. The Dulcamara headache is very severe, is accompanied by tremendous pains, and he may go to the doctor with the idea of getting rid of the headache, but it is a catarrhal state that is suppressed, that has slackened up, and the nose becomes dry. As soon as the flow starts up his headache is relieved. Then headache of this catarrhal kind that comes on from every cold, damp spell, or from getting overheated, from getting into a cold draft after being overheated, or getting overheated with too much

clothing and then throwing the coat off, will also belong to the Dulcamara
state.

A form of eruption that is very likely to be a Dulcamara eruption is the
ringworm, herpes circinatus. It comes sometimes upon the face and scalp
Children sometimes have ringworms in the hair. Dulcamara will nearly always
cure these ringworms in the hair.

The Dulcamara child is very susceptible to earache.

"Coryza dry, relieved by motion, worse during rest, and renewed by the
slightest exposure, and worse in cold air." Some coryzas cannot tolerate the
warm room, and others want a warm room. The Dulcamara coryza is worse
going out in the open air and better from motion. The *Nux vomica* coryza is
better in the open air. The patient feels much aching distress in the nose. The
Nux vomica patient ordinarily wants warmth and warm air and a warm room
but with the coryza he is the very opposite; he, wants motion in the open air
he looks for cool air, for it relieves the distressing sensation. In the warm
room there is a tickling sensation in the, nose, and the nose will drip, night
and day. The *Nux vomica* coryza is worse in the house, and worse in the
night, and worse in the warm bed, so that the discharge will run all over the
pillow. In Dulcamara it is more fluent in the house, in the warmth, and less
fluent in the cold air in a cold room. With the Dulcamara coryza, if the patient
should go into a cold room pain will commence in the nasal bones and he will
begin to sneeze, and water will be discharged from the nose. That very state
would relieve a *Nux vomica* patient. *Allium cepa* is made worse in a warm
room; like *Nux vomica,* is better in cold, open air. Commences to sneeze as
soon as he gets into a warm room. So that we see the meaning of such things
the necessity of going into particulars and examining every case.

Here is a state that you will often find in the fall of the year, somewhere
about August 20th. They sometimes call it hay fever. Every year as the nights
become cold, and there is cold, damp weather and fall rains, he has a stuffing
up of the nose with constant sneezing and wants the nose kept warm. I have
known these cases at times to sit in a warm room with cloths, wrung out of
hot water, over the face and nose to relieve the distress, the catarrhal state of
the eyes and the stuffing up of the nose. Heat relieves the stuffing up of the
nose. These patients can sometimes breathe with these hot cloths over the
nose, but if they go out into the night air, or a cold place, and especially
there is a damp, fall rain, they suffer much. Other cases of hay fever suffer
during the day, and they go to as cold a place as they can find, and are even
driven to the mountains for a cool place. These things are indicative of
state of the constitution; the state gives out signs and symptoms to lead the
intelligent physician to cure. If that state had no means of making itself
known by signs and symptoms, there could be no curing it by remedies.

"Profuse discharge of water from the nose and eyes, worse in the open air," "better in a closed room, on awakening in the morning," etc. The Dulcamara patient is so sensitive to newly mown grass and drying weeds, that he is obliged to absent himself from the country where they are found. For hay fever we have especially to look up such remedies as have complaints worse in the fall of the year. There are other conditions that are just as much hay fever, for instance, "rose cold" that comes on in June. There are other conditions that come on in the spring, sometimes cured by *Naja* and *Lachesis*. So that we have to observe the time of the year, the time of the day, night or day aggravations; the wet and the dry remedies, the hot and the cold remedies. We have to study the remedy by circumstances.

The Dulcamara patient often becomes a sickly patient, with threatening of the catarrhal discharges to centre in the bronchial tubes, *i.e.*, in the mucous membrane of the breathing apparatus. Many adults die of acute phthisis that might have been cured by Dulcamara, and you will find very commonly among this class of patients those that are worse from every cold, damp spell of weather. Such enter right into the Dulcamara sphere. They are better by going South where there is a continuously warm climate. The Dulcamara patient is a sickly patient, threatened with acute phthisis; pallid face, sickly yellow and sallow. This shows that it goes deeply into the life, creating such disorders as are found in very sick patients, *i.e.*, those chronically sick, in persons whose vital economy is so much disordered that it cannot keep the body in repair.

The throat comes in for its share of trouble. Persons who in every cold damp spell have a sore throat, from getting overheated, throwing off the wraps, getting into a cold place. The Dulcamara patient says: "Well now, I know I am fixed; I am now chilled; I begin to feel hoarseness in my throat." On comes the sore throat; it fills with mucus, with yellow slime; the tonsils become inflamed; even quinsy comes on. Or it may affect the throat uniformly; it may become red and inflamed and dry at times, and at other times filled with mucus, and at night the throat fills with thick, yellow, tough mucus, which is hawked up in great quantities. These colds that settle first in the nose and throat, post-nasal catarrh, of the very worst sort, gradually creep on until the whole respiratory apparatus is in a state of catarrhal inflammation. Every cold that he takes aggravates his catarrh wherever that may be. If it be in the nose, then the nose is aggravated; if in the chest, then those parts are aggravated. A continual rousing up. Every experienced physician must have met with many cases where for a time he felt unable to cope with the case because of his inability to reach the constitutional state that underlies this continual taking cold. So he puzzles, for a long time, and prescribes on the immediate attack and palliates it. For instance, the immediate attack might look like *Belladonna* or *Bryonia, Ferrum phos.* or *Arsenicum,* etc.; he treats that attack without taking into consideration the underlying constitutional state of the patient. It is quite a profitable business for one who has not much conscience and not much intelligence. But a conscientious physician feels worried and knows he is not doing what he ought to do by his patient, unless he reaches out for the remedy which touches the constitution. It is far more useful to keep people from taking colds than to cure colds.

There is a form of acute Bright's disease that Dulcamara cures. You can probably now surmise from what we have said of the nature of the remedy, that in cases of Bright's disease following scarlet fever, or from malaria, or in any acute disease that has ended badly, *i.e.*, the patient has been exposed to the cold too soon, and has taken "cold," or from sudden change of weather, damp and cold, the feet commence to swell, there is albumin in the urine, the limbs are waxy, the face becomes waxy and sallow, and there is constant urging to urinate. Dulcamara, with other constitutional symptoms, will be suitable.

In bladder catarrh, where there is a copious discharge of mucus, or muco-pus in the urine; when the urine stands, a thick, purulent sediment, yellowish-white, and a constant urging to urinate; every time he takes a little cold, the urine becomes bloody, the frequency of urination is increased, the urine becomes irritating, the catarrh of the bladder rouses up like a flame, all the symptoms are worse in cold, damp weather, and from getting chilled; better from becoming warm. So you see whether it is a catarrh of the kidney or a catarrhal state of the bladder, or an attack, of dysentery, or an attack of sudden diarrhœa, every cold spell of the weather brings on an increase of the trouble.

There is another Dulcamara symptom which will often be expresses suddenly in the midst of a lot of other symptons. After you have been hunting for a long time, the patient will say: "Doctor, if I get chilled, I must hurry to urinate; if I get into a cold place, I have to go to stool, or to urinate." So we see that the symptoms come on when the patient is cold and are better when he is warm. Any catarrhal trouble of the bladder that is better in the summer and worse in the winter.

In dry, teasing coughs that are winter "colds," that go away in the summer and return in the winter. *Psorinum* has a dry, teasing, winter cough. *Arsenicum* has a winter cough.

"Rash comes out upon the face before the menses." "As a forerun of catamenia, with extraordinary sexual excitement, herpetic eruptions." Its "cold" sores are very troublesome. The patients are subject to these "cold" sores upon the lips and upon the genitals. Every time he takes "cold," herpes labialis, herpes preputialis. "Catarrhal ailments in cold, damp weather." "Mammæ engorged, hard, sore and painful." "Mammæ glands, swollen, inactive, painless, itching, in consequence of a 'cold' which seems to have settled in them."

"Cough, from damp, cold atmosphere, or from getting wet." "Cough, dry, hoarse and rough, or loose, with copious expectoration of mucus and dull tearing; catarrhal fever." The cough is worse lying and in a warm room and better in the open air.

Rheumatic lameness and stiffness in the back from taking cold better by motion. Drawing pain in the lumbar region extending to the lower limbs during rest. Stiff neck from every exposure to cold. Stitching, tearing, rheumatic pains in limbs after exposure to cold, better by motion, worse at night or in the evening, with some fever. Sore, bruised feeling all over the body. Warts on hands, fingers and face.

EUPATORIUM PERFOLIATUM (BONESET)

Every time I take up one of these old domestic remedies I am astonished at the extended discoveries of medical properties in the household as seen in their domestic use. All through the Eastern States, in the rural districts, among the first old settlers, Boneset-tea was a medicine for colds. For every cold in the head, or running of the nose, every boneache or high fever, or headache from cold, the good old housewife had her Boneset-tea ready. Sure enough it did such things; and the provings sustain its use. The proving shows that Boneset produces upon healthy people symptoms like the colds the old farmers used to suffer from.

The *common winter colds* through the Eastern States and the North are attended with much sneezing and coryza, pain in the head, as if it would burst, which is aggravated from motion, chilliness with the desire to be warmly covered; the bones ache as if they would break; there is fever, thirst, and a general aggravation from motion. Such common everyday colds correspond sometimes to Eupatorium and sometimes to *Bryonia.* These two remedies are very similar, but the aching in the bones is marked in Eupatorium. If this state goes on for a few days the patient will become yellow, the cold will settle in the chest, a pneumonia may develop, or an inflammation of the liver,. or an attack commonly called a bilious fever. Such fevers frequently call for *Bryonia* and Eupatorium, each fitting its own cases. These remedies are especially useful throughout New England, New York, Ohio, the North and Canada. They do not have this kind of a cold very frequently in the warmer climates, but Eupatorium is often indicated in the warmer climates for fevers, yellow fever, bilious fever, break-bone fever and intermittent fever. It seems to be useful in one kind of complaints in one climate and in another kind of complaints in another climate.

In the Southwest and the West, in the valleys of the great rivers, Eupatorium cures complaints beginning as if the back would break, great shivering from head to foot spreading from the back, great sensitiveness to cold, congestive headaches, flushed face, yellow skin and yellow eyes, pain in the abdomen, and in the region of the liver, inability to retain any food, nausea from the sight and smell of food; the bones ache as if they would break, the fever runs high, the urine is of a mahogany color, the tongue is heavily coated yellow, and there is nausea and vomiting of bile. That gives the picture of Eupatorium in the Mississippi Valley, in the Ohio Valley, in Florida and Alabama, and all through the Southern States. The most prominent symptoms are the *vomiting of bile, the aching of the bones as if they would break,* the pains in the stomach after eating, and the nausea from the thought and smell of food. The stomach is very irritable; the thought of food gags him. The patient desires to keep still, but the pain is so severe that he must move and so he appears restless. These are among the acute manifestations, and are things only very general that we must take up and apply to sick people.

Eupatorium has been a very useful remedy in *intermittent fever,* when epidemic in the valleys. Among the first signs is nausea some time before the attack, and there are sometimes spells of vomiting of bile. About seven or nine o'clock in the forenoon, he commences to shudder, the shivering runs down the back and spreads from the back to the extremities; he has violent thirst, but the shiverings are made worse from drinking so that he dare not drink cold water. There is soreness and pulsation in the back of the head, violent pain in the occiput and back before and during the chill. During the chill he wants to cover up and the clothing needs to be piled on. The thirst extends through all the stages. At the close of the chill there is vomiting; often it does not occur until the heat, but before the sweat fairly sets in he vomits copiously, first the contents of the stomach and then bile. When the heat is on he seems to burn all over, sometimes as though with electric sparks. Intense heat, burning in the top of the head, his feet burn and his skin burns. The burning is more intense than the heat would justify. It is characteristic of this remedy for the sweat to be scanty; a violent chill, intense fever which passes off slowly, and very scanty sweat. The bones ache *as if they would break.* During the chill his head aches as if it would burst, it throbs, it tears, it stings, it burns; he describes the headache in terms expressive of violence, as if probably a congestive headache. One would think after the fever subsides and he commences to sweat a little that he would get relief, which is true excepting the headache, which often gets worse clear through to the end of the attack, and sometimes it will last all day and night; then he will have a whole day free from the headache, but on the third day at seven or nine o'clock on will come the same trouble with increasing violence. At times these attacks are prolonged, the one will extend into the other, that is enter into a sort of remittent character with no intermission. The longer this runs the more the liver becomes engorged, and finally the urine is loaded with bile, the stool becomes whitish, the fever increases, the nausea increasing, the tongue becomes pointed and enlongated, and is dry, the headache is extremely painful, and a state of masked fever comes on.

In those intermitent fevers that begin with violent shaking, and the headache continues without sweat, or, if with sweat the headache is made worse, thirst during all stages, vomiting of bile at the close of the heat or during the heat, with the awful boneaches, the Western men, who study their Materia Medica, know that they have a sure cure in Eupatorium. The time for the administration of this dose is at the close of the paroxysm. You get the best effect when reaction is at the best, and that is when reaction is setting in, after a paroxysm has passed off. That is true of every paroxysmal disease, where it is possible to wait until the end. You cannot mitigate them very much during the attack, indeed, if the medicine is given then it very often increases the difficulty, but if you wait until the close of the paroxysm you get the full benefit of your medicine, and the next paroxysm will not develop, or will be lighter, or, if another attack is brought on immediately, you may rest assured there will he no more. It is not an uncommon thing in intermittent fever, when the remedy has been administered at the close of the paroxysm, for the next paroxysm to come within twenty-four hours after the administration of the medicine; these mixed cases are often in a state of disorder. One who does not know this would immediately show the white feather, would be alarmed, would be afraid the patient was getting worse, but you have only to wait for the subsidence of the attack and you will see that you have broken its cycle and periodicity.

When this remedy has been apparently indicated by intermittents, and it has not proved of sufficient depth to root out the intermittent, there are two remedies, either of which is likely to follow it, and these are *Natrum muriaticum* and *Sepia*. These two remedies are very closely related to Eupatorium and take up the work where it leaves off, when the symptoms agree.

This medicine has also a chronic constitutional state, viz.: *its gouty nature*. It is a very useful medicine in gout. It has gouty soreness and inflamed nodosities of the finger joints, of the elbow joint, pain and gouty swelling of the great toe, red tumefaction of the joint of the great toe. It establishes, in persons who are subject to chalk stone, deposits around the finger joints. These gouty subjects take cold, the bones ache, the joints become inflamed, the patient will say he is chilly, the skin becomes yellow, the urine is charged with bile, the stool becomes whitish, and he becomes weak. In many instances these patients have been for years resorting to Burgundy for relief of their gouty joints and the weakness. Some one of our homœopathic remedies will relieve the suffering, but in those old gouty subjects who have been always drinking wine, you cannot take the wine away from them at once; you cannot do it while they are having the attack, because they have become so accustomed to it. Burgundy is the kind of wine very commonly used by the gouty, but the Scotchman with his gout thinks he must always have a little Scotch whiskey, and in the attack it is quite impossible to take it away from him. What has been his custom must be followed out for a while because he would grow weaker, but it is damaging him, and hence it is difficult to contend with gouty subjects who have been taking stimulants. You do not get the full benefit of Homœopathy and you cannot stop his stimulants because weakness will follow. Persons who have not taken wine as a regular beverage can and should do without it, as it interferes with the action of the hommœopathic remedy.

These gouty patients have terrible *sick headaches.* Pain in the base of the brain and back of the head, associated with gouty joints. These are often referred to as *arthritic headaches,* that is, gouty headaches, headaches associated with painful joints. Or the headaches may alternate with pains in the joints. Congestive headaches, the pain being in the base of the brain, with more or less throbbing; the pain spreads up through the head and produces a general congestive attack. Sometimes these headaches come on when the joints are feeling better, and the more headache he has the less pain he has in the extremities; and again, when the gout affects the extremities, then the headaches diminish. Headaches, having a *third and seventh-day aggravation,* coming with more or less periodicity. With the headache there will be nausea and vomiting of bile, nausea at the thought and smell of food. This gouty individual is also subject to vertigo, and the sensation as if he would fall to the left is especially noted with the coming on of the headache. The vertigo comes on in the morning; when he gets up he feels as if he would sway to the left, and he has to guard himself in turning to the left. Sometimes in intermittent fever this symptom of swaying to the left and vertigo ending in nausea and vomiting, violent pain in the back of the head and pain in the bones, are the first threatenings.

We have in this remedy also other gouty manifestations: shooting through the temples, shooting from the left to the right side of the head; shooting all through the head; stitching, tearing pains in the limbs as well as the bone aches. The headaches are so violent that they make him sick at the stomach. In gouty headaches, in intermittents at the close of the intense heat, in periodical headaches, the course is the same, the pain is so intense that nausea is soon brought on and then he vomits bile. Eupatorium has not been used on its symptoms in gouty states as often as it might have been. In intermittent fever it is well known; in headaches it is only occasionally used.

Only occasionally does a man realize its great benefit in headaches and in remittent fevers. In gouty and rheumatic affections it may be suited to the symptoms and is more useful than is generally known. It is not the purpose of our talks to point out ultimates of disease. I do not look upon gout as a disease, but as a great class of symptoms of a rheumatic character that occur in the human family; a great mass of symptoms that may be called gouty, a tendency to enlargement of the joints and gouty deposits in the urine. The ordinary so-called lithæmia is a gouty constitution. The gouty state of the economy is the superficial or apparent cause; the real cause rests in the miasm. So when I speak of gout I do not mean the name of a disease, but a class of manifestations that are met in large cities especially, less frequently in the country where the people live on farms and take plenty of exercise and have wholesome food and are not housed up. It is supposed to be due to wine drinking. Often when I say to patients that the symptoms are somewhat gouty, they reply, "I am not in the habit of drinking wine. I have not been a high liver." Such conditions of course bring on a tendency to gout.

Painful soreness in the eyeballs like *Bryonia* and *Gelsemium*. The eyeballs are very sensitive to touch and sore to pressure; feel as if he had been struck a blow in the eye; sore, bruised, pain in the eye. Coryza with aching in every bone.

With the bilious attacks there often may be an ending in a diarrhœa; copious green discharges, green fluid or semi-fluid stools, but after the attack has lingered until there is one grand emptying out of the bowels, this symptom will disappear and the secondary state comes on in which there is constipation and a light-colored stool, or bileless stool.

Boneset has a dry, hacking, teasing cough, that seems to rack the whole frame, as if it would break him up, it is so sore, and he is so much disturbed by motion. A great amount of tribulation is found in the respiratory tract, in the bronchial tubes. We find a cough in capillary bronchitis that shakes the whole frame, analogous to *Bryonia* and *Phosphorus*. The subject is extremely sensitive to the cold air, as much so as in *Nux vomica*. *Nux vomica* has aching in the bones as if they would break; he wants the room hot, and wants to be covered with clothing which relieves; often the slightest lifting of the covers increases the chilliness, which is true also of Eupatorium, so they run close together. In *Nux vomica* we have the dreadful irritability of temper; in Eupatorium we have overwhelming sadness. The *Nux vormica* patient is not likely to say much about dying, he is too irritable to go into the next world; not so with Eupatorium, he is full of sadness.

There are other states that come on secondarily in this medicine. After malarial attacks and in gouty affections, etc., there is bloating of the lower limbs, œdematous swelling. It is not an uncommon thing for a malarial fever

EUPHRASIA

that has lingered a long time to be attended with swelling of the lower limbs. Eupatorium very strongly competes with *Natrum muriaticum, China* and *Arsenicum* in such lingering malaria. When the symptoms have largely subsided and left only this state of anæmia and dropsy of the lower extremities, in the badly treated cases, it is very difficult to find what medicine to administer, and the course that the homœopath must pursue is to go back and examine the patient to find the symptoms he had at the time of the intermittent fever, before he was meddled with. If now there is swelling of the extremities, and you get symptoms to show you that he needed Eupatorium in the beginning, Eupatorium will still cure the dropsy of the extremities. It may bring back the chill, it may bring back an orderly state that you can prescribe on. If in the beginning he needed *Arsenicum,* that remedy will bring back the chill, turn it right end to and cure his symptoms. The trouble is that the symptoms were only suppressed, had not been cured. So the medicine he needed, but has never had for the chill, may be the medicine that he needs now. Then think of Eupatorium in dropsical swellings of the feet and ankles, and in gouty swellings also. The gouty swellings are all of an inflammatory character. Very commonly these are closely related to hydrarthrosis, and here Eupatorium is to be compared with *Arsenicum.* Gouty inflammation of the knee. All the way through this remedy you read about bone-aches and bone-pains.

It is peculiar that medicines come around on time with an exactitude. Diseases do the same thing, and we must see that it is also peculiar that they come with a regular cycle, a regular periodicity. We meet with headaches that come every seven days, headaches also that come once in two weeks, and there are remedies that have seven-day aggravations and fourteen-day aggravations and three-day aggravations, remedies that bring out their symptoms just in this form. Do not be surprised when your patient is perfectly under the influence of *Aurum* if he has a characteristic aggravation every twenty-one days. There are quite a number of remedies having fourteen-day aggravations, *e.g., China* and *Arsenicum.* Again, there are autumnal aggravations, spring aggravations, winter aggravations, aggravations from cold weather and aggravations in the summer from heat. Some remedies have both the latter.

EUPHRASIA

Euphrasia is a short acting remedy of great usefulness in acute catarrhal affections with or without fever. Headaches that occur with coryza and eye symptoms, head aches in the evening as if bruised. Stitching pain in the head. Head aches as if the head would burst with dazzling of the eyes from sunlight. These are catarrhal headaches with profuse watery discharge from the eyes and nose. The eye symptoms of Euphrasia are its most prominent feature. Catarrhal condition of the eyes with copious, acrid, watery discharge with or without coryza. Cutting pain in the eyes extending into the head, pressure in the eyes as if caused by sand. Sensation of dryness, burning, biting in the eyes. Sensation of dust in the eyes. Violent itching of the eyes obliging rubbing and winking, with copious lachrymation. Pupils much contracted and much tumefaction of the mucous membrane with redness and enlarged blood vessels and smarting. Iritis from rheumatism or in connection with rheumatic joints. Copious thin or thick discharges. General inflammation of all the tissues of the eyes. Ulceration of the cornea. It has cured Pannus. Pustular inflammation. Opacity of the cornea after injuries of the eye. It is suitable in the most violent acute conjunctivitis. Amblyopia with inflammation of conjunctiva and lids. Copious lachrymation and burning. The mucous membranes of the lids and eyeballs are injected, red, and vascular. Glutination of the lids in the morning. Copious, acrid lachrymation with fluent discharge from the nose during coryza. Dryness of the lids and the margins of the lids red, swollen, and burning. The lids are very sensitive and swollen. The margins of the lids itch and burn. Suppuration of the margins of the lids. Much swelling of the lids with inflammation. Fine rash about the eyes with puffiness of the lids. Blurred vision. Paralysis of the third nerve.

The next most important group of symptoms is in connection with the nose. Sneezing and fluent coryza. The discharge is bland and this occurs with acrid lachrymation. The nasal mucous membrane is swollen. Profuse, bland, fluent coryza. After this coryza has existed for a day or two it extends into the larynx with a hard cough. The coryza is worse during the night while lying down. The cough is worse in the daytime and *ameliorated by lying down.* The remedy has a rash like measles and it has febrile symptoms; therefore, when these symptoms are duly considered, it will be seen that Euphrasia is similar to the symptoms that occur in measles. It is a wonderful medicine in measles though not so frequently indicated as *Pulsatilla* owing to the fact that this combination of symptoms does not often come. Hoarseness in the morning. Irritation in the larynx compelling him to cough, followed by pressure beneath the sternum. Abundant secretion in the larynx causing loose cough with rattling in the chest. Deep inspiration is difficult. The cough, considered by itself, furnishes a very rare group of symptoms. Cough with copious expectoration along with or following coryza. Difficult respiration ameliorated at night while lying down. Worse in the morning when moving about with copious expectoration. Violent cough from tickling in the larynx. No cough at night causes the remedy to resemble *Bry.* and *Mang.* The dyspnœa and cough are *ameliorated by lying down.* The coryza symptoms, otherwise, are worse at night and from lying down. When these symptoms occur in grippe or influenza, this becomes a very suitable remedy. The abundance of mucus scraped from the larynx and trachea is often like the ending of bad colds. The expectoration is easy and almost without cough. It comes up without much effort. Pressive pain beneath the sternum showing that the trachea is especially involved in the catarrhal condition. The pain in the eyes is worse in the open air. The coryza is worse in the open air. The cough sometimes comes on in the open air. Windy weather causes fluent coryza. Cold air and windy weather cause lachrymation. He is a chilly patient and cannot get warm in bed. There is chill, fever, and sweat in this remedy. The chill predominates. The fever occurs mostly during the day with red face and cold hands. The heat descends the body. The perspiration is often confined to the front part of the body. Perspiration during sleep at night. Strange odor sometimes very offensive and most profuse upon the chest. It is especially suitable in catarrhal fever, influenza and measles. When the symptoms agree, it will make a violent attack of measles turn into a very simple form, making the patient feel better, bring out the eruption, control the fever, and relieve the cough, coryza, and other catarrhal symptoms. Streaming, hot, burning tears with rash, photophobia, running from the nose, intense throbbing headaches, redness of the eyes, photophobia from fever, dry cough during measles.

FERRUM ARSENICUM

Complaints in general are aggravated in the morning, on waking; afternoon; evening; night, before midnight, after midnight. Aversion to the open air; aggravation in the open air. General physical anxiety. Chlorosis, Anæmia. Chorea in anæmic subjects. In a general way cold air aggravates, and the patient is very sensitive to cold; aggravation from becoming cold, in a cold room. Takes cold easily. In low vitality from malaria, and inherited phthisis, Epileptiforrn convulsions; tonic spasms. Blood vessels distended. Internal and external dropsy. Many complaints come on, or are worse after eating. Emaciation. She faints easily. Must select the most digestible foods. Butter disorders his whole system. Cold drinks aggravate, fat food aggravates, sour things aggravate, vinegar aggravates. Sensation of fulness. Subject to hemorrhages. Inflamed parts indurate. Inflammation of glands and organs. Increased physical irritability. Sensitive to jar. Jerking in muscles. Languid and must lie down. After hemorrhage or loss of fluids. Lying aggravates many symptoms. The longer he lies the more restless he becomes; must get up and walk about. Motion aggravates inflamed parts, but ameliorates the patient. Desires to move. Catarrhal conditions. Numbness of hands and feet, and painful parts. Surging of blood in the body and head. Aching in the bones. Drawing, pressing paralytic pains. Sore; bruised; stitching; tearing pains. Periodical complaints. Perspiration gives no relief of symptoms. Plethoric subjects. General pulsation, pulsation in parts, and pulsating pains. This is a deep acting antipsoric. Most complaints grow worse during rest. It is useful in malaria cases when much quinine has been taken. Relaxation of the whole muscular system, with a sensation of heaviness or weight in the whole body. Physical exertion or running aggravates, but moderate motion ameliorates. Sensitive to pain. Sitting still aggravates. On first sitting down, amelioration. Some complaints come on during sleep, or on waking. Standing still long aggravates. Much swelling of affected parts. Dropsical swelling. Swelling of glands. Trembling. Varicose veins. Walking long causes weakness. Walking slowly about ameliorates. Walking in the cold air aggravates. Walking fast aggravates. Great general weakness; evening; from malarial influences, or loss of fluids; paralytic weakness, from exertion or walking. Complaints worse in cold weather or winter. Complaints aggravated in cold wind.

Irascible from contradiction. Anxiety at night. Anxiety as if guilty of a crime, with fear, during fever. Mirthful. Concentration difficult. Confusion of mind in the morning on waking; in the evening. Conscientious about trifles. Thinks of death. Discontented. Distraction. Excitable. Fear of a crowd, of death, of some mischief, of people. Forgetful. Hysterical. Indifference. Irresolution. Irritability. Laughing and mirthfulness. Alternating moods, and change of mental symptoms. Obstinate. Quarrelsome. Religious affections of the mind; remorse. RESTLESSNESS at night, driving out of bed. Tossing about the bed, during heat. Extreme sadness, in the evening, when alone. Oversensitive to noise. Serious mood. Stupefaction of mind. Indisposed to talk. It disturbs him to hear people talk. He is sensitive to their voices. Tranquility. Unconscious. Weeping.

Vertigo; tendency to fall, during headache, looking downward, with nausea, on rising up. When walking he staggers, with obscuration of vision

Sensation of coldness of scalp. Hyperæmia of the brain. Tension of the scalp. Sensation of emptiness in the head. Fulness in the head. The hair falls out. Heat in the head, with cold feet. Flushes of heat in the head. Heaviness of the head, of the forehead. Itching of the scalp. Violent headache; morning, afternoon, evening; aggravated in cold air, ameliorated in open air. Catarrhal headaches. Pain in head during chill. Cold applications ameliorate. Headaches with coryza. Pain when coughing; after eating, HAMMERING HEADACHES. Headache before and during menses; motion of head. Paroxysmal pains. Periodical headaches. Pulsating pains. Riding in a carriage aggravates. Shaking the head aggravates. Sitting aggravates.

Pain in the forehead; worse right side; evening; above the eyes; occiput. Sides of head; right; temples; right side. Temple and forehead. Vertex. Boring in temples. Bursting. Drawing. Pressing outward. Pressing in the forehead;

temples. Vertex. Soreness. Stitching in temples. Tearing pains. Pulsating in head; forehead, occiput, temples, vertex. Shocks in the brain.

Lids stick together at night. Discharge of mucus from the eyes. Eyes lusterless. Inflammation of the eyes; scrofulous. Blood vessels injected. Lachrymation. Difficult to open lids. Pain in the eyes; aching; burning; as if sand. Paralysis of optic nerve. Protrusion of eyes. Redness of eyes; of lids. Looks sunken about the eyes. Eyes swollen; lids swollen. Sclerotics yellow. Dim vision.

Discharge from ear, offensive. Itching. Noises in ears; humming, ringing, roaring, singing. Pain in ear. Stitching. Hearing impaired.

Chronic catarrh. Coryza. Discharge bloody; crusts; excoriating; greenish; purulent; watery. Nosebleed. Sneezing.

Dark circles around eyes. Pale, sickly, earthly, waxy face. Greenish. Sickly, suffering expression. Lips pale. Red face during chill. Sallow; jaundiced. Dryness of lips. Heat of face. Flushes of heat. Hippocratic countenance. Pain face. Perspiration of face. Swelling of face.

Bleeding mouth and gums. White tongue. Dryness. Numbness of tongue. Burning tongue. Increased saliva. Gangrenous sore mouth. Swollen gums. Taste bitter, insipid, putrid. sweetish.

Constriction and choking in throat. Throat feels hot. Lump in throat. Pain in throat on swallowing. Burning, rawness, soreness. Swallowing difficult.

Anxiety in stomach. Appetite increased, or ravenous; yet he does not relish his food. Appetite wanting. Aversion to food; to meat. Constriction. Craves bread, sour things. Distended stomach. Eructations after eating; abortive, bitter, empty; of food; foul; sour. Waterbrash, fulness. Heart-burn. Heat. Nausea, before eating, after eating, during pregnancy. Pain, after cold drinks, after eating. Burning; cramping; pressing after eating. Soreness. Pulsating. Thirst extreme. Also thirstless in chronic troubles.

Vomiting, morning, night, after drinking, coughing, after eating; with headache; during fever; during pregnancy. Blood, FOOD SOUR.

Constriction of abdominal muscles. Distension of abdomen from flatus. Ascites. Flatulence. Fulness. Gurgling. Hardness of abdomen. Sensation of heat in abdomen. Weight in abdomen. Inflammation of bowels. Itching of skin of abdomen. Congestive, sluggish and swollen liver. Pain in abdomen at night, on coughing, after eating, during menses. Paroxysmal pains. Warmth ameliorates. Pain in hypochondria, in hypogastrium, in the liver, sides of abdomen. Cramping before stool, from flatus. Soreness; hypogastrium. Liver. Nervous uneasiness in abdomen. Rumbling. Spleen enlarged. Swollen liver and spleen. Tension of abdomen.

Constipation. Constriction. DIARRHŒA; morning, afternoon, NIGHT, AFTER MIDNIGHT; colliquitive; during dentition AFTER DRINKING. after cold water, after eating; aggravated by motion. Painless. Flatus. Hemorrhage from anus.

Hemorrhoids, external, large. Involuntary stool. Itching of anus. Moisture at the anus. Pain during stool. Burning during and after stool. Stitching. Tenesmus during stool. Paralysis of rectum. Prolapsus during stool. Urging to stool; ineffectual; after stool. Stool excoriating, bloody, brown, frequent, hard, UNDIGESTED, mucus, watery, brown, watery.

Pain in the bladder. Tenesmus. Constant urging. Involuntary urination at night.

Pain in the kidneys.

Burning in urethra during urination.

Urine albuminous, bloody, burning; cloudy on standing; dark, red, copious, scanty; mucous sediment.

Seminal emissions.

Inflammation of female genitals. Uterus. Itching genitals. Leucorrhœa, EXCORRIATING, thin, white. Amenorrhœa. Menses bright red, copious, dark, too soon, painful, pale, protracted, scanty, suppressed. Uterine hemorrhage. Pain in uterus. Burning in labia. Prolapsus uteri.

Catarrh of larynx and trachea. Mucus in larynx and trachea. Burning in air passages. Roughness in air passages. Hoarseness. Voice lost. Respiration arrested on coughing; asthmatic; difficult, evening, night, during cough; lying; rattling; short; suffocative. Subject to asthma after midnight.

Cough morning on rising, evening in bed, lying down, at night, before midnight; cold air, open air, walking in open air; asthmatic; deep breathing aggravates; after drinking. Dry cough in the evening. Cough after eating. Exhausting cough. Cough during fever; from irrtation in trachea. Loose cough; lying aggravates; cough in bed, motion aggravates; on rising; must sit up. Spasmodic cough. Talking aggravates the cough. Tickling cough. Tickling in larynx and trachea. Whooping cough.

Expectoration in daytime, morning, night; bloody, blood streaked, copious, difficult; greenish mucus; offensive, purulent; nausiosis; putrid, sweetish, thick, viscid, whitish, yellow.

Anxiety of chest in heart symptoms. Catarrh of chest. Constriction of chest; constriction of heart. Fulness of chest. HEMORRHAGE OF LUNGS. Heat in chest. Inflammation of lungs. Cardiac and anaemic murmurs. OPPRESSION OF CHEST in the evening. Pain in the chest, during cough; in sides of chest; sternum. Soreness in chest on coughing. Stitching on coughing. Palpitation at night with anxiety. Spasms of chest.

Coldness of back. Pain in the back at night, during menses, during stool. Pain in cervical region, between shoulders, in lumbar region. Aching in back. Bruised pain in lumbar region. Tearing in back. Pulsating in back. Stiff neck.

Cold extremities, hands and feet. Contraction of fingers and toes. Cramps in hands, thighs, calves, feet, soles. Blueness of finger nails. Heaviness of limbs, feet. Numbness of hands and fingers; legs, feet. Pain in limbs;

rheumatic; joints. Gouty pains. Pain in upper limbs, rheumatic, shoulders, elbow, wrist, hands. Pain in lower limbs. Sciatica, worse at night. Pain in thighs; paralytic; knee, ankle, foot, heel. Aching in limbs. Drawing in upper limbs; thighs. Sore pain in limbs, upper limbs. Stitching in limbs; shoulders; hip, thigh. Tearing in shoulders, upper arms; thighs. Paralytic weakness of limbs. Restlessness of all the limbs, especially of the legs. Stiffness of joints of upper limbs, hands and fingers; of lower limbs, knees and feet. Swelling of upper limbs, hands; of knees, ankles and feet. Varicose veins of lower limbs. Weakness of limbs, joints; knees, legs, ankles.

Dreams anxious. Sleep restless. Sleepiness afternoon and evening. Sleeplessness before midnight. Sleepless with sleepiness. Waking early.

This remedy has chill, fever and sweat. Chill in morning, noon, evening, NIGHT. Chill even in bed. Quotidian; tertian. Chill with trembling. The fever is intense, and follows chill; aggravated in afternoon, evening, and highest at night. Fever after midnight. Fever without chill in afternoon, evening, night. Fever intermingled with chill. Dry heat. Heat in flushes. The flushes rush upwards. Chronic intermittent fevers with enlarged spleen and liver. Internal heat and external coldness. Heat comes on after sleep. Perspiration day and night. Perspiration morning, night; during anxiety; in bed; CLAMMY, cold, on coughing, with great exhaustion, after eating, during slight exertion; long lasting; while lying; on motion; PROFUSE, morning. Perspiration during sleep, after sleep; offensive, sour, staining linen yellow; during stool. Symptoms aggravated while perspiring.

Burning of the skin. Coldness of the skin. Liver spots. Pale skin. Red spots. Yellow. Dryness of the skin. Sensitive skin. Sore feeling in skin. Swollen skin. Œdema. Ulcers burning. Withered warts.

FERRUM IODATUM

Morning, afternoon, *evening*, NIGHT, after midnight. The patient feels better in the open air. Anæmia in a marked degree. General physical anxiety; *chlorosis;* choreic twitching of the muscles; constantly taking cold; congestion of organs and glands; external and internal dropsy. Symptoms are worse after eating. Emaciation. Markedly worse from exertion. Fainting in anæmic patients. Hemorrhage from many parts. Induration of glands. Lack of physical irritability. Lying down and lying in bed increases many symp-toms. Sensation as of lying in a cramped position. Worse before, during and after menses. Motion increases many symptoms; desire to move. Catarrhal condition of all mucous membranes. Orgasm of blood even when quiet; pulsation in body and limbs; on waking from sleep; fast pulse. Many symptoms are worse from touch. The glands are swollen. Walking aggravates many symptoms. Worse from warmth and warm clothing. Weakness from slight exertion; during menses; from walking.

Very irritable and easily angered. Anxiety and aversion to company. Dullness of mind and concentration difficult worse when reading; confusion of mind in the evening; over-conscientious about small matters; very excitable; hysterical conduct and hilarity; changeable mood; indifference; irresolution; *sadness.* Restless at night; starting from sleep. Stupefaction. Weeping. Vertigo while walking.

Heat and hyperæmia of the head; heaviness of the head; worse in a warm room; better in the open air; in the forehead. Itching of the scalp. Pain in the head in the morning; in the afternoon; better in the open air and worse in the house; worse coughing; with coryza; worse from the pressure of the hat; compelled to lie down; better lying; before menses; worse moving the head; better from pressure of the hand; *pulsating;* worse when reading; worse from smoking; worse from walking; worse from writing; worse in a warm room. Pain in the forehead; worse on the right side in the evening; better in the open air; better when standing in a draft; worse from coughing, from pressure of the hat, when reading, when writing, from motion, in a warm room, from smoking, above the eyes; above the left eye extending to the top of head. Pain in the occiput; in the sides of head; worse on left side, in temples, in vertex. Cutting pain from bridge of the nose to the occiput. Pressing pain in forehead; worse in right side; worse in a warm room; in temples; in vertex. Sharp pain from below the eyes up through to vertex. Stitching pain in head; in temples. Tearing pain in head. Pulsation in head; forehead; temples.

Inflammation of the conjunctiva, with copious pus. when forcibly opened; conjunctiva bluish-red; itching of eyes; lachrymation Pain in eyes from light; aching, burning of lids; cutting, as from sand; stitching. Photophobia. Protrusion of eyes; exophthalmic goitre. Redness of eyes; bluish-red, of lids; *swollen lids.* Weak eyes. The eyes are jaundiced. A cloud of sparks before the eyes after breakfast.

Noises in the ears; humming, ringing, *roaring.* Cutting pain in ears. Hearing impaired.

Catarrh of the nose; morning; post-nasal discharge bloody, copious *crusts;* EXCORIATING, greenish, *purulent, thick, watery* yellow. Fluent coryza, worse in the morning, with copious mucus from larynx. Sensation of dryness in nose. Epistaxis on blowing nose; from coughing. Obstruction of nose; morning, night; better after blowing; cutting pain in root of nose extending to occiput. Sneezing at night. The nose is swollen; ulceration in nose.

The face is *pale, earthy,* even *chlorotic;* RED; circumscribed redness; sallow; sickly; YELLOW. Eczema and vesicles on the face; expression sickly. Countenance hippocratic; swollen, puffed, bloated face; swollen submaxillary glands.

Bleeding gums. Coated thick, yellow tongue. Dryness in the mouth and throat; burning tongue; salivation; taste bad in the morning; bitter, insipid, metallic, offensive, putrid, like peppermint, sour, sweetish. Pain in the teeth.

Scraping of mucus from throat and nose; viscid mucus. Food seems to push up to throat as though it had not been swallowed; reversed action of *œsophagus*. Burning and pressing in the throat. Tickling and scraping throat and larynx. Swollen cervical glands. Exophthalmic goitre.

The appetie is variable; diminished, *increased, insatiable,* ravenous wanting, without relish of food, easy satiety. Atonic condition of the stomach; aversion to food; to meat. Distension of stomach from gas. Eructations; bitter, after eating; empty, greasy, of food, rancid, sour, violent, waterbrash. Feels as though he had eaten too much, even after small meal. Flushes of heat in the stomach. Heartburn. Heaviness after eating. Loathing of food. Nausea after eating. Pain in stomach; after eating; burning; cramping, after eating; distress with nausea and headache; pressing after eating; soreness in pit of stomach with pinching in back behind stomach. *Pulsating* in stomach. Tension. Thirst in evening; strong thirst; extreme thirst. *Vomiting;* on coughing; after drinking; after eating; of blood; of food. A feeling as of a cord drawn, connecting anus and navel, with a cutting pain every time he straightens up from a bent position. Distension of abdomen after food or drink. Enlarged liver and spleen without fever. Flatulence. Fulness or "stuffed" feeling. Heat in abdomen. Pain in abdomen; after eating; during menses; in hypochondria; in inguinal region extending across hypogastrium; in liver; spleen; in umbilicus; cramping before stool; pricking in sides of abdomen, worse raising arms and worse walking. Stitching in hypochondria and in inguinal region when walking; soreness in inguinal region when walking. Rumbling in abdomen before stool. Abdomen feels like a rubber ball when pressed; swollen abdomen.

Constipation; no stool for a week, alternating with diarrhœa; difficult stool, ineffectual straining. Constriction of anus. DIARRHŒA; stool frequent; morning; after eating; bloody stool; mucus; watery. Flatus; external piles; itching of anus; sensation as though anus were compressed; as of worms in rectum; as though a screw were boring in anus; crawling in anus; pain in anus; burning after stool. Stitching during hard stool; tenesmus; urging after stool; stool bloody; brown, *hard* mucus, scanty, soft, watery.

Urination frequent, involuntary, with tenesmus. Pain in both kidneys but worse in left. Gonorrhœal discharge from urethra; with itching crawling. Burning on urination. Sensation as if drops of urine remained in fossa navicularis and could not be forced out. Urine albuminous and of low specific gravity. It has cured where sugar was found in the urine. Urine; dark, red, copious and pale, scanty, white. *Urine smells sweetish.*

Erections troublesome and painful at night; wanting. Relaxed scrotum. Seminal emissions. Sexual desire increased. In the female it has been used to prevent abortion. Itching and soreness of the swollen vulva. it has cured dropsy of the ovaries. *Leucorrhœa;* acrid, hot, copious, *like starch;* before and after menses; thin and watery; menses absent, copious, too frequent or late, painful, SUPPRESSED. Metrorrhagia. *Bearing down feeling in the pelvis; while sitting she feels something pushing up.* It is a most useful remedy in prolapsus and displacements of all kinds.

Irritation and much mucus in the larynx and trachea. Pain in the larynx; burning. Tickling in the air passage. Hoarseness and aphonia.

Respiration asthmatic; difficult at night and on motion; rattling, short, suffocative, wheezing.

Cough in the morning, afternoon, evening, asthmatic, *dry,* during fever, from irritation in larynx and trachea, loose, from motion, short, spasmodic, from talking, from tickling in the air passages. Expectoration in the morn-ing; bloody, *copious,* difficult, greenish, hawked, bloody mucus, offensive, purulent, tasting putrid, *viscid,* whitish, grayish-white, yellow.

Anxiety in chest and heart. Cancer of right breast was greatly benefited. Catarrh of chest. Congestion of chest and *heart.* Hemorrhage of lungs and air passages. Inflammation of bronchial tubes; of lungs. Cardiac murmurs. Oppression of chest. Pain in chest during cough; in sides of chest; in right side, from heart to axilla; stitching on coughing. *Palpitation at* NIGHT; *from least exertion; on motion;* on rising up; on turning in bed; during sleep.

Pain in the back during menses; in dorsal region; in lumbar region during menses; in sacrum; aching, as if broken, in lumbar region, at night; dull pain in dorsal region, each side of spine; extending through chest; stitching pain in back. Stiffness in back on rising from bed.

Cold hands and feet at night; cramps in feet. Heat of hands; heaviness of limbs; lower limbs; of feet. Numbness of fingers, legs, feet. Pain in the limbs; in the joints; gouty, rheumatic; rheumatic in upper limbs; rheumatic in right upper arm; in elbow, in *hip,* in thigh, in right tibia; rheumatic pain extending upward from back of left foot, in evening. Aching in the shoulder. Drawing pain in lower limbs; in the thighs; in tendons of back of right hand and left foot. Sore, bruised lower limbs, thighs, legs, stitching upper limbs and shoulder; tearing upper limbs and hips. Paralysis of upper limbs; sensation of paralysis of shoulder; in right arm in evening when writing. Restless feet. Dropsical swelling in lower limbs; legs and feet. Weakness of limbs, of lower limbs. Trembling and weakness in limbs on using hands and on walking.

Dreams anxious; confused; of dead people; of fighting; of previous events; fantastic; of robbers; nightmare; unpleasant; *vivid.* Dreams that he is from

thirty to sixty feet tall. Restless sleep. Sleepiness morning and evening
Sleeplessness; frequent waking.

Chill at *night;* coldness in and better rising from bed; chilliness in eve
ning followed by heat and sweat; shaking chill; warm room does not ame
liorate the chill. Fever in the afternoon and evening with chilliness. Dry heat
Flushes of heat; internal heat, with chill. Intermittent fever with desire t
uncover.

Perspiration in the morning; in afternoon at *night;* in bed; *clammy, cola
copious,* on least EXERTION, worse on motion.

The skin burns or is cold; jaundiced; liver spots. Dry skin. Urticaria
Swollen skin.

FERRUM METALLICUM

We will take up the study of Ferrum metallicum. The Old School has bee
giving Iron for anæmia throughout all tradition. They have given it in grea
quantities, in the form of the tincture of chloride, and the carbonate. Wheneve
the patient became anæmic, pallid, waxy and weak, Iron was the tonic. It i
true that Iron produces anaemia, and it would be astonishing to any one wh
ever read the provings of Ferrum if the allopaths did not create additiona
bloodlessness with the doses of Iron they administer. It is true that under th
provings, and under those circumstances where Iron has been given in exces
the patient becomes greenish, waxy, yellow and pallid, with a sickly an
anæmic countenance. The lips become pale; the ears lose their pink colo
the skin of the body becomes waxy, and there comes a tendency t
hæmorrhage, at times with clots, but commonly with copious, thin, liqui
blood, very dark. The clots will separate and the fluid parts look brown, dir
and watery. The patient gradually emaciates. He is pallid and waxy; his muscl
become flabby and relaxed; he is incapable of endurance. All the muscul
fibres become tired from any exertion. Rapid exercise, or any unusual exertio
is impossible. Any rapid exertion or motion brings on weakness, dyspnœ
sinking and fainting.

A strange thing running through all the constitutional conditions
Ferrum is that the *pains and sufferings come on during rest.* The palpitatic
sometimes comes on during rest, the dyspnœa comes on during rest, an
even the weakness. The patient is ameliorated by moving gently about, b
any *exertion* tires and causes faintness. Any *rapid* motion aggravates t
complaints. The pains are ameliorated by moving about the house so that t
exertion does not excite or fatigue. In many cases the patient is dropsic
The skin pits upon pressure and is pale, yet the face shows an appearance

ple⌐¹ ora. From every little excitement the face becomes flushed. During the chill the face becomes red. From taking wine or stimulant the face becomes flushed, and the patient, though flabby, relaxed and tired, does not get credit for being sick. She fails to get the sympathy of her friends. She is feeble, she suffers from palpitation and dyspnœa, she has great weakness with inability to do anything like work, she feels that she must lie down—yet the face is flushed. This is called a pseudo-plethora. The blood-vessels are distended, the veins varicose, and their coatings relaxed. On this account bleeding takes place easily; capillary oozing; hæmorrhage from all parts of the body; haemorrhage from the nose, the lungs, the uterus. Women suffer much from hæmorrhage from the uterus, especially during and after the climacteric period. Ferrum will be found of great value—when the symptoms agree—in that wonderful anæmic state called "green sickness," that comes on with girls at the time of puberty and in the years that follow it. There will be almost no menstrual flow, but a cough will develop, with great pallor. So common is this sickness among girls that all mothers are acquainted with and dread it. In a large practice you will have a number of cases of chlorosis.

Sometimes the early menstrual period is attended with a copious flow, and then a great weakness occurs, and this goes on for a number of years before anything like menstrual regularity is established. In these cases the Old School always used to feed their patients Iron in great quantities, but the more Iron the patient took the worse she grew.

Congestion, tending upwards, with red face, hot head and coldness of the extremities. But the heat of the head and face is not at all in proportion to the red appearance. It will be found that this congestion upward in Ferrum will take place during a chill, in septic fevers or in other forms of fever, and the head is not always hot, but sometimes cool. The face may be red and cool.

Another grand feature of Ferrum is that, like *China,* it has complaints from loss of animal fluids; from prolonged hæmorrhage, with weakness remaining a long time. There is no repair no assimilation. The bones are soft and easily bent; they take on crooks. Emaciated and feeble children. Dryness of the joints, causing cracking on motion. Sudden emaciation, with false plethora.

Redness of face—a healthy looking bloom—in one who is unable to walk fast on the street, or to stand any exertion. Yet some of the complaints of Ferrum are better from occupation, from doing something, from taking a little exercise, because the complaints come on during rest. Over excitability and sensitivity of the nerves; over-sensitiveness to pain. The sensitive woman who needs Ferrum has a flushed face and is often complaining because she gets no sympathy. She does not look sick, yet she puffs on going up stairs; she feels weak and wants to lie down.

Restless when keeping still; must keep the limbs moving. Rending pains in the limbs; dull aching in the limbs. These pass off when moving about quietly and gently, like *Pulsatilla.* But Ferrum is a very cold remedy, and is ameliorated by warmth, except the pains about the neck, face and teeth, which are ameliorated by cold. But most of the pains are ameliorated by heat; the patient wants to keep warm and dreads anything like fresh air or a draught.

Weakness and prostration; weakness even from talking. Prostration with irregular pulse and rapid pulse, or with too slow pulse; palpitation. And then comes paralytic weakness; the limbs give out. Paralytic conditions from anæmia or hæmorrhage. Fainting spells from hæmorrhage. Jerking and twitching of the muscles; chorea; catalepsy. ,

You may easily imagine something of the character of the mental symptoms, for they are like the physical. The mind is confused and the patient tearful. Depression of spirits; mental weariness and depression. The highest degree of depression and despondency. Anxiety from the slightest cause; irritability. The least noise, like the crackling of paper, sets the patient wild. It brings on nervous excitement and restlessness; she must get up and move. Excitement from the slightest opposition. Any sudden or rapid motion, or the least hurry, causes blackness before the eyes; dizziness; things turn in a circle; she must sit down. And with all this the face is red When alone and at rest, the face becomes pale and cold, but the least excitement brings a flush to the cheeks.

The headaches are congestive in character, with mounting of blood upwards. There is a sense of fulness and distension, with red face. Fulness and distension of the eyes; fulness of the neck. Palpitation of the heart. Exophthalmic goitre. The headaches are ameliorated by pressure. Ferrum wants to be pressed to support the veins. Throbbing like hammers in the head. Every quick motion aggravates the headache. Coughing aggravates the headache; pain in the head and *occiput from coughing.* These pains are sometimes ameliorated by walking gently. Going up stairs, sitting down, rising from a seat—unless it is done very deliberately—will arouse all the pains of Ferrum. Any sudden motion will bring on hammering and a feeling of great expansion in the head. And then will come more or less shooting, tearing pains. Beating in the back of the head from rising or from coughing, because coughing is a sudden motion. Confusion of mind with hammering headache. Rush of blood to the head. Congestive headaches from excitement; from taking cold; from exposure; lasting three or four days or a week. The face is flushed and perhaps cold, the head somewhat hot, but not as hot as would be expected.

Redness of the eye; engorged vessels. Great weakness, dyspnœa and palpitation. Writing—a mental operation—causes the headache to reappear.

Great sensitiveness of the scalp. The patient must let the hair hang down. Mental disorders and headaches accompanying or following hæmorrhages, and in lying-in women. Bloated appearance about the eyes. All sorts of disturbance of vision from congestion. Venous stasis; swelling of the eyelids; pus-like discharge. Over-sensitiveness to sound; ringing in the ears.

The symptoms of the nose are numerous. Colds and catarrhal troubles, ending in nosebleed. Nosebleed on slight provocation, with headaches at the menstrual nisus. Scabs form in the nose. Extreme paleness of the face; face becomes red and flushed on the least emotion. Flushed face with dropsy of the lower limbs; flushed face with chill. Thirst during the chill is a striking feature of Ferrum. During the menstrual period there are violent pains, and as soon as the pain starts the face becomes flushed.

Nothing taken into the stomach digests, and yet there is no special nausea. It is the exception to find nausea in Ferrum. Food goes into the stomach and is vomited without nausea—simply emptied out. Sometimes there are eructations of food by the mouthful, like *Phosphorus*. *Phosphorus* was the remedy with all the old masters for spitting up of food by the mouthful until the stomach was empty. Canine hunger. It says in the text: "Double the amount of an ordinary meal in the evening was hardly sufficient." All food tastes bitter; solid food is dry and insipid. After eating there are eructations. Heat in the stomach; *regurgitation of food.* Spasmodic pressure in the stomach after the least food or drink, especially after meat. Aversion to meat, to eggs, to sour fruit. Aversion to milk, and to his accustomed tobacco and beer. Sweet wines agree, but sour wines and all sour things disagree. The tongue feels as if burnt. As soon as the stomach is empty vomiting ceases until he eats again. Vomiting of food, immediately after midnight. Vomitus tastes sour.

Ferrum is occasionally indicated during pregnancy. A few weeks after becoming pregnant the woman commences to throw up her food by the mouthful. There is no nausea, but the face is flushed and the woman is flabby and weak. She vomits without becoming sick. Fulness and pressure in the stomach; pressure in the stomach after eating. Ferrum is an unusually interesting remedy because of this peculiar stomach. It is like a leather bag; it will not digest anything. Fill it up and it empties itself just as easily as it was filled.

Ferrum has a troublesome diarrhœa, with acrid watery excoriating stool. Morning diarrhœa. Many of these patients are old sinners with broken-down constitutions, who have suffered long from constipation. Chronic constipation with ineffectual urging and hard, difficult stools.

Relaxation runs through the remedy. From this relaxation there is prolapsus of the rectum, vagina and uterus. Dragging down in the lower part of the body as if the organs would come out—and sometimes they do come out.

The bladder is also relaxed. Its sphincter is weak, and there is no regularity of its muscular action. Hence, we have involuntary urination from sudden motion, from walking, or from coughing. In little children the urine dribbles all day. Just as long as the child plays the urine dribbles and keeps the clothing wet, but this is better while keeping perfectly quiet. The bladder is so relaxed and tired that it cannot hold the urine, and as soon as it is partially filled it allows its contents to escape. This relaxation runs through the remedy and gives it character, just like a human being. You know what each one of your friends is likely to do on every occasion. So it is with a remedy. You ought to know what it is most likely to do, in order to know what it will accomplish in curing the sick.

Weakness and relaxation of the genital organs is common to Ferrum. The menstrual flow comes in for its share. Copious, watery flow; hæmorrhage or suppression—amenorrhœa—no flow at all, only a leucorrhœa. Suppression of the menses with great nervous excitement; with flushed face; with weakness and palpitation. Prolapsus of the vagina. Insensibility of the vagina during coition. Metrorrhagia. Menses too soon, too profuse and lasting too long.

Difficult respiration; pains and disturbances in the chest. Difficult breathing, with a sense of a great load on the chest. Suffocating fits at night; catarrhal conditions of the respiratory tract; congestion of the chest; dyspnœa. Spasmodic cough, such as we find in whooping-cough, coming on in violent paroxysms. Cough after every meal, with gagging, emptying the stomach of its contents. Cough felt in the head. Cough worse from the abuse of brandy, tobacco or tea. Cough coming on after the loss of fluids, as after hæmorrhages. Chest troubles following uterine hæmorrhage, and after other hæmorrhages. Coughing up blood; bleeding from the lungs, Persons deblitated by secret vices, with a tendency to go into tuberculosis.

Palpitation of the heart from fear, excitement, or exertion. Rapid action of the heart, or sometimes slow action. Fatty degeneration of the heart. Pulse accelerated *toward evening*. Pulsations throughout the body, feeling like little hammers.

Rheumatic pains in the extremities, ameliorated by heat and by gentle motion; aggravated by cold, by exertion, or by rapid motion. Pains through the deltoid muscles are spoken of more prominently than pains in other parts, but these pains are no more striking than the pains anywhere in Ferrum. Tearing pains through the limbs. *Inability to raise the arm;* paralytic pains— that is, pains that are benumbing. Pains that make him feel as if he were going to lose the power to move the part. Violent pains in the hip-joint are just as common as the pains in the shoulder. Lippe says, "Rheumatism in the left shoulder," but it is just as common in the right. *Rheumatic pains in the deltoid muscle of either side.* Violent pain in the muscles and along the nerves. Pinching in the right deltoid; boring in the right shoulder; aggravated by motion and by the weight of the bed-clothes; ameliorated by heat. Tearing and stinging pains. The Ferrum pains come on in the night, because the patient attempts to keep still in bed. *Rest brings on the Ferrum pains.* When moving gently about in the daytime he will not have so much pain. Coldness of the limbs; and again, heat of the soles and palms—they change about. With all this weakness and prostration dropsical conditions come on, so that the feet and hands become bloated.

Evening chill or chilliness with fever, cold hands and feet and red face. Icy cold feet with the chill. Chill ameliorated after eating. Thirst with the chill. Copious sweat which stains yellow. All symptoms worse while sweating. Strong-smelling night sweats. All the febrile symptoms are better by slowly moving about. In intermittent fever after the abuse of quinine.

We read in the text that Ferrum is a remedy for diarrhœa in the last stages of consumption. Well, sometimes it is—if the patient is prepared to die. Ferrum will stop the diarrhœa, but after it is stopped the patient will not live long. The diarrhœa is not usually painful. It is annoying, but it is painless, and the night sweats are painless. Do not suppress them; they had better be let alone. Let the patient go on to a peaceful termination. The best remedy for diarrhœa in the last stages of consumption is *Saccharum lactis* in the crude form, given in very small quantities and repeated as often as is required by the patient and the bystanders.

FERRUM PHOSPHORICUM

Great weakness, and desire to lie down. Nervous at night. Rheumatic conditions. While it has been used by Schüessler's followers for the first stage of inflammatory fevers, it is useful in the higher potencies in chronic diseases, and is a deep acting anti-psoric. It could not be less than the Ferrum and Phosphoric acid that form it. For many years I followed the Schüessler indications, but by the aid of new provings, homœopathic aggravations, and clinical experience the present arrangement of symptoms furnishes my guide for this valuable homœopathic remedy.

The time of aggravation of some complaints is in the morning, some in afternoon; others come in the evening and night, and after midnight. The patient is sensitive to the open air, and many symptoms are aggravated in open air. The most noticeable feature are anæmia and chlorosis (*like Ferrum*). The general physical anxiety is more like *Phos. acid.* Lack of vital heat, and aggravation in cold air and from becoming cold. Always taking cold. Congestion of head and organs; with fever and red face. The general weakness is like the low vitality of the phthisical inheritance. Dropsical conditions. Symptoms worse after eating, from physical exertion. Fainting spells. Cold drinks bring on symptoms. Sour food aggravates. Vascular fulness and distension of veins. The hæmorrhagic condition is a strong feature, as it is in *Ferrum, Phos. acid* and *Phos.* The nervousness of hysteria and hypochondriasis is found in this remedy. Soreness through the body, especially in congested parts; with aggravation from jar and walking. Complaints from lifting and straining muscles, and from sprains. Many symptoms are worse lying in bed and from rest, and ameliorated by moving slowly about (*like Ferrum*), but the great lassitude compels him to lie down. Motion that is a real exertion aggravates, but slow motion ameliorates. Numbness of parts and suffering parts. Surging of blood in body and head. Stitching, tearing pains. Tearing downwards. False plethora. Strong pulsation over body, and in head. Strong, full, frequent pulse. Generally oversensitive, and sensitive to pain. Standing aggravates many complaints. Trembling limbs. All combine to give us a remedy broad and deep acting.

This remedy has marked anger, even to violence; producing weakness, headache, trembling, sweat, and other nervous manifestations. Anxiety at night, as if he had done a great wrong to somebody; after eating; with apprehensiveness; during fever; about the future; hypochondriacal. Cheerful, talkative and hilarious; unnatural excitement, mingled with sadness. This remedy has been used in delirium tremens. Aversion to company and feels better when alone. He is unable to concentrate the mind, or reflect ordinary questions; cannot study. Confusion of mind when trying to think, in the morning, in the evening, after eating; ameliorated by washing the face in cold water. He is dissatisfied with everything he possesses, and with his surroundings. Very excitable in the evening. The fulness in his head makes him fear apoplexy. Fear of going into a crowd, or death, that some evil will come to him, of misfortune, of people. Forgetful. It is an excellent remedy for hysterical girls, when other symptoms agree.

His ideas are abundant, and there is unusual clearness of mind (*Coff.*). Again, extreme indifference to all pleasure and exciting events. Aversion to work. It might well be thought of for puerperal mania from the note, "Sows eat up their young." It has plenty of cerebral hyperæmia, then why not madness? Irritability. Alternating moods. Morose. Obstinate. Restlessness at night in bed, tossing about much during fever. Sadness in the evening before menses. Extremely sensitive to noise. Stupefaction. Indisposed to talk. Aversion to thinking. Weeping. Aversion to mental work.

Vertigo in afternoon from hyperæmia of brain, during chill, on closing the eyes; tendency to fall forwards; during headache; as if intoxicated; looking downwards; during menses; with nausea; on rising up; on rising from bed. Staggering when walking, with vanishing of sight. Sensation as if the head were pushed forward while walking.

The head feels cold and the vertex is sensitive to cold air. Hyperæmia of ʌe brain. Constriction of the scalp. Empty sensation in the head; during ᴉenses. Sensation of fulness in the head. The hair falls out. The heat feels ery hot. Flushes of heat, and red face. Heat in head; in vertex; during menses. ʾhe head feels heavy during menses. Weight in forehead and occiput. Itching f the scalp. Headache, in morning in bed, in afternoon, in evening. Cold air ᴉmeliorates the general headaches; ascending steps aggravates; blinding eadache; catarrhal headaches. Headache during chill, aggravated on closing ʌe eyes; cold applications ameliorate; with coryza; aggravated on coughing, fter eating, excitement. Headache during menses, worse from light and noise. ᴉammering headaches. Headache aggravated from a jar. He is compelled to e down. Lying ameliorates. Headache during menses; on motion, and on ᴉoving the head; noise. Paroxysmal pains. Pressure ameliorates. Pulsating ains. Riding in a carriage aggravates. Sitting. Stooping; walking. Wrapping p the head brings on or aggravates the headache. Pulsating in head and ᴉmples, worse on right side. Headache with hot, red face and vomiting food. evere frontal headache with epistaxis, which ameliorates. Predominance of ᴉffering on right side of forehead, aggravated in the morning on waking, vening; ameliorated in open air; aggravated on coughing. Pain above the yes. Pain in the occiput, on coughing, jarring; during menses. Pain in sides f head and temples, in vertex. Pain in vertex during profuse menses. Boring ain in temples. Bursting pain in head. Pressing pain in whole head, pressing ᴉtward, forehead, in frontal eminence, temples; vertex like a stone. Soreness f the scalp, of occiput, vertex. Stitching pains in head, in forehead, over yes, occiput extending to forehead, on stooping; sides of head, temples, ᴉrtex. Tearing pains in head. General pulsation in head, aggravated by motion, ᴉd stooping; strong in forehead; in occiput on coughing, in temples; in ᴉrtex. Shocks in the head.

Discharge of mucus from the eyes. Conjunctivitis with photophobia. ᴉannot see on stooping. Blood vessels enlarged. Lachrymation. Half open ᴉds. Pain in eyes; aching, burning; sand. Stitching. Sensation of protrusion. ᴉedness of conjunctiva, of balls and lids. Sunken eyes. Swollen lids. Sclero-ᴉs jaundiced. Vanishing of sight as from fainting.

Purulent discharge from the ear. Itching in ear. Noises in the ear; roaring, ᴉzzing, humming, ringing and singing. Catarrh of Eustachian tubes. ᴉflammatory pains in the ear. Otitis media. Pain deep in the ear. Drawing. ᴉitching. Pain and swelling of the parotid gland. Sensitive to noise. Impaired ᴉaring.

Catarrh of nose. Coryza; discharge bloody. Crusts form in the nose. ᴉscharge excoriating, purulent. When this remedy has been given on the ᴉochemical theory in the low potencies its use has been limited to the acute

stage of coryza, but when used homœopathically this limitation does no
hold good. Who would think of limiting *Ferrum* or *Phos. acid* or *Phos.* to the
acute or first stage of an acute disease?

Epistaxis with coryza, during fever, or headache when the head is hot and
full. Epistaxis in the morning, on blowing the nose, with cough. Sneezing.

Chlorotic face. Dark circles under the eyes. Earthy, pale, sallow face. Pale
lips. Red face alternating with paleness. Circumscribed redness of cheek
Red during fever; during headache. Yellow. Liver spots. Dryness of lip
Heat of face; flushes; while sitting; with toothache; with pains. Hippocrat
face. Inflammation of the parotid. Pain in face, from inflammation of teeth
neuralgia, ameliorated by cold applications, aggravated by motion. Pulsatir
pains. Stitching. Perspiration of face. Sunken face. Swelling œdematous, fro
toothache. Swollen parotids.

Bleeding from mouth and gums. Tongue dark red and swollen. Tongu
white. Dry mouth. Inflammation of gums, fauces, tongue and tonsils. Pains
teeth, with red, hot, swollen gums; ameliorated by holding cold water in th
mouth, and aggravated by warm things. Pains in the teeth after eating. Burnir
of the tongue. Salivation. Taste insipid, putrid, sweetish.

Constriction of throat. Redness in throat and tonsils. Swollen tonsil
Heat in throat. Inflammation of throat and tonsils. Lumps in throat. Pain o
swallowing. Burning. Soreness.

Appetite diminished. Ravenous appetite without relish of food. Appeti
entirely gone. Aversion to food, meat, milk. Desires sour things. Distensio
of stomach after eating. Eructations, after eating, bitter, empty, of food, fou
sour. Water-brash. Fulness after eating. Heat in stomach. Hiccoug
Indigestion. Inflammation of stomach. Nausea after eating, during pregnanc
Sudden attacks of nausea, coming at any moment; sometimes waking her o
of sleep, lasting a short time. Nausea felt in the throat. Nausea while walkir
Pain in the stomach after eating. Burning in the stomach. Cramping. Pressi
after eating. Soreness. Great thirst for much water. Vomiting, morning,
rising, on coughing, after drinking, after eating, during fever, during headacl
during pregnancy, riding in a carriage. Violent vomiting; blood, food, gree
sour. Vomiting with inflammation and pain in the stomach.

The abdomen is distended, and the liver and spleen are enlarged. Mu
flatulence, fulness and rumbling, gurgling. The abdomen is hard. Weight
the abdomen. Inflammation of the peritoneum. This remedy is curative
many complaints of the liver. Severe pain in the bowels, in the mornir
evening, night; on coughing; during diarrhœa; after eating; during mens
as if menses would come on; paroxysmal, before stool, when walking. Pain
hypochondria, in liver. Cramping, colicky pains. Dragging; pressing. So
bruised pains. Tension.

Constipation; difficult stool. Constriction of anus. Diarrhœa, in morning, afternoon, night, after midnight; after eating; painless. Flatus. Hæmorrhage from anus, from piles. Hæmorrhoids, external. Involuntary stools. Itching of anus. Moisture about the anus. Pain in rectum during stool; with dysentery, and fever. Burning during stool, after stool. Tenesmus. Pain in rectum from inflammation, constant, aggravation by pressure on stomach. Prolapsus of anus, during stool. Ineffectual urging to stool. Stool is excoriating, bloody, brown, frequent, hard, lienteric, slimy, green mucus, thin watery, green watery.

Hæmorrhage from the bladder or urethra. Inflammation of the bladder with fever. Pain in the bladder and neck of the bladder. Tenesmus. Urging; constant; frequent; with pain in neck of bladder and end of penis, must urinate immediately, which ameliorates the pain; aggravated standing; only in the daytime. Sudden urging. Must hasten or urine will escape. Frequent urination. Involuntary urination in the daytime, ameliorated lying down; at night in sleep; on coughing; while walking. Pain in the kidneys with fever.

Gleety discharge from the urethra. Gonorrhœa with heat in urethra in inflammatory stage; scanty, watery or mucous discharge. Hæmorrhage from urethra. Burning in urethra during flow of urine.

Urine albuminous, bloody, burning, cloudy on standing, dark, red, copious with headache; ammoniacal, scanty; much sediment, mucus, much uric acid; high specific gravity.

Troublesome nightly erections and seminal emissions. Erections feeble, or entirely wanting. Sexual passion increased, or entirely absent. In the woman here is slight change of symptoms; predisposition to abort, aversion to coition, or desire much diminished. Leucorrhœa, excoriating, before menses, milky, thin, white. Chlorotic girls, Menses absent. Menstrual flow bright red, clotted, copious, dark, too frequent, intermittent, irregular, late, painful, pale, protracted, scanty, suppressed, thin, watery. Uterine hæmorrhage. Pain in vagina during coition. Dysmenorrhœa with fever and red face. Bearing-down in pelvis with dull pain in ovarian region. Prolapsus of the uterus. Sterility. Sensitive vagina.

Acute catarrh of air passages. Inflammation of the larynx, with mucus, raw feeling and rattling in chest, fever, red face. Mucus in larynx and trachea. Dryness in larynx. Burning in larynx. Roughness in larynx. Hoarseness during coryza. Voice lost, weak.

Respiration asthmatic. Spasmodic asthma. Dyspnœa, evening, night, with cough, while lying. Rattling. Short. Suffocative respiration. Stitching in chest in deep inspiration.

Cough, daytime, morning on rising, evening, night; cold air aggravates; asthmatic; acute. Short, spasmodic and very painful cough. Deep breathing aggravates. Constant cough, with coryza. Dry cough. Cough after eating;

exhausting; with fever. Hacking cough. Cough from irritation in larynx and trachea. Loose cough. Lying aggravates cough. Cough in bed. Paroxysmal cough. Rattling cough. Spasmodic. Talking aggravates. Tickling. Tormenting cough, aggravated on walking. Whooping-cough. Touching larynx on bending head over. Increased cough from taking cold in phthisis.

Expectoration in daytime, morning, bloody, bright red, dark, copious difficult, frothy, greenish, mucus, offensive, purulent, scanty, putrid, thick viscid, whitish, yellow.

Anxiety in chest and region of the heart. Catarrh of the chest. Congestion of the chest. Constriction of chest and heart. Sensation of fulness. Hæmorrhage of lungs. Heat. Inflammation of bronchial tubes, lungs and pleura; oppression of chest. Pain in chest during cough, during inspiration; in sides of chest during deep inspiration. Soreness in chest on coughing. Stitching in chest, in sides of chest, on coughing. Right-sided pleuritis. Stitches, aggravated coughing and breathing. Palpitation at night with anxiety, on exertion and motion, while sitting, walking rapidly. This is a valuable temporary remedy in the acute colds during the course of phthisis. In acute phthisis. Spasms of the chest with suffocation, fever and red face. Rheumatism in the upper thorax.

Coldness in back. "Crick" in the neck or back. Pain in the back at night during menses, on motion, rising from a seat, while sitting, while walking cervical region, between shoulders, lumbar region during menses. Aching Stitching pains in back. Tearing. Stiffness in back of neck.

Cold extremities. Cold hands and feet. Cold feet evening in bed. Cold feet during headache. Contraction of fingers, result of rheumatism. Cramps in thighs legs, calves, feet. Blueness of finger nails. Hot hands, palms; soles. Heaviness of the limbs, upper limbs; legs. Inflammation of joints. Numbness of hand and fingers, legs and feet. Rheumatic pain in right shoulder and upper arm, of a drawing, tearing character, aggravated by violent motion of arm, ameliorated by gentle motion (*Ferr.*), part sensitive to touch. Deadness of the right hand could not lift with the hand. Acute rheumatism of right shoulder joint, red swollen and sore. Rheumatism of right deltoid. Rheumatism of Wrist Rheumatism of knee joint with fever. Gouty affection of joints. Sciatica. Pain in thighs. Sore bruised pain in limbs. Stitching pains in limbs, upper limbs shoulders; hips. Tearing pain in shoulders, upper arms, hips. Shooting pain in both knees, extending down legs, with fever. Restless legs. Stiffness of lower limbs, of feet. Swollen joints, upper limbs, forearm, hands; feet. Dropsical and rheumatic swelling. Great weakness of limbs, of joints, knees, legs. The rheumatism goes from joint to joint, aggravated by the slightest motion.

There are many dreams, anxious, confused, of falling, nightmare, vivid Late falling-asleep. Restless sleep. Sleepiness in the evening. Sleepless before midnight, with sleepiness. After once waking up he is sleepless.

Chill afternoons; 1 P.M. daily. Chill A night in bed. Chilliness. Shaking chill. The fever predominates. Fever at any time with inflammation of organs, joints, or mucous membranes. Fever without chill. Dry heat with thirst. Flushes of heat. Hectic fever and night sweats. Internal heat. Remittent fever. Heat after sleep. Perspiration in daytime, morning; clammy; with great weakness, on slight exertion, following the fever; copious; during sleep.

Burning skin. Coldness. Desquamation. Pale, red skin. Dry skin. Formication. Great sensitiveness of the skin. Skin feels sore. Ulceration. Small withered warts.

FLUORIC ACID

It takes a long time for this remedy, in the proving, to develop its symptoms. It is a very deep-acting medicine, and an antipsoric, anti-syphilitic and anti-sycotic. It is insidious in its action and its symptoms are slow in approach; it is like the deepest and slowest and most tedious diseases, the miasms, and hence it is suitable in the very slowest and lowest forms of disease. While it has in its nature some febrile action, it is not for this purpose that it is oftenest called for; its most typical febrile action is very slow and insidious. It corresponds to overheated states of the system, old cases of nightly fevers, coming on week after week and year after year.

It is an unusually hot-blooded remedy at times, and again it has conditions of coldness. In the evening and night great heat seems to evolve from the body without increase of temperature. The skin becomes very hot. That patient is often < from warm things, < from covering, < from warm air; suffocates somewhat like *Puls.* in a warm room. He wants to bathe the face and head in cold water; such bathing is grateful. The feet burn and are put out of bed in the night; he hunts around in bed for a cool place for the feet and hands. The soles perspire, and the palms perspire, and the sweat is acrid, making the parts sore; excoriation from the sweat between the toes. The perspiration is offensive; offensive, acrid sweat between the toes. Burning, unusual heat and acridity are words that modify a great many symptoms; an acrid lachrymation or other discharge from the eye; acrid discharge from the nose, acrid sweat, etc. Sensation of burning and burning pains in parts; heat evolved from the body as a chronic state. Aggravation from heat, from outward heat and from inward heat, belongs to this remedy. It is a strong feature of this remedy to be worse from drinking tea and coffee. Warm drinks bring on diarrhœa, or flatulence, or disturbance in the stomach, and cause indigestion to manifest itself in various ways. The symptoms are worse standing and sitting and better in the open air.

It is a remedy of great depth of action. It so disturbs the functions that there are peculiar outward signs in the nails, in the hair, in the skin; they are all imperfectly developed. Whenever such is the case, we know that a remedy has great depth of action and that it is very long acting. It forms little incrustations here and there upon the skin that seem to have no tendency to heal. A crust forms, but there seems to be no healing beneath the crust. The hair loses its lustre; it falls out, and if examined closely under the microscope it is seen to be necrosed; little ragged ulcers will be found along the course of the hair. The ends of the hair are dry, the hair mats and splits and breaks, becomes ragged in masses and lustreless. The nails are crippled, likewise corrugations in the nails; the nails grow too fast and grow awkwardly; that is, they are deformed and crippled, too thick in some places, and too thin in others; break easily, brittle. There is a tendency to breaking down of a slow character, where the circulation is very feeble, and the skin is near bone or cartilage, as in the cartilages in the ears, and in the cartilages of joints. Ulcers develop over the tibia. There is feeble circulation in the hands and feet, and they become cold. In the evening the extremities burn and are feverish, because that is the time of the feverish state; but in the morning and in the daytime there is coldness of the extremities. The patient is pallid and sickly, and at times becomes waxy and dropsical; œdema of the extremities, and particularly of the lower extremities; œdema of certain parts; œdema of the prepuce. When a debilitated subject, one suffering from bone and cartilaginous troubles contracts gonorrhœa, with it he will have enormous swelling of the prepuce and nothing seems to act upon it. Fluoric acid will cure œdema of the prepuce with gonorrhœa in such a subject. *Cannabis sativa* has the same symptom but it is especially useful in robust cases. Fluoric acid will prevent the manifestation of disease in sycotic subjects, will prevent formation of fig warts. It cures fig-warts. It produces hardened, dry warts, and dry crust upon the skin, and crusts not unlike rupia. It is useful in syphilitic rupia.

Bone affections stand out prominently. Necrosis, especially of the long bones, but also of the bones of the ear. It creates an offensive acrid discharge from the ear. It establishes an offensive ozæna, an acrid discharge with necrosis of the nasal bones. It is very analogous to *Sil.*, and it is one of the natural followers of *Sil.* where *Sil.* has been too frequently repeated by persons who do not know that *Silicea* does its best in a single dose and that it is a long acting and slow medicine. It not only antidotes the abuse of *Sil.* but also follows *Sil.* After practicing a while you will be surprised to observe the pendulum-like action between heat and cold in various complementary remedies. To make that clear I will illustrate it by using the series in which this remedy is set and to which it naturally belongs. You take a patient who is hot-blooded, who is always suffering from the heat, from too much clothing and too warm a room especially in the evenings, a patient that is tearful and sad, and may be a blonde. Why you say, I am trying to describe a *Pulsatilla* patient. Well, yes; anyone can see that. *Puls* is a hot-blooded patient, but after using that remedy a while you notice that the patient goes to the other extreme and becomes chilly, and wants much clothing; the heat is taken out of the case. *Sil.* is the natural follower of *Puls.*, and you would be astonished to know how often a patient leaving *Puls.* runs toward *Sil. Sil.* goes deeper into the case, it does more curing, and it is the natural chronic of *Puls.* Other remedies of course follow *Puls.*, but *Sil.* more frequently than any other medicine. Now, that is the second step; the patient has gone from a warm to a cool state; the overheated state has been lost and he has gone into *Sil..* but when S*il.* has been administered for a while it cures the cold state, and removes the chilliness of the patient (remember, however, that *Sil.* has at times something of *Puls.* in it; in some of its complaints it is < from being over-heated) and the patient under *Sil.* goes back to the warm state again, becomes hot-blooded, wants the warm covers thrown off, wants to be lightly covered. Then it is that this medicine comes in the series. Fluor. ac. follows *Sil.* as naturally as *Sil.* follows *Puls.* They exist in threes. There arc other remedies that exist in threes, but the most common ones you will think of will be *Sulph., Calc.* and *Lyc., Sulph., Sars.* and *Sep.*, and *Coloc., Caust.* and *Staph.*, which often follow each other and rotate in this way. Do not let these facts make you give a routine remedy unless the symptoms agree, but it does help to remember that remedies are somewhat similar. It is true that *Puls., Sil.* and Fluor, ac. are similar all along the line as to the nature of their symptoms. *Puls.* corresponds to more acute disturbances, or to the earlier stages of chronic disease; the more active or violent operations of chronic disease. It will take off the wire edge of the disease, and it will be followed by some medicine that is complementary to it, always to be determined by the symptoms that arise. There are cases that would be greatly injured by so deeply acting a remedy as *Sil.* if given in the beginning, that is, the suffering would be unnecessary; but if you commence with *Puls.* you can mitigate the case and prepare it to receive *Sil.*, providing the two would appear to be on a plane of agreement. A very serious case had better first receive *Puls.*, and the way being paved by that remedy follow it up with *Sil.*

Think of the remedy, then, in vicious bone diseases, in necrosis and caries, in fistulous openings, fistula leading to the teeth, fistula lachrymalis and fistula *in ano;* in calcareous degenerations; in deformity of the nails, hair and teeth; in affections of the thigh bones and leg bones, with chronic fistulous openings leading co bone discharging pus which excoriates the parts all around.

The patient is over-sensitive; is made worse if the bowels do not move regularly; is distressed if the menstrual flow is slightly delayed; suffers if the call to urinate cannot be immediately attended to, hence, as in the text, "headaches > by micturition." That symptom is all that is given in the text; but remember something that is analogous to it, viz.: If the call to urinate be not attended to the headache will continue to grow < until the urine is voided. That is a peculiar symptom, and it sometimes leads to the study of Fluor. ac. Violent congestive headache with heat and fulness. Violent occipital headaches, worse from motion.

Now, if we take into consideration its great depth of action, we will see furthermore that it is suitable in some brain diseases. In persons who have overworked, who have been working day and night to establish a business, or to keep it up, and when there has been constant use of the brain it is suitable. In mental depression and melancholy, with great sadness, in young men who have destroyed the nervous system by vicious practices, by secret vice. It is particularly suitable for that disorder of the human economy where men have continuously changed their mistresses. There is a state in which a man is never satisfied with one woman, but continually 'changes and goes from bad to worse until he is a debauchee. If a young man cannot keep away from women, he is not so bad off if he will only keep to one, but he goes from one to many, until he stands upon the street corners and, in his lust, craves the innocent women that go along the street. Fluoric acid is suitable in that state, like *Picric acid* and *Sepia,* and these medicines are particularly suited to that condition of enfeeblement of the mind and that disorder of the human economy that makes man so low, that we have the state described as "low mindedness." It takes that form in one who is a sort of debauchee, running after all sorts of things to tickle his fancy, but it takes another form in a man who stays at home with his good wife. He takes an aversion to his children and to his dearest friends and his wife, that is, he has lost that true and noble and orderly affection and friendship and companionship which ought to exist, and he fights against it. An orderly man considers his wife his best friend and he would rather stay with her than go anywhere else. To him there is no place like home. Now, when man arrives at the state when he wants to go somewhere else, that he wants to go away from home, that he is disturbed at home, that everything annoys him at home, that he no longer loves his children as he once did, he needs Fluoric acid. "Feeling of indifference towards those he loves best." The *Sepia* state is like this, but *Sep.* is more frequently indicated in women. The woman will say, "Doctor, there is one thing that I regret very much, and that is, I do not seem to enjoy my chilldren, my home,

my companions, my husband and my friends. There is a sort of alienation."
Such is the way it is told where it is *Sepia*. In the man it is more commonly
Fluoric acid, in the woman more commonly *Sep.,* but this need not necessarily
be so. *Sepia* corresponds more closely to the condition of the uterus and
ovaries, and such conditions, as the woman alone can have. (Compare
Calcarea.)

Fluoric acid has with this state an overwhelming sexual erethism. He is
kept awake nights by erections. This state of desire forces itself upon him,
not only when he is with the opposite sex, but at all times. At times, in the
beginning of a gonorrhœa, this condition of priapism and intense
uncontrollable sexual desire, with swelling of the foreskin, is overcome by
Fluoric acid. There are times when this priapism demands *Canth.,* but that
remedy differs wholly in its nature from this.

Reticence and silence; sitting and saying nothing. This reticence is like
Puls., and often belong to the insane who will sit in the corner and say
nothing all day, never uttering one single word, and hardly answering when
spoken to. A patient sits in the corner and says nothing and does nothing,
eats when food is offered, is led to her room when the time comes, resists
nobody, answers nothing; such a state is found in *Pulsatilla,* and is closely
allied to this remedy. There is some insanity in it, but especially the fatigue
and mildness of a tired brain. Mental exhaustion from overwork or from vices.

It is suitable after *Sil.* in the spinal affections that are attended with
paralysis, trembling and numbness in the soles of the feet. It will often stop
the progress of structural nervous diseases and prevent the case from getting
worse.

An excellent and very useful feature of this remedy is its ability to produce
varicose veins and varicose ulcers. The veins become varicosed anywhere,
but particularly upon the lower limbs, especially following pregnancy.
Hæmorrhoids protrude after a stool; the anus and rectum protrude, and there
is some bleeding, because of the hæmorrhoidal condition. Varicose conditions
with very old ulcers upon the lower extremities; the varicose veins ulcerate.
You might predict what kind of ulcer and what kind of a margin Fluoric acid
would produce. We see the feebleness of its circulation, we see its tendency
to create hard crusts, and hardened, horny skin and eruptions. We might
now easily assume that the inflamed borders of an ulcer would become
indurated, hard and glassy. The margins of ulcers are indurated and the ulcer
is an old, indolent ulcer. Parts once broken will not close up. Union will not
take place between the broken ends of bones, there is no repair. From bones
and from ulcers, we have the fœtid, acrid, thin, watery discharges, or at times
very scanty discharges, but acrid, burning the parts all around, raising
eruptions and scurfs around the ulcers.

From the feebleness of the circulation one might suppose that numbness would naturally be present, and it is true. The ears become numb, the scalp becomes numb, there is a sensation as if the back of the head were made of wood. The scalp loses its sensation, the hair falls out and crusts form. The extremities become numb and there is numbness of the feet and hands extending upwards; numbness, with or without dropsy; numbness in spinal affections; numbness in brain diseases. Numbness of the limb not laid on.

"Crusra lactea; dry scales; itches very much, bald places. Caries of the temporal bone; discharges offensive smelling pus periodically." "Whole left side of the head retarded in growth, left eye seems smaller." That is a clinical state, but it is significant.

Its use in syphilis must not be overlooked. In old cases with exostoses, caries and necrosis, cases that have been mercurialized, and treated by other drugs until ulcers have developed or those affections of the nose that we have often observed in syphilitic states. He blows small pieces of bone out of the nose; great pain in the nose; nasal bones all destroyed, and the nose becomes flat as though only a soft piece of flesh with perforations. The uvula is eaten off and the tonsils become honeycombed by syphilitic ulcers. Lingering, low forms of ulcers and eruptions. The teeth decay or break off or ulcerate at the roots; fiustulous openings from the root of the tooth, continuing to discharge. Many a time has this remedy taken away that ulcer of the root, closed up that fistulous opening, cured the pain, saved the tooth.

"Craves cold water and is continually hungry." Often that "all gone" sensation in the stomach. Is always eating and is relieved from eating, but like *Iodine* it does not last long, for soon he becomes hungry again. Such medicines are very deep. We see that they go to the very root of assimilation and nutrition.

Chronic ulcers of the throat not necessarily syphilitic, but it is particularly useful in the old forms of syphilis; not generally so suitable in the earlier ulcers as in those that are associated with the tertiary forms, with debilitated states, with brain disease, with nervous symptoms that go on for years when the patient is supposed to be cured. Very often the trouble will come back in the throat, and the ulcers consist of little gummatous growths. *Sil.* especially covers such a condition, and *Sil.* is also one of the most useful medicines for rooting out *Mercury.* In potentized form *Sil.* and *Merc.* are inimical, yet the high potencies of *Sil.* will antidote crude *Mercury.*

This patient craves pungent, spicy, highly seasoned things. The appetite must be tickled; there must be some inducement to eat. At times the appetite is changeable in spite of the fact that he is overwhelmingly hungry; he cannot eat, yet he is > when the food is in the stomach. > after eating.

The most vicious kind of chronic diarrhœa with this low feeble constitution, in insidious complaints. "Morning diarrhœa." *The itching of the anus is sometimes intense;* protrusion of the anus during defæcation; profuse hæmorrhage after stool; constipation with piles; itching around and in anus, in perineum, etc.

This drug is also suitable in the dropsy of drunkards. They are very often liver dropsies. Old cicatrices become red around the edges, surrounded by itching vesicles, itching violently; squamous eruptions upon the body; dry, cutaneous eruptions upon the body, very scaly.

"Sensation as if a burning vapor were emitted from the pores of the body." Especially under the covers there is this sensation of great heat, tremendous, like steam. It is not in fever. He has no fever but it is a chronic state of giving out heat without thirst, or increase of temperature.

GELSEMIUM

If you will observe the weather conditions in sharp climates, such as Minnesota, Massachusetts and Canada, you will find that the cold spells are very intense and that people, when exposed, come down with complaints very rapidly and violently. That is the way the *Bell.* and *Acon.* cases come on, but Gelsemium complaints do not come from such causes nor appear that way. Its complaints are more insidious and come on with a degree of slowness. A Gels. cold develops its symptom several days after the exposure, while the *Acon.* cold comes on a few hours after exposure. The *Aconite* child exposed during the day in dry, cold, weather will have croup before midnight. But in the South diseases are very slow. Like the people themselves, their organs are very slow, and their reaction is slow. Their colds are not taken from the violent cold, but from getting overheated. Hence, they take colds and fevers of a low; malarial type; they have congestive headaches and congestive complaints that do not come on suddenly. When we think of the climate, and consider the people, and the pace of remedies, we see that Gels. is a remedy for warm climates, while *Acon.* is a remedy for colder climates. Certain acute complaints in the North will be like *Aconite,* while similar complaints will have symptoms in the warmer climate like Gels. The colds and fevers of the mild winters will be more likely to run to this medicine, whereas the colds and fevers of a violent winter will be more likely to run to *Bell.* and *Acon.* It is true that *Acon* has complaints in hot weather, fevers and dysentery of hot weather, but they are different from the complaints of winter.

Gels. has been used mostly in acute troubles. In lingering acute troubles and in those resembling the chronic it is very useful, but in chronic miasms it is not the remedy. It is only a short-acting remedy, though slow in its beginning. In this it is like *Bryonia. Bry.* complaints come on slowly, and hence it is suitable for fevers coming on in the southern climates, but it also has sudden violent complaints, though not to the extent we find in *Bell.*

The complaints of Gels. are largely congestive. Cerebral hyperæmia, determination of blood to the brain and to the spinal cord. The extremities become cold and the head and back become hot. The symptoms are manifested largely through the brain and spinal cord. In connection with brain affections there are convulsions of the extremities, crampings of the fingers and toes and of the muscles of the back. Coldness of the fingers and toes; sometimes the extremities are icy cold to the knees, while the head is hot and the face purple. During the congestion the face is purple and mottled. The eyes are engorged, the pupils dilated (sometimes contracted), the eyes are in a state of marked congestion with lachrymation and twitching. The patient feels dazed and talks as if he were delirious; incoherent, stupid, forgetful. It is like this in intermittent fever that gradually develops towards a congestive chili. Great coldness running up the back from the lower part of the spine to the back of the head. Shuddering, as if ice were rubbed up the back. The pains also extend up the back. With the coldness of the extremities, the very dark red countenance, the dazed condition of the mind, the glassy eyes and dilated pupils, we have the neck drawn back and rigidity of the muscles of the back of the neck, so that the neck cannot be straightened, and there are violent pains up the back and coldness in the spine. This state would remind one of cerebro-spinal meningitis. Pain in the base of the brain and in the back of the neck. With all states there is a very hot skin and a high temperature, with coldness of the extremities. Sometimes the troubles are ushered in with a violent chill. This is a very important remedy to study when such symptoms are present in intermittents and in a few days the tongue begins to coat, nausea comes on, ending in vomiting of bile, and instead of there being an intermission a continued fever extends from one paroxysm into another, with a higher temperature in the afternoon. The chill practically subsides, leaving a state which has the appearance of typhoid, with dry tongue, not much thirst and marked head symptoms, dazed in mind. If this continues many days delirium and all the features of typhoid will come on and the fever will change its type altogether from the intermittent to the continued. In congestive chill with high temperature occurring in the afternoon, the chill part of it subsiding and the fever becoming continued, Gels. is a useful remedy. It is also a very important remdey in afternoon fevers without chill in infants and in children. You will find in malarial districts that it is a common thing for the infants to have remittent attacks, while the adults are having intermittents. It is only occasionally that you will see a child or infant shake with a distinct chill, but they often go into a remittent fever, an afternoon fever which will subside along towards morning, to be followed the next after-noon by fever. With Gels, the child will lie as still as in *Bry.* but there is more congestion to the head; there is the dark red face and duskiness like *Bry.*

Running through the febrile complaints, in the spinal meningitis, in congestion of the brain, in intermittents or remittents that change to a continued fever, and even in a cold when the patient is sneezing and has hot face and red eyes, there is one grand feature, viz., a feeling of great weight and tiredness in the entire body and limbs. The head cannot be lifted from the pillow, so tired and so heavy is it, and there is such a great weight in the limbs. The *Bry.* patient lies quietly because if he moves the pains are worse. He has an aversion to motion, because he is, conscious that it would cause an increase of suffering.

The heart is feeble and the pulse is feeble, soft and irregular. There is palpitation during the febrile state. Palpitation, with weakness and irregularity of the pulse. There is a sense of weakness and goneness in the region of the heart, and this weakness and goneness often extend into the stomach, involving the whole lower part of the left side of the chest and across the stomach, creating a sensation of hunger, like *Ignatia* and *Sepia.* There is a hysterical element running through Gels. and it has the nervous hunger, or gnawing.

There are cardiac nervous affections like *Digitalis, Cactus* and *Sepia.* *Sepia* is not known to be as great a heart remedy as *Cactus.* but it has cured many cases of heart troubles. *Sepia* has cured endocarditis, and a remedy that will take hold in endocarditis and root it out must be a deep acting remedy. He feels that if he ceases to move the heart will cease to beat.

The headaches are of the congestive type. The most violent pain is in the occiput, and it is felt sometimes as a hammering. Every pulsation is felt like the blow of a hammer in the base of the skull. These headaches are so violent that the patient cannot stand up, but will lie perfectly exhausted, as if paralyzed from the pain. There is an occipital headache that compels walking or rolling the head. There is commonly relief from lying in bed, bolstered up by pillows, with the head perfectly quiet. The face is flushed and dusky and the patient is dazed. After the headache progresses a while, the whole head seems to enter into a state of congestion, there is one grand pain, too dreadful to describe, and the patient loses his ability to tell symptoms and appears dazed; lies bolstered up in bed, eyes glassy, pupils dilated, face mottled, and extremities cold. Gels, has also headaches of a neuralgic character in the temples and over the eyes. With nausea and aggravation from vomiting. The headache is relieved by passing a copious quantity of urine; that is, the urine which has probably been scanty becomes free and then the headache subsides.

There is much nervous excitement. Complaints from fear, from embarrassment, from shock that is attended with fear, from sudden surprises that are attended with fright. A soldier going into battle has an involuntary stool; involuntary discharges from fright and surprises accompanying fright. On becoming suddenly overwhelmed by some surprise he becomes faint, weak and exhausted, he becomes tired in all the limbs and unable to resist opposing circumstances. His heart palpitates. This is similar to *Arg. nit. Arg. nit.* has the peculiar condition that when dressing for an opera a sudden attack of diarrhœa comes on, causing more or less sudden exhaustion, and she must go several times before she can finish dressing. They who are to appear before an audience are detained because of a sudden attack of diarrhœa. A lady has an attack of diarrhœa when about to meet friends over whom she expects to become excited at the meeting. The anticipation brings on the diarrhoea. Such a state is *Arg. nit.* These medicines are so closely related to each other that there are times when they will appear to do the work of each other.

Then we have paralytic affections of the sphincters, and so with the febrile conditions there is involuntary loss of stool and urine. There is also paralytic weakness of the extremities and of the hands. With paralytic states there is aching along the spine and in the muscles of the back; drawing, cramping in the muscles of the back and aching under the left shoulder blade.

There are many disturbances of vision; double vision, dimness of vision, appearance of a gauze before the eyes; confusion of vision and blindness. These symptoms come on before going into attacks, in connection with chill, at the coming on of sick headaches and congestive headaches.

All sorts of objects are seen; the field of vision appears full of black spots, or full of smoke or little waves of various colors. It is useful in inflammation of all the tissues of the eye and of the eyelids. The eyeballs oscillate laterally when using them. Drooping of the eyelids or ptosis is a marked feature and is in its paralytic nature. The muscles are relaxed, they do not hold the lids up. The lids close when he is looking steadily; they simply fall down over the eyes.

The patient in general is thirstless, and it is the exception that there is much thirst. It has a profuse, exhaustive sweat and is aggravated from motion, or rather motion seems to be impossible. It seems that he is unable to move, that he is too weak to move, and this runs through all complaints. At times it is a remedy for coryza, with sneezing and running of water from the nose, with coldness in the extremities, and the trouble will go down into the throat and produce sore throat, with redness, tumefaction, enlargement of the tonsils, hot head and congested face. With this, as with the other febrile conditions, there is heaviness of the extremities. The red face, the heaviness

of the extremities and sore throat that has come on gradually, a little worse
from day to day, until it has become a severe throat, will lead you to Gels.,
especiallly if there is paralytic weakness all over, and as the throat trouble
progresses the food and drink come back through the nose. This is due to a
paralysis of the muscles of deglutition. The tongue also becomes paralyzed
and does not perform its work in an orderly way. There are times when the
paralytic weakness is not sufficiently marked to account for things seen, but
there is an incöordination of muscles and he is awkward. He undertakes to
take hold of an article and takes hold of something else. When he does grasp
his hands feel weak. He is awkard and clumsy and the muscles do this and
that and something not ordered to do. The trembling, incöordination and
paresis are especially noticed during high excitement and afterwards, and
these states occur with the febrile condition and remain sometimes after.
Useful in paralytic cases that begin with fevers. Tearing is felt in the nerves
all over the body and seems to be due to an inflammatory condition. It has
cured sciatica, with tearing pains, associated with great weakness of the
limbs. Loss of sensation is sometimes found; numbness of the end of the
nose, of the ears, of the tongue, of the fingers, of the hands and feet,
numbness, here and there, of the skin.

In the male, the sexual organs are in the same condition as the patient in
general. The semen dribbles away; there is impotency, no ability to perform
the sexual act; the sexual organs are relaxed.

The sleep is greatly disturbed. He cannot go to sleep; every excitement
keeps him awake. During marked febrile conditions he has a profound sleep
or coma. When he is not in this comatose sleep during congestion he is in a
state of nervous excitement in which he lies awake thinking, and yet thinks of
nothing in particular, because his mind will not work in an orderly way.

The symptoms of Gels. may be present in inflammation of any organ,
uterus or ovaries, stomach, the lungs and of the rectum. It has congestion of
organs, but it has also high grade inflammation. There is nothing peculiar in
the inflammation itself that would indicate Gels., neither should Gels. ever be
given because there is inflammation, but when the mental symptoms are
present, the delirium, the flushed face, the determination of blood to the head
with the cold extremities, the *great heaviness of the limbs,* the disturbance of
sensation, the paralysis of sphincters, then Gels. would be good for
inflammation of any organ of the body. In a most distressing and violent,
rapidly spreading erysipelas that seems destined to cause death in a few
days all the symptoms point to Gels., and though Gels. may not have produced
erysipelas it will stop the progress of the disease in a few hours and the
patient will go on to a quick recovery. Many times when erysipelas has spread
over the face and scalp and in the most dangerous manner with the dusky red

color that belongs to Gels., and other symptoms such as I have described in a general way, Gels, has taken hold of the erysipelas and cured. If we master thoroughly the Materia Medica we do not stop to see if a remedy produces certain kinds of inflammation, etc., but we consider the state of the patient.

GLONOINUM

The most common feature in this remedy is the surging of blood to the head and to the heart. A patient often describes the state as a feeling as if all the blood in the body must be rushing around the heart, with a sense of heat or a boiling sensation in the region of the heart, or in the left side of the chest. Again he complains of a surging in the head, a warm glowing sensation in the head or a feeling of intense glowing from the stomach or from the chest up into the head, attended at times with loss of consciousness. There are also wave-like sensations in the head, as if the skull were being lifted up and lowered, or as if it were being expanded and contracted. Along with this there is most intense pain, sometimes as if the head would burst, sometimes great soreness. in the head, or a sense of soreness felt in the skull. Another accompaniment of the surging is great throbbing, synchronous with the heat of the heart, and when the skull has this soreness then the throbbing is like the beating of hammers, and every pulsation is painful, so that there are painful pulsations and sometimes painless pulsations. The pulsations are tremendous, and when they are greatest in the head they are felt also in the extremities. The fingers and toes pulsate, there is pulsation throughout the back, and it seems that the whole body throbs. If this continues a while the soreness in the skull is likely to come on and with it the painful throbbing, every throb is a pain. In this state, with every jar in stepping, and every motion, it seems as if the head would be crushed. The throbbing becomes more painful from motion. The vomiting which attends this condition relieves. The head is relieved in the open air, it is worse in the warmth, and is often relieved from the application of cold. It is made worse by lying down, or lying with the head low. In the extremities we have great coldness. The extremities cold, pale and perspiring, the head hot and the face flushed and purple or bright red. The pupils are dilated and the eyes red. Now, if this progresses only a little while, the tongue becomes dry, red and then brown. There is no great thirst, but the mouth is very dry. The eyelids become dry and stick to the eyeballs. At times the skin becomes dry and hot, and the face is red and glistens. All degrees of confusion of mind, even loss of consciousness, will be present.

Have I not described to a great extent that which is seen in a typical sunstroke? It is noticeable also that Glonoine symptoms are worse in the heat of summer and relieved in winter. The dull headaches and the continuous headaches are aggravated from warm weather and ameliorated from cold. They are worse in the sun and better in the shade. All sorts of contrivances will be resorted to by Glonoine patients to keep the sun's heat from the head. When he has had these troubles for years, and it has become a chronic state, he will never go out in the warmth of the sun without an umbrella.

Glonoine corresponds to congestive states in the head that come on suddenly, especially from heat, but also from gaslight, or from any bright light. The headaches that book-keepers are subject to, especially in those that have at their desk, or over the head, a hot gaslight. The bright light accompanied by the heat so close to the head will make this individual subject to headaches. These headaches are relieved by going into the cold air. The head aches all day when he is at his books, and when he goes home at night and lies down the headache comes on again, and he has to be bolstered up in bed. He wants the head high, and cold applications to the head; the headache is relieved from a long sleep, not generally relieved from siesta. From lying down and taking a nap the headache is sometimes aggravated, but from a good long sleep, a night's sleep, he is refreshed. His feet and hands become warm, the feverish state, and the throbbing all over the body subsides and he wakes up in the morning comfortable; but if he goes out in the sun, or goes to the gaslight, he comes home with the headache again. Since electric lights have been brought into use there is not so much beat in the light, but gas throws out an immense amount of heat in its light.

The child comes down with cerebro-spinal meningitis, the neck is drawn back, the face is intensely hot, red and shiny, the eyes congested or glassy, the head and upper part of the body are very warm, the feet and hands and lower portions of the body and the extremities are cold and covered with cold sweat. It is a most violent congestion to the brain and spinal cord. Convulsions come on, convulsions throughout all the limbs, the neck and whole body drawn back, opisthotonos. Cold feels good to the head; heat feels good to the extremities. The warm room increases the convulsions. When the lower limbs are covered with clothing in a cool room and the windows open the convulsions are relieved and the patient breathes more easily. With this head congestion there is difficulty in breathing and audible palpitation.

The head is made worse from shaking or jar, from stooping, from bending head backwards, after lying down, when ascending steps. It is aggravated in damp weather, and in the sun, while working under the gaslight, after overheating with copious sweat, and from the touch of the hat. The weight of the hat is a very common aggravation in headaches in school children. The little ones work all day in a hot stuffy room and feel better in the open air, but the weight of the hat seems an encumberance as in Nitric acid and Calc. phos.

The Glonoine patient is also worse from wine and from stimulants, and from mental application. When the headache is on he cannot think, and he cannot write. An additional hindrance to writing is that he trembles so that he cannot write. Trembling and throbbing of the fingers so that he is unable to do his work or perform any delicate work with the fingers or hands.

We have puerperal convulsions with such an appearance as I have described. We may have the same violence in congestive chills, or in any type of congestion of the brain.

There is a milder form of trouble that calls for its use, a condition corresponding to the chronic types of disease. This milder form exists where the patient has simply what might be called a hyperæmia of the brain, a rush of blood to the head when able to be about. It comes in spells, comes in moments when he least expects it; while walking on the street he feels a surging to the brain like a flush of heat and a flush on the face, his hands tremble, and the hands and feet become cold, he breaks out in a sweat; he looks around him and does not know which way to go home, he does not know where his dwelling is. He looks in the faces of friends and they seem strange, he loses his way when he is near home. It is a confusion which soon passes away, and he feels better again. But these spells come closer together, and constitute the earlier stages of softening of the brain. This surging of blood to the brain is attended with dizziness; he rolls and staggers, and must take hold of things, and especially does he suffer in this way from a warm day, or from the heat and light of the sun.

In threatened apoplexy, and when apoplexy has taken place, if the violent pressure keeps on, think of this remedy. The clot may not be at first in the place to take life, it may be outside of the life line, but if the congestion continues that blood clot will increase. Such medicines as *Opium* and Glonoine relieve the blood pressure when the symptoms agree. They equalize the circulation, and the patient may not die. A paralytic condition in one arm or leg may go on for a while, and at the end of many weeks or months the motion may be regained, and the patient recover; whereas if the suitable remedy had not been administered to reduce that blood pressure the continued congestion would certainly have ended in death in a few days. The stertorous breathing, the coma, the history, and the general appearance of an apoplectic patient are found in this remedy, but the intense heat that comes on in many cases of apoplexy along with the shiny skin and coldness of the extremities are the guiding features. *Opium* is the most frequently indicated medicine, but it must not be administered in large doses. The highest potencies are the best and one single dose is enough.

In a case noted it says, "frantic attempts to jump from the window". The headache was so intense that the patient became violent and attempted to jump from the window. You may rest assured that with his headache there was all this determination of blood to the head. It is enough to make one frantic to feel this continued hammering upon every fraction of the skull. He cannot lie down, and he cannot walk, because every step increases the jar, so you see why it is that the word "frantic" is used there. The patient becomes frantic with the pain. Another expression used is "disinclination to step around". The patient wants the room perfectly still. If sitting up in bed, you will often find a Glonoine patient with both hands pressing upon the head with all the power possible until the arms are perfectly exhausted. He wants the head pressed upon all sides. Wants it bandaged, or a tight cap fitted down upon it. The headache is worse from bending backward and from stooping forward. There are times when the headache is so severe that lying back upon the pillow cannot be tolerated. There is a sense of great heaviness in the head. You will notice, in reading over these congestive headaches as reported, that each patient has a different way of describing his headache and yet all have the same story to tell, that of violent determination of blood to the head.

"Some months after being violently jarred by being thrown from a carriage, a sensitiveness of the upper part of the back and neck came on." There are two strong characteristics of Glonoine in that cure, viz.: "< from wine and the < from lying down". The other symptoms might have pointed to other remedies, but these two features are there. It is interesting when reading a case; if you have first a knowledge of the Materia Medica, to note what symptoms are verified; when you do not know the Materia Medica then the case is confusing. Now, as we glance over that description we see at once these two things verified and the rest is fairly consistent. Very commonly the pain begins in the occiput and goes to the forehead, but the whole head is in a state of throbbing. But, we notice more particularly, the "aggravation from motion and the least noise". This patient will sit in perfect quietude and silence for hours. You will he astonished to know how long a Glonoine patient can sit without moving a muscle, because motion is so painful. Also "aggravation from lying with the head low and after sleeping." It is important for you to know what that sleeping means. As I have said before, the patient very often is worse after a little sleep, but the common state is relief after a prolonged sleep. If he can sleep long enough it will subside, unless it be the congestive sleep, or coma, and then it is a different thing. "Amelioration from

cold and external pressure." "Vertex burning hot, likewise upper part of back."
The whole crown of the head feels as if it were covered by a hot iron, as if an
oven were close by. Hot, especially in the back of the neck and between the
shoulders. The burning heat seems to appear at the top of the head and
extend down between the shoulders; a sensation of heat, as from a band.
"Face bluish, with a heavy, stupid expression." The face is bright red, but if
the condition becomes severe the face assumes a dusky appearance, and the
longer this state lasts the more dusky it becomes; that is true with apoplexy
and also with sunstroke. When the sunstroke first comes on the face is
bright red, intensely hot and shiny, but as the heat increases the face grows
dusky, even to purple. In all of these cerebral congestions there is a stupid,
heavy expression, even going on to coma. "Frequent deep inspirations."
With this congestion of the head there is commonly vomiting, palpitation of
the heart, pain in the stomach, great difficulty in breathing and finally loss of
consciousness. In another clinical case reported we read: "Every pulsation
is felt as if the head would burst." Now, suppose the head bones were already
intensely sensitive and sore and the head filled as full as possible with blood,
and then you commenced hammering upon the, blood column you can
understand that the pain would be most intense and would soon end in
stupefaction. "Sunken eyes, bluish pallor under the eyes." "Red eyes, with
photophobia; optical illusions. Black specks before the eyes; blindness."
"Face pale, in spite of high fever." In all of these cerebral congestions of
great violence the pulse fluctuates; it even becomes fine and wiry and hard;
sometimes becomes irregular and also slow.

Another common accompaniment of these congestions is tumefaction
about the neck. The neck feels full. The collar must be opened as it causes
choking, as if he would suffocate. Even in the chronic state in the one who
stands upon the street corner not knowing his way home because of the
surging of blood in the head, that state is accompanied by choking and the
collar causes uneasiness about the neck like *Lach*. He chokes and swells up
under the ears. There is not only a sensation, but with the sensation there is
actual swelling. Tumefaction about the neck and throat, under the chin, and
the glands become swollen.

The next circumstance in the text that brings forth the general aspect of
the remedy is in connection with the catamenia. The menstrual flow does not
appear, it is delayed, with violent congestion to the head, violent headaches
and these symptoms already described. These congestions may also come
on during the menstrual period. Again, if a uterine hæmorrhage stops
suddenly, or a copious flow from any part stops suddenly, the patient comes
down with great violence and the blood rushes to the head.

There are many conditions and complaints in life where we have surging of blood to the head, when this will he the remedy wanted. Persons who are subject to palpitation with dyspnœa, upon any effort. he cannot go uphill, he cannot walk along the pavement without bringing on palpitation and dyspnœa; any little exertion or excitement brings on the rush of blood to the heart and fainting spells; fainting spells in women, who are not supposed to be subject to fainting. Great weakness, palpitation, trembling of the limbs, shaking of one or both hands as with palsy. "Laborious action of the heart" is a strong feature of the remedy; pulsation all over. Fluttering in the region of the heart. Pulse quick, irregular, slow or quick and wiry. There are some persons that are apparently plethoric; very much affected by the slightest exertion and who have pulsation all over; pulsation in a warm room. They are sometimes relieved by opening the window if it is cool, by fanning, by cold air, by cold applications to the head. In keeping with the remedy, this is a clinical application of it: "Children get sick in the night after sitting up at an open fire or falling asleep there." "Bad effects from having the hair cut." Bell is generally thought of for taking cold in the head from having the hair cut. "Bad effects from being exposed to the sun's rays." "Bad effects from sunstroke."

GRAPHITES

The complaints of Graphites are worse morning, evening and during the NIGHT, especially before midnight. It is useful in people who are morbidly fat, or have been fat and are now emaciating; with constipation more commonly than diarrhœa; in women in these conditions whose menstrual habit is pale, late, short and scanty; catarrhal discharges that are albuminous and viscid represent to the mind some peculiar general states of the sick man not explainable and not common to diseased conditions nor to many remedies; hence, strange, rare and peculiar. Raw surfaces upon the skin are generally marked by such viscid glutinous discharges.

It is a very deep acting remedy, like all carbons, and is accompanied with induration and burning in the base of the ulcers, inflamed tissues and old cicatrices; hence, its great usefulness in cancerous growths and ulceration. Cancerous development in old cicatrices is a strong feature of this remedy. Contraction of tendons, especially behind the knee. It has hæmorrhagic oozing of pale blood. In the higher sense the patient is anæmic and chlorotic. From eruptions, catarrhal discharges, menstrual flow, ulcers, breath and perspiration there is marked offensiveness (like *Carbo v., Psorinum, Kali phos., Kali ars.*). When eruptions or discharges have disappeared suddenly from any cause and grave chronic phenomena have followed Graphites is one of the medicines to be studied. Scrofulous conditions and swelling of glands; recurrent herpes upon all parts of the body and especially about the anus and genitals; burning in many parts and especially in old cicatrices; general dropsical tendency; weakness in muscles and tendons after straining them by overlifting.

The patient is very sensitive to cold and needs warm clothing; he is sensitive to the cold in winter and to the heat in summer; he is sensitive to a warm room and desires open air which is grateful. Worse in a warm bed; complaints come on from becoming cold or heated; the headaches are worse in a warm room and better in the open air. Graphites has cured deep seated spinal complaints, and in such cases the patient delights to lie heavily covered in a cold draft from an open window. It is easy to see in this, the resemblance to *Carbo veg.*, which often cures when the patient wants to be fanned *Craving for air is strong in the carbons*, yet often easily chilled and just as *easily overheated* and complaints that come from overheating are related to the carbons. This one becomes ill from being overheated; exertion makes all symptoms worse. Motion increases all symptoms except the *numbness* and general feeling of stagnation which come on during rest. Extreme weakness. Weakness and desire to lie down. Paralysis in any part but especially in the lower limb's; sensation of paralysis or stagnation creeps over the body and limbs. He is made sick by bathing and is sensitive to cold, damp weather. What there is in the general life to cause eruptions to come out in the bends of the joints must be left for others to explain, but such is the case with this wonderful remedy. The same may be said of rawness and excoriation in the same regions. Cataleptic conditions are very marked in which the patient is conscious but without power to move or speak; tremulous sensation throughout the body; sudden sinking of strength; sudden weakness. Constriction in many parts. It has cuerd many kinds of convulsions. It is not the remedy for the convulsion, but in chronic sickness where the convulsion is but one of many elements it is often suitable. It has cured epilepsy and hysterio-epilepsy and epileptiform spasms many times when the totality of symptoms furnished the basis for the prescription. A careful comparison of the symptoms shows that this remedy acts predominantly on the left side of the body. The patient is oversensitive to pain and outer parts are very sensitive.

The pains are *burning*, drawing, pressing. Soreness. Stitching and tearing. Numbness is more characteristic than pain. The formation of fissures in all the commissures and in the anus with cracked and bleeding skin in many parts with much hardening; the tendency to grow wens on the scalp and elsewhere are features of this remedy not to be overlooked, and when coupled with the mental symptoms form such a strong and striking image of perverted vital action that the neophyte should not overlook Graphites. It is as broad and deep as *Sulphur*, showing the great similarity to this great remedy in chronic cases.

The patient becomes very restless when attempting close mental work and there is a marked dread of mental work. The mental depression is extreme, and it is made worse by music; her sadness is so great that she thinks only of death and salvation. Grief and vexation cause a recurrence of all her distressing mental sufferings. Her moods are constantly changing; while she may recall all the events of youth, recent events are forgotten; slow of thought and weakness of mind worse in the morning; Often excited, hurried and exhilarated in the evening; extremely fretful and impatient; irritable about trifles and very, critical. Irresolution is a marked symptom. She cannot make up her mind to do or not to do. Extreme activity of mind in the evening and first half of the night, which prevents sleep until midnight; apprehensive and distressed in the morning and excited in the evening; extreme anxiety even to desperation.

Vertigo in the morning on waking; in the evening; on looking upwards; on rising from stooping; compelled to lie down; with inclination to fall forward.

When the above general symptoms strongly predominate in any given sickness the following particulars will be cured by this remedy.

Hyperæmia of the brain in the evening in a warm room; frequent moments of congestion to head and face with faint feelings; numbness felt in whole head; burning spot on the vertex; drawing, pressing and tearing in forehead over the eyes; stitching pains in the temples; pain from temples to side of face and to shoulders; one-sided headaches in the morning on waking; tearing on one side of head extending to teeth and side of neck; pressing pain on the vertex and occiput; compressing, constricting pain in occiput and back of neck; pain as though the head were numb; violent headaches during menses. The headaches are brought on from becoming cold and from looking into a bright light; are worse in a warm room, and better in the open air. There is marked soreness in the scalp; itching of the scalp with or without eruptions; eczema of the scalp oozing a glutinous fluid; eczema behind the ears; fissures that bleed behind the ears; scaly eruptions on scalp; falling out of the hair; bald, shiny patches on the scalp.

Extreme photophobia in the sunlight with copious lachrymation. No remedy has photophobia more marked than Graphites. Pain in the eyes and over the eyes by looking long toward a sunlighted window; complaints from eyestrain. Letters appear double when writing, letters run together when reading; flickerings and fiery zig-zags just outside the field of vision in the evening; misty vision; vanishing of sight during menses. Burning, pressing, stitching pains in the eyes. It has cured ulceration of the cornea. Recurrent pustular inflammation of the cornea. Keratitis pustulosa in children with fissures in the canthi, extreme photophobia and eczema on the face. Marked congestion and injected veins of the conjunctiva. Chronic lachrymation in open air, tears acrid. The fissured canthi bleed easily and itch violently. Purulent discharges from the eyes; the lids are stuck together at night; the eyes feel hot; the lids are much swollen and the margins are red, raw and bleed easily—sometimes hard; ulcers on the margins of lids; the lids are covered with crusts; eczema of the eyelids and about the eyes; dry mucus in the lashes, styes on the lids, with drawing pain, especially when they recur frequently. Cystic tumors on the lids.

Discharge from the ear of sticky, viscid pus; bloody, offensive. Noises in ears; cracking; humming; hissing; ringing; rushing; roaring; reverberations. Violent roarings at night and the ears feel stopped; thundering, rolling sounds in ears. Deafness in various degrees and he hears better in a noise. He can hear better when riding on the cars in the roaring of the train. Deafness with eczematous eruptions on and behind the ears. Stitching pains in ears in cold air. Marked swelling of the ears.

Smell very acute; she cannot tolerate flowers; loss of smell with dryness in the nose; with coryza. Discharge from nose bloody mucus or pus, very Offensive, viscid, thick, sometimes yellow. It is a most useful remedy in chronic nasal catarrh. Very painful dryness in the nose. The bones and cartilages of the nose become very sore to touch. Sneezing and fluent coryza as marked as in *Carbo veg.* Frequent attacks of coryza all winter, worse in cold air; the coryza extends to larynx, like *Carbo veg.;* the excoriated, sore, cracked nostrils are plugged with scabs and hard mucus far up in the nose. Ulcers in the nose. Fissures in the nostrils that burn and indurate.

The face is pale, waxy and sickly. Eczema and herpes are found on the face with glutinous moisture. Itching with or without eruptions. A sensation as of a cobweb on the face. The commissures of mouth are fissured and the fissures ulcerate and the edges become hard and there is great burning in them. The skin chaps and cracks and often becomes excoriated and bleeds. Erysipelas of the face, spreading from right to left. The beard falls out. Crusts form on the lips and the chin is covered with eczema. The submaxillary gland is swollen and indurated. The gums are settling away from the teeth; the teeth burn and sting; drawing pain in teeth in cold wind; tearing in teeth worse from warmth. Taste in the mouth is bitter, salty, sour and like spoiled eggs; nauseating taste in the morning; sour taste after eating. The tongue is coated white; burning blisters on lower lip and on tip of tongue, painful ulcers on under surface of tongue, putrid odor from gums and mouth; breath smells like urine. Dryness of the mouth in the morning on waking; also in the night on waking; saliva flows from the mouth during the night. Chronic sore throat with ulceration and swelling; swollen tonsils; nightly pain in throat; copious white, viscid mucus; a continuation of the nasal and post-nasal catarrh. Constant choked feeling or constriction in the throat that makes swallowing difficult. Constant spasms in the throat compelling swallowing.

Ravenous appetite. Violent thirst in the morning with dry mouth and internal fever. Aversion to meat; to cooked food; to fish; to salt, to sweets. He is driven to eat to relieve a feeling of suffocation and burning gnawing in the stomach. *Pain in the stomach, relieved by eating.* Eructations bitter; sour; putrid; tasting of food eaten; of greenish water. Rancid heartburn after eating; nausea much of the time during menses, with trembling; vomits all she eats; vomiting, purging and cold sweat. The stomach feels constantly in a spoiled state or as from indigestion. Flatulence is as marked as in *Carbo veg.,* and the relief from belching is just as great. Burning, constriction, pulsation and cramping are frequent symptoms. Fulness, distension, pressure are constant features of Graphites. Retching on swallowing food (like *Mere. c.*). Gastric catarrh with internal heat drive him to eat and drink. Gastric pains worse from cold drinks and better by warm milk; periodical gastralgia with vomiting of food soon after eating. It is a wonderful remedy for old drunkards when the gastric symptoms agree (like *Carbon bisulphide*).

It is a most useful remedy in hard, swollen, sore liver with weight and distress in the liver; stitches in both hypochondria, burning in left hypochondrium when lying on it; sensitive to clothing in the liver region. Great suffering in the abdomen from flatulence; incarcerated flatus causes cramping pains, distension, and is a continual source of distress. Everything eaten seems to ferment and turn to gas; rumbling and movements felt in the abdomen; there is great burring and griping; cramping in the abdomen soon after eating; the clothing distresses the abdomen. The slightest indiscretion in eating causes increased flatus, rumbling and diarrhoea; the abdomen is distended with dropsy. Herpes zona on the side of abdomen; herpes over lower abdomen and groin; hard swelling of inguinal glands; œdema of the abdominal walls.

From the anus there is copious discharge of very offensive flatus day and night. While diarrhoea is not so common as constipation, yet it is a marked condition in some patients. The diarrhoea is painless with much flatus, with watery, brown, putrid, lienteric stools; excoriating stools, extreme soreness of the anus; fissures of the anus; great burning. Chronic diarrhoea; from the lightest indiscretion in eating on comes a renewed attack. With the loose stools, and with the constipated stools copious white jelly-like mucus is often found: Discharge of mucus from anus and a constant moisture about the outside parts. Large hæmorrhoids extremely sore with fissures.

Constipation with large, hard, knotty, difficult stools passed with extreme pain from soreness and fissures of the anus. Long narrow stools (like *Phos.*). Violent burning in the anus, prolapsus of the anus. It has cured many cases of bleeding piles of long standing where there was extreme soreness and fissures and great burning. Violent pains during stool. No desire to go to stool for many days. It requires a long time with hard straining to pass the stool. It often suits patients who have no stool except by injection or cathartic. Violent itching of the anus; eczema and herpes near the anus or involving the anus. It has cured the stomach and abdominal conditions that favor the tapeworm.

The urine flows in a feeble stream, becomes very putrid after standing and deposits much red or white sediment; after standing the urine is covered with an iridescent cuticle. After urination there is some dribbling; burning in the urinary passages and neck of the bladder when not urinating; pain in the sacrum and coccyx when urinating.

Violent sexual excitement and nightly emissions; the excitement is so strong that ejaculation comes instantly after intromission. The opposite State is also found where there is aversion to coition and erections are wanting. It is a most useful remedy for impotency following secret vice and sexual excesses. Emissions with feeble erections. Herpes on the prepuce; excoriated and fissured glans penis; dropsical swelling of the scrotum and penis, hydrocele in small boys and baby boys. Itching and moist eruptions on the scrotum. It has cured gleety, viscid discharge from the urethra. It has cured swollen testes.

In the female it causes aversion to coition; enlarged, hard ovaries; great tenderness in uterus and ovaries. It has cured ovarian tumor. Pain in the uterus when reaching high with hands; bearing down in uterine region. I cures cauliflower excrescence of the uterus; it has restrained the growth o cancer in the cervix uteri, when there was burning and putrid bloody discharge in this it resembles *Carbo an.* Menses late, irregular, scanty, pale or mixed with scanty dark, small clots, short duration. Menses six or eight week apart. Menses suppressed or very late in chlorotic girls. First menses delayed Leucorrhœa instead of the menses (*Cocculus*). Œdema of the vulva Leucorrhœa in gushes day and night. Dryness and heat in the vagina; cold ness in the vagina. Extreme lassitude during the menses. Many symptom come during menses; dry cough, copious sweat; œdema of feet; hoarseness coryza; headache; nausea;. morning nausea. Violent itching of the vulv before menses; marked excoriation of the genitals and between the thigh during menses; excoriating leucorrhœa before menses. Leucorrhœa white yellowish-white; thin; viscid; offensive. Sore, cracked nipples in nursin Women. Cancer of the breast coming in the cicatrix of an old cancer.

Larynx sensitive to touch. Hoarseness in the evening (like *Carbo veg.* Dryness in the larynx in the night; copious glutinous mucus in the daytime

He suffocates when falling asleep (like *Lachesis*) and often wakes up i the night gasping for breath; constriction of the chest.

Paroxysmal cough like whooping cough, cough is followed by expec toration of copious white viscid mucus; paroxysms come at any time. It has cured whooping cough. Cough from tickling in the larynx or trachea; violent night cough; deep inspiration causes cough. Rawness in the trachea; stitching pains in the chest. Constriction of the heart; electric shocks in the heart; palpitation on motion or exertion with strong pulsation all over the body and in the extremities, pulse full and hard, slow during day but fast in the morning; fast pulse in evening after eating, with fever. Itching herpetic eruption on the chest; herpes zona on left side of chest with pain. It is a useful remedy to ward off phthisis.

Enlarged hard painful glands of neck. Painless swollen glands of neck. The spine is very sensitive to the jar of the bed; pain in lumbar region as if "spine were broken;" pain in sacrum with numbness down the limbs; pain in sacrum and coccyx while urinating; itching and moisture over the coccyx. Drawing and tearing pains in limbs; weakness of all limbs; sensation of paralysis of limbs; herpes and eczema on the limbs; marked numbness of the upper limbs, during rest and when lain on; numbness and coldness of fingers and hands. Rheumatic and tearing pains in shoulders, worse in left. Herpes in axilla and bend of the elbow; horny callosities on the palms; skin of the hands hard, fissured, hot and bleeding. Psoriasis of the hands and fingers; raw, moist places between the fingers; the fingers nails thick and brittle; the finger nails become black and fall off. Great heat of palms.

Smarting and sore between the nates; excoriation from walking. Many eruptions on the thigh, but especially herpes and eczema; eruptions that ooze a glutinous fluid. Numbness of lower limbs during rest; the legs are weak and heavy as if paralyzed; oedema of the legs and feet. Herpes in the groin and hollow of the knee. Cold feet in evening in bed; copious, offensive sweat of the feet; ulcers on the feet and legs; tearing in thighs, legs, feet and toes; burning heat in soles and heels; gouty tearing in the toes; spreading blisters on the toes that become ulcers; the toenails become black; thick and crippled toenails; the nails are painful; ingrowing toenails.

Dreams vivid; anxious, horrible, vexatious. Sleepless before midnight; sleepiness during the day. Nightly pains in sleep. Frequent waking. Unrefreshed in the morning.

Graphites should be used more frequently in chronic recurrent intermittent fever. Chill in the evening with tearing in the limbs; chill intermingled with the fever; wants to be covered in all stages; chill worse after eating, better after drinking and in open air. Nightly fevers with chilliness but no sweat; dry heat evening and night, especially before midnight; anxiety and restlessness during the fever, hands and soles very hot; even burning heat. It has chill with fever followed by sweat; sweat from slight exertion; sweat on front of body; the sweat is offensive, cold and stains yellow; copious night sweats in weakness and during phthisis; entire inability to perspire in many chronic complaints.

Itching of the skin all over the body, with or without eruptions; itching worse at night in the warm bed; itching and burning with eruptions; the skin is very hot at night; excoriation of the skin in the bends of joints. Every injury festers. Fissures on ends of fingers, on nipples, labial commissures at anus and vulva, between the toes. Itching blotches. Erysipelas beginning in face and spreading to other parts; erysipelas beginning in face and going from right to left. Itching over varicose veins; itching piles. Herpes and eczema oozing a glutinous moisture. Crusty and scabby ulcers: Hard, painful cicatrices; old ulcers with proud flesh and burning, itching and stinging ulcers with indurated base and margins.

GRATIOLA

It is a great remedy for nervous prostration; marked lassitude, with mental and bodily weakness. It is closely related to *Coffea* and *Nux vomica* and especially useful for the weakness of the will and neuralgic pains in coffee drinkers. In hypochondria and in the female it has melancholia and nymphomania. Convulsive conditions without loss of consciousness. Complaints are better in the open air, but he is chilly in a warm room (like *Pulsatilla*); complaints predominate on the left side; constant vaporous exhalations from the body. Catarrhal conditions of the stomach and intestines with spasmodic ailments. There is a lack of will power and aversion to work; mental depression and capriciousness; he is very irritable and hypochondriacal; fear of the future. Complaints from pride. Bad effects from coffee and alcohol; nervous complaints associated with stomach and bowel troubles. Vertigo during and after eating; on closing the eyes; while reading; on rising from a seat; on motion; vertigo with cerebral hyperæmia. Heat and fulness of the head; sensation as though the head grew smaller; pulsation in head; in temples; rush of blood to head, after rising from stooping. The head symptoms are better in the open air and worse or come on in warm room. Pain in the occiput in the morning on waking, better rising or lying on the face. Sick headaches, nausea, vomiting or disgust for food, with vertigo, better in the open air.

Pain in occiput from sneezing. The head feels cold and is sensitive to cold air. Cold sensation of vertex. Corrugated forehead during the headache. Itching of the scalp; itching of the eyes and ears. Mist before the eyes while reading and green objects appear white.

Pain in eyes as from sand; itching in the nose. There is a sensation of burning heat in the face, but it feels cold to the hand.

Swelling of the upper lip in the morning. There is a sensation of tension of the face and tingling and it feels swollen. The face is red; the teeth ache from cold things taken in the mouth. Grinding of teeth in brain affections.

Pain in the throat, compelling constant swallowing; much mucus in the throat, which he cannot eject. Violent thirst; *emptiness in the stomach after eating;* emptiness when he does not need or desire food. Craves nothing but bread.

Nausea better after eating and by eructations. Vomiting of bitter, sour water and mucus. A feeling of anxiety in the stomach. Cramping in the stomach after food and a heavy load that seems to go from side to side as he turns from side to side, with nausea and eructation. Distension after eating. Pressure in stomach, after eating. *Marked coldness in stomach.* Cramp and hard aching in stomach, pain grows rapidly worse and seems to extend to back and kidneys.

Cold feeling in abdomen. Cramping like colic with nausea. Rumbling in abdomen with distension in afternoon and evening. Swelling of mesenteric glands. Pinching in abdomen, better by passing flatus. Diarrhœa, with copious gushing, yellow or yellowish-green, frothy, watery stools; copious watery vomiting and purging, like cholera morbus; copious green watery stools. The diarrhœa is brought on from drinking large quantities of water, due to the violent thirst. During the diarrhœa he is often sensitive to draft and open air which give him urging to stool. It has cured fully developed, rapid Asiatic cholera. Green stools and green vomiting, unconscious stools.

Before stool, nausea; rumbling, cutting; tenesmus. During stool, nausea; burning in rectum; straining, After stool, burning in rectum; tenesmus; pain in coccyx; creeping chills; pain in abdomen. Protrusion of stinging, burning hæmorrhoids. Tearing and pricking in anus. Constriction in anus; itching anus. Ascarides. Burning in the urethra during and after urination; scanty urine becomes turbid on standing; unconscious discharge of urine. Stitching in left spermatic cord to abdomen and chest.

It is a most useful remedy in the female when there is marked irritability of the sexual organs, if the sexual desire is greatly excited; it is one of our best remedies for nymphomania. When the desire is so violent that it drives her to secret vice the remedies are: *Gelsemium,*Gratiola,*Origanum, Nux vomica, Phosphorus, Platina* and *Zincum.*

The menses are too early and profuse; darting pain in right mamma when stooping and during menses worse on rising; leucorrhœa with pains in sacrum.

Violent palpitation after stool (*Conium*) with oppression of chest; heat in chest, head, hands, with red face.

Rheumatic pains in upper limbs; sore bruised pains in lower limbs, after walking; tearing in the tibia while sitting, better while walking.

Sleepiness after eating; deep sleep.

Itching and burning of the skin, after scratching.

GUAIACUM

This is a very deep acting remedy, even deep enough to cure the symptoms of and turn into order a constitution that is *rheumatic, gouty,* and *has inherited phthisis.* These patients are subject to diarrhœa; the tendons are too short, or they have abscesses, catarrhal troubles, bronchitis. Drawing, tension and contractions of muscular fibre. Sore swollen joints. The rheumatic joints are more painful from warmth (*Lac c., Led., Puls.*) and more comfortable when cool. Gouty abscesses of joints. The bones become spongy, or suppurate. The leg and ankle bones are especially affected. Sensitive periosteum. Stitching pains are characteristic, and burning is as marked as in *Arsenicum.* Limbs contracted and stiff. The excretions are all offensive. Drawing, tearing pains. His cold settles in the limbs, and the joints become sore and the muscles draw. His suffering is increased by the *slightest motion.* or *exertion.* Gradually increasing exhaustion. Progressive emaciation. In the first stage of phthisis it is a wonderful remedy, when the symptoms agree. The progressive character of the sickness, the weakness of mind and body, and such symptoms as belong to deep constitutionsal troubles. In psoric cases complicated with syphilis and mercury and other violent drugs we find use for this most neglected remedy. It is closely related to *Causticum, Sulphur,* and *Tuberculinum.*

Absent minded in the morning. Indolent, and low spirited. Obstinate; fretful, and forgetful.

Vertigo on rising.

Rheumatic pain in one side of the head, extending to the face. Gouty headaches. Sensation of looseness of the brain. Stitching in the head. Pain in forehead, occiput, and deep in the brain. Tearing pain in the head. Sensation as if blood vessels were distended. Neuralgia on left side of face and head. Pulsating pain, ameliorated by pressure and walking; aggravated by sitting and standing. This is an exception to the general rule, as most symptoms are aggravated by motion. Perspiration on head and face, when walking in the open air.

Sensation of protrusion of the eyes. Swelling of the eyes. Dilated pupils. Tearing in left ear. Paroxysmal pain in ear.

Pain in the bones of the nose. Nose swollen. Fluent coryza.

Pain in the bones of the face, nose and teeth. Face red and swollen, spotted. Heat in the face in the evening. Sharp pain in right malar bone. Paroxysmal pain in face, head and neck, every day at 6 P.M., lasting until 4 A.M. Dull ache in left of jaw. Tearing, stitching in teeth. Pain in teeth when ɔiting jaws together. Inflammation of the tonsils, worse from warm drinks, and there is much burning.

Perverted taste. Tongue coated thick white, or brown.

Burning in throat. Tonsillitis; it prevents suppuration.

Aversion to food, to milk. Much thirst.

Vomits a mass of watery mucus, followed by exhaustion. Nausea from sensation of mucus in throat.

Burning in stomach and abdomen.

Constrictive sensation in stomach, with anguish and dyspnœa.

Much flatulence in abdomen.

Morning diarrhœa (*Sulph.*). Stools watery. Constipation, with hard, crumbling, offensive stool.

Urging to urinate, even after micturition. The urine is profuse, and foetid. Cutting in urethra while urine flows.

Stitching in neck of bladder after ineffectual urging to urinate. Emissions without dreams. Discharge from urethra.

Chronic inflammation of ovaries. Menses absent. Membranous dysmenorrhœa. Shuddering in mammæ; with gooseflesh.

.Spasms of larynx. Difficult breathing. Palpitation.

Dry, hard cough with fever, finally relieved by expectoration. Copious, putrid expectoration, like pus. Expectoration of blood.

Rheumatism of the muscles of the chest, with great pain on motion. Stitching pains in chest from motion and breathing. Stitching pains seem to be in the pleura. Chronic bronchial catarrh with putrid expectoration, when rheumtaism extends to chest. *Phthisis pituitosa* in rheumatic and gouty patients. Chest pains after riding in open air.

Palpitation of the heart. Rheumatism of the heart; frequent weak pulse.

Rheumatic stiffness of back of neck and back. *Stitching in neck and back.* Drawing pains in back between scapulæ. All pains *aggravated from motion* and ameliorated during rest; *aggravated from heat.*

Drawing, tearing, stitching pains in upper limbs. Rheumatic pains in upper arm and shoulder. Pains in finger joints, and then in whole hand. Hot hands. Stitching in right thumb. Pains all aggravated from motion; aggravated from heat.

Shortening of the hamstrings. Pain in thighs extending to knees. Tearing, drawing pains in legs. Pains in the *tibia.* Gouty abscess of knee. Shooting pains in legs from feet to knees. Softening of tibia and ankle bones. The knee s flexed from the contraction of hamstrings. The right leg swollen and drawn close to the thigh. Pains in all the limbs, aggravated from motion and heat. Weakness of arms and legs. Numbness of lower limbs. Stiffness of limbs. Weakness of limbs after exertion. Rheumatism of joints, aggravated from heat and motion. Pain in limbs after taking cold.

Restless sleep. Sleeplessness. Wakens from sleep as if falling. Nightmare while lying on the back. Unrefreshing sleep.

Chilliness followed by fever in the evening. Burning fever. *Hot hands. Night sweats.* Copious perspiration.

The provers that perspired had no urinary symptoms.

HAMAMELIS VIRGINICA

The striking features of this remedy are venous congestion and hemor-rhages. Veins are distended in all parts, or only in single parts. Varicose veins of many parts, marked soreness in the varices. Bloody discharges from all mucous membranes. Purpura hemorrhagica has often been cured with this remedy. Dusky purplish appearance of the skin, with full veins. Inflammation of veins of any part, especially lower limbs and anus. Varicose veins about ulcers that bleed, a dark blood. Ulcers are dark, even black, and discharge black blood. Dark blood flows from any part. Bright red fluid blood is the exception, but has been recorded. Especially suitable in very nervous, sensitive, excitable patients. Sore, bruised feeling as in Arnica, all through the body, not only in single parts. Veins are especially sensitive to pressure. Extremely sensitive to a jar as in Belladonna, but only in the muscles and veins that are inflamed and swollen. Much weakness with or without bleeding: out of proportion to the loss of blood. Vicarious hemorrhages are a strong indication. The patient is tired mentally' and physically; aversion to mental work; he forgets the word when talking; irritable, depressed and stupid, with recurrent hemorrhages. Pulsating pain over the left eye. Feeling of a bolt from temple to temple. Bursting headache in the morning when waking, worse when stooping. Headaches are connected with venous congestion in other parts. The strange part of these cases and conditions is that the patient is often sensitive to cold and to cold air. Ecchymosis with extreme tenderness of head, eyes or face. Headache from straining eyes. Ecchymosis of eyeballs. Sore pain in the eyes. Congested veins of eyes with oozing blood. Inflammation and ulceration of eyeballs. Epistaxis of dark blood recurring frequently. With the menses also when the menses fail. Epistaxis sometimes copious and clotted and very dark. Gums bleed easily and are very vascular. Throat is dark red, chronically congested and covered with varicose veins. Tonsils are covered with varices. Suffers much from soreness in the throat with oozing of dark blood. No thirst and aversion to drink. Nausea, vomiting blood, tenderness in the stomach. Pulsating in the stomach. Vomiting black clots. Over the abdomen are found varicose veins that are tender to touch. Burning in stomach and abdomen. Dysentery when the stool is much blood rather than the scanty, bloody, mucous stool that belongs to dysentery. Copious dark blood from piles. Constipation a usual condition. Ulceration of intenstine, rectum and anus; with copious dark blood. Portal congestion and hemorrhoids, with much bleeding. Hemorrhoids that protrude, pulsate, and bleed much; also after confinement. The anus contracts spasmodically with intense burning pain. Itching of the anus. Urine; much blood every day, for weeks, was cured at once. Much urging to urinate. Much sexual excitement (male). With dreams and emissions; pain down spermatic cord to testes. Varices in spermatic cord. Tenderness in ovaries and uterus. Uterine hemorrhage with copious dark clots; sometimes with bright red blood. Active or passive uterine hemorrhage. Paroxysmal pain in left ovary. Vicarious menstruation from nose, stomach or lungs. Subinvolution with much uterine tenderness, and occasional bleeding. Menstrual flow copious, dark, clotted. Acute vaginitis with contraction and bleeding. Tenderness of vagina during coition. Spasms of the vagina. Recurrent hemorrhages in pregnant women. Hemorrhage occurring during parturition. Varicose veins during pregnancy. Has been useful in milk-leg. Most useful in the cough accompanied by expectoration of much dark blood. Cough from varicose condition of throat. Scraping blood from larynx and trachea by the mouthful. Hæmoptysis in phthisis, especially recurrent. Tenderness of spine, cervical region. Breaking and tearing pain in lumbar region of spine. Bruised pain in all the limbs. Aching bruised feeling in thighs. Soreness in veins of thighs and legs. Varicose veins of legs; with or without ulcers; worse during pregnancy can neither walk nor stand, limbs so painful during pregnancy. Pricking, stinging in the congested veins.

HELLEBORUS NIGER

In all the complaints of Helleborus stupefaction occurs in greater or less degree. Sometimes it is a complete stupor, sometimes a partial stupor, but it is always stupefaction and sluggishness.

Hellebore is useful in affections of the brain, spinal cord, the general nervous system and mind, but especially in acute inflammatory diseases of the brain and spinal cord and their membranes, and in troubles bordering on insanity. There is a peculiar kind of imbecility or stupefaction of the body and mind. The extreme state is unconsciousness. Complete unconsciousness in connection with cerebral congestion, or inflammation which has gone on to hydrocephalus, cerebro-spinal meningitis, or inflammation of the brain, with stupefaction. Even early in the disease Hellebore lacks the wildness and acute delirium found in *Stramonium* and *Belladonna.* It is passive. Again, it fits in after the wildness of the delirium has passed away and the patient has settled down into a state of stupefaction. The patient lies upon the back, eyes partly open, rolling the head, mouth open, tongue dry, eyes lusterless staring into space. Staring at the individual talking. Waiting a long time to answer, or not answering at all.

Violent attacks of brain trouble frequently come to a sudden end, but those that are more passive linger, and that is where Hellebore comes in. The Hellebore case will linger for weeks and sometimes months in this state of stupefaction, gradually emaciating. He lies upon the back with the limbs drawn up; he looks pale and sickly. When questioned he answers slowly. The text says: "Stupefaction bordering on insensibility." Another common expression is: "Diminished power of the mind over the body." The muscles will not act; they will not obey the will. It is a sort of paralytic state, but "stupefaction" expresses it. Cannot project ideas; cannot rivet the attention cannot concentrate the mind. The patient appears semi-idiotic.

Delirium is not common, and when present it is muttering. There is more stupefaction, more "do nothing," more "say nothing," than delirium. Yet there is evidently confusion of mind; he cannot think. In many instances very late in the disease, the patient can be roused up, and he will act as if he were attempting to think, as if he were attempting to answer, attempting to move. But he simply stares at the doctor with eyes partly open, with a dazed expression on his face, and picks his finger ends.

When questioned the Hellebore patient is not able to tell you what he has in mind, unless considerably aroused and agitated. But when so aroused he will talk about spirits, or say that he sees devils. He sees in his imagination those images that he has read about, or seen pictured, as the devil, with horns and a tail. A young person who has never heard of the devil, or of spirits, would not have that form of hallucination in his delirium. The hallucinations are shaped in accordance with what he has been taught to imagine.

Hellebore has a peculiar quasi-hysterical condition—a form of insanity. She imagines she has sinned away her day of grace. Like *Aurum,* she believe that she is doing wrong, that she is committing an unpardonable sin. That is as near as the remedy approaches to insanity.

"An old woman having been accused of theft by the women around took it so much to heart that she hanged herself. This suicide produced such an effect on the women of the village that one after another accused herself of having caused the death of the old woman."

The most striking type in Hellebore is the sick child. It comes in especially in children between two and ten years of age. The staring—lying on the back and staring with half-closed eyes—is typical of the remedy. Sometimes the lips move without any sound. The lips move as if the child wished to say something, but on further questioning the words he wished to speak are lost, forgotten.

In hydrocephalus there is a sharp scream, the brain cry. The child will cry out in sleep. He will carry the hand to the head and shriek, like *Apis*. But the *Apis* hydrocephalus is far more active and acute. The *Apis* patient kicks the covers off; this patient does not mind the covers, he does not mind anything. He is not easily disturbed. He lies upon his back with the limbs drawn up; often making automatic motions with the arms and legs. Sometimes one side is paralyzed, but the other keeps up automatic motions.

Hellebore is useful in the low form of disease known as "apathetic typhoid". These same symptoms guide to the remedy. Indifferent to all external impressions. Rarely much disturbed by being touched, or by being covered too warmly, or by not being covered at all. He does not seem to be sensitive to heat, or cold, or pricking, or handling or pinching. Listlessness. What is called in the text "stubborn silence" is more an apathetic silence, an inability to speak. It appears as if he refused to answer, but he does not, he does not know how to answer; he cannot think.

Fixed ideas in persons who are said to be just a little "off their balance," a little queer. And that fixed idea will stay; there is no use trying to argue him out of it. The woman gets a fixed idea that she is going to die on a certain day—and nothing can get it out of her head. This is not like *Aconite*, because there is no fear of death. *Aconite* has fear of death and fixes the time of death. Fixed idea that she has committed some sin, which she will at times name and describe, or perhaps only mention vaguely—but it is very real to her.

When able to be about the patient appears to be sad, because she sits and says nothing, and seems to be in a woeful mood. But there is not that great lamentation, with walking the floor and wringing the hands, that we find in *Aurum*. It is an apathetic state; she appears sad and melancholy, whereas perhaps she does little thinking. Any attempt at consolation, so long as the patient is able to think, only aggravates the trouble. Like *Natrum muriaticum,* the complaints are aggravated by consolation, but the complaints of *Natrum muriaticum* are not at all like these. If the Hellebore patient is able to meditate upon his symptoms, they seem to grow better.

Sometimes there are convulsive motions in this remedy, but they are more likely to be automatic. Motions that seem to have nothing to do with the will. He simply makes motions, like one moving in an absent-minded state.

The Helleborus patient is benumbed everywhere. The whole sensoriurm is in a benumbed state, a stupefaction, a blunting of general sensibility. The text says: "Vision unimpaired." Nevertheless he sees imperfectly; he does not regard the object his gaze is fixed upon; that is, his range of vision appears to be correct, yet if questioned a little as to what he saw, he has no recollection of it; it has made no impression upon his memory or his mind.

Vertigo, with nausea and vomiting. Vertigo from stooping. With the general stupefaction the head rolls and tosses. The child lies upon the back and rolls the head from side to side. The eyes are partly open, and he keeps boring the back of the head into the pillow. This is partly unconscious and partly to relieve the drawing in the muscles of the back of the neck. These muscles keep shortening, as the disease progresses, just as they do in cerebro-spinal meningitis; until the head is drawn back as far as it can go.

There is burning heat in the head; shooting pains; pressive pains in the head from congestion. Violent occipital headache. Dull aching in the occiput; benumbed feeling in the occiput. A feeling like wood; fulness, congestion and pressure. The headaches, the motions of the head and the appearance of the face are those occurring in congestion of the brain. I have seen children, after passing through a moderately acute but rather passive first stage, lie in this stupid state, needing Hellebore for weeks before they received it. When it was given, repair set in; not instantly, but gradually. The remedy acts slowly in these slow, stubborn, stupid cases of brain and spinal trouble. Sometimes there is no apparent change until the day after the remedy is administered or even the next night, when there comes a sweat, a diarrhœa, or vomiting—a reaction. They must not be interfered with no remedy must be given. They are signs of reaction. If the child has vitality enough to recover, he will now recover. If the vomiting is stopped by any remedy that will stop it, the Hellebore will be antidoted. Let the vomiting or the diarrhœa or the sweat alone, and it will pass away during the day. The child will become warm, and in a few days will return to consciousness—and then what will take place? Just imagine these benumbed fingers and hands and limbs, this benumbed skin everywhere. What would be the most natural thing to develop as evidence of the rousing up of this stupid child? It is necessary for you to know this. It is not really a part of the teaching of the homœopathic materia medica, but you must know what to expect after giving this remedy. It is a clinical observation which you will see if you see Hellebore cases, and *Zincum,* cases. *Zincum* is, if possible, even more profound in its dreadful state of stupefaction than Hellebore. Well, that child's fingers will commence to tingle. As he comes back to his normal nervous condition, the fingers commence to tingle, the nose and ears tingle, and the child begins to scream and toss back and forth and roll about the bed. The neighbors will come in and say, "I would send that doctor away unless he gives something to help that child;" but just as sure as you do it you will have a dead baby in twenty-four hours.

That child is getting well; let him alone. You will never be able to manage One of these cases if you do not take the father into a room by himself and tell him just how the case will proceed. Do not take the mother; do not tell her a word about it, unless she is an unusually excellent mother, because that is her child, and she is sympathetic, and she will cry when she hears that child cry; she will lose her head and will insist upon the father turning you out of doors. But you take the father aside beforehand and tell him what is going to happen; explain it to him so he will see it for himself; and tell him that if this is not permitted to go on, that if the remedy is interfered with, he will lose his child.

It is not so much the awful pains, but it is the itching, tingling and formation that cause the appearance of extreme agony. Sometimes in every part of the child's body it is a week before all these symptoms go away of themselves— but they *will* go away, if left alone.

All this will make you nervous. Do not stay and watch the case too long, because if you do you will change the remedy. I never heard of one solitary cure like these in the hands of an Old School doctor.

The face has a very sickly appearance; sunken; gradually emaciating. It has a sooty appearance, just as if soot had settled in the nostrils and in the corners of the eyes. You will say that the patient is going to die. Quite likely —without Hellebore. The remedy fits the kind of cases that the allopath knows nothing about and has no remedy for. His prognosis is always unfavorable. The face, of course, expresses the mental symptoms. Wrinkled forehead, bathed in cold sweat. Paleness of the face and heat of the head. Twitching of the muscles of the face. We find that knitting of the brow and wrinkling of the forhead in just this kind of brain trouble. We find a similar kind of wrinkling in *Lycopodium,* but the trouble is in the lungs. In this remedy the nostrils are dilated and sooty. Not much flapping, but extremely dilated. The eyeballs are glassy and the lids sticky.

There is violent thirst in these fevers, and unusual canine hunger. The nausea and vomiting are nondescript. In the early part of the proving there are diarrhœa and dysentery; with copious white gelatinous stool; stool consisting solely of pale tenancious mucus. And then comes paralytic constipation, and these prostrated, emaciated brain cases, such as described, will lie for days without stool, or any action of the bowels. After a day or two they will not even respond to injections. Little, hard, dry stool. Again, when reaction comes, it very commonly comes with a diarrhœa, or a sweat, or vomiting; perhaps with all three of these conditions.

The urine is retained or suppressed; sometimes it dribbles away—passes unconsciously. Urine passed in a feeble stream; bloody urine.

The patient lies on the back, with his limbs drawn up; or slides down in bed. Great debility; great relaxation; the muscles refuse to act. Convulsions of sucklings. Epilepsy with 'consciousness. Traumatic tetanus. Constant somnambulism; cannot be roused to full consciousness. Soporous sleep.

HEPAR SULPHUR

The Hepar patient is *chilly*. He is sensitive to the cold and wants an unusual amount of clothing when in cold air. He wants the sleeping room very warm and can endure much heat in the room, many degrees warmer than a healthy person ordinarily desires. He has no endurance in the cold and all his complaints are made worse in the cold. If he becomes cold in sleep his complaints come on; or if he is out in the cold, dry wind, complaints come on inflammatory and rheumatic complaints appear. The exposure of hand or foot at night in bed brings on symptoms. He wants the covers drawn close about the neck when in bed.

This patient is also *oversensitive* to impressions, to surroundings and to pain. What with an ordinary person would only be an ache or disagreeable sensation becomes with Hepar an intense suffering. But the pains of Hepar may be very severe, very sharp. Inflamed spots, eruptions, boils or suppurations are full of sharp pains. This is so intense that it is described at times as a sticking and *jagging like sharp sticks*. The pains in ulcers are often felt like sticks; intense and sharp as if sticks were jagging the ulcer. This sensation is often expressed by the patient suffering from sore throat. He feels as if he had swallowed a fish bone or stick. This is in keeping with the general character, because it is present everywhere, in inflammations, ulcers, pustules, boils and eruptions; all seem to have sticks in them or something jagging. Eruptions are *sensitive to touch*. This accords with the oversensitiveness of the nerves found everywhere. The Hepar patient *faints with pain*, even from slight pain.

This remedy belongs to patients that are called delicate, that are oversensitive to impressions. The *mind* takes part in this over sensitiveness and manifests itself by a state of extreme irritability. Every little thing that disturbs the patient makes him intensely angry, abusive and impulsive. The impulses will overwhelm him and make him wish to kill his best friend in an instant. Impulses also that are without cause sometimes crop out in Hepar. A man may have a sudden impulse to stab his friend. A barber has an impulse to cut the throat of his patron while in the chair. Mothers may have an impulse to throw the child into the fire or an impulse to set herself on fire; an impulse to do violence and to destroy. These symptoms increase to insanity and then the impulses are often carried out. It becomes a mania to set fire to things.

The patient is *quarrelsome, hard to get along with; nothing pleases; everybody disturbs; oversensitiveness to persons, to people and to places.* He desires a constant change of persons and things and surroundings and each new surrounding or person or thing again displeases and makes him irritated. With this irritability of temper and physical irritability there is a tendency to suppuration in parts. Localized inflammations incline to suppurate, especially in glands and cellular tissue do we have suppuration and ulcers. The glands of the neck, axilla and groin and the mammary glands swell, become hard and suppurate. First the hard swellings with the feeling as if they had sticks jagging in them, then it becomes highly inflamed and red over the part and ultimately it suppurates, discharges and heals slowly. The bone even suppurates and takes on necrosis and caries. Felons around the root of the nail and ends of the fingers. The nail suppurates and loosens and comes off. Sensation of splinters under the nails, even when they do not suppurate. The nails become hard and brittle. Warts crack open and bleed, sting and burn and suppurate. Hepar is especially useful in felons in such a constitution as described, but sometimes you will have nothing more than the fact that the patient is a scrawny, chilly patient, who is always taking cold and subject to felons. I have often had to give Hepar on no better information and have known it to stop the tendency to felons. It also competes with *Silica.*

The patient is often scrawny, and has a tendency to enlargement of glands. The lymphatic glands are generally hard and enlarged. They are chronically enlarged without suppuration, and at any cold that comes on some particular gland may suppurate.

The catarrhal state is general. There is no mucous membrane exempt, but especially do we have catarrh of the nose, ears, throat, larynx and chest. The Hepar patient is subject to coryza. In some instances the colds settle in the nose and then there will be much discharge, with sneezing every time he goes into a cold wind. The cold winds bring on sneezing and running from the nose, first of a watery character and finally ending in a thick, yellow, offensive discharge. These offensive discharges smell like decomposed cheese, and this characteristic runs through the remedy. The discharges from all parts of the body smell like old cheese. The discharges from ulcers are offensive, and have a decomposed, cheesy smell. It has discharges running through it also that smell sour, and this is also a general because it modifies all things that can be sour. The babies are always sour in spite of much washing. Or it may be noticed by the members of the family that one of the family always smells sour, has a sour perspiration. The discharges from ulcers are sour, and also discharges from mucous membranes. The discharge from the nose becomes copious, and causes ulceration in patches. The throat has a catarrhal condition; the whole pharynx is in a catarrhal state with copious discharge. Throat extremely sensitive to touch; *pain as if full of splinters;* pain on swallowing. The larynx also is painful on talking; painful as a bolus of food goes down behind the larynx, and painful to touch with the hand. There is a loss of voice, and a dry, hoarse bark in adults, especially in the mornings and evenings. Every time he goes out in the dry, cold wind, he becomes hoarse, loses the voice and coughs. It is a dry, hoarse, barking cough. Inspiring cold air will increase the cough and putting the hand out of bed will increase the pain in the larynx or cough. *Putting the hand or foot out of bed* brings a general aggravation of all the complaints of Hepar. Putting the hand out of bed accidentally when sleeping will bring on cough, and cause sneezing. The larynx has its catarrhal state, and in oversensitive children this catarrhal state becomes a croup. Sensitive children that are exposed during the day in a cold, dry wind, or cold air, come down next morning with a violent attack of croup. The Hepar croup is worse in the morning and in the evening; evening until midnight. Sometimes cases that at first call for *Aconite* run into Hepar. The *Acon.* croup comes on with great violence, worse in the evening before midnight. The child wakes up from its first sleep with a hoarse, barking croup. A dose of *Aconite* may prove entirely sufficient; or it may be only a palliative. The child goes to sleep and along towards morning, or at least sometime after midnight, there is another attack, which shows that *Acon.* was not sufficient. Such a case will be controlled by Hepar. When the croup comes on after midnight and the child wakes up frightened, suffocating, rouses up in bed with a dry, hoarse and ringing cough, which rings like a dry whoop, the *Spongia* will nearly always be the remedy, and again if *Spongia* palliates it and it is not sufficiently deep and there is a morning aggravation which shows that the trouble is returning Hepar follows. *Acon.*, Hepar and *Spongia* are closely related to each other and they are truly great croup remedies.

Dry, paroxysmal cough from evening until midnight and sometimes lasting all night, with choking, gagging and crouping; some loose coughing in the daytime; rawness and scraping the larynx; worse in cold air or uncovering hand or foot in bed.

The catarrhal state is sometimes lower down in the trachea, and the trachea becomes extremely sore from much coughing. The patient has been coughing days and weeks and has the morning and evening aggravations; a rattling barking cough with great soreness of the chest in an oversensitive and chilly patient. The cough is attended with choking and gagging, even to vomiting; it is worse in the cold air, and from putting the hand out of bed. He coughs and sweats. There is much sweating the whole night, without relief. Sweating all night without relief belongs to a great many complaints of Hepar. He sweats easily, so that with the cough and on the slightest exertion he is fairly drenched with perspiration.

It has catarrhal affections of the ear. A sudden inflammation comes on in the middle ear, an abscess forms, the drum of the ear ruptures and there is a bloody discharge and sticking, tearing pains in the inflamed ear. There is first a sensation of stooping up of the ear, then bursting and pressure in the ear, and then perforation of the drum. There is also an inflammatory condition causing a discharge that is foetid, or a bloody yellow, purulent discharge, thick, with cheesy particles and smelling like old cheese.

Hepar sometimes is bad on the oculist. When it is indicated, it cures eyes very quickly, so that the oculist does not have a very long case and it does away with the necessity for washes in the hands of the specialist. From the eyes we have the same offensive thick, purulent discharge. Inflammation of the eyes attended with little ulcers. Ulcers of the cornea, granulations, bloody, offensive discharge from the eyes. The eyes look red, the lids are inflamed, the edges are turned out and the margin of the lids become ulcerated. In all sorts of so-called scrofulous affections, the eye conditions may be covered by Hepar when the constitutional state is present. The constitutional state of the patient is the only guide to the remedy. Many times the eye symptoms are nondescript. You have only an inflamed eye with catarrhal discharge, and for this you could give a large number of the anti-psorics; but when you go into the state of the patient and find these general symptoms, then this remedy will cure. *The general symptoms will guide to the remedy that will cure the eyes.* You will see that the specialist for the eyes is often limited unless he knows how to secure all the symptoms of the patient and selects the remedy upon the totality of the symptoms.

There are other catarrhal conditions. Catarrh of the bladder, with purulent discharges in the urine and copious muco-purulent deposits. Ulcers of the bladder. The walls of the bladder become hardened, so that it has almost no power to expel its contents, and the urine passes in a slow stream or in drops, or in the male the stream falls down perpendicularly. No ability to expel the urine with force. It is a paresis. There is burning in the bladder and frequent, almost constant, urging to urinate. It has also a catarrhal state of the urethra that resembles gonorrhoea, and it has been a very useful remedy in chilly patients with gleety discharge of long standing. Thick discharge of white, cheesy character. Ulcers and little inflammatory spots along the urethra. There is a sticking sensation here and there along the urethra and when passing urine a sensation of a splinter in the urethra. Copious leucorrhoea with the same offensive, cheesy smell. The leucorrhoea is so copious that she is compelled to wear a napkin, and the napkins, I have been told by women who have been cured by Hepar, are so offensive that they must be taken away and washed at once because the odor permeates the rooms. This horribly offensive odor that is so permeating is often cured by *Kali phos.* It has really one of the most penetrating of odors, so much so that when a woman suffers from this leucorhœa the odor can be detected when she enters the room.

A very important sphere for Hepar is after mercurialization. Many old people are walking the street at the present day who have been the victims of *Calomel,* who have been salivated, who have taken blue pill for recurrent bilious spells, to "tap the liver," until finally they get into a state of chilliness felt, as it were, in the bone. They sweat much about the head, they ache in the bones, and every change of weather to cold, and every cold, damp spell affects them. They are like barometers. Hepar is the remedy for that state. They go into diseases of the bone easily and are always shivering. While they have periods of aggravation from warmth, as a general rule they are chilly subjects and feel the cold easily. In the more acute affections of *Mercury* there is an aggravation from the warmth of the bed, but the old subjects who have been years ago poisoned with it get almost bloodless, and they become chilly; they cannot get clothing enough to keep them warm. They become withered and shrivelled, and have rheumatic affections about the joints. Then it is that the symptoms of Hepar agree and it becomes a valuable antidote to that state of mercurialization. Hepar is also a complement and antidote to potentized *Mercury.* When *Merc.* has been administered and has done all it can do as a curative remedy, or when it has acted improperly and has somewhat mixed up the case and it is necessary to follow it with the natural complement or antidote and prepare for another series, Hepar is to be thought of as one of the natural followers of *Merc.* It is well known that *Merc. is* not followed well by *Silica. Sil.* does not do useful work when *Merc.* is still acting or has been acting. This is the time that Hepar becomes an intercurrent remedy. *Sil.* follows well after Hepar, and Hepar follows well after *Merc.,* and thus Hepar becomes an intercurrent in that series.

In old syphilitic cases when the symptoms agree Hepar a very full and complete remedy. It corresponds to the majority of symptoms of syphilis and it only needs to correspond to the symptoms of the individual patient when he is syphilitic to be indicated. Thus in old cases who have been mercurialized, who have had the symptoms suppressed so that the disease is latent and ready to crop out at any time, Hepar will come in and have a decided effect upon the syphilis and upon the mercury. It will straighten matters out and cause a development that will lead to clear prescribing. In this relationship to syphilis and mercury Hepar is closely allied to *Staph. Asaf., Nit. acid, Sil.,* etc. Especially is Hepar the remedy in those cases of syphilis where great quantities of mercury have been taken, until it is no onger able to suppress the symptoms of the disease; in old cases when the syphilitic miasm attacks the bones of the nose and they sink in, or a great ulceration takes place; those cases you sometimes see walking around the street, with a big patch over the nose or over the opening that leads down into the nasal cavity. When there is severe pain in the region of the nasal bones, the bridge of the nose is so sensitive that it cannot be touched and in the root of the nose there is a sensation as if a splinter were sticking in. For offensive discharge from the nose, fœtid ozæna in an old case, which has been mercurialized, who is chilly in his very bones, think of Hepar. It has cured many such cases; it has healed up the ulcers; it has cured the catarrhal state, and it has hastened the healing up of the portions of diseased bone, by hastening the suppuration and has returned the patient to an orderly state.

As we go into the syphilitic affections that lead into the throat, we find ulcers of the soft palate which eat away the uvula, small ulcers which finally unite and destroy the soft palate and then commence to work upon the osseous portion of the roof of the mouth. The odor that comes from that mouth when it is opened to show the throat is extremely offensive; very often like spoiled cheese. The medicines that are especially related, or especially useful in this form of ulceration in old syphilitics, will be *Kali bi., Lach., Merc. cor., Merc.* and Hepar, but in those syphilitic cases that have been mercurialized Hepar and *Nitric acid* should be thought of. *Nitric acid* is very closely related to Hepar; it is just as chilly; it has the sensation of sticks in the throat and in inflamed parts. It has fine ulcers in the throat, upon the tonsils and in the larynx. *Nitric acid* competes with Hepar. You think of the two together. Both have sensation of a fish bone or stick in the throat.

The cartilages of the larynx become attacked in syphilitic affections and old mercurial affections. When the case is not of syphilitic origin but is of sycotic origin, small or large white gelatinous polypi form in the larynx and they are sore, causing loss of voice, or cracked voice; when they cause choking or uneasiness, Hepar is one of the remedies. Hepar, *Calc., Arg. nit.* and *Nit. ac.* and sometimes *Thuja* are the remedies related to such conditions.

Again, in the earlier syphilitic manifestations, the chancre has the feeling of a stick in it; then comes the formation of a bubo that may be either non-suppurative or a suppurating gland, associated with a chancre or a harmless ulcer upon the penis. These conditions are often indications for Hepar, when the constitutional state is present. Hepar has also sycotic warts. It is useful in old cases of gleet; also when there is a sensation of a splinter in the urethra. In strictures and constrictions of inflammatory character during the

inflammation there is a tendency to ulcerate, and with this the sensation of a
stick is felt. *Arg. nit., Nit. ac.* and Hepar run close together for this kind of
inflammation, and will cure the inflammatory stricture before it becomes a
complete and permanent fibrinous stricture. It is only very rarely that you will
be able with your medicines to cure a stricture after it has taken on permanency,
after it is many years old, but as long as the inflammation keeps up there is
hope. I remember one very old one that was cured by *Sepia*. I did not know at
first of its presence, but prescribed *Sepia* on the symptoms of the case, and
the patient came back with great suffering in the urethra, and then confessed
to me that he had had gonorrhœa and had been troubled for years with a
stricture. That inflammation was aroused anew and after it ran its course it
really left the passage clear and there was never any more trouble with the
stricture. That was a very unusual result. I have many times prescribed for
patients with the utmost endeavors to do the same thing, and have cured the
patient in other respects, but the stricture would remain. Remember then that
Hepar has fig-warts, chronic sycotic discharges, or chronic gonorrhœa,
offensive, cheesy discharges, the sensation of sticks in the urethra,
inflammatory stricture, which will be associated with difficulty in passing
urine, to the extent that there is a weakness of the bladder and the urine falls
perpendicularly.

Hepar has served a valuable purpose in its ability to establish suppuration around foreign bodies. For instance, a foreign body is under the skin or
is somewhere unknown. Perhaps it is the tip end of a projectile after the
projectile itself has been taken away, or under the nail a Splinter is forming a
suppuration. It is so small that it is hardly observed and it is supposed often
that the splinter has been entirely removed, but an inflammatory condition
starts up. Hepar if *indicated by the general symptoms of the patient* hastens
the suppuration and heals up the finger, for it has all such things. *Silica* is
another remedy capable of establishing inflammation and suppuration and
removes little foreign bodies that cannot be located. Of course it is
understood that if the physician knows the location of a splinter, he will take
such steps as are necessary to remove it, and not wait for the action of a
remedy. But at times a needle point breaks off against the bone of the finger
of a seamstress, or small portions of the needle may exist where they cannot
be found without an immense amount of slashing which the patient refuses.
Hepar or *Silica* will remove it. A little abscess will form, and the little mite will
be discharged. Knowing that these two remedies have this tendency to
establish a suppuration wherever there are foreign bodies, it is well to be
reminded that if a bullet were encysted in the lungs it would be well, if the

symptoms called for Hepar or *Silica,* to consider whether it might not be injurious to give a remedy that would establish a suppuration. It might be that the bullet is resting in a vital place, in a network of arteries, and it would be well not to establish suppuration in this vital region. Deposits of a tubercular character are often located in a place that they can easily be suppurated out, and the action of the remedy on them would be the same as a foreign body. Hence it is that Hepar, after its administration, will very often abolish a crop of boils all over the economy because in the skin there are small accumulations of sebaceous matter and these will be suppurated out. *Sulphur* also does this; so that it may be well to be careful and not give *Silica* or *Sulphur,* or Hepar too often, or too high, in patients that have encysted tubercle in the lungs. Rokitansky in his numerous post-mortems found a large number of encysted caseous deposits in the lungs, in cases that had lived and outgrown these troubles; they had become encysted and therefore perfectly safe and the patient had died of something else. It might be dangerous to administer these medicines that have a tendency to cause suppuration in such, and you should at least proceed cautiously in using them. After you have seen a great many cases you will find that you have killed some of them. If our medicines were not powerful enough to kill folks, they would not be powerful enough to cure sick folks. It is well for you to realize that you are dealing with razors when dealing with high potencies. I would rather be in a room with a dozen negroes slashing with razors than in the hands of an ignorant prescriber of high potencies. They are means of tremendous harm, as well as of tremendous good.

In contrast with Hepar (although Hepar is a form of *Calcarea*), *Calc. carb.* has no such tearing down nature in it. It does not establish inflammation around foreign bodies and tend to suppurate them out, but causes a fibrous deposit around bullets and other foreign substances in the flesh. It causes tubercular deposits to harden and contract and become encysted.

Many excellent homœopathic physicians have said to me, "I do not agree with you as to the danger of *Sulphur* in phthisical cases. I have cured cases of phthisis with *Sulphur.*" So Have I, many of them. But I did not refer to curable cases, but to those cases which are well developed and have grave symptoms. It is well to know all the elements in the case; then if you have administered a remedy and killed your patient, you know at least what you have done. It is better to know what you have done if you have killed your patient, than to be ignorant of it and go on and kill some more in the same way.

HYDRASTIS CANADENSIS

Hydrastis is a slow, deep acting remedy, required in many trophic disturbances, where there is emaciation, catarrhal conditions and ulceration, even malignant ulceration. Defective assimilation. When it is noticed that the stomach is the centre of most of the symptom complex. The desires and aversions often give the key to a very complex totality of symptoms. In this remedy the sinking empty hunger with loathing of food is striking, strange, rare, and therefore peculiar. It is characteristic because it is a general of the remedy, and is predicated of the patient. Great weakness prevails at all times. Catarrhal symptoms with thick, viscid, ropy, *yellow* mucus, sometimes white, from any mucous membrane, with or without ulceration. Deep eating spreading ulcers upon the skin or mucous membrane, with thick, viscid, yellow pus. Induaration in glands, in base of ulcers. False granulations that bleed much and easily, on the slightest touch. This remedy has been very useful in the treatment of malignant ulcers. In such ulcers it is often a great comfort to the patient, even when it does not cure, as it removes the offensiveness, modifies the pain and restrains the destructiveness. The burning so commonly found in such ulcers is a strong symptom of Hydrastis. When the weakness and emaciation have progressed together for months and years in chronic stomach disease, fainting comes on, and this is also found in Hydrastis. In chronic cases, when the tissues have suffered and not the mind. The astonishig absence of mental symptoms except the general discouragement incidental to long suffering and weakness is striking. If it were carefully proved, most likely the mental loves and hates would come out. The symptoms are better during rest. Small wounds bleed and suppurate.

The headaches are only such as generally belong to stomach dis-orders, and prolonged nasal catarrh. They are not distinctive. It has cured eczema with thick crusts.

The eyes and face jaundiced. Ulceration of the cornea. Thick, yellow, viscid, mucous discharge. Chronic inflammation of lids. Inflammation, thickening, redness of margins of lids.

Otorrhœa with thick, viscid, purulent discharge. Copious mucous discharge. Catarrh of the Eustachian tubes with many noises in ears. Ears red, swollen, covered with scales; fissured behind where connected with head.

The nose is obstructed with stringy, yellow or white mucus. The air feels cold in the nose, and the membrane is raw and ulcerated. Ropy mucus is drawn from posterior nares into the throat. Rawness in both nares with constant urging to blow the nose. Coryza with discharge, scanty in room and profuse in open air. Bloody, purulent discharge from nose. Thick, white, or yellow mucous discharge. Large crusts constantly form in the nose.

The face is sickly, shrunken, pale, waxy, cachectic, jaundiced. It is of great service in epithelioma of face, nose or lip.

The tongue is yellow, large, flabby and spongy. Feels as if burnt.

Ulceration of mouth, gums, tongue; spreading and burning. Aphthæ in children and nursing mothers. Excessive secretions of ropy mucus, golden yellow. Excoriation of mouth. In old mercurial cases.

Catarrhal sore throat of long standing, granulated and ulcerated; excoriated and burning. Thick, viscid, yellow mucus that can be drawn out in ropes.

No appetite; no thirst; loathing of food. Nearly all foods disorder the stomach. Spitting up the food by the mouthful (like *Phos.* and *Ferr.*). Vomits all food. Retains only water and milk. Eructations, sour, putrid, of food eaten. *Empty, faint feeling in stomach with loathing of food and obstinate constipation with no desire for stool* is a combination that must generally have Hydrastis. Pulsation in the stomach. Ulceration of the stomach with burning. For suspicious lump in region of pyloris. Weight in stomach after eating. The stomach seems to be only in ordinary sack; digestion is slow, and tedious. Fulness after eating, lasting a long time. The empty, sinking feeling is not ameliorated after eating. Sour vomiting. Chronic gastric catarrh. Slow digestion.

This must be a useful liver remedy for the following reasons. The skin is jaundiced; the stool is light, even white, showing the absence of bile, and there is distress in the region of the liver. In chronic derangement of the liver. Liver enlarged, hard and nodular.

Cramping pains. Colic, flatulence and distended abdomen. It has cured many of the usual conditions that generally attend bad digestion and torpid liver. Intestinal catarrh and ulceration. Sharp pain in region of spleen.

It has cured obstinate piles, ulceration and fissures of anus. Relaxation and prolapsus of anus. Chronic diarrhœa with yellow, thin fæces, even watery. Inflammation of anus. Stools, bileless, white soft, acrid, greenish, much viscid mucus. Hard, nodular stools. Most obstinate constipation; no desire for stool for days. Paresis of the rectum. It cures constipation, when the stomach symptoms agree. In old cases when enemas no longer act, when the fæces remain high up, or do not come down into rectum to excite desire, this remedy has been of great service. In constipation or diarrhœa with "goneness" in stomach, trembling in the abdomen and palpitation.

Urine scanty or suppressed. Chronic catarrh of bladder with much viscid mucus in urine, causing difficulty in flow of urine.

Catarrh of the urethra. Chronic gonorrhœa when the discharge remains yellow in spite of time. Copious, painless discharge. Relaxed scrotum and testes. Offensive sweat of genitals.

Thick, yellow, viscid leucorrhœa, sometimes white, sometimes offensive. Excoriation of vagina. Soreness in vagina during coition. Bleeding after coition. Uterine hæmorrhage. Menses copious. Relaxed dragging feeling in pelvis. Intense itching of vulva. Epithelioma of mamma.

Most obstinate catarrh of larynx, trachea and bronchial tubes, with copious, thick, ropy mucus and ulceration. Rawness in air passages. Catarrh of chest in old people.

The cough is dry, hard; from tickling in larynx. Rawness in chest. Rattling cough. Thick, yellow, viscid, sometimes white, expectoration in old people, or when very chronic.

Palpitation from slowly progressing weakness.

Weakness and stiffness in back in lumbar region, must walk about before he can straighten up the back. Must use the arms to rise from a seat.

Rheumatic pains in upper limbs. Weakness and rheumatic pains in lower limbs. Ulcers on legs and about ankles, with stinging, burning pains; high, hard edges; painful at night in warm bed; sensitive to touch. Œdema of feet.

Warmth and washing aggravate ulcers and eruptions. The skin excoriates easily. Urticaria over body, aggravated at night. Fissures about mouth and anus. *Ulceration. Bed sores.* Lupus evedens.

HYOSCYAMUS

Hyoscyamus is full of convulsions, contractions, trembling, quivering and jerkings of the muscles. Convulsions in vigorous people, coming on with great violence. Convulsions that involve the whole economy, with unconsciousness, coming on in the night. Convulsions in women at the menstrual period; and then the lesser convulsions of single muscles, and contractions of single muscles. Little jerkings and twitchings. In low forms of the disease it takes on the latter, jerkings and twitchings of muscles. In low typhoid states where there is great prostration with twitching. He feels it himself if conscious enough to realize it, but others see it. An evidence of great prostration of the nervous system. Sliding down in bed, twitching of the muscles. All the muscles tremble and quiver, a constant state of erethism throughout the economy. A state of irritability and excitability. Convulsive jerks of the limbs, so that all sorts of angular motions are made, automatic motions. Choreic motions. But angular motions of the arms, and picking at the bedclothes. Picking at something in delirium. Gradually increasing weakness, whether it be in a continued fever where there has been a delirium or excitement, or in a case of insanity with erethism of the nerves and mind; excitability and gradually increasing weakness. Complete prostration, so that the patient slides down in bed, until the jaw drops. So the intermingling of jerkings and quiverings and tremblings and weakness and convulsive action of muscles are all striking features. Infants go into convulsions. "Falls suddenly to the ground with cries and convulsions. Convulsions of children, especially from fright. Convulsions after eating." The child becomes sick after eating, vomits and goes into convulsions. "Shrieks and becomes insensible." Goes into convulsions, such as the old books used to say, from worms; and the mother goes into convulsions soon after the child is born, called puerperal convulsions. "Convulsions during sleep. Suffocating spells and convulsions during labor. Toes become spasmodically cramped."

The mental state is really the greatest part of Hyoscyamus. Talking, passive delirium, imaginations, illusions, hallucinations; talking, rousing up and talking with a delirious manifestaton, and then stupor. These alternate through complaints. And during sleep talking, crying out in sleep; but, talking and mumbling and soliloquizing. Then, there are wakeful periods, in which there are delirium and illusions and hallucinations all mingled together. Sometimes the patient is in a state of hallucination, and the next minute in a state of illusion. Which means that a part of the time what he sees as hallucinations he believes to be so; and then these hallucinations become delusions. Again, the things he sees he knows are not so, and then they are illusions. But he is full of hallucinations. He sees all sorts of things, indescribable things in his hallucinations. He imagines all sorts of things concerning people, concerning himself, and he gets suspicious. Suspicion runs through acute sickness; it runs through the mania in insanity. Suspicion that his wife is going to poison him; that his wife is untrue to him. Suspicious of everybody. "Refuses to take medicine because it is poisoned." "Imagines that he is pursued, that the people have all turned against him, that his friends are no longer his friends. He carries on conversations with imaginary people." Talks as if he were talking to himself, but he really imagines that some one is sitting by his side, to whom he is talking. Sometimes he talks to dead folks; recalls past events with those that have departed. Calls up a dead sister, or wife, or husband, and enters into conversation just as if the person were present.

Hyoscyamus has another freak in this peculiar mental state. Perhaps there may be a queer kind of paper on the wall, and he lies and looks at it, and if he can possibly turn the figures into rows he will keep busy at that day and night, and he wants a light there so he can put them into rows, and he goes to sleep and dreams about it, and wakes up and goes at it again; it is the same idea. Sometimes he will imagine the things are worms, are vermin, rats, cats, mice, and he is leading them like children lead around their toy wagons—just like a child. The mind is working in this; no two alike; perhaps you may never see these identical things described, but you will see something like it that the mind is revelling in, strange and ridiculous things. One patient had a string of bedbugs going up a wall, and he had them tied with a string, and was irritated because he could not make the last one keep up. Hyoscyamus did him a great deal of good. You do not find that expression in the text, but I will speak of it as analogous to the things that belong to the text. He is in alternate states. One minute he raves, and another he scolds in delirium, in excitement; the next he is in a stupor. Finally, in a typhoid state, after he has progressed some time, he passes into quite a profound stupor. Early in the case he can be roused, and he answers questions correctly, and he seems to know what you have said to him; but the instant he finishes the last answer he appears to be sound asleep. Then you shake him and ask him another question, he answers that, and again he is sound asleep. The delirium that belongs to typhoid grows more and more profound, more and more passive, more and more muttering, until he passes into a complete unconsciousness from which he cannot be roused; in which he will lie for days sometimes, and weeks, becoming more and more emaciated; lying there in profound stupor unless this remedy is administered. Lying there picking the bedclothes, and muttering. Even when he is in a stupor and realizes nothing, apparently, that is going on, he makes passive motions, mutters, talks to himself, and once in a while utters a shrill scream. Picking his fingers, just as if he had something in his fingers when there is nothing there. He picks at the bedclothes the same way. Picking at his nightshirt, or picking anything he can get his fingers on. Or, picking in the air, grasping as if he were grasping at flies. This passive delirium goes on until he is in a profound stupor, and lies as one dead. In an insane state it sometimes takes on something of wildness, but not often. It is more passive, talking and prattling, sitting still in one corner and jabbering, or lying down, or going about. "Undertaking to do the usual things, the usual duties." That is, the housewife will want to get up and do the things she is used to doing in the house; the cooper will want to make barrels and the unusual things belonging to that business. Wants to carry on the usual occupation in his mind, talks about it, carries on the things of the day, and he keeps busy about it, so it is a busy insanity. Also, the delirium takes on the type of a busy delirium.

Now, to give you something of an idea as to the grading of this general type of insanity it should be compared with *Stram.* and *Bell.* You heard in the lecture on *Bell.* that it is violent, its fever most intense. There is much excitement. In *Stram.*, when we reach that you will see that his delirium, his insanity, is expressed in terms of extreme violence. These three run so close together that something can be brought out by associating them together. When considering Hyoscyamus in its mental state it is well to realize that it seldom has much fever in its insanity. It has a fever sometimes in the low form, but when Hyoscyamus is thought of in relation to a febrile state the intensity of the heat would be this order: *Bell., Stram.,* Hyoscyamus. Now, *Bell.* is very hot in its mental states. *Stram.*, most violent and active, murderously violent, is moderately hot in its fever, as a rule. Hyoscyamus has a low fever, not very high, sometimes none at all, with its insanity. When one comes to take into consideration the violence of its delirium, or the maniacal actions, then it changes the order. The order as to violence of conduct would be: *Stram, Bell.,* Hyoscyamus. That brings you to see that even when associated with those medicines that look most like it, it is at the bottom of the list. It goes as a passive medicine, while the upper ones are more active. Hyoscyamus has a passive mania. Does not go into violence. That is, the patient will sometimes become murderous, but it is more likely to be suicidal. Sometimes the patient will talk and prattle, sometimes sit and say nothing. "Full of imaginations and hallucinations when asleep and when awake. Religious turn of mind" with women who have been unusually pious; they take on the delusion that they have sinned away their day of grace. They have done some awful things. "She imagines that she has murdered, that she has done some dreadful thing. She cannot apply the promises that she reads in the Word of God to herself." She will say: "They do not mean me, they do not apply to me, they mean somebody else."

"Thinks he is in the wrong place. Thinks he is not at home. Sees persons who are not and who have not been present. Fears being left alone. Fears poison or being bitten." These phases sometimes take on fear in the sense of fear, but it comes from that suspicion that was spoken of; he suspicions or fears these things will take place. He imagines these things are to take place, and hence he is suspicious of all his friends.

Another thing running through the remedy, in insanity and in the delirium of fevers, is a fear of water, fear of running water. Of course. hydrophobia, which is named because of that symptom being a striking feature, has fear of water, but some remedies also have that fear of water. "Anxiety on hearing running water. A fear of water." That runs through *Bell.,* Hyoscyamus, *Canth.,* and, of course, the nosode *Hydrophobinum. Stram.* has the fear of water. *Stram.* has the fear of anything that might look like water, shining objects, fire, looking-glass. Fear of things that have in any manner whatever the resemblance of fluids, and hence the sound of fluids. *Hydrophobinum* has cured "involuntary urination on hearing running water. Involuntary discharge from the bowels on hearing running water." It has cured a chronic diarrhœa when that symptom was present. Hyoscyamus "makes short, abrupt answers to imaginary questions." Imagines that somebody has asked a question, and he answers it; hence, you will find a patient with typhoid fever answering questions that you have not asked. He imagines that persons are in the room and asking him questions. You hear nothing but his answers; he is in delirium or insane. "Mutters absurd things to himself. Cries out suddenly."

There is another form of his delirium, and there are two phases of this. He wants to go naked; wants to take the clothing off, and this must be analyzed. At first you might not understand that. Hyoscyamus has such sensitive nerves all over the body in the skin that he cannot bear the clothing to touch the skin, and he takes it off. That occurs in insanity and sometimes in delirium, and he has no idea that he is exposing his body. He appears to be perfectly shameless, but he has no thought of shamelessness, no thought that he is doing anything unusual, but he does it from the hyperæsthesia of the skin.

There is another phase running through the insanity, which is salacity, and it is violent at times, so violent that nobody but the old doctor can form any conception of the awfulness of it, and the dreadfulness of its effects upon those in the room. With a woman, a wife or a daughter, this state of salacity is manifested in this way: she exposes her genitals to the view of everybody coming into the room. There are instances where in violent attacks of salacity a woman has gathered her clothing up under her arms to expose her genitals to the doctor as he walked into the room.

"Violent sexual excitement and nymphomania. Obscene things. Speech illustrated by urine, fæces and cow dung," and all sorts of things come out in this state of insanity and delirium—and yet this is only sickness.

."He is violent and beats people. Strikes and bites. Sings constantly and talks hastily. Erotic mania, accompanied by jealousy. Lascivious mania. Sings amorous songs. Lies in bed naked, or wrapped in a skin during summer heat." Not because he is cold, but because of a fancy. Complaints involving any of these mental phases may come on in a young woman from disappointed affections, from coming to the conclusion that the young man in whom she has reposed her confidence has become wholly unworthy of her. It drives her insane, and she may take on any of these phases.

Patients who have come out of continued fevers, convulsions, or insanity have paralytic condition of the eyes, of the muscles of the eyes. "Disturbances of vision. Far-sightedness. Drawing tension in some of the muscles, and paralysis in others. Strabismus." This is one of the most frequently indicated remedies. The strabismus that comes on from brain disease should be cured with a remedy.

In the Hyoscyamus fevers there is so much brain trouble, and there is left behind a tendency to muscular weakness of the eyes, disturbances of the eyes, and congestion of the retina, and disturbances of vision. Double sight. "Obscuration of vision. Night-blindness. Distorted appearance of the eyes. Spasmodic action of the internal recti." "Pupils dilated and insensible to light." Sometimes contracted, but in these low unconscious states of typhoid it is likely to be dilated. Then again, after he recovers from these low forms of disease there is quivering of the lids, and jerking of the lids, jerking of the muscles of the eye, so that the eyeball is unsteady. It moves from little spasms of the various muscles of the globe of the eye. All of these symptoms occur either along with the fever, or afterwards. The child goes into convulsions, or has periods of convulsions, where, during the course of a week or ten days, there have been from fifteen to fifty convulsions, and it may be the convulsions have been remedied with *Bell.* or *Cuprum,* or any one of a number of remedies, and afterwards these eye troubles, strabismus and disturbances of vision. "An object looked at jumps." The letters jump while reading. Spasmodic complaints, periodical complaints, paroxysmal complaints of a nervous character will run through the remedy in various regions, and especially in its cough, its stomach troubles and abdominal conditions.

The mouth brings forth a lot of symptoms. The mouth is very dry, "as dry as burnt leather." The tongue tastes like sole leather, because of dryness. Sometimes the patient will say, "My tongue rattles in my mouth, it is so dry." Very great dryness of the mouth, throat and nose, wherever the mucous membranes are. Dry, cracked, red, will bleed in low forms of typhoid. About the second week, going into the third, the teeth are covered with black blood, lips cracked and bleeding. "Tongue cracked and bleeding. Patient unconscious, except by much shaking or repeated calling he is roused" and slowly puts out that trembling tongue, which is covered with blood, cracks, and is dry. "Sordes on the teeth" in low forms of fever. "Twitching of the muscles of the face upon attempting to put out the tongue." It trembles like it does in *Lach.,* catches on to the teeth from its great dryness, and the jaw hangs down, relaxed, the mouth wide open. The whole mouth is dry and offensive. Sometimes during fever the jaw becomes fixed as if it were locked, and it is with great difficulty that it can be moved. "Closes the teeth tightly together. Pulsating pains in the teeth. Jerking, throbbing, tearing in the teeth. Sordes on the teeth;" and in sleep in these low forms of fever he is grinding the teeth. Children, either in convulsions, or between convulsions, in congestion, also grind the teeth in the night, and in this comatose state. It says in the text, "The tongue is red, brown, dry, cracked, hard. Looks like burnt leather. The tongue does not obey the will. Difficult motion of the tongue; it is stiff, protruded with great difficulty. Biting the tongue in talking."

The tongue becomes paralyzed. "Loss of speech. Utters inarticulate sounds. Speech embarrassed. Talks with difficulty." The muscles of the throat, of the tongue, those that take part in swallowing, the muscles of the œsophagus, of the pharynx, become stiff and paralyzed so that swallowing is difficult. "Food taken into the throat comes up into the nose." Fluids come out of the nose, or go down into the larynx. "The sight of water, or the hearing of running water, or the attempt to swallow water produces spasmodic constriction of the œsophagus."

The next very important feature of this medicine is its stomach and abdominal symptoms. Vomiting. Dread of water. Unquenchable thirst. Aversion to water, as it were, from the stomach; a mental fear of water. The stomach is distended. Great pain in the stomach. Dryness evidently in the stomach like there is in the mouth, because it occurs along with it. Burning and smarting in the stomach; and when there is no inflammation there is vomiting of blood. Stitching pains, colicky pains, distension. The distension of the whole abdomen. "Abdomen wonderfully distended, almost to bursting." Feels like a drum, tympanitic. "Great soreness; can hardly touch the abdomen because of the soreness. Cannot be handled, cannot be turned except with great difficulty, very slowly, and with caution. Cutting pains in the abdomen." Inflammation of all the viscera of the abdomen in low typhoid state, with great distension. Petechia upon the abdomen, such as is found in a typhoid.

Then comes the diarrhœa, very much like that which is found in low forms of continued fever. "Bleeding from the bowels; ulceration of Peyer's glands," and the yellow, cornmeal mushy stool. In Hyoscyamus there is that mushy stool that occurs in typhoid fever, pappy consistency. Again, a watery, horribly offensive, bloody fluid. Most of the time the stools and the passages are painless. "Painless discharges from the bowels. Watery mucus, sometimes odorless, but commonly very offensive." Then, another part of it is that the patient has no realization of the passage. It is involuntary. Both the urine and the stool are passed without his knowledge. Watery, bloody, or mushy. Hysterical females and young girls, who are subject to attacks of diarrhœa and bloody stools. Relaxed state of the bowels connected with relaxation of the uterus. "Diarrhœa during pregnancy. Diarrhœa during typhoid fever. Paralysis of the sphincter ani. Paralysis of the bladder after labor, so that the urine remains in the bladder, with no desire to urinate." The routine remedy for retention of urine after labor is *Caust. Caust.*, like *Rhus,* is a great remedy for the effect of strain upon muscles and parts, and the violent effort that a woman passes through in expelling the child in many instances leaves all the pelvic muscles tired, relaxed, paralyzed.

Then comes that which was mentioned, which really belongs to the general state more than the local; violent sexual desire. Violent sexual desire in girls who never had that desire. Coming on and manifesting itself only during the inflammation of the brain.

"Labor-like pains from taking cold." A cold settles in the uterus, bringing on painful menstruation. Hyoscyamus has various crampings; cramps in the fingers and toes and of the muscles here and there; temporary paralysis, etc. It has suppressed menstruation. There are many conditions belonging to menstruation, pregnancy and parturition that are hysterical in character. Twitchings, cough, constipation, diarrhœa, etc., that belong to a hysterical nature. "Puerperal convulsions. Jerks violently at the on coming of the convulsions. After miscarriage, hæmorrhage of bright red blood. No desire of the bladder to expel the contents."

And then comes the voice, the larynx, respiration, and cough. Constriction of the larynx. Much mucus in the larynx and air passages, makes the speech and voice rough. Hoarseness with dry and inflamed throat. Speech difficult. Hysterical aphonia. Hyoscyamus and *Veratrum* are two medicines that cure and make a nervous hysterical woman a great deal more sensible.

"Difficult spasmodic respiration from spasms of the chest. Apparently loss of breath; rattling in the chest." Hysterical cough. Sensitive, hysterical girls, or sensitive women, with spinal irritation, have paroxysmal cough, coming on periodically, coming on from excitement. When this patient lies down in the daytime, at night, any time, on will come the spasmodic cough with contractions in the larynx, spasms in the larynx, choking, gagging, and vomiting. "Redness of the face, and suffocation." It is a dry, hacking, choking cough, that racks the whole body, in spinal affections. "Tickling in the larynx. Dry, hacking, and spasmodic cough, worse lying, better sitting, worse at night, after eating, drinking, talking and singing. Dry, spasmodic, persistent cough." But its characteristic cough is a dry, racking, harassing cough, worse lying down. Those young women and girls with sore spots on the spine from the coccyx to the brain, sore places that manifest themselves when leaning back against a chair. These take a little cold in the larynx, and sometimes it is purely from a nervous attack. Sometimes spinal irritation, spinal cough in those that have curvature of the spine. "During cough, spasms in the larynx. Cough worse after midnight; wakes the patient from sleep. Cough in cold air, and from eating and drinking. Cough after measles. Violent spasmodic cough." The cough is most exhausting. A cough will sometimes last until the patient is covered with sweat and is exhausted, and leans forward to get a little relief; and he coughs until he is exhausted. "Spasms of the muscles of the chest. Contraction of the muscles of one side of the neck. Spinal meningitis with convulsions."

Paralytic weakness of the limbs: Convulsions of the muscles. Twitching. Frequent twitchings of the muscles of the hands and feet.

Many complaints come on during sleep. The sleep is a great tribulation to this nervous patient. There are times of sleeplessness. Again, profound sleep. "Sleepless, or constant sleep." Either awake or asleep, there may be muttering. "Long continued sleeplessness. Lascivious dreams. Lying on the back he suddenly sits up and then lies down again." That means that the patient wakes out of sleep, looks all around, wonders what terrible thing he has been dreaming about; his dreams seem real. He looks all about and sees nothing of the objects of his dream, he lies down and goes to sleep again. He keeps doing that all night. Starts up in a fright. Jerks in sleep, and cries out. Grates the teeth. Laughing during sleep. With so much brain trouble as belongs to this medicine, we would expect the dreams and the fright, the disturbances, the twitching and trembling in sleep.

Its fevers are low forms of fever, the continued fever, the typhoid.

HYPERICUM

One who makes a study of the proving of Hypericum will be reminded of a class of injuries involving sentient nerves, and it is not surprising that this remedy has come into use for the results of such injuries. The surgery of Homœopathy largely involves the use of *Arnica, Rhus tox., Ledum, Staphisagria, Calcarea* and Hypericum. These remedies are used in a routine way when a physician runs into semi-surgical conditions, or the results of injuries. For the bruised, "black-and-blue," sore apperance and sensation *Arnica* comes into use; it corresponds especially to the acute stage until the soreness and bruised condition have disappeared from the parts injured or from the whole body; but for the strains of muscles and tendons *Arnica* proves insufficient and a thorough study of *Rhus* will show that that remedy is suitable for the resultant weakness of tendons and muscles, and the bruised rheumatic feelings that come on in every storm and often wear off on continued motion. For the final weakness that persists even after *Rhus* we have *Calcarea carb.*

In these three remedies we have a series, but to distinguish these from Hypericum is the important thing. Hypericum is only a minor remedy for bruised and strained tendons and muscles; it goes into a different class of complaints. Hypericum and *Ledum* run close together, and they have to be compared. *Ledum* has much of the sore bruised feeling of *Arnica* and will often take its place; but Hypericum and *Ledum* come together for consideration when an injury to a nerve has taken on inflammatory action. Instead of th muscles and bones and bloodvessels, as in *Arnica, Rhus* and *Calcarea,* the nerves are the sphere for these two remedies. When the finger ends or toes have been bruised or lacerated, or a nail has been torn off, or when a nerve has become pinched between a hammer and the bone in a blow, and that nerve becomes inflamed and the pain can be traced up along the nerve, and it is gradually extending toward the body from the injured part with stitching, darting pains, coming and going, or shooting up from the region of the injury toward the body, a dangerous condition is coming on. In this condition Hypericum is above all the remedies to be thought of and hardly any other medicine is likely to come in. It hardly need be said that lock-jaw is threatening.

Sometimes a vicious dog will take hold of an individual through the thumb, or through the hand or the wrist and run one of his great teeth through the radial nerve or some of its branches in the hand, causing a lacerated wound. You may not find in the earlier stages the symptoms of Hypericum, but they will develop gradually and you will have them to treat. Do not cut the arm off, but cure it. We cure all these injuries with medicines—punctured, incised, contused and lacerated wounds, painful wounds.

A wound will sometimes yawn, swell up, no tendency to heal, look dry and shiny on its edges; red; inflamed; burning, stinging, tearing pains; no healing process. That wound needs Hypericum. It prevents tetanus. Every practitioner knows that lock-jaw may develop after an injury to sentient nerves. The old school doctor is frightened by these shooting pains up the arms after an injury. A shoemaker may stick his awl into the end of his thumb or a carpenter may stick his finger with a brass tack and he does not think much of it, but the next night shooting pains extend up the arm with much violence. The allopathic physician looks upon that as a serious matter, for he sees lock-jaw or tetanus ahead. When these pains come on Hypericum will stop them, and from this stage to advanced states of tetanus with opisthotonos and lock-jaw Hypericum is the remedy. It is full of just such symptoms as are found in tetanus and such symptoms as lead to tetanus and it is full of all the manifestations of an ascending neuritis.

Again, you may have an old scar, and it comes in contact with a hard body and is injured, bruised, torn internally, smashed, and stinging, tearing pains come in that cicatrix, and it burns and stings, and there is no relief, and the pain runs toward the body along the course of nerves. A painful cicatrix with pain shooting up toward the centre of the body following up the nerves. Hypericum is the medicine for that.

Now there are other remedies—all know about *Arnica,* but be sure you keep it in its place. The first stage of the injury, where much bruising has been done, and there are none of these pains that I have described, for the first hours for bruised conditions and concussions and shocks *Arnica* is routine, because it produces states upon the human body like it had been bruised. But you will find *Arnica* only fits into that one place. *Arnica* should never be used for wounds the way the lay people use it, because if it is used in full strength it may bring on erysipelas.

Again, for bruises of bone, cartilages, tendons, insertion of tendons, bruises about cartilages and about joints, *Ruta* is better than any other remedy and if we study the proving of *Ruta* we will not be surprised, because it produces symptoms like those found in such conditions. Lingering, sore bruised places on bones, in joints and upon cartilages. But *Ledum* comes in very often as a preventive medicine. It is a preventive medicine when an accident happens to the ends of the fingers, if a patient steps on a nail or tack or sticks a splinter under a finger-nail or into the foot. If a horse picks up a nail, pull it out and give him a dose of *Ledum;* there will never be trouble, he will not have lock-jaw. These punctured wounds, rat bites, cat bites, etc., are all made safe by *Ledum;* i.e. *Ledum* prevents the shooting pains that naturally come and the nerves will never be involved. We will have no trouble if we can give it at once. Again, if the pain is a dull aching in the part that was injured, in the wound, *Ledum* is still the remedy; if it shoots from the wound up the nerve of the arm it is more like Hypericum.

A sensitive nervous woman steps on a tack during the day, and she feels all the day where the tack went in, lies down in bed and it aches so violently she cannot keep it still. *Ledum* will prevent any further trouble, but if that goes on until the morning the pains will be shooting up the leg, calling for Hypericum. I mentioned the use of *Ledum* when a horse picks up a nail. Now if a nail goes through the thin part of the hoof and strikes the coffin bone that horse is almost sure to die with tetanus; the veterinarians know nothing for it; though they poultice it and put on liniments, etc., that horse will die with tetanus; but if a dose of *Ledum* is given before the tetanus comes on it will save the animal from tetanus; after the jerking comes on *Ledum* will not do but Hypericum must be given. Hypericum belongs to lacerated wounds and when there is laceration of parts that are full of small nerves, sentient nerves give it at once. Do not waste time with *Arnica* because there is soreness, for the soreness is of much less importance than the danger from nerves in lacerated wounds. In punctured wounds give *Ledum* at once. Whatever sequences come on, of course, have to be met in accordance with the state and symptoms of the case.

Injuries of the spine give us another class of troubles requiring Hypericum. I remember a case such as has been met with quite often and such as we read of and hear about, one, however, that was not saved. A sudden lurch the car caused a man who was standing on the rear end of the car to be hurled back on his coccyx. He did not think much of it, went home, had pains in the head and various parts of the body. Several physicians were called; nobody could find out what was the matter with him, and at the end of ten days he died. They turned him over and found that his coccyx was black and an abscess was threatening in the muscular region. If it had been known Hypericum would have saved his life. Many times I have seen Hypericum cure similar conditions. Injuries of the coccyx are among the most serious and troublesome injuries that the physician comes in contact with; injuries just like that, falling back and striking a stone, or something that bruises the coccyx. Very little is found immediately in the coccyx; close examination reveals nothing more than soreness upon pressure, but many times we do have the description of pains shooting up the spine and down the extremities, shooting pains over the body and often convulsive movements. When such symptoms are present any physician ought to be wise enough to find out an injury, but even very astute physicians are blinded over injuries of the coccyx. Many a woman sustains an injury of the coccyx during labor, and however slight, soreness remains for years afterwards, and she is always in trouble, always hysterical and nervous, from this injury of the coccyx. Such injuries, if taken early, can be cured by Hypericum. It is in the remedy. Slight inflammation or irritation of the lower part of the cord; it feels lacerated, and sore, and aches and never passes over until the results of the injury right in the spot have been removed. These injuries have been cured in after years by *Carbo animalis, Silica* and *Thuja* and other remedies as indicated.

It is related also to injuries of the spine higher up. It is not an uncommon thing for a man, while going down stairs, to fall backward, his feet to slip from under him and he strikes his back upon one of the steps and undergoes a sharp injury. Some will at once give *Rhus tox.;* I have known others to give *Arnica.* Hypericum is to be given at once to prevent the kind of inflammation that may come from such an injury. Then there will be other tendencies, such as drawings and rheumatic symptoms, that will come on, calling for *Rhus* and finally *Calcarea.* Old weaknesses of the back, with painfulness on rising from a seat, are often cured by *Rhus,* followed by *Calcarea,* but Hypericum must first of all take care of the condition of the fibres of the cord and meninges. Meningeal troubles are common from injuries of that class, with drawing of the muscles of the back, a feeling of contraction or tightening. Stitching, shooting pains in the back in various directions; they shoot down the limbs. Injuries of the back are not so likely to end in tetanus as the injuries of the sensory nerves; but they are sometimes even more troublesome because they linger so long.

Persons who have been injured in the spine or about the coccyx linger along for years with symptoms that would lead to many remedies. We find in the provings such symptoms as occur after these injuries, and, of course, this remedy will cure anything that its proving justifies. Its action is upon the nerve sheaths and meninges, with stitching, tearing, rending pains along the nerves, wherever there are injuries. Now, there is another remedy that we want to know. If you have a clear-cut or incised wound made with a sharp instrument, or if you have made such an opening with your knife while practicing surgery, if you have opened the abdominal cavity and the walls of the abdomen take on an unhealthy look, and there are stinging, burning pains, *Staphisagria* is the remedy that will make granulation come immediately. *Staphisagria* is also a wonderfully useful remedy where the sphincter stretchers have been. *Staphisagria* is the natural antidote to stretching. When the urethra of a woman has been stretched for stone in the bladder, *Staphisagria* is useful. I remember a case of stretching of the urethra; after the operation the patient was in great distress, screaming and crying, bathed in a cold sweat, head hot and body in cold sweat. *Staphisagria* was given to her, and in a few minutes she went to sleep. She had been six hours in that suffering without any relief whatever. Where coldness, congestion of the head, and rending, tearing pains occur from stretching sphincters, or from tearing parts, for the purpose of operation, death is likely to occur, and *Staphisagria* is closely related to that tearing, lacerating and stretching of fibres which causes such suffering.

After a surgical operation, where there has been much cutting, a great state of prostration, coldness, oozing of blood, almost cold breath, of course the Materia Medica man, if there is one around, will say, "Why, give him *Carbo veg.,* of course." Yes, you will, but it will not help him. It may, disappoint you. But if you are a surgeon, know your surgical therapeutics better than a Materia Medica man, you will say, "No, *Strontium carb,* is what I want." It relieves that congestion all over the body; he gets warm and has a comfortable night. *Strontium carb.* is the *Carbo veg.* of the surgeon.

Lastly, we sometimes have to antidote chloroform, and because there are pains and aches you will get no action from these medicines; you can antidote your chloroform almost instantly by a dose of *Phosphorus,* because it is the natural antidote of chloroform. *Phosphorus* will stop the vomiting. *Phosphorus* has vomiting like that of chloroform. *Phosphorus* likes cold things, cold water in the stomach, and vomits as soon as water has become warm in the stomach. So does chloroform. Why should they not antidote each other?

IGNATIA

Ignatia is frequently required and is especially suited to sensitive, deli-cate women and children; to hysterical women. You will not cure the natural hysterics with Ignatia, but you will cure those gentle, sensitive, fine fibred, refined, highly educated, overwrought women in their nervous complaints with Ignatia when they take on complaints that are similar to such symptoms as come in hysteria. The hysterical diathesis is one that is very singular and difficult to comprehend. But a woman, when overwrought and overexcited and emotional, will do things that she herself cannot account for. She will do things as if she were crazy in her excitement. Will do things she regrets, while the hysteric is always glad, of it. No matter how much foolishness there is in it she has only made an exhibition that she is proud of. But our efforts go out for those who imitate them unconsciously. Those who will to do well.

A woman has undergone a controversy at home. She has been disturbed, is excited, and goes into cramps, trembles and quivers. Goes to bed with a headache. Is sick. Ignatia will be her remedy. When she has great distress; unrequited affections. A sensitive, nervous young girl finds out that she has misplaced her affections; the young man has disappointed her; she has a weeping spell, headache, trembles, is nervous, sleepless; Ignatia will make her philosophical and sensible. A woman loses her child, or her husband. A sensitive, delicate woman, and she suffers from this grief. She has headaches, trembles, is excited, weeps, is sleepless; unable to control herself. In spite of her best endeavors, her grief has simply torn her to pieces. She is unable to control her emotions and her excitement. Ignatia will quiet her and tide her over the present moment. In all of these instances where all of these conditions brought on from such troubles keep coming back, where your patient dwells upon them, dwells upon the cause, and the state. keeps recurring, *Natrum mur.* will finish up the case. It will nerve her up and help her to bear her sufferings. Especially useful in constitutions that have been overwrought at school, in science, music, art. Of course, it is natural for very sensitive girls to go into the arts, such as music, painting, etc. A daughter comes back from Paris after a number of years close application to her music. She is unable to do anything. She flies all to pieces. Every noise disturbs her. She cannot sleep nights. Excitable, sleepless, trembles, jerks, cramps in the muscles; weeps from excitement, and from every disturbing word. Ignatia will tone her up wonderfully. Sometimes it will complete the whole case. But especially in these oversensitive girls is *Natrum mur.* very commonly the chronic. It is the natural chronic of Ignatia. When the troubles keep coming back, and Ignatia comes to a place when it will not hold any longer.

Another place where Ignatia and *Natrum mur.* run close together. A sensitive, overtired girl, after she has been working in music, and in art, and in school, and has tired herself out, is unable to control her affections. Her affections rest on some one whom she would despise: That may be a singular thing, one may not be able to undestand it. A sensitive girl, though she would not let anyone but her mother know of it, falls in love with a married man. She lies awake nights, sobs. She says, "Mother, why do I do that, I cannot keep that man out of my mind." At other times a man entirely out of her station, that she is too sensible to have anything to do with, she just thinks about him. Ignatia, if it is very recent, will balance up that girl's mind. If not, *Natrum mur.* comes in as a follower. We do not know half as much about the human mind as we think we do. We only know its manifestations. These little things belong to this sphere of the action of this medicine. The one who knows the Materia Medica applies it in its breadth and its length, and sees in it that which is similar.

Ignatia has quivering in the limbs. Nervous, tremulous excitement. "Weakness of the body coming on suddenly. Hysterical debility and fainting fits. Fainting in a crowd." It is especially useful in the tearful, nervous, sad, yielding, sensitive minds. "Jerking and twitching. Convulsive twitchings." Children are convulsed in sleep after punishment. "Convulsions in children in the first period of dentition. Spasms in children from fright." The child is cold and pale, and has a fixed staring look, like *Cina.* "Convulsions with loss of consciousness. Violent convulsions. Tetanic convulsions. Tetanus after fright. Emotional chorea. After fright, or grief." Choreic girls. Emotional epilepsy, or epileptiform manifestations. Paralytic weakness. "Great mental emotion." Nursing; night watching. A loss of one arm with as perfect paralysis as if it had come from a cerebral hæmorrhage. In a few hours this passes off, and the arm is as well as ever. That is a hysterical paralysis. "Numbness of one or the other arm. Tingling and prickling in the arm."

Ignatia is full of surprises. If you are well acquainted with sickness, well acquainted with pathological conditions and their manifestations, you are then able to say whether you should or should not be surprised. You are then able to say what is unnatural, what is common to sickness. In Ignatia you find what is unnatural, and what is unexpected. You see an inflamed joint, or an inflamed part where there is heat, redness, throbbing, and weakness; you will handle it with great care for fear it will he painful. Ordinarily you have a perfect right to expect it would be painful. But you find it is not painful, and sometimes ameliorated by hard pressure. Is not that a surprise? You look into the throat. It is tumid, inflamed, red; the patient complains of a sore throat and pain. Naturally you will not touch it with your tongue depressor for fear it will hurt. You have every reason to suppose that the swallowing of solids will be painful. But you ask the patient when the pain is present, and the patient will say: "When I am not swallowing anything solid." The pain is ameliorated by swallowing anything solid, by the pressure. It pains all other times.

Mentally, the patient does the most unaccountable and most unexpected things. Seems to have no ruic. to work by, no philosophy, no soundness of mind, and no judgment. The opposite of what would be expected, then, will be found. The patient is better lying on the painful side. Instead of increasing the pain, it relieves the pain. "Pain like a nail sticking into the side of the head." The only comfort that is felt is by lying upon it, or pressing upon it, and that makes it go away.

The stomach is just as strange in its indigestion. Some day or other you will have a queer patient, vomiting everything taken into the stomach, and you will have her try gentle food, a little toast, and the simplest possible things, because she has been vomiting for days and people begin to worry about it for fear she will starve to death. You try this, and you try that, and she can keep nothing down. Finally she says, "If I could only have some cole slaw and some chopped onions, I think I could get along all right." It is a hysterical stomach, and the patient eats some raw cabbage and some chopped onions, and from that time on she is well. Those strange things that are ordinarily hard to digest ameliorate the nausea rather than increase it. While milk and toast, and delicate things, and warm things, such as are usually taken, disturb the stomach and increase the nausea. Cold food is craved, and cold food will be digested when warm food will be disturbing and create indigestion.

The cough has similar features in it. An irritation will come in the throat, as a rule, that is why people cough. People cough from smarting in the larynx and trachea, from irritation, from tickling, and from a sensation of fulness or a desire to expel something, and this is better by coughing. But when the irritation in the larynx and trachea comes in the Ignatia patient you have the unexpected again; because the more she coughs the more the irritation to cough is observed, until the irritation is so great and the cough is so great that she goes into spasms. It has been known of an Ignatia patient, that the more she coughed the greater the irritation to cough, and she was drenched with sweat, sitting up in bed with her night-clothes drenched, gagging and coughing and retching, covered with sweat and exhausted. When you are called to the bedside of such a patient, don't wait. You cannot get her to stop coughing long enough to say anything to you about it, only you will see the cough has grown more violent; Ignatia stops it at once. Without any provocation whatever a spasmodic condition will come on in the larynx. Any little disturbance, a mental disturbance, a fright, or distress, or a grievance, will bring a young, sensitive woman home and to her bed, and she will go on with a spasm of the larynx. It is a laryngismus stridulus that can be heard all over the house. Ignatia stops it at once (*Gelsemium, Moschus*).

Nervous affections and troubles of all sorts come on at the menstrual period. The mind is always in a hurry, in a state of excitement. No one can do things rapidly enough. The memory is untrustworthy. The mind flies all to pieces. It is a sort of confusion. No longer able to classify the things that have been classically put into the mind. Cannot remember her music, and her rules, and her scholastic methods. They have all vanished, and she is in a state of confusion. She is a worn-out, nervous person.

Then come fancies, vivid fancies, that are like delirium. Without fever, without chill. Just after excitement. She comes home from some great disturbance of her emotions, and goes into a state that, if looked upon, *per se,* would appear to be a delirium such as appears in a fever. But upon close examination it is not a delirium. It is a momentarily hysterical excitement of the mind, in which the balance is lost, and she talks about everything. Sees every manner of thing; it is a hysterical insanity, because after she rests or the next morning it has vanished. But these spells come oftener and oftener after they have once begun, and she gives way to them easier and easier, and, if they are not remedied, she becomes a lunatic, a confirmed mental wreck, so that excitement, grief, insanity, all intermingle together as cause and effect. These come first at the menstrual period, and then they come at other times, until they come from every little disturbance. Whenever she is crossed or contradicted. "She desires to be alone and to dwell on the inconsistencies that come into her life. Sits and sobs. At times she is taciturn; again, she prattles and is loquacious, and talks to herself." She comes into a state in a little while where she delights to bring on her fits and to make a scare The natural hysteric is born with that, and Ignatia will do her no good. But when this is brought on from conditions described, Ignatia is of the greatest benefit. It runs closely along by the side of *Hyoscyamus.* "A feeling of continuous fright, or apprehensiveness that something is going to happen."

With all these mental states she has a feeling of *emptiness in the stomach* and abdomen. Emptiness and trembling. "Melancholy after disappointed love, with spinal symptoms." "Great grief after losing persons or objects very near. Trembling of the hands disturbs her very much in writing. Dread of every trifle." She goes into a state where she is utterly unable to undertake anything, even to write a letter to a friend.

The Ignatia patient is not one that has been a simpleton, or of a sluggish mind or idiotic, but one that has become tired, and brought into such a state from over-doing and from over-excitement. From going too much. If rather feeble in body, from too much social excitement. Our present social state is well calculated to develop a hysterical mind. The typical social mind is one that is always in a state of confusion. Asks questions, not waiting for the answer. A good many remedies have this state; a lack of concentration of mind, that is what it is, but this is a peculiar kind of lack of concentration of mind. Dread, fear, anxiety, weeping, run through the remedy. "Sensitive disposition; hyperacute." Overwrought; intense.

Ignatia has another thing: "Thinks she has neglected some duty." That is very much like *Puls., Hell.* and *Hyos.,* only *Aurum* believes that she has committed a great wrong. "Thinks that she has neglected some duty." Dwells upon that much. "Melancholy after great grief."

It is full of headaches, and they are all congestive, pressing headaches, or tearing headaches, or headaches as if a nail were sticking into the side of the head or temple; ameliorated from lying upon it. The headaches are all ameliorated by heat. The patient generally is ameliorated by warmth and aggravated by cold. Wants cold things in the stomach, but warm things externally. Jerking headaches, throbbing headaches, congestive headaches. Headaches in nervous and sensitive temperaments Those whose nervous system has given way to anxiety, grief or mental work. "Headaches from abuse of coffee, from smoking, from inhaling smoke, from tobacco or alcohol." Headache from close attention. "Headache ameliorated by warmth and rest; worse, from cold winds and turning the head suddenly; worse when pressing at stool, or from jar, from hurrying, from excitement". Looking up increases the pain; moving the eyes; worse from noise, from light. "Pain in the occiput; worse from cold, better from external heat. Headache better while eating, but soon after it is worse."

"Disturbance of vision. Zigzags. Confusion of vision." Excessively nervous eyes. "Acrid tears. Weeping."

The face is distorted, convulsed, pale and sickly. Pains in the face. "Violent reading, tearing pains in the face." Let me put it this way: Some of these overwrought girls that come back from Paris, that I described, overworked in their music, will have violent face-ache, pains in the face, or some other hysterical pains. Others will come back with violent headaches; others with the mental state and confusion; others with all the hysterical manifestations. Prolonged excitement. Musical excesses. Yes, other girls come back fairly crippled with painful menstruation, ovarian pains, hysterical conditions, displacement; prolapsus of the vagina and of the rectum. "Tearing, shooting pains upwards from the anus and vagina up into the body towards the umbilicus."

Strange antipathies run through the remedy. It will be impossible for you to ever form any conclusion what one of these sensitive women will think of any proposition that is presented. You cannot depend upon her being reasonable or rational. It is best to say as little as possible about anything. Make no promises, listen, look wise, take up your travelling bag and go home after you have prescribed, because anything you say will be distorted. There is not anything you can say that will please.

Thirst when you would not expect it. Thirst during chill, but none during the fever, if she has a feverish state. It is suitable in intermittent fever. Excitable, nervous children and women with intermittent fever.

598

IODINE

This remedy, in all of its complaints whether acute or chronic, has a peculiar kind of *anxiety* that is felt both in mind and body. It seems also that this state of anxiety is attended with a thrill that goes throughout his frame unless he removes it by motion or change of position. The anxiety comes on when trying to keep still, and the more he tries to keep still the more the anxious state increases. While attempting to keep still, he is overwhelmed with impulses, impulses to tear things, to kill himself, to commit murder, to do violence. He cannot keep still and so he walks night and day. This remedy carries the same feature with it into the *Iodide of Potassium,* so that it makes the *Iodide of Potassium* patient walk. But there is this difference, the *Kali iod.* patient can walk long distances without fatigue, and the walking only seems to wear off his anxiety, whereas in Iodine there is great exhaustion; he becomes extremely exhausted from walking and sweats copiously even from slight exertion. Iodine corresponds to those cases in which it seems that there is some dreadful thing coming on; the mind threatens to give out, Insanity threatens, or the graver forms of disease are threatening, such as are present in the advanced stages of suppressed malaria, in old cases of chills, in threatened phthisis, especially abdominal.

Hypertrophy runs through the remedy. There is enlargement of the liver, spleen, ovaries, testes, lymphatic glands, cervical glands, of all the glands except the mammary glands. The mammæ dwindle while all other glands become enlarged, nodular and hard. This enlargement of the glands is especially observed among the lymphatic glands of the abdomen, the mesenteric glands.

There is this peculiar circumstance also in Iodine, viz., that while the body withers the glands enlarge. That is peculiar and will enable you to think of Iodine, because the glands grow in proportion to the dwindling of the body and the emaciation of the limbs. We find this state in marasmus. There is withering throughout the body, the muscles shrink, the skin wrinkles and the face of the child looks like that of a little old person, but the glands under the arms, in the groin and in the belly are enlarged and hard. The mesenteric glands can be felt as knots. We see the same tendency in old cases of malaria coming from the allopaths in which *Quinine* and *Arsenic* have been extensively used and the chills have kept on; the face and the upper part of the body are withered, the skin looks shrivelled and yellow; a diarrhœa has come on, the liver and spleen are enlarged and the lymphatic glands of the belly can be felt. Even in the earlier stages, when these states are only threatening, we may look forward and see that the case is progressing toward an Iodine state.

Now take a patient that is suffering from intermittent fever brought on from malaria, or damp cellars. The patient grows increasingly hot; it is not always a febrile heat, but a sensation of heat; he wants to be bathed in cold

water, wants the face and body cooled by cold sponging; he suffocates and
coughs in a. warm room, dreads heat, sweats easily and easily becomes
exhausted. It is in this kind of a constitution that acute complaints will come
on, such as acute inflammatory conditions of the mucous membranes and
gastritis, inflammation of the liver, inflammation of the spleen, diarrhœa, croup,
inflammation of the throat. The throat even becomes covered with white
spots and is tumid and red, and this extends down into the larynx; it may
even have a deposit upon it like diphtheria. Iodine has cured diphtheria,
when the exudation resembling the diphtheria exudations was present in the
stool. A constitution tending this way may bring on croup with an exudate,
and we can see that it is going towards Iodine. In every region of the body
peculiar little things come out. If we do not see to the full extent the
constitution of the remedy, we will not recognize the tendency of the patient
when progressing unfavorably.

The *mental state* of this patient is that of excitement, anxiety, impulses,
melancholy; he wants to do something, wants to hurry; he has impulses to
kill. In this it is very closely related to *Arsenicum* and *Hepar.* The *Arsenicum*
and *Hepar* patients also have impulses to commit murder without being
offended and without cause. The sensitiveness to heat will at once decide,
for while Iodine is warm-blooded the *Arsenicum* and *Hepar* patients are
always chilly. The impulse to do violence is sudden. There are remedies that
have peculiar impulses, impulses without any cause. These impulses are
seen in cases of impulsive insanity; an insanity in which there is an impulse
to do violence and strange things, and when the patient is asked why he
does these things he says he does not know. The patient may not be known
to be insane in anything else; he may be a good business man. Remedies also
have this. These things are forerunners. It is recorded under *Hepar* that a
barber had an impulse to cut the throat of his patron with the razor while
shaving him. The *Nux vomica* patient has an impulse to throw her child into
the fire, or to kill her husband whom she dearly loves. The thought comes
into her mind and increases until she becomes actually insane and beyond
control and the impulse is carried into action. A *Natrum sulph.* patient will
say, "Doctor, you do not know how I have to resist killing myself. An impulse
to do it comes into my mind." Iodine has the impulse to kill, not from anger,
not from any sense of justice, but without any cause. An overwhelming
anger is often a cause for violence but the impulses are not of that sort in
Iodine. While reading or thinking placidly at times a patient may have an
impulse to do himself violence, and this finally grows until the end is a form
of impulsive insanity.

The Iodine patient becomes weak in mind as well as in body; he is forgetful,
cannot remember the little things, they pass out of the mind. He forgets what

he was about to say or do; goes off and leaves packages he has purchased
The forgetfulness is extensive. But with all these states, do not forget one
thing, that the patient is compelled to keep doing something in order to drive
away his impulses and anxiety. The anxiety is wearing and distressing unless
he keeps busy. Though mentally prostrated, he is compelled to keep busy to
continue the work, which increases the prostration of mind. You tell a man
who is threatened with softening of the brain, from overwork, from anxiety
and labor in literary work, "You must stop working, you must rest." "Why,"
he will say, "if I do I would die or go mad." Such a state comes under Iodine
and *Arsenicum,* but there is one grand distinction by which the two remedies
are seen to part company at once. The Iodine patient is warm-blooded, wants
a cool place to move in, and to think in, and to work in, whereas the *Arsenicum*
patient wants heat, wants a warm room, wants to be warmly clothed, and
suffers from the cold. Iodine suffers from the heat. So that while the
restlessness and anxiety, which are both of body and mind in each remedy
loom up before the mind as one, if the patient is a hot-blooded patient we
would never think of *Arsenicum;* if a cold-blooded and shivering patient we
would never think of Iodine.

Among the generals we first mentioned was the tendency to enlarged
glands. Iodine has often cured a group of symptoms coming in the consti
tution that I have named, viz.; enlargement of the heart, enlargement of the
thyroid and protruding eyeballs. Now, if you have one of these patient
(suppose it has been sent to you by somebody who knows no better than to
call it exophthalmic goitre), those things that are so essential to the name of
the disease, as they call it, would not be an indication for the remedy, but the
indications would be found among those circumstances that I have given you
that are outside of the projection of the eyes, the enlargement of the thyroid
the hypertrophy of the heart and the cardiac disturbances. If the patient i
emaciated, is sallow, suffers from heat, has enlarged glands, and the othe
symptoms of this medicine, you may expect after its administration an ultimat
cessation of the group of symptoms that are selected to name the disease by

Brain troubles, acute and chronic, sometimes call for Iodine. The hea
throbs, the body throbs, there are pulsations all over, and the throbbin
extends to the finger ends and the toes; throbbing in the pit of the stomach
heavy pulsations felt in the arms, pulsations in the back, throbbing in th
temporal bone. There are congestive headaches with violent pain. The hea
pains are aggravated from motion, but the *patient* is relieved from motion
The patient moves because his anxiety is relieved by motion, but every motio
increases the head pains and the pulsation. Such distinctions are necessary
To distinguish between what is predicated of the patient and what is predicate
of a part is an essential in the study of the Materia Medica. Everything tha

is predicated of the patient is general, everything that is predicated of a part is particular. The two may be opopsite, and hence the student of the Materia Medica will sometimes be worried because he will find aggravation from motion and relief from motion recorded under the same remedy. It is only from the sources of the Materia Medica, *i.e.*, the provings, and from the administration of the remedy that we may observe what is true of a part and what is true of the whole. We find at times a patient wants to be in a hot room with the head out of the window for relief of the head. In that case the head is relieved from cold and the body is relieved from heat. This is a typical symptom of *Phosphorus*. which has relief from cold as to the head and stomach symptoms, but aggravation from cold as to its chest and body symptoms. So, if the *Phosphorus* patient has vomiting and head symptoms, he says: "I want to go. out in the open air and I want to take cold things into my stomach;" but if he has chest symptoms and pain in the extremities, he says: "I want to go into the house and keep warm." And just as we see this in patients it is so in the study of a remedy; we must discriminate.

As you may expect, all sorts of *eye troubles* are present in this debilitated constitution. The so-called scrofulous affections of the eyes, with ulceration of the cornea, catarrhal troubles, discharge from the eyes, with ulceration of the cornea, catarrhal troubles, discharge from the eyes, enlargement of the little glands of the lids, come along with the emaciation and yellow countenance in the constitution described. Optical illusions in bright colors. An œdematous state is in keeping with Iodine. There is œdematous swelling of the lids and œdematous swelling of the face under the eyes. Iodine has also œdema of the hands and feet, and carries this tendency with it into the *Iodide of Potassium*, which has œdematous swellings like those we find in kidney affections. It is capable of putting a stop to cases of Bright's disease in the early stages.

Another grand feature that runs through the complaints of Iodine is *hunger*. He is always *hungry*. The eating of the ordinary and regular meals is not sufficient. He eats between meals and yet is hungry. Moreover the complaints are better after eating. All the fears, the anxiety and distress of Iodine increase when he is hungry. There is pain in the stomach when the stomach is empty, and he is driven to eat. While eating he forgets his complaints, because it is like doing something, it is like moving, his mind is upon something else. He is relieved while eating and he is relieved while in motion. In spite of the hunger and much eating *he still emaciates*. "Living well yet growing thin," was one of Hering's key-notes of Iodine. As in *Natr. mur.* and *Abrotanum*, he emaciates while he has at the same time an enormous appetite. The nutrition is so disturbed that there is no making of flesh, and hence the emaciation.

The *catarrhal condition* of the nose is worthy of notice. The Iodine patient has loss of the sense of smell. The mucous membrane is thickened;

he takes cold upon the slightest provocation; is always sneezing and has from the nose a copious watery discharge. Ulceration in the nose with bloody crusts; he blows blood from the nose. The nose is stuffed up so that he cannot breathe through it. This increases every time he takes cold, and he is continually taking cold hence he becomes a confirmed subject of catarrh. I have described the general state. The patient is the first to be thought of. His constitution is the first thing to know, *i.e.*, what is true of the patient as a whole. After that we can find out what is true of each of his parts. The mucous membrane of the nose is constantly in a state of ulceration, or has a tendency to ulceration. Sometimes these little ulcers are deep.

There are aphthous patches along the tongue and throughout the mouth. The whole buccal cavity is studded with aphthous patches. I have mentioned already the tendency to exudation; white velvety, or white greyish or pale ash-colored exudations come upon the sore throat, all over the mucous membrane of the nose and all over the pharynx. The pharynx seems to be lined with the velvety, ash-colored appearances. With these throat symptoms and the tendency to ulceration it has a wide range of usefulness in throat affections. It is useful in enlargement of the tonsils when the tonsils are studded with exudations and in the constitution described. Enlarged tonsils in hungry withered patients. We often see one who is subject to quinsy progressing toward the Iodine state. He is always suffering from the heat like a *Pulsatilla* patient; at times in the earlier stages, before any organic changes have taken place, you may mistake Iodine for *Pulsatilla*. But if you watch the patient you will observe the tendency to emaciation and see that the two remedies soon part company. They are both hot, they are both irritable, they are both full of notions. The *Pulsatilla* patient is far more whimsical, more tearful, has greater sadness, and has constant loss of appetite, while the Iodine subject wants to eat much. The *Pulsatilla* patient often increases in flesh, although growing increasingly nervous. The Iodine, patient becomes thin, has a ravenous hunger cannot be satisfied, suffers from his hunger; he must eat every few hours and feels better after eating; he has also great thirst. If he goes long without eating, no matter what the complaints are, the suffering will increase. Any of the complaints of Iodine will likely be increased by fasting.

Iodine has also an indigestion that comes from overeating. The food sours, he is troubled with sour eructations, with much flatulence, with belching, with undigested stools, with diarrhœa, watery, cheesy stools, and he digests less and less. The digestion becomes more and more feeble until he digests almost nothing of what he eats, and yet the craving increases. He vomits and diarrhœa comes on and so he increasingly emaciates; because it is like burning the candle at both ends. It is not surprising that he is extremely weak because he is assimilating very little of what he takes. The articles of food act as foreign substances to disorder his bowels and stomach. Now, with this trouble going on, the liver and spleen become hard and enlarged, and the patient becomes jaundiced. The stool is hard, and lumpy and white, or colorless, or clay colored, sometimes soft and pappy; there seems to be little or no bile in it. This stage gradually increases until hypertrophy of the liver comes on. Finally the abdomen sinks in and reveals this enlargement of the liver and the enlarged lymphatic glands. These are very knotty and as hard as in tabes mesenterica. Iodine is indicated in the tubercular condition of the mesenteric glands with diarrhœa, emaciation, great hunger, great thirst, withering of the mammary glands, a dried beef-like or shrivelled appearance of the skin and sallow complexion. If the remedy is given early enough, before the structural changes have occurred, it will check the progress of the disease and cure.

This is a very useful remedy in the *chronic morning diarrhœa* of emaciated, scrofulous children.

When the constitutional state is present it is primary to the varying kinds of stools that it is possible for the patient to have. So if you have a marked state of the constitution, a case in which there are a great number of general symptoms for you to associate the remedy with, the little symptoms of the diarrhœa cease to be important. The constitutional state in that patient is that which is "strange, rare and peculiar". Almost any kind of diarrhœic stool will be cured if the constitutional state is covered by the remedy. When it is an acute diarrhœa and it occurs in a vigorous constitution, and there is nothing but the diarrhœa, then it is necessary to know all the finer details, and the characteristics of the diarrhœa become the rare, "strange" and "peculiar" features.

Incontinence of urine in old people. In the male with all these constitutional symptoms Iodine is especially suited when the testes have dwindled, when there is impotency, when there is flowing of semen with dreams, when there is loss of sexual instinct or power, or with an irritated state, an erethism of the sexual instinct; also when the testes are enlarged and hard, indurated and hypertrophied like the other glands, or when there is an orchitis, an inflammation and enlargement of the testicles.

Swelling and induration of the uterus and ovaries. Iodine has cured tumors of the ovaries in such a constitution as I have described. It has cured the dwindling of the mammary glands and caused them to grow plump with an increase of flesh upon dwindling patients.

Its nature to produce the catarrhal state is illustrated in the *leucorrhœa* that it produces. Uterine leucorrhœa with swelling and induration of the cervix. Uterus enlarged, tendency to menorrhagia. Leucorrhœa rendering the thighs sore. The discharges of Iodine are acrid. The discharges from the nose excoriate the lip, the discharges from the eyes excoriate the cheek, the discharges from the vagina excoriate the thighs. The leucorrhœa is thick and slimy and sometimes bloody; "chronic leucorrhœa, most abundant at the time of the menses, rendering the thighs sore and corroding the linen."

This remedy has a cough that is violent; it has grave and severe difficulties of respiration, dyspnœa, with chest symptoms. Croupy, suffocating cough in this delicate constitution. Again we say if you do not hold in mind the constitutional state while reading these very numerous respiratory symptoms, you will not be able to apply them because they are extensive and include a great many so-called complaints and would give you difficulty in individualizing them.

Now, there is one more complaint that I wish to call your attention to. In old gouty constitutions, with enlargement of the joints, the history is that the patients were once in a good state of flesh, but they have become lean, and although they are hungry, the food does not seem to do them good. The joints are enlarged and tender. Many gouty constitutions want a warm room, but the Iodine patient wants a cool room. His joints pain and are aggravated from the warmth of bed. He cheers up in a cool place and likes to be in the open air. He is growing increasingly weak; he is generally ameliorated on moving about and eating, he has the anxiety of body and mind. Iodine will put a check on his gouty attacks and cause him to go on comfortably for a while.

IPECACUANHA

Ipecac. has a wide sphere of action among acute sicknesses. Most of its acute complaints commence with nausea, *vomiting*. The febrile conditions commence with pain in the back between the shoulders, extending down the back, as if it would break, with or without rigors, much fever, vomiting of bile and seldom any thirst. This is the general aspect of the beginning of an Ipecac. fever or gastric trouble or chill in intermittents or bilious attacks.

The stomach is disordered. There is a sense of fulness in the stomach, cutting pains in the stomach and below the stomach, going from left to right. The cutting pain in colic goes from left to right. The patient is unable to stir or breathe until that pain passes off. It holds him transfixed in one position coming like the stabbing of a knife in the region of the stomach, or above the navel, going from left to right, and is attended with prostration and nausea.

All the complaints in Ipecac. are attended more or less with *nausea;* every little pain and distress is attended with nausea. The sufferings seem to centre about the stomach, bringing on nausea. There is continuous nausea and gagging. The cough causes nausea and vomiting. It is a dry, hacking, teasing suffocative cough, accompanied by nausea and vomiting. He coughs until his face grows red, and then there is choking and gagging. With every little gush of blood from any part of the body there is nausea, fainting and sinking. Hence its value in uterine hæmorrhages; bright, red blood with nausea; a little blood is attended with fainting or syncope, but the great overwhelming nausea runs through the complaints of this remedy. Though there is sometimes thirst, it is usually absent. When Ipecac. does its best work, there is thirstlessness. With the Ipecac. fever, or with the chill, there is likely to be pain in the back of the head, a bruised pain through the head and back of the neck and sometimes down the back, and drawing in the muscles of the back of the neck. A congestive fulness in the head, a crushed feeling in the head and back of the head; the whole head aches and is full of pain.

Ipecac. is sometimes as restless as *Arsenic,* but the Ipecac prostration comes by spells, whereas the *Arsenic* prostration is continuous. You will see Ipecac. patients tossing over the bed as much as they do when they need *Rhus,* turning and tossing, and moving the hands and feet, with restlessness. This is especially the case when the spine is somewhat involved. Ipecac. has symptoms that look like tetanus; it has opisthotonos, and it has been a useful remedy in cerebro-spinal meningitis with vomiting of bile, with pain in the back of the head and neck, and drawing of the muscles of the back, retracting the head. When cerebro-spinal meningitis has gone on until the patient is emaciated, when remedies have seemed but to palliate momentarily, and the whole body is inclined backwards, and there is vomiting of everything, even the simplest article taken into the stomach, the tongue is red and raw, and there is constant nausea and vomiting of bile, Ipecac. will cure. Ipecac. cures inveterate cases of gastritis when even a drop of water will not stay down; everything put in the stomach is vomited, continuous gagging, sharp pain in the stomach, pain in the back, below the shoulder blades, as if it would break, vomiting of bile, continuous nausea and great prostration. Irritable stomach. It also cures when the abdomen is distended, and sensitive, a tympanitic state, when there is vomiting of bile. Ipecac. has proved a useful remedy in epidemic dysentery, when the patient is compelled to sit almost constantly upon the stool and passes a little slime, or a little bright red blood; inflammation of the lower portion of the bowel, the rectum and the colon. The tenesmus is awful, burning, and continuous urging with the passage of only a little mucus and blood. With this there is constant nausea; while straining at stool, the pain is so great that nausea comes on, and he vomits bile. At times, whole families are down with it. It runs through a whole valley and may be epidemic; but it commonly relates to endemics. In infants it is indicated when a cholera-like diarrhœa has been present and it ends in a dysenteric state, with continued tenesmus, and the expulsion of a little bloody mucus, the child vomiting everything it takes into the stomach; nausea, vomiting, prostration and great pallor. It is also useful in such conditions when the stool is more or less copious, and is green, and the child passes, frequently, copious quantities of green slime. Much crying when at stool, much straining, with passages of green slime, vomiting of green slime, and vomiting of green curds; milk turns green and is vomited.

The chest complaints of Ipecac. are interesting. Ipecac. is especially the infant's friend and is commonly indicated in the bronchitis of infancy. The usual bad cold that ends in chest trouble in infants is a bronchitis. It is very seldom that an infant gets a true pneumonia, it is generally a bronchitis with coarse rattling. The child coughs, gags and suffocates, and there is coarse rattling which can be heard throughout the room, and the trouble has come on pretty rapidly: The child is pale, looks dreadfully sick, and sometimes looks very anxious. The nose is drawn in as if dangerously ill, and the breathing is such as appears in a dangerous case. Ipecac. will sometimes modify this into a very simple case, break up the cold, and cure the child. In the old books; the pneumonia of infancy had a distinct and separate description, and the typical symptoms were those of Ipecac. You will see a great similarity of symptoms when you study Ipecac. and *Ant. tart.* together in chest troubles. If you have been studying them together, you will say, "How do you distinguish them; they both have rattling cough and breathing, and both have the vomiting?" Well, the Ipecac. symptoms correspond to the stage of irritation, while the *Tartar emetic* symptoms appear in the stage of relaxation. That is, the Ipecac. symptoms come on hurriedly, come on as the acute symptoms, whereas the *Tartar emetic* complaints come on slowly. The latter is seldom suited to symptoms that arise within twenty-four hours, or at least the symptoms of *Tartar emetic* that arise in twenty-four hours are not of this class. This group comes on many days later, comes on at the close of a bronchitis when there is threatened paralysis of the lungs; not in the state of irritation, not the dyspnœa from irritation, not the suffocation of that sort, but the suffocation from exudation, and from threatened paralysis of the lungs. When the lungs are too weak to expel the mucus, the coarse rattling comes on. Then there is the great exhaustion, deathly pallor of the face and sooty nostrils. We see now that these two remedies do not look alike. If we observe the pace of the two remedies, we see that the complaints differ. It is not so much that they belong to stages, although they do, but rather that Ipecac. brings on its symptoms rapidly and effects a crisis speedily, and that *Ant. tart.* brings on its symptoms slowly and effects a crisis after many days.

You can readily see the value of Ipecac. in whooping cough, for it has the paroxysmal character, the red face, and vomiting and gagging with the cough. The red face, thirstlessness, violent whooping, with convulsions, with gagging and vomiting of all that he eats are the symptoms that you will generally find.

I have hinted at the hæmorrhages, and these open out a great field for Ipecac. I could not practice medicine without Ipecac., because of its importance in hæmorrhages. When I say hæmorrhages, I do not mean those from cut arteries, I do not mean hæmorrhages where surgery must come in; I mean such as uterine hæmorrhages, hæmorrhages from the kidneys, from the bowels, from the stomach, from the lungs. You must know your remedies in hæmorrhages; if you do not, you will be forced to use mechanical means; but the homoeopathist who is well instructed is able to do without them. In the severest form of uterine hæmorrhages the homœopathic physician is able to do without mechanical means, except when mechanical means are causing the hæmorrhage. This does not relate to hourglass contractions, it does not relate to conditions when the after birth is retained, or when the uterus has a foreign substance in it, because under such circumstances manipulation is necessary. A distinction must be made. But when we have simply the pure dynamic element to consider, simply and purely a relaxed surface that is bleeding, the remedy is the only thing that will do the work properly. When the uterus is continuously oozing, but every little while the flow increases to a gush, and with every little gush of bright red blood the woman thinks she is going to faint, or there is gasping, and the quantity of the flow is not sufficient to account for such prostration, nausea, syncope, pallor, Ipecac. is the remedy. When with the gushing of bright red blood there is an overwhelming fear of death, *Aconite*. If your patient while going through the confinement has had a hot head, an uncontrollable thirst for ice cold water, and after the confinement, everything has gone on in an orderly way, and the placenta has been delivered, and although you have no reason to expect such hæmorrhage it comes on, *Phosphorus* will nearly always be the remedy. In those withered women, lean and slender, who are always suffering from the heat, who want the covers off and want to be cool, who have had a tendency to ooze blood from the uterus, and now have a hæmorrhage that is alarming, either with clots, or only an oozing of dark, liquid blood, you can hardly do without *Secale*. A single dose of any one of these medicines on the tongue will check a hæmorrhage more quickly than large doses of strong medicine. The hæmorrhage will be checked so speedily that in your earlier experiences you will be surprised. You will wonder if, it is not possible that it stopped itself. In copious menstruation Ipecac. is often indicated when the woman has taken cold, or has a shock. In cases where she is not especially subject to copious uterine flow at the menstrual period, she is naturally alarmed, for it is something she has never had before, and the flow is likely to continue for many days, attended with this weakness. All her power seems to go with a little gush of blood. Ipecac.

will cure and end the menstrual flow normally. A fortunate thing in nature is the tendency to check hæmorrhage, which is always good. There are a large number of medicines that control hæmorrhage, and these you must keep at your finger's ends. They belong to emergencies. You must know the remedies that correspond to violent symptoms and violent attacks. Ipecac. is full of hæmorrhage. Vomiting of great clots of blood, continuous vomiting of blood in connection with ulceration. In persons who are subject to violent attacks of bleeding, who bleed easily, who have a hæmorrhagic tendency, Ipecac. will control temporarily the hæmorrhage when the symptoms agree.

Severe pain in the back in the region of the kidneys, shooting pains, frequent urging to urinate, and the urine contains blood and little clots of blood. The urine is extremely red with blood, which settles to the bottom of the vessel, and lines the whole commode with a layer of blood the thickness of a knife blade. Every pint of urine that it contains will have that coating of blood in the vessel; every attack of pain in the kidney is attended with that condition of the urine. Ipecacuanha will stop that bleeding. It is true that when patients have bled until they have become anæmic, and are subject to dropsy, Ipecac. ceases to be the remedy; its natural follower then is *China,* which will bring the patient in a position to need an antipsoric remedy.

Then there are the "colds". Simple, common coryzas among the children. When a cold settles in the nose, and the nose is stuffed up at night, or when the adult has a coryza, with much stuffing up of the nose, blowing of mucus and blood from the nose, much sneezing, and the cold goes farther down and is followed by hoarseness, extending into the trachea with rawness, and finally into the bronchial tubes with suffocation and settling in the chest, think of Ipecac. The Ipecac. colds often begin in the nose and spread very rapidly into the chest. With these colds in the nose there is copious bleeding of bright red blood. Every time he takes cold in the nose he has copious bleeding; a tendency to nosebleed with the colds. The inflammation that comes upon the mucous membrane in Ipecac. is violent. The irritation comes on suddenly, and the mucous membrane inflames so rapidly that the parts become purple, turgescent, and bleeding seems to be the only natural relief. Stoppage of the nose and loss of smell; the nose becomes so stuffed up that he cannot breathe through it.

With the head symptoms, with the colds, with the whooping cough, with the chill, and with many of the inflammatory complaints, the face becomes flushed, bright red, or bluish red, and the lips blue; with the chill the lips and the finger nails are blue. The chill is violent, sometimes congestive in character and often a rigor. The whole frame shakes, and the teeth chatter.

There are old incurable cases of asthma that are palliated by Ipecac and carry around a bottle of it from which they say they get much relief. It is useful in cases of humid asthma, in cases of asthmatic bronchitis, when they suffer from the damp weather and from sudden weather changes; every little cold rouses up this bronchial attack, and he suffocates and gags when he coughs, or spits up a little blood. He has to sit up nights to breathe, and the attacks are common and frequent. These patients say they get relief from Ipecac., and it is not surprising that Ipecac. relieves that state of asthmatic breathing, because it has such symptoms. Some of these cases are incurable, they are people advanced in life. This remedy, more wisely administered, will give more relief. A powder of Ipecac. will break up the attack, so that the patient is comfortable, and then will go on in an ordinary sort of asthmatic way, until catching another cold. The cough is rattling and asthmatic.

As a convulsive medicine Ipecac. is not well enough known. Convulsions in pregnancy. Convulsions in whooping cough; frightful spasms, affecting the whole of the left side, followed by paralysis; clonic and tonic spasms of children and hysterical women. Tetanus, rigidity of the body, with flushed redness of the face. These are strong features of Ipecac., and they have not been sufficiently dwelt upon, and the remedy is not sufficiently known as having these states so prominently. Medicines like *Belladonna* are more frequently spoken of in the books and in treatises of spasms, yet Ipecac. is just as important a remedy to be studied in relation to spasms, and its action upon the spine.

In suppressed eruptions, the symptoms will very commonly point to Ipecac. When the eruption does not come out, or an eruption has been driven back by cold, sometimes acute manifestations of stomach and bowels follow and colds settle in the chest from suppressed eruptions. Ipecac. will also cure erysipelas, when there is the vomiting, the chill, the pain in the back, the thirstlessness and the overwhelming nausea.

Ipecac is often sufficient for the nausea and vomiting, when the scarlet fever rash is slow to come out. Instead of the rash coming out as it should, Ipecac. symptoms come on in the stomach with nausea and vomiting. Ipecac. will check the nausea and vomiting, will bring out the eruption, and the disease will run a milder course.

KALI ARSENICOSUM

This is a very deep, long acting remedy, and one greatly abused by traditional medicine in the form of Fowler's Solution. It was used extensively as an antiperiodical after quinine had failed, and as a tonic, for skin diseases of all sorts, for syphilis, for anæmia, etc. It is a most positive remedy in all of these complaints, when it suits the patient's symptoms. The toxicological symptoms following the traditional abuse have furnished a broad beginning for the homœopathist to build upon. How well it was known to the good old doctor that Fowler's Solution must be stopped if the patient became pale, waxy, puffed under the eyes and was weak. Who does not knew the "fattening" powers of this drug! Horses become fat and shiny of coat after taking Fowler's Solution for a while. The jockey knew this too well. He traded off a broken-down horse as a fine animal, but the horse soon gave out; his wind was short; he would sweat easily, become weak and incapable of work. It was then said "That horse must have been jockeyed up on arsenic." The old medical journals are full of effects of overdosing with this drug. A summary of old school drugging, a few pathogenetic symptoms, and extensive clinical observation with the use of this remedy in potentized form, have given the basis of this study. Not too much reliance should be' placed upon the writer's clinical opinion; let the remedy be tested along the lines indicated until provings shall fix the finer action.

While it has morning and evening aggravation, the nights are full of sufferings; midnight especially, and from 1 to 3 a.m., there are many sufferings. The chilliness is very marked. Extreme sensitiveness to cold, and complaints are aggravated from cold, from cold air, from becoming cold, from entering a cold place. Aversion to open air. Takes cold from a draft, and from being heated. Anæmia. Chlorosis. Pale, waxy, and covered with sweat. Ascending brings on suffocation, cough, and manifests the weakness of body and limbs. Glands dwindle and the extremities become numb and prickly. Molecular death prevails extensively. Cancerous ulceration has been restrained by this remedy many times. It has cured lupus.

The weakness that it has produced is much like that found in patients looking toward phthisis and Bright's disease. Clonic spasms have been produced by it. Convulsive action of muscles with full consciousness is not uncommon. It has cured epilepsy and hysterio-epilepsy. It has caused abdominal dropsy and œdema of all the limbs, face and eyelids. While taking it there is an increase of flesh and weight, but after stopping it the prover emaciates. Most complaints are aggravated after eating and after exertion. The muscles are flabby. Faintness and fainting spells. Eating ice cream when overheated brings on many complaints. Aggravated from cold foods, cold drinks, milk and fat food. There is formication all over the body. It sets up inflammation in many organs and glands, especially the stomach. liver and kidneys. Great dread of motion. All mucous membranes become catarrhal. It is a most painful remedy; burning, stitching and tearing. The most marked periodicity is every third day. Pulsation felt all over the body. It is a deep acting antipsoric, and often useful in rheumatic and gouty affections. It has cured syphilis in the hands of the traditional doctor, and in the highest potencies it cures many specific complaints—when the symptoms agree.

Some symptoms come on first falling asleep, but during and after sleep are also marked times of aggravation. Rheumatic and gouty stiffness of all the joints and œdema of legs and feet. Swelling from inflammation of joints and glands. Trembling from noise, or sudden unexpected motion. Tension of muscles. Twitching of muscles. Extremely sensitive to touch. Ulceration of skin, especially of legs and mucous membranes, with burning and spreading. Uncovering brings on the pains, and increases many complaints. Symptoms aggravated on waking. Walking fast aggravates most symptoms, especially the breathing and weakness. Warmth ameliorates most complaints. He is so weak he cannot sit up in bed. The restlessness of arsenic is often present.

Arsenicum is stamped upon the mental symptoms. Anxiety even to great anguish, with great fear. Anxiety in the morning on waking, but most marked in the evening and during the night. He is anxious without cause, about his health; anxious before stool; wakens during the night with anxiety and fear. He fears to go to bed. He fears death, or a crowd of people, yet equally dreads being alone. Fear that something will happen. Fear of people. He is very easily frightened and startled. He has frightful delusions and sees images. He despairs of recovery. He sees dead people in his nightly delirium. His thoughts dwell upon death, and he is sure is going to die. He is very fretful, and dislikes to answer questions. He behaves like a crazy man. Fickle-minded, with confusion. Constantly discontented. Very excitable. Mental exertion intensifies mental and head symptoms. Always in a hurry, and very excitable. Many hysterical symptoms, with cramps and fainting. Indifference to all pleasure. Cannot settle upon what he wants to do. Wakens up in the morning very fretful. He is irritable during chill, and during headache. He has impulses to do violence to his friends, to kill somebody. Lamenting and bewailing. His memory is weak. He grows morose and quarrelsome, fault-finding, and scolds those about him. She is restless of mind and body, evening and night; anxious tossing all night, during chill and heat; also during menses. Sadness in the evening when alone, and during the fever. Oversensitive to noises, and especially to voices. Becomes so besides herself that she shrieks. There are long spells of silence in which she refuses to answer questions; at these times she sits even with others near her and refuses to speak. Easily startled from noise, on falling asleep and during sleep. Thinks of death and suicide. Suspicious of all her best friends. Persistent tormenting thoughts often keeping him awake at night, with feet and legs icy cold and head hot. He becomes increasingly timid. Weeping at night without cause. Weeping in sleep.

Vertigo in the evening, during headache, with nausea, and when walking in the open air.

The forehead perspires easily and complaints and pains come on from uncovering the head. There are congestive, pulsating headaches, with electric shocks through the head. The head feels cold, and is sensitive to cold air and to drafts. The neck is stiff, and the head is drawn to one side. During the headache the head feels heavy and enlarged. Eruptions with crusts, dry or moist, form upon the scalp. It has cured many cases of eczema. From the suppression of eruptions on the scalp, many chronic periodical sick headaches have come, lasting a lifetime, or until cured with a similar remedy. These headaches begin in the afternoon and evening, very severe after midnight, worse from cold air and from a draft. Headaches caused by checking a chronic catarrh, or such as come with coryza, or with gastric disturbances. Rheumatic headaches. Congestive headaches during chill, during fever and during menses. All headaches of this remedy are aggravated after eating, while lying, during motion, from noise, after sleep, from standing, and walking in cold air; ameliorated from sitting, external heat and hot drinks, and wrapping up the head. The pains are paroxysmal, and the headaches are often periodical. The pains come in the forehead, over the eyes and in occiput, and in parietal bones. Sides of head become sore. Burning, stitching and tearing are most common pains. Pressing outward over the eyes, and stitching on coughing. Tearing over eyes and in occiput. Many of these headaches come from suppressed malaria, and it will be stated that these headaches began after having been cured(?) of ague. This remedy is an excellent antidote to the abuse of quinine.

Catarrhal conditions of the eyes, excoriating mucous discharges, and the lids stick together in the morning. The veins are injected, the balls feel enlarged, and there is free lachrymation. The eyes look glassy, pale, fishy. Opening of the lids difficult because of dryness. Œdema under the eyes, and the lids are swollen. Ulceration of the cornea. The eyes are jaundiced, and tears acrid. Staring, fixed, startled look. Spots on the cornea. Redness of the eyes and lids. Pains at night, worse from motion and reading, and ameliorated from warmth. The pains are burning, tearing and pressing. Sensation of sand in the eyes. Smarting in eyes while reading. There are colors in the field of vision, green and yellow. Vision is dim and foggy. Sparks before the eyes. Asthenopia. Vision lost.

The ears tingle, and are hot. Ears swollen. Eruptions on ears. Ears cold. Otorrhœa, bloody, fetid and yellow. Itching deep in auditory canal. Noises in the ears; buzzing, cracking, humming, ringing, roaring, rushing; after quinine. Earache evening and night, ameliorated by heat; aggravated in cold air. The pains are burning, stitching and tearing. The hearing is at first acute, later impaired, and finally lost.

This remedy cures chronic nasal catarrh that has lasted from childhood, when the discharge is excoriating, bloody, burning, greenish, thick or yellow. It is purulent and offensive. Dryness in nose nights. The nose is obstructed. Epistaxis. Itching of nose, and inside of nose. Sneezing, frequent and violent.

Cachectic, anxious, frightened look. Pale, waxy and chlorotic. Lips pale. Lips bluish, or even black. Dark circles below the eyes. The face is sunken and pinched. Face covered with eruptions; eczema, herpes, scurfs, vesicles. Furfuraceous eruption in the beard. Eruptions on nose, and about the mouth. The face is sickly, haggard and suffering. Itching of the face. Inflammation of the paratoid and submaxillary glands. Much perspiration on face. Twitching of the muscles of the face. Ulcers on face and lips. Epithelioma of lips. Œdema of face. Swollen lips. Pain in face in cold air, ameliorated by heat. Rheumatic and neuralgic pains, coming periodically. The pains are burning, stitching and tearing.

Aphthæ and ulcers in mouth. Dryness of mouth and tongue. Tongue is red, and coated white. Inflammation of tongue. Bleeding gums. Offensive odors from mouth. Burning, raw mouth and tongue. Excoriation of tongue. Swollen gums and tongue. Taste bad, bitter, insipid, putrid, sour, sweetish. Vesicles in mouth and on tongue.

The teeth are sore, and there is pain on masticating. Pain in teeth from cold drinks, during menses, extending to ear, head and temples; ameliorated by warmth. Pulsating, tearing pains in teeth.

Sensation in throat and larynx as if forced asunder. Inflammation, with heat and dryness. Lump rising from stomach to throat, like globus hystericus, ameliorated by eructations. Choking, with copious flow of saliva. Roughness, and scraping in the throat. Spasms of the œsophagus. Swallowing is very difficult and painful. There are burning, soreness and stitching in throat. Ulcers in throat.

A multitude of sufferings is found in the stomach. Great anxiety. An anxiety from stomach to spine, with palpitation. Appetite ravenous, or wanting. Aversion to food and meat. Coldness in the stomach. Desires sour things, sweets, warm drinks. The digestion is poor and the stomach is easily disordered, with distension from flatulence. Empty, sinking sensation and faintness. Eructations after eating, bitter, empty, of food, or sour fluid; waterbrash. Fulness after eating. Heaviness after eating like a stone. Heartburn. The most obstinate form of gastritis, acute and chronic. Loathing of food. With most complaints there is intense nausea. It has nausea during chill, after cold drinks, during cough, after dinner, after eating, during headache, during menses, and during stool. It has cured nausea during pregnancy. The pains are burning, cramping, cutting, pressing, soreness, stitching; and they come on at night and are worse after food, and cold drinks; and ameliorated by heat. Retching on coughing. Pulsating in stomach. Tightness felt in stomach. Thirst extreme during heat, and for warm drinks during chill. In chronic complaints it is thirstless, like Arsenicum. Vomiting bile, food, mucus, sour, watery; aggravated morning and during night, on coughing, after drinking cold water, after eating, with headache.

Coldness felt in whole abdomen; must have much warmth. Distension of abdomen after eating. Tympanitic distension and dropsy. Flatulent distension. Inflammation of intenstines with ulceration, and of peritoneum. The abdomen is very painful at night. Pain on coughing, during diarrhœa, after eating, during menses, during stool. Pains all paroxysmal and violent, ameliorated by warmth. Pain in liver, hypogastrium. Gall-stone colic. The whole abdomen burns. Cramping before stool, and constant desire for stool. Cutting in abdomen and liver. Pressing pain in liver. Soreness in abdomen and liver. Stitching in abdomen, liver and groin. Pulsating in abdomen. Great uneasiness in abdomen. Rumbling before stool. Twitching of the muscles of abdomen.

There is some constipation, alternating with diarrhœa. Constriction of the anus. Violent diarrhœa at night, after midnight, after cold drinks, after eating, after milk. Much pain during and after stool. Involuntary stool. Itching and excoriation about the anus. Hemorrhoids, and bleeding from the anus. External and internal piles, aggravated walking. Burning as with a red hot iron, with piles, and diarrhœa, during and after stool. The pains are cutting, pressing, soreness, stitching. There is tenesmus during and after stool. Paralysis and ineffectual urging for stool. Catarrh of the colon.

Stool is acrid, black, bloody, brown, copious, frothy; or scanty, watery, white and frothy; or hard, dry, dark, knotty. Sometimes light colored, offensive, or purulent, yellow.

Inflammation of the bladder. Retention of urine. Urging to urinate at night, constant, frequent, ineffectual. Urination is dribbling, or difficult and painful. Urination frequent at night. Incontinence. He feels that he had not finished.

Inflammation of the kidneys. Pain, cutting and stitching. Cutting along the ureters. It has been of service in Addison's disease.

Hemorrhage from the urethra, and burning during urination.

Urine albuminous during pregnancy. Urine bloody, burning, cloudy. Color of urine is black, greenish or red. Urine copious. Urine scanty with pellicle on surface. Sediment copious, mucus, pus, red. Specific gravity diminished. Urine watery and clear.

The testes are hard, painful and swollen. Seminal emissions, Erections feeble.

This remedy has greatly restrained the development of cancer of uterus. It is mentioned for cauliflower excrescence with putrid discharge. Itching of vulva, Leucorrhœa excoriating, burning, offensive, putrid, yellow; aggravated after menses. Menses absent, acrid, bright red, copious, frequent, offensive, painful, pale, protracted, scanty, suppressed. Uterine hemorrhage. Burning in the genitalia. Pain in uterus. Stitching in ovaries. Prolapsus.

Catarrh of larynx and trachea. Sensation in throat and larynx as if forced asunder. Dryness in larynx. Rawness, soreness and scraping in larynx. Hoarseness, and voice lost.

Respiration is rapid, anxious and asthmatic at night, aggravated from 2 to 3 a.m. Difficult evening and night, and aggravated 2 to 3 a.m., on coughing, on exertion, on lying, on motion, when walking. Respiration rattling, short, suffocative, wheezing and whistling.

In the cold anæmic patient there is a morning cough with copious expectoration, and a night cough that is dry. The cough is aggravated after midnight, and at 2 a.m., and 3 a.m. The cough is a hacking cough during the afternoon and evening. The cough is aggravated in cold air, on becoming cold, after cold drinks; aggravated lying in the evening, and on motion. The cough comes during chill, and fever, and with coryza. It is a choking asthmatic cough sometimes It is spasmodic and suffocative. Irritation to cough is felt in the larynx and trachea, and he coughs until exhausted.

Expectoration morning and evening, bloody, copious, difficult, greenish, purulent, viscid and yellow. It tastes bitter, sickening, putrid or sweetish.

In the chest there is great anxiety and oppression. It has cured obstinate cases of catarrh of the chest. It has constriction of chest and heart. Effusion of the pleural sac. Hemorrhage of the lungs. Inflammation of bronchial tubes, endocardium, pericardium, lungs and pleura. Cardiac and anæmic murmurs. Oppression of heart and chest. Anxious and violent palpitation. Weak feeling in chest. A most useful remedy in threatened phthisis, and especially when there are cavities in the lungs, and the patient cannot get warm even with warm clothing and in a warm room. Cannot get warm in summer; and when cold drinks bring on many symptoms. The pain in the chest is aggravated from coughing, and from inspiration. It is felt most in the sides of chest, and in the heart. The pain is burning, cutting, soreness and stitching. The stitching pains are aggravated on coughing, and on the left side.

The back is cold, and sensitive to cold air and drafts. Pain in the back during heat, and during menses. Pain in the cervical region, scapulæ and between the shoulders. Pain in lumbar region and sacrum. Aching, bruised, burning, drawing in back. Tender spine. Stiffness in the back.

Cold hands and feet. Cold feet evening in bed. Cold extremities during fever. Knees bent up by muscular contractions so he could not move his feet. Corns on the palms, and soles. Cramps in the thigh and calf. Blueness of the nails during chill. Herpes on the shoulders. Pimples and vesicles on the extremities. Fissures on the elbows and wrists. Vesicles on the upper limbs. Pimples and vesicles on the hands. Eruption on thighs and legs. Vesicles on the soles. Excoriation between the thighs. Formication of the limbs. Burning heat of feet. Heaviness of lower limbs. Insensibility of the fingers. Itching of hands, lower limbs and feet. Numbness of the extremities, hands, fingers and feet. Rheumatic and neuralgic pains in the limbs during chill, in cold air, ameliorated by heat. Aching in the shoulder. Sciatica, extending downwards.

Pain in hips, thighs, knees and legs. Pain in the knee as if bruised. Burning in hands and fingers, feet and soles. Drawing in lower limbs, knees, tibia, and feet. Stitching pains in the limbs when the legs are cold; especially knee, foot and heel. Tearing pains in shoulders, upper arms, elbows, wrist, hand and fingers; also in hip, thigh, leg and foot. Paralysis of limbs, upper and lower. Perspiration of feet. Restlessness of the lower limbs. Stiffness of knees. Dropsical swelling of hands and knees, legs and feet. Tension in the hollow of knee and hamstrings. Trembling limbs. Twitching in the thighs. Ulcers on the legs. Varicose veins on lower limbs. Weakness of all the limbs, but greatest in lower limbs.

The sleep is much disturbed by dreams, amorous, anxious, of the dead, of death, fantastic dreams, of fire, frightful, misfortune, nightmare, vivid. He is late falling asleep. The sleep is restless; he tosses and turns all night. Sleepiness afternoon and evening. Sleepless before midnight, but worse after midnight. Sleepiness, but cannot sleep. If he wakens cannot sleep again. Wakens early and cannot sleep again. Distressing yawning.

Constitutional coldness is a marked feature of this remedy. It has intermittent fever with chill, fever and sweat. The chill may come at any time, but most likely in the afternoon. Chilliness from drinking cold water, from walking in the open air, and from motion. The periodicity is not very regular. It has chill with perspiration. The paroxysm may be daily, tertian or quartian. It has a violent shaking chill. The time most common is 4 p.m., 8 p.m. and 1 p.m. Warm room ameliorates the chill. This remedy has fever without chill. It has fever with chilliness. Dry external heat. Flushes of heat. It has been helpful in hectic fever. The heat is intense. It has internal heat with external chill. The perspiration is often absent. It is a very useful remedy in chronic intermittent fever. He sweats copiously at night from great weakness, as well as from fever. He sweats while eating, from slight exertion and from motion, and during sleep. The sweat is cold and offensive. When the sweat has been suppressed, from entering a cold damp room or cellar, complaints come on much like this remedy.

There are blotches on the skin. There are burning spots, and the skin burns after scratching. It is an excellent remedy to be used against the spread of malignant disease, as so often the symptoms are found in this remedy. The skin is cold. Desquamation, with or without eruptions. Pale waxy skin, or yellow skin. Liver spots, red spots and yellow spots. The skin is dry and burning. Inability to perspire. The complaints of this remedy are often associated with eruptions. It has moist, and dry eruptions. Blisters, and bloody eruptions. The eruptions burn. Eruptions that are furfuraceous and powdery, mealy. It has cured eczema many times. Itching, scaly herpes. The eruptions itch and burn violently. They are painful, and spread rapidly, often turn into phagadenic ulcers. Psoriasis must scratch until moist Pustules. Rash. Scabby, scaly eruptions. Stinging in the skin after scratching. Nodular urticaria. Vesicular eruptions. Vesicles come after scratching.

It cures erysipelas, when the symptoms agree. Intertrigo. Itching when undressing, and when warm in bed. Itching, burning, crawling, and stinging. Sensitive skin, sore to touch. Sticking after scratching. The dropsical swellings burn. Pain in the skin as if an ulcer were forming. Ulcers; bleeding, burning, indolent, phagadenie, suppurating, with ichorous bloody discharges, and turned up edges. Warts grow easily.

KALI BICHROMICUM

This remedy is recognized by most physicians by the copious ropy mucous discharges from all mucous membranes, but it is also a most important remedy in rheumatic affections of the joints with swelling, heat and redness, whenever these conditions wander around from joint to joint. The bones all over the body feel bruised, and caries is reckoned among its symptoms. A marked feature of this remedy is the alternation between catarrhal symptoms and rheumatic pains. Exudations from mucous membranes, somewhat like croup, are found in the larynx, trachea and in the rectum. It is not surprising, therefore, that it has proved a very effective remedy in diphtheria. It emaciates, like the rest of the *Kali* salts. We have running through it the cachectic conditions, or malignant diseases with ulceration; and especially is it indicated when the ulceration period is present. Ulceration is a striking feature of this remedy. Its ulcers are deep; are said to be as if punched out and are very red. Gouty conditions are as common in this remedy as in the other *Kalis*. It is especially like *Causticum* with its cracking in the joints. Syphilitic conditions have been cured in the most advanced stages. It has the sharp stitching pains like *Kali carb*. It has one feature quite its own—very severe pain in small spots that could be covered by the end of the thumb. It has wandering pains from place to place, and *wandering rheumatism from joint to joint*. There are pains in all parts. Pains are sometimes very violent; sometimes shooting; sometimes stitching, stinging; again aching. Burning is a very marked symptom of the remedy. The pains appear rapidly and disappear suddenly.

The patient is sensitive to cold. There is a lack of vital heat. In fact, he wants to be wrapped up and covered warmly, and many of his complaints are much better when he is perfectly warm in bed. All the pains and his cough are relieved from the warmth of the bed, and yet there are other complaints, like rheumatic conditions, that come on in hot weather. The cough is better in warm weather and worse in winter. Catarrhal conditions of the larynx and trachea are worse in winter, especially in the cold, damp weather, like *Calc. phos.,* when the snow melts. Sensitive to cold winds. *Causticum,* it will be remembered, is sensitive to cold, dry winds. The *Kalis* generally are sensitive to cold, dry weather, but Kali bichromicum throat troubles are continuous in the winter and during cold, damp weather, and are worse in cold, damp winds. It is a most useful remedy in septic and zymotic fevers. Many of its symptoms are aggravated about 2 or 3 A.M., like *Kali carb.* Most of the symptoms are worse in the morning, yet some come on in the night. A marked feature of Kali bichromicum is a feeling of great weakness and weariness. When the pain has passed off, if in the limbs, the limbs are felt very weary. Great prostration and cold sweat. It has neuralgia every day at the same hour, showing its periodicity. Like the rest of the *Kalis* it has cured epilepsy. Ropy saliva and mucous discharges from the mouth during the convulsion has led to its use in epilepsy. The symptoms generally, especially the pains, are worse from motion, except the sciatic and some of the pains in the lower limbs, which are better from motoin. The patient pulsates all over the body.

There are very few mental symptoms owing to the fact that the remedy has been proved only in crude form. It needs to be proved in potencies to bring out the mental symptoms.

It has violent headaches and its headaches are mostly associated with catarrhal conditions. A Kali bichromicum patient always suffers more or less from catarrh of the nose, and if he is exposed to cold weather the catarrhal condition will turn to dryness; then will come on violent headache; also headaches during coryza. Headaches during coryza when the discharge of the coryza slacks up a little. Headaches often begin with dim vision. Pains are violent. Headaches are better from warmth, especially warm drink; better from pressure; worse from stooping; worse from motion and walking; worse at night and still much worse in the morning. Pain is pulsating, shooting and burning. Headaches come on with vertigo. Headaches are often one-sided. It has been a very useful remedy in syphilitic head pains. Pains over the eyes and in the forehead. It is very useful when the headaches are with retching and vomiting; when the pain is confined to a very small spot that could be covered with the thumb and is violent; when the headaches come periodically and with dizziness. Headaches are somewhat ameliorated in open air if it is not too cold.

It has cured eczema of the scalp with thick, heavy crusts from which ooze a yellow, thick, gluey substance.

Daylight brings on photophobia. There are sparks before the eyes; dim vision before the headache, as mentioned above. Rheumatic conditions affecting the eyes, hence it is said rheumatic affections of the eyes. Granular lids. Ulceration of the cornea. The ulcer is deep with pulsation in it. The eyes are much inflamed and red. The lids are red and swollen. Eyes and lids are injected. Croupous inflammation of the eyes. Burning and itching in the eyes. Inflammation of the mucous membrane of the eyes with copious flow of thick mucus. Margins of the lids are red and swollen. It has cured polypus on the conjunctiva, swelling of the lids and stringy mucus.

There are yellow, viscid discharges from the ears, with stitching pains and pulsating in the ears. Chronic suppuration of the middle ear with perforated tympanum; eczematous eruptions on the ears; itching of the whole external ear.

The symptoms of the nasal passages are very numerous. The most prominent are the catarrhal symptoms. It has catarrhal symptoms both acute and chronic, with copious, thick, viscid, yellow or white mucus. Fœtid odor from the nose. Troubled much with a sensation of dryness in the nose. Loss of smell, and the nose is obstructed nights with thick yellow mucus, too viscid to be blown out. Accompanying this catarrhal condition there is a hard pain at the root of the nose. Ulcers form all over the nasal mucous membrane. There are ulcers, crusts, mucous plugs; must blow the nose constantly without success, but finally blows out large green crusts or scabs from high up in the nose. Sometimes they are drawn into the posterior nares. There is burning and pulsating in the nasal cavities. When the nasal cavity is in this state of ulceration and catarrh there is shooting pain from the root of the nose to the external angle of the eye through the whole forenoon. Extreme soreness inside of the nose. Expired air feels hot and causes a sensation of burning. He has snuffles and increased catarrhal conditions in damp weather. There are also burning, excoriating, watery discharges from the nose, as in acute catarrhal conditions. Coryza is fluent, excoriating, with loss of smell. With the chronic condition there comes perforation of the septum and pressing pains of the frontal sinus. A very strange condition then is observed. Scabs form upon the nasal septum; when these are removed there comes photophobia, then dimness of vision, followed by hard frontal headache. The septum is sometimes destroyed by ulceration. Much thick blood is blown out of the nose: Now, it has cured these conditions when they were syphilitic. It has cured nasal polypus. It has cured lupus of the nose.

The bones of the face are often very sore, with shooting pains in the malar bones. Pain in the malar bones on coughing. With the catarrhal conditions there is much suffering from the malar bones, like *Merc.* It has cured lupus exedens. It has cured ulceration of the lip. Swollen parotid is quite a common feature in its proving. It has cured impetigo.

The tongue is smooth, shiny, sometimes cracked. This is especially observed in low forms of fever, like typhoid. The tongue is often coated, thick and yellow at the base. Papillæ raise on the dorsum of the tongue, making it look like strawberry tongue. Again, the tongue is coated a thick brown. The provers seemed to be much annoyed by a sensation of a hair on the base of the tongue. It has produced and cured ulceration of the tongue; even when syphilitic it is a useful remedy. Ulcers deep as if punched out, with stinging pains.

There is great dryness of the mouth; ropy saliva and mucus; ulcers anywhere in the mouth; aphthous patches; ulcers of the roof of the mouth; even when these are syphilitic it is a most useful remedy; deep, punched out ulcers.

The throat symptoms are very numerous. I will only mention a few of the most characteristic ones.Inflammation of the throat in general; involving all the tissues in it, extending up into the nose, and down into the larynx, even with a high degree of ulceration with copious, ropy mucus. It has cured diphtheria exudation in the throat when it is confined to the throat, and also when it has extended to the larynx. A marked feature of the Kali bichromicum throat is its œdematous uvula. This symptom is also found in *Apis, Kali i., Lach., Mur. ac., Nit ac., Phos., Sulph. ac.,* and *Tab.* Deep ulcers in the throat and ulcers on the tonsils. Ulceration so extensive that it has destroyed the whole. soft palate. Inflammation of the tonsils when they are swollen and very red, when the neck is swollen; inflammation of the tonsils with suppuration. In this sore throat there is quite commonly a shooting pain extending to the ears. There are also enlarged veins in the throat: Like the sensation of the tongue as if a hair in various places in the fauces and nose. Dry, burning sensation in the throat is very common. Quite a characteristic symptom of Kali bichromicum is the intense pain in the root of the tongue, when putting the tongue out. It has much exudation in the throat that is not diphtheria, but resembles it.

The stomach symptoms are also very numerous. There is aversion to meat, and, strange to say, he craves beer, which makes him sick, brings on diarrhœa. Food lies like a load in the stomach; digestion seems suspended; there is a pressure as of a load after eating and much fœtid eructation. Nausea comes on very suddenly, sometimes while eating, soon after eating; vomits all food and it is sour as if it had turned sour very rapidly; so that there is vomiting of sour, undigested food, bile, bitter mucus, blood, yellow mucus and ropy mucus. It is a very useful remedy in nausea and vomiting of drunkards and beer drinkers. When a beer drinker has arrived at a point where he can no longer tolerate his beer but it makes him sick, Kali bichromicum is a useful remedy. In the stomach there is also soreness and coldness. It is a very useful remedy in ulceration of the stomach; and when such ulcer is cancerous it relieves the pain, stops the vomiting, makes the patient comfortable for a long time. In other words, it palliates him. There are some pains in the stomach that are ameliorated by eating; nausea sometimes is ameliorated, but such is the exception. He has a faintness in the stomach which drives him to eat often. Chronic catarrh of the stomach is a strong feature and perhaps is a condition that is generally present with Kali bichromicum patients.

There is pain in the liver, hard contracting pain extending to the shoulder, resembling *Crot. h.* Pain in the liver from motion. Dull, aching pain in the liver. It is a useful remedy in liver conditions associated with gall-stones. It corrects the action of the liver so that healthy bile is formed and the gallstones are dissolved. Stitching pain in the liver, and also in the spleen, on motion.

The abdomen is very tympanitic, with tenderness. There are stitching, cutting pains. Sinking in the abdomen with nausea after eating, then comes vomiting, then comes diarrhœa. This is the order in which these symptoms generally appear. It is a very useful remedy in gastro-intestinal cases. Ulcers of the intestines in typhoid conditions. This remedy has also a morning diarrhœa like *Sulphur.* It has diarrhœa in phthisis. It has diarrhœa in typhoid fever. Watery stools. Stools are brown and watery, or may be blackish watery. There is often much tenesmus at stool. Chronic diarrhœa in the morning. Diarrhœa after beer like *Aloe, China, Gamb., Lye., Mur. ac.,* and *Sulph.*

Frequently there are clay colored stools. Again there are bloody stools, as in dysentery. It has both diarrhœa and dysentery after rheumatism has disappeared. It seems rheumatic conditions are inclined to alternate with diarrhoeic conditions. In hot weather it has diarrhœa and dysentery; in winter it has chest troubles and catarrh of the air passages. There is pain in the abdomen before the stool; much pain during the stool, cramping and tenesmus. After stool it has tenesmus like *Merc.* It has constipation with hard, knotty stool, followed by severe burning in the parts. Burning in the anus after stool. Prolapsus of the rectum. After dry hard stool there is burning in the rectum. Patient suffers from a sensation of a large plug in the rectum and there is great soreness in the anus. He suffers much from hæmorrhoids which protrude after stool and are very painful.

Pain in the back with bloody urine. Shooting pains in the region of the kidneys, also aching in the region of the kidneys with urging to urinate in the day time. There is suppressed urine with aching in the kidneys. Ropy mucus in the urine. Pain in the coccyx before urination, relieved afterwards. Burning in the fossa navicularis during urination.

In the male the sexual desire is generally absent. There is a strong constricting or contracting pain in the end of the penis and much itching of the pubes. Deep punched out chancres, very hard. Stitching in the prostate gland when walking. Ropy, viscid, mucous discharge from the urethra.

As there is much relaxation in the remedy during hot weather it especially affects the woman. She suffers from prolapses in the summer time, during hot weather. It is a very useful remedy in the woman for subinvolution. In the menstrual flow there are often membranes that cause her to suffer. The menstrual flow is too soon, excoriates the parts, causes the labia to swell and itch. Like the catarrhal conditions of other mucous membranes, there is leucorrhœa that is yellow and ropy.

It has been a most useful remedy in the vomiting of pregnancy when the other symptoms agree and also where the milk becomes stringy.

There are numerous symptoms connected with the larynx and as is usual copious, thick, ropy mucus. Chronic hoarseness, rough voice, dry cough, swollen feeling in the larynx and sensation as if there was a rag in the larynx. Catarrh of the larynx, croup, cough when breathing, membranous croup, diphtheria, burning, smarting and rawness of the larynx, rattling in the trachea. Now these symptoms come in the cold, damp weather, in the winter. They are associated with much coughing and uneasiness. Sometimes these symptoms are entirely relieved and he is comfortable in a warm bed at night; and he is worse always in cold weather; they come on when the cold weather comes in the fall and last all winter. He has much wheezing when breathing; tightness at the bifurcation of the trachea. Quite a characteristic pain in the chest is the pain from the sternum to the back, associated with catarrhal conditions and with cough. Cough is caused from tickling in the larynx and at the bifurcation; dry, frequent, hard cough; great soreness in the chest when coughing and breathing deep. Cough with pain in the sternum through to the back. Cough with stitching pain in the chest. Loud, hard cough. When he wakes up in the morning he begins this hard coughing. He is often ameliorated by lying down and is ameliorated by the warm bed; is worse undressing, from exposure to the air, worse after eating, aggravated by taking a deep breath, ameliorated by getting warm in bed. The irritation and the cough is increased very much by exposure to cold air. The cough is also a choking cough at times; sometimes a hoarse cough. It is sometimes much like whooping cough, spasmodic and constrictive.

The expectoration connected with the chest cough is ropy, yellow, or yellowish green, sometimes bloody, sometimes expectorates quantities of clotted blood. There is much rattling in the chest, catarrhal conditions in the winter, last all winter, with rattling catarrhal conditions in old people, rattling in the chest.

It is a most useful remedy in phthisis and hæmorrhages from the lungs and cavities in the lungs. There is a cold sensation in the chest which is generally felt in the region of the heart. There is a pressure in the chest after eating also near the heart or supposed to be about the heart and there is palpitation. It has cured and been a very useful remedy in hypertrophy of the heart with palpitation.

In all parts of the body there is chilliness, in the back, especially in the back of the neck. Stabbing pains in the neck and in the dorsal region. Sharp pains in the region of the kidneys. Dull ache in the back. Many of the symptoms in the back are of a rheumtaic character and wander from place to place. The rheumatic pains are worse stooping, and, like other pains, worse from motion. An exception to this is in the sacrum where there is an aching pain at night when lying and is better in the day time on motion. There is pain in the sacrum on straightening up from sitting. Pain in the coccyx from rising after sitting; pain in the coccyx on first sitting down and in the act of sitting down.

The limbs are stiff in the morning on rising and the pains wander about, especially in the joints. Rheumatic pains that wander about. Pains in the limbs are worse from cold and worse from motion. They are better from heat and better in rest. Periodical pains, coming at regular times. The bones feel sore to the touch or on deep pressure. There is cracking in the joints. Rheumatic pains are very common in the shoulders; lameness; there is burning in the forearms; rheumatic pains in the elbows; weak feeling in the hands and fingers with much clumsiness; spasmodic contraction of the fingers. Bones in the hands and fingers feel bruised and very tender to hard pressure. Rrheumatic pains of the fingers are very common to this remedy. In the lower limbs we have marked rheumatic pains through the hips and knees, worse walking and on motion. Then comes the exception: pains in the sciatic nerves, very severe, worse in hot weather; these are better in motion, better in the warmth of the bed, worse from changes in the weather and better on flexing the leg. Drawing pains in the tibia are very common. It has cured ulcers on the legs, deep as if punched out. Burning on the ankles, soreness of the heels. It has cured ulcers on the heels.

The sleep is most restless. Starting in sleep and turning and tossing. Its chest symptoms are worse on walking.

Upon the skin we have pustules, boils, eczema, blisters, herpes, shingles, ulcers on the skin, tubercles, suppurating tubercles and eruptions that are syphilitic in character.

KALI BICHROMICUM

The following symptoms have recently been cured by Kali-bi. They are found under Kali-bi. in Allen's Encyclopædia of Pure Materia Medica, page 237:

Weakness of digestion, so that the stomach was disordered by any but the mildest food (chrome washers). Incarceration of flatulence in stomach and whole lower portion of abdomen. (Zlatarovich).

Great feebleness of stomach in the morning. (Lackner).

Feeling of emptiness in the stomach, though want of appetite at dinner. (Marenzetler).

Feeling of sinking in the stomach before breakfast. (Dr. R. Dudgeon).

The patient wakes in the night with great uneasiness in the stomach, and soreness and tenderness in a small spot to the left of the xiphoid appendix, which is very similar to symptoms in Drysdale's proving.

Sudden violent pain in the stomach, in its anterior surface, a burning constructive pain. (Zlatarovich).

The same patient complaints of repletion after a mouthful of food; and he had taken Lycopodium without benefit.

There was also cutting as with knives, and he was unable to digest potatoes or any starchy food.

There were no catarrhal symptoms of nose or chest, and no thick, ropy, mucous discharges, therefore Kali-bi, was neglected. The stomach symptoms alone guided to its use, as he had no other symptoms of importance.

The relief is marked. and I think permanent.

It will be seen that I have made use of the language of the prover mostly, as it so perfectly describes the symptoms of the patients.

In looking over the proving, the patient underscored such symptoms as he had suffered from, and the remedy was furnished on these symptoms, which really lends value to the provings. Especially are these provings the more beautiful, as they are by several provers.

KALI CARBONICUM

The Kali carb. patient is a hard patient to study, and the remedy itself is a hard one to study.

It is not used as often as it should be, and the reason is that it is a very complex and confusing remedy. It has a great many opposite symptoms, changing symptoms, and thus it is related to patients that withhold their symptoms and have many vague symptoms.

The patient is whimsical, irascible, *irritable to the very highest degree,* quarrels with his family and with his bread and butter. He never wants to be alone, is *full of fear* and imaginations when alone, "fear of the future, fear of death, fear of ghosts". If compelled to remain alone in the house he is wakeful, sleepless, or his sleep is full of horrible dreams. He is never at peace, is full of imaginations and fear. "What if the house should burn up!" "What if I should do this or that!" and "What if this and the other thing should happen!"

He is oversensitive to everything, *sensitive to every atmospheric change;* he can never get the room at just exactly the right temperature; he is sensitive to every draft of air and to the circulation of air in the room. He cannot have the windows open, even in a distant part of the house. He will get up at night in bed and look around to see where that draft of air comes from. His complaints are worse in wet weather, and in cold weather. He is *sensitive to the cold* and is always shivering. His nerves feel the cold; they are all painful when it is cold. The neuralgias shoot here and there when it is cold, and if the part affected be kept warm the pain goes to some other place. All his pains change place and go into the cold part; if he covers up one part, the pain goes to the part uncovered.

This remedy is full of sticking, burning, tearing pains, and these fly around from place to place. Of course Kali carb. has pains that remain in one place, but usually *the pains fly around* in every direction. Pains cutting like knives. Pains like hot needles, sticking, stinging and burning. These pains are felt in internal parts and dry passages. Burning in the anus and rectum, described as if a hot poker were forced into that passage; burning as with fire. The hæmorrhoids burn like coals of fire. The burning of Kali carb. is like that of *Arsenicum.*

Again from studying the text it will be seen that it is a common feature of this medicine to have its symptoms come on at 2, 3 *or 5 o'clock in the morning.* In Kali carb. the cough will come or have its greatest < at three or four or five o'clock in the morning. The febrile state will occur from 3-5 in the morning. The patient, who is subject to asthmatic dyspnœa, will have an attack at 3 o'clock in the morning, waking him out of sleep. He will wake up with various symptoms and remain awake until 5 o'clock in the morning, and after that to a great extent they are relieved. Of course, there are plenty of sufferings at any time in the twenty-four hours, but this is the worst time. He wakes up at 3 o'clock in the morning with fear, fear of death, fear of the future, worries about everything and is kept awake for 2-3 hours and then goes to sleep and sleeps soundly.

His body is cold and requires much clothing to keep it warm, but in spite of the fact that he is cold he sweats copiously; *copious, cold sweat* upon the body. Sweats upon the slightest exertion, sweats where the pain is, sweat over the forehead; cold sweat on the forehead with headache.

Neuralgia of the scalp and the eyes and the cheek bones in association with the nervous shooting pains. Violent pains here and there in the head, as if the head would be crushed. Cutting and stabbing in the head. Violent congestive headaches as if the head were full. Head hot on one side and cold on the other; forehead covered with cold sweat.

It has *catarrhal congestive headache.* Whenever he goes out in the cold air, the nose opens up and the mucous membranes become dry and burn; when he returns into a warm room the nose commences to discharge, and the nose stuffs up so that he cannot breathe through it, and then he feels most comfortable, so that it has stuffing up of the nose in a warm room, and opening up of the nose in the open air. When the nose is open so that he can breathe through it, that is the time the head is most painful it is painful to the cold air and the cold air makes it burn. The cold air feels hot. All these patients suffer from a chronic catarrh and when they ride in the wind the catarrhal discharge ceases and then will come on a headache, and thus he has headache from riding in the cold wind. Whenever the discharge ceases from taking cold in a draft on comes headache, and as the discharge becomes free again the headache is relieved. Neuralgic pains in eyes and scalp and through the check bones from a cessation of chronic catarrhal discharge, and when the discharge starts up again, these pains cease.

With the chronic catarrh of the nose there is a *thick, fluent, yellow discharge;* dryness of the nose, alternating with stuffing up. The one who suffers from a chronic catarrh will also have the discharge in the morning, which will fill up the nose with yellow mucus. In the morning he blows out and hawks up dry, hard crusts that fill up the nasal passage, clear over into the pharynx and down into the throat. These crusts become dry as if they were partly formed upon the mucous membrane and when they are blown out there is bleeding. The bleeding starts from where the crusts are lifted up.

He is subject to sore throat, is always taking cold, and it settles in the throat. He is also subject to enlarged tonsils and with these has enlargement and chronic hardness of the parotid glands—one or both. Great knots below the ear, behind the jaw. These grow and become hard, and at times, painful; shooting, darting pains when he is moving about in the open air. When air strikes these enlarged glands they are sore and painful, and he is ameliorated by going into a warm place. The acute colds extend into the chest, but Kali carb. has been found most suitable in the chronic catarrh of the chest, chronic bronchitis.

The *chest* is very often affected in just the same way as the nose. There is the dryness and dry barking, hacking cough in cold air, but a copious expectoration of mucus when it becomes warm, and that is the time he is most comfortable, for the expectoration seems to relieve him. He suffers mostly from a dry, hacking cough with morning expectoration. The cough begins with a dry hacking, increases gradually and sometimes very rapidly to a violent, *spasmodic cough with gagging or vomiting,* and when coughing it feels as if his head would fly to pieces. The face becomes puffed, the eyes seem to protrude and then there is seen that which is commonly present in Kali carb., a peculiar sort of a *swelling between the eyelids and eyebrows* that fills up when coughing. Your attention is called to that peculiar feature, for although there may be bloating nowhere else upon the face that little bagging will appear above the lid and below the eyebrow. It fills up sometimes o the extent of a little water bag. Such a swelling has been produced by Kali carb., and sometimes that symptom alone guides to the examination of the remedy for the purpose of ascertaining if Kali carb. does not fit all the rest of the case. Bœnninghausen speaks of an epidemic of whooping cough in which the majority of cases called for Kali carb., and this striking feature was present. No remedy should ever be given on one symptom. If you are led to a remedy by a peculiar symptom, study the remedy and the disease thoroughly to ascertain if the two are similar enough to each other to expect a cure. Any deviation from that rule is ruinous and will lead to the practice of giving medicines on single symptoms.

Dry, hacking, incessant, gagging cough with whooping, blowing of blood from the nose, vomiting of everything in the stomach, and expectoration of blood-streaked mucus, is a whooping cough that will be commonly cured by Kali carb., but especially if there is present that peculiar and striking feature of a bag-like swelling below the eyebrow and above the lids, puffiness of the eyes.

There are some cases of pneumonia that need Kali carb., in the *stage of hepatization* (*like Sulph.*) Again, when pneumonia has passed away think of Kali carb. if every time the patient takes a little cold it settles in the chest with these symptoms that I have described. There is sensitiveness of the body to weather changes, to cold air and to wet, a continuous dry, hacking cough, with gagging, the aggravation from three to five in the morning. and the patient has flying neuralgic pains. These symptoms gradually increase and the patient dates them back to his pneumonia. He says: "Doctor, I have never been quite well since I had pneumonia." The catarrhal state has settled in his chest and there is a chronic tendency to take cold. These cases are threatening to go into phthisis and will hardly be likely to recover without Kali carb, In this tendency for catarrhal states to locate in the chest, Kali carb. should be thought of as well as *Phosphor., Lycopod.* and *Sulphur.*

Another general state that belongs to this remedy is a tendency to *dropsies.* It has dropsies all over the body. The feet bloat and the fingers puff; the back of the hands pit upon pressure, the face looks puffy and waxy. The heart is weak. I can look back upon quite a number of cases of fatty degeneration of the heart in which I could have prevented all the trouble with Kali carb. if I had known the case better in the beginning. These cases are insidious, and the indications calling for Kali carb. must be seen early or the patient will advance into an incurable condition. That peculiar state of weakness and feeble circulation that finally ends in dropsy and many other complications has its likeness in Kali carb. There is an insidiousness about Kali carh. in the approach of all of its complaints. He has a sort of nondescript appearance, he is withered, has much dyspnœa upon going up hill or even walking on the level.

Examination of the lungs shows them to be in very fair condition, but finally complications come on, there is a breakdown and organic changes and you look back over these cases and say, if I had only seen in the beginning of this cast what I see now it seems as if the patient ought to have been cured. We learn the beginnings of remedies as we learn the beginnings of sickness. It is a prudent thing for a homœopathic physician to glance back over a case that he has failed on, or someone else has failed on, to study its beginnings and see what the manifestations were. This kind of study to the homœopathic physician is as delightful as post mortems are to the old school.

The *teeth* present a peculiar state. The gums take on a scorbutic or scrofulous character. The gums separate from the teeth and the teeth decay and become discolored and loose, so that they have to be extracted early in life. He suffers from pain in the teeth whenever he takes cold from riding in the wind and raw weather. The pains come on even when the teeth are not yellow or decayed; stitching, tearing, rending pains in the teeth. Offensive smell from the teeth; pus oozing out from around the teeth. The mouth is full of little ulcers, little aphthous patches. The mucous membrane is pale and ulcerates daily. The tongue is white with offensive taste; coated gray, with sick headaches.

While many of the symptoms of Kali carb. are aggravated after eating, some symptoms are relieved after eating. There is throbbing in the pit of the stomach when the stomach is empty. There is also throbbing all over the body, pulsation to the fingers and toes; there is no part that does not pulsate, and he is kept awake by this pulsation. Pulsation even when there is often no feeling of palpitation in the region of the heart. It has also violent palpitation of the heart.

Kali carb. fits many *old dyspeptics.* After eating he feels as if he would burst, so bloated is he. Great flatulence; belches wind upwards and passes flatus downwards; offensive flatus. The belching up is also attended with fluid eructations, sour fluids that set the teeth on edge; they excoriate, or cause smarting in the pharynx or mouth. Pain in the stomach after eating; burning in the stomach after eating. Gone feeling in the stomach, that is not even relieved by eating. A peculiar condition in Kali carb., is a state of *anxiety felt in the stomach,* as though it were a fear. One of the first patients I ever had expressed it in a better way than it is expressed in the books; she said, "Doctor, somehow or other I don't have a fear like other people do, because I have it in my stomach." She said when she was frightened, it always struck to her stomach. "If a door slams, I feel it right here" (epigastric region). Well, that is striking, that is peculiar. It was not long before I developed another feature of Kali carb. By a little awkwardness on my part my knee happened to hit the patient's foot as it projected a little over the edge of the bed, and the patient said, "Oh!" Sure enough that was Kali carb. again, for you will find in Kali carb. a patient that is afraid and everything goes to the stomach and when touched upon the skin there is an anxiety or fear or apprehension felt in the region of the stomach. You might imagine that it is connected with the solar plexus, but the symptom is the all in all to the physician. A Kali carb. patient is so *sensitive in the soles* of the feet that the mere touch of the sheet brings a sensation of thrill throughout the body. Hard pressure is all right, it does not disturb, but something that comes unawares excites. The Kali carb. patient is oversensitive to all the surrounding things, oversensitive to touch; shivering from the simplest and lightest touch, even when hard pressure is agreeable. Violently ticklish in the soles of the feet. I have often examined the feet when a patient would shiver and draw up the feet and scream nut, "Don't tickle my feet." I had probably touched it so lightly that I did not know that I had touched it at all. In *Lach.* also gentle touch is painful, while hard pressure is agreeable, but here it is not so much the ticklishness. In *Lach. the* abdomen is so sensitive that the touch of the sheet is painful. I have seen *Lach.* patients using a hoop to keep a light sheet from touching the abdomen. You may know then that you are in the realm of *Lachesis,* and that it is like those persons who are unable to hear the slightest touch upon the neck and suffer from uneasiness on wearing a collar. All that, however, is different from this state of ticklishness. I have seen patients who are really so sensitive in the skin that I would not dare touch it, unless they knew just where I was going to touch. "Now I am going to feel your pulse, hold still." If I were to touch the hand, or reach out to feel the pulse without warning there would be a thrill. Such a state is in keeping with Kali carb. These things often have to be dug out by observation in studying the nature of provings, and associating things. These things that run into the oversensitiveness of patients are of great value clinically. The capabilities of our Materia Medica are something wonderful, but they could be developed much more rapidly if a number of homœopathic physicians would make application of the Materia Medica with accuracy and intelligence, observing what they see and relating it literally. At the present day there is only a very small number of homœopathic physicians that can come together in a body and say things that are worth listening to, a shamefully small number when we consider the length of time Hahnemann's books have been before the world.

There are many old chronic *liver subjects* who talk about nothing else but the liver. Every time they go to the doctor's office they talk about the liver, and about a condition of fulness in the region of the liver and pain through the right shoulder blade and up through the right side of the chest, with a good deal of oppression and distension; vomiting of bile and a good deal of stomach disorder, fulness after eating; attacks of diarrhœa, alternating with constipation lasting for many days with great straining at stool. Periodical bilious attacks, when a constipated state is present; cannot lie down at night; difficult breathing at night or at 3 o'clock in the morning, especially when it is in a patient oversensitive to cold, damp weather, one who wants to sit by the fire all the time. These liver subjects are often thoroughly cured by Kali carb. Sometimes they have been resorting to all sorts of liver tappings, taking such medicines as purge or cause vomiting, drugs that really aggravate the trouble. Kali carb. goes to the bottom of these cases, and roots out the evil.

In the abdomen we have many Kali carb. symptoms. Persons subjected to repeated attacks of *colic,* cutting pains, with distension, with pain after eating constipation or diarrhœa. Colic, with cutting, tearing pains, doubling him up coming on every little while. Tremendous flatulence. When the attack of colic is on it might remind you of *Colocynth* or of some other of the acute remedies that cure colic in two or three minutes, but you will find that these acute remedies that relieve colic so speedily when given the second or third time do not produce so marked an effect. You will find it necessary to hunt for an antipsoric, remedy that will control the whole case. In the study of the colic alone during its attacks you only get a one-sided view of the case, and after the colic is over (say he has been cured by *Colocynth*) you now study the patient and go over the case, and behold all the symptoms are covered by Kali carb. After giving that remedy you may expect that the patient will not have another attack. Such is the nature of Kali carb. It is deep-acting, long-acting, goes deep into the life. It cures conditions due to psora, or to the suppression of eruptions in childhood, or to the closing up of old ulcers and fistulous openings with history of troubles ever since. All these wandering pains and the chilliness are again relieved by eruptions, by the outbreak of discharges, by hæmorrhages, by ulcers that eat in deep and flow freely and fistulous openings.

"Cutting in abdomen, as if torn to pieces." "Violent cutting, must sit bent over pressing with both hands, or lean far back for relief; cannot sit upright. "Cutting and drawing like false labor pains." There is great coldness with the pains; with the cutting in the abdomen; he wants heat, hot drinks, hot water bags. A chronic coldness is felt in the abdomen, cold externally and internally. It would sometimes be cruel to give a dose of Kali carb. when the colic is on because if the remedy fitted the case constitutionally, if all the symptoms of the case were those of Kali carb., you would be likely to get an aggravation that would be unnecessary. There are plenty of short acting remedies that would relieve the pain speedily, and at the close of the attack the constitutional remedy could then be given. If the patient can bear the pain to the end, it is better to wait until it passes off without any medicine. That sometimes is cruel, and then the short acting medicines should be given. All recurrent troubles, those that come periodically, or after eating certain articles or from exposure, or with a periodicity that belongs to time—all these states are chronic; they are not acute troubles. They are simply a small portion of chronic miasm, a side view, and all such cases must have a constitutional emedy sooner or later. You can, it is true, relieve violent pain at the first visit, but then you must look deeper and prevent your patient having more trouble. Otherwise, if you should give *Bell.* or *Colocynth* or any medicine that simply fits the colic, the trouble will come back again; you have not cured your patient; you have only palliated. But, on the other hand, you take such a colic as is described here and Kali carb. fits just these symptoms alone and does not fit the whole constitution of the patient. Then it is that a constitutional and long-acting remedy like Kali carb. acts in fulness. It does not take the usual long time to act and is not attended with an aggravation.

"Abdominal muscles painful to touch; swelling of glands." In the abdomen, also, following troubles in the bowels, or following peritonitis, we have effusion into the peritoneal sac, which is usually associated with dropsy of the extremities, but not always. In liver dropsies especially is this remedy useful.

It has a great many complaints of the rectum and anus and of the stool. It has most persistent and enormous *hæmorrhoidal tumors* that burn, that are extremely sensitive to touch, that bleed copiously, that are extremely painful, making it impossible for him to sleep. He is compelled to lie upon the back and hold the nates apart, because the pressure is very painful to the external piles. The piles cannot be put back; there is great distension and swelling inside. Hæmorrhoids that come out after stool and bleed copiously and are very painful; they must be pushed back, and long after going to bed they burn like fire. There is great aggravation from stool, which is hard and knotty and requires great straining to expel. Fistulæ of the anus. Burning temporarily relieved by sitting in cold water.

It has *chronic diarrhœa* and also diarrhœa alternating with constipation. Many times where there are numerous particulars, we have to rely upon the generals that are characteristic of the remedy. The text gives much less of diarrhœa than has been developed by clinical uses. "Diarrhœa painless, with rumbling in the abdomen and burning at stool, only by day; chronic cases with puffiness under the eyebrows." It gives few symptoms, but it is a large and extensive remedy in diarrhœas that are chronic. In old, broken down subjects, in weakly, pallid subjects, with poor digestion, with great flatulence, with much distension, with disordered liver.

Then the kidney, bladder and urethra come in for their share of trouble, which is of a catarrhal nature. Discharges from the bladder, purulent discharges of a thick, tenacious, copious mucus deposited in the urine. In keeping with this there is much burning; burning in the urethra, during and after micturition. "Urine flows slowly with soreness and burning." Kali carb. runs very close to *Natr. mur.* in many of its old, long-standing bladder troubles. In old cases of gleet and long-standing cases of urinary troubles that follow gonorrhœa these two medicines are useful, both suitable in the scanty, white,

gleety discharge that remains. In both, the urination is painful. In *Nat. mur.*
the burning is *after urination.* Where there is scanty, gleety discharge and
the burning is very marked and only *after* urination, and the patient is
extremely nervous and fidgety, *Natrum mur* will cure. If the burning is *during
and after* urination and you have the broken down constitution we have
described then the remedy may be Kali carb. Some of these old cases are
entirely painless, having no pain either during or after micturition. Then you
get an entirely different class of remedies. The old chronic discharges
following a gonorrhœa are as troublesome for the young doctor as anything
that will ever fall into his hands. The remedies are numerous, the symptoms
are scanty, and many times the patient has not been long under the doctor's
care, therefore he does not know the patient's constitutional state well and
the patient can only tell him of the discharge. "Nothing but the discharge,
doctor." You cannot get his mind on his symptoms; he has forgotten that he
wakes at *3* o'clock in the morning and cannot get to sleep until 5 o'clock, he
has forgotten all the nervous manifestations. With the patient you have had
under control, whose constitutional state you get before this condition comes,
you ought not to have much difficulty.

One of the evidences that the Kali carb. patient is of a weakly constitution and is on the road to a break-down is that all of his symptoms are
aroused and brought into action after coition, after sexual excitement. Now
you will take notice in practice and remember it, that coition is a natural thing
with man, when it is carried on in order, and when that which is natural is
followed by prostration, and this has been so for a long time, there is a break
in the constitution, there is something radically wrong. All the symptoms are
likely to be *worse after coition* in Kali carb. He has weak vision, weakness of
the senses, tremulousness, and is generally nervous; he is sleepless, and
weak, and he shivers and trembles for a day or two after coition. Similar
symptoms are observed in the woman. In spite of the fact that the patient is
weak, the sexual desire is excessive. It is not orderly. There is a sexual
erethism, which is not under the command of the will, and in the male he is
subject to copious and frequent pollutions, nightly dreams, sexual prostration.
Young men who have abused themselves, or who have indulged excessively
in sexual pleasure, go into marriage with weakened genitals, incapacitated,
and then there comes a disgust, and it is not strange that there are so many
divorces in the world. When the patient is young, some of this trouble can be
overcome by living an orderly life and correct Homœopathy.

In Kali carb. there are many complaints affecting the male genital organs,
uneasiness and sensitiveness of the testicles. One is in a state of swelling
and hardness. Itching and smarting and annoying sensations in the scrotum
and sensations that constantly remind the patient that he has genital organs.

Constant irritation calling his attention to the genitals, brought on from abuse, from vice, from excesses. *Phosphorus* is a medicine that is abused in this sphere. Many physicians look upon it as one of the great remedies for the weakness of the genital organs. In *Phos.* the genital indications are extreme excitement, too active erections, a disorderly strength of the genital organs. Beware of giving it in impotency or in weakness, as this is often associated with very feeble constitutions, and *Phos.* not only fails to cure, but seems to add to the weakness. It is a weakness that you will learn is a vital weakness. *Phos.* will set patients to running down more rapidly who are suffering from a vital weakness, who are always tired, simply weak, always prostrated and want to go to bed.

The female has a great friend in Kali carb. It is full of her complaints and has many symptoms likely to be found in a sick woman. It is useful in cases of *uterine hæmorrhages* that have been incessant in pale, waxy, hæmorrhagic women; incessant hæmorrhage following an abortion. She has been curetted and has had all sorts of treatment, but still that oozing keeps right on. At the menstrual period the flow is very copious and clotted, and then after prolonged menstruation of ten days or so, during which she has had a copious flow, she settles back into a state of oozing and flowing until next month and then it rouses up into another ten days of copious menstruation. Kali carb. has cured a number of cases of fibroid tumor long before it was time for the critical period to cure. You must remember that there is natural tendency for a fibroid to cease to grow at the climacteric period, and afterwards to shrivel and that this takes place without any treatment, but the appropriate remedies will cause that hæmorrhage to cease, will cause that tumor to cease to grow and after a few days there will be a grand shrinkage in its size.

Kali carb. is often a remedy for *vomiting in pregnancy,* but to find out when it is *the* remedy for vomiting of pregnancy we have to go to the whole constitutional state. Vomiting of pregnancy is not cured, although it may be temporarily relieved, by *Ipecac.,* as this is a medicine that corresponds merely to the nausea itself. In a large number of instances gagging and nausea are only a second or third grade symptom in the remedy that will cure. The condition really depends upon the constitutional state, and the remedy that is to cure must be a constitutional remedy. *Sulphur, Sepia* and Kali carb. are among the remedies commonly indicated. Sometimes *Arsenic* is needed. Of course, if a pregnant woman has simply disordered her stomach and has vomited bile a few times the remedy might be *Ipecac.* When a pregnant woman has no constitutional symptoms at all, and upon examining the case you find nothing but the nausea, overwhelming deathly nausea, with continuous vomiting day and night, a single dose of *Symphoricarpus rac.* will help. That is prescribing upon very limited information, and should only be done in circumscribed or one-sided cases. It is not a long acting remedy it is not a constitutional remedy and acts very much like *Ipecac.*

At times you will go into the confinement room when the woman ha pains in the back below the waist line. The pains in the uterus are very weak they are not sufficiently expulsive to make progress in the labor, the kind o pain that makes the woman utter the cry, "My hack, my back!" The pain extend down the buttocks and legs. Pains in the back as if the back woul break. Under good prescribing these pains are changed into contractions which prove sufficient to expel the contents of the uterus. When you hea such things you will look back over the history of the case. You will lool back for weeks as the woman has been drawing near the end of gestation an see that the vague things, the chilliness and other features in he constitutional state for which you have been trying to find a remedy nov culminate at the time of her confinement into a class of pains. Had you seer that six weeks before and given her Kali carb. you would have prevented th severe labor. It is a severe labor, a prolongd labor; the uterus appears to b weak, and the pains are feeble; they are all in the back, and do not go to th centre of operation as they should. Now, this same kind of a pain may deceiv you in taking another form. The pains begin in the back, and appear to go t the uterus and then run up the back, which would turn you aside entirel from the Kali carb. pain into a pain that would indicate *Gelsemium.* Sometime these pains are so severe that they actually seem to prevent rather tha encourage the contractions of the uterus; when the contractions of the uteru cease, and the woman screams out and wants her hips rubbed, and scream out with pain in each side of the abdomen rather than in the centre, pains i the region where the broad ligaments ought to he, *Actæa racemosa* will mak the pains regular. *Puls.* is the medicine for absence of marked contraction, i cases inclined to do nothing; in a case that is inactive when the os i sufficiently dilated and the parts relaxed, and the prediction is an easy an simple labor, but the patient does not do anything. It is a state of mildness o inactivity. *Puls.* will very often cause in five minutes a very strong contractio of the uterus, sometimes almost in a painless way.

"The back aches so badly while she is walking that she feels as if sh could lie down on the street," etc. etc. The pain seems to take the force an vigor all out of the patient. After delivery there is a tendency to prolong th flooding, rousing up at every menstrual period, as described.

Weakness of the heart, *cardiac dyspnœa;* the breath is short and th patient cannot walk or must move very slowly. It is the coming on of a fatt heart. With the suffocation and dyspnœa the breathing is so short that th patient cannot stop to take a drink or eat; the breathing is rapid, not deep but weak. Dyspnœa with violent, irregular palpitation of the heart, throbbin that shakes the whole frame, pulsation that can be felt to the ends of the fingers and toes. Violent pulsations; patient cannot lie on the left side; accompanied by stitching pain through the chest, and cough. In old asthmatic patients with weak pulse, with the same pulsations and palpitation and cannot lie down. The only position it seems that he can find any comfort in is leaning forward, with his elbows resting upon a chair. The attack is violent and continuous, especially worse from 3 to 5 A.M., and worse from lying in bed. He is aroused at 3 o'clock in the morning with these asthmatic attacks. Asthmatic dyspnœa, when the state is that of humid asthma or filling up Of the chest with mucus, coarse rattling in the chest, loud, rattling breathing. In patients who always have rattling in the chest, rattling cough, stuffy breathing; with every rainy spell or misty spell, or in cold, foggy weather, the condition becomes that of a humid asthma; asthmatic breathing, with much weakness in the chest, worse from 3 to 5 in the morning. The patient is pale, sickly and anæmic, and complains of stitching pains in the chest.

The *cough* of this medicine is one of the most violent coughs of all the medicines in the Materia Medica. The whole frame is racked. The cough is incessant, attended with gagging and vomiting, comes on at 3 o'clock in the morning, a dry, hacking, hard, racking cough. "Suffocative cough and choking cough at 5 A.M. Great dryness in the throat between 2 and 3 A.M." Think of Kali carb. when, after troubles like measles, a catarrhal state is left behind, due to lack of reaction, the psoric sequelæ. The cough following measles is very often a Kali carb. cough. Kali carb., *Sulphur, Carbo veg.* and *Drosera* are perhaps more frequently indicated than other medicines in such coughs as follow measles or pneumonia.

The *expectoration* is copious, very offensive, tenacious, lumpy, blood-streaked or like pus, thick yellow or yellowish-green. Very often it has a pungent, cheesy taste, strong taste, as of old cheese. Catarrh of the chest. Dry cough day and night, with vomiting of food and some phlegm, worse after eating and drinking and in the evening.

Nothing is more striking in Kali carb. than the *wandering stitching pains through the chest*, and *the coldness of the chest*. The great dyspnœa, the transient stitches, the pleural stitches are important features of this remedy. A great number of the cases in which Kali carb. is suitable are those where the trouble has spread from catarrhal origin and from the lower portion of the lungs upwards. It is not so commonly indicated in those cases where the dullness has begun at the apex of either or both lungs. It will very often ward off future sickness where the family history is tuberculous. Do not be afraid to give the antipsoric remedies when there is a history of tuberculosis in the family, but be careful when the patient is so far advanced with tuberculosis that there are cavities in the lung, or latent tubercles, or encysted caseous tubercles. Your antipsorics might rouse him into a dangerous condition. Do not suppose, however, that it is dangerous to *give Sulphur* because one's father and mother have died of phthisis. *Sulphur* might be just the remedy to prevent the child from following the father and mother. Kali carb. is often suitable, and will act as an acute remedy in the advanced stages of phthisis in cases in which it was not indicated primarily as a constitutional remedy. In such instances it will act as a palliative in phthisis, whereas if it were indicated primarily as a constitutional remedy it would do damage in the last weeks. The fortunate thing is that a great many homœopaths are not able to find the homœopathic remedy. If the patient has yet lung space enough to be cured Kali carb. will do wonders where the symptoms agree.

I want to warn you in one respect concerning Kali carb. It is a very dangerous medicine in gout. When you get an old gouty subject who has big toe joints and finger joints, and they are sore and inflamed every now and then, you might think that Kali carb. covers the case very suitably; he is disturbed in just such weather, he is pallid and sickly, his complaints come on at 2 to 3 o'clock in the morning, he has the shooting pains. But these gouty patients are often incurable, and, if so, to undertake to cure them would be a dreadful calamity, because the aggravations would last so long. If you give Kali carb. to one of these incurable patients in very high potency it will make your patient worse, and the aggravation will be serious and prolonged, but the 30th may be of great service. *Kali oid.,* when it is indicated in the gouty state, acts as a soothing and palliative remedy. But Kali carb. seems to be a dreadful medicine to handle, it is a sharp and a two-edged sword. Do not undertake to give medicine with a view to curing these old cases of gout when the nodosities are numerous. Do not give that constitutional medicine that should have been administered to these patients twenty years ago because there is not reaction enough in the life of the patient to turn him into order, and he will be destroyed. It seems paradoxical to say it, but to cure him is to kill him. The vital action that is necessary to restore him to health would practically tear his framework to pieces. You need not believe these things, you are not obliged to. But think about them, and some day after practicing awhile and making numerous mistakes in attempting to cure incurables you will admits the awful power of homœopathic medicines. They are simply dreadful. In old gouty cases, in old cases of Bright's disease, in advanced cases of phthisis where there are many tubercles, beware of Kali carb. given too high.

While studying the text book, look over the sensations. They are very numerous. Of course, those most striking are the stitching, and tearing pains, shooting, sticking and wandering pains.

KALI IODATUM

This remedy is an antipsoric and antisyphilitic. It has been used very extensively by the old school as an antisyphilitic, but in the very large doses which they used it became to a great extent allopathic to the disease, because of the tremendous effect it produced upon the economy, and implanted its own miasm, and thereby in a measure it suppressed many cases of syphilis. The medicines that are the most powerful substances are really those that sustain a homœopathic relation to the disease in general, and of these the very smallest dose will cure when similar. When the remedy is not similar enough to cure in such a form the increasing of the dose does not make it homœopathic. There is an idea in vogue that increasing the dose makes the remedy similar. That is going away from principle. If the remedy is not similar there is no form of dose that can make it similar.

It affects the glandular structures and the periosteum after the manner of syphilis. It produces catarrhal inflammations. It is a deep-acting medicine and closely related to *Mercurius.* It has ulcerations and catarrhal states and glandular affections like *Mercurius.* It is similar in its action to *Mercurius* and is an antidote to it.

The old subjects who have always been taking *Calomel* or *Blue Mass* for their bilious complaints will in time become subject to frequent coryzas, constipation, pains and aches, and disturbance of the liver, and disordered stomach, and must have another dose of *Mercury.* Some of these cases need this remedy. If you practice medicine in a neighbourhood where there is a very poor homœopath you will find that he is giving the *Biniodide,* or some other preparation of *Mercury,* for almost all of the colds or sore throats. This establishes upon all of these patients an over-susceptibility to the weather changes, and they keep taking these red mercurial powders. Some of them carry them around in their pockets. But the more they take of these red powders the more frequently they have sore throats and colds. Many times they will not get over these troubles without Kali iod. in potentized form, or *Hepar.* *Hepar* and Kali iod. are the two principal medicines that such patients need. Individuals with this susceptibility to colds and sore throats and weather changes, that is, from the effects of *Mercury,* who have been led into a *Mercurial* state, run two ways. Those who are invariably shivering and cold, and want to hover around the fire, and cannot keep warm, will need *Hepar,* and those that are always too warm, that want the covers off, and want to be in constant motion, extreme restlessness, very tired when keeping still, will have their *Mercury* antidoted by Kali iod. The *Mercurial* state will be antidoted, but it sometimes takes several prescriptions and sometimes a series of carefully selected remedies. The psora, that is, his chronic state, will not manifest itself until you have lifted off this miasmatic state, which has been caused by *Mercurius*. It is astonishing what a great number of men, women and children are bowed down by the miasm that *Mercury* produces, and yet those prescribers go on giving this form of *Mercury* and say it is practicing Homœopathy. I am led to remark that there is yet much to be learned about the art of prescribing.

This remedy has a peculiar mental state. There is a very strong degree of *irritability, cruelty, and harshness of temper.* He is harsh with his family and with his children; abusive. It will take all the sense of refinement out of his mind and then he will become sad and tearful. Extremely nervous, and must walk and be on the go. If he remains in a warm room he becomes weak and tired, and feels as if he could not stir, does not want to move, and does not know what is the matter with him. He is worse in the warmth of the house, but as soon as he goes into the open air he feels better, and as soon as he begins to walk he feels still better and can walk long distances without fatigue; goes into the house again and becomes weak and tired and exhausted. A nervous and mental exhaustion comes on from resting.

The head manifests some peculiar things, such as we sometimes see in syphilis, which the remedy controls when the other symptoms agree. Bi-parietal head pains of nerve syphilis, old, long standing cases. Pains through the parietal bones, through the side of the head, as if crushed in a vise; awful crushing, pulsating, pressing, rending pains on both sides of the head. These are worse in the house, and better from warmth and from motion, better walking in the open air. All through the head there are pains like knife stabs, like nails driven in; lancinating pains, cutting pains in the scalp, in the temples, over the eyes, through the eyes. The pericranium becomes sensitive and filled with nodules. The scalp breaks out with nodular eruptions, tuberculous eruptions, syphilitic eruptions. "Scalp painful on scratching as if ulcerated." "Great disposition for hair to change color and fall out." Coldness of the painful parts

In watching a syphilitic case, there is often noticed disturbance of vision and finally iritis. They can be treated homœopathically. I have seen syphilitic iritis of the most severe character cured with *Staphisagria, Hepar, Nitric acid, Mercurius,* Kali iod. and many other remedies. The inflammatory process stops at once, there are no adhesions, no deformity, and no troubles remaining behind. If you consider that a case of inflammation *must* run its course, and will be associated with fibrinous exudations, and adhesions most probably follow, of course you must adopt the plan of dilating with *Atropine,* and hold the iris so until the disease has run its course. But the disease *does not* run its course after a proper remedy, and as that is the last symptom to appear, it will be the first to go, and you may expect the eye symptoms to disappear within twenty-four hours after the administration of the homœopathic remedy

This remedy has marked conjunctival trouble, with green catarrhal dis charges from the eyes. This green character applies whenever you can find discharges. *There is copious, thick, green expectoration, green discharges of muco-pus* from the nose, from the eyes, from the ear, thick, greenish leucorrhœa, green discharge from ulcers. These thick green or yellowish-green discharges are sometimes very fœtid.

At times when you examine the conjunctiva it seems to puff out as though water were behind it, a chemosis. Iodide of potash produces that state. "Chemosis, purulent secretion." In olden times when I used to give Iodide of potash to rheumatic patients, according to the prevailing craze, I would notice, after a day or two, chemosis coming into the eyes and the patient beginning to ache in his bones all over, while the rheumatism of the joints would disappear. An allopathic effect was taking root upon that patient which would last for years. I have noticed that a large dose of Kali iod. in syphilitics would make the patient get up the next morning with difficulty in opening the lids, and upon opening the eyes the conjunctiva would form water bags, as though water were behind them and they were bagged out. Kali iod. also produces œdema of the lids and injection and tumefaction of the conjunctiva. The mucous membrane becomes red, raw and bleeding. The vessels are enlarged and the surface is very sore, inflamed and smarting. He is compelled to hold the eyelids during winking; the winking is painful and causes scratching, as from sand. Acute conjunctivitis, especially when it occurs in patients who have rheumatism, who have been abused with *Mercury,* or those afflicted with syphilis. Syphilitic and rheumatic affections of the eye.

Old gouty subjects who must keep in motion, and must keep in the open air, who are always too warm, and cannot endure any degree of warmth in the room, who suffer more from their gouty pains when keeping quiet, those who are fatigued when keeping quiet and can walk and move without fatigue in the open air, especially when it is cold, with enlarged joints, with restlessness, anxiety, nervousness, harshness of the temper and great irritability, alternating with weeping. This relief from motion will make the routinist give *Rhus* in many instances, but *Rhus* would have no relation to the case whatever. Remember, *Rhus* is a cold patient, who is always shivering and wants to be by the fire, whose complaints are > by the heat, he is > in a warm room and becomes fatigued from motion, whereas Kali iod. does not become fatigued from continued motion.

The nose comes in for much trouble. In old syphilitic catarrhs they blow out great crusts and pieces of bone; syphilitic ozæna; the bones of the nose are very sensitive to touch and become necrosed, and the nose flattens down and becomes soft. It is deprived of the bony framework that holds it in shape and settles down flat, leaving only the red tip. Extreme pain at the root of the nose like *Hepar.* Thick, yellowish-green, copious discharge from the nose. Every change of the weather brings on catarrhal states. He is constantly taking cold, sneezing continuously. Copious, watery discharge from the nose, excoriating the passage, and causing burning in the nose. This coryza is < in the open air, but all the rest of the patient is > in the open air. Consequently, when a patient has two such conditions that operate against each other he suffers much, because he cannot find quarters for relief. In a warm room his nasal catarrh, or his coryza, is > but in the open air he feels > as to the rest of his complaints. "Repeated attacks of violent, acrid coryza from the least cold." With the coryza the frontal sinuses become involved, and there is great pain through the forehead; pain in the eyes, pains through the cheek-bones.

In the throat, as you might suppose from its relations to syphilis and *Mercury*, there is much trouble. Deep ulcers in the throat, old syphilitic ulcers; perforating ulcers, eating away and destroying all the soft tissues, the uvula and the soft palate. Ulceration upon the tonsils; enlarged tonsils; very painful sore throat. Knots and knobs in the throat upon the mucous membranes. "Dryness of throat and enlarged tonsils." "Terrible pain at the root of the tongue at night." The whole pharynx, larynx, trachea and bronchial tubes suffer from catarrhal conditions. Inflammatory conditions with greenish discharge.

While all the external symptoms and the rest of the body symptoms are relieved in the cold air and by the contact of external cold, internally cold things aggravate. Cold milk, ice cream, ice water, cold drinks and cold food, cold things in the stomach < all the symptoms. Though he has an excessive thirst and will drink large quantities of water, if very cold it will make him sick.

Kali iod. has all the flatulence and belching of *Carbo veg.* and *Lycopodium*.

The glands all over the body become tumid, enlarged and hard. It has cured enlargement of the thyroid gland; it may take this from *Iodine*.

Very characteristic is the chronic inflammation of the urethra, following gonorrhœa, where the discharge is thick and green, or greenish-yellow, *without pain*. Inflammation of the testicles, syphilitic in character.

Pain and rawness in the larynx, with hoarseness; awakens from constriction of the larynx. It is very useful in phthisis of the larynx. Cough from constant irritation in the larynx. Dry, hacking cough, hoarse cough with copious greenish expectoration. Catarrhal phthisis with thick, copious, greenish expectoration. Pleuritic effusion. Fluttering of the heart. Palpitation on slight exertion or when walking. Rapid pulse.

Not only in old gouty troubles, but in patients threatening phthisis, and in old malarial troubles this medicine will be of great service.

It cures sciatica when the pain is sharp from the hip down, worse lying, sitting or standing and better walking.

You may go to the bedside of a patient who is suffering from what she calls "hives;" you will find she is covered from head to foot with an eruption that forms great nodules; she is fairly burning up from head to foot. She cannot endure any covering; the heat of her body is intense, yet she has no rise of temperature. Rough nodular manifestations all over the skin; a condition that will go away in a few hours, but in a few days, weeks or months come back again. A single dose of a very high potency of Kali iod. will turn things into order in persons subject to these hives and they will not come again.

KALI MURIATICUM

Symptoms appear in the morning; forenoon; afternoon; evening; *night;* before midnight; after midnight. Aversion to the open air and sensitive to drafts. The open air aggravates many symptoms. Asleep feeling in single parts. Dread of bathing and worse from bathing. Cold in general makes the symptoms worse; worse from cold air; worse from becoming cold; worse from cold, wet weather. It has been a useful remedy in many kinds of convulsions; clonic; *epileptic;* epileptiform; internal. Worse after eating and from exertion. Fainting spells. Worse from cold food, fat food, cold drinks. Formication in many parts. Sensation of fulness. Easy bleeding of any part; blood dark and clotted. Heaviness external and internal. *Induration of many tissues;* in glands; in muscles. Inflammation and the results of induration; infiltration following inflammation; hepatization after pneumonia (Calc. Sulph.). Marked lassitude. Desire to lie down. Complaints from lifting and straining of muscles and joints. Lying makes many symptoms worse; worse after lying; worse lying in bed; worse lying on the right side. Wore lying on the painful side; better lying on the painless side. Worse before and *during* menses; worse from motion. Increased mucous discharges *viscid and milk-white.* The pains are biting, bruised, burning, *cutting,* jerking, pinching, pressing, stitching. Stitching pains, outward, transversely in glands, *in muscles.* Tearing downward in muscles Twinging and ulcerative pains.

Paralysis one-sided; of organs. Pulse full, hard, intermittent, irregular, slow; small, soft. General pulsation. Marked relaxation of muscles. Rising from sitting increases or brings on symptoms. Rubbing ameliorates symptoms. Sensitive to pain. Complaints one-sided; either side; mostly *left side.* Complaints worse while sitting: Sluggish patients; feeble reaction; slow repair; slow convalescence. Swelling of parts; of glands. Feeling of tension in muscles. Aggravation from touch. Twitching of mucles. Warmth of bed makes some symptoms worse. Weakness of the whole body; in the morning; in the evening; after acute catarrhal diseases; from walking. Worse in wet weather.

Irritability and anger in the evening; anxiety: in the evening; about trifles. She has a delusion that she must not eat. Discontented and discouraged. Dullness of mind. Mental exictement. Fear that some evil will come to him. It has been used with benefit in imbecility. Indifference to all pleasure. Insanity and irresolution. Loathing of life. Moaning, MANIA. Obstinate. Restlessness. *Sadness.* Silent. Inclination to sit in complete silence. Talking in sleep. Unconsciousness in advanced states of brain and meningeal diseases. Vertigo; when rising or stooping; when walking.

Constriction of the scalp. Dandruff, copious, white. Eczema. Heaviness of the head; of the forehead; in the *occiput* with aching in trachea and hard cough; in the *occiput* as if full of lead; in occiput as if head would sink backwards; in *occiput* with hard cough. Sensation of looseness of the brain. Sensation of movements in the head. Pain in the head in the morning on walking; in the afternoon; *evening;* in cold air; in the open air; worse from binding up the hair; worse after eating; paroxysmal; worse from pressure; worse from stooping; worse from touch; worse walking; worse walking in the open air; worse from wine; better from wrapping up the head. Pain in the forehead. Pain in occiput, like a weight holds head fast to pillow (like Opium). Pain in the sides of head; temples; boring, bruised, burning in forehead; cutting; gnawing in occiput; jerking. Pressing pain in whole head; in forehead, outward; in *occiput;* in temples, outward. Shooting pain in head, in occiput. Stitching pain in head; worse stooping; in forehead; in *occiput;* in sides of head; in temples. Stunning pains in head. Tearing pains in the head; in the forehead; in the occiput and sides of occiput; in *sides of head;* in the temples; in the *vertex.* PERSPIRATION ON THE HEAD. Pulsation in the head. Shocks in the head.

Catarrhal discharges with milk-white mucus or greenish or yellow purulent. Inflammation of the conjunctiva with thickening; PUSTULES; of the *cornea.* Burning in the eyes; in the canthi. Pressing: Pain as if sand in the eyes. STITCHING pain in eyes. Photophobia. Protrusion of the eyes. Redness in the evening with pain. Staring. Swollen lids. Twitching inner canthi. Vesicles on the cornea. Vision dim. Double vision. Lights before the eyes when coughing or sneezing.

Closure of the eustachian tubes. Discharge from ears of milk-white mucus. Dry catarrh of the middle ear; the ears are hot. Stitching in the ears. Noises: buzzing; cracking on blowing nose and on swallowing; humming; reverberations; ringing; roaring; singing; snapping; tickling; whizzing. Pain in the ear; behind the ear; drawing; pressing; *stitching;* stitching behind the ear; tearing; tearing behind the ear. Pulsation behind the ear. Tingling in the ears. Twitching. Hearing acute; for noise; for voices; impaired.

Nasal catarrh; discharge copious; *excoriating;* purulent; thick; *white; milk-white;* viscid; yellow; posterior nares. *Coryza;* with cough; fluent, dry; *thick* and *milk-white discharge.* Dryness in the nose. Epistaxis in the afternoon; evening. Itching in the nose. The nose is obstructed with mucus. Frequent sneezing.

Epithelioma of the lips and lupus of the face. The face is bluish; pale; red. Dryness of the lips. Eruptions on the face; cheeks; lips; *around the mouth;* pimples. Suffering, sickly expression. Flashes of heat in the face. The face is hot. Pain in the face; worse in the right side; drawing; *stitching; tearing.* Paralysis of the face. Perspiration. *Sunken face.* Painful, swollen face; lips; glands of jaw. Tension. Twitching. Ulceration of face; lips.

Aphthæ in the mouth of children and nursing mothers. Bleeding gums. Gum boils. The tongue is red or *white.* Dry mouth and tongue. Heat in the mouth. inflammation of gums and tongue. *Mapped tongue. Milk-white mucus in the mouth.* Odor from the mouth offensive, even putrid. Burning mouth and tongue. Sore gums and tongue. *Scorbutic gums.* Salivation. Speech wanting. Swollen gums and tongue. Taste; *bad, bitter;* metallic; *putrid; saltish; sour; sweetish.* Ulceration of *mouth* and tongue; *syphilitic.* Vesicles in the mouth. Teeth on edge and become loose. Pain in the teeth; stitching.

The throat is dry and red and there is choking. Heat in the throat and much mucus. Inflammation of throat; tonsils; *chronic.* White exudate in the throat; gray patches. It has many times cured diphtheria. Mucus: VISCID; thick; *milk-white;* covers pharynx; adherent. Pain in throat; on swallowing; burning; pressing; rawness; *sore.* Scraping in the throat. Swallowing very difficult. Swollen throat; *tonsils; uvula,* œdematous; parotid gland. Ulceration of the throat.

Anxiety of the stomach. The appetite is diminished or entirely lost or it is increased, even ravenous, after eating. Aversion to food; to meat. Constriction of the stomach. Emptiness not ameliorated by eating. Eructations: after eating; ineffectual; bitter; empty; of food; sour; waterbrash. Flashes of heat; heartburn, and sensation of fulness. Weight in stomach worse at night. Hiccough. Inflammation of the stomach. Loathing of food. Nausea after fats and rich food. Nausea and shivering. Pain in the stomach; aching; burning; cutting; pressing with emptiness; sore to touch; stitching. Tension. Thirst extreme; during chill. Vomiting; bile; blood; *food;* mucus, milk-white and dark green; morning diarrhœa with vomiting white mucus; sudden; incessant.

Distension in abdomen after eating. *Emptiness.* Ascites. Enlarged spleen. Flatulence; in day time; afternoon; night; prevents sleep. FULNESS; AFTER EATING. Pain in abdomen; night; colic; griping with diarrhœa; during diarrhoea; after eating; as if menses would appear; before and *during* stool; in hypochondria, especially the right, burning in right hypochondrium. Cramping in abdomen; before stool; in hypogastrium with diarrhœa. Cutting in abdomen, in umbilical region. Pressing in hypochondria; in right better by passing flatus. Sore bruised abdomen; in right hypochondrium; in inguinal region. Rumbling before stool. Tension in abdomen.

Constipation; stool difficult; from inactivity of the rectum. The stool is dry, *hard,* large, light colored, clay colored. Diarrhœa; painful; morning, evening; after fats. The stool is excoriating; bloody mucus; copious; green; offensive; watery; white mucus. Dysentery with slimy stool or pure blood. Flatus during diarrhœa. *Formication of the anus.* Hemorrhage from rectum. Hemorrhoids; congested; *external;* large; SORE; worse walking. Involuntary stools; when passing flatus. Itching of the anus; *after stool. Pain* in rectum and anus; during and after stool. Burning during and *after stool.* Pressing in the anus. SORENESS; *after stool.* Tenesmus. Paralysis of the rectum. Urging with normal stool; constant.

Catarrh of the bladder with much mucus in the urine. Retention of urine. Urging to urinate; at night; constant; *frequent;* ineffectual. Urination *dribbling;* feeble stream; frequent, at night; involuntary at night; retarded. Must press long to start the urine. Inflammation of the kidneys. Pain in the kidney's. Suppression of urine. It has been used much in chronic gonorrhœa with gleety, milky discharge. It has cured violent chordee. Itching of the urethra. Burning and cutting during urination. Urine: albuminous; black; greenish-black; *bloody;* burning; cloudy; dark; pale; red; copious at night; scanty; containing sugar; thick.

Inflammation of glans penis and testes. Indurated testes. Erections troublesome; violent. Stitching of the scrotum. Drawing pain in testes. Seminal emissions. Ulcers on the penis; chancres.

Leucorrhœa: excoriating; MILKY; white; VISCID. Menses bright red; clotted, *frequent;* late; painful. Metrorrhagia. Labor-like pain.

Irritation of larynx; inflammation; dryness; croup. Mucus in the larynx. THICK MILKY Larynx sensitive to touch. Tickling in larynx. Hoarseness; voice finally lost. Respiration rapid; *asthmatic;* deep; *difficult;* rattling; snoring. Cough day and night; asthmatic; barking; from deep breathing; croupy; dry; hacking; after eating; harsh; from irritation in larynx and trachea; loose; paroxysmal; racking; short; violent; whooping cough. Expectoration morning; bloody; mucus; white; gray; *milk-white;* yellow.

Catarrh of the chest and anxiety of the heart. Coldness in the region of the heart. Congestion and flashes of heat in chest. Constriction of the chest; of the heart; as from sulphur fumes. Hemorrhage of the lungs. Hepatization of lungs after pneumonia. Inflammation of *bronchial tubes; of lungs; pleura.* *Oppression of the chest. Pain* in chest; on respiration; sides of chest, on respiration; heart; cutting; pressing; *soreness.* Stitching on breathing; stitching in the heart. Violent palpitation.

Coldness in the back. Stitching of the back. Pain in the back; on breathing; better lying; while sitting; while standing; while walking. Pain between the scapulæ. Pain in the lumbar region; better lying; while sitting and standing. Pain in the *sacrum;* better lying. Pain in the coccyx. Aching in the back; lumbar region; sacrum. Burning in the back. Drawing pain in lumbar region; in sacrum. Lightning-like pains in small of back to feet, must get out of bed and sit up. Pressing pains in back; in lumbar region. Stitching pains in scapula:; in sacrum.

Cold extremities; HANDS; *feet.* Cracking in joints and tendons of back of hand. *Cramps* in *limbs;* thighs; LEGS. Eruptions in limbs; pimples; vesicles. Heat of hands and feet: burning soles. Pains in the limbs; nightly; rheumatic worse from the warmth of bed; rheumatic in joints; rheumatic left shoulder and elbow. Drawing pains in wrists; thighs; knees; legs. Pressing pains in shoulders. Stitching pains in knees, in legs. Tearing pains in shoulders; hands; fingers; in thighs, worse from heat of bed; in *knees; calf.* Paralysis of one side; perspiration of feet; *cold.* Stiffness of knees. Swelling of legs and ankles; œdematous. Tension in knees; calf. Twitching in limbs; in *thighs.* Ulcers on legs, warts on hands. Weakness of the limbs; of thighs.

Dreams; amorous; *anxious;* of depth; of previous events; frightful; of misfortune; pleasant; vexatious; vivid. Restless sleep. Sleepiness afternoon; evening; after dinner; *after eating.* Sleeplessness all night. Waking early.

Chill morning; afternoon; evening; in *open* air; in bed; chilliness in evening; external coldness; shaking chill. Fever evening in bed. Perspiration morning; *night;* midnight.

Burning or coldness of skin. Dryness of skin. Eruptions; eczema; herpes; pimples; scabby; scaly; white, thin bran-like scales; vesicles. Jaundice. Erysipelas. Excoriation; intertrigo. Formication. Itching in evening in bed; night; burning; crawling; better by *scratching;* stinging. *Ulcers* burning; suppurating, warts.

KALI PHOSPHORICUM

The symptoms of this remedy are worse morning, evening, and during the night. The over-sensitive, nervous, delicate persons, worn out from long suffering, much sorrow and vexation, and prolonged mental work; also such as are broken down from sexual excesses and vices. It is a long-acting

antipsoric. Anæmic and chlorotic patients. Most complaints are worse during
rest, and ameliorated by gentle motion and slowly walking about. The patient
in general, and his pains, are aggravated in cold air, from becoming cold, after
becoming cold, from entering a cold place, and in cold, wet weather. He takes
cold easily. Aversion to the open air. Draft of air aggravates, and open air
aggravates. Numbness in the extremities. Great lassitude. Aggravated by
ascending stairs, and by physical exertion. Glands dwindle. Choreic
movements. Complaints are worse after coition. The weakness, emaciation,
and anæmia and tubercular tendency are strong features of this wonderful
antipsoric remedy. Œdema of the limbs and dropsy of serous sacs. Complaints
aggravated after eating. Emaciation, wasting diseases with *putrid discharges
and putrid stools.* Fainting spells. Fasting ameliorates. Fatty tendency of
muscles and organs. Aggravated after cold drinks, milk. This remedy has
been used in gangrenous condition. Parts become black. Septic, *putrid
hæmorrhages,* and great prostration. All forms of nervous weakness.
Hypochondriasis and hysteria. Inflammation of glands. Complaints from loss
of fluids. Orgasm of blood. The pains are aching, pressing, stitching, tearing,
tearing downwards, paralyzing. Chronic neuralgia, ameliorated by gentle
motion, aggravated from cold. One-sided paralysis from a gradually
Increasing weakness. Paroxysms of pain followed by exhaustion Pulsation
felt all over the body and in the limbs. Symptoms are often *one-sided.* Many
symptoms come during and after sleep. Twitching of muscles, and jerking of
limbs. Ulcers with putrid discharges. Offensive catarrhal discharges. Walking
fast aggravates; walking in open air aggravates. Warmth of bed ameliorates.
Complaints worse in winter. Too many cures have been made by the followers
of Schuessler to permit this remedy to remain unexplained. Good provings
are found in our literature. The high and highest potencies have served the
best. and it should be used in the single dose.

Flies into a passion and can hardly articulate. Aversion to answering
questions. Apprehensive anxiety, in the evening in bed, and during the night;
anxiety after eating, about the future, about his health, about his salvation.
Whenever he wakens it oppresses him, and he becomes hypochondriacal.
She takes an antipathy to her husband. She is cruel to her baby and husband.
Perverted affections. Broods over his condition. Aversion to company.
Complaints come on from bad news. Confusion of mind morning and evening.
Contrary humor. Low form of delirium in typhoid and septic fevers. Delirium
tremens. Imaginations. Sees dead people. Sees figures, frightful images.
Discontented and sad. Dullness of mind in the morning. Discouraged. He
refuses to eat. He is very excitable and greatly wrought up from bad news;
then follows palpitation and many nervous symptoms. Exhaustion after
exertion of mind. He dwells much in fancy. Fear in the evening. Fear of a

crowd, of death, of *disease,* of evil, of people, *of solitude.* He is easily frightened, which increases his many nervous and mental symptoms. *Weak memory. Forgetful.* Cannot recall words. Home-sickness. Effects of grief and prolonged sorrow. A nervous hurry is noticed in action and speech. Nervous excitement has increased until hysterical conduct is present. It is a great remedy for *imbecility.* She is impatient and impetuous. Indifference to surroundings, to joy and to her family. Indifference to his business matters, and then comes indolence and lassitude. Insanity; melancholia; thinks she has sinned away her day of grace and refuses to eat. She does not recognize her surroundings. Shrieks and acts like one insane. Quarrels with her family. The irritability is very marked, in morning on waking, in the evening, after coition, during headache, during menses, when spoken to, on waking at any time, after becoming exhausted from a diarrhœa. There is laughing and crying, lamenting and wringing the hands. There is loathing of life; moaning during sleep. *Dullness of the senses.* Weakness of memory for words, and great *prostration of mind. Sadness* in morning on waking, in the evening, and also day and night. Obstinate; morose; mood changeable. Mistakes in speaking and writing. In many cases cured a mild mental state was noticed. Over-sensitive in general, and especially to noise. Restlessness during menses. The numerous cases of nervous prostration from mental work, prolonged anxiety, much sorrow, and sexual excesses and vice are likely to require this remedy. Incoherent speech. Starting; *easily startled* from fright, during sleep, *from touch* and *from noise.* Stupefaction and *suspicious.* He is indisposed to talk, or to be talked to. Talking in sleep. Vanishing of thought. Becomes timid and bashful. Vexation brings on many complaints. *Weeping* and weary of life.

Vertigo afternoon and evening, ameliorated in open air, aggravated after eating, with a tendency to fall forward: aggravated on looking upwards, compelling him to lie down; with nausea and with headache; objects turn in a circle on rising up, when standing, when stooping, on turning the head, when walking in open air.

The head is cold, and sensitive to cold air. Congestion; fulness of the head felt on coughing. Heat in head evening, flushes of heat in the forehead. The head inclines to fall forward. Tension of scalp. Heaviness of the head, morning on rising, in forehead and occiput. This has been a useful remedy in hydrocephalus and many brain affections, when associated with putrid diarrhœa. Itching of the scalp morning on waking, in the night in bed, aggravated 3 to 5 A.M. Movements felt in the head. It has much pain in the head. Pain *morning* in bed, on rising, on waking, and *passes off on moving about.* Pain afternoon, evening and *night.* Worse in very cold air, but ameliorated in open fresh air. She must let the hair hang down. The headache comes with coryza, comes from taking cold. The pain is worse on coughing, and ameliorated by eating; aggravated from becoming over heated, from disordering the stomach, from excitement, and from physical exertion. Weight in occiput with exhaustion. Must lie down and shun the light, lying on back ameliorates; aggravated from jarring and stepping, aggravated before and during menses. The headaches from mental work, in students, brain-fag from overwork are cured by this remedy—when the symptoms agree. Nervous headache during menses. Paroxysmal headaches. The pains in head are ameliorated by gentle motion; aggravated from noise, riding in a carriage, after sleep, sneezing, stepping, stooping, touch, pressure, walking and writing. Headache comes from eye-strain, and is ameliorated by wrapping up the head. Violent pulsating pains. Pain in forehead before menses, above the eyes extending to occiput; across forehead into both temples. Pain in occiput lasting all night; frequent waking, with pain on rising; wakens with pain in occiput and loins ameliorated lying on back, passes off after rising. Pain in occiput as if hair were pulled; must let hair hang down. Violent headache in *sides of head.* Neuralgia of left mastoid process, aggravated by motion and in open air. Pain in temples. The pains are aching, boring; burning. Burning in forehead during stool. Bursting in forehead. Drawing in forehead, sides of head and vertex. Jerking pain, pressing pain. Forehead as though bored, ameliorated by eating. Pressing *outward* in *forehead* over eyes as if brain would expand. Pressing in occiput, ameliorated by eating. Pressing in temples and vertex. Soreness in occiput. Stitching in the head, forehead, over eyes, in occiput, sides of head, right frontal eminence and in temples. Stunning pains. Tearing pains in the head, in forehead before menses, ameliorated lying and on appearance of the flow. Tearing in occiput, sides of head, temples, and vertex. Perspiration on mental exertion, of the forehead; cold sweat. Pulsation, forehead and temples. The brain is very sensitive to jar, and to sounds. Shocks felt in the head. Softening of the brain. Complaints come on from uncovering the head.

Anæmia of the optic nerve. Lids agglutinated in the morning and a discharge of mucus, aggravated in the evening. Dryness and dullness of the eyes. Falling of the lids. Inflammation of the conjunctiva, injected blood-vessels and lachrymation. Paralysis of the optic nerve. Photophobia. Redness of the eyes. Staring, restless, excited look. Strabismus following brain diseases. Sunken eyes. Swollen œdematous lids. Twitching of eyes and lids. Weak eyes. Pain in eyes on motion of eyes, on reading, on waking; aggravated in sunlight. Aching. Smarting of eyes and margins of lids. Drawing, pressing. The balls are sore to touch. Sharp pains from eyes to temples in the morning. Stitching. Sticks. Sensation of sand. Tearing pains. Blurred vision. Colors before the eyes, floating black spots, dark colors; halo around the light. Dim vision after *coition.* Vision is foggy. Exertion of vision brings on eye troubles and headaches. Vision weak.

Discharge from the ear, bloody, *offensive, putrid, purulent.* Eruptions on the ears. Pimples in the canal. Fulness in ears. The ears are hot. Itching in the ears, aggravated lying. Noises from nervous exhaustion and cerebral anæmia, with vertigo. Buzzing, fluttering, humming, ringing, roaring, rushing, *singing,* whizzing. Pain deep in ear. Cramping, drawing, pressing. Stitching in left ear down to cheek, and behind the ear. Stinging in ear, aggravated lying. Tearing in ear. Pulsation in ear. Stopped sensation. Singing in ear. Ears swollen. Twitching. Hearing acute to noises and voices, but impaired as to the articulation of the human voice. Deafness.

Coryza, fluent or dry, with cough, with *headache.* Hay-fever with great nervous weakness. Obstinate catarrh. Discharge bloody, excoriating, greenish *offensive,* purulent, stringy, thick, watery, white, *yellow,* worse in the morning. Yellow crusts, worse in right nostril. He suffers much from dryness in the nose. Epistaxis in the morning, on blowing the nose, in low fevers. The nose is obstructed. Itching and burning in the nose. Pressing pain at the root of the nose. Much soreness inside of the nose, with yellow crusts and dark blood. Smell at first acute, later wanting. Sneezing frequent; violent at 2 P.M., from slight exposure. Ulceration in the nose. The nose is swollen.

Brown patch from the edge of the brows to the eyebrows, three inches wide, lasting three months. Chlorotic face. Dark circles under eyes. Cracked lips. Face pale, sickly and dirty. Circumscribed red cheeks. Jaundiced face. Herpes on the lips. Sore crusts on lips. Vesicles on lips. The expression is haggard, sickly and suffering. Flushes of heat in face. Inflammation and swelling of the parotid gland. Itching of the face, in the whiskers, on right cheek, on temples. There are drawing, stitching, tearing pains in the face, aggravated in cold air. Cold applications ameliorate pain in right side of face from a hollow tooth. Pain in jaw bones, ameliorated after eating, speaking, waking and touch. Neuralgia of face followed by great weakness. Neuralgic stitch riding in cold air, ameliorated by heat of hand. Paralysis of one side of face (*Caust.*). The face perspires. Swollen lips, parotid and submaxillary glands. Tension of the face. Ulceration of lips.

The tongue is dark coated and bleeding. The gums bleed, and are covered with sores. The typhoid mouth, tongue and teeth in septic fevers when there are putrid odors. Redness of gums and edges of the tongue. The tongue is white, slimy, greenish yellow. Dry mouth and tongue in the morning. Inflamed mouth and gums. *Offensive odor, putrid morning,* like spoiled cheese. Sore burning mouth and tongue. Receding gums. Thick salty saliva. Scorbutic,. spongy gums. The roof of the mouth swollen in ridges, feels as if lined with grease. Taste bad, bitter, insipid, *putrid,* sour; bitter in the morning. Grinding teeth in sleep. Nervous chattering of teeth. Pain in teeth from taking cold, aggravated by cold things, aggravated masticating, aggravated after sleep.

Pulsating, aching, jerking, pressing, sore, stitching, *tearing.*

This remedy has been used with some success in diphtheria with *putrid odor.* Dryness in throat in evening. Fulness and constriction of the throat. Inclination to clear the throat by hawking. Mucus in the throat in the morning, sometimes tasting salty. Lump in throat. Pain in throat on swallowing. Pain in right tonsil. Burning, rawness, soreness. Stitching on swallowing. Stitching pain from left tonsil to ear, while driving in forenoon. Inflammation and swelling of throat and tonsils, with white deposits like membrane.

The appetite is increased and sometimes ravenous, but goes on the sight of food. Hunger soon after eating, from nervous weakness. Hunger during menses. Aversion to food, to bread, to meat. Sensation of coldness in the stomach. Desires *cold drinks,* sour things, sweets. The stomach is commonly disordered. *Fulness* and distension. Emptiness with nausea, during menses, after eating. Eructations, after eating, ineffectual, of bile, bitter, empty, of food, sour; waterbrash. Heartburn. Weight in stomach after eating. Loathing of food. Nausea on coughing, after eating, during headache, during menses, during pregnancy; ameliorated by eructations. Retching. Pain in stomach after eating and during menses. Burning, cramping, cutting, *soreness.* Stitching. Gnawing pain at 5 A.M. on waking. Pressing after eating. Sensation of a stone in the stomach. Extreme thirst for cold water. Thirst during heat. Thirstlessness sometimes. Vomiting in the morning, on coughing, after eating, during headaches, during menses, during pregnancy. Vomiting bile, blood, *food,* mucus, sour.

The abdomen feels cold, and is sensitive to uncovering. Distension after eating, during menses. Tympanitic with great pain, in *typhoid fever.* Distended with dropsy. Sensation of emptiness. Fermentation with distress in heart. Flatulence, *obstructed, noisy.* Sensation of fulness after eating. Heat in abdomen and heaviness. Inflammation of intestines, peritoneum, and liver. Pain in abdomen agravated at night; across the abdomen left to right; bending double ameliorates; during cough, during diarrhœa, *after eating, before* and during menses; paroxysmal; before stool. Pain in region of liver. Bearing down, ameliorated sitting, aggravated lying on left side, aggravated after drinking. Seems as though sides of abdomen would burst when sneez-ing. Burning. Cramping after eating. Cutting. Griping in hypogastrium with ineffectual urging to stool. *Soreness* in abdomen and liver. Stitching in abdomen and liver. Stitching, catching in spleen, aggravated from motion, Rumbling and tension.

Constipation with very difficult stool; hard, large, knotty. Diarrhœa, morning, 6 A.M., evening, *night,* during or *after eating;* colliquative; from fright or excitement, during menses, painless, with vomiting and cramps, with *great exhaustion,* in *typhoid.* Dysentery Offensive flatus which ameliorates the symptoms. Formication of the anus. Hæmorrhage from intestines in typhoid. Hæmorrhoids, external and internal, itching, painful with burning and swelling. Inflamed piles with offensive moisture. Inactivity of the rectum. Involuntary stools. Pain in rectum during and after stool. Burning during and after stool. *Soreness* and pressing pains. Stitching pain. Tenesmus after stool. Paralysis of the rectum. Relaxed anus. Ineffectual urging to stool. The stool is excoriating; bloody mucus or pure blood, brown, clay colored, watery stool; putrid flatus followed by tenesmus after breakfast. Stool *copious,* dark, frequent; large,, light colored. Lienteric stools. Stools OFFENSIVE PUTRID, purulent, watery, like rice water, yellow or yellowish green mucus.

Chronic catarrh of the bladder in old people and nervous wrecks. Pressing and stitching in the bladder. The urging to urinate is frequent, or ineffectual, and worse at night. The urine dribbles. Dribbling after urination; feeble stream, frequent, copious at night. Stream *stops and starts. involuntary at night,* in old people, in typhoid, in nervous prostration. In obstinate cases of enuresis, in excitable sensitive children. Unsatisfactory urination. Inflammation and stitching in the kidneys. Burning in the urethra during and after urination. Stitching in the urethra. The urine is albuminous, burning, cloudy, *copious,* offensive, scanty, watery, yellow like saffron. Sediment is flocculent, mucous, red and sandy. Specific gravity increased. Sugar in the urine.

Erections very troublesome in the morning and during the night without sexual desire; violent in the morning. *Impotency. Frequent* seminal emissions with erections. Inflammation of glans penis. Sexual passion obliterated.

In tired out nervous women who are subject to abortion. Aversion to coition. Desire increased, intense for four or five days after menses. Inflammation of uterus. Itching from leucorrhœa. It cured a chronic abscess discharging periodically through the vagina and rectum a copious orange-colored fluid. Leucorrhœa *acrid, burning, copious,* greenish, yellow, offensive, putrid; after menses; in young girls. Menses absent, black, *copious, dark,* delayed, frequent, irregular, late, *offensive, painful,* pale, protracted, *scanty, short,* suppressed, *thick.* Uterine hæmorrhage. Pain in ovaries, in left, ameliorated lying on the back and bending double, during menses. Pain in ovaries on going to sleep. Stitching pain in ovaries. Pain in uterus and ovaries at night during pregnancy. Labor-like pains. Prolapsus of uterus.

Irritation of the larynx and trachea in cold air. Catarrh of the air passages, with thick, yellowish white mucus. Soreness and scraping in the larynx. Tickling in *larynx and trachea.* Voice hoarse, *lost from paralysis of the vocal cords;* hoarse from over-exertion of vocal cords.

Respiration difficult at night; rattling, short; difficult on going upstairs. Nervous asthma, aggravated after eating.

Cough in daytime, morning, evening in bed and during the night. Dry cough at night during fever. Hacking cough. Cough from irritation in larynx and trachea. Loose cough. Paroxysmal cough. Racking cough. Rattling cough. *Short,* spasmodic. Cough in cold air, from deep breathing, during chill and fever, after eating; aggravated lying. Asthmatic cough. Cough from tickling in larynx and trachea. Whistling cough. Whooping-cough with great nervous exhaustion.

Expectoration in *morning,* bloody, frothy, greenish, mucous, *offensive, purulent,* putrid, salty, thick, sweetish, viscid, *yellowish* white.

This remedy has been favorably mentioned in angina pectoris. Anxiety in the chest in the morning. Catarrh of the chest. Spasmodic constriction. Constriction of the heart. Fatty degeneration of the heart. Hæmorrhage from the lungs. Hepatization of the lungs. Inflammation of the bronchial tubes, lungs, pleura. Oppression of the chest. Itching of the skin. Pain in chest during cough, on inspiration, on motion, on breathing. Pain lower part of chest on coughing, inside of chest, in heart. Aching in left side of chest through to scapula. Burning in chest. Cutting under right breast. Soreness in chest. Stitching in chest on coughing, during respiration, in mammæ, sides of chest, in heart. Tearing pains in chest. *Palpitation, anxious,* ascending steps, aggravated by motion. *Violent.* Perspiration like onions in axilla. It is a very useful remedy in catarrhal phthisis. Suffocation of lungs. Swelling in axilla; abscess. Weakness of chest. *Weak heart.* Pulse intermittent and irregular; feeble circulation.

The back feels cold. Eruptions on the back, pimples. Weight in lumbar region. The nape and back lame. Itching. Pain in the back during rest, ameliorated by motion, respiration aggravates, during menses. Pains in occiput and loins morning on waking, ameliorated lying on back, passing off after rising. Pain in back of neck. Pain in dorsal region. Pain in scapulæ morning on waking, had to sit up to turn over. Pain first in right, then left scapulæ. Pain between scapulæ. Pain in lumbar region during menses, while sitting, ameliorated by motion. Pain in sacrum during menses. Intense pain along spine. Pain in coccyx. Aching between scapulæ. Sore, bruised spine. Burning in back, in lumbar region. Drawing in back, lumbar region. Lameness and stiffness of whole back, ameliorated by gentle motion. Stitching pains in the back, in dorsal and lumbar regions. Stitching toward front of chest with dyspnœa, ameliorated leaning back against chair, aggravated lying on the back, sitting or walking. Tearing pains in the back, in lumbar region. Softening of the spinal cord. Weakness with stumbling when walking. Swollen glands of neck. *Weak* back. Cannot sit erect without a chair back to lean against. This remedy cures many nondescript spinal affections.

Cold hands and feet. Feet cold and damp. Cramps in thighs, calves and soles. Eruptions on limbs, pimples. The hands are hot. Heaviness of limbs, of lower limbs and feet. It has been of great service in hip joint disease. Itching of the limbs, of *palms* and *soles.* Numbness of the limbs, upper and lower; hands and finger tips, feet and legs. Rheumatic and gouty pains in limbs and joints, ameliorated by motion and warmth. Pain in back and limbs, ameliorated by motion. Pain in shoulders and arms, in arms when raising them. Sciatica, ameliorated by gentle motion. Pain in hip and knee. Pain in legs 5 A.M. on waking, ameliorated by gentle motion. Bruised knees and legs. Burning feet, soles and toes. Paralytic drawing in limbs,, ameliorated by warmth and gentle motion. Drawing in upper limbs, in the thighs, knees and legs. Drawing laming pain in soles. Pressing pain in shoulder and thighs. Stinging in soles. Stitching in joints, shoulders and knees. Tearing in the limbs; shoulders, upper arm, elbow, forearm, hand, fingers. Tearing in lower limbs; hip, knee, legs, feet. Paralytic tearing in limbs, ameliorated by motion. *Paralysis of limbs. Hemiplegia.* The, feet perspire. The lower limbs and feet are restless. Rheumatic stiffness after resting. Œdema of hands and feet. The hands tremble. The limbs twitch. Weakness in all the limbs, especially the lower.

Profound sleep. Dreams anxious, *amorous,* of falling, frightful, of being naked, nightmare, vivid; night terrors in children (*Borax*). Restless, nervous and hot in sleep. Sleeps on the back. Sleepiness early in evening, after eating. Sleepless after midnight, after mental exertion, after excitement, after vexation. Sleepless with sleepiness. Waking early, as from fright. Walking in sleep. Very troublesome yawning.

Chill, morning, forenoon, noon, afternoon, evening. Chilliness in the open air, in bed. Could scarcely get warm in bed. Chilliness ascending spine in evening. Cold all day. Chilliness after eating. External and internal chill. Nervous shivering and shuddering. Shaking chill. One-sided coldness.

Fever in afternoon and evening. Heat all night, with hunger. Fever alternating with chill. Fever at night in bed. Typhoid fever, low, putrid type. Dry heat. Flushes of heat: It has been a very useful remedy in hectic fevers when there is putrid sweat and putrid expectoration and great nervousness and excitement. Internal heat. Fever with no sweat. Scarlet fever. skin dusky and throat putrid and dark red. Sweat mornings and nights. when eating and drinking, and on slight exertion, during sleep offensive. profuse night sweats.

Dusky spots on calves. Burning after scratching. The skin is cold, jaundiced, dry. Eruption moist, and the moisture is bad smelling. Herpes. Eruptions, itching, pimples, psoriasis, scabby, urticaria; vesicles, bloody, chorous. It has cured erysipelas that was almost gangrenous with putrid odor. *Inactivity of the skin.* Itching, crawling, stinging in the skin. Very sensitive skin. Sticking in skin. Ulcers, burning, offensive, even putrid, with yellow discharges.

654

KALI SILICATUM

The silicate of potassium is a very deep acting remedy. Some of the symptoms are worse or come on in the morning, a few in the forenoon and afternoon, many in the evening, and very many in the *night,* and especially *after midnight.* Aversion to the open air and worse from the open air and from draughts He dreads bathing and is worse from bathing. *He is sensitive to cold weather and worse from becoming cold;* after becoming cold complaints come on; worse in cold room and in dry, cold weather; cold, wet weather also makes him worse. He takes cold easily. After eating complaints are all worse; worse after slight exertion. Faintness, *emaciation.* He is worse after *cold drinks,* cold food, milk and fat food. Creeping feelings all over the body, but especially in the limbs. Induration in glands and muscles. His painful parts are very sensitive to a jar. Lassitude is very marked and quite constant. *Desire to lie down* all the time. After straining muscles the weakness lasts long. He dreads to move or walk and he is worse from motion.

Mucous secretions all increased. The blood surges from the body to the head. Stitching, tearing pains are numerous; he suffers if the perspiration is suppressed from a draft, or from insufficient clothing; he is worse from pressure and very sensitive to touch.

Pulsation in head and limbs; stiffness all over the body and in the limbs; he trembles all over, especially in abdomen; twitching of muscles. Symptoms all *worse from uncovering the body;* worse walking and from walking fast. Great weakness in the morning on waking, also in the evening; also after eating and after walking. *Weariness.* Worse in winter, in cold weather and better in summer.

Absent-minded and becomes angered over trifles; anxiety in the evening in bed and during the night; anxiety with fear; anxiety after eating, about his health; during menses, about trifles, carpriciousness. It is a very useful remedy for children in school when they cannot learn their lessons. Difficult concentration of mind; he has lost confidence in his own ability. Confusion of mind in the morning on arising, in the evening, *after mental exertion,* while sitting. Consolation aggravates the mental symptoms; contrary and cowardly. His mind is full of imaginations; about dead people; illusions of fancy; sees images in the night; sees frightful images; sees ghosts and thieves He is discontented and discouraged. Dullness of mind when reading and writing; in the morning on waking. Much excitement. Mental exertion aggravates many symptoms. Fear with anxiety; fear and dread of work; easily frightened; forgetful and heedless, which looks like approaching imbecility many hysterical manifestations. He is very impatient, and indifferent to his friends and to pleasure; he takes pleasure in nothing. *Irresolution.* He seem not to care how things *go,* one way is as good as another. Has no opinions on prevailing questions. Extremely irritable; worse in morning and evening; *worse after coition;* worse from any attempt to console him. Memory very feeble; mistakes in speaking and writing; misplaces words. He is very obstinate and his moods are constantly changing. *Mental prostration.* Great restlessness during the night. Very sad in the morning. Seems at times to lose his senses. At times he is very sensitive to noises. It is a very useful remedy where these symptoms have been brought on by sexual excesses. Wants to sit still or sit around and do nothing; *very indolent.* Startled easily, from fright; from noise, on falling asleep, when touched. *Wonderful timidity.* Indisposed to conversation. Talking in sleep. Weeping much; weeping evening and night; weeping in sleep. Will-power feeble; aversion to mental work.

Vertigo morning, afternoon, evening; inclination to fall backwards vertigo during headache, as if intoxicated; must lie down; vertigo with nausea; objects seem to turn in a circle; vertigo almost constant; while rising, *while sitting, while stooping,* while walking, while walking in open air. Coldness of the head, of vertex; the head is sensitive to cold and must be covered. Boiling sensation in the brain; anæmia of the brain; congestion of head at night on coughing; constriction of the scalp, especially of the forehead. Eruptions in margin of the hair, back of head moist-like eczema; fulness of the head and the hair falls out; heat in the whole head; worse in forehead; heaviness in the forehead in the morning; sensation of movements in the head. Pain in the head *morning,* afternoon, evening, *night; after midnight;* pain *worse in cold air* and from a draft; *after coition;* from head becoming cold; from coryza; after eating; when hungry; from being overheated; *worse from a jar;* from light; from *mental exertion;* from motion; from motion of head or eyes; from noise; during menses. Compelled to lie down. *Applied heat relieves.* The pains are pulsating, periodical and paroxysmal. Headache came on from sexual excesses; worse after sleep; from stepping heavily; *from stooping* and from *straining the eyes.* The pain is violent, worse from touch and when walking, *wrapping up the head relieves.* Pain in forehead daytime; morning; *afternoon* evening, night, above the eyes; pain in occiput; pain in sides of head, worse on right side; pain in temples. Boring pain in forehead; bruised pain in the whole head; bursting pain in forehead; drawing pains in whole head and in *forehead;* pressing pains; pains pressing outward; pressing in forehead, *outward over* eyes, occiput, temples and vertex; shooting pains in forehead and occiput; *stitching pains in head,* forehead, occiput, sides of head and temples; stunning pains in head; tearing pains in head, forehead, occiput, sides of occiput, *sides of head, temples* and vertex. Perspiration of whole scalp; perspiration of forehead. Pulsating in the head, in forehead. Shaking or trembling sensation in the brain; uncovering the head in cool air brings on many symptoms.

The eyelids are stuck together in the morning. Cataract has been cured by this remedy. Discharges yellow and thick; dryness in the eyes; eczema around the eyes and in the eyebrows; the eyes feel hot; inflammation of the eyes, of the conjunctiva, of the lids; psoric complaints of the eyes; infected blood vessels; lachrymation in cold air. It has cured opacity of the cornea. Pain in the eyes, right most affected, better by warmth; the pains are *burning, pressing, stitching,* tearing; pain as if sand in eyes. It has cured paralysis of the optic nerve. Photophobia marked in daylight; redness of the eyes; spots on the cornea; staring, swollen lids; ulceration of the cornea; weak eyes. In the field of vision there are many colors, *floating spots* and black flies; dark colors, yellow. Dim vision. *Dazzling.* Complaints from *exertion of vision;* flickering before the eyes; thinks he is going blind; sparks before the eyes and weak vision. Discharge from ear, bloody, offensive, purulent, *thick, yellow.* Scurfy eruption behind the ear; flapping sensation in the ears; the ears are hot; inflammation in the middle ear; intense itching deep in the ears; noises in ears with dizziness; flapping sounds, ringing, *roaring.* Pain in ear, mostly right, better by warmth; pain behind the ear and deep in the ear; aching, boring, cramping pain; drawing, *stitching, tearing;* drawing and tearing behind the ear. Pulsating pain deep in the ear; the ear feels stopped; ulceration in the ear. Hearing is acute for noise, later impaired. It has cured deafness from catarrh of the eustachian tubes and the middle ear.

Catarrh of the nose and posterior nares in chilly people who are weak and want to keep still and rest; very offensive discharge, offensive breath in syphilitic subjects; the discharge is bloody, crusty, acrid, *greenish,* purulent, thick, yellow. He is subject to frequent coryzas as he is taking cold constantly. Dryness in the nose; bleeding of the nose on blowing it; itching deep in the nose where many crusts form; the nose is constantly obstructed; pain in the nose, and in the bones of the nose; great soreness in nose; burning pain in nose. Smell acute, later diminished, finally lost. Frequent violent sneezing; the nose is greatly swollen; much swelling inside of nose; ulceration in the nose.

Discoloration of the face; bluish, red, pale; circumscribed red cheeks; the face is jaundiced; the lips are cracked and dry; face looks sickly and drawn with *suffering* expression. The face, chin, lips, upper lip, around the mouth, nose, extending down on the neck, covered with moist eczema. She was a sight to look upon and her friends all shunned her; she was comfortable only when in a very hot room. Herpes and pimples on the face. Indurated parotid gland; inflammation of the parotid gland. itching of the face; drawing, stitching, tearing pain in the face; much sweat on the face; swelling of the cheeks, lips, parotid and submaxillary glands; ulceration of the lips; hard crust continues to form on the under lip.

Dry mouth without thirst; bleeding gums and white tongue; apthæ in the mouth; copious mucus forms in the month; odor from mouth offensive. The tongue is very sore, copious saliva flows into the mouth; swollen gums and tongue; taste is bad, bitter in the morning, bloody, sour.

Sensation of dryness in the throat with copious mucus; sensation of a lump in the throat; pain in the throat on swallowing; stitching pain in throat on swallowing; burning, rawness and soreness in the throat; much swelling in the throat and tonsils and swallowing is difficult. Swelling of cervical glands.

Sensation of anxiety in the stomach with aversion to food and especially to meat; ravenous appetite; appetite entirely lost; sensation of coldness in stomach; most troublesome eructations, worse after eating; bitter, empty, sour, waterbrash; eructations ameliorate the stomach symptoms; heartburn and fulness of the stomach; hiccough and weight in the stomach. Loathing of food. Nausea after eating and during headache; nausea with dizziness. Pain in the stomach at night, after eating; the pains in stomach are cutting, burning, cramping, gnawing, *pressing* and stitching; sore, bruised feeling in stomach; pressing in stomach after eating; pulsating in stomach after eating; retching when coughing. Sensation of tightness in stomach from flatulence. Thirst during chilliness and during fever; extreme thirst. Vomiting night and morning; of bile, of food, mucus and watery fluid; vomiting on coughing, after drinking *cold water, after eating,* and during headache.

The abdomen is distended after eating with obstructed flatulence; fulness, hardness and heaviness in abdomen; great heat in abdomen; pain in abdomen at night, during cough, after eating, before and during menses, after stool; warmth ameliorates. Pain in right hypochondrium, in the hypogastrium, in the inguinal region and in the liver; the pains in the abdomen are burning, cramping, *cutting, pressing, stitching* and *tearing;* pressing and stitching pains in the liver. Rumbling and tightness in the abdomen. *Constipation with very difficult stool;* difficult soft stool; insufficient stool. Constipation during menses. Stool dry, *hard, knotty, large,* light colored. Diarrhœa in the morning and at night; painful diarrhœa during menses, with stool bloody, frequent, offensive, purulent, watery; dysentery with scanty mucus, purulent and bloody stool; constriction of the anus. It has cured fistula in ano. Passing flatus ameliorates; formication of the anus. Hemorrhoids that protrude, ulcerate and bleed; inactivity of the rectum; itching of the anus after stool; ineffectual urging of stool; pain in anus during stool; burning during and after stool; burning after a hard stool. *Cutting,* pressing, sticking, stitching, pains in the anus; tenesmus, *extreme soreness* in the anus.

Catarrh of the bladder. The urine is cloudy, red, copious or scanty, with much mucous sediment; pressing pain in the bladder; urging to urinate; night, constant, frequent, ineffectual; the urine dribbles; urination frequent during the night; feeble stream; he cannot quite empty the bladder; slow in starting; he feels that he has not finished; involuntary at night. Burning in the urethra during urination.

Erections in the morning and during the night, painful, even violent, without desire; induration of the testes; itching of the scrotum; *seminal emissions.* Sexual desire at first increased, then diminished, later lost; swelling of the testes.

Eruptions and itching of the vulva; leucorrhœa, *excoriating* and *yellow;* worse after the menses. Menses bright red, copious, *frequent, intermittent, late, offensive,* painful, pale, scanty, short, *suppressed;* metrorrhagia between the menstrual periods; dragging down feeling in the pelvis; burning in the genitals; labor-like pains at the menstrual period; soreness in the genitals; prolapsus of the uterus.

Catarrh of the air passages; irritation of the larynx and trachea; much mucus in the air passages and especially in the larynx; scraping in the larynx, tickling in the larynx and trachea. The voice is hoarse and rough. It is a very useful remedy in asthma. Difficult breathing from exertion, while lying and when coughing; rattling in the chest; short, suffocative, whistling breathing; cough in daytime, morning, forenoon, evening and most severe and constant during the night; cough worse after eating, during fever, lying; the cough is asthmatic and suffocative, racking and spasmodic; dry cough during the night; hacking cough during the night; cough from irritation in larynx and trachea; cough from tickling in the larynx and trachea; the cough is violent, spasmodic and paroxysmal, like whooping cough. Expectoration in the morning, bloody, copious, greenish, mucus, *purulent,* putrid-looking, tough, *viscid,* yellow.

Catarrh of the chest; abscess of the lungs; abscess of the axilia. Tightness of the chest. Dropsy of the pleura. Hollow sensation in chest; hemorrhage of the lungs; chronic inflammation of bronchial tubes; weight on the chest; pain in chest during cough on deep inspiration; pain in the sides of chest on deep inspiration; burning, pressing, stitching pains. Rawness on coughing, soreness in chest, stitching on coughing and on inspiring, extending to back, stitching in sides of chest on breathing; stitching in mammæ; tearing pain in the walls of the chest. Palpitation on excitement and on slight exertion. It has been a most useful remedy in phthisis. Swelling in the axillary glands. Feeling of great weakness of the chest much like Stannum.

The back feels cold. itching of the back. Pain in the back *during menses,* while sitting and when stooping; pain in the back of the neck, between the scapulæ, in the *lumbar region* and in the sacrum; pain in coccyx; the whole spine is painful. Aching in lumbar region and sacrum; burning in the lumbar region; drawing pain in cervical region, lumbar region and sacrum; pressing pain in lumbar region. The whole spine is sore. Stitching pains in scapulæ, *lumbar region* and sacrum; tearing in the cervical region; stiffness of the neck; tension in the back; weakness in the lumbar region.

The hands are chapped in cold weather; the hands and feet are cold; cramps in hands and calves. There are vesicular eruptions on the hands; pimples on the lower limbs; many eruptions on the thighs. Felons on the fingers. The hands are hot. Marked heaviness of the lower limbs, legs and feet. *Hip joint disease.* Itching of upper limbs, hands and palms; itching of lower limbs, thighs and legs. Jerking of the muscles of lower limbs; numbness of upper limbs, hands and fingers; numbness of lower limbs, legs and feet. Pain in limbs during chill, better by warmth. Rheumatic pains in limbs; hard pain in the joints; gouty pains in joints; pains in shoulder and fingers, in hips, thighs and knees; pain in the sciatic nerve. Aching in the legs; burning soles; drawing pains in limbs; upper limbs, shoulder, elbow, forearm, wrist, hands, fingers, lower limbs, thighs, knee, leg, ankles, feet; pressing pains in thighs; sore, bruised pain in all the limbs; upper limbs, lower limbs, hip, leg; sprained feeling in all the joints; stitching pains in all the limbs and in the joints, stitching in shoulder, upper arm, wrist, hand, fingers; stitching in thighs, knees, legs, ankle, *foot, heel,* toes, first toe; tearing pains in all the limbs and joints; tearing in shoulders, upper arm, elbow, forearm, wrist, hand, fingers, finger joints; tearing in hip, thigh, knee, leg, calf, ankles, foot, soles, toes, first toe; paralysis of upper and *lower limbs.* Sweat of palms; profuse, cold, *offensive* sweat of feet and between the toes. Stiffness of the joints, shoulders, knees; swelling of feet, legs and knees; tension in the knees and calves; trembling of all the limbs, of hands and legs; twitching of all the limbs, *thighs.* Ulcers on the legs; weakness of the joints, thigh, knee and ankles.

Dreams *anxious;* of dead people; of death; events of the previous day; horrible, fantastic, fire, *frightful,* ghosts, nightmare, visionary, vivid, of water. Sleep is restless, sleepiness in the afternoon, *evening, after* dinner. Sleepless before midnight, after midnight, after 2 a.m., with sleepiness. Sleeplessness from thinking, after waking. Waking frequently and too early; frequent yawning.

Chill morning, forenoon, noon, afternoon, evening, night, in open air, in cold air, in a draft of air; chilliness in evening in bed, after eating; chill external and internal, worse from motion; chilliness with pain; *one-sided chill;* shaking chill in the evening; better in a warm room, external heat ameliorates.

Fever afternoon, evening and during the night, alternating with sweat;

dry heat, external heat; flushes of heat; perspiration absent; *night sweats.*
Perspiration morning, daytime and *during night*. Perspiration during and
after eating, from slight exertion, from motion; *profuse at night;* sweat during
sleep; offensive while walking. If perspiration is checked in cool air, many
complaints come on.

   Burning after scratching; old scars become painful. The skin is cold much
of the time. The skin cracks; discoloration of the skin; blotches, liver spots,
red spots, yellow skin; dry skin, dry, burning skin with inability to perspire.
Blisters on the skin; burning eruptions; chafing skin; desquamating eruptions;
eruptions moist and eruptions dry. It has cured most stubborn cases of eczema
where Sulphur and Graphites seemed indicated and failed. Herpes that burn
and are corrosive, scabby and itch and sting; eruptions that the painful,
itching and spreading; itching pimples and pustules; scabby eruptions after
scratching; scaly eruptions dry or moist; smarting after scratching; stinging
after scratching; *nodular urticaria*. Vesicular eruptions; excoriation after
scratching. Erysipelas. Indurations in the skin. *Intertrigo*. Itching, burning,
crawling, smarting and stinging after scratching. It has cured lupus. Moisture
of the skin after scratching, he scratches the skin until it is moist or bleeds;
sore sensation of the skin. After scratching, the skin is swollen and burns,
looks œdematous; sensation of tension in the skin; ulcerative pain in the
skin. The ulcers that form upon the skin are characterized by *bleeding,*
burning, spreading, pulsating, smarting and suppurating; ulcers are very
indolent; the discharge from ulcers is bloody, copious, ichorous and thin.
Tearing pain in the ulcers. Injuries and small wounds of the skin refuse to
heal and suppurate. Warts that are painful, stinging, suppurating and withered.

KALI SULPHURICUM

   Two very deep acting remedies unite to form this one. It was left to
Schüessler to show its first curative powers. Dewey's work on the "Tissue
Remedies" gives the best presentation from the biochemic view. The writer
gathered the symptoms from reported cures for many years, and found that
they were justified by the study of the two remedies entering into the formation.
Many of these symptoms come out upon the sick as aggravations. Some of
these are only cured symptoms. This arrangement could be improved upon
much by provings. If the reader will carefully use this remedy as herein directed
he will be astonished at its depth of action, and if he uses it high he will be
surprised at the length of action of every dose. It has cured epilepsy, lupus

and epithelioma, and many desquamating skin affections. It has cured most obstinate cases of chronic intermittent fever. It is useful in catarrhal affections with thick yellow or greenish pus, viscid or *thin yellow watery discharges.* Most symptoms are aggravated in the evening. The patient craves fresh and even cold air, and he is ameliorated in open air and cool air. Aggravation by exertion and becoming heated. Complaints come on during rest, and are ameliorated by motion. Complaints aggravated in warm room. Takes cold from being overheated. When once heated he cannot cool off without taking cold. *Predisposition to phthisis.* It is frequently indicated after *Tuberculinum.* Epileptiform convulsions. Jerking of the limbs and twitching of muscles. Dropsical condition of the extremities. Loss of flesh, and complaints aggravated after eating. Fasting ameliorates many symptoms. Flabby muscles. Fatty degeneration of glands, liver and heart. Heaviness of limbs and weariness of the body. Hysterical symptoms. Sluggishness of the body and lack of physical irritability. Well selected remedies fall short in action. Wants to lie down, but lying in bed aggravates; he must walk about to ameliorate his sufferings. Surging of blood in the body. Pain in the limbs, bones and glands. *Wandering pains.* Pains ameliorated by motion, ameliorated walking, ameliorated in open air; aggravated in a warm room, aggravated sitting or lying, or rest in any form. The pains are burning, *cutting,* jerking, STITCHING and TEARING. ULCERATIVE PAINS. Tearing downward in the limbs. Tearing in glands and muscles. PULSATION ALL OVER THE BODY. Touch aggravates many symptoms. Many symptoms appear *on waking.* Trembling and quivering. Walking ameliorates. Warm coverings aggravate, warm room aggravates, warm bed aggravates, warm wraps aggravate; bathing aggravates. Complaints dating back to suppressed eruptions. Post scarlatinal nephritis. One does not need to reflect to perceive this is *Pulsatilla* somewhat intensified. It takes up the work and finishes as a complement of *Pulsatilla,* unless, as in some instances, the patient becomes a cold and chilly subject and is better during rest, and then *Silicia* often will be found to have what symptoms remain. It is usual for a patient under a deep acting remedy to go to opposite modalities, and hence *Puls.* is so often followed by *Silicea;* but this is not always true. When *Puls.* has acted well for a time and because of opposite modalities *Silicea* does good work for a while, and then the patient swings back to the original state, symptoms and modalities, then it is that Kali sulph. is of great usefulness. What occurs is the same as when *Sulph., Calc.* and *Lyc.* have rotated in a given case too deep to be cured by a single remedy and a series of remedies has been what was required because the symptoms changed in such a manner that such a series was homœopathically suited.

Quite unlike *Pulsatilla,* this patient is easily angered and obstinate and VERY IRRITABLE. Seems to be thinking of something far away. ANXIETY in *evening* in bed, during the night and on waking. Aversion to work, to business and to company (like *Puls.*). Concentration of mind difficult, and want of self-confidence. Confusion in the evening and in the morning, in a warm room, ameliorated in open air. *Dullness of mind,* discouraged and discontented with everything. Extremely *excitable,* and *mental exertion aggravates.* Fear at night of death, of falling, and of people. Frightened at trifles, and forgets what he was going to do and to say. He is always in a hurry, as if excited. Impatient and impetuous. Hysterical and excited in the evening, and mind active. Cannot make up his mind to do and act. Very irritable in the morning on waking, in the evening and during menses. Misplaces words in writing. Alternating moods. Changeable disposition. Restlessness during menses. Low spirited morning and evening. *Oversensitive* to noise. *Mental* symptoms from sexual excesses. Walking in sleep, Shrieking. Easily startled, from fright, on falling asleep, and *during sleep.* Indisposed to talk. He talks in sleep. *General timidity.* Weeping.

The vertigo in a prominent feature in the evening, in a warm room, aggravated after eating, aggravated during headache, aggravated looking upwards; with nausea; must lie down; objects turn in a circle; aggravated sitting, aggravated rising up, and standing; ameliorated in open air. Feels he is falling forward. He staggers.

Boiling sensation in the head, and coldness of vertex. Hyperæmia in bed, on coughing, and in a warm room. Constriction like a band or close fitting cap. Constriction of forehead. Much dandruff. Eruptions on scalp, crusts, eczema, moist, sticky, pimples, scaling. Fulness in head and *hair falls out.* *Heat* in head in a warm room. Heat in *forehead.* Flushes of heat. Heaviness of head, morning, in forehead, in occiput. Itching of the scalp in the morning. The brain feels loose. Sensation of movements in head on moving the head. There are numerous headaches. Pain *morning* on waking, EVENING and *night,* aggravated from a draft, during chill, taking cold, during coryza, on coughing, after eating, when heated, from *warm room,* jarring, during menses, motion of the head, pressure. It is ameliorated in open air, in cold air, lying. Rheumatic headache in evening, aggravated in warm room, aggravated moving head from side to side or backwards. Catarrhal headaches. Gastric headaches. The aggravation of headaches by motion is an exception, and it will be interesting to learn what further provings and observations bring forth. The pains are pulsating, aggravated shaking head, after sleep, sneezing, standing, stepping heavily, stooping, straining the eyes; aggravated in a *warm room.* The pains are violent. Walking in open air ameliorates. Pain extends to eyes and forehead. Pain in forehead, morning, evening; aggravated after eating. *Pain over eyes.* Pain in *occiput, sides of head,* temples. The pains are *boring,* burning, bursting, drawing, *jerking. pressing,* STITCHING in head and SIDES of head.

Stunning. Tearing. Pulsating in occiput, sides of head, temples, vertex. Shocks in head, in sides of head, mostly in *right side*.

The eye symptoms are numerous. Lids agglutinated. Dryness. Discharge, yellowish, greenish. Inflammation of conjunctiva, of lids. Dark veins. Eruptions about the eyes and on the lids. Lachrymation and itching. Opacity of the cornea. It is recommended for cataract. Pain, *burning,* pressing and tearing. Photophobia, redness of eyes and edges of lids. Spots on the cornea; ulceration of the cornea. Swollen lids. Dark colors, variegated colors, yellow. Halo around the light. Black floating specks. Dazzling. Dim vision. Exertion of vision brings on many complaints. Foggy vision. Sparks before the eyes. Weak vision.

Catarrh of Eustachian tubes and middle ear. Dryness of the middle ear. Discharge from ear, *yellow,* thin, *bright yellow* or greenish, bloody, *offensive,* PURULENT. Eruptions, eczema, excoriated, pimples. Eruptions behind ears. *Itching in ears.* Noises; buzzing, chirping, cracking, crackling humming, RINGING *roaring, rushing,* whizzing. Flapping sensation in the ear. Pain in ear, evening, aching, boring, cutting, pressing, stitching, tearing. It has cured polypus. The ears feel stopped, and pulsate. The hearing is impaired.

Fluent coryza. Catarrh with discharge, bloody, burning, excoriating, greenish, offensive, purulent, *thin,* YELLOW slimy, or thick and viscid. Dryness in the nose. Bleeding in morning on blowing. *Itching in nose.* Obstruction. Pain, burning. Soreness in nose, of septum. Smell acute, later *lost.* Sneezing. Swollen nose.

Sickly, yellow, *chlorotic* face. Cracked lips. Sometimes pale. Sometimes circumscribed redness. Drawn face. Suffering, sickly expression. Eruptions on face, lips and nose. Herpes, pimples and scales. Desquamating face. Flushes of heat. Itching. Inflammation of the submaxillary gland with swelling. Prosopalgia, aggravated when the room becomes too warm, and in the evening; ameliorated in the open air. The pains are drawing, stitching and tearing. Perspiration of the face. Swollen glands of jaw, swollen lips. Twitching face. It has cured a wart on the lip, and will cure epithelioma when the symptoms agree.

Aphthæ in mouth. Dryness of mouth and bleeding gums. Mucus in mouth and on the tongue. Sore burning tongue. Salivation. Taste insipid, putrid, sour, sweetish, wanting.

Coated yellow slimy tongue, mostly at the base. Toothache aggravated in a warm room, ameliorated in cool fresh air.

Dryness and *constriction of throat.* Frequent hawking of mucus. Heat and inflammation of throat. Sensation of a lump in the throat. *Mucus in the throat* in the morning. Painful sore throat. Pain on swallowing. Rawness, burning and sticking. The tonsils much swollen. Swallowing difficult.

Great anxiety and distress in the stomach. Appetite is increased, ravenous, or *wanting*. Aversion to bread, to eggs, to food, to meat, to hot drinks and warm food. Coldness in stomach. Catarrh of stomach. Desires sour thing, SWEETS, cold drinks and cold food. Distension of stomach. Irritable, easily disordered stomach. Sensation of emptiness and faintness in stomach. *Eructations,* after eating, bitter, empty, of food, SOUR, waterbrash. Eructations ameliorate. Gastroduodenal catarrh with jaundice. Fulness after eating *ever so little* (*Lyc.*). Heartburn, *heaviness* and flushes of heat. Hiccoughing. Loathing of food. Nausea during chill, during cough, after cold drinks, after eating, *with headache,* on motion. Pain in stomach after eating and drinking. Burning, cramping, cutting, pinching, pressing, soreness, stitching. Pulsating in stomach. Retching when coughing. *Burning thirst.* Vomiting on coughing, after eating, during headache, during menses. Vomiting bile, food, mucus, *sour.*

Coldness in the abdomen. *Distension* after eating. Dropsy. Enlarged liver. Obstructed flatulence. Sensation of fulness after eating. Sensation of emptiness in lower abdomen after stool ameliorated by displacing flatus. Heat and heaviness. Complaints of the liver. Itching of the skin. Pain in abdomen at night. Cramping during diarrhœa, after eating, before the menses, during menses, aggravated by motion. Pain in inguinal region and in the liver. Burning, cutting, pressing. Pressing in hypogastrium and liver. Soreness in abdomen and in the liver. Stitching in the abdomen, in the sides of the abdomen, in the inguinal region, in the liver. Pulsating. Rumbling before stool. Trembling in abdomen. Tympanitis.

Constipation that is very obstinate, alternating with diarrhœa. Stool difficult, soft or *hard,* insufficient during menses, from inactivity of the rectum. *Diarrhœa* in the morning, evening, night, after *midnight,* painless, or with cramps, during menses. *Chronic diarrhœa.* Offensive, putrid flatus which ameliorates many abdominal symptoms. Hæmorrhage from the anus. *Hæmorrhoids,* external, internal, large and bleeding. Involuntary stool. *Violent itching of the anus. Pain* in the *rectum and anus,* during stool, after stool; BURNING during diarrhœa, during stool, after stool. Cutting, pressing, smarting and great SORENESS Parts *excoriated..* STITCHING *in anus.* Tenesmus after stool. Urging to stool, ineffectual, absent in constipation.

Stool is excoriating, black, thin and offensive. Stool bloody, frequent, offensive, purulent, watery, yellow slime. When constipated the stool is dry, hard, knotty, LARGE, like *sheep dung,* small. The stool is light colored and bileless.

Chronic catarrh of bladder. The pain is pressing, sticking. It has urging to urinate aggravated at night, constant or frequent, ineffectual. Urination is painful, frequent at night, dribbling when walking. Inflammation of the kidneys with stitching pains.

Gonorrhœa in the advanced stage, with green or yellow thin or viscid discharge. Hæmorrhage from the urethra. Burning during urination, and in the meatus. Cutting.

The urine is albuminous, and this remedy has been especially useful in albuminuria following scarlet fever. The urine burns and is cloudy, high colored, *copious,* or *scanty,* offensive, with red and purulent sediment. Copious viscid mucus in the urine.

Impotency. Induration of testes. Inflammation of glans penis. Orchitis after suppressed gonorrhœa (*Puls.*). Itching of genitalia and scrotum. Drawing in testes. Sexual desire diminished or entirely lost. Swollen testes.

It builds up women who have been subject to abortion. Aversion to coition. Excoriation of the genitalia, with *itching. Leucorrhœa,* burning, excoriating, *greenish, yellow,* purulent, thick or *watery.* Menses absent; bright red, *copious, too soon,* or *too late,* offensive, *painful,* protracted, scanty, suppressed. Hæmorrhage from the uterus. Pain in uterus, during menses. Bearing down in the pelvis. Burning in the genitalia. Labor-like pains during menses. Prolapsus of the uterus.

Catarrh of the air passages with thick greenish, yellow or white mucus. Dryness in the larynx. Rawness in the larynx. Soreness and roughness. Almost constant *scraping in* the larynx, aggravated after eating, at night in bed, until midnight; almost driven to distraction by the necessity to clear the larynx and gets up only white thick mucus. Tickling in the larynx. Hoarseness. Recurrent coryza with irritation in larynx. Voice lost. Every cold settles in the larynx.

Asthma aggravated in a warm room, ameliorated in open air. Dyspnœa evening, night, *with cough,* when lying, walking, ameliorated in open air. RATTLING BREATHING. Short, suffocative breathing in a warm room. Wheezing in a warm room. Whistling.

Coughing in *morning, evening,* in bed, NIGHT; ameliorated in cold air, ameliorated in open air, ameliorated by cold drinks.. Cough with coryza, aggravated lying. Dry, hoarse, croupy cough at night. Cough aggravated after eating, during fever. Exhausting cough. Hacking cough. Loose cough. Paroxysmal, racking cough. RATTLING cough. Suffocating cough. Tickling in larynx, trachea and deep in chest. *Warm room aggravates cough.* Whooping cough *with yellow slime* or *yellow watery* expectoration. Expectoration bloody, *difficult,* must be swallowed, or *slips back, purulent, yellow* or *greenish, slimy, watery,* viscid.

Anxiety in the chest. It is one of the most surprising remedies in catarrh of the chest. Rattling in chest from every cold change in the weather. Constriction of the chest. The last part of pneumonia and pleurisy will bring out symptoms for this remedy. Itching of the skin of the chest. Eruptions, eczema, pustules. *Oppression* of chest and hæmorrhage. After bronchitis in children, when every cold causes rattling in chest and there is no expectoration. Burning, cutting, *stitching* and soreness in chest. Pain in heart. Stitching in the heart. Palpitation with anxiety of heart. Tumultuous palpitation. Perspiration in axillæ. Weak chest. This remedy has saved many people from *phthisis.* It has cured swollen sensitive mammæ coming every month before menses.

Coldness in the back. Pain in the back on breathing, during menses, periodical, aggravated sitting, aggravated standing; ameliorated walking; aggravated in a warm room. *Wandering pains.* Pain in cervical region, *dorsal region,* between the shoulders. Pain in lumbar region *during menses,* while sitting, and walking. Pain in sacrum. Aching, bruised, burning, drawing, STITCHING. Tension in the cervical region. Weakness in the lumbar region.

Arthritic nodosities. Coldness of upper limbs and hands. COLD FEET evening in bed, and during fever. Cracked hands. Cracking in joints. Pimples and vesicles on limbs. Desquamation on legs above the shoe tops in a young woman. Heat of hands. Hip joint disease. Heaviness of lower limbs. Itching of the skin. Jerking of the limbs. Numbness of *hands, lower limbs* and feet. Pain in the limbs during chill. *Rheumatic* pains in limbs. Cramps in muscles. Drawing in knees and legs. Rheumatic pains aggravated in a warm room; ameliorated walking in open air; aggravated sitting; ameliorated moving about. Sore bruised pain in tibia. STITCHING in the joints, in lower limbs, knees, legs; WANDERNIG STITCHING Tearing pains during chill, in joints, upper limbs, lower limbs, thighs, legs. Wandering tearing pains, ameliorated by motion, and walking in open air. Perspiration of palms, of feet. Cold sweat of feet. Restless legs. Stiffness of joints. Swelling of knees, legs, feet. Trembling of limbs, hands and feet. Twitching *thighs. Ulcers on leg.* Weakness of joints, upper limbs, of knees.

The sleep is full of dreams. He has nightmare. Dreams anxious, of death, of being in an accident and nearly killed, of robbers, of sickness, *frightful,* of *ghosts.* Late falling asleep. *Restless sleep.* Sleepiness in afternoon and *evening,* and after eating. Sleepless before midnight. Waking early, and frequently.

Chill EVENING and night. Chilliness in the evening. Chilliness after exertion. Coldness of the skin. Quotidian chill. *Shaking chill* EVENING, 5 P.M., 6 P.M.. Fever without chill, evening until midnight. Fever, dry heat, flushes. Hectic fever. Intermittent. Perspiration in morning, NIGHT, after midnight. Perspiration on slight exertion; copious.

Sensation of burning in the skin; burning after scratching. The skin is often cold. DESQUAMATION. Discoloration; liver spots; red spots. Dry skin; inactivity of skin. Dry, burning skin. Epithelioma. Eruptions, blisters, burning, dry, *moist;* eczema with yellowish green, watery, discharge, herpetic. Itching and stinging eruptions. Rash like measles. Eruptions painful, pimples, psoriasis, pustules, red eruptions. *Scabby eruptions.* Scabby after scratching. *Scaly* eruptions on a moist base. Smarting, suppurating eruptions. Tubercular eruptions. Urticaria, nodular. Vesicular eruptions. Erysipelas with blisters. Easy excoriation of the skin. Intertrigo. Formication. Itching, *burning,* crawling, *stinging;* aggravated when warm in *bed;* ameliorated scratching. Moisture of the skin after scratching. Neuritis. The skin is very *sensitive* : a sore feeling in the skin. Sticking after scratching. Skin swollen and dropsical. Sensation of tension. Ulcerative pain. Ulcers, bleeding, burning, bloody discharge, stabbing, yellow discharge, *indolent,* pulsating suppurating, tuberculous. Painful warts.

KALMIA LATIFOLIA

The symptoms that indicate this remedy show themselves especially in the muscles, in the tendons, in the joints, along the course of the nerves, in rheumatic complaints. The pains change about, wandering pains, and they are aggravated from motion. The sharp pains spread from the centres to the extremities, the wandering pains go downwards, down the arms, down the back and down the legs; from the shoulder to the fingers, and from the hips to the toes. These pains sometimes shoot like lightning, again they tear along the nerves, along the sciatic and crural nerves, down through the calves. In rheumatic constitutions the pains are dull, tearing, crushing and pressing, and are aggravated by motion and go from the lower to the upper limbs. Motion will bring on the pain or aggravate it when it is present. The head pains are very severe. They often begin in the back of the neck or back of the head, and extend to the top of the head. There are also pains in the front of the head, pains over one or both eyes, tearing neuralgic pains aggravated by heat and motion.

Pains come and go with the sun, that is, they begin in the morning at the rising of the sun and increase till noon, then gradually decline and disappear at sunset. He is incapacitated for mental work when in motion and even when sitting up, but, when lying upon his back perfectly quiet, making no motion, the mind works well and with clearness; with the slightest motion, however, even of the hand, on comes vertigo and confusion of mind. Moving about disturbs him, makes him incompetent. The pains are also worse the first half of the night.

With these symptoms there is cardiac trouble of rheumatic origin. The condition has increased until organic disease has come, even hypertrophy of the heart and valves. This remedy has cured that state. Palpitation very marked when lying on the left side, > when lying on the back, sometimes >

when sitting erect, < when bending forward. These symptoms alone cause this remedy to stand out in relief. It is useful in rheumatic patients where syphilis is at the bottom, syphilitic rheumatism that has taken the course described until finally the heart has become affected and there is thickening of the valves. Shooting pains through the heart, pains in the chest, intermittent pulse, pulse skipping a beat now and then. Either the arterial or venous system, or the valves of the heart, or both, may be affected. Dyspnœa from any kind of exercise, cardiac dyspnœa. You have in this a remedy for such complaints. It goes to the bottom in old cases of rheumatic syphilis, and has cured many a cardiac complaint that was the result of syphilis. You will be guided to it especially if the pains wander from place to place, and if they go from above downwards, if they go from the shoulder down toward the fingers, from the hips toward the feet, or down the spine. It is also suitable in old cases of gonorrhœal rheumatism when the symptoms agree.

The slightest motion, the slightest effort or exertion brings on the vertigo, and this is due to disturbance of the circulation. The heart is so susceptible to any exertion that disturbance of the circulation of the blood in the brain comes on from the slightest motion. "In a recumbent posture mental faculties and memory perfect, but, on attempting to move, vertigo." If the patient persists in moving, nausea and vomiting will follow. It has palpitation, shaking the whole frame, audible, vehement palpitation. He cannot lie on his left side.

It is suitable in old, troublesome, recurrent headaches associated with cardiac affections. A headache will come on daily if the sun comes out, but it will not come on if the day is clouded. He is aggravated from the light of the sun and the increasing brightness of the sun's rays.

In addition to these there are paroxysms of pain that are nightly. These are the bone pains, pains in the shin bones as if the periosteum would be torn off; these pains come on at night, or the first half of the night. It is well known in syphilis that the < is at night. It is an antipsoric, antisycotic and antisyphilitic, it can be selected when the symptoms agree with any of the three miasms. Pains in the pericranium, pains in the bones nearest to the surface. In bed at night the pains become very severe and last all night. This night aggravation is especially true of the marked antisyphilitic medicines. It is found under *Hepar* and *Mercurius;* but in none of the remedies do we find it so strikingly manifested as in the disease, or miasm, syphilis itself. In syphilis the < comes with the setting of the sun. It is one of man's enemies that does its work in the night. Many of the complaints of sycosis conform to the day hours, and the pains are < from the rising to the going down of the sun. Medicines also have such queer whims. We must study remedies as we would human character. Some, of them seem to be extremely whimsical, and it is by knowing these whimsical, strange and peculiar things that we are able to mark the character of the remedy. When we know these peculiarities we have found the circumstance under which the remedy works best.

There are kidney affections. All the organs are related to each other, but especially the heart and kidneys. When the kidneys are not working well, the heart is very often troublesome. All through the varying forms of Bright's disease the heart is troublesome. Difficulties of breathing, difficult heart action, with albuminuria. It will relieve the breathing. Again. associated with kidney affections, we have many eye complaints, difficulties of vision, and these also especially call for this remedy. It is often indicated in Bright's disease, with disturbance of vision, occurring during pregnancy. For the pains in the eyes, the stitching, tearing pains that occur during kidney disturbance in pregnancy, or during albuminuria, kalmia becomes a remedy. This remedy is useful in neuralgia; neuralgia of the eye, neuralgia of the face, violent, tearing pains in the face. Sometimes it takes the form of a nightly < and sometimes it takes the form of daily <. The aggravation in the daytime comes and goes with the sun. The < at night time comes with the lying down. "Anxious expression of countenance" associated with rheumatism of the heart. "Flushing of the face, with vertigo."

After the disappearance of a herpetic eruption, violent neuralgic pains, shooting, tearing pains in those nerves that supply the part where the eruption was. When shingles, ring-worm, cold sore, or isolated vesicular eruptions disappear, suddenly from some violent cause or inappropriate treatment, or from catching cold, violent neuralgias come in their place and continue until the eruption comes out again. This remedy becomes suitable if the symptoms agree; that is, if the whole patient is in agreement with the state of the remedy. The pains are stitching and tearing, very severe, sometimes cutting and shooting when this remedy is most useful. The pain will seem to take hold of a nerve and will hold on to it for many minutes, coming with violence, coming suddenly and letting loose suddenly. Pains come in the extremities in the same way, taking hold as if the nerve were being pinched by nippers, or as if it were being torn to pieces. "There, now it is gone!" says the patient. Pretty soon, again, you will see his face in a state of horrible distress. The pain is there again and he cannon move a muscle, and "there, it is gone!" he says, and it remains away for some minutes and sometimes for hours.

The heart has many symptoms which should be studied. "Fluttering of the heart, palpitation of the heart." "Palpitation up into the throat, after going to bed, trembling all over." *Very slow pulse.* I remember a patient, an old syphilitic, who was told if he ever, made a violent move he would die, the valves of his heart were so badly affected. He had all the murmurs that it seemed possible from the heart valves. He had travelled all over and had taken large doses of *Mercury,* and his syphilitic condition had to a great extent been suppressed, until finally the whole trouble had located in the heart. Kalmia removed all the dyspnœa and palpitation in a few months, and it was nearly two years before there was a marked return of the symptoms and a repetition put him in a state of health, so that he needed no more medicine. This shows what a deep-acting remedy Kalmia is, how long it may act, what wonderful changes it may effect. A remedy must be capable of going deep into the life to do such things.

"Wandering rheumatic pains in the region of the heart." "When articular rheumatism has been treated externally and cardiac symptoms ensue." Rheumatism that goes from the lower to the upper limbs. Not uncommonly you will meet such things. These "rubbers" that go around the streets with a strong liniment and considerable magnetism frequently do cause a rheumatism to leave the knee joint, and, when it does that, the heart is likely to be the organ that suffers. Then Kalmia, *Aurum, Bryonia, Rhus tox., Ledum, Calc.* and *Abrotanum,* and sometimes *Cactus,* are remedies that prove suitable for such cardiac affections. Rheumatic affections that are driven away in this manner are changed without being cured. The people cannot realize the danger of merely removing symptoms. Every removal that is not in accordance with cure affects the centres of man, that is the heart and brain. Rubbing is a dangerous thing. When you are importuned with the question, "Doctor, will it hurt me to have this rubbed?" you reply, "If rubbing does not affect any change in the symptoms, it will do not harm." In proportion as it mitigates the symptoms or relieves, just in that proportion it does the patient harm, for the whole vital economy is weakened. There are instances where rubbing is of benefit, but not in rheumatism. In paralyzed muscles it is a beneficial exercise for then rubbing can take the place of exercise of the patient himself, of the muscles. But rubbing is not admissible if it is used to reduce pain. The more agreeable it is, the worse it is for the patient. In a *Phosphorus* patient you would be astonished what wonderful relief they can get from rubbing. There is no person more inclined to be weak in the vitality, in the internal economy than the *Phosphorus* patient. He is an excitable, weakly patient, and feels better by rubbing and craves it, but if he has rheumatism in the knees and the knee is rubbed the rheumatism may go to the heart. The *Phos.* patient love to be rubbed, because rubbing relieves the symptoms; he loves to be magnetized.

Weariness of all the limbs; shuns all exertion." "Weakness the only general symptom with neuralgia." This weakness is a state that you can glea something from. When severe pain is fatiguing the economy the heart is threatened. A general weakness, prolonged weakness after confinement, or from the pain, as we find in *Hepar,* but with the weakness, these pains are threatening to leave their parts and go to the heart. He is perfectly exhausted and continuously tired.

The text speaks only of *Aconite* and *Belladonna as* the antidotes. *Spigelia* follows this remedy very well and antidotes it. *Benzoic acid* is a natural complement to it. *Calc., Lith. carb., Lyc., Nat. mur* and *Puls.* are the remedies that are closely related and should be compared.

KREOSOTUM

There are three things that stand out most prominently in Kreosotum, and when they appear together the symptoms in minor degree will be likely to be associated. These three characteristics are: 1. Excoriating discharges; 2. Pulsations all over the body, and 3. Profuse bleeding from small wounds.

When these three things are associated in a high degree Kreosote should be examined. A prick of a pin will cause the oozing of bright red blood, and mucous membranes bleed easily. Any pressure upon the mucous membranes will cause oozing. Bleeding here and there about the body. The lachrymation is excoriating. It excoriates the margins of the lids and cheeks, and they become red and raw, and smart. If there is a purulent discharge it is acrid. The corners of the lips and mouth are red and raw, and the saliva burns and smarts. The moisture about the mouth, whatever it may be, excoriates and the mouth is raw. The eyes smart and burn as if raw. The leucorrhœa causes smarting and burning about the vulva, so that the mucous surfaces of the labia are red and raw, sometimes inflamed, but always burning. The vagina burns during coition, and there is bleeding after coition; granulations of the vagina and os uteri, so that the pressure of the act of coition brings on bleeding and burning, smarting and excoriation. And the male organ will smart and burn after coming in contact with the secretion of the vagina during coition. The urine burns and smarts. This tendency to excoriation from the excretions and secretions applies to all the tissues of the body.

Every emotion and exciting circumstance is attended with throbbing all over the body, pulsations to the ends of the fingers. Every emotion is attended with tearfulness. Music that will in the slightest way excite the emotion, minor strains and music that strikes home to the heart, pathetic music, will bring out tears that are acrid, and palpitation and pulsations that are felt to the extremities.

When the Kreosote sore throat is present the least pressure of the tongue depressor will establish oozing, little drops of blood will appear. During the coryza there is nosebleed. When the eyes are red and raw and inflamed, they will bleed easily. If an individual pricks the finger the blood will not merely be a single drop, but a good many will flow. Prolonged hæmorrhage from the passages; hæmorrhage from the kidneys, from the eyes, the nose, the uterus. Hæmorrhage after coition. Tumors bleed easily.

These are the most marked features of Kreosote. If these are fixed in your mind, we have what may be known as a Kreosote constitution, out of which may come all the rest of the symptoms in all their minutiæ, and little symptoms and fragments in every organ. You have in this one group the strong features of Kreosote. No matter how many particulars you may have in a case, if you do not have something of these general features you need not expect to find your patient constitutionally cured or relieved by Kreosote. These may be considered essentials.

Mentally the patient is so irritable that there is nothing that will suit him. The wants are so numerous that nothing satisfies. The patient wants everything and is satisfied with nothing, that is, he wants something and when he has it he does not want it. That is the state of irritability and lack of satisfaction in a chronic condition. You see the child in the mother's arms. It wants a toy, and when given it throws it in the face of somebody; it wants this and that and is never satisfied, always wanting something new —a new toy which it throws away the moment it gets it and then calls for something else. The lips are red and bleeding, the corners of the mouth are raw, the eyelids red and the skin excoriated. If it has, in connection with all this, loose passages from the bowels and you examine the fissure between the nates, you will find it is red and raw. If the child be old enough to make such motions he will put the hands upon the sore genitals and fissures and cry out in a most irritable way, because of the smarting. Such is the Kreosote baby. It may be suffering from cholera infantum; it may be subject to wetting the bed; it may have spells of vomiting, in which it vomits all its food; it is a Kreosote baby. Kreosote has attacks of diarrhœa and vomiting; all sorts of disturbances of the urine; great distension and trouble with the bowels; abdomen distended from flatus. You look over the whole case at once as a Kresote case, because of these general features that can be summed up in the aspect of the child.

The Kreosote face has a yellowish pallor; it is a sickly countenance, semi-cachectic, intermingled with blotches that are reddish looking, as if erysipelas were going to set in. In olden times this countenance was called a scorbutic countenance.

Take a woman with this kind of countenance; at every menstrual flow she complains of much swelling and rawness of the genitals; the flow is copious, clotted, stops and then starts again, comes too soon and lasts too long; at times it is black, very fœtid, produces rawness upon the thighs and the genitals, with much swelling; at every menstrual period there is rawness of the lips and fissures in the corners of the mouth; the tears become acrid; at the menstrual period all the fluids of the body seem to be acrid and they burn wherever they touch. Very often there is a loose stool. which is also acrid and smarts the anus at the menstrual period. All the symptoms are worse at the menstrual period, sometimes in the early part, sometimes at the middle, sometimes all through, and sometimes at the close. Something more about the scorbutic constitution is brought out in relation to the gums; the gums become puffed and red and tumid and settle away from the teeth. They become spongy and bleed easily. In the mouth there is much ulceration and little ulcers spread from aphthous patches, smarting and burning; the tongue has ulcers upon it, which bleed easily upon touch.

At the close of a typhoid fever hæmorrhage from the bowels, bleeding from the mucous membranes. The mouth becomes raw, and wherever there is a mucous membrane there is a rawness, and the fluids that ooze continue to eat and cause ulceration. If at the close of a typhoid fever, when the time comes for convalescence, vomiting comes. Vomiting, bleedings, diarrhœas. The fluids vomited from the stomach are so acrid that they seem to take the skin off from the mouth, set the teeth on edge, make the lips raw. So excoriation from acrid fluids, as well as throbbing all over the body, are features that you must bear in mind with Kreosote.

The discharges from the body are offensive; offensive, bloody, acrid discharges from the nose; offensive, watery discharges from any part of the body; sometimes even putrid; the leucorrhœa is very offensive. Rapid emaciation, with spongy, burning ulceration, pus acrid, ichorous, fœtid and yellow. Sometimes the inflammatory condition will run so high in an ulcer, only a small ulceration, that gangrene will set in, and hence we have a gangrenous ulceration; gangrene of parts that are inflamed. Very low formations occur upon the margins of mucous membranes; crusts form. Indurations under the crusts, and the crusts continue to form. The circulation is so poor, so feeble in the parts all about the margin of the lips and the corners of the mouth, and corners of the eyes, and eyelids, and upon the genitals, and there is so much venous engorgement that crusts form and ulcerate and bleed and pile up, and this continues until a phagedenic spot comes. This condition is so much like epithelioma that Kreosote has cured epithelioma.

The next striking thing in Kreosote is its stomach symptoms. Soon after eating there comes a burning pain in the stomach, and then a sense of fulness and an increasing nausea, ending in vomiting of the food, which looks as it did when taken; it looks undigested, but it is sour and acrid, coming up an hour or two after eating. Vomiting, the stomach seems unable to digest, and after the patient empties it there is constant nausea. After a swallow of water a prolonged bitter taste remains in the mouth. There is aggravation from eating cold things and relief from warm diet. In malignant diseases of the stomach when this symptom is present. Kreosote becomes a great palliative; it relieves the burning and improves the digestion for a while, but the trouble comes again. Many times our remedies furnish us the greatest known palliation in cancerous affections. Homœopathy should at all times furnish a degree of palliation in cancerous and other incurable malignant diseases of the stomach. This palliation will bring more comfort to the stomach than can possibly be brought about by *Morphine*. I have watched patients under *Morphine* and under homœopathic medicine, and as a mere matter of comfort I will take the homœopathic medicines. This has been the experience of many. When you hear a homœopath say that he prefers anodynes in cancerous affections of the stomach and in other painful affections, it is pretty sure evidence that he is not able to find the medicines that are suitable for the patient. These cases test the ability of the physician.

Kreosote is a great remedy for diarrhœas in the summer, especially for infants. The infant that I described as to his temper may be the infant suffering from the worst form of summer complaint, or having a light attack of cholera infantum. Or he may be "teething," and suffering from the troubles that are sometimes associated with teething. Infants have troubles at the time of teething only because they are sick, and if the child were not in disorder he would not have trouble when teething. Teething is a crisis, and the things that are within will come out at the time, just as there are troubles that are likely to come out at the time of puberty and at the climacteric period.

A marked feature of the Kreosote constitution is that when the desire to urinate comes he must *hurry or the urine will escape*. The urine is passed during sleep. Bloody urine; clots in the urine; acrid and excoriating urine; weakness of the bladder; inability to hold the urine. Smarting and burning in the pudenda, during and after micturition. "Sugar in the urine." It has cured diabetes. Generalize the symptoms given and you will see what kind of a diabetic patient will need Kreosote.

LAC CANINUM

A beginning in this remedy was made by Dr. Reisig, and after Reisig it was used by Bayard. After Bayard's death Dr. Dyer gave me a vial of the 30th potency, made by Reisig, from which the potencies have mostly been made.

All the milks should be potentized, they are our most excellent remedies, they are animal products and foods of early animal life and therefore correspond to the beginning of our innermost physical nature. If we had full provings of monkey's, cow's, mare's and human milk they would be of great value. *Lac defloratum* has done excellent work, and so has this remedy. Lac caninum is in its beginnings yet, although it has made some marvellous cures, but many of its symptoms are doubtful and it would take a century to confirm them. Some may think because the milks are only food for the young they are not medicine, but let one who is made sick from milk take it in potentized form and report the result. Provers who dislike milk will become sick from taking it in potencies in a few days, and their symptoms are very numerous.

This remedy abounds in nervous symptoms, although it has no doubt tissue changes as well. It is deep and long acting; the provers felt its symptoms for years after the proving was made. The mental symptoms are prolonged and distressing. It has cured enlarged glands. It makes ulcers very red, and it has cured such ulcers. Ulcerated areas have a dry, glistening appearance as if coated with epithelium. It is an important remedy in complaints following badly treated diphtheria, in paralysis and other conditions dating back to diphtheria. The greater number of its symptoms belong to the nervous system. An oversensitive state prevails, a general hyperæsthesia of the skin and all parts. It makes women violently hysterical, and causes all sorts of strange and apparently impossible symptoms. For example, a woman lay in bed for days with the fingers abducted and would go wild if they touched each other. The fingers were not aggravated from hard pressure, but she would scream if they touched. This state is difficult to cure outside of Lac can. and *Lach. Lach.* has produced a similar condition. The sensitiveness of the abdomen so that the sheet cannot be permitted to touch the skin belongs to both.

Another strange state is a peculiar vertigo, a condition, when walking, in which she seems to be floating in mid-air, or, when lying, as if she were not on the bed. Other remedies have this. The sensation as if floating, or not touching the bed, or sinking down, belongs to *Lach.* The sensation of gliding while walking is strong under *Asarum Europæum.*

The complaints, almost regardless of kind or quality, *change sides.* The rheumatism is first found in one ankle and then in the other, and then back again to the original site. If in the knee or hip or shoulder the *rheumatism alternates sides.* The headaches and neuralgias do the same thing. The ambulating erysipelas first attacks one side, then the other. In inflammation and neuralgia of the ovaries the same alternation is observed. Sore throats affect alternately the sides of the throat or tonsils. Many cases of this sort have been cured by this remedy. The trouble commenced on the right and went to the left and *Lyc.* failed but when it returned to the right the alternation was noticed and the remedy revealed. Only a limited number of remedies have alternating sides.

One or two provers had many symptoms, and so not all are reliable; but this remedy *so intensifies the imagination and senses* that it would be easy for them to imagine symptoms, and that itself is suggestive. Full of imaginations and harassing, tormenting thoughts. Wandering features in the mental sphere, wandering and alternating states. Cannot collect the thoughts. She wants to leave everything as soon as it is commenced, a condition of irresolution common to quite a number of remedies. She is impressed with the idea that all she says is not so, thinks everything she says is a lie, as if there is no reality in the things that be. In this it is somewhat analogous to *Alumina*, in which the patient feels as if someone else and not himself were saying everything, a lack of consciousness of the reality of things.

Every time a symptom appears she thinks it is a settled disease; fear and anxiety that some horrible disease has come upon her, a delusion that she was suppurating and in a loathsome state; infested with snakes. Horrible sights are presented to the mental vision, not always snakes, and she fears the objects will take form and present themselves to her eyes. This is analogous to *Lach.*, which has the feeling that the atmosphere is full of hovering spirits, although he never sees them.

Imagines he wears someone else's nose. Imagines she is not herself and her properties not her own. Imagines she sees spiders, snakes, vermin. She cannot bear to be alone. In *Lach.* the patient wants to be alone to indulge the strange fancies, and when alone she feels as if she were floating out of the window and over the grassy plains, but a sound will bring her back to the world again. This is on the borderland of insanity or delirium.

Although the patient has all these strange feelings, yet she goes around all day about her business, and no one knows them unless she confesses them. Chronic sadness, everything so dark; irritable, ugly, hateful. Full of vertigo, but it is a sensorial symptom, unusually refined; not the vulgar swaying or tossing or feeling as if things were going round. It affects the whole body, as if she were swimming or floating in the air, spirit-like.

The headaches are violent and are mostly frontal, but it has also occipital headaches. Headeache above the eyes from riding in the cold wind, ameliorated in a warm room. Both the frontal and occipital headaches are aggravated by turning the eyeballs upwards and using the eyes for fine work. Pains in the head during the day, first on one side then on the other, either side being first affected. Pains in the face or eyes, alternating sides, perfectly unbearable, ameliorated going into the open air. The rheumatic symptoms are ameliorated by cold and cold applications, thus classifying it with *Puls.* and *Led.* Some headaches are noted as relieved by warmth.

Sensitiveness is marked; sensitive to light and noise. The page is not clear when reading. She sees faces before her in the dark. Old, troubled, distorted, disagreeable faces come to the vision or imagination. Dark, hideous faces she has seen come up, and she is tormented by them. This is not really a symptom of the vision, but a state of the brain.

Sounds seem far off. Paralysis of the throat with diphtheria; fluids return by the nose when drinking. Coryza, with sore throat and sneezing. Stuffed nose; discharge of thick white mucus. Faceache; pain aggravated by exertion, ameliorated by warm applications, but only cold applications relieve the soreness.

Putrid mouth is a strong feature. The mucous membrane and teeth are coated with a fuzzy, shining, silvery substance, somewhat like milk. In the throat there is a felt-like exudation, ashy gray or *silvery shiny deposit.* It has been used in diphtheria for the class of cases taking alternate sides, and it has also cured paralysis following diphtheria. The pain in the throat pushes toward the left ear. Pains take alternate sides. The throat is ameliorated by cold or warm drinking, and aggravated by empty swallowing. It is indicated especially in a glazed, shiny, red appearance of the throat like *Kali Bich.* The diphtheritic membrane is also white like silver. Lac c. has cured most alternating cases, with patches first on the right tonsil, then on the left. Membranous croup. Wherever there is mucous membrane there will be exudate, a gray, fuzzy coating, like that piling up on the tongue. I once cured with Lac c. a chronic affection in which the whole buccal cavity had a white exudate without inflammation or ulceration, an apparent infiltration which dipped down everywhere extending under the tongue. It was white and silvery, looking as if a mouthful of carbolic acid had been swallowed, and the mouth was so sensitive that the patient could not swallow anything but milk.

The abdomen is full of distress. Pressive pain in the pelvis; acute pain in left groin. Constant urging to urinate. Irritable bladder.

The female sexual organs furnish a mass of symptoms. Severe pain in the region of the right ovary, ameliorated by the flow of bright red blood, is again somewhat like *Lach.* These pains take alternate sides. *Zinc.* also has pain in the ovaries ameliorated by the flow; she never feels well except when menstruating; hysterical at all other times but well at the menstrual period, is *Zinc.* Membranous dysmenorrhœa is another example of the exudative tendency of Lac. c. Sore throat beginning and ending with the menstrual period. *Mag. carb.* has sore throat before the menstrual period and *Calc. c.* has cured painful throat when menstruating.

Escape of *gas* from the vagina. The fermentation of mucus and other substances in the bladder causing the escape of gas when urinating is found only under *Sars.;* the urine flows with a loud noise. It is not uncommon for a child to break wind when urinating, and the urine is passed with a gurgling noise; this is cured by *Sars.*

Much trouble with the mammæ; they feel as if they would suppurate. When a mother has lost her infant and it is necessary to dry up the milk, Lac c. and *Puls. are* the best remedies for this purpose, when no symptoms are present. They will do it speedily. The Lac c. patient is imaginative and sensitive to pain and her surroundings, hyperæsthesia and touchiness. *Puls.* will he called for in the *Puls.* constitution.

Rheumatism with swelling of the lower extremities, especially when it affects the limbs alternately; aggravated by motion and heat, *ameliorated by cold.* Pains in the limbs as if beaten. Rheumatic swellings of joints.

LAC VACCINUM DEFLORATUM

The untrained mind naturally rebels at the idea of giving skimmed milk to sick people as a remedy, but when potentized like any other substance it becomes one of the most useful remedies. Every physician has seen a few cases in his practice; men, women and children who cannot drink milk. They say they are made sick by drinking or using milk, and that milk is poison to them.

It is the work of the true physician to study cases and ascertain in each case what symptoms are observed after taking milk These symptoms constitute a proving of it and it is the best kind of a proving as it is produced upon sensitive persons.

The writer has made it his duty to study each and every one of these cases until the image of the sickness produced by milk *has dawned upon him* both from the individual symptoms and from a collective view.

Much can be learned by meditating upon the milk constitution; some may think there is a difference of importance between milk skimmed and new milk, but for all practical purposes the skimmed milk is sufficient and cures the oversensitiveness to milk, if used in a high potency. It is useless in low potency.

It is a useful remedy as it may demonstrate to the unbeliever the wonderful power of the high potency. It has aggravation during the whole twenty-four hours; some cases manifest symptoms only during the day-time, and amelioration comes with the going down of the sun—but this is uncommon.

The chronic milk subject is very cold and bloodless and cannot get warm even in a warm room and by warm clothing; she is so chilly and so sensitive to cold that she feels the air blowing on her in the room as if she were fanned, even where there is no possible draft and others feel the room to be very warm. She is very sensitive to wet weather. She is subject to neuralgic and rheumatic pains all over the body but more especially in the head. The pain in the head is better from cold applications, but the pains elsewhere are better from heat. The sufferings are all worse by motion and better by rest; pains are better by pressure. The bones are sore to touch. Great lassitude and even weakness, can endure no exertion. There is marked restlessness and she is unable to hold up after loss of sleep; extreme weariness from a short walk. She looks and acts as though she had been suffering long or as if she were going into a decline. The skin all over the body is violently sensitive to cold objects and touch of cold sponge. There is marked periodicity in the nature of the remedy, most noticed in the recurrent headaches. This remedy has had a reputation for curing diabetes and this is not to be wondered at When it is known to have cured the weakness, anæmia and copious, watery urine and great thirst; also copious, dense urine. Many invalids cured by this remedy have appeared to the writer much like the typical diabetic patient; but it can cure only where the peculiar symptoms agree. It will not cure simply when the common symptoms are present. Let all observers faithfully and minutely study all patients who have an aversion to milk; all who have diarrhœa, nausea, vomiting, sick headaches, eructations, foul stomach after drinking milk and in time the general idea of the milk sickness will be known.

It is a most useful and frequently needed remedy for infants and children who cannot take milk, not always as their specific remedy, but as one of the remedies that will help many infants to grow up; some grow morbidly fat and others become lean when fed on milk.

It has been useful in dropsy from weak heart; from liver complaints and from suppressed malaria. People who drink milk habitually become anæmic and catarrhal; fatty degeneration of muscles, heart and liver. Malassimilation is the most marked feature of milk poison.

The pains become violent in many parts; in the spinal cord; in eyeballs; in supra-orbital nerves; in forehead and through the head; in the stomach; in lower part of the abdomen. Many people are made sick by milk who use cream with safety and delight. Lac defloratum is often the remedy for such patients and after a careful examination their symptoms appear like the proving of skimmed milk.

Loss of memory, listlessness and aversion to mental work; sadness, desires death and meditates upon the easiest method of self-destruction; sadness with weeping and palpitation; aversion to seeing and talking to people; weakness and vacillating mind. He is sure he is going to die. She imagines that all her friends will die and that she must go to a convent; a horror when in a small closet lest the door will be closed and she will suffocate. She becomes faint and dizzy when raising her hands high to thread her needle; vertigo on turning in bed; on moving the head from the pillow; on opening the eyes when lying; in the act of lying down. Faintness and nausea when stepping upon the floor in the morning. Vertigo when reaching up with the hands; tendency to fall to the right when standing or walking.

In sickly, pale, careworn women, when the headache is over the eyes and through the frontal region and the pain is violent; is better from pressure and tight binding up, is better lying down in a dark room; is better from cold applications; is better from perfect rest; is worse from least motion, worse from light, noise, and conversation; when the headache comes on from drinking milk and is attended with *copious, pale urine;* with nausea and vomiting of food, mucus and bile. Violent pain in occiput, vertex and sides of the head; marked pulsation in the head with all headaches; during the headaches the face is pale and cold. There is also marked congestion with heat of the head and flushed face; the headache often comes with marked periodicity though sometimes not with regularity. Weekly headaches are the most common. Great soreness all over the head on jarring or coughing; sensation as if top of head was lifted off; pain first in the forehead extending to occiput, making her nearly frantic. Intense headache in forehead and through head, worse in vertex—afterwards head felt bruised. With all the frontal headaches there is strong pulsation in temples. It has cured many violent, periodical, sick-headaches, that have been present since childhood and said to be inherited. During these violent headaches there is sometimes a sensation as though the head were expanding; it has cured headaches that come before and after menses. Morning sickness during pregnancy.

Dim vision before the headaches; can only see light, not objects; sensation as if eyes were full of stones; *extreme photophobia;* dull pain in eyes, worse in left, even while lids are closed; better by cold applications, better by closing eyes, in a dark room; drawing pain in eyes when reading—could only read a few minutes at a time; great pain in eyes on first going into the light; pain in and above eyes, worse by heat and motion. Lids feel heavy, sleepy and dry. Pain most marked over left eye with lachrymation.

Painful pressure or tightness at the root of the nose.

Deathly paleness of the face; wasted, thin and excessively sallow, with dark stains beneath the eyes. Sallow complexion with eczema. Flushes of heat in left side of face; sensation as if flesh was off the bones of the face and edges were separated and sticking out.

Grinding teeth during sleep, with pain in stomach and head, with vomiting.

Taste insipid, sour; mouth dry; breath offensive; mouth clammy and frothy especially, during conversation.

Globus hystericus; sore throat, worse when swallowing. The mucous membrane of the throat is very pale.

Entire loss of appetite; great thirst for large quantities of water; eructations empty or *sour;* distension from gas; nausea after drinking cold water in the evening—worse after lying down; nausea from a recumbent position or from motion or on rising in the morning; deathly nausea, but cannot vomit, with groans and cries of great distress; great restlessness and sensation of coldness although the skin was hot and pulse normal. Vomiting, first of undigested food intensely acid, then of bitter water and, lastly, of a brownish clot which in water separated and looked like coffee grounds. Incessant vomiting which has no relation to her meals; vomiting of bile, with headaches; violent pain in stomach. It is a very useful remedy for vomiting in pregnancy in women who loathe milk. Cramping in the stomach.

Chronic gastro-enteritis with chronic diarrhœa and vomiting; tenderness of abdomen; flatulence and distension. Heaviness and feeling of stone in abdomen. Severe pain across the umbilicus, with headache.

Chronic constipation where rectum seems paralyzed and injections and cathartics have failed; the stool is large, hard and difficult; after prolonged straining the stool recedes. It has cured after *Silica* failed. Constipation in very chilly patients; constipation with periodical headaches and vomiting; frequent but ineffectual urging to stool; diarrhœa from drinking milk.

Frequent scanty urination; profuse, pale, watery urine with headache; urine very dark and thick; *albuminous urine*. It cured involuntary urinations when walking in cold air, or when riding on horseback and when hurrying to catch a train; it cured dribbling after urination; it cured a lack of sensation when the bladder was full.

It cured a yellow-brown leucorrhœa, worse before and after menses; it cured a profuse yellow leucorrhœa. Bearing down in ovarian region; menses too late and scanty; menses too late, pale and watery. Pain in back and ovarian region during menses; sudden suppression of menses after putting hands in cold water; pains all over, especially in head; when the milk is diminished or fails it is of great service. The breasts are dwindling.

Asthma with bloating of stomach; cardiac dyspnœa.

Short, dry cough; worse in a cold room or in cold air.

Soreness of chest with oppression; rheumatic pains in chest in cold, damp weather; tubercular deposits in apices of both lungs.

Pressure in the region of the heart with dyspnœa and a feeling that he must die; cutting as with a knife apex of the heart. Pulsation of the heart and flashes of heat *in the left side of face and neck;* palpitation from least exertion or excitement.

Heat up and down the back and across from shoulder to shoulder; extreme sensitiveness of back to cold sponge. Herpes on side and neck; itching and burning after scratching; hard pressive pain at fourth cervical vertebra; chills creeping along back between scapulæ; intense burning pain in small of back and sacrum; constant pain in small of back.

Ends of fingers icy cold—rest of hand warm; numbness and loss of sensation over outer and anterior surface of thighs; pain pressing down sciatic nerve and heel; morning on rising, with nausea and faintness; weakness and aching in the swollen ankles. Skin thickened on edges of foot; feet cold as ice. Aching pains in wrists and ankles; cold hands and feet during headache.

Great restlessness; extreme and protracted suffering from loss of sleep at night; sleepy all day; extreme insomnia.

Fever at 9 A.M., until morning; wakes in profuse sweat, which stains linen yellow. Hectic fever sensation as if sheets were damp.

The skin is so very sensitive to the touch of a cold hand or sponge that the prover could bathe only in very warm water. The skin is cold and pale and veins look blue and very prominent. Herpetic eruptions; itching of the skin; burning, after scratching.

LACHESIS

Lachesis is a frequently indicated remedy, and one that you will need to study much in order to know how to use. Lachesis seems to fit the whole human race, for the race is pretty well filled up with snake as to disposition and character and this venom only causes to appear that which is in man.

We will first give a survey or the *general symptoms,* those which characterize the remedy and are of greatest importance, and the circumstances under which the symptoms appear, are brought out, or are aggravated.

One who is a constitutional Lachesis patient will find himself suffering from an aggravation of his symptoms in the *Spring,* when he goes out from the cold weather into the milder weather, and especially is that so if it is mild and rainy, or cloudy weather. Or if he goes from a cold into a warmer climate the symptoms of Lachesis will come out. The warm south winds excite the Lachesis symptoms.

The symptoms of Lachesis are worse on entering *sleep.* He may have felt nothing of his symptoms when awake, but when sleep comes on they are aroused, and they gradually increase as the sleep is prolonged, so that a very long sleep will aggravate all the state and condition of a Lachesis patient, and when awakening from sleep he looks back on that sleep with sorrow. The sleep has been disturbed by attacks of suffocation and by awful dreams, and now, after having slept a long time, he arouses with dreadful headaches, with palpitation, with melancholy, with sorrows from head to foot. His body is full of suffering and his mind sees no brightness in anything. There is a cloudy state, sadness, melancholy, insane notions, whims, jealousy and suspicion. When taking *a warm bath,* or applying warm water to places that are inflamed, his mental symptoms are aggravated. After a warm bath or after getting warmed up, or, if he becomes chilled from being out on a cold day and then goes into a warm room the symptoms come on. After going into a warm bath, palpitation comes on; it seems as if his head would burst, his feet become cold, and he is shocked all over, pulsation all over, or feeble heart. Fainting in a warm bath. Girls sometimes faint when going into a warm bath. The patient may be cold and chilly yet the warm room increases or brings out the symptoms.

The general aspect of the patient and the localities will point sometimes to Lachesis. Upon the face there is an appearance of anxiety, of unrest and distress. The face is spotted or *purple* and the eyes are engorged. The eyes look suspicious. If there is an inflamed spot, it is purple. If there is an inflamed gland, and Lachesis is full of inflammation of the glands and cellular tissues, there is a purple or mottled appearance. If there is an ulceration the ulceration bleeds black blood, which soon coagulates and looks like charred straw. From the wounds there is much bleeding. *Small wounds bleed much* like *Phosphorus* and *Kreosote.* A prick of a pin *will* ooze great drops of blood. Ulcers eat in, have false granulations, are putrid, bleed easily, and the blood is black, and all round the ulceration there is a *purple, mottled appearance,* looking as if about to become gangrenous. Often gangrene does come; gangrene of parts that have been injured. Sloughing with great offensiveness. The parts turn black and slough. The veins become varicose. These are found upon the limbs, having the appearance of the varicose veins that come after gestation. Enlargement of the veins is a prominent condition of Lachesis.

From the slightest exertion of the mind or from the slightest emotion the extremities become cold, the heart becomes very feeble, the skin is covered with sweat and the head is hot. Warmth does not seem to relieve the coldness of the feet and hands; they are so cold. They may be wrapped up in flannels and still they remain cold, but suffocation is brought on. He cannot breathe and wants the windows open. It is weakness of the heart; sometimes so weak that it can hardly be heard or felt, and the pulse is feeble and intermittent. At other times there is audible palpitation of the heart.

As we go over the symptoms of the text we will notice something singular about the complaints, that is, their tendency to affect the *left side,* or to begin on the left and extend to the right. The paralysis begins by gradually appearing weakness upon the left side. Which extends to the right side. It has a strong affinity for the ovaries, and in this it will be found that the left ovary is affected first. So, in inflammation of the ovaries, the left will be affected first, and later the right. The inflammation begins on the left side of the throat and gradually goes to the right. The left side of the head is commonly most affected. The left eye becomes painful and the pain extends to the right. The left side of the back of the head, in the occipital headache, will be more affected than the right. This does not always follow, and if the reverse is true it does not contra-indicate Lach., but such is the common feature of it. Left upper and right lower has been observed.

In many symptoms of Lachesis, there is *morning aggravation.* This is the well-known Lachesis *aggravation after sleep;* the patient will sleep into the aggravation. In the milder symptoms this aggravation is mild and is not felt until after the patient wakes up from a long sleep, but if the aggravation is one that is of considerable violence, the patient may feel it immediately on going to sleep, and it arouses him; for instance, the heart symptoms. As soon as he goes into a sleep he rouses up with palpitation, with dyspnœa, with suffocation, with exhaustion, with vertigo, with pain in the back of the head, and many other circulatory disturbances.

The next most important thing to be studied is the *mental state.* Nothing stands out more boldly than the self-consciousness, the self-conceit, the envy, the hatred, the revenge and the cruelty of the man. These things, of course, are matters of self-consciousness, an improper love of self. Confusion of the mind to insanity. All sorts of impulsive insanity. The mind is tired. The patient puts on an appearance like the maudling of a drunkard, talks with thick lips and thick tongue, blunders and stumbles, only partly finishing words; the face is purple and the head is hot. There is choking and the collar is uneasy about the neck; and the more uneasiness about the neck, the more choking, the more confusion of mind and the more appearance of intoxication. You will see if you talk with one who is intoxicated with whiskey symptoms like Lachesis, he stumbles through, hardly realizing what he says, half finishing his sentences and his words, leaving his "g's" off all the present participles; he stumbles and blunders, he mutters, and tells you first one thing and then another. These symptoms are increased under the circumstances mentioned in the Spring; in the warm weather following a cold spell; in rainy weather; after a warm bath; after sleep. The mental state is large. Jealousy without any reason. Unwarranted jealousy and suspicion. Many times this medicine has cured *suspicion* in girls, when they were simply suspicious of their girl friends. She never sees a whispered conversation going on but they are talking about her, to her detriment. Suspects that they are contriving to injure her, and she will resort to any scheme to see if they were not talking of her to her detriment. A woman imagnies that her friends, husband, and children are trying to damage her; that her friends are going to put her in an insane asylum. Apprehension of the future. Thinks she is going to have heart disease, and is going insane; and that people are contriving to put her in an insane asylum. Imagines her relatives are trying to poison her and she refuses to eat. She thinks sometimes that it is only a dream and she can hardly say whether she dreamed it or whether she thinks it. She thinks she is dead, or dreams that she is dead, and in the dream preparations are being made to lay her out, or that she is about to die.

Thinks she is somebody else, and in the hands of a stronger power. She thinks she is *under superhuman control.* She is compelled to do things by spirits. She hears a command, partly in her dream, that she must carry out. Sometimes it takes the form of voices in which she is commanded to steal, to murder, or to confess things she never did, and she has no peace of mind until she makes a confession of something she has never done. The torture is something violent until she confesses that which she has not done. Imagines she is pursued. Imagines that she has stolen something, or that somebody thinks she has stolen something, and fears the law. She hears voices and warnings, and in the night she dreams about it. The state of torture is something dreadful, and it then goes into a delirium with muttering. The delirium is carried on like one muttering when drunk. This state increases until unconsciousness comes on and the patient enters into a coma from which he cannot be aroused. The patient also goes through periods of violence and violent delirium.

It is full of *religious insanity.* You will find a dear, sweet old lady, who has always lived what would be called an upright and pious life, yet she is not able to apply the promises that are in the Word of God to herself; these things seem to apply to somebody else, but not to her. She is full of wickedness and has committed the unpardonable sin. She is compelled to say these things; she is overwhelmed by these things and she is going to die and going to that awful hell that she reads about. The physician must listen to this with attention. The physician might make the mistake in this instance of making light of such feelings. If he does, the patient will not return, and he will be deprived of the chance of benefiting her. No matter what her whims are, no matter what her religious opinions are, her state of mind must be treated with respect. It must be treated as if it were so.

She must have sympathy and kindness. It is an unfortunate thing for a doctor to get a reputation of being an ungodly man, among pious people, as he will be deprived of doing these people an immense amount of good. He must be candid with all the whims and notions of the people that he visits in the world. He must be everybody's friend, and he can be such without any hypocrisy if he is simply an upright and just man.

The state of religious melancholy, with religious insanity, is not uncommonly attended with much *loquacity,* with talkativeness, which Lachesis is full of. It is commonly among women, very seldom among men, that we find this religious melancholy. Now, this woman is impelled to tell it; she will annoy her intimate friends, day and night, with this story of the damnation of her soul and her wickedness and all the awful things she has done. If you ask her what things she has committed she will say everything, but you cannot pin her down to the fact that she has killed anybody. If you allow her to go through with her story she will tell you all the crimes in the calendar that she has committed, although she has been a well behaved and well-disposed woman. There is another kind of loquacity belonging to Lachesis. The patient is impelled to talk continuously. It is found in another state in which the patient is compelled to hurry in everything she does, and wants everybody else to hurry. With that state of hurry is brought out the loquacity, and this is something far beyond comprehension until you have once heard it. There is no use attempting to describe it, it is so rapid, changing from one subject to another. Sentences are sometimes only half finished; she takes it for granted that you understand the balance and she will hurry on. Day and night she is wide awake, and with such sensitiveness to her surroundings that you would naturally think, from what things she hears and how she is disturbed by noise, that she can hear the flies walk upon the walls and the clock striking upon the distant steeple. You do not get all these things in the text, you have to see them applied. But the things I give you that are brought out clinically are those things that have come from applying the symptoms of the remedy at the bedside to sick folks. "Most extraordinary loquacity, making speeches in very select phrases, but jumping off to most heterogeneous subjects." "One word often leads into the midst of another story." These states may come on in acute diseases like typhoid, when it will take the usual typhoid delirium, or they may come on in conditions like diphtheria, or in any of the diseases that are characterized by blood poisoning; they may come on in the puerperal state, or may take the form of insanity. It is a long acting remedy, and if it has been abused its effects will last a life time.

In many cases a close connection between the mental symptoms and the heart symptoms will be noticed, especially in young women and girls who have met with disappointment, who have been lying awake nights because of disturbance of the affections, or from disappointment, or from shattered hopes, or from grief. Prolonged melancholy, mental depression, hysterical symptoms, weeping, mental prostration and despair, with pain in the heart, with a gone sensation or sensation of weakness in the heart, with difficult breathing. She meditates upon suicide, and finally settles back into an apathetic state, in which there is an aversion to everything, to work, and even to thinking.

I might impress upon your mind the head symptoms if I related the case of a patient who described her symptoms probably more typically than you can find in the books. She was sitting up in bed and unable to lie down; she was worse from lying down, her face was purple, her eyes were engorged, the face puffed and tumid and the eyelids bloated. She sat there perfectly quiet in bed and described the pain as a surging sensation, which came up the back of the neck and head and then over the head. That is a typical feature of Lachesis. A surging in waves. *Waves of pain* that are not always synchronous with the pulse. They may not relate to the flow of blood at all. The surging is aggravated by motion, not so much in the act of motion, but after moving. It is sometimes felt after walking or changing to another place, and sitting down again; that is, a few seconds after the motion is completed the pain begins, and it comes to its height instantly and then gradually subsides into a very steady surging or a more steady ache. In the head there is a continuous steady ache, which may be aggravated or aroused into a surging which is so violent that it seems as if it would take the life of the patient.

The headache begins in the morning on waking. The milder Lachesis headaches begin in the morning on awaking and wear off after moving about a while. With the headaches and complaints in general there is a momentary vanishing of thought; all sorts of vertigo. Vertigo with nausea and vomiting. The vertigo inclines the patient to turn to the left.

Lachesis has *bursting* pains in the head; congestive pains with a feeling as if all the blood in the body must be in the head, because the extremities are so cold and the head pulsates and hammers. This pulsating headache is part of a *general pulsation* from head to foot. In all arteries and inflamed parts, there is pulsation. The inflamed ovary pulsates, and it feels at times as if a little hammer were hammering upon the inflamed part with every pulsation of the artery. Lachesis has a number of times cured fistula in ano when associated with this feeling as if a hammer continually hammered the little fistulous pipe. It has cured fissure of long standing when it felt as if the inflamed part were being hammered. Hæmorrhoids have been cured when this sensation of hammering was present. So that we see this pulsation in the head is not a special symptom, but is a general symptom, brought out in relation to the head.

Some symptoms are valuable because of the frequency of their association, and when such is the case their concomitant relation becomes important. The cardiac symptoms are frequently connected with the headache symptoms in Lachesis. It is seldom that you will see Lachesis headaches without cardiac difficulty. A weak pulse, or the pulsation felt all over the body, is more or less associated with violent Lachesis headaches.

In the text we find *weight* and *pressure as a* strong feature of the Lachesis head symptoms. With almost any complaint of the body, with typhoids, at the menstrual period, during the congestive chill, it seems that the body becomes cold, the extremities become cold, the knees are cold, the feet are cold, and it is impossible to keep them warm, while the face is purple and mottled, the eyes are protruding and engorged, and this awful pain in the head, with a tendency to become unconscious, incoherent speech, difficulty of articulation, and finally actual unconsciousness.

In relation to the head symptoms and mind symptoms and the sensorium in general, the *oversensitiveness* that is found in Lachesis ought to be mentioned. His symptoms become very intense. The vision becomes very intense; the hearing becomes intense; the sense of touch especially is over wrought. The touch of the clothing becomes very painful, while hard pressure may be agreeable. The scalp becomes so sensitive to the touch of the hand that it is painful, while the pressure from a bandage is agreeable. Oversensitive to noise, oversensitive to motion in the room, to conversation and to others walking over the floor. By these circumstances the pains are increased. The patient becomes extremely sensitive throughout all the senses of the body. The *oversensitiveness* to touch is probably extensively in the skin, because of the fact that hard pressure often gives relief. In one who is suffering from peritonitis, from inflammation of the ovaries or uterus, or any of the abdominal viscera, the skin is so sensitive to the clothing that contrivances are sometimes necessary to relieve the suffering from the touch of the bed clothing. Something in the form of a hoop will be found in the bed, or the patient will have the knees drawn up, or with the hands will hold the clothing from touching the body. The ordinary weight of the hand may bring out the soreness that is in the abdomen, which is an entirely different soreness, whereas the clothing touching the abdomen only brings out the oversensitiveness of the skin. The mere touch of the skin with the finger or hand is unbearable.

There are many inflammatory and congestive conditions of the *eyes*. The eye symptoms are worse after sleep, and the eyes are oversensitive to touch and light. With the eye symptoms we have headaches, because the brain and eyes are so closely associated. In the sore throats, when the spatula or tongue depressor happens to touch the wall of the throat, the tonsil, or the root of the tongue, there is a feeling as if the eyes would be pressed out. Violent pain in the eyes from touching the throat. Lachesis is a great jaundice medicine, because it produces much disturbance in the liver. Yellowness of the skin and whites of the eyes, and thickening of tissues about the eyes. "Fistula lachrymalis," which is accompanied by long standing eruptions about the face.

Oversensitiveness of the meatus auditorus externus. Anything introduced into the canal of the *ear* will cause violent, spasmodic coughing and tickling in the throat. So sensitive is the mucous membrane of the ear that a violent cough, like whooping cough, will come on from touching the mucous membrane of the ear. This only shows the oversensitiveness of reflexes, and the oversensitiveness in general. With the hearing there is the same over-sensitiveness that we have spoken of elsewhere. The Eustachian tube becomes closed with- a catarrhal thickening, stricture of the Eustachian tube.

The catarrhal symptoms of the *nose* are prominent. Frequent bleeding of the nose and body, watery discharge from the nose. Always taking cold in the nose. Stuffing up of the nose, with disturbance of smell. Oversensitiveness to smell, and oversensitiveness to odors, finally loss of smell. Lachesis has inflammatory conditions, very chronic in character, with crusty formations in the nose, sneezing, watery discharges from the nose and catarrhal headaches. Sometimes the headache goes off when the catarrhal discharge comes, and when the catarrhal discharge stops the headache comes on. Violent headache with discharge, with sneezing and coryza. Congestive headaches with coryza. This catarrhal condition has fed to the use of Lachesis in syphilis. It is sufficiently similar to cope with the severe forms of nasal syphilis; syphilis where it has affected the nasal mucous membrane, producing crusts and finally affecting the bones. Fœtid ozæna; very offensive discharges from the nose. Bleeding from the nose need not surprise you, because Lachesis is a hæmorrhagic remedy. The blood from the nose or any part, when it dries or clots, looks like charred straw or becomes black. Parts bleed easily. Copious and prolonged uterine hæmorrhage, copious and prolonged menstruation, bleeding from the nose, vomiting of blood, hæmorrhage from the bowels in typhoids. "Great sensitiveness of the nostrils and lips, swelling of the lips, great swelling and tumefaction of the nose in old cases of syphilis." The nose swells up and becomes purple. The nasal bones are very sore, soreness upon sides of the nose. Lachesis is an especially useful medicine in old drunkards who have red nose, and in heart affections with red nose. A red knob on the end of the nose, a strawberry nose.

The face is purple and mottled, the eyelids are tumid, very much puffed; not bloated as in œdematous subjects, but puffed. There is not the pitting upon pressure that we find in œdema, although Lachesis has that, but there is a puffiness peculiar to Lachesis, the face looks swollen and inflamed, due to a venous stasis is, so that the face is purple and mottled. The nose is tumid, yet it will not remain pitted upon pressure. The lips feel as if inflamed, yet are not inflamed, simply sensitive to pressure. The face has also an œdematous appearance in which there is pitting upon pressure, in cardiac affections, in cases of Bright's disease. On the other hand the face becomes very pale, pale and cold; the skin covered with scaly eruptions. Eruptions that bleed easily, with crusty eruptions, with vesicular eruptions. Eruptions that fill with blood, bloody vesicles and large blood blisters, such as occur sometimes in burns, with burning. The face becomes jaundiced and very sallow. At times it takes on the appearance also of a chlorosis. If you have once seen the chlorotic color, it need not be described. It is a condition of anæmia, with yellowish pallor, ash colored or grey, intermingled with a sort of greenish color, so that the ancients often referred to it as green sickness. Again the face becomes livid and puffed like the bloated aspect of drunkards, the mottled purple appearance of drunkards who have been drinking for years, until they are bloated and broken down and have a besotted aspect. You see that in Lachesis.

In Lachesis we have a remedy for erysipelas and gangrenous affections, and about the affected part there is the Lachesis appearance, that is the mottled, purplish appearance. Lachesis has become clinically a marked remedy for erysipelas and for gangrene. As provers do not follow up remedies until they produce these things, we have to gather them from the poisonous effects and clinical observation.

In Lachesis there is oozing of blood around the *teeth,* the *gums* bleed easily. Dry crusts appear upon the teeth in zymotic diseases, often black formiations, sordes, and the tongue takes part in the appearance of the mouth and becomes slick. This occurs in typhoid conditions when there is a total loss of assimilation, the appetite is entirely gone, the stomach will not take food, and when food is put into the stomach it is rejected. There is also paresis of the tongue. The tongue seems to be like leather in the mouth, it is moved with great difficulty. And the speech is like that of one half intoxicated; he is unable to articulate. The tongue swells and is protruded very slowly. It is dry and catches on the teeth and seems to have lost its stiffness. Seems like a rag, or as if the muscles did not act upon it so that it cannot be protruded, or if it is protruded it trembles and quivers and jerks and catches on the teeth. Again it is swollen, it is denuded of its papillae, and smooth, shiny and glassy as if varnished. In the mouth there is a soapy appearance of the saliva. The saliva runs into the mouth copiously and the patient will often lie with the head over the side of the bed, and the saliva dripping into a pan or commode. The saliva is stringy and can be pulled out of the mouth in strings; white mucus or saliva. This is not an uncommon feature in diphtheria, in sore throat, in inflammation of the tongue and mouth and gums, and in inflammation of the salivary glands. When this mucus is thick, tough, yellow, stringy and ropy it is like *Kali bichromicum.* You will often find in severe sore throat that the patient will lie and gag, and cough, and attempt with difficulty to protrude the tongue to expel the saliva from the mouth. Very often the pain is so severe in the root of the tongue that he cannot expel the saliva by the tongue and he will lie with the open mouth over a commode, or with a cloth over the pillow, to receive the thick, ropy saliva. In such a state with sore throats, especially those that commence on the left side and go to the right, you hardly need to question longer, for it is the aspect of Lachesis. This state of affairs would lead to Lachesis in ordinary inflammatory conditions of the tongue and in cancerous affections of the tongue. Lach. has in its nature the tendency to formation of malignant scabs and malignant ulcers, such as we find in epithelioma. It has cured a number of cases of epithelioma. It has been a very useful remedy in lupus. It is an important remedy in syphilitic sore throat, in syphilitic ulceration of the throat, tongue and roof of the mouth with this copious, stingy saliva.

The, muscles of the pharynx become paralyzed and will not act, and hence the food will collect in the pharynx, that is, the bolus to be swallowed goes to the pharynx and stops, and then a tremendous effort at swallowing, with gagging and coughing and spasmodic action of the chest, takes place in order to carry on respiration, and he will not again attempt it. This state often occurs with diphtheria. I have a number of times seen it brought about by the physician, who has, instead of giving just enough Lachesis, high enough and similar enough to the disease to cure, given it as low as he could get it, the 8th or 10th, dissolved it in water and fed it all through the diphtheritic state. When you come across cases that have been treated in this way you need not be surprised if a post-diphtheritic paralysis comes on, because Lachesis will produce it. It may cure the diphtheria, but it will leave its poisonous effects which will last that patient a lifetime. Every spring the symptoms of Lachesis will crop out. In all the circumstances of aggravation described the symptoms of Lachesis will crop out if he has once been poisoned by it.

In the sore throat we have a combination of symptoms. Lachesis has produced this state, going from left to right; but with the sore throat there is a sensation of fulness in the neck and throat, difficult breathing, pallor or plethoric appearance of the face, choking when going into sleep, the peculiar kind of saliva and aggravation of the throat symptoms *from warm drinks*. There is not always an aggravation of the pain itself from warm drinks, but the patient is often unable to swallow warm fluids. The swallowing of warm fluids often causes choking, and after a swallow of warm tea is taken the patient will clutch at the throat and it seems as if he would suffocate. He says, "Oh do not give me any more warm drinks." Something cold will relieve. The dyspnœa and the distress about the throat is increased by swallowing something warm. Now, in the sore throats of *Lycopodium,* warmth often benefits, but it is also true in some cases of *Lycopodium* sore throat, they want cold drinks and cold feels good to the throat.

Very often in the more acute symptoms of Lachesis a warm drink in the stomach is hurtful and causes nausea and suffocation and increases the choking and palpitation and the fulness in the head, whereas in the chronic cases of Lachesis, those that have been poisoned years before, there will be a sensation of nausea and tendency to vomit from taking a drink of cold water and then lying down. The nausea comes on after lying down, that is, let the patient take a drink of ice cold water and go to bed and nausea will come on. Such a state is peculiar to Lachesis. It has been a later observation of those who have long before proved Lachesis. The symptoms of Lachesis have sometimes to he taken years after.

Lachesis has ulcers in the throat. It has aphthous patches, it has red and grey ulceration, it has deep ulceration. The tendency to ulceration upon the margins of mucous membranes is peculiar to Lachesis. Also ulceration upon the skin, where the circulation is feeble. It seems that the pain in the throat is particularly marked between the acts of swallowing, and the pressure of the bolus going over the inflamed tonsils relieves the pain. Always choking when swallowing, choking and gagging in the throat. The cough is a choking cough and produces a sensation of tickling. This is like the *Bell..* cough. *Bell.* antidotes a Lach. cough, it has a cough so much like Lach. that no one can tell them apart. Again the throat takes on extreme dryness in Lach., and this dryness is without thirst, dryness with aversion to water. Much inclination to swallow; the tendency is to continuously swallow, yet it is painful. Empty swallowing is more painful than the swallowing of solids. Sonic Lach. patients suffering from cardiac affections are annoyed with constriction of the throat, choking in the throat when anything warm is swallowed, and sometimes when going into a warm room, choking and palpitation of the heart. Tendency to chronic sore throat or recurrent sore throat and ulceration with every recurring sore throat. Liquids, of course, you will see, are analogous to empty swal-lowing, and empty swallowing causes more pain than the bolus which presses upon the sore throat, because it is of the nature of a slight touch. The slight touch increases the soreness and pain in the throat. Slight pressure of the collar increases the pain in the throat. With the sore throat the muscles and glands about the neck become painful, inflamed and swollen, and very tender to the touch. With the sore throat, very commonly, there is pain in the base of the brain or in the back of the head, and soreness of the muscles of the back of the neck, which is often relieved by lying on the back and aggravated by lying on either side. If you look into the throat it has *a* mottled, purplish appearance. Put all these things together, with the copious flow of tenacious saliva, and you will be able to manage cases of diphtheria that commence on the left side and spread to the right, whether the membrane is scanty or copious. Tonsillitis with suppuration of the tonsils, when the left tonsil becomes inflamed and after a day or two the right one becomes inflamed and swollen, and they both finally go on to suppuration, or when one swells and suppurates and the other swells and suppurates. Diphtheritic appearances of the throat, *spreading from left to right.* The pharynx is full of thick, white; ropy mucus in the morning; must hawk out a mouthful of mucus in the morning.

The abdomen is distended with flatus. The abdomen is tympanitic in typhoid condition, much rumbling in the distended abdomen. The clothing cannot be tolerated, not even the slightest touch of the clothing, and yet it may require hard pressure to bring out soreness that is deep in the abdomen. This state is as it is in inflammation of bowels, ovaries and uterus, the patient lies on the back with the clothing lifted from the abdomen. Violent, labor-like pains, menstrual colic, present in typhoid, in puerperal fever, in malignant scarlet fever, in the more malignant affections of zymotic forms of the continued fever.

Lach. has a series of liver troubles with jaundice; congestion of the liver, inflammation of the liver, enlarged liver and the nutmeg liver. Cutting like a knife in the region of the liver. Vomiting of bile; vomiting of everything taken into the stomach. Extreme nausea; continuous nausea with jaundice. White stool. It has cured cases with gall stone. "Cannot. endure any pressure about the hypochondria." In the chronic state the, sensitiveness of the skin is so great over the abdomen, and about the waist and hips, that the wearing of the clothing creates pain, great restlessness and uneasiness, the patient grows increasingly nervous and finally goes into hysterics. Sensitiveness over the lower abdomen; can scarcely allow her clothes to touch her.

It seems strange at first reading that Lachesis can be such a common remedy at the *menstrual period.* It is also laid down as a remedy for the *climacteric period.* Now if you will study the cases of many women at the climacteric period you will find that many of them have the flushes of heat and the surgings in the head and the great circulatory disturbances that are found under Lachesis. This is also true of the complaints, the headaches, etc., that come in women at the climacteric period and at the menstrual period. The Lachesis symptoms are strong in women during menstruation. There is violent headache, boring pain in the vertex, nausea and vomiting during menses.

The discharge in the female, either as a menstrual flow or as a hæmorrhage, is black blood. Pain in the left ovarian region, or going from left to right. Induration of one or both ovaries. It has cured suppuration of the ovaries. The uterine region is very sensitive to touch, to the slightest contact of the clothing; in inflammation of the ovaries, pains in the ovaries and uterus going from left to right. Pains in the pelvis going upwards to the chest, sometimes a surging of pain going upwards, grasping the throat. Labor pains surge up, with clutching at the throat, or the labor pains cease suddenly, with clutching at the throat. The menstrual pains increase violently until relieved by the flow. The menstrual sufferings are before and after the flow, with *amelioration during the flow.* The menstrual flow intermits one day and then goes on for one day, and during the intermission there is likely to be pain or headache. Menorrhagia with chills at night and flushes of heat in the daytime. During the menstrual period violent headache, especially at such times as the flow slackens up. *It is a general feature of Lachesis to be relieved by discharges.* Catamenin flow but one hour every day; on stopping, violent pains follow in region of left ovary, alternating with gagging and vomiturition.

It is especially useful at the menopause, because of the flushes of heat. Uterine hæmorrhage, fainting spells, suffocation in a warm room; orgasm of blood most violent. Complaints during pregnancy. Inflammation of the veins of the leg. Varicose veins, blue or purple, extreme sensitiveness along the veins; sensitive to the slightest touch, though relieved by pressure.

The study of Lachesis is only a commentary on some of its important parts.

LAUROCERASUS

The many strange constitutional symptoms indicate feeble circulation and weak heart. Great general coldness, that is not ameliorated by external warmth. It is like wrapping up a dead man. Yet if he approaches a warm stove nausea comes on. If he is in a warm room the sweat breaks out on the forehead and the forehead is cold; but if he moves about slowly in the open air the sweat ceases and the forehead warms up. Want of animal heat. Want of reaction. Remedies act only as palliatives, act only as short acting remedies in constitutional disease, or the symptoms partially subside but the patient does not react. The patient does not convalesce. It often cures the heartfailure due to *Digitalis* in Old School hands, or when convalescence is attended by weak heart if there is cold skin and external heat is objectionable. It should be compared with *Camph., Am. c.* and *Secale.* A prolonged fainting spell; twitching of the limbs, gasping for breath. Complaints after deep sorrow or fright. Chorea after every excitement. Spells of profound sleep, with snoring or stertorous breathing. In the spells of suffocation he must lie down (*psor.*) but the dry, hacking cough comes on as soon as he lies down.

Weakness of body and mind. Fainting. Motionless. Apprehensiveness, Vertigo in the open air; he must lie down.

Coldness of the forehead in a warm room, ameliorated in the open air. Stupefying pains in the head, with pulsation. Stitching pains in the head. Periodical paroxysms of aching pain under the frontal bone. Sensation as if brain fell forward on stooping. Tension in the brain. Headache is sometimes ameliorated by eating. The scalp itches.

Dim vision. Veil before the eyes. Objects larger.

The face is blue, sunken, bloated, and expressionless; jaundiced; yellow spot. *Formication of the face.* Lockjaw.

Mouth and tongue dry. The tongue is dry, cold and numb; stiff and swollen.

Spasmodic contraction of throat and œsophagus; drink rolls audibly down the œsophagus and through the intestines.

Emptiness in stomach after eating (*Dig.*) *as* if he were still hungry. Violent thirst. Loathing of food. Nausea on coming near a warm stove. Vomiting of food with the cough. Eructations, tasting like bitter almonds. Violent pain in stomach, with cold skin. Coldness in stomach and abdomen. Contractions like cramps in stomach and cutting in abdomen. Pain in liver as though an abscess were forming. Stitching pain in liver on pressure. Rumbling in bowels.

Diarrhœa, with green mucus, and green watery stools, with tenesmus. Constipation, with difficult stool. It cures cholera infantum with green watery stools when drinks gurgle down the œsophagus and there is general coldness, blueness, and fainting spells.

The whole urinary apparatus is in a paralytic state. Suppression of urine or retention, or urine passed in a very feeble stream. Involuntary urination. Pain in stomach when passing urine. These urinary symptoms sometimes come with palpitation and suffocation, and fainting spells, or other cardiac symptoms and Laurocerasus must be consulted.

Menses too frequent, profuse, thin, with tearing in vertex at night. Uterine hæmorrhage, with flow dark and clotted during climaxis. Fainting spells with coldness during menses. Pain in sacrum during menses.

Heart patients that often suffer much from constriction of the larynx are helped by this remedy. Laryngismus stridulus.

Difficult breathing. Suffocation, oppression of chest, gasping in heart complaints, ameliorated by lying down. Clutching at the heart and palpitation. It has cured mitral regurgitation many times.

Short, hacking, dry, nervous cough. Cardiac cough. Whooping cough in puny children when there is a history of feeble heart, blue cold skin, and laryngeal spasm. Paralytic chest symptoms.

Irregular action of the heart, slow pulse, fluttering heart. Sitting up causes gasping; lying ameliorates the oppression. Feeble pulse, cold blue surface, twitching of muscles of face and limbs. Slight exertion aggravates all the symptoms, *Cyanosis neonatorum.* Burning in chest on inspiration.

The veins of the hands are distended. Cold clammy feet and legs. Painless paralysis of limbs. Stinging and tearing in limbs. Feet numb from lying with limbs crossed.

LEDUM PALUSTRE

This remedy comes up well after the study of *Lachesis,* for we find in the pathogenesis many features similar to those in *Lachesis.* It has the mottled aspect and the same puffed and bloated appearance of the face. It is antidotal to *Lachesis,* to the poison of insects, to the poison of *Apis* and to animal poisons.

Ledum is a remedy for the surgeon, and is closely associated in traumatism with *Arnica* and *Hypericum.* The symptoms very much resemble such as follow certain kinds of injury, for instance an injury from stepping on tacks, from puncturing with needles, wounds that bleed scantily but are followed by pain, puffiness and coldness of the part. Stepping on a nail and it pierces the sole of the foot or the heel, or he receives such a wound in the palm of the hand from a splinter, or he runs a splinter under the nail. If, after such punctured wounds, the *part becomes cold* and then pale, paralyzed and mottled think of Ledum. The horse sometimes steps on a nail. If that nail goes through and strikes the margin of the coffin bone, tetanus will folow. It is known to be almost sure death. Put Ledum on the tongue of that horse and there will not be any trouble for it prevents such conditions.

When tetanus comes on from punctured wounds in the palms or soles, or in other parts, think of *Hypericum,* or when you have a punctured wound to treat, give Ledum at once and you will prevent tetanus. When the finger nails have been torn, or the nerves in sentient parts like the ends of the fingers have been torn and lacerated, *Hypericum* becomes the remedy. For bruising of various parts, and when the patient feels as if bruised all over, no matter how extensively he is bruised, *Arnica* is generally the remedy. It may be said, for punctured wounds study Ledum; for lacerated wounds of sentient nerves, study *Hypericum;* for bruises, study *Arnica;* for open lacerations and cuts, study *Calendula.* The conditions that come from the external ought to be remedied to a great extent by external means. A solution of *Calendula* is excellent in conditions that come from the external, and it should he applied externally. When you have lacerated wounds and cuts with knives or other sharp instruments, apply *Calendula,* because the injury is external without internal effects. The symptoms that arise from internal cause, treat with internal remedies, and symptoms that arise from external cause, when all that there is of the case is external, treat locally; in other words, for local causes use local means, and for internal or dynamic causes, use internal means. Let internal wrongs be treated by the homœopathic remedy and external or local conditions be treated by such soothing dressings as are most comfortable. Always protect surfaces that are exposed, and raw, and bleeding with something of a bland and superficial character. Wounds must be dressed with as simple a means as possible, and there is no simpler dressing than *Calendula,* one part to four or six of water. The tincture will smart too much. Your open wounds will granulate most beautifully under *Calendula,* and you will have no constitutional effects. When the constitutional state is orderly and there is an open injury let the constitution alone, but put on some soothing application externally. In doing this there is no law to govern the action of the physician. Air is an irritant to a raw part and will keep up an unnecessary discharge of pus, even from a perfectly healthy sore. *Calendula* will keep it protected. The sides of a cut must be drawn together, and if it is perfectly tight it will heal itself by first intention. If it does not, then you may know there is a constitutional condition that you must ferret out and find remedy for. Local treatment must then be suspended. These remedies that I have mentioned, to a great extent, cover the management of wounds, and it is simple. Anyone has sense enough to draw together and close up a yawning wound, and to properly dress it. The muscles that naturally draw a wound open have to he overcome by stitches or by strappings. They do not belong to prescribing, they belong to the surgeon.

The Ledum patient is very often subject to what may be called constitutional coldness, coldness to touch, coldness in the body and coldness in the extremities with hot head, and again we see the other extreme, where the whole body is overheated, and the head also is in a state of great heat. There is throbbing and pulsating all over the body; the skin is purple or is too highly colored;.he wants the covers all off at night. It is not uncommon to hear a patient, who has a Ledum headache, say that she wants the head out in the cold air, wants to put it out of the window, does not want any covering upon the head; delights to bathe it with very cold water.

Ledum has a bloated condition of the hands, face, and feet; bloated and purple from the knees down in certain dropsical conditions. With this purple, mottled, bloated condition from the knees to the feet the swelling as big as the skin will allow, and the pain excruciating. The only relief that patient gets is by sitting, with the feet in a tub of ice cold water. I remember the first time I ever saw this in a patient. He was an old syphilitic, whose nasal bones had been eaten out by syphilis, and his nose was a flabby piece of skin; it had no stiffening in it. He was a drunkard, and was extremely abusive to his family when drunk. He had been for several years unwilling to work, having lost his ambition, and he would sit in the house and allow his wife to wait upon him. He had practically become a tramp, only he could not tramp, for this dropsical condition had come on and his feet were so badly swollen and sensitive that he sat in the house day after day. When I first saw him he had before him a good-sized old-fashioned wash-tub, and there he sat with the ice water two-thirds up to his knees and pieces of ice floating around on the top of the water, which he liked to have coming in contact with the skin. When that ice was out he would put in more. The wife described his sufferings by saying he "suffered agonies something dreadful". Ledum took his feet out of the ice water so that he never used it afterwards. It caused the purpleness to disappear, the bloating went out of his feet, and he quit drinking. Ledum cured him of his syphilitic trouble, and he never had a return of that original state. *Pulsatilla* and Ledum are the two principal remedies that want the feet in very cold water. But Ledum suited that man.

Where there are inflamed surfaces the tendency in Ledum is to bleed, and the blood is black. Ledum patients are full-blooded and plethoric, of a robust character. Such plethoric patients bleed easily, have red faces; they are fleshy, strong and of robust constitution. Hæmorrhages sometimes occur in the chamber of the eye, hæmorrhage of the nose, hæmorrhage in cavities, bloody urine.

Old painful ulcers that spread, that are mottled round about, in a constitution that always wants to be cold. The ulcers are relieved by cold.

This remedy is of a rheumatic nature, rheumatic and gouty. It is a gouty medicine, having complaints in persons who suffer from gout, and have chalk stones in their joints, deposits in the wrists, fingers and toes. The deposits go from below upwards. The gouty joints become suddenly inflamed and are relieved by cold. Ledum especially singles out the knee; it is suitable in old prolonged cases of inflammation of the knee-joint, of rheumatic knee-joint. You will find such patients sitting with the joint exposed to the cold, fanning the joint, or putting evaporating lotions upon the joint, such as chloroform, or ether, which give relief to the joints while evaporating to dryness. Rheumatic and gouty extremities with pain and swelling; pain worse from motion, worse at night and from warmth of bed; better from cold applications with copious pale urine. The pains and swelling go upwards and the heart becomes affected.

The face I have already described as puffy or bloated like the *Lachesis* face. It is a besotted face and looks very much like the face of an old drunkard. Ledum counteracts the effect of whiskey, and takes away the appetite for whiskey. Ledum is to whiskey what *Caladium* is to the smoking habit. You can break patients from the habit of smoking so that they go to the other extreme, and have an aversion to it.

It has erysipelas, as you might expect. It has a blue, mottled and puffed and sometimes œdematous appearance. It takes on an acute character and becomes burning. Phlegmonous erysipelas of any part of the body, but particularly of the face, or the injured part.

You might naturally suppose that a medicine that has such a gouty nature in it would have more or less kidney symptoms. "Urination frequent, quantity diminished or increased, stream often stops during the flow." "Burning in the urethra after urinating." "Itching redness and discharge of pus." It has red sand in the urine as marked as *Lycopodium*. It has great quantities of sandy deposit of various colors. When the patient is feeling at his best, there are great quantities of sandy deposits passing away. When there is little deposit in the urine, the gouty deposits in the joints become marked, and he does not feel so well. It has another symptom that was verified by Lippe: Copious clear, colorless urine, light in specific gravity and from its being light or deficient of salts in the urine we have an aggravation of the gouty manifestations. Remember, that the rheumatic tendency spreads upwards from the lower extremities, from the circumference to the centre.

"Menstruation too early, too profuse, bright red; absence of vital heat." Great coldness of the body at this time, yet the patient wants the cold air. Copious menstrual flow. Old gouty subjects, with mottled face with the puffiness that is not œdema, simply a venous stasis, with copious menstrua

flow, with great pain during menstruation. The uterus is extremely sensitive
to touch, and the pelvic organs are so sensitive that any deep touch becomes
painful to the patient. Dysmenorrhœa in gouty subjects. It turns the
constitution into order, and prevents the after-formation of gout. When such
cases are very deep-seated the uterine troubles will be cured in middle life,
and the gouty appearance will come separately. The better the internal is, in
an incurable disease, the worse the external becomes, and, when this is so,
the external trouble is essential to health, and so long as the external
manifestations are in the extremities, and the joints are being increasingly
affected, so long the internal is in a state of order. When the remedy works in
that way, do not change it and try to get something that will drive the external
away. So long as the patient is improving and the external is glowing worse,
that is the right direction. Ledum acts in this direction. Its tendency is to
make complaints go away from the centre, for its complaints begin in the
circumference and go towards the centre. It is sometimes impossible to manage
a gouty patient without giving him some sort of explanation. *Lycopodium*
also keeps conditions coming to the surface. It will send them back to their
own place in the externals when they have a tendency to go in. *Lycopodium*
often causes a return of the red sand in the urine.

"Emaciation of suffering parts." A nerve is injured by a puncture and a
slight infection takes place, so that the wound becomes congested, with a
mottled, œdematous appearance, and the part becomes cold, just such a
condition as Ledum will cure. The nerve that supplies that part takes on an
ascending neuritis, pains shoot along the nerve, the muscles that are supplied by that nerve dwindle and the part withers. We have in *Pulsatilla* a
similar state. "The diseased limb withers."

LILIUM TIGRINUM

So far as proved Lilium tigrinum has shown itself adapted to the complaints
of women. It is especially suited to hysterical, women, who suffer from uterine
troubles, cardiac troubles and various nervous manifestations; suitable to a
woman who is extremely irritable, full of fanciful notions, insanity, religious
melancholy and imaginations, with cardiac affections and prolapsus. These
conditions often alternate; when the mental symptoms are most marked the
physical symptoms are relieved. The "dragging down" that is associated with
prolapsus seems to be a dragging down from the region of the stomach, and
even sometimes from the throat. A bearing down, as if all the interior organs
were dragging down. With this state of extreme relaxation there is great
fidgetiness and, most marked of all, palpitation. She can lie only on the back,

and is aggravated from lying on either side. From every emotion the heart flutters, and is irregular and excitable. These mental symptoms and heart symptoms and uterine symptoms often rotate or alternate, and constitute the principal features.

She can hardly speak a decent word to anybody. She will snap even when spoken to kindly. She is so irritable that her friends cannot pacify her. Even consolation aggravates. When spoken to she is irritable. She lies awake nights, and is tormented either by fanatical religious ideas, or a religious melancholy, and seems inclined to dwell upon insane ideas concerning religion and modes of life, unreasonable, illogical and fanciful. Has wrong ideas concerning everything. Receives wrong impressions and everything is inverted. It is impossible to please her. Now these states are present with a state of irritability of the sexual organs, nymphomania; violent sexual excitement associated with spasms, with palpitation, with sweats, with periods of exhaustion. She sits alone and broods over imaginary troubles, and when spoken to is crabbed. "Ideas not clear; they become more so if she exercises her will." "Makes mistakes in writing, in speaking, cannot apply the mind steadily; tormented about her salvation."

The patient tries to describe an indescribable feeling by saying she has a "crazy feeling" in the head, as if the ideas scattered, and the more she attempts to think rationally the more irrational she becomes. The more she attempts to think of something the less likely she is to recall it. When putting the mind upon something else it comes back again. This remedy has all kinds of symptoms from sexual excesses in overwrought and nervous women, from sexual excitement, causing confusion of mind with palpitation.

It says in the text: "Listless, inert, yet does not want to sit still." This patient will sit still and brood and think over the past, and when spoken to will jump up and run hastily and excitedly and slam the door without any cause; when spoken to kindly by members of the family, or a friend, it seems that she will go wild. A patient once under an aggravation from this remedy said to me: "I was spoken to to-day in a street car, and I was so mad I wanted to fling something at his head." She was thinking over something about herself, and did not want to be disturbed. It is a violent state of temper, a violent state of irritability, a loss of balance. She says: "It seems as if I must fly when spoken to or disturbed." When coming in contact with her friends she has these feelings. The contact seems to arouse her out of a state of lassitude and quietness. Strange things occur in this remedy. The sensation described in the text are so vague and so varied that you can see that it is an effort on the part of the provers to describe what they feel. The sensations are numerous and indescribable.

This patient very commonly is a warm-blooded patient. She is like the *Pulsatilla* patient; warm-blooded, wants a cool room, likes to walk in the open air, except at times when the prolapsus is aggravated by walking. The head is generally relieved by moving about in the open air, > when walking.

in the open air. The headache and most of the complaints are relieved from cold, or from a cool room, and aggravated from a warm room. The dyspnœa comes on in a warm room. The patient suffocates in a crowded room, in the theatre, in church, like *Apis, Iodine, Kali i., Lyc.* and *Puls.*

A crazy feeling comes up from the back of the head to the top of the head. What that is only one that feels it can describe. It is described sometimes as a tingling, or an electric sensation. A slight tingling comes up the back of the head and goes to the top, and is associated with vertigo. When you come to sift that thought it really brings nothing to mind. Very often you have to get those things clinically, and think about them to get at the idea. The pains in the forehead are very marked, and they are associated with great disturbance of vision, a loss of vision, the room looks dark, or the eyes are unable to focus. Nervous disturbance of vision, photophobia, twitching of the lids, jerking about the eyeballs, and inflammation of the mucous membrane of the eyes, of the lids and balls, conjunctivitis. Very often with the complaints of the head the eyes are turned in, a convergent strabismus, or there is threatened syncope, with the pain in the forehead. By all these things mentioned it may be known what an over-sensitive, extremely nervous, hysterical person the Lilium tig. patient must be. These things are commonly associated with patients who are extremely nervous, who have fluttering of the heart, who have pain down the spine, and more or less prolapsus, with a great sense of dragging down. When one condition is present, the other is commonly absent; they alternate, or they may exist all together.

"Wild feeling in the head, as tho' she would go crazy, with pain in the right iliac region." These provers seemed to like the expression "crazy feeling in the head, as if she would go crazy". That crazy feeling is a confusion of mind, as if the mind were quite unable to concentrate itself. That is what is interpreted by this crazy feeling the patients have. It is sometimes like a vertigo, as if things were going round, or as if she would lose her mind. Then it comes again as a terrible, tearing headache, described as a crazy headache in the forehead. Headache in which there is confusion of the mind, or as if the mind would go crazy.

The abdomen, stool, urinary and sexual organs, furnish us a field for the use of this medicine. The whole abdominal viscera seem to be dragging down from the stomach. The patient wants to hold up the abdomen, pendulous abdomen. It seems as if the pelvic organs would protrude. The patient must lie down, wants to wear a T bandage. Wants to grasp the abdomen from the sides and lift up for support. It is a sensation of weakness or bearing down in the pelvis as if everything were coming into the world through the vagina.

This remedy has a very urgent diarrhœa, driving out of bed in the morning; he must make great haste. You may get this confused with *Sulphur,* because

Lilium tig. has great heat in the head, emptiness in the stomach, and great burning of the palms and soles. It has also a dysentery that you will, hardly be able to distinguish from *Merc. cor.,* so marked is the tenesmus, mucus and blood. The stool is merely mucus mingled with blood, and the tenesmus is as great and the burning in the anus as marked as in *Merc. cor.* It is especially suited for those attacks of dysentery that come on as an occasional chronic manifestation in nervous patients such as I have described. Now, do not think that because this patient is nervous that she is weak, or liliputian, or lean; for it is especially suitable for those with full veins; apparently plethoric, full blooded, fleshy, rotund women who are very nervous, and especially at the change of life. Recurrent dysenteric attacks with every cold in those who suffer from pelvic and abdominal relaxation, mental irritability as described, palpitation and fluttering of the heart, with nervous constitutions. You do not see *Merc. cor.* in such a picture. If it were a dysentery alone I would not be able to tell which it was. All of these dysenteric manifestations have been left out of the *Guiding Symptoms,* yet I have seen them verified over and over. Again, it has a most inveterate and troublesome constipation.

It has also a tenesmus of the bladder and rectum. Teasing to urinate, as well as urging to stool. Sits a long time with much urging, and after long straining no stool. Frequent urging, with a sensation as if a ball were in the rectum. When the fundus of the uterus is turned back to the rectum it gives a sensation as if the rectum were full of fæces; it brings on urging to stool and the patient will sit and strain, and the tenesmus of the bladder and rectum is unbearable. Constant urging to stool, and no stool in the rectum. You will be astonished to know that the remedy that is indicated with such symptoms will relieve the patient of all distress in a short time. But you ask, will this remedy put the uterus right again? Well, the patient will get relief of her sufferings and will not feel this uncomfortable state after the administration of the remedy. The bowels become regular, the disturbance of micturition is relieved and the patient gradually returns to health and later the uterus will be found in place.

"Pressure in the rectum, with almost constant desire to go to stool." Lilium tigrinum has cured the most inveterate protruding hæmorrhoids with burning. "Hæmorrhoids after delivery, sore to touch, bearing down after stool as if all would protrude from the vagina." It does not mean that we shall apply that simply to hæmorrhoids that come after delivery, but it has cured hæmorrhoids in such a constitution, and not only hæmorrhoids, but relaxed uterus and vagina.

A paralytic relaxation is present in all the abdominal tissues. I have mentioned the uterine symptoms incidentally in connection with other parts. "Menses scanty, flow only when moving about." This will make you think of *Puls.,* the menses being so scanty, and because the *Puls.* patient is of similar nervous temperament. *Puls.* has scanty menstruation and relief in the open air. It has also much dragging down in the pelvis, though not so extreme as a rule as in this medicine. But there is much in this medicine quite different from *Puls.*

Then come the heart symptoms. "Seems as if the heart were grasped or squeezed in a vise, hard, as it violently grasped." "Constrictive pain in the heart." "In fresh air, chilly, but vertigo is >."

Pain in the back and down the spine; irritable and sensitive spine with trembling. It competes very closely with *Platina*.

LYCOPODIUM

Lycopodium is an antipsoric, anti-syphilitic and anti-sycotic, and its sphere is broad and deep. Though classed among the inert substances, and thought to be useful only for rolling up allopathic pills, Hahnemann brought it into use and developed its power by attenuation. It is a monument to Hahnemann. It enters deep into the life, and ultimate changes in the soft tissues, blood-vessels, bones, liver, heart, joints. The tissue changes are striking; there is tendency to necrosis, abscesses, spreading ulcers and great emaciation. There is a predominance of symptoms on the *right side* of the body, and they are likely to travel from *right to left* or *from above downward, e.g.* from head to chest. The patient emaciates above, especially about the neck, while the lower extremities are fairly well nourished. Externally there is *sensitiveness to a warm atmosphere* when there are head and spine symptoms. The head symptoms also are worse from the warmth of the bed and from heat, and worse from getting heated by exertion. The patient is sensitive to cold and there is a marked lack of vital heat, and worse in general from cold and cold air and from cold food and drinks. The pains are ameliorated from warmth except of the head and spine. Exertion aggravates the Lycopodium patient in general. He becomes puffed and distressed, and dyspnoea is increased by exertion. He cannot climb, he cannot walk fast. The cardiac symptoms are increased as well as the dyspnoea by becoming heated from exertion. The inflamed parts are sometimes relieved from the application of heat. The throat symptoms are generally relieved from the application of heat, from drinking hot tea or warm soup. The stomach pains are often *relieved by warm drinks* and taking warm things into the stomach. Nervous excitement and prostration are marked.

In the rheumatic pains and other sufferings the Lyc. patient is *ameliorated by motion*. He is extremely restless, must keep turning, and if there is inflammation with the aches and pains the *patient is better from the warmth of the bed* and relieved from motion, and he will keep tossing all night. He turns and gets into a new place and thinks he can sleep, but the restlessness continues all night. He wants cool air, wants to be in a cool place with head symptoms. It is true that the headache is worse from motion enough to warm the patient up, but not from the motion itself. The headache is worse from lying down and *from the warmth of the room, and better in cold air and from motion* until he has moved and exercised sufficiently to become heated, when the headache becomes worse. That is quite an important thing to remember concerning Lycopodium, because it may constitute a distinguishing feature. The head symptoms are worse from warm wraps and warm bed.

The complaints of Lyc. are likely to be worse at a fixed *time,* viz., *from four till eight o'clock* in toe evening. An exacerbation comes on in the acute complaints and often in the chronic complaints at this time. The Lyc. chill and fever is worse at this time, and in typhoid and scarlet fever the patient is especially worse from 4-8 P.M. In gouty attacks, in rheumatic fevers, in inflammatory conditions, in pneumonia, in acute catarrhs, which are complaints especially calling for Lycopodium, it is always well to think of this remedy when there is a decisive aggravation from 4-8 P.M.

The Lycopodium patient is *flatulent,* distended like a drum, so that he can hardly breathe. The diaphragm is pushed upwards, infringing upon the lung and heart space, so that he has palpitation, faintness and dyspnœa. It is not uncommon to hear a Lycop. patient say, "Everything I eat turns into wind." After a mere mouthful he becomes flatulent and distended, so that he cannot eat any more. He says a mouthful fills him up to the throat. While the abdomen is distended he is so nervous that he cannot endure any noise. The noise of the crackling of paper, ringing of bells or slamming of doors goes through him and causes fainting, like *Ant. crud., Borax* and *Natr. mur.* These general conditions go through all complaints, acute and chronic. There is an excitable stage of the whole sensorium in which everything disturbs. Little things annoy and distress.

The Lyc. patient cannot eat oysters; they make him sick. Oysters seem to poison the Lyc. patient, just as onions are a poison to the *Thuja* patient. The *Oxalic acid* patient cannot eat strawberries. If you ever have a patient get sick from eating strawberries, tomatoes or oysters, and you have no homœopathic remedies at hand, it is a good thing to remember that cheese will digest strawberires or tomatoes or oysters in a few minutes.

The *skin ulcerates.* There are painful ulcers, sloughing ulcers beneath the skin, abscesses beneath the skin, cellular troubles. The chronic ulcerations are indolent with false granualtions, painful, burning, stinging and smarting, often relieved by applying cooling things and aggravated by warm poultices. It is somewhat a general in Lycopodium that warm poultices and warmth ameliorates; warm applications ameliorate the pain in the knee, the suppurating condition and the gouty troubles. In an unusually warm bed, and in a warm room hives come out. The hives come out either in nodules or in long and irregular stripes, especially in the heat, and itch violently. Lyc. has eruptions upon the skin, with violent itching. Vesicles and scaly eruptions, moist eruptions and dry eruptions, furfuraceous eruptions, eruptions about the lips, behind the ears, under the wings of the nose and upon the genitals; fissured eruptions, bleeding fissures like salt rheum upon the hands. The skin becomes thick and indurated. The sites of old boils and pustules become indurated and form nodules that remain a long time. The skin looks unhealthy, and it will slough easily; wounds refuse to heal. Surface wounds suppurate as if they had contained splinters, and this suppuration burrows along under the skin. Ulcers bleed and form great quantities of thick, yellow, offensive, green pus. Chancres and chancroids often find their simillimum in Lyc.

The Lyc. state when deciphered shows feebleness throughout. A very low state of the arteries and veins, poor tone and poor circulation. Numbness in spots. Emaciation of single members. Deadness of the fingers and toes. Staggering and inability to make use of the limbs. Clumsiness and awkwardness of the limbs. Trembling of the limbs.

The *mental* symptoms of Lyc. are numerous. He is tired. He has a tired state of mind, a chronic fatigue, forgetfulness, aversion to undertaking anything new, aversion to appearing in any new role; aversion to his own work. Dreads lest something will happen, lest he will forget something. A continually increasing dread of appearing in public comes on, yet a horror, at times, of solitude. Often in professional men, like lawyers and ministers, who have to appear in public, there is a feeling of incompetence, a feeling of inability to undertake his task, although he has been accustomed to it for many years. A lawyer cannot think of appearing in court; he procrastinates, he delays until he is obliged to appear, because he has a fear that he will stumble, that he will make mistakes, that he will forget, and yet when he undertakes it he goes through with ease and comfort. This is a striking feature also of *Silicea.* No medicines have this fear so marked as these two.

Lyc. also has a religious insanity, which has a mild and simple beginning, a matter of melancholy. This religious melancholy grows greater and greater until he sits and broods. He has very often aversion to company, and yet he dreads solitude. "Dread of men and dread of solitude; irritability and melancholy." This dread of men is not always a state of dread in women. It is a dread of people, and when that is fully carried out in the Lyc. patient you see that she dreads the presence of new persons, or the coming in of friends or visitors; she wants to be only with those that are constantly surrounding her; does not want to be entirely alone; wants to feel that there is somebody else in the house, but does not want company; does not want to be talked to, or forced to do anything; does not want to make any exertion, yet at times when forced to do so she is relieved. "Taciturnity, desires to be alone." Now, let us follow that out a little further. The taciturnity is because the patient does not want to talk, wants to keep silent, yet, as I have said already, very glad to feel there is somebody else in the house and that she is not alone. She is perfectly willing to remain in a little room by herself, so that she is practically alone, yet not in solitude. If there were two adjacent rooms in the house you would commonly find the Lyc. patient go into one and stay there, but very glad to have somebody in the other.

The Lycopodium patient often weeps in the act of receiving a friend or meeting an acquaintance. An unusual sadness with weeping comes over this patient on receiving a gift. At the slightest joy she weeps, hence we see that the Lye. patient is a very nervous, sensitive, emotional patient. Here it is: "Sensitive, even cries when thanked."

When lying in bed suffering from the lower forms of fevers, there is delirium and even unconsciousness. He picks at imaginary things in the air, sees flies and all Sorts of little things flying in the air. "Excessively merry and laughs at simplest things." A condition of insanity. "Despondent." The Lyc. patient wakes up in the morning with sadness. There is sadness and gloom. The world may come to an end, or the whole family may die, or the house may burn up. There seems to be nothing cheering, the future looks black. After moving about a while, this passes off. This state precedes conditions of insanity, and finally a suicidal state comes, an aversion to life. See how this remedy takes hold of the will and actually destroys man's will to live. That which is first in man is his desire to be, to exist, and to be something, if ever so small. When that is destroyed, we see what a wonderful thing has been destroyed. The very man himself wills then not to be. It is a perversion of everything that makes the man, the destruction of his will. "Apprehensiveness, difficult breathing and fearfulness." "Anxious thoughts as if about to die." "Want of self-confidence, indecision, timidity, resignation." Loss of confidence in himself and in everything. "Misanthropic, flies even from his own children." "Distrustful, suspicious and fault finding." "Oversensitive to pain; patient is beside himself."

Lyc. is subject to periodical headaches, and headaches connected with gastric troubles. If he goes beyond his dinner hour a sick headache will come on. He must eat with regularity or he will have the headache which he is subject to. This is somewhat like a *Cactus* headache. *Cactus* has a congestive headache which becomes extremely violent with flushed face if he does not eat at the regular time. One distinguishing feature is that with the Lycopodium headache, if he eats something, the headache is better while the *Cactus* headache is worse from eating. Lyc. and especially *Phos.* and *Psorinum* have headaches with great hunger. At or about the beginning of the attack there is a faint all-gone hungry feeling which eating does not satisfy. Such is the nature of *Phosphorus* and *Psorinum* when the appetite and headache are associated. The Lycopodium headache is < from heat, from the warmth of the bed, and from lying down, > from cold, from the cold air, and from having the windows open. Lean, emaciated boys are subject to prolonged pains in the head. Every time this little fellow takes cold he has a prolonged, throbbing, congestive headache, and from day to day and from month to month he becomes more emaciated, especially about the face and neck. This same trouble is present when a narrow-chested boy has a dry, teasing cough, without expectoration, and emaciates about the neck and face. This remedy is especially suitable in these withered lads, with a dry cough or prolonged headache. In children who wither after pneumonia or bronchitis, emaciate about the face and neck, take cold on the slightest provocation, suffer with headache from being heated, have nightly headaches, and a state of congestion that affects the mind more or less, in which they rouse out of sleep in confusion. The little one screams out in sleep, awakes frightened, looks wild, does not know the father and mother, or nurse or family until after a few moments, when he seems to be able to collect his senses and then realizes where he is and lies down to sleep again. In a little while he wakes up again in a fright, looks strange and confused. That repeats itself. The headaches are throbbing and pressing, as if the head would burst; but this is not so important as the manner in which they come on, the circumstance of their cause, the things that the child does and the fact that they are better from cold, worse from noise and talking, worse from 4 to 8 P.M., and he emaciates from above downward. These are more important than the quality of the pain that the patient feels, but if he describes the quality of the pain it is spoken of as a throbbing, pressing, bursting or as a fulness.

Upon the scalp we find eruptions in patches, smooth patches with the hair off. Patches on the face and eczematous eruptions behind the ears, bleeding and oozing a watery fluid, sometimes yellowish watery. The eczema spreads from behind the ears up over the ears and to the scalp. Lyc. is a very important remedy to study in eczema of the infant. Eczema in a lean, hungry, withering child with more or less head trouble, such as has been described, with a moist oozing behind the ears, red sand in the urine, face looking wrinkled, a dry teasing cough, in a child that kicks the covers off, a child whose left foot is cold and the other warm, with capricious appetite, eating much, with unusual hunger at times and great thirst, and yet losing steadily, will often be cured by Lyc. It will throw out a greater amount of eruption at first, but this will subside finally and the child will return to health. The head in general is closely related to one symptom, viz., red sand in the urine. As long as the red sand is plentiful, the patient is free from these congestive headaches, but when the urine becomes pale and free from the red pepper deposit, then comes the bursting, pressing headache, lasting for days. It might be said that this is a uræmic headache; but it does not matter what you call it, if the symptoms are present the remedy will be justified. In old gouty constitutions, when the headache is most marked, the gout in the extremities will be > and *vice versa*. The headache is present only in the absence of pain in the extremities. Again, when there is a copious quantity of red sand in the urine the gouty state, either in the head or extremities, will be absent, but whenever he takes cold the secretion seems to slacken up with an < of the pain. There is another feature of the Lyc. headache related to catarrhal states. The headache is < when the catarrh is slacked up by an acute cold. The Lyc. subject often suffers from thick, yellow discharge from the nose. The nose is filled with yellow, green crusts, blown out of the nose in the morning and hawked out of the throat. Now, when the patient takes cold the thick discharge to a great extent ceases, and he commences to sneeze and has a watery discharge. Then comes on a Lyc. headache, with great suffering, with pressing pains, with hunger, and finally the coryza passes away, and the thick yellow discharge returns and the headache subsides.

We have many *eye* symptoms in Lycopodium, but most prominent are the catarrhal affections of the eyes. The symptoms are so numerous they describe almost any catarrhal condition of the eyes, so that you cannot discriminate upon the eye symptoms alone. Inflammatory conditions with copious discharge, with red eyes, ulceration of the conjunctiva and lids, and granular lids.

For the *ears* Lyc. becomes an important remedy, because this self-same emaciating child, with the wrinkled countenance and dry cough, has had, since an attack of scarlet fever, a discharge from the ears, thick, yellow and offensive, with loss of hearing. If the suitable remedy be given in a case of scarlet fever, there will be no ear trouble left, because ear troubles do not necessarily belong to scarlet fever. They are not a part of scarlet fever, but are dependent on the constitutional state of the child. Lyc. has also most painful eruptions of the ears, otitis media, abscess in the ear, associated with eczema about the ears and behind the ears.

The *nose* symptoms I have only partly described in association with the head. The trouble often begins in infancy. The little infant will lie at first with a peculiar rattling breathing through the nose, and finally it will breathe only through the mouth, as the nose is obstructed. This goes on for days and months. The child breathes only through the mouth, and when it cries it has the shrill tone, such as is found when the nose is plugged up. If you look you will see the nose is filled up with a purulent matter and hanging down the throat is a muco-purulent discharge. Much stuffing up of the nose is a chronic state of Lyc. The child will go on with this trouble until it forms into great crusts, yellow, sometimes blackish, sometimes greenish, and the nose bleeds

It is most useful in those troublesome catarrhs associated with headaches; in such patients as lose flesh about the neck. It may seem strange and unaccountable that Lyc. can cause emaciation about the neck and shrivelling of the face when the lower limbs are in a very good state of preservation. In old chronic catarrhs of adults they must keep continually blowing the nose. He cannot breathe through the nose at night, as crusts form in all portions of the mucous membranes. Crusty nostrils with eczema, with oozing eruptions about the face and nose. The mucous discharge is almost as thick and tenacious as in *Kali bi.*

The *face* is sallow, sickly, pale, often withered, shrivelled and emaciated. In deep-seated chest troubles, bronchitis or pneumonia, where the chest is filled up with mucus, it will be seen that the face and forehead are wrinkled from pain, and that the *wings of the nose flap with the effort to breathe.* This occurs with all forms of dyspnœa. We see something like it in *Ant. tart.,* the sooty nostrils being wide open and flapping. In *Ant. tart.* the rattling of the mucus is heard across the room and the patient is seen to be in distress, but if you see the patient lying in bed with the nose flapping and the forehead wrinkled, with rattling in the chest, or a dry, hacking cough and no expectoration, you will often find the particulars of the examination confirm your mind that it is a case for Lyc. In the exudative stage of pneumonia, the stage of hepatization, Lyc. may save the life of that patient. It is closely related in the period of hepatization to *Phos.* and *Sulph.* The *Sulph.* patient is cold; there is no tendency to reaction; he feels the load in the chest, and examination of the chest shows that hepatization is marked. He wants to lie still and is evidently about to die. *Sulphur* will help him. It does not have the flapping of the nose, nor the wrinkles upon the forehead, like Lyc. In the brain complaints of *Strammonium* the forehead wrinkles, and in the chest complaints of Lyc. the forehead wrinkles, and their wrinkles are somewhat alike. You go to a semi-conscious patient suffering from cerebral congestion and watch him, he is wild, the eyes are glassy, the forehead wrinkled and the tendency is to activity of the mind. That is not Lyc. but *Stram.* By close observation these practical things will lead you to distinguish, almost instantaneously, between *Stramonium* in its head troubles, and Lyc. in the advanced stage of pneumonia.

The face is often covered with copper-colored eruptions, such as we find in syphilis, and hence it is that Lyc. is sometimes useful in old cases of syphilis, cases which have affected the nose, with necrosis or caries of the nasal bones, and the catarrhal symptoms already described. About the face also there is much twitching. You will see by the study of the face that his face conforms to his sensations. He is an over-sensitive patient, and at every ear or noise, such as the slamming of a door, or the ringing of a bell, he wrinkles his face. He is disturbed, and you see it expressed upon his countenance. He has a sickly wrinkled countenance, with contracted eye-brows in complaints of the abdomen as well as in chest complaints. We also see that the jaw drops as in *Opium* and *Muriatic* acid. This occurs in a state marked by great exhaustion and indicates a fatal tendency. It is especially marked in typhoid when the patient picks at the bed clothes, slides down in bed, wants almost nothing, and can hardly be aroused. It is the expression of the last stage of the disease, a low type of fever, typhoids, septic and zymotic diseases. Under the jaw there is often glandular swelling, swelling of the parotid and submaxillary glands. The swelling is sometimes cellular and the neck muscles are involved. The tendency is to suppuration of these glands, and swellings about the neck in scarlet fever and diphtheria.

The next important feature we notice are the *throat* symptoms. It was mentioned when going over the general state that the striking feature of Lyc. in regard to *direction* is that its symptoms seem to spread from right to left; we notice that the right foot is cold and the left is warm; the right knee is affected; if the pains are movable they go from right to left. Most complaints seem to travel from right to left, or to affect the right side more than the left. This is also true of sore throats; a quinsy affecting the right side will run its course, and when about finished the left tonsil will become inflamed and suppurate if the appropriate remedy be not administered. The common sore throat will commence on the right side, the next day both sides will be affected, the inflammation having extended to the left side. This remedy has all kinds of pains in the throat and fauces. It is useful in cases of diphtheria when the membrane commences on the right side of the throat and spreads over towards the left. Patches will be seen one day on the right side and the next day on the left side. We have noticed also that complaints in Lyc. spread from above down, so it is with these exudations. They often commence in the upper part of the pharynx and spread down into the throat. Lyc. has cured many such cases. It is the case sometimes that Lyc. is better by holding cold water in the mouth, but the usual Lyc. sore throat is better from swallowing warm drinks. It is a feature whereby it is possible to distinguish *Lachesis* from Lycopodium. *Lachesis* is better from cold and has spasms of the throat from attempting to drink warm drinks, while Lyc. is better from warm drinks, though sometimes better from cold drinks. Lyc. does not sleep into the suffocation and constriction of the throat and dyspnœa as in *Lach.* The throat is extremely painful, it has all the violence of the worst cases of diphtheria. It has the zymosis.

The *stomach* and *abdominal* symptoms are intermingled. There is a sense of satiety, an entire lack of appetite. He feels so full that he cannot eat. This sense of fulness may not come on until be has swallowed a mouthful of food he goes to the table hungry, but the first mouthful fills him up. After eating he is distended with flatus, and gets momentary relief from belching, yet he remain distended. Nausea and vomiting; gnawing pains in stomach as in gastritis; catarrh; burning in ulcers and cancer; pains immediately after eating; vomiting of bile, coffee ground vomit, black, inky vomit. Under Lyc. apparently malignant cases have their life prolonged. The case is so modified that, instead of culminating in a few months, the patient may last for years. Right hypochondrium swollen as in liver troubles. Pain in liver, recurrent bilious attacks with vomiting of bile. He is subject to gall-stone colic. After Lyc. the attacks come less frequently, the bilious secretion becomes normal and the gall-stones have a spongy appearance as though being dissolved. Lyc. patients are always belching; they have eructations that are sour and acrid like strong acid burning the pharynx. "Sour stomach," sour vomiting, flatus, distension and pain after eating, with a sense of fulness. Awful "goneness," or weakness, in stomach, not relieved by eating (*Digit.*). The stomach is worse *by cold drinks, and often* relieved by warm drinks. In the stomach and intestines there is a great commotion, noisy rumbling, rolling of flatus as though fermentation were going on. Lyc., *China* and *Carbo veg.* are most flatulent remedies and should be compared. The stomach symptoms are worse or brought on from cold drinks, beer, coffee or fruit, and a diarrhœa follows. Old chronic dyspeptics, emaciated, wrinkled, tired and angular patients, everything eaten turns to wind. Lycopodium is useful in old tired patients with feeble reaction and feebleness of all the functions, with a tendency to run down and not convalesce.

This patient has most troublesome constipation. He goes for days without any desire, and although the rectum is full there is no urging. Inactivity of intestinal canal. Ineffectual urging to stool. Stool hard, difficult, small and incomplete. The first part of the stool is hard and difficult to start, but the last part is soft or thin and gushing followed by faintness and weakness. Lyc. patients have diarrhœa and all kinds of stool. So you will see from reading the text that the characteristic of Lyc. is not in the stool. Any kind of diarrhea, if the other Lyc. symptoms are present, will be cured by Lyc. It has troublesome hæmorrhoids, but they are nondescript. Any kind of hæmorrhoids may be cured by Lyc. if the flatulence, the stomach symptoms, the mental symptoms, and the general symptoms of Lyc. are present, because the hæmorrhoidal symptoms are numerous.

The kidneys furnish many symptoms and may be the key to Lycopodium in many instances. There seems to be the same inactivity in the bladder as in the rectum. Though he strain ever so much, he must wait a long time for the urine to pass. It is slow to flow, and flows in a feeble stream. The urine is often muddy with brick dust, or red sand deposits, or on stirring it up it looks like the sediment of fermenting cider. We find this state in febrile conditions. In acute stages of disease, where the red sand appears copiously, Lyc. is often the remedy. This is a very prominent symptom. In chronic symptoms when the patient feels best the red sand is found in the urine. Lyc. has retention of urine and suppression of urine. It has "wetting of the bed" in little ones, involuntary micturition in sleep, involuntary micturition in typhoids and low fevers. A marked feature of Lyc., and one of the most prominent of all remedies, is polyuria during the night. He must arise many times at night and pass large quantities of urine, although in the daytime the urine is normal. Enormous quantities of urine, very clear and of light specific gravity.

Male sexual organs. One of the most prominent remedies in impotency. Persons of feeble vitality, overwrought persons, overtired persons, with feeble genital organs, seldom need *Phosphorus,* but Lycopod. is a typical remedy where the young man has abused himself by secret vices and has become tired out in his spine, brain and genital organs. If this patient makes up his mind that he will live a somewhat decent life and marries, he finds that he is impotent sexually, that he is not able to obtain erections, or that the erections are too feeble, or too short, and that he is not a man.

Lyc. has inflammation of the mucous membrane of the urethra, with a gonorrhœal discharge. It is anti-sycotic and has troublesome fig-warts upon the male and female genitals. "Moist condylomata on the penis, enlargement of the prostate gland."

It is a great friend of the woman in inflammation and neuralgia of the *ovaries,* and in inflammation of the *uterus.* The neuralgia especially affects the right ovary, with a tendency to the left., Inflammation of the ovaries, when the right is more affected than the left. It has cured cystic tumors of the right ovary.

Lycopodium produces and cures dryness in the vagina in which coition becomes very painful. Burning in the vagina during and after coition. It has disturbance of menstruation. Absence or suppression of menses for many months, the patient being withered, declining, pale and sallow, becoming feeble. It seems that she has not the vitality to menstruate. It is also suitable in girls at puberty when the time for the first menstrual flow to appear has come, but it does not come. She goes on to 15, 16, 17 or 18 without development, the breasts do not enlarge, the ovaries do not perform their functions. When the symptoms agree Lyc. establishes a reaction, the breasts begin to grow, the womanly bearing begins to come, and the child becomes a woman. It has a wonderful power for developing, and in that respect it is very much like *Calc. phos.* "Discharge of flatus from the vagina." "Varices of the genitals."

In the respiratory organs Lyc. furnishes a wonderful remedy. Dyspnœa and asthmatic breathing in catarrh of the chest. The colds settle in the nose, but nearly always go into the chest, with much whistling and wheezing and great dyspnœa. The dyspnœa is worse from walking fast, after exertion and from going up a hill. Throbbing, burning and fielding in the chest. Dry, teasing cough. *Dry cough in emaciated boys.* After coming out of pneumonia, the dry, teasing cough remains a long time, or there is much whistling and asthmatic breathing. The extremities are cold while the head and face are hot, with much coughing and troubles in the chest. He wants to go about with the head uncovered, because there is so much congestion in the head. This patient has a feeble reaction. There is no tendency to repair and the history of the case is that the troubles have existed since an attack of bronchitis or pneumonia. Besides the dry, teasing cough, Lyc. goes into another state in which there is ulceration, with copious expectoration of thick yellow or green muco-pus, tough and stringy. Finally night sweats, with fever in the afternoon from 4 to 8 o'clock, come on. Its use in the advanced stage of pneumonia, in the period of hepatization, with the wrinkled face and brow, the flapping wings of the nose and scanty expectoration, we have already spoken of. Then it has marked catarrh of the chest with much rattling, especially in infants. *Rattling in the chest, flapping of the wings of the nose and inability to expectorate.* The right lung is most affected, or more likely to be affected than the left, or it is affected first in double pneumonia and troubles that go from one side to the other. Think of Lyc. among the remedies for neglected pneumonia, in difficult breathing from an accumulation of serum in the pleura and pericardium'.

I have mentioned sufficiently the gouty tendencies of the limbs and that nerve symptoms. But there is a restlessness of the lower limbs which comes on when he thinks of going to sleep and this prevents sleep until midnight. Much like *Arsenicum.* It is often a very distressing feature. *Numbness of the limbs.* Drawing, tearing in the limbs at night; better by warmth of bed and motion. These pains are sometimes found in chronic intermittent fever and are cured by this remedy. Sciatica that comes on periodically, better by heat and walking. Varicose veins of the legs. One foot hot, the other cold.Œdema of the feet.

It has all manner of fevers, continued, intermittent and remittent. It is especially suitable in old age, and in premature old age, when a person at 60 years appears to be 80 years, broken down, feeble and tired. It is eminently suited in complaints of weakly constitutions. It is suitable in various dropsies, associated with liver and heart affections. Scabs remain upon the skin, do not separate; they crust over and the crust does not fall, or may become laminated like rupia. *Sulphur, Graph.* and *Calc.* are not longer acting or deeper acting than Lyc. These substances that seem to be so inert in their crude form come out strongest when potentized and form medicines of wonderful use.

MAGNESIA CARBONICA

This remedy has only been partially proved; and comes to us now as Hahnemann left it. The mental symptoms and symptoms of sonic portions of the body and particulars have not been fully brought out. The remedy really needs reproving with high potencies upon sensitive provers that the finer shades may be understood. I would not speak of it but for the fact that it relates to a class of cases so very important that you will not be able to get along without it. It is related to the older and deeper psoric sickness. It is deep acting and long acting and permeates the economy as thoroughly as *Sulphur.*

Some of the most striking general features are: Amelioration from motion; desire for open air, yet very sensitive to cold air; wants to be covered during all stages of fever; daily evening fevers; symptoms recurring every twenty-one days. Sensation of heat and even sweat from eating and drinking warm things; evening thirst.

Like other *Magnesias* it has most violent neuralgic pains, pains along the course of nerves, pains so violent that he cannot keep still, and he moves about and *is relieved by motion.* The provers felt these pains mostly in the head and face, but clinical experience has demonstrated that it has violent neuralgia everywhere. We are justified, from the proving, in considering it as especially related to the *left side of the face; neuralgia in the night; driving him out of bed,* keeping him in constant motion. As soon as he stops moving the pain becomes very severe, shooting, tearing and cutting.

It has varied eruptions upon the skin; dry, scaly, dandruff-like eruptions upon the skin, very unhealthy hair and nails. Particularly does it affect the teeth and roots of the teeth. In every change of the weather the roots of the teeth become violently painful, burn, shoot and ache continuously. Toothache before and during menstruation. During pregnancy she suffers all the time with toothache, tearing pains in the left side of the face, although the roots of the teeth are perfectly sound. The hollow teeth are unusually sensitive, and painful. The teeth are so sensitive that they cannot be manipulated by the dentist. This is like *Ant. crud.,* but Magnesia carb. especially affects the roots of the teeth, while *Ant. crud.* affects the dentine more particularly. Sensitiveness of the teeth, so that he cannot bite upon the teeth, and the teeth feel too long. Magnesia carb. and *China,* when no other symptoms are present, are prominent remedies among the affections of the teeth during pregnancy.

There is a kind of marasmus that you will puzzle over if you do not know this remedy. If we analyze the remedy in general, we will see that it produces a state of the body like that prior to tuberculosis. He does not undergo repair, he loses flesh, and the muscles become flabby as if some serious disease were coming. In children of tuberculosis parents there is that tendency to go into marasmus. The child's muscles are flabby, the child will not thrive in spite of feeding and medicines. It seems to be laying the foundations for some serious trouble. Finally, it emaciates and the back of the head begins to sink in, as if from atrophy of the cerebellum. The appetite increases for milk and meat and animal broths, and yet they are not digested, and when the milk is taken it continually passes the bowel in the form of white potter's clay, or like putty. The stool is soft and of the consistency of putty. If you go through a china factory where the men are forming with their hands, in such wonderful manner, all sorts of beautiful dishes, and moulds, you will see that the original clay, as they are manipulating it, is white. It is a perfect picture of the Mag. carb. stool, composed of putty-like undigested milk.

I have observed, especially among illegitimate infants, those that have been conceived by clandestine coition, that they have a tendency to sinking in the back of the head. The occipital bone will sink in, and the parietal bones jut out over it, and there will be a depression. That is not an uncommon thing in children that go into marasmus. They are very likely to have a potter's clay stool. It does not run, and it is not hard. The white, hard stool is quite another symptom, and the soft, semi-fluid white stool leads to another class of remedies, but this pasty stool, looking as if it could be moulded into any kind of shape, is a Magnesia carb. stool. I once had in charge an orphanage, where we had sixty to one hundred babies on hand all the time. The puzzle of my life was to find remedies for the cases that were going into marasmus. A large number of them were clandestine babies. It was a sort of Sheltering Arms for these little ones. The whole year elapsed, and we were losing babies every week from this gradual decline, until I saw the image of these babies in Magnesia carb., and after that many of them were cured.

The Mag. carb. baby *smells sour like the Hepar baby.* Wash it as you will and it smells sour; the perspiration is sour, and the whole baby smells sour. It is not especially the stool. The stool smells strong and pungent, putrid, and very often the whole child has a pungent odor, like an unclean baby, though it be well washed.

The *Magnesias* produce inactivity of the rectum and anus—a paresis. The stool is large and hard, requiring great straining to expel. It is dry, hard and crumbling. The stool will remain partly expelled and then crumble, breaking up in many pieces. Another stool that is laid down in the books as a most striking condition of Magnesia carb. is green; it is the diarrhœic stool, and the green part floats upon the watery portion of the stool. The stool is often lumpy, and liquid. The lumps lie in the bottom of the vessel, but floating upon the liquid portion of the stool is the green like the scum of the frog pond. This is recognized as one of the most striking features. "Stools green, like scum on a frog pond; sour, frothy; with white floating lumps like tallow, bloody, mucous." Floating like lumps of tallow, is more characteristic of *Phosphorus,* and many a time has *Dulcamara* cured it.

The face of the chronic adult case is pale, waxy, sickly and sallow, and you wonder why this patient will not right up, and will not thrive. She has a sickly countenance, *her muscles are lax,* she becomes so tired and sweats upon little exertion. She is disturbed in every change of the weather, and is worse at the beginning of menstruation. She seems to take cold whenever menstruation is coming on. She says: "I know my menstrual period is coming on, because I have a cold in my head." Magnesia carb. has coryza every month before the monthly period. These patients take on an appearance as if going into decline, and yet they go on year after year unable to do anything, not able even to keep house, have a violent craving for meat and an aversion to vegetable food, grow thin and increasingly flabby, muscles relaxed, and with tendency to prolapsus. The walls of the abdomen have a tendency to fall down and to be relaxed, and the rings favor the formation of hernia. That is the kind of relaxation. The nerves are painful, and the muscles are tired. When you have such a case and have prescribed, and they persist in spite of every remedy, you know that the case does not well indicate a remedy, that the conditions are latent and there is a tendency to some grave internal disorder. The organs are threatening to break down; the kidneys, the heart, the lungs, or the brain are about to undergo organic change.

We have a catarrhal state in this remedy, but it is a dry catarrh, not much discharge. An old ulcer will dry up and become shiny and discharge almost nothing. The nose is dry and the eyeballs are so dry that the lids stick together and it is difficult to open the eyes. The skin becomes dry and itches and burns. Tendency to dryness of the mucous membranes and dryness of the skin. Dryness is a marked feature of this medicine.

"Inordinate appetite for meat in children." The stomach is a troublesome organ. The Magnesia carb. patient is always complaining of a sour stomach; sour eructations. Food comes up sour. There is nausea and coming up in the throat of sour food. Pains in the stomach after eating an ordinary amount of food; bloated after eating; much flatulence after eating. The stomach digests the food slowly and it becomes sour.

This remedy is especially useful if the history has been a tubercular one. Losing flesh and craving for meat in those who are tubercular or in those that are from tubercular parents. Patients suffering from a dry cough. Dry cough before the evening chill like *Rhus tox.* There are persons who have simply this tendency who go along year after year in this withered state, with the little hacking cough, not rousing up into much. Finally some favorable circumstance arises and the tuberculosis comes on rapidly after it has remained in a sluggish state for a long time. There are a few remedies more likely to be associated with that condition than any others, *Arsenicum, Calc. carb., Lycopodium,* Magnesia carb. and *Tuberc.* They fit into this lingering state, this prelude to active phthisis. They sometimes set a patient thriving, but, mind you, these cases are hard cases to manage.

They are difficult, to find remedies for. Their trouble is so latent, the symptoms do not come out, and sometimes you have to read between the lines. They are the one-sided cases spoken of by Hahnemann.

In addition to this dry, tickling cough, which is not mentioned in the books, we find "Cough, spasmodic at night from tickling in the larynx." "Sleepiness during the day and sleeplessness at night." When you have seen many of these cases that are threatening to go into phthisis, you will notice that it is a general feature with all of them. "Doctor, I am so tired in the morning; while I sleep some in the night, in the morning I feel as if I had not slept." Always tired and relaxed. Most of these subjects are cold and chilly. This state has not been brought out yet in the remedy, but clinically it relates to *cold and chilly patients*. Patients who say that they have not much blood.

MAGNESIA MURIATICA

It would seem rather strange that the two remedies to which Hahnemann gave such a good start by proving and use should be so neglected and forgotten as *Magnesia carb.* and Magnesia mur. have been. These two, if used, would cure many of the liver troubles that are not now cured. Magnesia mur. could cure many conditions in nervous, excitable women that now go uncured. These remedies are neglected, while *Phosphorus* and *Sulphur* are prescribed for almost everything.

Magnesia mur. is a deep-acting antipsoric suited to nervous patients with stomach and liver troubles. It has enlarged glands and irritation of the nerve centres and brain. This patient is often sensitive to cold, chilly, but he desires fresh air and open air. Many of the complaints are ameliorated by the open, fresh air, but some head symptoms are an exception. The head must be covered, as it is so sensitive to the open air. He is extremely restless; only with great difficulty can he keep still, and if forced to keep still he becomes anxious. Anxiety is the marked feature. Restlessness, fidgetiness throughout the body, coupled with anxiety. This comes on at any time, but it is worse at night in bed and still worse on closing the eyes to go to sleep. When he closes the eyes he becomes so anxious, restless and fidgety that lie must throw the covers off, take a long breath or do something. He is kept awake at night by the anxious feeling. It was described originally by the prover as an uneasiness, but in the Guiding Symptoms it is spoken of as a restlessness in bed. If you study the hysterical nature, the anxiety and restlessness, you will see it is throughout the whole economy and should be classed under mind and nerves. Some remedies have vertigo on closing the eyes, some have anxiety on closing the eyes. *Conium* has sweat on closing the eyes. These were the points used by keynote prescribers and some times good results were obtained. I remember once curing an organic stricture, which had been dilated but was no better. The patient described his symptoms and like the stricture was all he could think of. I did not see his remedy and gave everything without relief. One day, however, he told me he could not close his eyes to go to sleep without having a profuse sweat. I gave him *Conium* on that keynote alone, but it cured him of the sweat and the stricture, brought back an old gonorrhœal discharge and resorption of the inflammatory material took place. A scientific prescriber would not do that; but when he heard that symptom he would not know it was in the nature of *Conium* to have the stricture, and in another case he would see that *Conium* did not suit, and he would know when and when not to give it.

Anxious in the room, ameliorated in the open air. Anxiety at night in bed on closing the eyes. While reading she felt as if some one were reading after her and she must read faster and faster. That occurs in patients who are tired from being worked up to the highest pitch and it seems as if they would fly to pieces. Any thought that comes into the mind tends to repeat itself.

Vertigo, ameliorated walking in the open air. Vertigo in the morning on rising. The head symptoms are troublesome. *Silicea* will be given in cases where this remedy should be given, because the *Silicea* headache is ameliorated from wrapping up the head. This remedy has it also. Soreness of the hair follicles. Sensation as if the hair were pulled. Headache ameliorated from tying a bandage tight around the head or wrapping up the head.

Yellowness all over the body. Yellow eye in jaundice and liver troubles. Eyes inflamed. Margins of lids and eyelashes crusty; fine pimples and eruptions. After leaving the heats symptoms, which are relieved by warmth, we find many symptoms worse in the warm room.

Pulsation in the ears. Ulceration of the edges of the nostrils. Tongue has the appearance as if it had been burnt, excoriated and cracked in various directions. Fissures burn like fire. Hunger, but knows not for what. Ravenous hunger followed by nausea. Aggravation from salt things, from eating salt food, from salt baths, from sea bathing, and at the seashore from inhaling sea air. Chest complaints, liver complaints and constipation at sea. *Bromine* has complaints of sailors when they come on shore. Magnesia mur has complaints from going to sea. When a patient has urticaria at the seashore *Arsenic* will cure in *Arsenic* cases and will often mitigate when it is the only symptom:

Foul eructations tasting like rotten eggs. Disordered stomach. Stomach easily disordered. Waterbrash, vomiting. Like *Magnesia carb.*, it has inability to digest milk. Milk causes pain, and it is passed undigested—lienteric stools. Fainting at the dinner table in hysterical women.

It has many liver troubles. Enlargement and induration of the liver, with jaundiced skin. Right lobe of liver sore, painful while lying on it, and when he turns over to the left he is uncomfortable, as it feels as if the liver dragged over to the left. *Natrum sulph.* often cures that symptom, and *Ptelea* has a somewhat similar condition. These two symptoms, aggravation from lying on the right, that is, the soreness, and aggravation from lying on the left, that is, the dragging, come separately or together. It has much liver trouble from lying on the liver.

Tenderness in the region of the stomach and over the bowels. Attacks of gastralgia in the evening. A strong feature in this remedy is indigestion. The stomach becomes less and less able to digest and finally he cannot take a mouthful of food without distress. Abdominal dropsies. Colic, cramps, tearing pains. Great flatulence. With this kind of digestive disturbance we have a good home for tapeworm, it hatches out easily in this patient. The most troublesome patients I have are those who come after having had a tapeworm removed by violent drugs. It takes a long time to restore them. If a patient will come with his worm and all his symptoms, I will give him relief, and he will soon be turned into order and the tapeworm will cause no trouble.

Constipation of infants, as in *Magnesia carb.* Chalky stools like *Magnesia carb.* When the patient is an adult and yellow with jaundice, the stools are light colored, bileless and there is no expulsive power.

No power to expel the contents of the bladder, so he presses with the abdominal muscles on the full bladder and passes a little. Lack of sensation in the bladder, so that sometimes he cannot tell whether he has to urinate or not until the bladder is so full that it causes pressure. The inability to feel extends to the urethra, and he cannot tell in the dark whether he is passing urine or not.

Metrorrhagia, with backache which is ameliorated by pressing hard back in the chair or lying on a hard pillow. Bearing down pains in the pelvis, especially in hysterical women and girls.

Congestion of chest from sea bathing. Chest troubles and colds on the chest at the seashore and from salt baths. Palpitation of the heart, with anxiety. Anxiety and restlessness come on at rest; he must do something, must hurry. These symptoms are likely to come on again in the evening when he tries to go to sleep.

Shocks through the body, like electric shocks, when wide awake, jerking the whole frame; twitching and jerking. Numbness in the extremities. Tearing pains in the upper limbs and marked restlessness in lower limbs. Cramps in calves at night. Paralytic drawing and tearing in all the limbs. Burning of the soles at night in bed. Foot-sweat is another symptom like *Silicea.* Numbness of the arms in the morning on waking.

Hysterical and spasmodic complaints. Weakness from sea bathing or salt baths. It is the aggravation from salt. Sleep unrefreshing, anxious dreams.

Bodily state sensitive to cold, and great disposition to take cold. Some complaints are ameliorated by *fresh* air, if not too cold.

MAGNESIA PHOSPHORICA

Magnesia phos. is best known for its spasmodic conditions and neuralgias. The pains are very violent and may affect any nerve. A pain localizes itself in a nerve and becomes worse and worse, sometimes coming in paroxysms, but becoming so violent that the patient becomes frantic. The pains are *ameliorated by heat and pressure*. The patient feels better in a warm place; and his neuralgias are also better, he is miserable, and his pains are brought on when he becomes cold or is in a cold place. Pains are brought on from riding in the cold, and in cold, damp weather. Exposure for a long time to cold winds causes neuralgia of the face.

The pains are felt everywhere. Pain in the bowels, enteralgias, cramps in the stomach and bowels, with the same modalities. Pains in the spinal cord under the same rule—amelioration from heat. There are times when a nerve, in which there is considerable pain, becomes sensitive to pressure, becomes sore. The spinal cord becomes sore. Convulsions, with stiffness of the limbs. Convulsions in adults or children, followed by extreme sensitiveness to touch, to wind, to noise, to excitement, to everything. Such convulsions as children have during dentition. Colic; three months' colic, cramps, bilious colic. But the special feature is its power to debilitate, to cause irritation of the nerves and muscles. Cramps from prolonged exertion. Stiffness, numbness, awkwardness and deadness of a nerve from prolonged exertion. Thus it applies to long use of the hands and fingers in writing, and gives a fair sample of writer's cramp. It is especially useful in the cramps that come in the fingers, from writing, playing instruments and piano practice. Pianists suddenly break down, with stiffness of the fingers, after several hours' labor every day for years. The fingers give out. In playing the harp a cramp comes on and the fingers cannot perform their use. Other parts are affected in the same way from prolonged exertion. A laborer's hand will sometimes cramp and become almost useless. As soon as he undertakes to do that particular thing his hand cramps and he clutches the implement or loses hold. The carpenter after prolonged use of a tool has a cramp. This is a strong feature of the remedy in all sorts of over-exertion.

Violent cramps in dysentery and cholera morbus, that make him scream out. Twitching of the muscles all over the body, as in cholera. It was Schuessler's main remedy for chorea, but we only use it by its proving. Schuessler prescribed it in all nervous conditions, but its proving justifies its use in neuralgia ameliorated by heat and pressure, cramps and twitchings.

Shooting pains along the nerves, but these are not so common as violent pains in paroxysms—a tearing pain as if the nerve were inflamed and put on a stretch. Shaking as in paralysis agitans and complaints resembling it. Amelioration from heat and pressure, and aggravation from cold, cold bathing, cold winds, cold weather, lack of clothing. Pains all over, but more likely pain located in one part.

The mental symptoms have not been brought out to any extent. It has been used clinically when diarrhœas have ceased suddenly and brain troubles have come on. Congestion of the brain, but this is clinical. Neuralgia and rheumatic headaches ameliorated by heat. Excruciating pains. Violent attacks of headache ameliorated by hard pressure, heat and in the dark. I have seen this mitigation of the symptoms in chronic congestive headache, when the face was red and there was throbbing, almost like *Bell.;* those headaches give way to Magnesia phos., when there is relief by heat and pressure. He wants the head bandaged with a tight-fitting cloth, a warm room, and he is aggravated by cold.

Spasms and jerking about the eyes, or prolonged tonic spasms producing a strabismus. Violent supra and infra-orbital pains with amelioration from heat and pressure. It has cured more face-aches than other pains. Neuralgia of the face, worse on the right side, and ameliorated by heat and pressure, and aggravated by cold. Tic douloureaux. Chronic jerkings of the face. It favors rheumatic and gouty subjects who suffer with neuralgia. It is a wonderful remedy for spasmodic hiccoughing. I have sometimes given Magnesia phos. for hiccoughing when I could not get any other symptoms to prescribe on.

Pain at the pit of the stomach. Spasms of the stomach with clean tongue. Colic ameliorated by doubling up, like *Coloc.,* and ameliorated by heat. The colic is not so markedly relieved by heat in *Coloc.,* but is relieved by pressure. Distension of the abdomen and flatulence, with much pain. *Radiating pains in the abdomen.* Compelled to walk and groan from pain. Meteorism. It is said to cure cows of this condition. *Colchicum* will cure cows when they are distended with gas after being turned into clover patches.

Cutting, darting pains in hæmorrhoids. If well proved we would probably have many liver symptoms, because both *Magnes.* and *Phos.* have liver symptoms.

Violent pains in acute rheumatism, ameliorated by heat. Neuralgic pains in the limbs. Rest relieves many complaints, and the least motion brings them on. Pains changing place.

MANGANUM

Manganum is pre-eminently a drug that causes a species of chlorosis, and it is suitable for chlorotic girls, in broken down constitutions, waxy, anæmic, pallid, sickly, *threatening phthisis,* with necrosis and caries of bone and organic affections. There is the history of a long period of scanty menstruation, or the menses have been delayed until the patient was eighteen or twenty years of age.

A strong feature is the great soreness of the periosteum, and especially of the shin bone. Tendency to ulceration and eruptions, and around these there is thickening and infiltration. Chronic eruptions; inveterate like psoriasis. Small ulcers suppurate and infiltrate with purple hardness. It has a deep action, breaks down the blood corpuscles and lays the foundation for tuberculosis, especially in the larynx. Repeated attacks of laryngitis, each leaving the patient in a worse state than before. Tuberculosis that begins in the larynx. Aversion to food, no appetite, nothing will tempt him. This, with great soreness over the body, lays the foundation for some deep complaint. It is not an acute periostitis, but a passive soreness all over. Inflammation of the joints and swellings go on to suppuration and necrosis. Ulcerations and suppurative processes take on a quality of semi-malignancy and do not heal, presenting an erysipelatous appearance. Everywhere there is soreness to touch and soreness from jarring. The bones are sore from walking. *Arnica* relieves only a day or two; but in this remedy it is deep-seated and prolonged, and we would not think of *Arnica* or *Baptisia,* which would only give relief for a day or so. Vesicular eruptions, infiltrating. deep-seated, with tendency to crack and bleed. Roughness of the skin and psoriasis. *Complaints worse in cold, damp weather* and before a storm.

And now we will take up some of the mental symptoms. There are only a few of them, but they are striking, and these go deeper into the nature of the man himself, even than those we have been speaking about. Anxiety and fear. Great apprehensiveness. Something awful is going to happen. Restless and anxious. He walks the floor, and the more he walks the floor the more anxious he becomes. He attempts mental occupation; tries to occupy his mind, and the more he does this, the more anxious he becomes. He is tired and careworn. He cannot think; he cannot meditate. He has difficulties in his business because he cannot do good thinking. Anxious restlessness.

The queerest part of all is just how he gets relief. He lies down and it all passes away. You cannot find that in every medicine; that is rare, strange and peculiar. And yet, see how general it is; it defines the whole nature of the sick man. His very life is excited, tired and anxious. Great sadness and distress. He lies down and says, "Why did I not think of that before?" Perfectly comfortable now. He gets up, and the anxiety and restlessness come over him again, and he is fairly driven to distraction. See how unlike *Rhus* that gets relief from motion. See how unlike *Ars.* that is, the patient goes from one bed to another, from bed to chair and back again; he cannot sit still, or lie still; for his anxiety is worse keeping still. See how striking these symptoms are, and see what a contrast we have. The very innermost life of the patient is talking to us and asking for remedies. We must now read the signs and inner expressions of the disordered economy.

Then, he has these tormenting fears. Anxiety in the day time while moving about, better while lying down. Sad, weeping and silent. Can think of nothing to console him but to lie down and get peace. Is it any wonder, then, that some of these patients are driven to a bedridden state? And Manganum is a wonderful remedy for bedridden women who love to keep still, and it is said of them that they love to lie in bed. As far as we have gone we see that everything brings out that very idea and the nature of things that Hahnemann talks about in his first paragraph, that the sole duty of the physician is to pay his attention to the sick, to the patient himself; and who is this patient himself? This is what we have been talking about, this is what we have been trying to bring out here; and all the particulars that I shall take up corroborate these very things. These particulars are so linked with these generals talked about that they make a grand unity of thought, and we cannot separate them.

Irritability and low-spirited, like *Sulph.* and *Graph.* It is similar to *Arg. met., Phos., Graph.* and *Sulph.,* in its underlying tendency to tuberculosis. Fretfulness from small things.

Headaches as in anæmia. Dreadful headaches; head feels heavy; sticking pains; pressing, boring pains. Stitches like needles. Aggravation from jarring on stepping. Soreness in the brain and skull. Skull sensitive to touch and pressure. Red, sore spots here and there on the scalp (like *Phos.*), *as* if erysipelas would develop. Drawing, stinging headache in the open air, ameliorated in the house. Other headaches are ameliorated in the air. Aggravation from a jar, motion, and change of temperature and in cold, damp weather.

Agglutination of the eyelids. It is a suppurative and catarrhal remedy. The eye-lids are swollen. Aching of the eyes on looking at near objects, especially a near light. I have used this medicine often with that symptom and cured when there was pain in the eyes from sewing, reading fine print and doing anything that would concentrate vision. *Ruta* in nervous, gouty constitutions, when there is pain in the eyes and complaints from sewing and reading fine print for a long time. *Ruta* is especially a remedy for artists who work with a magnifying glass.

Offensive discharges from the ear. Dullness of hearing ameliorated by blowing the nose. Stopped sensation ameliorated by blowing the nose. Catarrh of the Eustachian tube. The external ear is painful to touch.

The ear symptoms are numerous. It seems to many patients that all their troubles settle in the ears. All the pains and aches in the upper part of the body settle in the ears. The pains in the throat shoot to the ears. There are pains in the throat, and pains in the teeth that go to the ears. Pains in the eyes that centre in the ears. That is strange. The ear is a centre of much tribulation. "Catarrhal conditions, with increasing deafness." From cold, damp weather. He is deaf whenever the cold rains come in the fall. Then there is a soreness, rawness and burning in the auditory canal, with much itching. *Silica* and *Kali carb.* are the two principal remedies for the paroxysmal cough that comes on from scratching the auditory canal. I have seen them choke and gag and vomit when they needed *Kali carb.* after scratching the auditory canal. Spasmodic cough from scratching the auditory canal belongs principally to *Silica* and *Kali carb.*, but Manganum has cured it. Itching in the ears from talking, from swallowing, from laughing, or doing anything that brings the throat into operation. From talking, which is using the larynx. When the bolus passes down behind the larynx is when it takes place. It is sometimes present in laryngeal phthisis, in chronic ulceration of the larynx, with burning, stinging pains in the larynx that shoot to the ears. In the proving of Manganum it is astonishing how many ear symptoms are recorded. And all these ear symptoms, like the others, are brought on, or increased, *in cold, damp weather.* "Catarrh of the Eustachian tube." Obstruction. Feels as if the ears were obstructed. "Feels as if there were a leaf before the ear." In cold, rainy weather.

A strong feature running through the remedy is similar to *Dule.*, in that it is worse from cold, cold air, and cold, damp weather. His catarrh rouses up in cold weather. Every cold, damp spell causes hoarseness and the formation of mucus in the throat. All of its complaints respond to the weather.

Wherever there is irritation there is great soreness. The eyes are red and sore. The throat is red and raw. Ear discharges are followed by great tenderness. Soreness and tenderness run all through. Chronic catarrh. Nose stopped up. Discharge yellow, lumpy and green in the morning. Bloody discharge. The nose and cartilages are sore. He avoids handling the nose.

No medicine will give you a sicklier face. When persons have bled out and have become waxy and pale the routinist thinks of *China,* but when there has been no bleeding and this same state is present from breaking down of the blood corpuscles Manganum is to be thought of. Chlorosis and pernicious anæmia would make one think of Manganum, and also *Picric acid* and *Ferrum.* Small wounds suppurate; every bruise remains sore for a long time. There is not much bleeding, for there is not much blood.

Infiltration is in keeping with this remedy. I have seen it cure inveterate ulcers, indurated and purple, in anæmic patients. Old "fever sores" can be cured with this remedy. Squamous eruptions.

All sorts of stomach disorders. Indigestion. Want of appetite. Drawing in the region of the stomach. Colic. All of these are worse from cold, damp weather. The pains are ameliorated from bending double. It is a very useful remedy for warding off *tabes mesenterica,* anæmic constitution, no appetite, diarrhœa, pain in the bowels, and, as the patient emaciates, the glands are felt. Useful in women who have been anæmic for some time from loss of blood, but it is not so great a remedy for anæmia following hæmorrhage as for that condition resulting from destruction of the blood corpuscles. Dreadful flushes of heat like *Psor., Lach., Sulph.* and *Graph.,* coming on in women who have been anæmic for some time.

It is also a great liver remedy. There is congestion and tumefaction of the liver. It has cured a tendency to fatty degeneration. It has cured jaundice; it has cured many cases of gall-stone; which means that the liver goes into such a sluggish state that the bile is unhealthy, the flow *is* impeded, and then little nodules form in it, and form gall-stones. It establishes a better working order of the stomach—a better working basis of the liver, the bile becomes healthy, and gall-stones are dissolved in healthy bile. Gall-stone colics are likely to occur along with gall-stones.

The abdomen may be said to be full of rumblings, and there are frequent griping pains—and these come on in cold, damp weather. They come on from eating cold food, like iced foods. Cold things create much distress in the region of the liver. Distress in the stomach, and distress through the bowels. "Pain and contraction at the navel;" something like *Plumbum,* although it is not said to draw like a string at the navel, like *Plumbum* and *Platinum.*

"Passes much flatus with the stool. Irregular action of the bowels." There may be periods of constipation, interrupted with every indigestion, causing diarrhœa—so that the bowels are always irregular. He is never quite safe, he has constipation or diarrhœa. As we might suppose, the stomach is the faulty organ.

"Cramps in the anus while sitting. Better lying down."

It is a useful remedy for those flashes of heat that occur at the climacteric period. The chlorotic state mentioned is closely related to the menstrual state. Disorders of the uterus, and of the stomach.

Very scanty menstrual flow. It lasts but a day or two, and it comes too soon. This is unusual in anæmic conditions, unusual in chlorosis. In women past the turn of life, every little while there will come a little hæmorrhage, a little watery flow. Anæmic old ladies, with a little watery flow from the uterus. We have had in the past to rely mostly on *Calcarea* for the old ladies with hæmorrhages of the uterus.

We are not surprised with all these weaknesses if we have muscular relaxation, and it is true in Manganum with these tired, weakly, anæmic women;

and also there is prolapsus of the uterus and prolapsus of the rectum. A dragging down of the intestines, and the whole abdomen feels heavy from a state of relaxation.

The region most threatened is the larynx, trachea and lungs. If this anæmic girl does not improve and get up a better reaction something serious Fill happen. Menstruation is merely a pale fluid or a little leucorrhœa. Rawness of the larynx. Hoarseness and loss of voice in a chronic state. It is suitable in recurrent cases coming with every spell of damp weather until finally tuberculosis starts. Every cold starts up additional trouble in the larynx, causing a laryngitis. It is a wonderful remedy in speakers and singers, as useful as *Argentum met.* Constant accumulation of mucus, more forms as soon as he clears it. Hemming all the time and annoying everybody. *Arg. met., Sil., Sulph., Phos.* and Manganum all do that. Each hem brings up a mouthful of mucus. Tubercular laryngitis. Rawness in the larynx. Expectoration of green mucus, great anæmia. Every spell of cold rouses up a bronchitis, like *Dulc.* Cold, dry weather sometimes relieves, but the patient is sensitive to cold; he is chilly and anæmic.

The cough is ameliorated by lying down. Most coughs are worse from lying down, and few remedies have amelioration from lying. In *Euphrasia* there is a cough coming from coryza, especially acute coryza in vigorous persons, and the cough is better while lying. Again there is a nervous spinal cough in spinal subjects, nervous girls, who have a cough as soon as they lie down, which is cured by *Hyos.* This remedy has a day cough—no cough at night because he is lying. *Arg. met,* has a day cough; like manganum it refers to the larynx, and is ameliorated by lying down. Cough worse from talking, laughing, walking, deep inspiration and cold, damp weather.

This remedy is most useful in recurrent complaints, and is hardly ever seen in first attacks. It is of great use in patients who are gradually declining. Ulceration and bleeding in the lungs. The hæmorrhage is watery, like bloody saliva or bloody mucus. The patient grows nervous, tremulous and has palpitation.

The limbs are full of distress, even to gout. Sore bones, burning in soles, arthritic enlargements, painful periosteum, sore joints. It has not rapid inflammatory rheumatism, like *Puls.* and *Bell.,* but tenderness of the joints, with not much swelling and aggravation from damp weather, like *Rhod., Rhus* and *Dulc.*

This remedy does not usually come up in fevers, but in cases of low typhoid, after the fever has somewhat abated, the bones are sensitive, sore all over, the patient does not rally, there is prolonged convalescence, especially in badly treated cases, who have been drugged until the blood corpuscles are ruined. You would think if he could only start up a big abscess he would be better, but he has not vigor enough for that. Some of these patients have "fever sores," and this acts as a seton and relieves them; but this patient cannot develop one, only the periosteum is sore and infiltrated.

MEDORRHINUM

One of the many uses of this remedy is in the inherited complaints of children. The physician of long and active experience meets many obstinate cases in children. The infant soon emaciates and becomes marasmic, or a child becomes asthmatic, or suffers with vicious catarrh of nose or eyelids, or has ringworm on the scalp or face, or is dwarfed; and after some waste of time it comes to mind that the father was treated for gonorrhœa that was obstinate and perhaps had condylomata on the genitalia. This remedy will cure, or begin the recovery. The woman married several years desires to become a mother. She was healthy when she married, but now she has ovarian pains, menstrual troubles, she has lost all sexual response, is growing pale and waxy, and becoming violently sensitive and nervous. The husband's history gives the cause, and this remedy will cure. The pale waxy young men, who crave stimulants and tobacco, who are sensitive to drafts, become stiff after exertion and walking, who perspire easily and are extremely sensitive to cold, who have never been well since having a gonorrhœa cured by injections. Rheumatic symptoms in every part of the body. Some symptoms are worse in the daytime. The usual comparison with *Syphilinum,* which reads, "Med. in daytime and *Syph.* at night," does not hold good as a sweeping statement. It is true that many *Syph.* pains are worse nights. It is true that some sycotic and Medorrhinum symptoms are worse daytimes. It is also true that many sycotic symptoms are violent day and night. It is also true that the mental symptoms of Med. are most violent at night. It will not do to be too sweeping with circumstances of this nosode. The rheumatic inflammations are worse from motion, but where swelling is not present these patients act like *Rhus* patients; they are sensitive to cold, suffer from aching and torturesome pains, and find relief only in motion—like *Rhus.* Most sycotic patients suffer from cold, sane are sensitive to heat. Sore, bruised and lame, as if he had taken a deep cold and was coming down with a fever. The pains come on with a feeling of general tension. Obstinate cases of rheumatism. Losing flesh. Walks stooped, becoming clumsy. Stumbles. Looks as if he were going into quick consumption. Intense nervous sensibility, respecting touch of garment or a lock of hair by any one not *en rapport.*

Trembling and quivering; growing steadily weaker. *Intense formication* all over the body. Starts from the slightest noise. Feels faint and wants to be fanned. Wants open air. Cold and pulseless, with cold sweat. *Œdema of the limbs* with great soreness and dropsy of serous sacs. Externally sensitive to cold damp weather. *Subject to neuralgias.* Stitching, tearing pains. The pains are ameliorated by heat. Drawing pains in back and limbs. The patient is extremely sensitive to pain. The remedy should never be used low.

Forgetful of facts, figures and names; of what he has read. Makes mistakes in writing, of spelling, and words. *Time moves too slowly;* everybody moves too slowly. He is in a constant hurry; in such a hurry that he gets out of breath. She is in such a hurry that she feels faint. Confusion of mind, dazed; fear of sensation; lasses the idea when speaking. Great difficulty in stating her symptoms, loses herself and must be asked over again. Thinks some one is behind her; hears whispering. Sees faces that peer at her from behind the furniture (*Phos.*). Everything seems unreal (*Alum.*). Wild desperate feeling as if incipient insanity. Weeps when talking. Exhilaration in evening. Changeable state of mind; one moment sad, the next mirthful. Presentiment of death. Frightened sensation on waking as if something dreadful had happened. *Fear* of *the dark.* Anxiety about her salvation.

Vertigo when stooping; ameliorated lying; aggravated on motion. Fear of falling.

Wandering neuralgia of head, worse in cold damp weather. Sharp pains come and go suddenly. No part of head is free from pain. Pain aggravated from light, and on coughing. Burning pains deep in, as if in brain. Extreme tension of scalp. Band across forehead. Pain in occiput and nape, aggravated on motion. Intense itching of scalp. Herpetic eruptions on scalp; ringworm. Copious dandruff. Hair dry and crispy.

Flickering before the eyes. Blurred vision, and black or brown spots in the field of vision. Objects look double, or small. Sees imaginary objects. Eyes feel drawn. Tension in the muscles. Pain in eyes on turning them. Sensation of sand in eyes. Sensation of sticks. Inflammation of conjunctiva with ulceration of the cornea. Blepharitis with much swelling. Lids stuck together in the morning. Margins red and excoriated. Ptosis. Smarting of lids. Eyelashes fall out. Swelling under eyes, as in Bright's disease.

Impaired hearing and total deafness. Imagines he hears voices or people in conversation. At first the hearing is very acute. Pain along Eustachian tubes into ears. Crawling in ears. Itching in ears. Stitching pains in ears.

This remedy cures obstinate nasal catarrh, also post nasal obstruction with loss of smell. Mucus, white or yellow. A middle aged man was cured of an obstinate nasal discharge by Med. very high and a discharge from the urethra which had been suppressed many years before came back and acted like a chronic gleet, and finally subsided without other treatment. Bleeding from the nose, and bloody nasal discharge. Nose sensitive to inhaled air. Itching and crawling in nose.

The greenish yellow, waxy, sickly face of the sycotic patient looks like that of the *Arsenic* patient, but strange to say, *Arsenic* does not otherwise correspond to the symptoms, but may be mistaken for it. The skin shines, and is often covered by blotches and there are fever blisters about the mouth. Herpes on the face. Epithelioma of wing of nose, or on lip. Rheumatic pains and stiffness of face. Swelling of the submaxillary glands. The teeth are always sensitive when chewing. The taste is perverted, and the tongue is foul and white at base. The mouth is full of canker sores. Ulcers in the mouth and on the tongue. The breath is foul. Stringy mucus in mouth and throat. Mouth dry and feels burnt. Catarrh of throat, and thick white mucus is constantly drawn from posterior nares.

Ravenous hunger, even after eating. Unquenchable thirst. Craves stimulants, tobacco, sweets, green fruit, ice, sour things, oranges, ale, salt. Nausea after eating, and after drinking water. Vomiting of mucus and bile. Sour and bitter vomiting. Violent retching. Vomiting without nausea.

Gnawing in stomach, not relieved by eating or drinking. Trembling in stomach. Clawing in stomach, aggravated by drawing up the knees. Sinking in stomach. Agonizing pains in stomach.

Terrible pains in liver. Grasping pains in liver and spleen. It has cured ascites. Pulsation felt in abdomen. Pain and swelling of the inguinal glands. A young man who had been in good flesh and health took gonorrhœa. He was treated by injection. Soon he began to lose flesh. He suffered from pain in the groin, which compelled him to walk bent. He became pale and waxy; stiff and lame all over, and was very sensitive to cold. Took cold frequently, which seemed never to get quite well. After Med. very high the discharge returned, and he seemed quite well. Pain in spermatic cords.

This remedy has cured many cases of marasmus in infants that had inherited sycosis from a parent. Children of a sycotic father are especially subject to attacks of vomiting and diarrhœa, and emaciation: They resist well selected chronic remedies, or are only palliated by well selected remedies. After Med. high they thrive, and remedies act better. Constipation. Can pass stool only by leaning far back when straining at stool. Inactivity of the rectum. Round balls, and hard lumpy stool. Ooozing of moisture at the anus, smelling like fishbrine.

Scanty, high-colored, strong-smelling urine in a patient suffering from rheumatic lameness and stiffness. Sensitive to cold, with tenderness of the soles. In albuminous urine with hyaline casts when the patient is waxy and there is œdema of feet and ankles, and the soles so tender he can scarcely walk on them, the skin of soles is bluish and hot; also when the swollen legs are so sore he cannot have them touched, or endure the pressure to ascertain whether the swelling will or will not pit on pressure. In the above conditions Med. will act promptly if there has been gonorrhœal history. Inflammation of bladder, prostate gland or kidneys. Copious mucus in urine. Renal colic.

Parenchymatic inflammation of the kidneys. Copious pale urine. Frequent urination at night. Loses urine in bed. Inactivity. of the bladder and feeble stream of urine. It has cured many cases of polyuria.

Nocturnal emissions and impotency in young men who have had gonorrhœa several times, especially if treated by injections. Prolonged gleety discharge with rheumatic symptoms and declining health. For gonorrhœal rheumatism it is a most important remedy. It controls the rheumatic symptoms and restores the discharge. It has cured induration of testes, and pain in the spermatic cords. Pain in left spermatic cord, left sciatic nerve and lumbago from every exposure to a draft in one who suffered from gonorrhœa several years ago and was cured by Med. 10 m. at long intervals.

Chronic pain in ovarian region. Sterility. Painful menstruation. Obstinate leucorrhœa. Enlarged ovaries. Violent itching of vulva and vagina. Profuse menses. Drawing in sacrum as if menses would come on. Cutting like knives in whole pelvic region. Burning in sacrum and hips during menses.

Respiration is difficult. Suffocation and short breath on slight exertion. Asthma in children of sycotic parents (*Nat. s.*). Spasms of the glottis with clucking in the larynx; air expelled with difficulty, but inhaled with ease. Several cases of asthma have been cured by this remedy. Dryness of the larynx causes spasms and cough on falling asleep. Most obstinate catarrh of air passages with copious viscid expectoration has been cured by this remedy. Cannot cough deep enough to reach the phlegm (*Caust.*). The cough is ameliorated by lying on the abdomen, is aggravated at night. The expectoration is yellow, white or green, viscid, difficult to raise. Cough worse in a warm room.

Many of the patients that need this remedy look sick, pale, and walk stooped as if about to go into phthisis. Dry cough, with rattling in chest. Great heat, even burning in chest. Many pains in chest. Rheumatic, sharp pains through chest on exposure to damp cold air. When patients who have suffered from gonorrhœa seem to be taking on a phthisical complex of symptoms and the paucity of individualizing symptoms makes the remedy doubtful, this remedy will bring better reaction, and sometimes be the remedy for many months. Intense pain in chest on coughing. Sensation of coldness in chest and mammæ. Stitching pain in chest. The chest is sore to touch, and aggravated by the motion of breathing.

The heart manifests all the symptoms usual to rheumatic constitutions. Dyspnœa; fluttering heart; palpitation. The pains are acute, cutting, stitching; aggravated by motion. Burning in heart, extending to left arm.

"Lame back" is the common complaint of these patients. It is generally a lumbago, or it is a lumbo-sacral pain, and often extends into the lower limbs. Crural or sciatic pains. Drawing in nape and back. Pain across the back, from left to right shoulders. Great heat in the upper part of spine. Stiffness in the back on rising, or beginning to move. Pains all aggravated in cold damp weather. Tender spine. Soreness in region of kidneys.

Chronic rheumatic pains in limbs in cold damp weather. The limbs are lame and stiff. Stitching pains all over the body, and in limbs Sharp pains. The patient is extremely sensitive to pain, and feels pain as sharp and stitching. Some of the pains come on during motion, and some are better from continued motion. Cold extremities. Burning palms and soles. Trembling of the limbs. Rheumatic pains in shoulders, aggravated from motion. Numbness of arms and hands, worse left. Trembling hands and arms. Burning palms, wants them fanned. Right hand cold, then left. Cold hands. Heat and numbness of back of hands.

Trembling weakness and numbness of lower limbs. Awkwardness of legs, they do not go where they are willed to go. Numbness of thighs. Must stretch the lower limbs constantly. Drawing pains and tension in legs. Rheumatic pains. Stiffness and soreness in flesh and periosteum. Shooting up the legs during a thunderstorm. Restlessness in legs, must move them constantly. Aching, drawing in legs and thighs, in sciatic and crural nerves, ameliorated by continued motion. Legs numb and heavy, like wood. Legs cold up to the knees. Contraction of muscles of posterior part of thigh down to knee. Cramps in soles and calves. Weak ankles. Burning feet, wants them uncovered and fanned. Legs swollen to knees, and pit upon pressure. Sore bruised legs, ankles and soles. Soles sore and bruised, look blue. He cannot walk on the soles. Swelling and itching of the soles. It cures the tenderness in the soles so common in chronic gonorrhœal rheumatism. Tenderness of soles so that he had to walk on his knees. Cold sweaty feet.

Can sleep only on the back with hands over head. Sleeps on her knees with face forced into the pilow. Terrible dreams of ghosts and dead people; he dreads the nights. Sleepy but cannot sleep. Sleeplessness fore part of night. Copious night sweats.

MERCURIUS

The pathogenesis of Mercury is found in the provings of Merc. viv. and Merc. sol., two slightly different preparations, but not different enough to make any distinction in practice.

Mercury is used in testing the temperature, and a Merc. constitution is just as changeable and *sensitive to heat and cold.* The patient is worse from the extremes of temperature, worse from both heat and cold. Both the symptoms and the patient are worse in a warm atmosphere, worse in the open air, and worse in the cold. The complaints of Mercury when sufficiently acute to send him to bed are *worse from the warmth of the bed,* so that he is forced to uncover; but after he uncovers and cools off he gets worse again, so that he has difficulty in keeping comfortable. This applies to the pains, the fever, ulcers and eruptions and the patient himself.

He is an *offensive* patient. We speak of mercurial odors. The breath especially is very fœtid, and it can be detected on entering the room; it permeates the whole room. The perspiration is offensive; it has a strong, sweetish, penetrating odor. Offensiveness runs all through; offensive urine, stool and sweat; the odors from the nose and mouth are offensive. When Merc. is used in large doses and the patient is salivated he gives off these odors. One who has once smelt a salivated patient will remember the mercurial odor. I remember when I was a student, almost every room had the mercurial odor. Mercury was given till the gums were touched and salivation was produced. That odor is often an index to the use of Merc.

He is *worse at night*. The bone pains, joint affections and inflammatory conditoins are all worse at night and somewhat relieved during the day. *Bone pains* are universal, but especially where the flesh is thin over the bones. Periosteal pains, boring pains, worse at night and from warmth of the bed.

The *glands are inflamed, and swollen;* the parotids, sub-linguals, lymphatic glands of the neck, groin and axilla are all affected; the mammæ swell and there is inflammation and swelling of the liver; It is pre-eminently a glandular remedy. *Induration* is also a general; *inflamed parts indurate.* If the skin is inflamed it is hard. Inflamed glands are hard. There is induration with ulceration

A *tendency to ulcerate* runs through the remedy. Ulcers are found everywhere, in the throat, nose, mouth, and on the lower limbs. Ulcers *sting and burn* and have a *lardaceous base,* an ashy-white appearance looking as if spread over with a coating of lard. It looks like a diphtheritic exudate, and Merc. has diphtheritic exudations on inflamed surfaces. Ulcers in the throat have this appearance. The mucous membrane sometimes inflames without ulceration, but with exudation, and hence it is useful in *diphtheria.* It has the same condition in ulcers; when the system is run down they exude a grey lardy or ashy deposit. *Chancres* take on that form, a whitish cheesy deposit on the base. When you realize that the complaints of Merc. are worse at night, and think of the bone pains, periosteal inflammations, etc., it is not surprising that Merc. sometimes cures syphilis. It is wonderful that the allopat hit upon it for this disease, and he cures or suppresses enough cases by similarity to justify its continued use. When given suitably it cures.

Another marked feature is the *tendency* to *the formation of pus.* With inflammation there is burning and stinging and the rapid formation of pus and the part is aggravated by both warmth and cold. Abscesses burn and sting; inflammation of joints is attended with pus formation; in inflammation of the pleura the cavity fills up with pus. The discharges of pus are yellow green. The Merc. gonorrhœal discharge is thick greenish-yellow, with stinging and burning in the urethra.

Rheumatic inflammation of joints and catarrhal inflammation of mucous membrane are features running through the remedy, and these are attended with sweat, and an astonishing feature is that the sweat does not relieve, and there is even an aggravation while sweating. Rheumatism in old syphilitic, gonorrhœal and gouty patients. It is similar enough to relate to some cases of psora, syphilis and sycosis. It partakes of the nature of all three miasms.

After a prover has taken Merc. a long time he emaciates. This is seen in old mercury takers and in syphilitics who have been mercurialized. It is a great remedy in this condition—steady emaciation with trembling, worse at night and from the warmth of the bed, great restlessness, can't find peace in any position. These miserable wretches, who are breaking down, are great sufferers, whether psoric, syphilitic or sycotic.

A strange feature is. repeated swelling and abscess formation without any heat. An abscess or swelling in a joint forms, and he sweats from head to foot, is worse at night, loses flesh, trembles and is weak, but there is no heat while the abscess goes on. Abscesses form when the life force is so low that there is no tendency to repair; a slow and prolonged pus formation, no irritability in the abscess, no tendency to granulate, it opens and keeps on discharging and seems dead. Merc. will warm it up, stop the sweat and favor granulation.

The superficial ulceration is inclined to spread and become phagedenic; it is not deep but grows larger. These open ulcers are especially seen in old syphilitics; lardaceous base; not much irritability, they are even numb, and if pus is discharged it is greenish-yellow; false granulations appear. Merc. con is a greater remedy for the superficial, eating, phagedenic ulcer. At times Merc. takes on a gangrenous condition. This may be seen anywhere, but especially on the lips, cheeks and gums. Cancrum oris. Gangrenous chancre, fœtid and black; a sphacelus forms in the chancre and the part sloughs off. All these conditions are aggravated by heat. A patient with a typical Merc. abscess rebels at times against the poultice, for it makes the trouble worse.

Trembling runs through the remedy, quivering all over. It has been used with benefit in paralysis agitans. Tremor of the hands so that he cannot lift anything or eat or write. Merc. is a great remedy in children with epileptiform fits, twitching and disorderly motions. It will help children to grow out of these incoordinate angular movements of the hands and feet. Jerking, twitching and trembling. The motions of the tongue are disorderly and the child cannot talk. Convulsions. Involuntary motions which can be momentarily controlled by volition. The restlessness is extreme.

The trembling, weakness, sweat, fœtor, suppuration and ulceration, the aggravation at night and from heat and cold, give the earlier impressions of the remedy.

The *mental* symptoms, which still more deeply show the nature of the medicine, are rich. A marked feature running all through is *hastiness;* a hurried, restless, anxious, impulsive disposition. Coming in spells, in cold cloudy weather, or damp weather, the mind will not work, it is slow and sluggish and he is forgetful. This is noticed in persons who are tending toward imbecility. He cannot answer questions right off, looks and thinks, and finally grasps it. Imbecility and softening of the brain are strong features. He becomes foolish. Delirium in acute complaints. From his feelings he thinks he must be losing his reason. Desire to kill persons contradicting her. Impulse to kill or commit suicide; sudden anger with impulse to do violence. She has the impulse to commit suicide or violent things, and she is fearful that she will lose her reason and carry the impulses out. Impulsive insanity, then, is a feature, but imbecility is more common than insanity. These impulses are leading features. The patient will not tell you about his impulses, but they relate to deep evils of the will, they fairly drive him to do something. Given a Merc. patient, and he has impulses that he tries to control, no matter what, Merc. will do something for him. During menses, great anxiety, great sadness. Anxious and restless as if some evil impended, worse at night, with sweat.

All these symptoms are common in old syphilitics, broken down after mercurial treatment and sulphur baths at the springs, with their bone pains glandular troubles, sweating, catarrhs and ulcerations everywhere.

Merc. is suitable to rheumatic troubles of the *scalp,* and neuralgias and brain trouble when there are burning, stinging pains and *pains affected by the weather,* and when there are head troubles that have come on from suppressed discharges, such as suppressed otorrhœa after scarlet fever, or when there are head troubles in scarlet fever. Think of Merc. if you are called to a child with *sweating of the head,* dilated pupils, rolling of the head, and aggravation at night, who has had scarlet fever or a suppressed ear discharge. Merc. cures lingering febrile conditions analogous to the typhoid state, but caused by suppressed ear discharge. I have cured cases that were due to packing the ear with borax, iodoform, etc., the patient having first a remittent and later a continued fever. This would go on for five or six weeks and be relieved only when the discharge returned after a dose of Merc. I remember a case of this type. It was called cerebro-spinal meningitis; the head was drawn back and twisted and held to one side. It began as an otitis media with discharge which was suppressed. Two or three doctors were called and could do nothing. In the night I went to the bedside and got the history and symptoms of Merc. Merc. re-established the discharge in twenty-four hours, the torticollis passed away, the fever subsided and the child made an excellent recovery. I can recall many such cases.

There is a tension about the scalp as if it were bandaged. Nervous girls have headache over the nose and around the eyes as if tied with a tape, or as if a tight hat were pressing on the head. Pressing, tearing pain in the eves. Burning pains in the temples ameliorated by sitting up and moving about, worse at night. Periosteal pains worse in *cold, damp weather,* in rheumatic and gouty constitutions, with sensitiveness in the eyes and ears, sore throat and glandular swellings. Headaches in old mercurialized syphilitics; they become barometers; sensitive to the weather. The catarrhal headaches are very troublesome; headache in those suffering from chronic catarrh with thick discharge. The thick discharge becomes watery and the pain in the forehead, face and ears very distressing. These headaches are violent. Chronic rheumatic headache from the suppression of a discharge from any part, or from foot sweat suppressed; alternation of foot sweat and headache. When the foot sweat is gone he has pain and stiffness in the joints. *Silicea* has that also. *Sil.* and Merc. do not follow each other well, when well selected; but if crude Mercury has been taken for a long time, *Silicea,* like *Nitric acid,* is a good remedy to eliminate it when the symptoms agree.

With all headaches there is much heat in the head. Bursting headaches, fulness of the brain, and constriction like a hand. Vise-like pressure. He is sensitive to the air when he has headache. This is true of Mere. all through. He is relieved in the room, but worse in a warm or cold room, and violently worse from a draught. He wants to he covered but is worse from heat. The hoop-like sensation is worse at night.

Merc. is a wonderful remedy to ward off *acute hydrocephalus* after measles and scarlatina; the child rolls the head and moans, and the head sweats. It is closely related to *Apis,* which is also a great remedy after scarlet fever to ward off or cure hydrocephalus.

Exostoses in old syphilitics. Lacerating, tearing pains in the pericranium. *The whole external head is painful to touch.* The scalp is tense and sore. Fœtid, oily sweat on the head. Children have moist eczema, an excoriating, offensive eruption.

Merc. is a wonderful *eye* remedy, especially for "colds". Every cold settles in the eye in gouty and rheumatic patients. Catarrh of the eyes worse from looking into the fire or rather from sitting close to the fire; the radiated heat causes smarting. Eyelids forcibly drawn together as if long deprived of sleep. Fog or mist before the eyes. Merc. cures iritis in syphilitics. The rule now-a-days is to use a mydriatic in iritis to prevent adhesions. I have treated many cases and I have no desire to dilate the pupil. I believe it is unnecessary. The homœopathic remedy will stop the iritis speedily so that no adhesions will form, and if they have begun the remedy will remove them. Pains tearing and burning around the eyes, in temples, etc. Tension of the scalp as if it were a tight fitting cap, or tension as from a tape. Ulceration and inflammation of the cornea. Vascular appearance of the cornea; inflammation, especially confined to the cornea, sometimes pustular, sometimes diffused. There is copious lachrymation with all eye symptoms, and the tears excoriate, causing a red line down the cheeks. Greenish yellow, or a green discharge. Lids spasmodically closed. Great photophobia. In inflammatory conditions of all the tissues of the eye lids, conjunctiva and deeper structures. Colds settle in the eye like *Dulc.*

Sometimes you will see a little fine growth on the iris, growing across the pupil and attached by a pedicle. It is really a syphilitic condyloma. Merc. cures it in a few days. Inflammation of the retina and choroid and of the optic nerve. All sorts of disturbed vision. It is useful in purulent ophthalmia, with swollen lids. Two kinds of constitution need it, the syphilitic and the rheumatic or gouty. He cannot open the eyes; they are spasmodically closed, and there is great tumefaction.

Ear troubles. Horribly stinking greenish discharge. Green, thick, acrid pus from the ears like the discharge from the nose and other parts. Stinking otorrhœa. In otitis media with ruptured drum, Merc. is a frequently required remedy. In Spring after a long, cold Winter, the cold, damp weather causes many cases of otorrhœa; it is almost endemic in large cities. The ear drum heals like any other place if the patient is put in good condition by the remedy. If not well treated a hole will be left. Ears inflamed, With cramp-like pains. Merc. has *stinging pain like Apis.* All routinists will give *Apis* for stinging pains, and yet it often is Merc. that the patient needs. Purulent, offensive otorrhœa. Enlargement of the parotid and cervical glands with all inflammations of the ears. Parotids sore and enlarged, neck stiff, and head sometimes drawn back. Furuncles in external canal. Fungous excrescences and polypi.

The *nose* troubles would take a long time to describe. Old syphilitics, with nasal bones affected, thick, greenish, yellow, acrid, stinking discharge. Nosebleed and bloody, discharge from the nose. Coryza acrid, watery, with pressure through the bones of the face, worse from heat or cold, worse at night; sensitive to every draught; must get up and walk the floor. has coryza with much sneezing with an opposite state, ameliorated lying, not at all during the night while lying in bed, only in the daytime while up and about. The inhalation of hot air feels good to the nose, but the heat aggravates the body. Incessant sneezing. Bleeding, scurfy, red nostrils. Old catarrhal smell in the nose. Rawness, burning and swelling. Inside of the nostrils smarting and burning. Aching, tearing and pressure in the bones. Bones of the face painful, feel as if pressed outward, and he wants to press, but it is painful.

Merc. is not deep enough to cure the whole constitution in psoric cases that are constantly taking cold. It cures the cold at once, but implants its own nature and the patient catches cold, oftener. It should not be given often, not oftener than twice in a winter. *Kali iod.* is better for the same burning in the face, running coryza, and aggravation from heat and warmth of the bed, and it will cure the coryza in a night when apparently Merc. is indicated. It is also an antidote to Merc. Don't give many doses of Merc. in psoric cases; look for a deeper medicine.

It has syphilitic eruptions and neuralgias of the *face* with or without catarrh. It is a great medicine for mumps; it is a routine remedy for this condition, which shows that it must be frequently indicated. It cures where the symptoms agree.

Scorbutic gums in those who have been salivated. Rigg's disease; purulent discharge from around the teeth. Toothache; every tooth aches, especially in old gouty and mercurialized patients. Looseness of the teeth. Red, soft gums. Teeth black and dirty. Black teeth and early decay of the teeth in syphilitic children, like *Staph.* Copious salivation. Gums painful to touch. Pulsation in the gums and roots. Gums have a blue red margin, or purple color, and are spongy and bleed easily. Gums settle away, and the teeth feel long, and are elongated. Teeth sore and painful so that he cannot masticate. Abscesses of the gums and roots of the teeth.

The *taste, tongue* and *mouth* furnish important and distinctive symptoms. As the tongue is projected it is seen to be *flabby,* has a mealy surface, and is often pale. The *imprint of the teeth* is observed all round the edge of the tongue. The tongue is *swollen* as if spongy, and presses in around the teeth and thus gets the imprint of the teeth. Inflammation, ulceration and swelling of the tongue are strong features. Old gouty constitutions have swollen tongue; the tongue will swell in the night and he will waken up with a mouthful. The taste is perverted, nothing tastes right. The tongue is coated yellow or white *as* chalk in a layer. *Offensive mouth; putrid odors* from the mouth especially the mercurial odor of the salivated patient. The tongue becomes clumsy; difficulty in talking; his speech is hardly intelligible. Awkwardness of the tongue as in persons intoxicated. Ulcers flat; eating ulcers; holes are eaten through the cheek. Eating away of the soft palate and the bone of the hard palate is often eaten away. Purulent formtion in the antrum of Highmore and fistula from the mouth to the antrum. *Fluoric acid* and *Silicea* are more frequently indicated in these fistula, especially if the bone is involved. *Copious flow of fœtid saliva.* Sore mouth of children and nursing mothers; little aphthous patches with the mercurial odor and flabby, spongy appearance of the mucous membrane and tongue. General diffused inflammation of the mouth. The whole mucous membrane is sensitive and painful, burning, stinging and smarting· dryness with or without aphthous patches. Thrush of children. Scorbutic gums.

Sore throat. It is a remedy for inflammation of the throat, with spongy appearance, general diffused tumefaction, swelling of the parotids, fulness and stiffness of the neck. Lardaceous base in ulcers; flat ulcers, spreading ulcers. Great dryness in the throat. The swelling impairs the motion of all the muscles that take part in swallowing. Swallowing is attended with difficulty, pain and paralytic weakness, and the effort to swallow forces the bolus up into the nose, and liquids come out through the nostrils. The mercurial odor is a strong feature, but Merc. often cures when that odor is not perceptible; it has such an affinity for the throat. It has chronic throat troubles and syphilitic ulcers and patches. The inflammation extends upwards and downwards, red and pale patches, the red looking as if they would suppurate or ulcerate. The red spots become quite purple, but the more purple they are the more they are like *Lach.* Tonsils dark red with stinging pains. Quinsy, after pus has formed. It is useful in diphtheria, and most cases are diffused, extensive patches or patches here and there, with spongy appearance, but no ulceration. Tumefaction; and the exudations are upon a tumefied base. Stiff neck. Erysipelatous inflammation of the throat. Dark, sloughing, eating, corroding ulcers in the throat.

He has aversion to meat, wine, brandy, coffee, greasy food, butter. Milk disagrees, and comes up sour. Sweets disagree. He is turned against his beer. The *stomach* is chronically disordered; eructations, regurgitations, heartburn, etc. Sour stomach; it is foul. He has nausea with vomiting and regurgitation of food. In such a stomach food is like a load. Bad taste; bitter mouth; he tastes the food; it comes up sour. With all this the saliva constantly runs from the mouth. It does not improve as digestion goes on. The half-digested substances are vomited. It is like the state in persons who have destroyed their stomach from crossing liquors, beer, wine and whisky.

The *liver* furnishes much trouble. Our forefathers for years took blue mass every Spring to regulate the liver. They physicked themselves with it and tapped their liver every Spring with it, and as a result they had worse livers than they would have had if the doctors had stayed at home. Constipation, bilious habits and disordered stomach. The fulness in the region of the stomach, coming in spells, worse in cold, damp weather and warm, damp weather, worse in the Spring, jaundiced condition, disordered stomach, the aggravation at night and, from the warmth of the bed, nightly feverishness and foul mouth, will give you the Merc. state. Stitches in the liver. Liver symptoms worse lying on the right side. Many complaints of Merc. are *aggravated by lying on the right side.* The lung symptoms and cough, liver, stomach and bowel symptoms are all worse while lying on the right side.

In the *abdomen* we find colic, rumbling, distension, aches and pains, stinging and burning. It has a great variety of stools, of diarrhœa and constipation. It has a well-defined dysenteric condition. Slimy, bloody stools with much straining, he feels as if he could never finish, even when no more is passing, a *"never-get-done" feeling.* This is the very opposite of *Nux* and

Rhus in *dysentery.* These are relieved if a little stool is passed, but Merc. and *Sulph.* will sit and strain, and all the salts of Merc. have the same state. *Merc. cor.* has a more violent attack, with violent urging to stool and to urinate, and intense suffering, with burning in the parts and the passage of pure blood. *Merc., Ipec.* and *Acon.* are frequently indicated in epidemic dysentery that comes in *hot* weather, and *Ipec., Dulc.* and Merc. are frequently indicated in the dysentery of *cold* weather. You should go to the bedside of a case of dysentery with the repertory or go home and send medicine. Your first prescription should cure in epidemic dysentery, and if you work cautiously you will cure every case. It is a very simple condition to cure, but a very bad thing to get mixed up. Do not give *Arsenic* just because it conforms to the dysenteric condition, for if it does not cure it will mix up the case. Hesitate about giving *Ars.* in dysentery until you are perfectly sure it is indicated. A few days ago I saw a patient who could not lie down because of pain in both hypochondria; he had incessant vomiting, inflammatory rheumatism of the ankles, hands, arms and shoulders, he had purpuric spots on the arms and legs, he had inflammation of the stomach, and was a perfect museum of diseases. He had had *Phos.* and *Ars.* and many remedies very high, all supposed to be well selected, but *Cadmium sulph.* put him to sleep in fifteen minutes. The point was that he wanted to keep perfectly still, and hence it was unlike *Ars.,* although all the other symptoms were like *Ars.* That is a strong feature of *Cadmium sulph;* he wants to keep as still as *Colch.* and *Bry.* For many years I have used it for such cases. I saw another case of cancer with coffee-ground vomit, and *Cadmium sulph.* stopped her vomiting, and she ate quite well until she died six weeks later. The doctor in charge had given her *Ars.* and *Phos.* and Morphine till she could take no more.

The *urine* burns and smarts. Frequent urging to urinate, dribbling a little; bloody urine, great burning. Hæmorrhage from the urethra. Itching worse from the presence of urine. *Gonorrhœa* which has existed for some time; discharge thick, greenish-yellow, and offensive. Smarting and burning in the urethra when urinating. Loss of sexual power. Lascivious excitement with painful erections. Ulcers on the prepuce and glands, making it suitable in *chancre* and chancroid. Flat ulcers; ulcers with lardaceous base. Inflammation of the inner surface of the prepuce. Balanitis, offensive pus. In chronic balanitis when pus forms behind the glans and under the fore-skin, gonorrhœal or psoric, consult *Jacaranda caroba.*

The woman has much tribulation. *Burning, stinging in* ovaries. Screaming from pain. Stinging, tearing, cutting pains in the ovaries; patient covered with sweat. Copious, excoriating leucorrhœa, parts raw, sore, inflamed and itching. Stinging, itching and boring pains in the uterus. Pains in the uterus and ovaries at the menstrual period. Milk in the breast of the non-pregnant woman at the menstrual period. Milk in the breasts instead of the menstrual flow. I once had a freak in a sixteen-year-old boy, who had milk in his breasts. I cured him with Merc.

Menstrual flow light red, pale, acrid, clotted, and profuse or scanty. The menses are sometimes suppressed. Women who have been in the habit of taking mercury for biliousness remain sterile. (Coffee drinkers often remain sterile also and you must stop their coffee.) Amenorrhœa with ebullitions. Chancres on the female genitals. Aged women have denuded genitals, rawness, soreness and false granulations, which are always bleeding. Burning, throbbing and itching in the vagina. Itching of the genitals from the contact of the urine; it must be washed off. In children, boys or girls, the urine burns after urinating and they are always carrying the hands to the genitals. Little girls have acrid leucorrhœa causing burning and itching and much trouble. Phlegmonous inflammation of the genitals. Boils and abscesses at the menstrual period; little elongated abscesses along the margin of the mucous membrane and skin, painful, aggravated by walking, forming during the flow and breaking after the period. This, with itching, causes great suffering.

Morning sickness. A woman, while pregnant, has œdematous swelling of the genitals. Diffused inflammation, soreness and fulness of the genitals and pelvis, causing difficulty in walking, and she must take to bed. In pelvic cellulitis in the early months of pregnancy Merc. is an important remedy. Repeated miscarriages from sheer weakness Merc. is a wonderful strengthener when properly used. Prolonged lochia. Milk scanty and spoiled.

Merc. is one of the best palliatives in cancer of the uterus and mammæ. It will restrain and sometimes cure epithelioma. I knew one case cured by the *Proto-iodide,* an ulcerated, indurated lump in the breast, as large as a goose egg, with knots in the axilla, blueness of the part, and no hope. The 100th attenuation, given as often as the pains were very severe, took it away and she remained well.

The effect observed on the nose is not all of the Merc. coryza. Most Merc. cases begin in the nose and travel down the throat, creating rawness and scraping of the larynx, and rawness and soreness in the chest; laryngitis, tracheitis and bronchitis. Loss of voice, complete aphonia. The course of the Merc. cold is downwards, even going on to pneumonia, with sweat restlessness and aggravation from the warmth of the bed. Of course many of the colds remain in the nose.

There are various conditions in the *chest*. Coughs; colds that remain in the chest, lack of reaction and tardy recovery. The colds finally settle in the bronchial tubes; the chest feels as if it would burst and the cough is *worse lying on the right side.* I look back over many cases of patients who took cold from exposure and now look sickly and sallow, with a dreadful cough and rattling on the chest; every change of the weather gives them a new cold, and they cannot lie on the right side; their tendency is to go into mucous phthisis or quick consumption. The cough is worse in the night air. There are many pains in the chest. He has a rheumatic constitution, is always sweating, worse while sweating and from the extremes of heat and cold. Stitching stabbing, rheumatic pains in the chest with night sweats. Bloody, thick green expectoration. Suppuration of the lung, great quantities of pus form. Tremendous orgasms, bubbling and flushes of heat in the chest. With many complaints there is sore throat and rheumatism and stiffness of the neck; stiff neck with swollen glands and goitre. Stiff neck with every cold; stiffness of the side and back of the neck. Induration and soreness of the cervical glands along with other complaints.

Merc. especially affects the *joints; inflammatory rheumatism* with much swelling, aggravated from the heat of the bed and from uncovering. It is difficult to get just the right weight of clothing. Rheumatic affection with sweat, aggravation at night, from the warmth of the bed and while sweating, with sickly countenance. It especially attacks the upper limbs, but is also found in the lower.

Tremulous condition of the extremities, like paralysis agitans. Trembling of the hands with great weakness. Paralysis of the lower limbs, and twitching, jerking and quivering of the paralyzed parts. *Arg. n., Phos., Stram., Secale* and Merc. have twitching of the muscles of the paralyzed limb.

Soreness between the thighs and genitals. Ulcers on the legs; abscesses. Edematous swelling of the feet. Cold perspiration. Copious sweat during sleep. Pain and sweat come on when comfortable in bed; bone pains. He covers up because he feels cold, but when he becomes warm the pains are aggravated.

Merc. is full of *fever.* Very seldom, however, has it a true, idiopathic, continued fever. It stands very low for continued fever alone, but it is especially indicated in surgical fevers, at first remittent, but later continued, such as come on from the suppression of discharges. The Merc. patient about to go into a chill is chilly even when the chill has not yet come on; sensitive to the moving air in a warm room; violently sensitive to a draught. Cold hands and feet. The sweat is profuse and offensive. The complaints in general are worse while he sweats, and the more he sweats the worse he is. He sweats copiously and his greatest sufferings are in the sweat. Merc. does not have a clear intermittent. Between the paroxysms he has fiver disturbances, diarrhœa, fever. In surgical fevers, bilious fevers, worm fever in children, and remittent fevers there is much aching in the bones, great sensitiveness to the air, aggravation at night in bed when the fever runs highest, mercurial breath and sallow skin. The fever does not go so high and the skin is not so hot as in *Bell.* The loaded tongue and the bilious fevers fade out after Merc. It is useful in hectic fever in the last stages of consumption, and in exhausting diseases with hectics, and in cancer when there is the aching, foul sweat, etc. It acts wonderfully in catarrhal fever, grippe, etc., and when colds extend to the chest and there are the copious discharges everywhere. It is suitable in quasi-typhoids that have come out of remittents, symptomatic typhoids, when the patient is icteric, low, prostrated, tremulous, with quivering muscles, great exhaustion and continued fever.

There are many *skin* symptoms; scurfy eruptions, vesicular eruptions, eruptions discharging pus. Vesicles burn and smart, with excoriating discharges, especially on the head. Much itching of the skin, violent, in all parts of the body, as from fleas, especially when warm in bed at night. Copper-colored eruptions as in syphilis, and mucous patches. The scurfy eruptions are especially marked. Ulcers on parts where the skin and flesh are thin over the bones. Offensive forms of eczema. Most eruptions are moist with copious oozing. It cures shingles. The skin is sallow. Excoriating wherever two parts come together. Rawness between the thighs and between the scrotum and thighs. Eruptions in such places. It has fissures at commissures, at the corners of the mouth and eyes; rawness and bleeding of the perinaeum rendering walking difficult.

This furnishes a basis for the Salts of Mercury.

THE SALTS OF MERCURY

After studying Merc., corrosive mercury, the proto-iodide and the bin-iodide, we may from some specific symptoms in the case say that we prefer one of the salts of Mercury. When we go to rheumatic and gouty cases with the aggravation from sweat, aggravation from the warmth of the bed, the mercurial odor, etc., we can commonly say that one of the *Mercuries* will cure this case.

MERCURIUS CORROSIVUS

Merc. cor. has more excoriation and burning, *more activity and excitement. Merc.* is slower and more sluggish. Merc. cor. is violent and active in its movements, it takes hold and runs its course with greater activity. So with a mercury base we have often to prefer this salt.

In the *eye* symptoms there is more excoriation. The pains, burning, smarting, etc., in the eruptions and ulcers are more violent. In *Merc.* we have slow spreading ulcers, but in Merc. cor. there is *great eating;* it will spread over an area as large as your hand in a night. He has the mercurial odor and sweat, and he is sallow; he needs mercury, but a more active preparation than *Merc. viv.*

Merc. cor. has decided symptoms of its own, but they are limited. You cannot tell the ptyalism, or the lardaceous ulcers apart. In *sore throat,* if it i a *Merc. case,* the ulcers are spreading rapidly and burning and smarting like coals of fire, you would say that *Merc.* is not so intense as this. You need Merc. car. for the *violence,* the *intense burning,* and the *rapid spread.* The throat is enormously swollen, the glands are swollen, and the thirst is insatiable.

In *dysentery* there is more violence; copious bleeding; great anxiety, can scarcely leave the stool a second, great tenesmus of rectum and bladder; urging to urination and stool is constant; great burning in the rectum. It is a violent case of dysentery. I would prefer *Merc.* in ordinary *Merc.* cases, but if this patient is not relieved he will not live, and Merc. cor. is needed here.

In the *urinary organs* the symptoms are violent. *Albuminuria* is more marked in Merc. cor. than in *Merc.* It is one of the most frequently indicated remedies in the albuminuria of pregnancy and a very useful remedy when gout is present.

From slight irritation of the foreskin of the male organ, the mucous membrane and skin contract and phimosis takes place. Merc. cor. relieves the itching and burning, and causes the purse-string to let up. It is seldom indicated in gonorrhœa, but is called for when there is greenish yellow or bloody watery discharge, with violent burning and urging to urination and to stool, and violent painful erections. Chancres spread with great rapidity.

Stitching, rending, tearing pains, here and there, especially in the chest.

MERCURIUS CYANATUS

Given a Merc. base and diphtheria, when the membrane is greenish and inclined to spread through the nose and involve a large surface, the Cyanide of Mercury is needed. It has exudation more marked than any other form of *Mercury.* Malignant forms of diphtheria, rapidly forming, and with phagedenic ulceration.

MERCURIUS IODATUS FLAVUS

(*Proto-iodide of Mercury.*)

There are sore throats that especially call for the proto-iodide. When in sore throats the inflammation and pain predominantly affect the *right* side, and there is a tendency to remain on the right side, or if the Merc. state is present and the sore throat goes from *right* to *left,* it is the proto-iodide you want. The patient that needs this remedy for constitutional troubles will be worse during rest and from a warm room and better in the open air.

This is especially true when the patient needs Merc. prot. in neuritis of the right arm that comes on in writers. The arm then is very painful when writing, from passive motion, from rubbing, from pressure, from both heat and cold, but better from walking in the open air. Complaints are nearly all worse on the right side of the body.

MERCURIUS IODATUS RUBER

(*Bin-iodide of Mercury*)

Again, if in a Merc. patient with diphtheria, tonsillitis, etc., the inflammation and pain begin on the *left* side, and incline to remain there or spread to the right, the bin-iodide is indicated.

These two iodides have more rapid and greater induration beneath ulcers and chancres than *Merc.,* and in old syphilitics the iodides are sometimes more useful.

MERCURIUS SULPHURICUS

(*Sulphate of Mercury. Turpeth mineral.*)

Merc. sulph. will sometimes help, when you have a case of hydrothorax with quick, short breathing, etc., and burning of the chest. If you go to an old case of hypostatic congestion, with dropsy, or a case of dyspnœa from hydrothorax, when the Merc. base is present, you will be astonished at the action of this sulphate.

CINNABARIS

(*Red Sulphide of Mercury.*)

The symptoms are worse at night from warmth of the bed, and when perspiring, like *Mercurius.* Worse from both heat and cold. Catarrhal inflammation. Fig-warts (*Thuja*). Ulcers. Many complaints from eating Syphilis in all stages. Suppurating glands; chancres. It is best to study this remedy as a form of *Mercurius,* which has a few cunning phases of its own. It is a deep acting remedy in sycosis.

The patient desires to be alone. Aversion to mental work. Forgets things which he intended to do. Mind crowded with thoughts preventing sleep.

The pains in the head are violent; worse after eating; better by heat and pressure. Fulness in the whole head. Constriction. Pain in the cold forehead which is ameliorated by heat. Tearing in the forehead before the menstrual flow. Pain in the forehead and vertex in the morning, worse lying on the left side and back, ameliorated lying on the right side, and it passes off after rising. Shooting pains in the left side of the head with flow of saliva and copious urine. Headache with nosebleed. Sensitive scalp and skull. Supra-orbital neuralgia.

Stitching, and dull pains in the eyes. Inflammation of the conjunctiva worse at night. Red, congested lids. Ptosis. Weak vision. Iritis of syphilitic origin. The symptoms are worse at night. Sharp paroxysmal pains from the warmth of the bed.

Roaring in the ears after eating. Itching in the ears.

Cold spot on root of nose. Pressure on the bones of the nose. Coryza with dirty yellow mucus drawn from posterior Nares. Epistaxis; pains in back and limbs.

The symptoms of the teeth are similar to *Mercurius*.

Tongue coated white every morning. Taste putrid, metallic and bitter. Sore ulcerated mouth. Salivation. Inflammation of mouth and throat with great thirst, worse at night. Dry mouth, and viscid mucus in the throat. Fulness in the throat, with constant desire to swallow. Dryness of the throat.

Aversion to food. Eructations, and vomiting. Tenderness of the stomach. Syphilitic buboes.

Dysentery, worse every night; bloody mucous stools; much straining. Diarrhœa, with greenish stools, worse at night. Protrusion of anus during stool.

Copious urine. Pain as from an ulcer in urethra when urinating; it wakes him also at night. Albumin in the urine.

Inflammation of glans penis with profuse secretion of pus. Increased sexual desire. Swelling of prepuce with much itching. Warts on the prepuce and fraenum, bleeding when touched. Chancres on the prepuce of gangrenous odor. Inflamed and swollen chancres, hard, discharging pus. Indurated, or neglected chancres;

Gonorrhœa, of yellowish green discharge, much pain during flow of urine. Symptoms worse at night, and from the warmth of the bed. The patient is sensitive to both a warm room, and to cold air. Induration of testes.

Syphilitic laryngeal ulcers in a tubercular patient. Hoarseness in the evening.

Pulse fast in the evening and night.

Stiff neck with pains shooting to occiput. Stitching pains each side of spine in dorsal and lumbar regions, worse on deep breathing.

Pain in the limbs at night. Sensitive to sudden changes in the weather. Lame, bruised and stiff in all the limbs. Pains worse from motion. Syphilitic nodes on tibia. Pain in tendo Achillis and os calcis after walking. Numbness in the feet. Cold feet, day and night. Wandering gout.

Burning itching of the skin, worse scratching. Itching all over. Redness; and red spots on the skin. Pustules. Gangrenous ulcers. Elevated ulcers. It is antidoted by *Hepar* and *Nitric acid*. It is closely related to *Thuja*.

MEZEREUM

The principal use of this remedy is in eruptions and ulcerations. The most violent and important of its symptoms are those of mucous membranes, skin and periosteum. The outer surfaces of the body are in a constant state of irritation; nervous feelings, biting, tingling, itching, changing place from scratching. Even when there is nothing to be seen, there is violent itching and the patient rubs and scratches until the part becomes raw and then burns; itching changes place; the part becomes cold after scratching, cold in spots. Itching changing place after scratching, especially when associated with no visible cause. As soon as he gets warm in bed or as soon as he goes into a warm room, the itching begins. Formication, itching, biting. The patient is so nervous that he is compelled to move, to change positions.

Vesicular eruptions upon the skin, running a certain course, itching, burning like fire; dries into a crust and disappears; a new crop appears near or in the same place. Vesicles form crusts beneath which is ulceration; these crusts turn white, chalk-like, are thick, tough, and leathery. They are often elevated; fluctuation beneath the crusts; pressure causes thick, white pus, sometimes yellow-white, to ooze forth; violent itching. The pains are aggravated by cold, but the itching and restlessness are worse from heat. A child tears at the eruption with its fingers when the crusts are present.

Scald-head; thick, white, elevated crusts; copious, white or yellow-white pus, often offensive, putrid; vermin are often found among the crusts. Acrid pus eating away the hair; the eruption spreads to any part of the scalp, especially to the top; it is also found beneath the ears, and about the face and chin.

Eruptions with much itching; dark, red rash with violent itching, biting, tingling, crawling, changing place by pressure, rubbing or scratching. Cases with a history of suppressed eczema or syphilis. Eruptions upon the legs and arms, on parts with poor circulation as the ears, wrists, backs of the hands; skin eruptions followed by ulcers; discharging a thick, white, offensive matter. Especially useful where eruptions have been suppressed by zinc ointment, mercurial salve, etc. Eruptions on the face, eyes, ears and scalp in child or adult, which have disappeared under the use of some ointment and inveterate catarrhal conditions have resulted, or in which eye symptoms have developed; conjunctiva chronically swollen, ectropion granular lids, conjunctival surfaces like raw beef; fissures in the corners of the eye; red cicatrices about the eyes where the eruptions have been; dry spots and enlarged veins about the eyes and nose; skin feels indurated.

Ear troubles from suppressed eruptions; thickening of the mucous membranes of the ears; degeneration of the drum of the ear; deafness, otorrhœa.

Offensive and troublesome catarrh of the nose; incrustations, thickening of the mucous membrane, ulceration; he hawks thick, yellow matter out of the throat; has been cauterized, atomized, etc., and yet the offensive ozæna remains. The periosteum is affected so that it breaks down. Advanced state of atrophic degeneration of the mucous membranes of the throat and nose.

In the throat, thickening, burning, chronic redness, tumefaction, smarting, soreness on swallowing; granulations and ulcerations of the throat. Perforating ulcers of the soft palate, all due to suppressed eruptions. Give the remedy and you will have a copious eruption in the original place; if not, there will be no relief. Often the deafness cannot be cured, because the drum of the ear or the whole ear is destroyed, is white, chalky, and contains no blood-vessels; a state of atrophic catarrh, so that there is too much structural change for hearing to be restored, yet the patient can be cured.

Has all the catarrhal states, the ulcerations and patches of copper-colored eruptions found in syphilis.

When outward manifestations are pronounced, its internal manifestations are scanty. It tends to manifest the sufferings of the body on the skin; it throws the physical evils to the surface, hence, the Mez. patient is in fairly good health when the eruptions are out; when they are suppressed, then catarrhal affections, bone diseases, nervous disorders, strange mental symptoms, constipation, rheumatism, and joint symptoms appear; he becomes a mental wreck.

Religious or financial melancholy; melancholy which shapes itself upon the patient's business; indifference to everybody and everything; irritable; thought is difficult; memory weak; absent minded; has no rest when alone, yet averse to talking. Insanity with melancholy, sadness, and a history of eruptions that have called for Mez.

Violent headaches and brain affections; pains rending, tearing; boring; head painful to touch; syphilitic affection of the brain; headaches through the sides of the head as if in the bone; feels as if the head would be crushed (closely related to *Merc.* and *Kali iod.*). Headache extending from the root of the nose to the forehead (*Merc.* and *Hepar*). Pains in the head cause faintness (*Hepar*). Pains in the bones of the skull aggravated by touch; bones feel as if scraped.

The hair mats together. "Head covered with thick, leather-like crusts, under which thick, white pus collects here and there, and glues the hair together. Scabs on the head look chalky and extended to the eyebrows and nape of neck. Elevated, white, chalk-like scabs with ichor beneath, breeding vermin."

Neuralgias, sciatica, pain in the spine, in the brachial plexus and down the arms; neuralgia of the face; all following suppressed eruptions.

The Mez. patient is sensitive to warm air as far as the skin and eruptions are concerned, but very sensitive to damp or cold weather as to the neuralgias. After the eruptions have given place to internal manifestations, the patient is chilly, sensitive to the changes of the weather, worse in stormy weather; worse after a bath, because he takes cold and his internal complaints are aggravated. The eruptions are aggravated after washing. When the eruptions are not out, the skin is hot and he wants something to cool it; he is better from cool water; there is simply a redness at this time. The itching is aggravated from bathing in warm water.

Ulceration about the roots of the teeth; a scrofulous condition of the gums, which bleed, settle away from the teeth; the teeth decay suddenly.

The face is sickly, full of ulcers, old scars, boils, etc. The anæmic face may flush up at times, but it is usually pale, gray, and waxy, expressive of a cachexia met with in some bone diseases.

Sensation of goneness, fear, apprehension, faintness in the stomach, as if something would happen; every shock, pain and hearing bad news, cause this apprehensive, hungry, faint, weak, all-gone feeling in the pit of the stomach. It comes on when the door-bell rings, if the patient is expecting the postman, while waiting at the depot for the arrival of a friend or the departure of the cars; on being introduced to sonic one, he experiences a thrill beginning in the stomach is "frightened in the stomach". *Calc., Kali carb., Phos.* and Mez have this. These "solar-plexus" individuals often have a deep cracked tongue and are hard to cure.

Worse from the warmth of the bed (hence related to *Merc.* and syphilis). Neuralgia worse in bed and at night, relieved by the external application of heat, but worse afterward; better in the open air.

Inflammatory rheumatism, worse from the warmth of the bed and at night; worse from touch; pains run down the bones; bursting sensation in the bones. They feel enlarged; tearing pains in the periosteum, necrosis, caries, fistulous openings discharging briny particles and large ulcers surrounded by pustules.

MILLEFOLIUM

This is a most useful remedy in varicose veins; especially are the capillaries spongy and enlarged. Veins break easily when congested. Wounds bleed easily and much. It favors apoplexy. Ecchymoses of the skin and eyes It favors local congestions. Hæmorrhage from any part, from wounds, from ulcers. *Atony of the blood vessels.* Hemorrhage from the lungs, stomach rectum, nose, after extraction of teeth. The blood is generally bright red Varicose veins on the limbs during pregnancy when *painful.* Hæmorrhage in malignant ulceration. After an operation and the wound has been properly closed the skin forming the edges of the wound continues to ooze a bright red blood. When a general hæmorrhagic condition prevails. These features are often associated with heart troubles that will be expected. If there has been a history of bleeding it should be given before a surgical procedure (*Lach.*). Violent congestion after hæmorrhage. No tendency to repair of vascular tissue. Hyperæmia of the brain and red face. Fulness and heat in head, but no fever. A rush of blood from chest to the head like a surging. Violent headache. Dull occipital pain. Pain in head aggravated by stooping.

Blood-shot eyes. Sharp pain in eyes and root of nose. Eyes red and congested. Foggy vision.

Noise in left ear startles her; later when laughing. Sensation as of cold air passing out of ear. Sensation as though ears were stopped. Sharp pain in ear. Earache.

EPISTAXIS, with congestion to head and chest.

Face red, without fever. Venous face. Flushes to face.

Pain in teeth from hot things. A hæmorrhagic patient should have a dose of Mill. or *Lach,*. before having teeth extracted. The throat is red, ulcerated and bleeds easily.

Empty hungry feeling in morning. Burning in stomach, aggravated bending forward. Burning in stomach and abdomen extending to chest. Vomiting blood.

Abdomen distended with flatus. Hæmorrhage from intestines and rectum. Hæmorrhage in typhoid fever. Internal hæmorrhage from lifting and from injuries. Prolonged bleedings. Bleeding piles. Bleeding condylomata of anus.

The urine is bloody, clots in the urine after standing. Pain in kidneys followed by bloody urine lasting many days. Incontinence of urine.

Want of ejaculation in coition. Hæmorrhage from bladder and urethra. Bleeding wounds.

Profuse menses, protracted, with cramps in uterus and abdomen. Uterine hemorrhage after slight exertion from abortion, or during labor; continuous, bright red blood. Varicose veins of legs ulcerate and bleed in pregnant women. After hard delivery prolonged obstinate bleeding. A woman predisposed to hæmorrhage should have a dose of Millefolium before going into confinement. Suppressed lochia. No milk in breasts. Inflammation of the uterus after a uterine hæmorrhage.

Oppression of the chest; palpitation; *surging of blood* from chest to head. Hæmorrhage from lungs. Congestion of lungs following bleeding of lungs. Bleeding from lungs from suppressed menses. Expectoration of blood 4 P.M. daily. Bleeding from the lungs in phthisis. Bleeding from lungs after exertion. A man thrown from a carriage had continued to cough up blood for many weeks was cured by this remedy very high. Orgasr)f blood about heart.

MOSCHUS

Moschus cures many hysterical girls who have come to adult age without ever learning what obedience means. They are self-willed, obstinate and selfish. When they have been encouraged to resort to crafty cunning, to have every whim gratified from infancy to eighteen years of age they, become fit subjects for Mosch., *Asaf., Ignatia* and *Valer.* They not only have volumes of real and imaginary symptoms, but they become adepts at producing at will a kaleidoscopic complex of symptoms, increasing in quantity and intensity until all their own desires are attained, and the onlooker, be he or she nurse, physician or bewildered mother, is overwhelmed, dismayed and in retreat. However much they pretend to be honest and truthful their reported sensations are untrustworthy. They have traded upon their sensations and imagination so long that a direct effort to give a truthful statement is unsuccessful. The most erratic and unexpected neuropathic phenomena are always in appearance. The physician cannot measure these cases by his experience and say what is common and uncommon. He is compelled to fall back upon the one word that covers a multitude of these manifestations viz., "Hysteria". Moschus is often indicated in these constitutions and cures much that is morbid, when its own peculiar symptoms agree. When one of these girls becomes sick from taking cold the acute symptoms will be told with a host of her imaginary sensations. The globus hystericus is generally present, hyperæsthesia of the skin, quivering of the muscles, wakefulness, palpitation, excitement, fainting and trembling. "Dreadful" pain all over the body, rush of blood to head, cramps in hands and feet, convulsions of whole body. It is not generally known that the morbid sensations and functions correspond with the mental state of the individual. When the functions and tissue symptoms are hysterical or erratic the mental state will be found to be correspondingly hysterical. When the peculiar Moschus symptom of the face is present, viz.: one cheek red and cold, the other pale and hot, there is certainly some hysterical perversion in the mind of that patient. Many times it is possible to suspect morbid mental states by knowing morbid sensations and functions. There is a kind of order in all morbid expressions seen in sick people. Sensitive to cold, and complaints come on from becoming cold. In addition to numerous hysterical mental symptoms she has violent fits of anger with rage and scolding until she is blue in the face and falls in a faint. Dread of death, and talks only of death when there is no serious complaint. Anguish and palpitation. Peevishness and quarrelsomeness. In a constant hurry, and lets things fall from her hands. Foolish gestures and complaint of pain. Apprehension, trembling and palpitation. Fear of lying down lest she die.

Sensation of falling from a height, or as if rapidly turned around.

Vertigo on moving head or eyelids, ameliorated in open air, with nausea and vomiting and fainting.

The headaches are ameliorated from becoming warm, and in the fresh air. Tension in back of head and nape. Aching in head, with cold feeling. Pressive, stupefying headache, mostly in forehead, with nausea, aggravated on motion, ameliorated in fresh air. Hysterical headaches, with copious colorless urine. Constriction as with cord. Pain as if a nail in occiput; aggravated in room, ameliorated in fresh air.

Eyes staring. Sudden blindness or dim vision, coming and going. Eyes turned up, fixed and glistening.

Rushing sounds in ears as from wind, or fluttering as the wing of a bird. Detonation in ears as from the report of a cannon, with a few drops of blood. Nervous deafness in paroxysms, or after a mad fit.

Epistaxis and illusions of smell.

One cheek is red and cool, the other is pale and hot. Heat in the pale face and dim vision. Tension in face. Pale face with sweat. Earthy pale face. Moving of lower jaw as if chewing.

Mouth and throat dry and hot; bitter, putrid taste; great thirst; especially in hysterical conditions.

Craves beer or brandy. Aversion to food. The sight of it makes her sick. Vomiting. Pressive, burning pain and distension of stomach. Fainting during meals. Water-brash. Hysterical hiccoughing. Nausea when thinking of food. Drawing in at the umbilicus (*Plb.*). Prolonged vomiting of food. Fulness in stomach after eating. Vomiting blood. Stomach easily disordered.

Tympanitic distension of abdomen with sharp pains. No flatus up or down, yet greatly distended. Cramping pains.

Involuntary stools during sleep. Copious watery stools during night. Stitching in anus to bladder.

Copious colorless watery urine. Urine passed during the night is offensive and full of mucus.

In the male, violent sexual excitement. Emissions without erections.

In the female, violent sexual desire. Menses too early and profuse, with drawing pains; tingling in genitalia and fainting. Bearing down sensation. Erratic nervous phenomena during pregnancy.

Laryngismus stridulus in self-willed girls when they fail to have their own way. Constriction of larynx as from vapor of sulphur. Spasms of larynx when becoming cold. Spasmodic croup in nervous children after punishment.

Dyspnœa and oppression of chest and heart. Spasmodic asthma in extremely nervous women and children.

Constriction of chest. Spasms of chest and diaphragm, turns blue in face and foams at mouth on becoming cold. Paralysis of chest, rattling, cannot expectorate; fainting.

Palpitation in hysterical girls. Palpitation, oppression of chest, fainting, excitement, with copious colorless urine. The heart seems to quiver when the pulse is normal.

Aching in limbs. Restlessness in legs, and tibia cold. One hand hot and pale, the other cold and red.

Heat in evening in bed, on right side only; wants to uncover. Perspiration smelling like musk in the morning.

Cold skin, trembling, fainting and palpitation.

MURIATIC ACID

When treating a low form of continued fever with extreme prostration *Arsenicum,* Muriatic acid and *Phos. acid* force themselves upon the mind. With *Arsenicum* there has been the anxious restlessness; with *Phos. acid* there has been the mental prostration, and then the muscular weakness; with Muriatic acid the muscular weakness comes first, and there has been history of restlessness and the mind has been stronger than could be expected. With this great muscular exhaustion with jaw hanging down and the patient sliding down in bed and soon the involuntary stool and urine, this remedy is forced upon the mind. Paralytic weakness is what it must be called. Soon the tongue is paralyzed, as well as the sphincters of the bladder and rectum. It seems to be eminently fitted for the lowest forms of zymotic fever when the above symptoms are present. He finally becomes unconscious. There has been some restlessness, but nothing like *Arsenicum* and *Rhus tox.* He refuses to talk because it frets him to do so. *Phos. acid* is slow answering questions because of exhaustion of mind which makes him unable to think.

The vertigo comes on moving eyes, and on lying on the *right side.* This vertigo is sometimes associated with liver disease. A stout, full-blooded jaundiced man about forty had suffered much from pain in the liver, with great soreness, was comfortable only when lying on left side; when he turned on his back or right side an anxious vertigo would come at once and be would break out in copious sweat, and be forced back to the left side. Muriatic acid made a complete cure of this liver trouble, which had been pronounced serious.

The headache is aggravated moving the eyes and rising up in bed, ameliorated by walking about slowly. Occipital headache with dim vision, aggravated by effort to see. Heaviness in occiput. Numbness in forehead. Soreness in occiput. Feeling as if hair were standing on end. Heat in top of head.

Perpendicular half sight. The eye symptoms ameliorated in the dark.

Stitching pain. Burning, extending left to right eye, ameliorated washing. Itching in the eyes.

Hardness of hearing; loud cracking sounds during the night. The sound of voices unbearable. Buzzing in the ears.

The nose is stopped. *Nosebleed* in whooping cough, in zymotic fevers, in diphtheria and scarlet fever. Dark putrid blood from nose.

The lower jaw hangs down in typhoid fever. Margin of lips dry, sore and cracked. Burning lips.

Mouth and tongue coated white.

Sordes on the teeth. Gums swollen and bleeding. Teeth become loose. Tongue dry, heavy, *stiff and paralyzed.* Mouth dry. Ulceration of mouth and tongue. Red tongue. Blueness of the tongue. Mucous membrane of lips denuded. Sore mouth of nursing infants. Mouth studded with ulcers. Deep ulcers with black base.

Violent inflammation of the throat. Dryness of the throat. Dark red throat with ulcers. Greyish white exudations. White exudations resembling diphtheria. Gangrenous sore throat. Hawks out fœtid mucus. Diphtheria with extreme prostration.

Great thirst. Thirst during chill and thirstless during the fever. Aversion to meat. Craves stimulants. Eructation bitter and putrid. Spasmodic action of œsophagus. Vomiting sour. Involuntary swallowing. Emptiness in stomach, not ameliorated by eating. Empty sensation in stomach and abdomen without desire for food. Emptiness in stomach from 10 A.M. till evening. Emptiness in abdomen in the morning after the usual normal stool. Indigestion; faintness; constipation; confusion; sleepiness after eating.

Pressing in the liver. Soreness, and enlarged liver. Fulness and rumbling in abdomen.

Watery stools, involuntary while urinating. Stools pass unnoticed. Dark brown stools, *with blood.* Much flatus with stools. Urging aggravated by motion. Dysentery, putrid blood and slime. Hæmorrhage from intestines of dark liquid blood. Prolapsus ani while urinating. Urging to stool while urinating. Marked relaxation and itching of anus.

Large, dark, purple hæmorrhoids, extremely *sensitive to touch.* Inflammation of the pile tumors, hot and pulsating; must lie with limbs wide apart. *Bleeding piles.* Burning and cutting during stool. Burning after stool, ameliorated by warm applications, aggravated from bathing with cool water. Excoriation of anus. Fissures.

The urine flows in a feeble stream. Must wait a long time for urine to start; must press so that anus protrudes. This is in keeping with the general paralytic muscular weakness in the body. Involuntary flow of urine and stool in low fevers. Burning and cutting in the urethra while urinating, tenesmus follows.

Impotency; desire weak. Bloody, watery discharge from the urethra. Scrotum bluish. Itching of the scrotum not ameliorated by scratching. Margin of prepuce sore.

Pressing in genitals as if menses would appear. Menses too early and profuse. Ulcers on genitalia with putrid discharges. Cannot bear least touch, not even of sheet on genitals. *Leucorrhœa* with backache. Puerperal fever with extreme prostration, dropped jaw, sliding down in bed, suppressed lochia. Stool and urine putrid and involuntary.

Short breath with rattling after drinking. Breathing seems to come from stomach. Oppression of chest.

Pulse slow and weak, intermits every third beat.

Pressing pain in back. Pressing, drawing, tired feeling in small of back. Burning in spine.

Heaviness of arms. Numbness and coldness of fingers at night. Lower limbs dusky. Putrid ulcers on legs, with burning margins. Swelling of right tendo Achillis. Feet cold and blue. Burning of palms and soles. Swelling and burning of tips of toes. Tearing in limbs, ameliorated by motion. Pain in the limbs, during intermittent fever.

Evening fever with chill with or without sweat. Chill mingled with fever. The image of this remedy is found in typhoid and yellow fever. Perspiration during first sleep. Symptoms worse when perspiring.

NAJA

The use of Naja has extended far beyond its proving. So many of the Ophidian family present symptoms in common with it, that much has been presumed—truly so. Many characteristics run through these remedies, each remedy having its own peculiar sphere. Taken together the family presents a wide range of curative action.

Mure, of Brazil, thought that the snake family presented curative powers for the healing of the nations.

In the mineral kingdom, man may find his remedy when sick, so in the vegetable and animal kingdom. It is possible that the product of the serpent may be everything needed for the healing of man. Extend this to the whole animal kingdom and it is probably so. There seems to be everything existing in one kingdom that exists in another. The lowest is the mineral, the next the vegetable, and last the animal kingdom. If we had a perfect knowledge of any one kingdom, we could probably cover the entire scope of curative possibilities. But we have only a knowledge of a few remedies in each kingdom.

Another idea has been advanced that in any particular region, the vegetable kingdom provides all that is necessary for curing in that region. If we were acquainted with all the vegetable growths, how much we would know in comparison with what we do know! It is highly probable that there is a throwing off from the sick human race of something that is absorbed by the plants. The evils that are thrown off by man may be absorbed by the vegetable kingdom. Plants will correspond to men in the region in which they grow, if there is anything in this. In two thousand years there might be a necessity for some kind of a check upon the growth, of plants. The absorption of these evils may cause them to vary in species, and if they continue to grow and each to absorb the evils from the human race, they will continue to differ. This favors evolution and explains it in a sense.

It is important to compare the symptoms of Naja with those of the other snakes. The patient is disturbed by closeness of the collar, < after sleep. There are exhaustion and trembling, trembling of the muscles. Its direction is somewhat like *Lach.*, from left to right, *i.e.*, the ovarian pains, the diphtheria, the joint affections go from left to right. Naja, like *Lach.*, is < in damp weather. On inflamed surfaces it produces grayish exudations. It does not partake so extensively of this character as do *Lach.* and *Crotalus.* There is only a shadow of the septic in Naja, but it is extensive in *Lach.* and extremely marked in *Crotalus.* Naja is not as subject to hæmorrhage as either *Lach.* or *Crotalus.*

There is trembling of the muscles, rheumatic diathesis, and tendency of all complaints to settle about the heart. It is used in valvular troubles of the heart, in young persons who grow up with cardiac valvular diseases. The whole trouble settled about the heart. This suggests Naja, and Naja has often cured. If the valvular trouble is congenital it cannot be cured; but if not, it shows that all the disturbing forces have settled about the heart. All the symptoms have settled about the heart; Naja has this. In school boys and girls who have no symptoms this is the generic remedy for this kind of complaint. Always prescribe Naja unless guided away from it by some specific symptom.

Naja has more nervous, *Lach.* more septic symptoms. Naja, marked agitation without sepsis, *Lach.*, all the nervousness with a tendency to hæmorrhage and sepsis; black blood, like charred straw; dark clotted blood.

Naja has surging of the blood upwards, like *Lach.*—a distressing symptom. There is marked dyspnœa, cardiac or otherwise. There is stuffing up of the chest; great rawness of the trachea and larynx, the whole passage is raw as if excoriated.

There is much sneezing, with running of water from the nose; inability to lie down at night; dryness of the air passages of the nose, hay fever. The patient has suffocative attacks in August.

The whole chest is in a state of congestion; emptiness of the left side of the chest; low pulse or intermittent pulse. With all the complaints of the chest there is inability to lie on the left side. Numbness of the left arm. There is dyspnœa; if he goes to sleep, he wakes up suffocating, gasping, choking, or he starts from sleep as if from a dream. In most complaints there is inability to lie on the left side.

There is a dry, hacking cough with sweating in the palms of the hands that is cured by Naja. These cardiac cases are often attended by a dry, hacking cough, a cough with every little exertion. It is not a catarrhal state, nor is it tubercular. The heart beats slowly and will not be urged to work, and a cough comes on from exertion. *Cactus* also, has a cardiac cough.

The extremities are cold and blue and the head hot. The head symptoms are < in a warm room; the head feels warm, fevered, yet the feet and limbs do not become warm. There is copious sweating of the hands and feet, causing the gloves and shoes to rot out; but the sweat is not offensive. There is a sense of fulness and puffiness of the hands and feet, showing a slow circulation in the veins which we might expect.

We might naturally expect that this patient would be intense and excitable, which is the case. There is a suicidal tendency.

The headaches are nondescript; of a congestive character all over the head, especially in the occiput. Headaches accompanied by a quick and nervous pulse.

Profound sleep is consistent with all the snakes. There is deep, profound sleep with stertorous breathing.

She wakes with a headache every morning. It is natural for the Naja headache to be present in the morning and wear off with exertion. The other complaints are < exertion. The mind symptoms are < exertion of the mind.

These are symptoms in connection with hay fever; The rawness in the throat and larynx; dreadful aching in the throat extending to the larynx, which swallowing does not relieve. The *Lach.* state is expressed more by a lump in the throat; grasping of the throat with a sense of choking.

The Naja patient is subject to severe attacks of bronchitis. There is rawness between the larynx and trachea, < after coughing.

This is a great remedy in asthma, especially cardiac asthma. The breathing is so bad that he cannot lie down.

Useful in chronic nervous palpitation; palpitation after exertion of any kind. Chronic nervous palpitation with inablity to speak on account of choking.

There is a continued, dull, aching pain through the back between the shoulders, associated with cardiac affections. Sometimes there is little beside this sensation of heat, of aching, to indicate the remedy; he is so tired in that spot that he wants to lie down or lean backwards to rest his back.

The palpitation is < lying on the left side, < walking.

This is the most useful of all the remedies we have in a cardiac state with very few symptoms. It is true that this region is particularly singled out by Naja to produce its symptoms.

NATRUM ARSENICOSUM

The symptoms of this remedy appear in the *daytime,* in the MORNING, in the *forenoon, evening, night* and after MIDNIGHT. The symptoms are worse in the cold air, but warm open air ameliorates; the mental symptoms are better in the open air; worse from cold in general; in cold air; *becoming cold;* in cold, wet weather; the patient takes cold easily. The symptoms are worse ascending. Anæmia and weakness and dropsy of the limbs. Complaints worse after eating. The body is losing flesh. The symptoms come on FROM EXERTION. Worse from butter, cold drinks, cold food, fats, *fruits, milk, pork,* vinegar. Formication all over the body and in the limbs; induration of glands; inflammation in any part. Marked physical irritability and irritable weakness. Jarring aggravates many symptoms. Lassitude prevails throughout the provings. Desire to lie down and not be disturbed; yet lying often makes the symptoms worse and aggravation is marked after lying Still many symptoms are worse from motion; there is a strong aversion to motion. Mucous secretions are copious. After exposure to cold he becomes rheumatic. Aching, burning and pressing pains; sore pains; stitching pains in all parts; darting pains in all parts; downward and upward. Perspiration does not ameliorate. Pressure aggravates. General pulsation.

Pulse irregular. Rheumatic and malarial patients, oversensitive, internally and externally. Electric shocks in the body. Symptoms predominate on the right side. Wants to sit or lie and not be disturbed. There are symptoms before sleep, during sleep, and on waking; trembling is a strong symptom. Twitching of the muscles. Walking in the open air increases the physical symptoms, but improves the mental symptoms; walking fast excites many symptoms. Weakness in the *morning,* during menses, on *slight exertion, while walking.* Wet weather brings out the symptoms. Worse from wine and in winter.

Anger at trifles; furious from contradiction; complaints are made worse from anger. Anxiety in the evening in bed; at night in bed; apprehensive anxiety; during fever; on waking. Concentration of mind difficult in the house, better in the open air; confusion of mind in the evening. Conscientious about trifles. Discontented; discouraged and, at times, in despair. He is easily distracted. Dullness of mind, better in the open air. Easily excited. Mental exertion makes the symptoms worse. Fear in the evening on going to bed; in a crowd; of impending disease; of some evil; that something will happen; of people. *Easily frightened;* forgetful; he feels constantly hurried. Hysterical and her mind is very active; ideas very active. Imbecility, irritability, impatience; indifferent to all joy. Aversion to mental work and to business; aversion to reading; indolence; *memory weak.* Lamenting, laughing, loathing of life, loquacity. The mental symptoms are all mild. Mirthful, hilarious; prostration of mind. She becomes quarrelsome. Restlessness; nights, tossing, anxious restlessness. Sadness in the evening; during fever. Sensitive to noise; startled easily, by noise, on going to sleep, from sleep. Suspicious. Indisposed to talk; disturbed by the conversation of people. Timidity with a vacant feeling of mind. Weeping. Vertigo while walking. When the above general symptoms are present in any considerable number the following particulars will yield to this remedy.

Hyperæmia of the brain with heat and fulness; fulness in the forehead. Subjective heat with objective coldness of forehead. Heaviness in the head, in the forehead. Empty feeling in the head. Numbness in forehead in the evening. *Pain in the head;* morning; afternoon; *evening;* night, night on waking; better in the open air; catarrhal headache; with coryza; worse after eating; from becoming heated; worse from heat; from a jar; from light; before and during menses; *from mental exertion;* moving head; every motion jars head; from NOISE; paroxysmal pains; *periodical headaches;* from pressure; pulsating; worse in a room; after sleep; from stooping; tobacco smoke; from walking; in a warm room; from wine. Pain in the forehead; in the morning on waking; during the whole day; above the eyes, extending to the temples. Pain in the occiput; pain in the sides of the head; pain in the temples; right side, from temple to temple; pain in the vertex. Boring in the temples; right to left; with nausea; bursting in the head, in the forehead; drawing in the head, *in the forehead; pressing* pain in the head; in the forehead, *in the occiput, in the temples;* in the vertex; sharp pains above the right eye; shooting pains above the right eye. Sore and tender scalp; forehead. Stitching pains in the head; *stunning* pains in the head; tearing in the head; in the forehead; in the sides of the head. *Perspiration on the forehead.* Pulsation in the head; forehead, temples, vertex; with fulness in the forehead.

The eye symptoms are worse in the morning; lids are stuck together in the morning; congested eyes and blood vessels; discharge of mucus from the eyes. Dryness. Sensation of enlargement of the eyes in the morning on waking. Granular lids. The eyes feel hot. Inflammation of the conjunctiva from cold or wind; worse in the morning, after night work; of the lids and margins. Injected veins. Lachrymation in the morning on waking, in the open air, on looking steadily, when reading, unable to open the lids. Pain in the eyes, worse in sunlight; from motion; while reading; while reading by gas light; while writing; *better by warmth.* Aching in and over the eyes; in the morning on waking. Burning in the eyes; in the evening, in the open air, while reading. Pressing pain in the eyes; smarting as from smoke; sore and tender when reading; stitching pains in the eyes.

Paralysis of the upper lids; of the optic nerve. Photophobia in daylight. Pupils dilated: left eye larger than right. *Redness of* THE VEINS. Staring eyes; stiffness of the lids; of the *eyeballs.* Strabismus. Swollen eyes; LIDS; *œdematous lids; supra-orbital œdema.* Ulceration of the cornea. Weak eyes and vision; vision blurred; tires out when reading. Dark colors before the eyes. Vision dim, on looking long; wipes eyes for relief. Flickering, foggy vision. Hemiopia. Myopia. Sparks before the eyes.

The ears are hot; itching in the ears. Noises: morning, evening, with vertigo, humming, ringing, roaring, rushing in the right ear; singing. Pain in ears: *morning, stitching,* tearing, behind the ears. The ears feel stopped. Hearing *acute;* for *noises; impaired.*

Catarrh with pain in forehead and root of nose, post-nasal with viscid mucus. Coryza: worse in open air, with cough, fluent or dry, fluent alternating with dry; discharge: *copious, crusts,* dry *bloody crusts,* hard bluish mucus, offensive, *purulent, suppressed, thick, viscid,* WATERY, *yellow.* Dryness in nose. Epistaxis after removing crusts from nose; bright red blood. Obstruction of nose at night (right); morning on waking; mucous membrane thickened and it is difficult to breathe through the nose. Ozæna. The nose is red. Pain in the nose, in the roof of nose; burning, pressing at root of nose; rawness in nose. Smell acute at first, later wanting. Frequent, violent sneezing.

Corners of lips cracked and indurated. Discoloration of the face; bluish, around eyes; earthy; PALE; red; yellow; liver spots. Face is drawn. Eruptions on the face; forehead and lips; AROUND THE MOUTH; on *the nose;* comedones; herpes on lips; moist eruptions; pimples, vesicles. The face is hot and itching. Pain on moving the jaw. The face feels puffed. Stiffness of muscles of mastication. Swelling in the morning on waking; molar bones feel swollen; œdematous; swollen parotids. Twitching of face. Ulcer on the lips. Aphthæ in the mouth; bleeding gums; cracked and corrugated tongue. Discoloration: redness of mouth and tongue; white tongue; yellow tongue. Dryness of mouth; *tongue;* flabby tongue. Inflammation of mouth and tongue. Salivation and saliva is viscid. Stammering speech. Taste bitter in the morning; *metallic,* saltish, SOUR, sweetish. Ulceration in mouth. Vesicles in mouth and on tongue; burning. The teeth become loose. Pain in the teeth; night; pulsating; warmth ameliorates; jerking pains, tearing pains.

Choking; constriction of œsophagus; dryness in throat; worse in the morning; after a cold. Throat red and glossy, purple red; hawks frequently to raise white mucus, worse in the open air. Inflammation; dark red, covered with yellow mucus. Sensation of a lump in the throat; gray exudation in the throat. It is said to have cured diphtheria. Mucus in the throat; tough gelatinous, greyish, yellow, white, from posterior nares. Pain in throat on swallowing, on empty swallowing, but no pain on swallowing food or drink; burning, sore, stitching. Roughness in the throat; scraping in the throat.

Swallowing difficult. Swollen pharynx, uvula and tonsils; œdematous; uvula hangs down like a water bag. Constriction in the region of the thyroid gland. Stiffness in the sides of the neck.

Appetite *increased, ravenous, wanting;* aversion to fats, to meat, to his cigar; sensation of constriction in the stomach. Desires beer, bread, cold drinks, sweet things. Disordered stomach; by milk. Stomach is distended; sensation of emptiness; eructations afternoon, after eating; *empty,* tasting of food, SOUR after eating, waterbrash. Fulness in the stomach after eating. Heartburn. Flushes of heat, heaviness after eating. HICCOUGH after eating, indigestion is very marked. Loathing of food. Nausea: after eating; con-stant; during cough; after cold drinks; with headache; during menses. Pain in the stomach: AFTER EATING; burning after warm things; *cramping;* CUTTING; gnawing; pressing after eating; soreness; stitching. Pulsation in the stomach. Retching when raising mucus from the throat. Sinking sensation. Sensation of a stone in the stomach. Tension in the stomach. Thirst; morning; evening; night; burning thirst; extreme thirst; unquenchable thirst; drinks often but small drinks. Thirstlessness. Vomiting: on coughing; after eating; *bile; bitter; blood;* mucus; *sour;* watery.

Distension of abdomen after eating; flatulence; fulness, gurgling, hardness. Heavy feeling in abdomen. Inflammation of liver; spleen. Liver affections. Pain in the abdomen; at night; after eating; *from flatus;* before a diarrhœa; before stool; better after stool and after passing flatus; in hypochondria; hypogastrium; in region of umbilicus. Cramping; before stool better by passing flatus and stool. Cutting; before stool. Drawing in abdomen; in hypochondria. Sore, tender abdomen; in hypochondria. Stitching in abdomen; in hypochondria; in inguinal region; in spleen. Nervous feeling in abdomen. Rumbling in abdomen; as if a diarrhœa would come on. Affections of the spleen. Swollen inguinal glands. Tension in abdomen, in hypochondria.

Constipation, alternating with diarrhœa; stool hard. Diarrhœa: evening; daytime; morning; drives him out of bed; NIGHT; after midnight; frequent stool during daytime; from becoming cold; from cold drinks; *from taking cold;* worse *after eating;* during menses; AFTER MILK; after vegetable; stool: bloody; copious, frequent, mucous, painless, pasty, *scanty,* soft, thin, watery, *yellow.* Excoriation of anus. Flatus copious and offensive. *Itching of anus.* Pain: BURNING during and after stool; cramping, better after stool; cutting, during stool and in the hypogastrium; before stool; soreness and stitching; tearing during stool; *tenesmus during stool.* Urging to stool; ineffectual; after stool.

Sore pain in bladder relieved by urinating; urging to urinate at night; constant; frequent. Urination difficult; frequent; *involuntary* at night in sleep; unsatisfactory. Burning and aching in the kidneys. Burning in the urethra when passing urine. Urine: ALBUMINOUS; burning; dark; pale; copious at night;

clear as water; *offensive;* scanty; with mucus and phosphate. Specific gravity decreased; 1010.

Morning erections; incomplete. Inflammation of glans penis, prepuce and testes. Stitching of the genitals, penis, scrotum. Soreness left testis. Seminal emissions. Swollen penis and testes.

In the female the desire is increased. Leucorrhœa; *copious; offensive;* thick; yellow. Menses: copious; too soon; *protracted; scanty.* Metrorrhagia. Pain in the uterus.

Dryness and constriction in the larynx; scraping slate-colored mucus from the larynx; mucus is detached with difficulty; burning and soreness in the larynx; roughness in larynx. The symptoms of the larynx are worse from dust, smoke or cold air. Voice: hoarseness with coryza; lost; weak. Respiration is fast and deep; miner's asthma from coal dust; difficult on ascending, short.

Cough: morning; afternoon; evening; *night;* from deep breathing;. dry at night; in the morning and from exertion; dry teasing cough all day; exhausting; hacking; from irritation in larynx and trachea; loose; racking; short, spasmodic; from tickling in larynx and trachea; violent; worse in a warm room. Expectoration: morning, evening, bloody, difficult, mucous, OFFENSIVE PURULENT, tasting bitter, flat, putrid, viscid, yellow.

Anxiety and constriction of the chest. Eruptions, pimples. Sensation of fulness in the chest. Hæmorrhage from the lungs. Pneumonia and phthisis in miners from dust of coal. Irirtation in the bronchial tubes in the morning. Oppression of chest on exertion and deep breathing; heart. Pain in the chest, during cough; in the heart; *burning,* cutting below the seventh rib; pressing; rawness; sore from coughing; *stitching.* Palpitation of the heart; night; *anxious;* assending steps; exertion; tumultuous. Sensation as if he had inhaled smoke.

Coldness of the back at night. Stitching of the cervical region. Pain in the back, evening; night; worse walking; in the scapulæ; between the scapulæ; on bending forward and on breathing in the lumbar region when stooping and walking; in the sacrum both when walking and sittting; aching in the back; drawing pain in the back; sore pain in the back; sore pain in the sacrum when walking and stooping; sore pain in cervical region; sore pain under scapulæ; sore pain in spine on pressure. Stiffness in the cervical region, *weakness* in the back.

Awkwardness of the limbs; cold *hands* and FEET; cramps in calf; in soles. Eruptions on limbs; thin white scales; vesicles. Excoriation between the thighs. Formication of the feet. Heaviness, a tired feeling in lower limbs, in feet. Itching of all the limbs. Jerking in the lower limbs. Lameness in the limbs. Numbness in the feet. Pain in the limbs; in the joints, during chill; neuralgic pain in limbs; RHEUMATIC; gouty pains; upper limbs; right arm *rheumatic;* shoulder; rheumatic pain in shoulder and elbow; palms painful; pain in fingers.

Pain in lower limbs; sciatica worse walking; in the hip; thigh when walking; knee. Aching down front of legs; bruised pain in limbs from continued motion; burning feet and soles, crampy pain in calf; flying pains in fingers, palms and forearms; drawing pains in lower limbs, thigh, knees, calf; neuralgic pain from axilla to little finger, stitching pain in hip, thigh, hip to knee on motion; knee, leg; tearing pains in upper limbs, in lower limbs, in thigh, legs, ankles, foot. Perspiration of hands, of feet. Pulsation of limbs. Restlessness of the limbs, upper limbs, lower limbs, legs. Stiffness of limbs, *joints,* wrists. Swelling of limbs: *dropsical;* legs; feet. Trembling hands; lower limbs. Twitching upper limbs; thighs. Weakness of the limbs; upper limbs; hands; *lower limbs;* thighs; *legs;* ANKLES; feet.

The sleep is deep. Dreams: amorous; *anxious; frightful;* of murder; nightmare; pleasant; vexations; vivid. Late falling asleep; restless sleep. Sleepi-ness in the afternoon. Sleeplessness before midnight; *after midnight;* with sleepiness. Unrefreshing sleep. WALKING EARLY, frequently.

Chill morning; *forenoon;* evening in bed; in cold air; coldness comes on at night in bed; chilliness, internal chill, shaking chill in the morning; chill at 2 A.M.; 1 P.M.; 2 P.M.; the chill is relieved in a warm room.

Fever at night, dry heat, flushes of heat, perspiration absent.

Perspiration: morning; *nights;* from anxiety; in bed; cold; on coughing; on slight exertion; following the fever; on motion; profuse at night; symptoms worse while perspiring; aversion to uncovering while perspiring.

Burning skin; cold skin; desquamation. Liver spots, red spots, yellow skin; dryness of the skin. Eruptions: blisters; boils; burning; moist; *herpes;* itching in warmth; painful; pimples; scaly; thin white scales; stinging, suppurating tubercles; urticaria; nodules; vesicular erysipelas, with swelling, worse after scratching; formication of skin; itching, crawling, worse after scratching. Swelling of skin with burning. Ulcers: burning; deep; yellow discharge; spreading; *stinging.*

NATRUM CARBONICUM

Proved by Hahnemann, Hering and others. Persons who are in the habit of taking carbonate of soda for sour stomach get a proving of this remedy. I have met some of these people and been able to confirm many *Natrum* symptoms.

Old dyspeptics who are always belching and have sour stomach and rheumatism; after twenty years they are stoop-shouldered, pale, sensitive to cold, chilly, aggravated by the least draft; require much clothing; unable to resist the cold or the heat; require a medium climate; are worse from the changes of the weather; their digestive, rheumatic, and gouty troubles are all worse from the weather changes. A state of trepidation from the slightest noise, the slam of a door; nervous excitement and palpitation with great prostration; nervous weakness with trepidation; weakness from slight exertion of mind or body; internal and external trembling. The rattling of paper causes palpitation, irritability and melancholy. Estrangement from family and friends. Aversion to mankind and to society; to relatives, to strangers; feels a great division between himself and them; sensitive to certain persons. Music causes a tendency to suicide, melancholy, weeping and trepidation; playing the piano is so exhausting that she must lie down; music causes great sadness which increases to religious insanity. This is true of all the *Sodiums,* but especially so of Natrum carb; aggravation from the slam of a door, a pistol shot, which causes headache and complaints in general, aggravated from music.

The more soda these patients take, the more flatulent do they become; they are stoop-shouldered; digestion is difficult, and finally milk will not digest at all, bringing on a diarrhœa with undigested, lienteric stools; also, starch causes flatulence and looseness of the bowels. Many symptoms from drinking cold water when overheated.

Urine offensive like that of a horse, from a vegetable or milk diet. This is not so marked as in *Nitric ac.,* but resembles it.

Natrum carb. throws out eruptions upon the knuckles and finger-tips; also the toes; vesicular eruptions open up and form ulcers on the joints or finger-tips. *Borax, Sepia, Ars.,* and Natrum carb. are the remedies most inclined to produce ulceration of the tips and kunckles of the fingers, and also the toes.

Vesicular eruptions on the body in patches and circles; the herpes family is especially related to Natr. carb.; zona, herpes labialis, herpes preputialis; patches as large as a dollar on the hips, thighs and back. Smaller patches show vesicles containing a white serum; burning, smarting and itching, better from scratching. The eruption passes away with a crust, but will often ulcerate, it does not heal and an ulcer forms. Circulation feeble; wounds suppurate. Feet and skin burn. Crusty eruptions on the skin that have not been vesicular; but most Natr. carb. and *Natr. mur.* eruptions are of the vesicular form. Tingling, biting, itching, changing place, now here and now there; cold skin; sweaty body.

Nervous exhaustion, physical exhaustion, weakness of mind and body. Bookkeepers lose the ability to add up figures. In reading a page, the one previous to it soon goes out of the mind. The memory will not hold out from the beginning to the end of a sentence. Forgets what he reads. Confusion of mind follows and then he is unable to perform any mental labor. Men become so fatigued from the details of business that a confusion of the mind comes over them, they get brain-fag.

Oversensitive to heat, especially after sunstroke, even some years after; has to be well shaded when walking in the sun, must seek a cool or dark place; the patient has not had the proper acute remedy during the attack; the remedy is aggravated by both cold and heat, but this is a special aggravation from the heat of the sun; head troubles are not worse from cold in Natr. carb. Old cases of brain-fag with weakness and trepidation. The body troubles are aggravated from cold and in the winter; as cold as if he had no blood in the body, extremities cold, and he cannot get them warm; cold as ice to the knees and elbows. The body and extremities are worse in winter, the head in summer.

Anxious trembling and sweating during pains.

The senses are all disturbed; oversensitive to light; pain in the eyes from a bright light.

Oversensitive hearing; little noises seem enormous, like thunder; the crumpling of paper seems like the crashing of a waterfall.

Taste perverted, too sensitive, so that the tasting of things ordinarily grateful becomes painful; sometimes loss of taste.

Loss of smell. Hay fever, catarrhal fever; where catarrhal conditions are present there is copious, thick, yellow, purulent discharge from the eyes, nose, vagina. The vesicles are filled with thin, white serum, but the pustule, when it ruptures, throws out a thick, yellow discharge. Leucorrhœa thick, yellow, ropy; gonorrhœa of the same character; thick, yellow, ropy, purulent discharge from the bladder which clogs up the urethra when urinating.

Otalgia, with sharp, darting, piercing pains; when the mental state, the chilliness and other generals are present.

The discharges are commonly offensive.

Coryzas trouble much; always has a cold in the head; the watery discharge is of short duration, and is soon followed by a thick copious flow of yellow mucus. Ulceration, thick crusts; sleeps at night with the mouth open; dry, yellow crusts are blown out with pain and bleeding. The catarrh increases with each fresh cold, until it becomes fœtid; the bones of the nose are affected; almost a constant headache over the eyes, in the forehead. at the root of the nose; congestive headaches, worse from change of weather, cold room, damp weather; increased by every storm. Most fœtid ozæna, mucous membranes ulcerated and destroyed.

Pale face with blue ring around the eyes, yellow blotches on the forehead, puffiness. There is puffiness in general; the hands, feet, face pit on pressure; infiltration of the cellular tissue; those states of the heart and kidneys that favour dropsies; old malarial cases, flesh doughy; urine albuminous.

Enlargement of the glands with induration, axillary, inguinal, abdominal, salivary Especially suitable for enlargement of the prostate in old men. Chronic enlargement of the parotids, slow and of long duration; of the tonsils.

Ulcerations of the mouth; nursing sore mouth in women; thrush in infants; little white aphthous patches, especially in nervous, withered infants who cannot stand any kind of milk, who have diarrhœa from milk; they thrive better on cereals; when asleep the child jumps, cries, springs up and grasps the mother; a nervous, cold baby, easily startled like the *Borax* baby. So are the *Natrum* babies in general.

Accumulation of mucus in the throat and posterior nares, generally yellow in color, while with *Natr. mur.* it is white; the latter spits up copious, thick, white mouthfuls.

Natr. carb. is ameliorated by eating; when chilly, he eats and is able to keep warm; the pains are ameliorated after eating; he has an all-gone feeling and pain in the stomach which drives him to eat; he gets hungry at 5 A.M. and 11 P.M., 5 A.M. Is the favorite time for the Natr. carb. aggravation; he becomes so hungry at this time that he is forced out of bed to eat something, which also ameliorates the pain. Headache, chilliness, and palpitation better from eating (*Ignat., Sepia, Sulph.*).

Nervous hunger in pregnant women, who cannot sleep unless they get up at night and eat crackers, calls for *Psorinum.*

Locomotor ataxia with its fulgurating pains, amel. by eating; gnawing, all-gone, hungry feeling in the stomach. Soles numb, in males erections and priapism, sensitive thighs, hypersensitive spine; the results of too much excitement. Emissions; ejaculation of semen premature.

Thirst in the afternoon, incessant; thirst between chill and heat; great desire for cold water a few hours after dinner. Extreme aversion to milk.

Flatulency and accumulation of wind in the bowels; diarrhœa; stool yellow, soft with violent tenesmus and urging; a yellow substance like the pulp of an orange in the stool; *diarrhœa from milk.* The most troublesome constipation; stool hard, dark, smooth and crumbling. All the *Natrums* take away the desire to go to stool; no ability to bear down; stool large and hard, great effort to pass it.

Prostatorrhœa after urinating and a difficult stool.

Sterility, a constitutional state in a woman where she is unable to conceive; she is nervous, cold to the knees and elbows; cold body in winter, hot head in summer; always tired; relaxation of the sphincter vaginæ causing the seminal fluid to gush out as soon as ejaculated by the male, thus causing sterility. There may be a spasm of the sphincter, producing the same effect, or a clot of blood or mucus shoots from the vagina with noisy flatus Nervous, fidgety, excitable, lean, dyspeptic women, not hysterical. Menses too soon or too late; neuralgias, oversensitive to drafts and dampness, sensitive spine, legs numb; leucorrhœa yellowish-green, copious.

Paralytic states; ptosis or spasms of the lids; difficult swallowing, must drink much water to wash the food down on account of paralysis of the pharynx; paralysis of the bowels, cannot bear down at stool; stool like sheep's dung; paralysis of the left lower extremity with tingling.

Palpitation at night when ascending and while lying on left side. Many spinal symptoms. Goitre. Stiffness of the neck, violent backache after walking. Rheumatic pains in the extremities. Jerking in all the limbs. Stumbling while walking. Weak ankles in children. Heaviness of the legs. Pains in the hollow of the knees on motion. Tension in the bend of the knee. Easy dislocation of the ankle. The soles burn while walking. Ulceration of the heel from blisters. Icy cold feet. Weakness of the legs. Vesicles on tips of fingers and toes. Spots and tubercles on the skin. Skin dry and cracked. Itching and crawling.

NATRUM MURIATICUM

Salt is so common an article of diet that it has been assumed that it could be of no use in medicine. This is only the opinion of men who operate entirely on the tissues. There are no constitutional effects from crude salt.

One may find an individual growing thin with all the symptoms of salt; he is taking salt in great quantities, but digesting none of it. Salt will be found in the stool, for it does not enter into the life. There is a Natr. mur. inanition, a starving for salt. The same is true of lime. Children can get plenty of lime from their food and that is better when the salt or the lime is given in such shape that it cannot be resisted by the internal man—aimed not at the house he lives in, but at the individual himself—then the bone, salt inanition, the Natr. mur. inanition, will soon pass away. We do not with our small dose supply the salt that the system needs, but we cure the internal disease, we turn into order the internal physical man, and then the tissues get salt enough from the food. Drugs must all be administered in suitable form. We may need to go higher and higher until the secret spring is touched.

Natr. mur. is a deep acting, long acting remedy. It takes a wonderful hold of the economy, making changes that are lasting when given in potentized doses.

A great deal is presented that can be seen by looking at the patient, so that we say: this looks like a Natr. mur. patient. Experienced physicians learn to classify patients by appearance. The skin is shiny, pale, waxy, looks as if greased. There is a wonderful prostration of a peculiar kind. Emaciation weakness, nervous prostration, nervous irritability.

There is a long chain of mental symptoms; hysterical condition of the mind and body; weeping alternating with laughing; irresistible laughing at unsuitable times; prolonged, spasmodic laughter. This will be followed by tearfulness, great sadness, joylessness. No matter how cheering the circumstances are she cannot bring herself into the state of being joyful. She is benumbed to impressions, easily takes on grief, grieves over nothing. Unpleasant occurrences are recalled that she may grieve over them. Consolation aggravated the state of the mind—the melancholy, the tearfulness, sometimes brings on anger. She appears to bid for sympathy and is mad when it is given. Headache comes on with this melancholy. She walks the floor in rage. She is extremely forgetful; cannot cast up accounts; is unable to meditate; forgets what she was going to say; loses the thread of what she is hearing or reading. There is a great prostration of the mind.

Unrequited affection brings on complaints. She is unable to control her affections and falls in love with a married man. She knows that it is foolish, but lies awake with love for him. She falls in love with a coachman. She knows that she is unwise, but cannot help it. In cases of this kind Natr. mur. will turn her mind into order, and she will look back and wonder why she was so silly. This remedy belongs to hysterical girls.

In a mental state where *Ign.* temporarily benefits the symptoms, but does not cure, its chronic, Natr. mur. should be given. It is as well to give Natr. mur. at once if there is an underlying constitutional state too deep for *Ign.*

Aversion to bread, to fats and rich things.

The Natr. mur. patient is greatly disturbed by excitement, is extremely emotional. The whole nervous economy is in a state of fret and irritation, < from noise, the slamming of a door, the ringing of a bell, the firing of a pistol, < music.

The pains are stitching, electric-like shocks, convulsive jerkings of the limbs on falling asleep, twitchings, shooting pains. She is oversensitive to all sorts of influences, is excitable, emotional, intense.

Complaints come on in the warm room, worse in the house, she wants the open air. The mental complaints are > in the open air. She takes cold easily from sweating, but is generally > in the open air, though worse on getting heated, < by sufficient exertion to heat up, but > by moderate exertion in the cold air.

Both *Natr. carb.* and Natr. mur. have the general nervous tension of *Natrum,* but one is a chilly patient, the other warm blooded.

The face is sickly looking, the skin greasy, shiny, sallow, yellow, often chlorotic, covered with vesicular eruptions around the edges of the hair, the ears and back of the neck. There are scaly and squamous eruptions, with great itching, oozing a watery fluid, or sometimes dry. An exfoliation takes place, a shining surface is left. In the meatus, scales form and peel off, leaving an oozing surface. Watery vesicles form about the lips and wings of the nose, about the genitals and anus. Vesicular eruptions, white, oozing a watery fluid, come and go. Great itching of the skin is present.

The skin looks waxy, dropsical. There is great emaciation, the skin looking dry, withered, shrunken. An infant looks like a little old man. There is a down on the face that passes away when improvement sets in. Emaciation takes place from above downward. The collar-bones become prominent and the neck looks scrawny, but the hips and lower limbs remain plump and round. *Lyc.* also has emaciation from above downward. The directions of remedies will often enable us to distinguish one from another.

The characteristic discharge from the mucous membranes is watery or thick whitish, like the white of an egg. There is a marked coryza with a watery discharge, but the constitutional state has thick, white discharges. He hawks out a thick, white discharge in the morning. There are gluey oozings from the eyes. From the ears flows a thick, white, gluey discharge. The leucorrhœa is white and thick. With the gonorrhœa the discharge has existed a long time and become gleety. There is smarting in the urethra only after urination.

The headaches are awful; dreadful pains; bursting, compressing, as if in a vise; the head feels as if the skull would be crushed in. The pains are attended with hammering and throbbing. Pain like little hammers in the head on beginning to move. Hammering pains in the head on waking in the morning. The pain comes on in the latter part of sleep. There is great nervousness during the first part of the night; she falls asleep late and awakes with hammering in the head. There are also headaches beginning at 10 to 11 A.M., lasting until 3 A.M. or evening. The headaches are periodical, every day, or third day, or fourth day. Headaches of those living in malarial districts, > from sleep; the patient must go to bed and be perfectly quiet, > from sweating, headaches associated with intermittent fever. During the chill it seemed as though the head would burst; he is delirious and drinks large quantities of cold water. There is no relief to the head until after the sweat. Sometimes all the symptoms are relieved by the sweat except the headache.

In another form of headache; the greater the pain the more the sweat; sweating does not relieve; the forehead is cold, covered with a cold sweat. When the head is covered warmly he is > moving about in the open air.

Headache due to disturbance of vision where there is inability to focus rapidly enough. Headache < from noise.

Headache involving the whole back of the head and even going down the spine in troubles following the brain diseases, hydrocephalus.

In spinal troubles, when there is great sensitiveness to pressure—an irritable spine. The vertebræ are sensitive and there is a great deal of aching along the spine. Coughing aggravates the pain in the spine, also walking makes it worse, but it is > from lying on something hard, or pressing the back up against something hard; they may sit with a pillow or the hand pressed against the back. In menstrual troubles you find the woman lying with some hard object under the spine.

A general nervous trembling pervades the body. There is jerking of the muscles, trembling of the limbs, inability to keep the limbs still, as in *Zincum.*

The stomach and liver are closely related. The stomach is distended with flatus. After eating there is a lump in the stomach. It seems to take a long time for food to digest. < from eating. Whitish, slimy mucus is vomited attended with relief. There is great thirst for cold water, sometimes there is relief from drinking, sometimes the thirst is unquenchable. We find fulness in the region of the liver with stitching, tearing pains. The bowels are distended with gas. There is slowing down of the action of the bowels, the stool being very difficult, in hard, agglomerated lumps. There is slowing down of the action of the bladder. Must wait before the urine will start, and then it comes slowly— dribbles; there is not much force in the flow. After urination there is a sensation as if more urine remained in the bladder. *If anyone is present he cannot pass urine,* cannot pass it in a public place. There is also continued urging, he must pass the urine often.

This remedy and *Natr. sulph.* were used by the homœopaths to clear up chronic diarrhœa, the old army diarrhœa.

Natr. mur. is useful in the complaints of women, in troublesome menstruation. There is a great variety of menstrual complaints: menses too scanty or too free, too late or too soon. We cannot individualize from the menstrual symptoms, we must do it from the constitutional state. Examine every possible function to be sure you have all the symptoms. Examine every organ, not by examining it physically, for results of diseases do not lead to the remedy, but examine the symptoms.

Observe the rapidity with which remedies affect the human system; there are some that are long acting, deep acting. Natr. mur. is one of these. It operates very slowly, bringing about its results after a long time, as it corresponds to complaints that are slow, that are long in action. This does not mean that it will not act rapidly; all remedies act rapidly, but not all act slowly; the longest acting may act in acute diseases, but the short acting cannot act long in chronic diseases. Get the pace, the periodicity of remedies. Some remedies have a continued fever, some a remittent, others an intermittent fever. In *Acon., Bell.* and *Bry.* we have three different paces, three different motions, three different forms of velocity; so in *Sulph., Graph., Natr. mur., Carbo veg.*—a different form, a different development. Some would not hesitate in a continued fever to give *Bell.,* but its complaints come on in great haste, with great violence and have nothing in their nature like a continued fever. This is not like typhoid. *Bell.* and *Aeon.* have no manifestations of typhoid, even if the symptoms are present. Be sure that the remedy has not only the group of symptoms, but also the nature of the case. The typhoid case has a likeness in *Bry.* or *Rhus*, but not in *Bell.* We owe no obedience to man, not even to our parents, after we are old enough to think for ourselves. We owe obedience to truth.

Natr. mur. is a long acting remedy; its symptoms continue for years; it conforms to slow-coming, long-lasting, deep-seated symptoms. It requires a long time for a map to be brought under the influence of it, even when moderately sensitive.

The chill comes in the morning at 10.30; every day, every other day, every third or fourth day. The chill begins in the extremities which become blue; there is throbbing pain in the head, the face is flushed; delirium, talking of everything, constant, maniacal actions. They grow worse until a congestive attack comes. During the entire attack there is thirst for cold water. During the coldness he is not > by heat, not > by piling on the clothing, but wants cold drinks. We would naturally suppose that a person freezing to death would want warm things, but the Natr. mur. patient cannot bear them. The teeth chatter, he tosses from side to side, the bones ache as if they would break, and there is vomiting as in congestive conditions. In the fever he is so hot that the fingers are almost scorched with the intense heat, and he goes into a congestive sleep or stupor. The sweat relieves him; the aching all over is > by the sweat, and in time the headache passes away. There is intense chill, fever and sweat. Sometimes the attacks are in robust, strong people, but usually in the anæmic, in emaciated people full of malaria; lingering, chronic cases. Complaints do not always have this long prodrome. Its most striking use is in cases that have been living a long time in malarial swamps; saturated with the malarial atmosphere; they are anæmic, often dropsical; in old cases that have been mixed with arsenic and quinine, the crude drugs used by the Old School to break the fever as long as the patient is under their sway, but the patient is sick internally even more than before, and when the condition comes back it is generally in its original form; the crude drug is usually unable to change the type of an intermittent fever. Remedies only partly related to the case will change the character of the sickness so that no one can cure the case. The homœopathic remedy will cure intermittent fever every time if you get the right remedy. If there is a failure the case is mixed up so that no one may be able to cure it. First of all a master must realize the case and turn it into order so that it can then be cured. There are few men who never spoil a case of ague, because many cases come from partly developed, masked cases, the symptoms not being all out, especially in cases that have taken homœopathic remedies. The homœopathic failures are the worst failures on earth.

Natr. mur. is irregular enough in its nature to develop the chills into regularity. When it has come into better order. wait: either the whole case will subside, or another remedy will be clear. There are other remedies that can turn cases into order. Often cases spoiled by homœopaths can be turned into order by *Sep.* Marked cases with congestion of the head, aching in the back and nausea are turned into order by *Ipecac.* The cure is permanent after homœopathic prescribing; the chills do not return.

Natr. mur. not only removes the tendency to intermittents, but restores the patient to health, and takes away the tendency to colds—the susceptibility to colds, and to periodicity. It is the susceptibility that is removed. We know that every attack predisposes to another attack. Each attack of ague is more destructive than the previous one. The drugs used increase the susceptibility; the homœopathic remedy removes the susceptibility. Homœopathic treatment tends to simplify the human economy and to make diseases more easily managed. Unless this susceptibility be eradicated, man goes down lower and lower into emaciation—emaciation from above downwards.

Children born in a malarial region are likely to go into marasmus. They have a voracious appetite, a wonderful hunger, eating much, but all the time emaciating.

Conditions of pregnancy. The mammary glands waste, there is wasting of the upper parts of the body. The uterus is intensely sore. The leucorrhœa, which is at first white, turns green. Women take cold in every draft of air. There is pain during sexual congress with dryness of the vagina; a feeling as though sticks pressed into the walls of the vagina; pricking pains. There is dryness of all mucous membranes; everywhere the membranes are dry. The throat is dry, red, patulous; a sensation of a fishbone jagging into it when swallowing; there is inability to swallow without washing down the food with liquids; there is sticking all the way down the œsophagus.

Most prescribers give *Hep.* for every sticking or fishbone sensation in the throat; this is the old keynote, the old routine. *Nitr. ac., Argent. nit., Alum.* and Natr. mur. all have it, but all differently.

Hep.—The tonsils are swollen, full, purple—quinsy. The patient is sensitive to the slightest draught, there is pain in the throat even on putting the hand out of bed; he sweats in the night with no relief; he is sensitive to every impression; feels everything ten times amplified.

Nitr. ac.—There are yellow patches in the throat; ragged, jagged ulcers in the throat, or it is inflamed and purple. The urine smells like horses' urine.

Argent. nit.—There is much hoarseness, the vocal cords being disturbed. The throat is swollen, patulous; the patient wants cold things, cold water, cold air. Adapted to those cases that have had ulceration of the os uteri with cauterization.

Natr. mur.—There is extreme dryness of the mucous membranes, as if they would break; chronic dryness without ulceration. There is much catarrhal discharge like the white of an egg, with dryness of the mucous membranes when not covered by this mucus. The patient is extremely sensitive, sensitive to a change of weather.

Every remedy has its own pace, its order of succession. We must bear in mind the order of succession.

Natr. mur. is useful in old dropsies, especially dropsy of cellular tissues. Sometimes there is dropsy of sacs, dropsy of the brain following acute diseases. In acute spinal meningitis with extreme nervous tension, where there is chronic drawing back of the head, chronic jerking of the head forward. Acute diseases that result in hydrocephalus, or in irritation of the spine. Sometimes useful in abdominal dropsy, but more often in œdema of the lower extremities. Acute dropsies after scarlet fever; the patient is oversensitive, starts in his sleep, rises up in the night with confusion; there are albumen and casts in the urine.

In dropsy after the malaria Natr. mur., when it acts curatively, generally brings back the original chill. The only cure known to man is from above down, from within out, and in the reverse order of coming. When it is otherwise, there is only improvement, not cure. When the symptoms return there is hope; that is the road to cure and there is no other.

The skin symptoms are sometimes very striking. In old lingering cases where the skin looks transparent as if the patient would become dropsical, a waxy, greasy, shiny skin; other remedies with greasy, shiny skin are *Plumb., Thuja, Selen.* These remedies go deep into the life. Any remedy that can produce such wonderful changes is long-acting.

Useful after labor when the mother does not progress well; she is feeble and excitable; the lochia is prolonged, copious and white; the hair falls out from the head and genitals; the milk passes away, or the child does not thrive on it. Useful in afterpains where there is subinvolution of the uterus, the uterus is in a state of prolonged congestion. She is < noise, music, the slamming of a door. She craves salt and has an aversion to bread, wine and fat things. Sour wines disorder the stomach. Natr. mur. will clear up the case, restore the milk, turn the case into order.

Natr. mur. is needed by those chlorotic girls who have a greasy skin, a greenish, yellowish complexion; who menstruate only once in two or three months. The menses are copious, or scanty and watery. Where the symptoms agree, this remedy can eradicate this chlorosis and turn the countenace into a picture of health, but not in a short time. It takes years to establish health in a typical chlorosis; the cut finger bleeds only water; the menstrual flow is only a leucorrhœa; there is pernicious anæmia. Natr. mur., goes deep enough into the life to restore the pink complexion.

NATRUM PHOSPHORICUM

We are not dependent upon Schüessler alone for indications for this remedy, as we have many pathogenetic symptoms. Schuessler's indications were good and mostly confirmed by clinical observations. The author has given this remedy for twenty years to many patients whose nerves were in a fret from mental exertion and sexual excesses and vices. The symptoms are worse in the *morning,* EVENING and *night,* and after midnight. There is marked *anæmia* and *aversion to the open air.* He is aggravated from a draft, from open air, from cold, from becoming cold and after becoming cold, and there is a tendency to frequent taking cold. He is worse from changes in the weather. Chlorosis. Aversion to bathing. Many symptoms come on after coition. He may be a sexual debauche. Many symptoms come on from fasting, and he is generally ameliorated after eating. He is aggravated from any physical exertion. His muscles are flabby, and he is losing flesh. He is disturbed by butter, cold drinks, cold food, *fats,* fruit, MILK, *sour things* and *vinegar.* Formication externally and internally. There is great physical irritability, and later a marked lack of reaction. Many symptoms are aggravated from a jar, or stepping. There is marked lassitude in the morning in hot weather. Constant desire to lie down. Prolonged weakness from loss of fluids. Lying on left side aggravates many symptoms. Worse before and after menses. During menses the symptoms are aggravated afternoon and evening. Numbness in single parts. Orgasm of blood. Stitching, tearing pains, aggravated during a thunderstorm. Pulsation all over the body. Sensation as though a shot was forced through the arteries is a verified symptom. *Oversensitive* in general, and to pain. Shocks through the body, in night while awake. Sitting aggravates. General aggravation during a thunderstorm. Tension in muscles and tendons. Trembling in thunderstorm. Twitching of muscles. *Nervous* and paralytic weakness aggravated in morning, and after exertion. The body smells sour (like *Hepar, Sulph., Lyc.*).

Anger over trifles, and complaints from vexation. Anxiety evening and night; in bed; before midnight; after eating; with fear; during fever; about the future; about his health; on waking. Complaints from bad news. Aversion to company. Concentration difficult. Confusion of mind in the morning; in the evening; after eating, from mental exertion; on waking. Delusions, frightful; thinks he sees dead people; imagines; thinks he is going to have typhoid fever; that he hears footsteps in the next room. Discontented, discouraged, and easily distracted. Dullness of mind while reading. Mental exertion brings on many complaints. He is very excitable. Fear at night; of impending disease; that something will happen; of misfortune; on waking. Fears bad news, *Forgetful.* Easily frightened, and heedless. She is hysterical, and in a hurry. No one works fast enough to suit him. Sometimes his ideas are abundant, and again deficient, and his mind grows sluggish. Impatience. He is indifferent to everything, even to his family. A gradually increasing indolence; a dread of mental and physical work. Irritability; in the morning; during menses; about trifles. Memory weak. Times of mirthfulness. GREAT PROSTRATION OF MIND. Restless and anxious evening and night. Sadness in evening, after emission, during fever, and from music. He is extremely sensitive to music and noise and to his surroundings. He grows serious and silent, and sits by himself quite still for a long time. He is easily startled, from fright, from noise, on falling asleep, and during sleep. Spells of stupefaction creep over him. His friends call him suspicious. Indisposed to talk. His thoughts wander. He is growing timid and bashful. Weeps easily. Mental work becomes impossible and he seems to be approaching imbecility.

Vertigo in the morning; aggravated from mental exertion, while sitting and walking. Tendency to fall.

Congestion in the evening. Heat in head in evening, in forehead and vertex. Flushes of heat after sweat. Tension in the scalp. Eruptions on the head of golden yellow scabs; eczema on the forehead. Fulness in forehead; over the eyes; in the morning; aggravated by mental exertion. Heaviness of the head, and the hair falls out. Pain in the head, morning, afternoon, evening and night, aggravated binding up the hair; *after eating;* must lie down; aggravated from light; lying; before, during and *after menses;* MENTAL EXERTION; after sour milk; motion; motion of head; noise; rising from lying; in a room; *sexual excesses;* after sleep; after stooping; straining eyes; *during a thunderstorm; ,* while walking; warm room; ameliorated in open air; by pressure. The headaches are periodical, pulsating. Pain in forehead aggravated from MENTAL EXERTION; from motion; *over eyes;* in *occiput;* sides of head; temples; in vertex on waking in morning; in vertex and forehead. The pains are bursting, cutting in temples and sides of head; drawing in head and occiput; pressing with sour slimy vomiting; pressing in forehead, outward, over eyes; pressing in occiput, and sides of occiput; pressing in temples; pressing in vertex as if it would open. Stitching in head, in forehead, in sides of head, in temples. Stunning in head and forehead. Tearing in head. Perspiration of forehead. Pulsating in head, forehead, temples and vertex. Shocks in the head. Twitching. Uncovering the head brings on the symptoms.

Dryness of the eyes. Creamy yellow discharges. Heaviness of the lids. Inflammation of the eyes. Scrofulous ophthalmia, and granular lids. Itching and burning of the lids and margin of the lids. Burning lachrymation. must rub the eyes. Pain in the eyes when reading. Burning and cutting. Pressing during menses. Pain as though sand in eyes. Sore, bruised feeling when reading. Stitching pain in eyes. Paralysis of the optic nerve. Photophobia. Pupils dilated. One pupil dilated. Quivering of right eyelid while reading.

Staring. Strabismus. Swollen lids. Yellow sclerotics. Colors before the eyes, dark. Halo around the light. Dim vision for distant objects. Foggy vision; blindness. *Exertion of vision* aggravates many symptoms. Flickering before the eyes morning on rising, at 5 P.M. Mist before the eyes aggravated in gaslight at 8 P.M. Myopia. Sparks before the eyes.

Eruption on the ears. Creamy yellow crusts on the ears. Fulness in ears. Heat and redness of one ear. Itching in the ears. Lobe of right ear burning and itching, must scratch it until it bleeds. Noises in ears, with vertigo, humming, ringing, *roaring,* rushing, singing, whizzing. Pain in ear. Aching in right meatus. Burning. *Stitching* in and behind ear. *Tearing.* Pulsation. Stopped sensation. The hearing is *acute,* acute for voices; impaired, lost.

The patient is subject to fluent coryza, and catarrh of the nose with *thick yellow purulent discharge.* Epistaxis on blowing the nose. Fulness at the root of the nose. The nose is obstructed with mucus and crusts, but the discharge is generally scanty. Offensive odors in the nose in the morning. Ozæna. Pricking in the left nostril brings tears to the eyes. Smell is acute. Soreness in the left nostril. He picks the nose constantly and scales form. Frequent sneezing. Tension over the root of the nose.

Discoloration of the face, bluish; circles around the eyes; earthy, PALE; red blotches but not feverish; red alternating with paleness; yellow, liver spots, white about nose and mouth. Eruptions on the face, on the chin, forehead, lips, about the mouth, ON THE NOSE. Pimples on the forehead. Pustules on the face. Heat in the evening, during chill. The face burns. Itching of the face and nose.

Pain in the face, burning, neuralgic. Shooting in the right cheek. Soreness in the right lower jaw at angle, darting through it. Stitching. Swelling of the glands of the lower jaw. Swelling of the sub-maxillary gland.

Bleeding gums. The tongue is coated yellow. *Yellow at the base,* or dirty white. Roof of mouth coated *golden yellow or creamy.* Dryness of mouth and tongue. Salivation. Sensation of a hair on the tongue, followed by prickly numbness of whole mouth. Speech difficult. Stinging on the tongue. Taste bad on waking, bitter, metallic, saltish, *sour.* Vesicles in mouth and on tongue.

Caries of the teeth. Grinding the teeth during sleep in children. Looseness of the teeth. Pain in the teeth, at night, ameliorated by pressure and external warmth. *Burning,* pressing and pulsating.

Throat and tonsils coated yellow. Dryness of the throat. Mucus forms in throat. Tough clear white mucus in posterior nares. Thick yellow mucus drops from posterior nares, aggravated at night, must sit up to clear the throat. Sensation of a lump in throat. Much hawking. Inflammation of throat. Pain in throat on swallowing. Sore throat on right side, aggravated swallowing. Burning, pricking, stitching. Pulsation in left tonsil. Scraping mucus from posterior tares. Swallows liquids better than solids in sore throat.

The appetite is *increased, ravenous or wanting.* Aversion to food, to meat, to milk, to bread and butter. Desires alcoholic drinks, beer, pungent food, eggs, fried fish, cold drinks. The stomach is disordered by fat and milk. Emptiness, aggravated after eating. Eructation after eating, empty, SOUR; waterbrash. Fulness after eating. Heartburn, heaviness and pressure. Heat in the stomach. Nausea in the morning, evening, during cough, and during headache. Pain in the stomach; after eating; two hours after eating; cramping; gastralgia, several attacks every day with vomiting sour fluids; over-secretion of lactic acid. Gnawing in the stomach. Pressing after eating. Soreness and stitching. Retching. Extreme thirst. Ulceration of the stomach. Sour vomiting. Creamy coating on the tongue. Sour odor of the body. Vomiting on coughing, with headache, of bile, bitter, frothy with headache, of mucus, SOUR in infants fed on milk, sour cheesy masses in intermittent fever; in pregnancy; vomiting yellow, green.

Distension of the abdomen after eating. Sensation of emptiness, after stool. Flatulence, obstinate, after eating. Fulness, gurgling and hardness. Pain afternoon and night, after eating, paroxysmal, before stool. Pain in hypochondria Burning in abdomen. Cramping before stool, causing urging to stool, while walking. Cutting in abdomen. Pressing in the hypogastrium. Soreness in the whole abdomen. Stitching in the abdomen and in liver. Torpid liver. *Rumbling.* Tension.

Constipation with difficult hard stool. Inactivity of the rectum; one day constipated, next day diarrhœa. Diarrhœa morning, night, with colic, after eating, in summer, with flatus. The anus is excoriated; *much flatus;* involuntary stools, involuntary when passing flatus. Sore, itching anus, aggravated in the warmth of the bed. Pain in the rectum after stool. Burning during and after stool. Painful contraction of anus. Cutting during stool. Stitching on walking. Tenesmus. Urging to stool after coition, in a man. Urging ineffectual, unsatisfactory. Weak feeling in the rectum before stool. The stool is bloody, cheesy, crumbling; light colored, bileless stool; *green;* jelly-like masses; pasty; sour-smelling stools; thin yellowish brown stool; watery; yellowish green; yellowish brown. Worms with the stool.

Paralysis of the bladder. Pressing pain in the bladder before urination. Urging to urinate at night, after coition (man); after eating; constant; frequent. Dysuria. Urination frequent, *at night,* during perspiration, involuntary, night, during sleep. Must wait for urine to start. Must press a long time before urine starts. Unsatisfactory urination. Stitching pain in the kidneys. Emission of prostatic fluid during stool. Enlarged prostate. Burning in the urethra during the flow of urine. After stool burning and itching of the meatus. The urine is *albuminous,* burning, cloudy, dark, pale, copious night and morning, offensive, scanty, with mucous sediment.

Erections are troublesome morning and night, continued, frequent, *incomplete,* painful, without desire, violent, *wanting.* Vesicles upon the genitalia. Itching of the scrotum, prepuce and anus. Pain in the spermatic cords and testes. Drawing in spermatic cords. Pressing in testes. Seminal emission *after coition,* without dreams, without erections, *frequent,* unconscious. Sexual passion diminished, or increased, *without erection, vomiting.* Swelling of penis and testes.

Desire increased in the female. Leucorrhœa *after menses,* acrid, *copious, creamy,* honey colored, *sour smelling,* yellow and watery. Menses absent, copious, too frequent, late, pale, painful, *protracted.* Prolapsus of the uterus with a weak sinking feeling after stool. Sterility.

Soreness in trachea. Hoarseness and loss of voice. Respiration is asthmatic, *difficult,* short and sighing.

Cough afternoon, evening in bed, night, during chill, constant, with coryza, after drinking. Dry evening cough with expectoration in the morning. Hacking, hollow, short, racking cough, with irritation in chest or larynx. Loose morning cough. Tickling in larynx and chest. Violent cough. Cough aggravated while sitting. Expectoration in the morning, bloody, greenish, mucous, *offensive,* purulent, thick, viscid, yellow; tasting flat, putrid, salty.

Anxiety in the chest; a bubble starts from the heart and passes through the arteries. Constriction of the chest. Empty sensation in the chest after eating. Pimples on the chest. Sudden feeling of fulness in the upper part of the chest. Oppression of the chest. Pain in the chest after dinner, from deep breathing, during cough. Pain in the heart. Aching, pressing in the chest. Burning deep in the chest, aggravated on the right side, evening in bed. Cutting, pressing. Rawness in chest on coughing. Soreness in chest. Stitching in the chest, sides of chest, aggravated in left side. PALPITATION, *anxious,* after eating; aggravated from *noise,* lying on the left side, *during a thunderstorm.* Phthisis florida in young people. Trembling of heart, after menses, on ascending stairs.

Heavy dragging in the back. Itching of the skin of the back. Pain in the back at night, during menses, on motion, from *sexual excesses,* while sitting. Pain in the dorsal region; left scapula, between scapulæ. Pain in lumbar region, during menses. Pain in sacrum, during menses. Aching in back during menses in lumbar region. Sore bruised back and spine. *Spinal irritation.* Burning in lumbar region and in the spine. Drawing in the back. Sharp in right sacro-iliac junction. Stitching in lumbar region.

Perspiration of the back. Stiffness both sides of neck. Swelling of the glands of the neck. Weakness of the back toward evening, in the lumbar region, after emissions.

COLD HANDS, *legs and feet.* Feet icy cold during menses, in daytime, burn at night in bed. Contraction of extensors in forearm while writing. Sore stinging corns. Cramp in calves and feet. Cramp in hands, while writing. Cracking in joints. Eruption on limbs, vesicles; pimples and vesicles on lower limbs; pimples on nates, eczema of ankles. Formication of upper limbs and of feet. Heat of hands and feet. Heaviness of limbs, of lower limbs, legs and feet. Itching of limbs, upper limbs, lower limbs, *ankles.* Numbness of limbs, upper limbs, right hand and arm, of fingers, right fingers, of feet. Pain in the limbs. Gouty, rheumatic joints, wrist. Rheumatic pain in shoulder (right). Pain in leg, calf, ankle, ball of foot, first toe. Bruised pain in limbs, lower limbs, knee, leg. Burning hands and soles. Crampy pain in left hand and index finger. Drawing in forearm, wrist during menses, hand, joints, left shoulder, hip and knee. Pressure in shoulder. Stitching in shoulder and fingers, in hip, *thigh,* knee, soles, heel. Tearing in limbs, joints, upper limbs, shoulder, upper arm, elbow, fingers; lower limbs, hip, knee, leg, foot, toes. Perspiration of hands and feet. Restless legs. Shortening of tendons in hollow of knee, also after menses. Stiffness of joints. Swelling of fingers; of lower limbs, of feet. Tension in hamstrings and calf. Trembling in hands, in knees after emissions. Twitching of muscles. Weakness of upper limbs, of hands, of right wrist and left ankle after menses; of lower limbs, thighs, ANKLES. Weakness of ankles in children (*Nat. c.*). Sudden giving way of legs while walking.

Very deep sleep. The patient is a great dreamer. Dreams anxious, amorous, of dead people, distressing, of previous events, of fire, *frightful,* nightmare, *pleasant,* vexatious and vivid. Falling asleep in the chair. The sleep is restless. Sleepiness all day and after dinner, most in *forenoon.* Sleepless before midnight, after, midnight, from crowding of thoughts. Sleepiness, yet cannot sleep. Unrefreshing sleep. Wakeful from 12 to 3 A.M. Waking early, 5 A.M. unrested. Waking late.

Coldness in evening in bed, in cold air. Chilliness in evening, during menses, after eating. Shaking chill. One-sided coldness. Internal chill. Fever flushes of heat and headache every afternoon. Cannot get to sleep, feels so hot. Fever with sweat during sleep. Intermittent fever with vomiting of sour masses. Perspiration in the *daytime,* morning, afternoon, during the night. Anxious sweat. Cold sweat. Perspiration on coughing, on *slight exertion.* Profuse sweat in the morning and during the night with great nervous weakness. Sour-smelling sweat. The infant smells sour.

Biting, burning, or coldness of the skin. Liver spots; red spots, yellow spots, and jaundiced skin. Dry skin. Dry, burning eruptions; blisters, boils, burning, desquamating, moist, dry, herpetic, painful, phagedenic, pimples, golden yellow scales; suppurating, urticaria, vesicular. Eczema with honey colored discharge. Erysipelas. Excoriation. Formication. Freckles. Gnawing pain in skin. *Inactivity* of the skin. Itching, biting, burning, crawling, creeping, stinging, ameliorated by scratching, aggravated by warmth of bed. *Sensitive skin.* Sore feeling in the skin. Sticking in skin. Swelling of skin, of affected parts. Dropsical skin. Ulcerative pain. Ulcers; biting, burning, crawling, deep; discharge offensive and yellow; fistulous, inflamed, red areola, sensitive, stinging, suppurating, swollen, unhealthy. Unhealthy skin. Warts.

NATRUM SILICATUM

The times of aggravation of the symptoms of this remedy are morning, *forenoon, evening, night,* and after midnight; he feels amelioration sometimes during the forenoon. Formation of recurrent abscesses; it relieves the pain and hastens the flow of pus in abscesses. AVERSION TO THE OPEN AIR; the symptoms are worse in the open air and he is extremely sensitive to a draft of air. The symptoms are worse from stimulants. He is sensitive to every change of weather from warm to cold and to cold damp weather. He feels all used up after coition. He is worse from cold in general, from cold air, from becoming cold, and after becoming cold; he is always taking cold. He feels worse and his symptoms are worse after eating. He is worse from slight exertion. He emaciates rapidly. Symptoms are worse after cold food, cold drinks, fat food, and milk. *There is a marked lack of vital heat.* Heaviness felt in body and limbs. Formication through the body. Induration of glands. Inflammation of external parts; of bone, excessive physical irritability and sensitiveness to jarring. Great *lassitude and desire to lie down;* lying ameliorates and motion aggravates. This remedy is full of pain; pain in the bones; the pains in the body are boring, burning, *cutting,* pressing, sore, *stitching and tearing.* Pressure ameliorates many symptoms. There is a marked pulsation felt all over the body and in the limbs. Pulse fast in the evening and until 2 a.m. There is marked sensitiveness in the remedy. The symptoms are worse after sleep, worse from touch, when walking and after wine. Trembling and twitching. Great weakness in the morning, from walking; NERVOUS WEAKNESS. He is weary throughout the proving.

He becomes angry when contradicted. Anxiety in the evening and during the night but especially before midnight; anxiety at night in bed; after eating; on waking; during the night. Concentration of mind is difficult. He has lost all confidence in his own judgment. There is confusion of mind in the morning and in the evening; after eating; FROM MENTAL EXERTION; on waking. He is over-conscientious and there are moments of being discouraged and sometimes despair. Dullness of mind on waking. Worse from reading or any *mental exertion;* all of the mental symptoms are worse from *mental exertion.* He is very excitable. He wakes up with anxiety and fear. His memory is very weak; he forgets almost everything. He is *easily frightened.* The female provers become quite hysterical. The first stage of imbecility is the general character of many mental symptoms. He is very indifferent to his friends and surroundings; irresolution is a strong feature and he cannot conclude to do one thing or the other. Irritability in the evening; after coition; after sleep. He no longer desires to live and seems to loathe life. A high degree of mental prostration prevails. Restless during the night driving him out of bed and with it there is great anxiety. Sadness during menses, with weeping. Extreme sensitiveness to noise. Starting from fright; *from noise;* from sleep. Indisposed to take a part in any conversation. Vertigo at night; with headache; from mental exertion; while walking; when turning in bed.

The following particulars will always yield to this remedy whenever the above generals strongly predominate.

There is tension of the scalp and especially of the forehead; *falling of the hair;* hyperæmia, fulness and heat of the head at night, felt especially in the forehead; heaviness of the head and forehead. It is wonderful headache remedy; the headaches are of many kinds and the circumstances numerous. Pain morning, afternoon, *evening* or night; pain worse after eating; from motion, *from exertion;* MENTAL EXERTION; before and during menses; binding up the hair in women; *from noise;* rising from sitting; sitting after sleep; stooping; straining eyes; walking; wine. Pressure ameliorates; very hot applications are grateful. It is very useful in periodical headaches. With coryza there is severe pain in the forehead especially on the left side; comes on in the morning; pain in forehead above the eyes; pain in OCCIPUT; sides of head; temples; pain bursting; drawing in forehead; dull, jerking. Pressing from mental exertion in forehead, as if brain would be forced out; pressing in occiput, temples, forehead; stitching in forehead; sides of head; temples; stunning pains in the head; forehead, sides of head, temples; perspiration of forehead; pulsation in head; forehead, vertex; twitching of the head. Uncovering the head brings on headache.

The lids are stuck together in the morning. Fistula lachrymalis. Heaviness of the lids; inflammation with ulceration of the cornea; inflammation of the lids; itching of the eyes and lachrymation. Biting, burning, pressing, sore, stitching pains in eyes. Paralysis of the optic nerve. Photophobia, especially in daylight. Staring appearance, swollen lids; dark colors before the eyes; sparks in the field of vision. The vision is dim. Symptoms are worse from exertion of vision.

Itching in the ears; noises in the ear with vertigo; humming, ringing and roaring in ears; pain in ears and behind ears; stitching. Tearing in and behind ears; pulsation in ears. Stopped sensation. Hearing is acute for noise. Hearing is impaired.

Fluent coryza with cough. It cures catarrh of the nose with crusts and greenish, *offensive, purulent, thick* or *yellow* discharges. Epistaxis in the morning and on blowing the nose. The nose is obstructed during the night. Smell acute at first, later lost. Much sneezing. Ulcer high up in nose.

The lips are cracked; the face is pale, even earthy, or red with headaches; sometimes yellow. Eruptions on face worse on nose; herpes around lips; vesicles on lips; itching. Some pain in face. The glands of lower jaw swollen; *swelling of the submaxillary glands* and lips; ulcer on the Iip.

Bleeding gums; *dryness of the mouth;* saliva flows freely; speech is difficult. Taste is bitter, bloody. Metallic; sour. The teeth are painful during the night, and after eating; better from warmth. The pains are boring, digging, pulsating and stitching. The teeth are sensitive.

The throat is inflamed and red, *very dry.* He hawks much to clear the throat of thick, yellow mucus; sensation of lump in the throat; pain in the throat on swallowing; burning and stitching in the throat. Swallowing is difficult. It cures goitre and swollen cervical glands.

The appetite is increased and even ravenous; aversion to meat; a sensation of emptiness in the stomach. Eructations after eating; empty, tasting like food, sour, waterbrash. Many symptoms of stomach are better after eructations. Fulness after eating. Heartburn. Weight in the stomach and hiccough after eating; loathing of food; nausea morning and evening, and during diarrhœa; pains in stomach after eating; cramping, pressing, after eating; stitching pain; sore and tender to touch. Pulsation in the stomach. Retching. Sensation of a stone in the stomach. Extreme thirst, worse at night; during chill. Vomiting on coughing; after milk; bile, bitter; mucus.

Distension after eating; obstructed flatulence; fulness and gurgling; a commotion in the abdomen. Hard, heavy abdomen. Pain in morning, afternoon, night; after eating; in hypogastrium; in hypochondrium; burning, cramping, cutting, stitching in hypochondria, liver and spleen; rumbling in bowels. Sensation of tightness in abdomen.

Constipation with difficult even soft stool; fruitless urging to stool; inactivity of the rectum; unsatisfactory stool. Constricted anus. Diarrhœa morning and evening, from milk, painless; stool bloody, frequent, slimy, thin, watery; constipation with stool hard, light colored, soft, scanty. Formication of the anus and much flatus. Itching. Pain after stool; burning during and after a hard stool; soreness of anus, with cutting, stitching and tenesmus.

Pressing in the bladder; tenesmus; constant or frequent urging to urinate; worse during the night; urination frequent during the night. Involuntary urination at night. Must wait long for urine to start in the morning. After urination he feels that he has not finished. Emission of prostatic fluid during a difficult stool; enlarged prostate. Burning during urination. The urine is hot, cloudy, *copious.*

Troublesome, painful, violent erections; the glans penis is inflamed; itching of the penis and scrotum; pain in the testes; seminal emissions. Sexual passion increased. Swelling of the testes. It greatly restrains the progress of cancer of the cervix uteri. The desire is much increased. Induration of the cervix. Leucorrhœa copious and yellow before menses; menses absent, copious; frequent or late; protracted, scanty. Bearing down in the pelvis as in prolapsus. Pain in left ovary during coition.

Irritation in the larynx; hoarseness; respiration is rapid; asthmatic, *deep, difficult, short.*

Cough in daytime, morning, afternoon, evening, *night;* dry, hacking cough in morning; lose cough in the morning; cough from irritation in the larynx; cough during chill, cough with expectoration morning and evening. Expectoration bloody, greenish; *offensive, purulent;* viscid, yellow, tasting putrid, salty.

Constriction and oppression of the chest; pain in chest on coughing. Pressing in the region of heart. Rawness in chest on coughing; chest feels sore and bruised on coughing; stitching in sides of chest, especially the right. Palpitation strong, worse at night, after eating. Swelling of the axillary glands.

Coldness of the back; itching of the skin of the back; pain in the back during menses; on motion; while sitting. Pain between the scapulæ; pain in lumbar region in stooping pain in sacrum; aching in back; lumbar region; burning in lumbar region; drawing in cervical region; soreness in spine; stitching between scapulæ; in lumbar region, in sacrum. Perspiration on the back; stiffness of the cervical region; during headache. Tension in the cervical region. Weak feeling in small of the back.

Awkwardness in using the hands and in walking. Coldness of hands, lower limbs, *legs.* FEET; evening in bed; corns that are sore and sting; cracked skin of hands and fingers. Cramp in calf, foot, toes. Vesicles on fingers and lower limbs. Hear of hands; of feet; of soles. Heaviness of upper limbs; *lower limbs;* feet. Itching of upper limbs; lower limbs; legs, *soles,* toes. Jerking of limbs during sleep. Jerking of lower limbs. Numbness of the right arm in the morning; of the arm lain on; of feet. Pain in joints, pain in shoulder. Bruised pain in limbs. Drawing pain in elbow; forearm; lower limbs; thighs; knee; leg Stitching in hip, thighs, knees, legs, ankles, soles, heels. Tearing in limbs joints; upper limbs; shoulders; upper arm; elbow; wrist; fingers. Tearing in *hip,* thigh, knee, leg, foot, toes. Paralytic weakness of the sides of body right arm and right lower limb. Perspiration of hands and *feet.* Restless arm and feet. Stiffness of the limbs. Œdematous swelling of feet and, legs. Tension of calf. Tingling of fingers. Trembling of hands and lower limbs. Twitching in limbs; upper limbs; forearm; thighs. Weakness of limbs; upper limbs; hand lower limbs; thighs, *legs,* ANKLES; feet.

Dreams ANXIOUS; previous events; frightful; of ghosts; nightmare; murder pleasant; VIVID,. Falling asleep late. Restless sleep. Sleeplessness before midnight, *after midnight;* with sleepiness. Sleep unrefreshing; waking too early: too frequent. Sleepless during nightly fevers.

Chill morning; forenoon; evening in bed. Chill in cold air; after eating; one-sided, chilliness. Shaking chill. Internal chill. Flushes of heat. Fever without chill or sweat from 9 p.m. until 2 a.m. with very red face and hot skin.

Perspiration nights; cold, on *least exertion; profuse.*

Biting of the skin after scratching. Blotches here and there in the skin. Burning skin. Coldness of the skin. Desquamation. Dry burning skin. Erup-. tions; boils; burning, moist; dry; herpetic; itching; painful; pimples; sting-ing; urticaria; vesicular. Formication. Itching, biting, burning, crawling, worse after scratching. Itching stinging. Moisture after scratching. Sensitive sore skin. Unhealthy skin.

NATRUM SULPHURICUM

This is one of our most frequently indicated constitutional remedies. The symptoms appear in the morning, evening and during the night, especially before midnight. Some symptoms are better after breakfast, during the daytime and after midnight, *except the sweat.* It is a very useful remedy for complaints following neglected gonorrhœa. The symptoms and the constitutional state of the patient are worse in wet weather. It is useful in patients who live near waterways and have suffered long from malarial influences. It is useful as an antidote to the abuse of quinine. It especially belongs to patients of the neuropathic and bilious constitution. He is extremely sensitive to the night air. He suffers from universal catarrh and the discharges are generally greenish. It cures dropsical conditions. Sensitive to touch and pressure; oversensitive mentally and physically. Very sensitive to pain. The pains are very numerous; dull pains, sharp pains, all better from motion. Bruised feeling all over. Strong desire for open air and better while walking in the open air. Sensitive to a warm room, though he is sometimes sensitive to cold and must have warm clothing. The feeling of fulness or distension is found in many places; in the head, in the ear, in the abdomen, in the veins generally. Complaints all worse in the spring and in warm weather. General physical restlessness and anxiety. Marked weakness and trembling with internal pulsations and rapid heart. Twitching of muscles. Complaints from injuries of head and spine. The symptoms all worse during rest. Rheumatic complaints all over the body. He is compelled to lie on the back. Convulsions from injuries of the head. Sycotic conditions with a history of warts and condylomata. Anxiety in the morning which passes off after breakfast; in the evening in bed; at night before midnight; during fever, about the future; anxiety and loathing of life with suicidal impulse, must use all self-control to prevent taking his life. A woman during gestation attempted several times to hang herself, after this remedy she was cheerful and there was no return of the suicidal disposition. Cheerful after stool. Music makes her sad. Sadness in the morning, which passes off after breakfast. Extremely irritable in the morning. Violent anger which is followed by jaundice. Aversion to company. Dislikes to speak or to be spoken to. Dullness of mind and excitability. Mental exertion brings on mental symptoms. Mental troubles come on from injuries of the head. A young man became very sad and subject to attacks of vertigo, and neglected his business after being hit on the side of the head by a base ball. He was entiraly free from all symptoms after taking this remedy. Fear of a crowd; of evil; of people. Forgetful, easily frightened, hysterical; indifferent; indolent; insanity. She is oversensitive and suspicious. Starting from fright or noise and in sleep. Subject to vertigo, congestive headaches with fulness and heat. Pressing outward in the head with pulsation. Periodical headaches with vomiting bile. The pains are worse when thinking of them and better by pressure in the open air and when lying. Pulsation in the temples when walking. Splitting pain in the vertex. Heat of the vertex. Headache in the morning on waking. Mental exertion brings on headaches. Sensation as of brain falling to side lain on. Headache with intermittent fever. Violent occipital headache with pain in the nape of the neck. Headache from injuries of the head. Itching of the scalp. Formication. Eczema of the scalp with much moisture.

Photophobia and head complaints from looking into the light. Lachrymation and dim vision, jaundiced eyes; inflamed eyes with many blisters. Burning in the eyes morning and evening. Greenish discharge from the eyes. Lids stuck together in the morning. Granular lids. Scrofulous inflammation of the conjunctiva. Redness, swelling and burning of the margins of the lids. Heaviness of lids. Pressing in eyes when using eyes. Itching of the eyes in the morning.

Chirping in the ears in the evening; during chill and fever. Flapping sensation in the ears. Ringing in the ears. Pressing out feeling in the ears. Earache as if something was forcing its way out. Stitching pains in ears, worse entering warm room from cold air; in damp weather. Earache. Complaint worse on right side. Heat in right ear in evening. Catarrh of right ear. Stopped sensation in right ear. Purulent discharge from the ears.

Catarrhal discharge from nose, yellowish green. Epistaxis before and during menses; in afternoon and evening. Dryness and burning in the nose. Obstructed with mucus in the night. Mucus drawn from posterior nares tasting salty. Sneezing with fluent coryza and influenza. Epidemic influenza. Chunks of dried mucus blow from high up in nose.

Itching of the face with eczema. Sickly expression and jaundiced skin. Vesicles and pimples on the face. Vesicles on the lower lip and around the mouth. Pimples on the chin burning on touch.

The teeth become loose and fall out in sycotic constitution. The gums separate from the teeth. Pain in the teeth worse from warm things, better from cold drinks and the cold air. Gums red, ulcerate and burn. Blisters on the gums. The mouth is always slimy. Much mucus forms in the mouth and throat. Taste is bitter and tongue is heavily coated a dirty greenish brown. Blisters on the tongue and roof of the mouth. Burning in the roof of the mouth during menses. Numbness in the mouth. Salivation.

Chronic inflammation of the throat with copious viscid white mucus. Dry sensation in throat. Pain in throat on swallowing food. Choking feeling in the throat when walking. It is often needed in goitre. Great thirst in the evening; for very cold drinks; during chill and fever. Aversion to bread and meat. Qualmishness after farinaceous foods; hiccough after bread in evening. Eructations of sour water; of bitter fluid. Nausea before breakfast. Constant nausea. Vomiting of sour or bitter fluid. Vomiting of green bile with colic. The stomach feels distended and heavy. Pulsation in the stomach after breakfast. Extreme cases of gastric weakness with acidity. Can digest only the simpler foods. Digestion very slow. This remedy has cured many complaints of the liver; congested, enlarged, sore liver. Pain in the liver from lying on the right side. Dragging in the right hypochondrium when lying on the left side (*Mag. m., Card. in., Ptel.*), soreness and itching in the liver when walking. Sharp pains in the liver on deep inspiration. The liver is disturbed by mental exertion and anger. The liver seems to manufacture an excess of bile. Perverted viscid bile that readily forms gall-stones. It causes the liver to make healthy bile which is the natural solvent of gall-stones, when given in homœopathic doses at long intervals. It has cured many cases of gall-stone colic. It has removed gall-stones in many cases. Sensitive to clothing over the hypochondria. The following three cases will testify:

Case I.—Woman, married, grown children. Aged 37. Headache followed by vomiting of bile for several years. Face purple. Heat ameliorates the pain. Pain begins in right eye, spreads over the forehead with a dragging feeling in back of head. Pain in sacrum extends to thighs, aggravated on right side. Nervous, easily startled, apprehensive. Intensely fastidious. Had gall-stone colic three months ago. Cold feet. Headache at menstrual period for sixteen years. Menstrual flow thick, clotted, dark, lasts one day. Stool, light color when sick, darker when in better health. Must restrain herself or she will commit suicide. Slow pulse at times. Tired all the time. Condemned to an operation by the surgeon for gall-stone. Fissured tongue. Natrum sulphuricum cured; the gall-stones disappeared.

Case 2.—Man actively engaged in business, weight 180 pounds. Age 40. Pain in region of gall bladder. Gall-stone colic. Came on after indigestion. Dull aching in that region. Must walk about the room, not ameliorated in any position. Only once has stool become light colored. Pain in region of kidneys, also through pelvic region and legs with a cloudy condition of the urine; dribbling of few drops of urine after urination. Dull heavy pain in right side behind the lower ribs, continuous pain; pain extends up right side as far as nipple; stabbing pains in breast. Pain in duodenum aggravated after eating. Natrum sulph. cured. The patient is in perfect health.

Case 3.—Woman. Age 64. Diarrhœa; stool watery, sometimes chalky; enlarged liver; clawing feeling in gall bladder; gall-stone colic, Had been condemned by a surgeon to the operating table. Sinking spells after stool; cold spells; vertigo, stooping, lying or walking; spells of rapid heating of heart; mental depression; thirstless; temperature sub-normal; sensitive to jarring abdomen; flatulence and rumbling in abdomen; cold legs to knees; cold hands; much belching, aggravated after meals; sensitive to weather changes; nervous and sleepless before a storm; sore dragging feeling in the liver; bowels sluggish; slow digestion; heaviness of arms and leg; chilliness down the back; unable to lie on right side with comfort; urine copious; strong; late going to sleep. Natrum sulph. made a radical change in her condition and there are no more signs of gall-stones.

Distress in the abdomen relieved by displacing flatus. Emptiness relieved by passing flatus and by eructations. Cramps and many pains from obstructed flatus. Pain and distension in the ascending colon from flatus. Pain in the region of the cæcum. It has cured many cases resembling the first stage of appendicitis. Pain and tenderness in the whole abdomen. Dull heavy pain from abdomen to back. Burning in the abdomen. Feeling in the abdomen as if a diarrhœa would come on, ameliorated by eructations and passing flatus. Distress in the abdomen that hurries him to stool but only flatus passes. Pain in the abdomen during menses. Cramp in morning before breakfast. Pain in abdomen, 4 to 8 P.M., and in evening. Constant distress in bowels and urging to stool. Fulness, rumbling, motions, gurgling with or without diarrhœa. Pain in right ascending colon when lying on the right side. Bilious colic with vomiting of bile. It has cured many cases of syphilis. It has cured enlarged abdominal glands. Morning diarrhœa with copious flatus soon after rising or soon after standing on the feet. Diarrhœa in wet weather. Stools gushing; copious; greenish; thin; very offensive; slimy, bloody; cramps in the abdomen before stool. Smarting in the anus during stool. Sometimes cheerful after stool. Often the diarrhœa is painless. Diarrhœa after farinaceous food; from vegetables; fruit; pastry; cold drinks; ice cream. Diarrhœa alternating with constipation. Diarrhœa with stools at any hour of the day or night, but especially *morning* and evening. It has cured many cases of chronic diarrhœa with stool involuntary and lienteric. Itching and crawling in the anus. Condylomata at the anus. It cured an ulceration in the rectum with copious bleeding in a lawyer who had long struggled with suicidal impulses. It has often cured bleeding piles.

It has cured parenchymatic inflammation of the kidneys following scarlet fever and from malarial influences. It has cured sugar in the urine and polyuria. It has cured brick dust sediment many times also where copious white sandy sediment was present. It has cured copious deposits of phosphates with copious jelly-like mucous sediment. Must rise often in the night to urinate. Burning during and after urination. Urine loaded with bile. Where these symptoms apear after neglected gonorrhœa.

In the male strong sexual desire and troublesome erections. Gonorrhœa when the discharge has a greenish yellow color and there is burning during and after urination. It has cured enlarged prostate many times. Condylomata, soft fleshy with greenish discharge. Œdema of the scrotum and prepuce. Itching of the penis and scrotum with burning after scratching.

The menstrual flow is copious, acrid and clotted. Leucorrhœa acrid greenish, purulent, excoriating the parts. It has cured milk leg.

Much thick, viscid white mucus forms in the larynx and trachea. Dyspnœa on exertion and while walking; with sharp pain in left chest. Stitching on deep breathing. Dyspnœa in damp weather. It is a most useful remedy in humid asthma in children of sycotic parents. Humid asthma with copious viscid mucus in every spell of hot weather. Chronic catarrh of the bronchial tubes.

Frequent attacks of paroxysmal cough from irritation in larynx ending in copious white, viscid expectorations. Expectoration bloody; greenish yellow; purulent; white; viscid. *Oppression of the chest front damp evening air* and in the morning on waking. Emptiness in the chest on inspiration. Soreness in the chest on coughing, better by holding the chest with the hands. Bronchitis and pneumonia are sometimes hard to cure in sycotic patients until they have received this remedy. Muco-purulent expectoration in old people. Eruptions on the chest every spring in sycotic patients. Swelling and suppuration in the axillary glands.

It has been the epidemic remedy in this country in cerebro-spinal meningitis, where the pain in the back of the head and neck was marked, "as the gnawing of a dog" and the head was drawn backward. Piercing pain between the scapulæ in the evening while sitting. Tenderness of the spine. Sore pain in the small of the back and sacrum. Pain in the small of the back during the night compelling her to lie on the right side; it passes away in the morning after rising. Pain in the small of the back from retaining the urine. Itching of the back when undressing. Pain in the sacrum, cannot lie on either side.

Trembling, twitching and weakness in the limbs, twitching in hands and feet during sleep. Pains in the limbs during rest. Rheumatic pains in the limbs in wet weather. Cracking in the joints. Warts on the arms and hands. Pains in the limbs during chill and fever, better by motion and walking. Worse in the lower than in the upper limbs.

Weakness in the hands; flexors pain on grasping anything. Trembling in the hands in the morning on waking and when writing. The tendency to suppuration around the nails is a marked symptom in this remedy. Palms raw and sore and exude a watery fluid. It has cured bad cases of psoriasis of the palms. Fingers swollen and stiff. Panaritium, pain more bearable in the open air.

Ulceration, pain under the nail and in the tips of the fingers.

Pain in the right hip joint on motion. Stitching in the left hip. Pain in the hip extending to the knee. Swelling in the left leg. Sciatica better in motion. Dull aching in the lower limbs during chill and fever, better when walking. Restlessness of the limbs at night in bed. Ulcers on outer side of thighs. Stiffness of knees. Weakness in lower limbs. Burning of feet and legs to the knees. Dry heat in feet at night. Œdema of the feet. Sharp pain in soles and heels.

Drowsiness in the forenoon when reading. Frightful dreams. Chill from 6 to 9 P.M., with fever, them dry heat until 1 A.M., sweat absent. Chill with icy coldness and gooseflesh from 4 to 8 P.M. during menses. Shaking chills. Chilliness with fever in the evening from night air. Perspiration after midnight or toward morning. Fevers with vomiting bile. Remittent and intermittent fevers. It is a much neglected remedy in chronic intermittent fever.

Eczema with watery oozing. Water blisters. Yellow scales after breaking the vesicles. Jaundice. Intertrigo. Wart-like, red excrescenses all over the body. Red, knotty eruptions on head above the ears; on the forehead and left side of nape of neck; in the middle of chest. Itching when undressing.

NATRUM SULPHURICUM AND SYCOSIS

As its name indicates, it is the chemical combination of Natrum and Sulphur, Glauber's salts, Sulphate of Soda. It partakes of the wonderful properties of both Sodium and Sulphur, and some day will become a very frequently indicated remedy. It is a remedy which typically corresponds to many of the complaints of a bilious climate. Natrum sulphuricum combines, in a measure, the wonderful effects of Natrum muriaticum and of Sulphur in the Western climate, as an active malarial agent. Malarial climates are all more or less bilious. Of course, I do not mean every man or every woman that comes to you and says: "Doctor, I am bilious." We never know what that means. It means more or less liver; it means more or less stomach; a general derangement of the system. Any kind of sickness may be called biliousness, but where the liver and stomach combine to effect disorders, we have true biliousness.

It is a most wonderful combination in its symptoms, because it not only pertains to muscular debility and disturbances of the general structures of the body, but also combines that which gives it consideration mentally. Its complaints are those that are brought on from living in damp houses, living in basements, and in cellars. They are generally worse in rainy, wet weather; hence it was called, primarily, by Grauvogl, one of his hydrogenoid remedies. It produces a profound impression upon the system in a general way like sycosis and a deep-seated or suppressed sycotic diseases. Therefore, it is one of the grandest remedies underlying asthma, asthmatic and inherited complaints. In fact, Natrum sulphuricum is one of the best, one of the clear-cut indicated remedies for those constitutional conditions in children that result in chest catarrhs and asthmatic complaints. This shows you only one of its hereditary features. Now, if we take into consideration the sycotic nature, the hydrogenoid condition of the constitution—always worse in wet weather—and this heredity, we have one of the grand features of this medicine.

Its next grand sphere is its action upon the liver and stomach, producing a bilious disturbance. We have, corresponding with this liver excitement a long list of mental symptoms marked with irritability, anxiety, desire to die, aversion to life and to things in life that would generally make people pleasant and comfortable. Now, if I begin on this mental state and go down through it, we will see more of it.

A good wife goes to her husband and says: "If you only knew what restraint I have to use to keep from shooting myself you would appreciate my condition!" It is attended with wildness and irritability. No remedy has that symptom like Natrum Sulphuricum. You may examine the various remedies in our drug pathogenesy and you will find almost every kind of mental symptom, but here is one that stands by itself—this wonderful restraint to prevent doing herself bodily harm, is characteristic of Natrum sulphuricum. The satiety of life, aversion to life; the great sadness, the great despondency. coupled with the irritability and dread of music—music makes her weep, makes her sad, makes her melancholy—this symptom runs through the Natrums which it receives from the Natrum side of its family; Natrum carbonate, Natrum muriaticum, Natrum sulphuricum, all have it. Anything like melancholic strains aggravate her complaints; mild music, gentle light, mellow light that pours through church windows, these little glimmers of light that come through the colored glass, all these make her sad. Now, such are the mental characteristics of Natrum sulphuricum.

With the constitutional troubles there are important head symptoms— mental symptoms from inujries of the head. A young man in St. Louis was hurled from a truck in the fire department. He struck on his head. Following this for five or six months he had fits; I do not know what kind of fits he had;

some said epilepsy. Some said one thing and some another, and some said he
would have to be trephined. He was an Allopathist, of course, as these firemen
all are, for it is hardly ever that you can get one to go outside of Allopathy
and try something else. He was a good, well-bred Irishman; so he had to have
some good stout physique. Some of his friends prevailed upon him to stay in
the country for a while. He did so, but he did not get better; he was irritable;
he wanted to die. His wife said she could hardly stand it with him; always
wanted to die; did not want to live. His fits drove him to distraction. He did
not know when he was going to have one, they were epileptiform in character.
Well, in the country he ran across a homœopathic doctor, because he had
one of these attacks and the handiest doctor at the time was a Homœopath.
That Homœopath told him that he had better come back to St. Louis and
place himself under my care. He did so. At that time it had been about six
months that he had been having these fits. When he walked into my office he
staggered; his eyes were nearly bloodshot; he could hardly see, and he wore
a shade over his eyes—so much was he distressed about the light—such a
photophobia. He had constant pain in his head. He had injured himself by
falling upon the back of his head, and he had with this all the irritability that
I have described. There was nothing in his fits that was distinctive of a
remedy, and the first thing that came into my head was Arnica; that is what
everybody would have thought. Arnica, however, would not have been the
best remedy for him. Had I known no other or better remedy, Arnica would
have perhaps been the best. As soon as he had finished his description, and
I had given the case more thought, I found that Natrum sulphuricum was the
best indicated remedy for injuries about the head, and I have been in the
habit of giving it. So I gave it in this case. The first dose of Natrum sulphuricum
cured this young man. He has never had any pain about the head since. He
has never had any mental trouble since, never another fit. That one
prescription cleared up the entire case. If you will just remember the chronic
effects from injuries upon the skull—not fractures, but simple concussions
that have resulted from a considerable shock and injuries without organic
affections—then Natrum sulphuricum should be your first remedy. Now, that
may not be worth remembering, but when you have relieved as many heads
as I have with Natrum sulphuricum you will be glad to have been informed of
this circumstance. Ordinarily, Arnica for injuries and the results of injuries,
especially the neuralgic pains and the troubles from old scars; but in mental
troubles coming on from a jar or a knock on the head or a fall or injury about
the head, do not forget this medicine, because if you do many patients may
suffer where they might have been cured had you made use of this remedy.

It has violent head pains, and especially so in the base of the brain;
violent pains in the back of the neck; violent crushing pains as if the base of

the brain were crushed in a vice, or as if a dog were gnawing at the base of the brain. These symptoms have led me to prescribe the medicine. In the spinal meningitis of today, if all the remedies in the Materia Medica were taken away from me and I were to have but one with which to treat that disease, I would take Natrum sulphuricum, because it will modify and save life in the majority of cases. It cuts short the disease surprisingly when it is the truly indicated remedy. In relation to the symptoms that you are likely to find in spinal meningitis, there is a drawing back of the neck and spasms of the back, together with all the mental irritability and delirium already described. The violent determination of blood to the head we find in this disease, clinically, is readily relieved.

The next most important feature is in relation to the eyes. That is characteristic, and is equalled only by one other remedy in chronic diseases where there is an aversion to life with photophobia, and that is Graphites. You take these cases of chronic conjunctivitis, with granular lids, green pus, terrible photophobia, so much so that he can hardly open his eyes; the light of the room brings on headache, distress and many pains. Here Natrum sulphuricum should be compared with Graphites, because Graphites has also an extreme aggravation from light in eye affections. Of course, this classes it entirely away from Belladonna and the other remedies that have acute photophobia, of acute determination of blood to the brain, because it gives you a chronic state and condition that you must study.

Natrum sulphuricum produces a stuffing up of the nose, red tongue, irritable mucous membrane of the eyes, nose, and ears, with great dryness and burning in the nose. Pus becomes green upon exposure to the light.

The mouth always tastes bad. The patient says: "Doctor, my mouth is always full of slime." That is a common expression of the patient when he comes to you. And the provers, all of them, said that they were troubled with a slimy mouth. Thick, tenacious, white mucus in the mouth. Always hawking up mucus; it wells up from the stomach; mucus from the œsophagus; mucus by belching; mucus coughed up from the trachea, and it is always foul and slimy.

There is a distended feeling in the stomach; a sense of a weight in the stomach; almost constant nausea; vomiting of slime, bitter and sour. These are the characteristics; bitter and sour.

A sensation of weight in the right hypochondrium, in the region of the liver; aching pains; sometimes cutting pains, and a great amount of distress in the region of the liver. Engorgement in the region of the liver. He can only lie on his left side, his complaints are aggravated from lying on his left side. When lying on the left side, the congested liver seems to pull and draw; the great weight increases the pain and uneasiness and he is compelled to turn back on the right side. Now, it is from these symptoms, whenever a patient comes into my office and says, "Doctor, my mouth is so slimy and tastes so bad, and I think I am bilious," that he always gets Natrum sulphuricum.

Natrum sulphuricum produces great flatulence, distension of the abdomen, cutting pains in the abdomen, associated with congestion of the liver. In this tympanitic condition of the liver that sometimes comes on in the inflammatory conditions in bilious fever, you will find Natrum sulphuricum your remedy.

I began the use of this remedy with Schüssler's remedies some years ago, and find the indications well carried out by the higher and highest potencies. Bell says that if the thirtieth potency of Arsenic is equal to a complete knowledge of the drug, crude Arsenic would be equal to complete ignorance.

There is a condition of the chest that is characteristic, and that is in relation to the cough. It has a cough with a sensation of "all-goneness" in the chest. In this it completes with Bryonia; both hold the chest when coughing. Bryonia holds the chest because he feels as if it would fly to pieces; there is such a soreness that he feels the necessity of steadying his chest. The complaints of Bryonia are relieved by pressure. Natrum sulphuricum has this same desire to hold the chest; but in Natrum sulphuricum the muco-pus that is expectorated is thick, ropy and yellowish-green, looking like pus—purulent—and there is an "all-gone", empty feeling in the chest. He feels a sense of weakness there; that his lungs are all-gone, that he must die in a few days with consumption or some other failing like that, and that it is coming on in a short time.

Bryonia corresponds more to the irritable states with the cough, where there is great rawness, great constriction, great sense of tearing in the chest; burning in the chest; while Natrum sulphuricum corresponds to a case that has been going on for perhaps a week; every cough brings up a mouthful of purulent sputa with a desire to press upon the chest to relieve the weakness; Natrum sulphuricum is then your remedy.

Another condition is that of humid asthma. If a child has asthma, give Natrum sulphuricum as the first remedy. Asthma, when hereditary, is one of the sycotic complaints of Hahnemann. You will not find that in your textbooks, so do not look for it, but it may be an observation worth knowing. I have cured a very large number of such cases of asthma, although the textbooks would discourage you if you should read them under asthma, because they will tell you that cases of asthma are incurable. For years I was puzzled with the management of asthma. When a person came to me and asked: "Doctor, can you cure asthma?" I would say, "No." But now I am beginning to get quite liberal on asthma, since I have learned that asthma is a sycotic disease, and since I have made judicious application of anti-sycotics I have been able to relieve or cure a great number of such cases. You will find in the history of medicine that wherever asthma was cured, it has been by anti-sycotic remedies. That is one of the first things I observed, that outside of sycotics you will seldom find a cure for asthma. There is that peculiarity that runs through sycosis which gives you a hereditary disease, and asthma corresponds to that disease. Hence it is that Silicea is one of the greatest cures for asthma; it does not cure every case, but when Silicea corresponds to the symptoms, you will be surprised to note how quickly it will eradicate it. While Ipecac, Spongia, and Arsenicum will correspond just as clearly to the supervening symptoms and to everything that you can find about the case, yet what do they do? They palliate; they repress the symptoms; but your asthma is no better off, your patient is not cured. Arsenic is one of the most frequently indicated remedies for the relief of asthma; so also are Bryonia, Ipecac, Spongia and Carbo veg., but they do not cure; though they relieve surprisingly at times. Where a patient is sitting up, covered with a cold sweat, wants to be fanned by somebody on either side of the bed, dyspnœa is so distressing that it seems almost impossible for the patient to live longer, to get another breath, then Carbo veg. comes in and gives immediate relief and the patient will lie down and get a very good night's rest. But what is the result? On comes the asthma again the very next cold. Natrum sulphuricum goes down to the bottom of this kind of a case. If it is hereditary, that is, not longlived, if it is in a growing subject, Natrum sulphuricum goes down to the bottom of such a case and will cure when its symptoms are present; and the symptoms will so often be present. It is because of this deep-seated anti-sycotic nature, we find in the combination of Natrum and Sulphur, that we have a new state and combination running into the life. When the chest is filling up with mucus, rattling of mucus, expectoration of large quantities of white mucus, with asthmatic breathing in young subjects, this remedy must be thought of.

In relation to the genito-urinary organs, we have some very valuable symptoms. In chronic gonorrhœa, with greenish or yellowish-green discharges. Instead of gonorrhœa running off into a white, gleety discharge, it keeps up a yellowish, thick, greenish discharge. It competes here with Thuja and Mercurius, both of which are anti-sycotics. When Natrum sulphuricum is indicated there is generally very little pain, it is almost painless. There is chronic loss of sensibility in the part.

The urine is loaded with bile, is of a pinkish or yellow color, with a "corn-meal" sediment, or it looks like stale beer and is extremely offensive. Offensive urine is not in the text.

Like sulphur, it has burning of the soles of the feet at night, and the burning extends to the knees; burning from the knees down. It has also, like sulphur, great burning in the top of the head; it has tearing, rending, cutting pains from the hips down to the knees; worse at night. The stomach symptoms are worse in the morning, and so also with the mental symptoms, they are generally worse in the morning.

Now, upon the skin we have some eruptions; we have those cases of so-called itch, scabies or vesicular eruptions, vesicular eczema, with a thin, watery discharge exuding from the fingers, and the fingers are swollen stiff and stand out stiffened by the swelling; they are swollen so stiff they can hardly be gotten together. (Baker's itch and barber's itch come under this head). Natrum sulphuricum cures where the palms of the hands are raw and sore and exude a water fluid. Also vesicular eruptions around the mouth and chin and various parts of the body; little, fine water blisters, very much like Natrum muriaticum and very much also like Natrum carb. So you see it runs into the Natrums. The other disease that I incidentally mentioned a moment ago—the barber's itch—is a sycotic disease, a sycosis menti, a disease of the hair follicles. It is sometimes even contagious. It is one of the highest types of sycosis; the next highest type of sycosis is the veneral wart known as the gonorrhœal warts. This medicine corresponds to this state and condition of the body.

Now, we have said considerable about sycosis. We know in sycosis, which is a constitutional miasm, that we have venereal warts or gonorrhœal warts; that we have another sycotic state that comes upon the female in cauliflower excrescences. We have also hereditary asthma, a constitutional disease that depends upon sycosis; and this peculiar barber's itch is one of the highest types of sycosis; they are all due to one cause, and some day this cause will be demonstrated to be latent sycosis. Gonorrhœa will some day be known to be the true offspring of this sycosis. It is the contagious part of the sycosis. It is the means by which the disease is handed from generation to generation. This thing you will not find in the books, and it is, perhaps, only a private opinion and, therefore, worthless. But some day you will remember that I told you this. I have seen things in my observation that astonished me. I believe I have solved what Hahnemann called sycosis, though he has never described it. To me it is very clear from the cases I have cured, with this theory in view or this doctrine in view. The cases I have cured lead me to believe that I am on the right track.

Now, I say that gonorrhœa and all of these latent conditions of the body are one and the same thing; that primarily they date back to one and the same source. Of course, the books will tell you that gonorrhœa is not a constitutional disease; but when gonorrhœa will produce warts, and gonorrhœal rheumatism, and will last throughout life, and children be brought into the world with the same disease, how are you going to get around it? There was a young man in the St. Louis City Hospital who had been there many months, and who was so sore in the bottoms of his feet that he could not get around; he had to

eave his business, he was a baker. Finally his old employer came to me and
wanted to know if I could do anything for that young man. I did not know
anything about the nature of his disease. I told him to bring the young man
to me. He was brought, and I learned from his history that years before he
had had gonorrhœa; that it had been suppressed with injections. I put him
under such constitutional treatment as these theories that I have just
mentioned guided me to, and I cured him. In our city I have cured twenty-five
or thirty cases of this peculiar kind of sycosis that dated back to a latent
gonorrhœa. Symptoms of a latent gonorrhœa are unknown to the books. You
will find nothing of it. It is known only to such observers as have been able
to make two out of two times one—by putting things together. By and by I
hall have a complete chain of evidence to show that gonorrhœa is a
constitutional disease and can be handed down from father to son, as can
yphilis. It is one of the chronic miasms, and one about which very little is
nown. If this be true, it is as dangerous to suppress a gonorrhœal discharge
before its time, as it is to suppress a syphilitic chancre before its time. You
will never know if you go on treating these constitutional miasms by
uppressing the primary manifestations—you will never know the harm you
re doing

The most of these are calculated by the process of evolution to wear
hemselves out, to roll out, or to evolve themselves into symptoms that are
o depleting to the disease that they leave of themselves, or leave the patient
ery nearly free from the disease. Such is the calculation of Nature in a
onorrhœal discharge, and such has been the intention of Nature in the
hancres that appear upon the genitalia. But poor ignorant man, believing he
ust do something, has made it his first business to cauterize these chancres—
o dry up these discharges—and he does not know how much harm he is
oing. But this is only a private opinion. I have observed this, that there are
vo kinds of gonorrhœa—one is a simple urethral discharge, which when
opped by injections, will not produce a constitutional taint, because that is
ot sycosis; and the other form is the sycotic gonorrhœa, which, if suppressed
ith injections, will appear in constitutional symptoms. Now, it is for you to
ve and think for yourselves. If you can make anything out of what I have
ld you, and it ever helps anybody, I shall be amply repaid. You will most
aturally see that all these thoughts are in furtherance of Hahnemann's
aching, based upon the facts observed by him and his faithful followers.
nless guided by the light of the dynamic doctrine of disease and cure,
ese things would scarcely be observed. For the study of this sycosis I
ight have taken up Thuja, but knowing how well the master has performed
s work. I have taken a remedy that is scarcely second in importance to
ing out as well the use of a remedy as a miasm in relation to it.

NITRIC ACID

Great general weakness; feeble reaction; extreme sensitivity, and nervous trembling, are marked features in this remedy. Patients greatly broken by long suffering, pain and sickness, physical more than mental suffering, finally anæmia and emaciation are marked. Sensitive to cold; always chilly. Symptoms are aggravated from becoming cold, and in cold air. Always taking cold. The walls of blood vessels are relaxed and bleed easily; profuse dark blood. Pains as if flesh were torn from the bones and a sensation as though a splinter felt in inflamed parts, in ulcers and in nerves. Inflammation of the periosteum, in bone, and in the nerves. Syphilitic bone pains. Caries of bone, and exostoses. The margins of orifices bleed and grow warts. Old scars become painful in cold weather and when weather changes to cold; pains like splinters. Inflammation of glands after the abuse of mercury in syphilitic subjects. Prolonged suppuration in glands, with no tendency to repair, when there are sticking pains. The discharges are thin, bloody, offensive and excoriating, sometimes a dirty yellowish green. Suppuration where there is no tendency to repair. This is often the case when the patient is syphilitic and has been surcharged with mercury. For suppuration and ulceration in cancerous affections with bloody, watery, offensive discharges and sticking pains. It has often been observed that the patient requiring Nitric acid is more subject to diarrhœa than constipation. It has cured many complaints in patients who are never so comfortable as when riding in a carriage. Twitching of muscles in all parts of the body. Many complaints are aggravated from a jar, and from noise. Even his pains are aggravated from noise. Nitric acid patients are often extremely sensitive to medicines, especially high potencies—indeed they prove every remedy given too high. Fissures form in many places; canthi, corners of the mouth, above the anus; the skin cracks—and all these have the splinter sensation. He finally becomes dropsical, especially in the extremities. Offensiveness is a marked condition of this patient, often putrid odors. The urine smells like that of a horse. Offensive leucorrhœa, offensive catarrh, and breath; fœtid foot sweat. Strong odors from the body. Too much weight must not be given to the dark, swarthy complexion so often mentioned as the one most likely to need this remedy. Nitric acid will cure blondes as often as brunettes, *if the symptoms agree.*

Prostration of mind. Any effort to reflect on certain things causes the thoughts to vanish. A general indifference to all matters; tired of life; has no enjoyment in anything; aggravated before menses. Mental depression in the evening. Anxiety about his failing health, with fear of death. Anxiety after loss of sleep; vexation and sorrow. He is angered over his own mistakes. Anger with trembling. Obstinate and refuses to be comforted about his misfortune. He is weary of life but fears death. Excitable and weeps. Despair of recovery. Hopelessness. Easily startled, frightened. Starts from fright on falling asleep. Cannot comprehend what is said to him. The whole mental state is better when riding in a carriage.

Suffers much from vertigo in the morning; must lie down.

His headaches are violent, aggravated from noise of wagons on the paved streets, but often ameliorated from riding in a carriage on a smooth, country road. The noise and jarring increase the pain. Pain as if in a vise from ear to ear. The biparietal syphilitic pain is often cured by this remedy. Pain as though the head were bound up. Painful drawing in head extending to eyes, with nausea. Stitching pains in the head. Hammering pain in the head. Pain in morning on waking, ameliorated after rising, aggravated by a jar, motion and noise, ameliorated riding in a carriage. Heat often ameliorates the head pains and cold aggravates. Wrapping up ameliorates. Pain as if constricted by a tape. Extreme sensitivity of the scalp and skull to combing the hair, and to the hat. The hair falls out in profusion, as in syphilis. Eruption on the scalp with sharp sticking pains as from splinters; moist; itching, offensive eruptions. Caries of bones of skull. Exostoses.

The eyes have lost their lustre, the pupils are dilated, and there is diplopia. There is inflammation of the conjunctiva with acrid tears. Ulceration of the cornea with pricking pain. Iritis with stinging, stitching pain, aggravated at night and changing from warm to cold room or in cold air. Spots on the cornea. Intense photophobia, burning, pressure and sensation as though sand in the eyes. Ptosis. Swollen lids, which are hard and burn. Small warts on upper lids. Warts that bleed easily, with sensation of sticks.

Deafness, ameliorated when riding in a carriage or train. Catarrh of the Eustachian tubes. Pulsating in ears. Discharge from ear, fœtid, brown, chorous, purulent—since scarlet fever. The auditory canal nearly closed. Swelling of glands about the ear. Caries of the mastoid.

Subject to coryza every winter; no sooner does he get over one cold than he has another. The nose is obstructed in the night during sleep. Sneezing in cold air, from every draft, must keep the room very warm. Bad smells in the nose, and the catarrh is offensive to others. Nose-bleed mornings and nights. Nasal catarrh, acrid, watery at night, yellow, offensive, excoriating, bloody, brownish, thin—since scarlet fever or in mercurio-syphilitic patients. The nose feels as if there were splinters in it. Large crusts from high up in nose. Green crusts blown out every morning. Ulceration high up in nose. Warts form in and about the nostrils. Red, scurfy tip of nose. Crusts form on the wings of the nose. Cracked nose.

Deep lines of suffereing characterize the Nitric acid face. The face is pale, yellow, sallow and sunken. The eyes are sunken. Dark rings about the eyes, mouth and nose. The face is bloated. The lids are tumid in the morning. There are brown spots. Pigmented warty spots on the forehead. The right parotid is large. The skin feels drawn over the face. Crusts and pustules form on the face. Cracking in jaw when chewing. Corners of the mouth cracked, ulcerated and scabby. The lips raw and bleeding. Painful swelling of the submaxillary gland. The expression is anxious, haggard, sickly.

Pain in the teeth, tearing, aggravated from cold or warm things. Pulsating evening and night, after mercury. Caries of teeth. Teeth become yellow, Gums bleed easily, scorbutic, swollen.

The tongue is excoriated, sore, red, yellow, white and dry, fissured, with sore spots. Ulceration of tongue with viscid mucus in mouth. Inflammation of the tongue.

Ulcers in mouth, on tongue or in throat, white, or dark and dirty, putrid, phagedenic, syphilitic, with sticking pains as from splinters. Sore mouth with stinging, burning pain. Excoriated, red, swollen membrane. Foul cadaveric odor from the mouth. Saliva flows from the mouth so acrid that it excoriates the lips.

Confusion of the muscular action in throat causes food to stop in throat and choking. Difficult swallowing. Violent pain in throat, extending to ear or swallowing. Stitching in throat like a splinter (*Hepar, Nat. mur., Alum., Arg n.*) on swallowing. Viscid mucus in throat. Mucus drawn from posterior nares Inflammation of throat, tonsils, uvula and soft palate. Uvula and tonsilsœdematous (*Apis, Rhus t.*), Great swelling of the throat and tonsils Ulceration of tonsils. "It has cured diphtheria where the splinter sensation was present," and the other symptoms agreed. Inflammation of the œsophagus.

Longing for fats, pungent things, herring, chalk, lime, earth; and aversion to bread and meat. *Generally thirstless.*

The stomach is disordered by milk. Food sours, and causes sour eructations and vomiting. Fats disagree. Nausea after eating, ameliorated by moving about or riding in a carriage. Vomiting bitter and sour, contents of stomach. Ulceration of stomach. Pain in cardiac opening of stomach on swallowing. Sticking pain in stomach. Catarrh of stomach. Weight after eating Sensation of rawness in stomach after eating.

Chronic inflammation of liver. Clay-colored stools. Enormously enlarge liver. Pain in region of liver with jaundice. Stitching pain in liver. Enlarge spleen.

Cramping pain in abdomen. Violent pain in ilio-cæcal region, sore and tender, aggravated from motion. Awakened at midnight with a crampy pain abdomen; chilly; pain aggravated from motion. Rumbling in abdomen Abdomen distended and tender. Great soreness in abdomen. Inflammatic and suppuration of inguinal glands. The relaxed condition in weakly infant boys, that so much disposes to inguinal hernia, is often overcome by Nitric acid and the hernia cured (*Lyc., Nux v.*).

Broken down subjects who are disposed to suffer from frequent attacks of diarrhœa, or from constipation alternating with diarrhœa, often need this remedy—when the urine smells strong like that of a horse, and he is pale and sickly, losing flesh and strength, subject to excoriation of orifices and excoriating catarrhs and ulcers. The stool is bloody, putrid, undigested, green, slimy, excoriating, sour, curdled if milk is used as a diet, black putrid blood. In dysentery. Cold changes of the weather bring on diarrhœa. Anus excoriated, burning, fissured, covered with warts. Membrane comes with the stool. Much pure blood with the stool not even clotted, very offensive. Ineffectual urging to stool. Sensation as if rectum were filled and he cannot expel it. Constipation, painful hard difficult stool. Drawing, cutting and pressing before stool; constant fruitless urging (*Nuv v.*). During stool there is colic, tenesmus, spasmodic contraction of anus, unsatisfactory straining. Splinters in rectum. After stool there is still urging (*Merc.*), exhaustion; soreness of anus; cutting pain; burning and shooting in rectum; constriction of anus; great nervous excitement; palpitation. The pain keeps her in bed for hours after every stool. Itching and burning in anus. Constant acrid moisture about the anus. Periodical bleeding of rectum and pain in sacrum. Fissures of anus. Painful prolapses of rectum. This has been a most useful remedy in fistula, fissures, condylomata, polypi, caruncles, cancer of the rectum and hæmorrhoids—*when the symptoms agree.* It has cured caruncles so sensitive that the patient would cry out when they were touched. Hæmorrhoids that are exquisitely painful to touch and at stool; that bleed, external or internal, with burning and sticking during stool. Piles that ulcerate and discharge copiously of blood and pus. When piles are so painful that she breaks out in sweat, becomes anxious, and pulsates all over, on the slightest touch or at stool, this remedy has been useful (compare *Pæonia* and *Staph.*). Fœtid moisture at the anus.

The male sexual organs are in a constant state of irritability. Sexual desire is increased and erections troublesome at night. Painful spasmodic erections at night; stitching pain in the urethra and chordee. It has been a useful remedy in gonorrhœa when the discharge is thin and bloody, later when it is greenish or yellow; burning and sticking on urination, and the urethra is swollen and very sore. It has cured condylomata which have the "splinter" sensation, and bleed easily, and extremely sensitive to touch. Condylomata on genitals and around the anus. Inflammation of the prostate gland with gonorrhœa, especially when the discharge becomes scanty from taking cold or from strong injections. It cures old cases of gleet when the urethra has pain in it like a splinter on touch or when urinating. Prolonged inflammation of the urethra with infiltration, making the urethra feel hard and nodular like a whip-cord (*Arg. n.*). *Sore spots* in the urethra, ulcers, with bloody pus, and the sensation of splinters. Itching in the urethra after gonorrhœa (*Petr.*). Pimples, vesicles, herpes and crusts on the prepuce. Small ulcers on the glans or prepuce. *Spreading ulcers.* The ulcers discharge a brown, bloody water, offensive. Phagedenic ulcers (*Ars., Aur. m. n., Caust., Merc. c.*). Inflammation of the prepuce. Ulcers that destroy the frænum. Inflamed and ulcerated parts have the splinter sensation and flow a bloody water. Paraphimosis and phimosis and great swelling. The hair falls off from the pubes.

The female is greatly troubled by the constant itching and burning and sexual desire. Excoriation of the parts from leucorrhœa and menstrual discharges. Every exertion brings on uterine hæmorrhage (*Calc.*). The menstrual flow is dark and thick. Menses too soon and profuse, like bloody water. Uterine prolapsus. Many and extreme nervous sufferings come during the menstrual period; flatulence, bruised pain in limbs, pain down thighs, "splinter" under the finger and toe nails, palpitation, anxiety, trembling, neuralgic pains in any part. After the menses there comes a muddy, watery flow, lasting many days, and extreme excoriation of the parts. Thin, bloody, excoriating leucorrhœa at all times or at any time. The vagina is excoriated and condylomata grow upon the genitalia. Erectile tumors. Caruncles at the orifice of urethra, exquisitely sensitive to touch. The itching is aggravated by cold. The parts are fissured and bleed easily.

Many troubles culminate during menses and lactation. Lumps in the mammæ. The nipples are fissured and tender, are excoriated and have "splinters". Tendency to abortion from general weakness and the ease with which a uterine hæmorrhage may set in.

Hoarseness, and ulceration of the larynx. Voice lost. Laryngitis in old syphilitic subjects. Oppression of the chest, ameliorated by expectoration. Shortness of breath. Intermittent breathing.

The cough is aggravated in winter, yet aggravated in a warm room and from becoming warm. The cough is dry, barking, aggravated during the night, aggravated lying, aggravated before midnight; comes on during sleep. Cough with hectic fever and night sweats. Paroxysmal cough with retching, like whooping cough, violent, racking cough. Hard, prolonged coughing spells with difficult expectoration. The irritation to cough is like a tickling in the larynx. The expectoration is greenish, viscid or thin, dirty, watery, bloody mucus, or dark clotted blood. Loose cough in daytime, dry at night. Rattling in daytime, but no expectoration. Cough in broken down constitutions, from liver and lung affections, in tubercular subjects. The sputum tastes bitter, sour or salty. It is offensive, even putrid. He is covered with sweat during efforts to expectorate. Stitching in the chest. In typhoid pneumonia, with rattling in the chest, inability to expectorate. or when he can expectorate the sputum is brown and bloody, and the urine smells like that of a horse. In tuberculosis with night sweats and hæmoptysis. Palpitation from excitement, on ascending stairs. The pulse is rapid, irregular, and every fourth beat is missed.

Swelling of glands of neck and axilla. Stiff neck. Stitching pains in back and chest. Burning spots in spine. Pain in back, nights, compelling him to lie on the abdomen. Sharp pains in back and limbs in tabes dorsalis. Sharp pains in back on coughing.

Rheumatic pains in limbs. Emaciation of upper arms, and thighs. Weakness of limbs. Dropsy of limbs. Crippled nails. Rheumatic pains in upper limbs. Stitching. Stitching pains in limbs in cold weather. Numbness of arms and hands. Copper colored spots on arms. Chilblains on hands and fingers. Cold, sweaty hands. Numerous large warts on back of hands. Herpes between the fingers. Vesicles on the tip of the thumb that open into ulcers, felons, distorted and discolored nails. Yellow curved nails, splintered sensation under nails. It is useful in wounds that inflame and have the "splinter" sensation. Tearing in the long bones of the lower limbs at night. The legs are weary and bruised. Pain in hip as if sprained. Sticking pains along the nerves as from splinters. Syphilitic nodes on the tibia with nightly pains. Chilblains on the feet and toes. Phagedenic blisters on the toes (*Graph.*). Extreme soreness of the tibia. Profuse, offensive sweat of feet.

Shocks on going to sleep (*Agar., Arg. m., Ars., Nat. m.*). The pain comes during sleep. Starting in sleep. Anxious, unrefreshing sleep, with frightful dreams.

Nitric acid is a very useful remedy in fevers. The thirstlessness during all stages has often called attention to it. Cold hands and feet. Chronic intermittent in cachectic constitutions, copious night sweats, extreme weakness, with the characteristic odor of the urine, and bleeding from some part a dark blood, this remedy will act well.

NUX MOSCHATA

This is not a very great remedy; it has not a very wide range of usefulness, but it is often overlooked when needed. We get into the habit of relying entirely on the polychrests.

The old women used to give nutmeg to hysterics, and wonderful to tell its provings justify its use. It must have had some palliative relation to the hysteria. The root is much stronger than the nut, in the same proportions, and contains the real medicinal qualities.

The patient appears to be dazed; there is a complete loss of memory; she is automatic in her actions. This is wonderful state of the mind. She goes about the house performing her duties, but if interrupted, forgets what she has been doing, forgets that she was all day in conversation with her son; she has no recollection of past events. This is a singular state of the mind sometimes found in hysterical women. Sometimes it is impossible to find out what state of the mind is present she is so forgetful. She lies with the eyes closed and yet knows everything that is going on, but remembers nothing. She speaks with intelligence about the things of the moment, but knows nothing of the past. She prophesies, predicts with a sort of clairvoyance. The mental state is the keynote. Sometimes she is < in the morning, sometimes in the evening, or on waking. She performs all her duties and yet seems to be in a dream—she seems not to know her friends.

The Nux mos. patient is always ready to go to sleep; it is with great difficulty that she can keep awake. She falls asleep on all occasions, in season and out of season. The eyes look heavy; she cannot keep awake; falls into a profound slumber, sometimes into coma.

Useful in the coma of typhoid and intermittent fever. When aroused she remembers nothing; looks dazed; looks about and wants to know who the people are around and what they are doing. It is a state in which patients answer questions slowly after a long interval, and then look confused again. They give an answer that has no relation to the question asked, or, answer correctly. We find such a state in typhoid, in hysteria, after shock, after fear, blighted affections, or the loss of a friend. It is more suitable after shock ending in this kind of trouble than in typhoid. It is also useful in typhoid, but where there is great weakness, sliding down in bed, and nervous trembling, *Phos. ac.* is a better remedy. Nux mos. does not relate so completely to the general image of a typhoid as does *Phos. ac.*

The sleepiness and the dazed state are two things combined, and when combined are difficult to cover by a remedy. This state is somewhat like *opium.*

Faintness and even fainting when standing long, such as occurs in a nervous woman standing to have a dress fitted.

There is a dry mouth, the tongue cleaves to the roof of the mouth in all complaints. There is great sleepiness and automatic conduct, especially in nervous women. It has cured petit mal.

The hæmorrhages stand out in bold relief; hæmorrhages from the nose, uterus and bowels. There is vomiting of blood.

The patient is sensitive to wind, to a draft, to damp air. She has a headache < walking against the wind; hoarseness from walking against the wind; she is so sensitive to cold weather that she comes home dazed and sleepy from walking against the wind; her mouth is dry but there is no thirst, she doesn't desire water (sometimes thirst is present). The patient may hold water in the mouth without desire to swallow it. Nux mos. holds ice water and succulent fruits in the mouth to relieve the sensation of dryness. Often there is a sensation of dryness when the mouth is moist.

In the extremities there is numbness, tingling, prickling, paralytic weakness; there is threatened paralysis; momentary hysterical paralysis; coming for a short time and then going away. Aphonia with a dry mouth, in hysterical patients; when walking out of doors. This aphonia passes away on going into the house.

The whole back is sensitive to pressure; the vertebræ are sensitive.

The remedy has prolonged and inveterate constipation; prolonged urging to stool followed by a soft stool. (*Alum., Psor., China.*) The stool is difficult but soft. He wonders why he has to urge for a soft stool.

In woman there are many troubles; menorrhagia lasting ten or fifteen days; the blood is clotted; the menses are too often, last too long, are irregular. The abdomen is full of colic; cramping pains extending to the broad ligaments and down the limbs; most distressing dysmenorrhœa from exposure to cold, riding in the wind or living in damp houses. With this there is a dry mouth and thirtlessness; she wakes at night with a dry mouth; it seems as if the tongue cleaved to the roof of the mouth.

This remedy is especially suitable for lean women, those who have lost flesh. The breasts are flat. I remember a case of a woman thirty-five years old whose breasts which were once well rounded became perfectly flat. Nux mos. restored the breasts.

This is a little remedy, but when wanted nothing will take its place.

NUX VOMICA

Everywhere in this remedy we observe the striking oversensitiveness of the patient; it is brought out in all the symptoms. Irritable; oversensitive to noise, to light, to the least current of air, to his surroundings; extremely touchy in regard to his food; many kinds of food disturb, strong foods disturb; he is aggravated by meat; craves stimulants, pungent, bitter, succulent things, something to brace him up. Oversensitive to medicines. One reason why

there are so many Nux patients is because people have been overdrugged by
the old school. When a patient comes from the old school and bad prescribing,
having had stimulants and tonics to brace him up, wine, and stimulants of all
sorts, it is sometimes impossible to get reliable symptoms, to get the patient
settled down, until we give Nux as an antidote.

It is useful in those overdrugged by tea, coffee, wine. Old coffee drinkers
become sensitive, oversensitive to noise, their symptoms are flitting; they
do not give their symptoms well. Such patients will do well for a few days on
Nux; some of their symptoms will drop out and they will settle down.

The mental state is varied, but they all show oversensitiveness; irritable,
touchy, sensitive conditions. They are never contented, never satisfied;
disturbed by their surroundings, and they become irritable, so that they
want to tear things, to scold. Impulses are strongly marked at times. The
woman has impulses to destroy her husband or to throw her child into the
fire; the impulse is intermingled with violent temper, cannot be contradicted
or opposed; if a chair is in the way he kicks it over; if, while undressing, a
part of his clothing should catch on a button he would pull it off because he
is so mad at it. (Like *Nit. ac.*). An uncontrollable state of irritability; it is a
weakness and is accompanied by physical weakness; a lack of balance. For
example, a business man has been at his desk until he is tired out, he receives
many letters, he has a great many irons in the fire; he is troubled with a
thousand little things; his mind is constantly hurried from one thing to
another until he is tortured. It is not so much the heavy affairs but the little
things. He is compelled to stimulate his memory to attend to all the details;
he goes home and thinks about it; he lies awake at night; his mind is confused
with the whirl of business and the affairs of the day crowd upon him; finally
brain-fag comes on. When the details come to him he gets angry and wants
to get away, tears things up, scolds, goes home and takes it out of his family
and children. Sleeps by fits and starts; wakens at 3 A.M.; and his business
affairs crowd on him so that he cannot sleep again until late in the morning
when he falls into a fatiguing sleep and wakens up tired and exhausted. He
wants to sleep late in the morning.

Melancholy, sadness, but all the time he feels as if he could fly to pieces,
jerks things about, tears things up; wants to force things his own way. Driven
by impulses to commit acts that verge upon insanity—the destruction of
others. *Natr. sul.* has a strong impulse to destroy himself: *Arg. nitr.,* also,
particularly by jumping from a height, but he avoids placing himself in such
a position.

He is oversensitive to the open air, to a draft of air; always chilly, always
taking cold and it settles in the nose and extends to the chest.

Skin oversensitive to touch, to draft. Full of pains and aches. He sweats easily on the slightest provocation. Brain-fag, fatigue, neuralgias; on the verge of insanity and this goes on to convulsions. Convulsions of single muscles and those of the whole body; muscular twitchings; weakness, trembling, and paralysis. This paralytic weakness and disordered state of the activity of the muscles and nerves are prominent.

Another state running through Nux is that actions are turned in opposite directions. When the stomach is sick, it will empty its contents with no great effort ordinarily, but in Nux there is retching and straining as if the action were going the wrong way, as if it would force the abdomen open; a reversed action; retches, gags, and strains and after a prolonged effort he finally empties the stomach. The same condition is found in the bladder. He must strain to urinate. There is tenesmus, urging. The bladder is full and the urine dribbles away, yet when he strains it ceases to dribble. In regard to the bowels, though the patient strains much, he passes but a scanty stool. In the diarrhœa at times when he sits on the commode in a perfectly passive way, there will be a little squirt of stool, and then comes on tenesmus so that he cannot stop straining, and when he does strain there comes on the sensation of forcing back; the stool seems to go back; a kind of anti-peristalsis. In constipation the more he strains the harder it is to pass a stool. In diarrhœa and dysentery there is straining without relief, but as soon as he passes a little stool there is relief. In dysentery, *Merc.* has the constant urging; *Merc. cor.* tenesmus with great desire to urinate. The reversed action of the various functions shows the spasmodic nature of this remedy. Pains shoot from the rectum up; burning.

Neuralgias about the eyes, face, and head; neuralgic headaches; the pains stick, and tear; they cause weeping, fainting; they burn and sting. Pains in the head and face and in the extremities, that sting and tear, but especially draw. Sensation of tension in the muscles. A drawing in the back like a pulling or tension in the muscles. The pain feels as if drawing, a spasm of the muscles; a drawing pain in the back; drawing pain in the back of the neck, forcing the patient to let the head go back; drawing pain down the spine; lumbago. Backache worse as soon as she lies down (pregnancy) as if it would break (*Bry., Phos.*—as if broken, *Kali c.*) must get up and walk. Neuritis with great soreness of skin. Pains in the regions of the kidneys and liver. Pains draw so that he cannot turn over in bed, and the only way he can get over is to lift himself up by his hands and then turn over and lie down. Drawing pains in the sacrum and hips; drawing pains in the sacrum in connection with dysentery. Rending pains in the bowels and every *pain causes desire for stool.* Such is the characteristic of all the abdominal pains. Drawing pains in the extremities, causing spasms in the calves, feet, and toes. Cramps in the abdomen *cause desire for stool;* after pains in the form of cramps urge to stool; menstrual colic, with urging to stool; pains in the stomach, after eating, urge to stool. After much straining no stool passes, but after going several times a small stool passes with relief. It is scanty and with reversed peristaltic action.

Oversensitive to stimulants. It is a routine remedy in men trying to sober up; even in delirium tremens. Old debauchees, broken down with stimulants, sexual excesses and the worry and fret of business; they work half an hour and then go out and get a drink, and this goes on until finally they must give up, go home and go to bed. He is on the verge of insanity, irritable, fatigued, sweats much, is aggrravated from the air, sensitive to noise and light; broken down. He must have Nux, rest and no stimulants.

In those drinking too much tea, coffee and stimulants, they stay awake day and night until the end must come; there is tension in all the nerves; he feels as if he must fly, as if he could no longer hold together; his muscles and hands tremble; there is jerking of the limbs on going to sleep and in sleep.

Full of anxiety, despair, and hypochondriasis; "oversensitive to impressions;" all the senses are in this condition; "cannot bear reading or conversation; irritable, and wishes to be alone." Everybody displeases or does something to annoy him. Everybody that attempts to soothe only angers him. He dreads the business affairs of the day. Finally this state comes on—"he quarrels, reproaches, scolds, insults from jealousy, mingled with unchaste expressions; soon afterwards howls and weeps aloud."

Patient is broken down sexually because he is unusually endowed with sexual desires and he indulges until broken down; sexually exhausted, impotent. Mental erethism but relaxation on intromission. Driven to suicide.

Nux is an old dyspeptic, lean, hungry, withered; bent forward; premature age; always selecting his food and digesting almost none; aversion to meat, it makes him sick; craves pungent, bitter things, tonics. Weak stomach; after meals pain in the stomach, nausea, retching; stomach sinks in; withers and loses flesh.

Tendency to take cold; gets coryza. Colds settle in the nose, throat, chest and ears. Takes cold from the least provocation; perspires easily and the least current of air causes headache with coryza. If he is in a heated room and is disturbed in his equlibrium he gets a coryza. *Cepa* coryza is also worse in a warm room. Much stuffing up of the nose in the house at night; nose feels completely filled up, particularly out of doors, but fluent in doors; thin, watery discharge during the day. Sensitive to the least draft; sneezing caused by itching in the nose. This itching goes to the throat and trachea. Cough; burning in the air passages; all the mucous membranes in a state of irritation; nasal tone to voice; loss of voice; sore throat; tickling cough. Dry, teasing cough with great soreness of the chest, like *Bry.*, the head feels as if it would split. Coryza goes to the chest. Grippe with fever and bone pains; must pile on clothing; the only relief is by keeping unusually hot, yet a warm room aggravates the coryza before the fever comes on; but after the fever comes on he must have heat; aggravated even from the movement of air under the bed clothes; lifting the covers aggravates the pains, cough, etc.

Sharp fever and sweat, or a hot sweat like *Opium* (but *Opium* in a hot sweat wants the covers off, while Nux cannot raise the covers). Chills and fever; heat and sweat intermingled. In chills the fingers and hands are cold, and purple; cold from head to foot; the chill begins in the extremities or back, and extends over the whole body and the patient must be covered up. Shortly there is a reaction and heat and sweat come on, but he must be covered through all the stages. Thirst is not a marked feature; sometimes it is found in the heat.

Tendency to jaundice in all the febrile states. Sclerotics become yellow. Skin becomes very yellow. Old intermittents with yellow skin. Runs close to *Bry.* in abdominal complaints with jaundice.

Nux suffers from a disordered stomach. A stasis of the portal system is present, portal congestion; stasis in the hæmorrhoidal veins with hæmorrhoids; constipation; dysentery; paralysis of the rectum. Stomach symptoms like *Puls.*; worse in the morning; foul mouth in the morning also like *Puls.* Bursting sensation in the head as if a stone crushed the vertex after disordered stomach.

Full of paralytic conditions. The bowels are in a state of excitement but this passes away and the time comes when the fæces remain in the rectum with no warning. This extends to the bladder, so that it becomes full of urine which cannot be voided; dribbling of urine in old men with large prostate, or in gonorrhœa. Paralysis of the extremities; of the face; one arm; one hand; single muscles; facial paralysis not uncommonly cured by Nux. The sticking pains in paralysis are important.

At times false plethora, with flushed face; excitement of face; blushing; great weakness and exhaustion, with irritability and the mental condition. When under no exertion with nothing to think of, patient appears to be well, but the thought of doing something exhausts him in a moment.

Headache from sweating; in wine drinkers; in those staying out at night; from night watching. The greatest relief in headaches is from perfect quiet. Headaches as if a stone pressed upon the vertex. Most symptoms better from heat, but the head is worse from heat. Acne from eating cheese.

It has most violent convulsions with opisthotonos; convulsions of all the muscles of the body, with purple face and loss of breath from the movements; conscious or semi-conscious during the whole spasm, aware of

the sufferings and contortions which are horrible; worse from the slightest
draft of air; tickling of the feet; the merest touch of the throat causes gagging.

It is given as a routine remedy for loss of appetite. It will increase the
appetite but do dangerous work to the patient. "Aversion to meat, usual food
and drink, and customary tobacco and coffee, to water, ale, food just eaten."

Pains particularly of the abdomen; pains cutting, causing the patient to
bend double, with nausea from overeating; bearing down; spasmodic pains
in the abdomen, often extend into the limbs, but more often towards the
rectum; colicky pains which urge to stool and urination; renal colic, especially
when each pain shoots to the rectum and urges to stool. Renal colic is caused
by a stone in the ureter, which by its irritation causes a spasmodic clutching
of the circular fibers of that canal; the proper medicine relaxes these fibers
and the pressure from behind forces these calculi out at once. The same is
true of gall-stone colic. The remedy that ameliorates, or some of its cognates,
will overcome the tendency to form stones. Healthy bile dissolves gall-stones
in the sac; healthy urine does the same to a stone in the pelvis of the kidney.
Nux runs close to *Bry* in abdominal complaints with marked yellowness of
the skin. *Bry,* is worse from motion and not better from heat—Nux is both and
is more suited to portal congestion, the neuralgias, etc.; is worse from slightest
pressure (*Coloc.* is better from the slightest pressure,—*Mag. ph.* is better
from pressure and heat). *Bry.* indicated more in peritonitis, lies with limbs
drawn up. Hæmorrhoids, portal congestion, cutting pains to rectum causing
urging to stool. *Cupr.* has cutting pains from front to back as if transfixed.
Abdomen sunken in Nux, while in *Calc.* and *Sepia* it is engorged. *Inula*
resembles Nux; has colic with urging to stool and to urinate.

"Milk sours on the stomach." "Heat in the head when eating." Bad effects
from coffee, alcoholic, drinks, debauchery. Sensation of phlegm in the throat;
worse from eating. *Aloe* has diarrhœa from leaving off beer. Nux has diarrhœa
from leaving off alcoholic drinks. Sensation of a lump in the stomach (*Bry.*).
In chronic cases *Sepia* is more apt to be indicated and follows Nux well, but
quarrels with *Bry.;* associate this with the pressure in the vertex and you
have the typical Nux condition. Sensation of stone comes an hour after eating,
showing that there has been an attempt at digestion, but in *Abies nig.* it
comes at once. *Kreos.* pains do not begin until three hours after eating and
then the food is vomited.

It is closely related to *Sulphur* and often antidotes the overaction of
Sulphur. It seldom goes to the bottom and antidotes the constitutional action
of *Sulphur,* but it will remove its exaggerated action, its superficial action.

Menses too soon; too long; flow copious; more strikingly prolonged;
flows and dribbles just enough to stain the linen, starting up now and again
with clots. One menstrual flow is prolonged into another. This will be

accompanied with the mental state; excitable; oversensitive to medicines. "Menses too early and too profuse; occur too soon and last too long; flow dark." At times attended with violent pains, cramps in the uterus, extending over the body, ameliorated from heat and pressure; aggravated by the slightest current of air or cold; pains and spasms ameliorated by the hot water bottle, clothing and heat. Labor pains with soreness like *Arn.*— urging, etc. Bearing down as if contents would protrude, with teasing to urinate and urging to stool. The flow may be scant and fitful. Itching of the vulva is prominent.

Full of hysterical manifestations. Europeans develop symptoms more often calling for Nux in their hysterical manifestations, while Americans oftener need *Ignatia.*

Has troublesome asthma. Useful in persons who say they have asthma from every disordered stomach. They may go free for a year after Nux is given, and then they eat something that disagrees, and they sit up all night with asthma. They need Nux. Asthma associated with cough; rattling in the chest; chest fills up with mucus; cough with gagging, retching; appears as if he had taken a fresh cold.

Coryza every time he disorders his stomach. I have a patient who has a coryza every time she eats sausage; there is no cure for her because she places her coffee, wine, and social matters above her health. She can eat steak; some cannot eat any meat. After a disturbed stomach coryza which goes to the chest and then asthma comes on.

Palpitation and excitement of the heart and circulation. Much throbbing.

Worse in the morning—mentally and physically. The coryza and some head symptoms are worse from the warmth of the bed like *Merc.*, yet worse uncovering; worse from eating and from motion; head is worse from heat.

Pressure and sense of weakness in the left inguinal ring—hence cures hernia in babies (*Lyc.*, right side). *Arn.* relieves soreness, etc. *Conium,:* also —it competes with Nux in sense of goneness in the groin.

Chills are not better from any amount of covers; *Ign.* chills are better uncovering. In intermittents, the chill and heat intermingle, the heat is short and dry, and followed by hot sweat and intense heat; worse in the morning, but the chill comes at any time.

OPIUM

Among the striking features of Opium is a class of complaints marked by painless, inactivity, and torpor. Many of the provers taking small doses had torpor, inability to realize or feel their surroundings, or to take in the nature of states and judge of things. Deception in vision, taste, touch; deception of

810 OPIUM

the state he exists in; in his own realization; a perversion of all the senses
with much deception.

The general characteristic is painlessness, but now and then an alternate
state is produced, in which a small dose of Opium will cause pain,
sleeplessness, inquietude, nervous excitability; the very opposite state from
that produced in the majority of cases. The majority are constipated, but in
some there is dysentery and tenesmus. The patient is sleepy, yet at times the
drug is characterized by sleepless nights, anxiety, increased sensitiveness to
noise, so that he says he can almost hear the flies walking on the wall, and
hears the clock striking in the distant steeple.

It is generally supposed that in these opposite conditions one is primary
and the other is secondary. This is true, *e.g.*, those exhibiting stupor and
painlessness will go into a state of increased insensibility, inquietude, anxiety,
and irritabliity, and also one who has a state of increased sensibility first will
have a docile state following. Some oversensitive provers will get a basilar
headache in the first hour after taking a dose, so that they cannot raise the
head from the pillow; they are paralyzed from it; the pain holds them down.
This does not come on in most provers until the waning of a large dose. This
has been debated over as the primary and secondary actions. What is the
action in one is the reaction in another, but all are the effects of the drug, and
all the actions that follow are the symptoms of the remedy.

The sluggishness and painlessness are most striking. The inaction is
shown in the lack of reaction to the properly selected homœopathic remedy.
It here competes with *Sulphur*. On studying the case you may find many
Opium symptoms, and when given thus indicated, it rouses the system out
of the state of sluggishness and causes reaction.

Ulcers which are perfectly painless, which do not granulate, and do not
eat or spread, with numbness or lack of sensibility in the ulcer that ought to
be sensitive; Opium will often heal. Insensibility in parts that are in a high
grade of inflammation.

Paralytic conditions or paresis, partial paralysis; inactivity, sluggishness.
Such a condition is found in the bowels so that they do not move, and the
rectum fills with round, hard, black balls, which can be dug out with the
finger or spoon. There is no activity, no ability to strain at stool.

The bladder is in a similar state. There is no ability to use the abdominal
muscles; he cannot strain to urinate; retention of urine; accelerator muscles
are in a state of paresis.

When drinking the œsophagus seems to have no action and the fluid
does not go down but passes out through the nose; a paresis; fluids go
down the wrong way or out through the nose.

Weakness of limbs and muscles; weakness and paralysis.

Often there is a state of peace. Wants to be let alone. She tells you she is not sick; and yet she has a temperature of 105°–106°, is covered with a scorching hot sweat, has a rapid pulse; is delirious. You ask her how she is and she says she is perfectly well and happy; no pains or aches; wants nothing and has no symptoms. But the nurse tells you that the patient has passed no stool or urine. The face looks besotted, bloated, purple; the eyes are glassy and the pupils contracted. The brain is in a state of confusion, yet she can answer questions. Or the mental symptoms may be more marked and the physical condition less prominent; there is confusion of mind, delirium, loquacity, but this is rare, more commonly only talks when aroused; a condition of stupor in which the patient will say nothing and do nothing. Delirium with a happy turn of mind.

The stomach is in a state of undue warmth, sinking, all-gone, hungry, and this is not relieved by eating. He fills the stomach full and yet the faint feeling remains. The food sours in the stomach and is vomited. He can take no more food. He becomes covered with a cold sweat; great exhaustion; nausea, retching and the vomiting continues. This nausea is a troublesome symptom following the administration of Opium or *Morphine*. It is a prolonged vomiting and nausea. He can take nothing into the stomach and nothing will stop the vomiting for him. The homœopath knows the use of *Chamomilla* and one dose will give wonderful relief at once and stop the deathly sinking and nausea.

There is never any use for the crude Opium in the sick room. In surgery at times it is admitted that something seems necessary, and we will not quarrel with the surgeon. But in disease, in sick people, it is not necessary. It performs no use and in the end it is an injury; it prevents finding the homœopathic remedy. It has masked the symptoms and spoiled the case, and you cannot do anything for days.

Opium has been much abused and much has been learned about it, but this abuse has not helped much in its proving, for the individualizing symptoms are not obtained. Big doses cause gross effects, and the symptoms thus obtained are sometimes useful, *e.g.*, in cerebral apoplexy with stertorous breathing, jaw dropped, pupils dilated or contracted generally the latter, face mottled, purple, or hot, hot sweat, one-sided paralysis. You would wonder on seeing such a case whether he had been paralyzed, had Opium, injured himself in a fall or had been indulging in the bottle, and you would examine the case to distinguish. This is a mechanical trouble, there is pressure of blood on the brain. This alone may not kill but later on inflammatory action is set up around the clot. Opium causes a flow of blood to the brain, and when given homœopathically it checks this, and in six hours he will become rational, his skin cool, face normal color, pulse normal. We thus see the usefulness of the crude effects of Opium in giving us a picture of apoplexy.

Nervous headaches beginning in the back of the head and spreading over the whole face; worse in the morning. He feels as if his head were held down to the pillow by the intense aching pain in the base of the brain, and yet when he gets up he is unable to lie down again. This is common in women; a false plethora; excitable; going through pregnancy or menstruation; headache. The patient sits up and is unable to lie down. The pain begins in the morning and is so violent that the patient cannot move, cannot wink the eye, turn the head, cannot bear the least jar or the ticking of the clock; face is mottled, purple, blue; eyes injected. It is difficult to get symptoms from her. Opium will relieve at once.

But most of the complaints are painless.

It takes on the appearance of drinkers, besotted; fever with besotted countenance. Delirium tremens with awful anxiety, vomiting, congestive headache, contracted pupils; violent headache after drinking, exhaustion; not able to get out of bed; delirium. Most of the complaints are attended with stupor; lies in a stupor like apoplexy, cannot be aroused.

The Opium patient is full of convulsions. The patient wants to be uncovered, wants the cool air, the open air. Convulsions if the room is too warm. Opisthotonos; head drawn back; cerebro-spinal meningitis. In a case of cerebro-spinal meningitis we find convulsions approaching, opisthotonos, head drawn back, kicks the covers off, wants a cool room; skin red; face red and mottled, pupils contracted. Now if the mother puts that child into a hot bath, to relieve the convulsions, it will become unconscious and cold as death. If you are called to see such a case be sure to give Opium, and in twelve hours you will be astonished to see the state of quietude. It competes here with *Apis.* Puerperal convulsions.

A mental state appears in these constitutions. Fear and its results. The Opium patient, when not too stupid, rouses up as if startled, rouses up with the appearance of awful fear or anxiety. The old Opium eater is overwhelmed with anxiety and fear. If a dog jump at him suddenly, he will be thrown into convulsions, have diarrhœa, fits of some sort, and it will be days and weeks before that fear is gone. Complaints from fear when the fear remains, or the idea of the fear remains, or the cause of it comes before the eyes. A pregnant woman is frightened and an abortion is impending, and the object of the fright continually looms up before her eyes. Epilepsy dating back to a fright, and that object comes up before the eyes before the attack comes on, and *the fear of the fright remains.* Hysterical attack; physical shock with diarrhœa and sometimes constipation; retention of urine or return of the menstrual flow as results, or it may stop the menses for months. In these conditions there is great fear and the object of the fear remains before the eyes.

An Opium prover, when coming out from under the influence of the drug, sees frightful images, black forms, visions of devils, fire, ghosts, someone carrying her off, murder. Imagines that parts swell and that he is going to burst.

There is also a sensation of bodily well being; great happiness; great state of confidence in the first hours of the drug. Hence, complaints from sudden joy, anger, shame, sudden fright. *Coffea* has a similar state of beatitude. It is both a physical and mental beatitude in Opium. Opium and *Coffea* are related; they antidote each other.

Opium eaters like whisky drinkers are constitutional liars. They have no conscience left.

"Great sensibility to sound, light, and faintest odors." "Drowsiness with headache, amounting almost to stupor." "Marasmus; child wrinkled and looks like a little dried up old man; stupor."

Old cases of lead piosoning. *Pulsatilla* cures the diarrhœa following the abuse of Opium.

OXALIC ACID

This remedy has been greatly neglected. It will cure many heart complaints that are treated with vague, crude, unproved remedies with indifferent results. The violent action upon the heart racks the whole system. Trembling, convulsions, loss of sensation; numbness of the body and limbs; blueness of the lower limbs, fingers and lips; paralysis of the limbs are symptoms showing how violently this remedy takes hold of the body, affecting the heart, spinal cord and brain. Symptoms are worse from exertion and motion. The patient is sensitive to cold air. Symptoms come on in paroxysms. Palpitation alternates with loss of voice. No remedy produces more violent pains; cutting, shooting, stitching, tearing pains in many parts; sores and bruises all over the body; burning in forehead, stomach, abdomen, throat, urethra, hands and feet; painful spots on the scalp, sore to touch, also in other places. The body is mottled in places. Complaints come on from eating sour fruits, such as strawberries, cranberries, apples, rhubarb, tomatoes, grapes; also from eating sugar and starchy foods. Wine and coffee disagree. The symptoms, and especially the pains, come on or are worse when thinking about them. At times there is great excitement and exhilaration—again there is loss of memory and dejection; maniacal conduct; aversion to conversation. Fainting during stool. There is marked hyperæmia of the brain and surging of blood from body to head; flashes of heat mount upward; he becomes dizzy and there is vanishing of sight. The head feels empty; dull aching in the head; in forehead and vertex; the brain burns; *headache in spots;* pressing pain in small spots; pressing pain behind ear; the headaches are worse from wine, lying, after sleep, and on rising and better after stool. *Sore tender spots on the scalp.* Type blurs when reading; vanishing of sight; small, especially linear objects seem larger and more distant; pain in eyes, especially the left; bleared eyes. Epistaxis with vanishing of sight. Face is pale and blue; sunken expression; heat in face; face covered with cold sweat; drawing pain with rigidity near the angle of lower jaw—first in left, then in right. Ulcers on gums; gums bleed and are painful in spots; sour taste in the mouth; tongue sore, red, dry, burning, swollen, with white coating; there is loss of taste; aphthæ in the mouth; much thick mucus compels him to constantly clear the throat; swallowing is painful in the morning; pain in throat; chronic sore throat.

Appetite increased; wanting, with loss of taste; thirst.

Pain in stomach better after eating; gnawing in stomach better after taking soup. After eating, eructations, nausea, pains at the navel, colic, rumbling in bowels, urging to stool, weakness. Sugar increases the pain in stomach; wine makes headache worse; coffee acts violently on the heart and causes diarrhœa; heartburn worse in the evening; eructation, sour, tasteless, after eating. Nausea and vomiting; nausea during pregnancy; thirst and colic after diarrhœa; nausea and cramp in calves after stool. Paroxysmal pains in abdomen in the night, relieved by passing flatus; burning in stomach and throat; extreme tenderness of stomach; inflammation of stomach and intestines; empty feeling relieved by eating. Cramping pains in abdomen. Burning in the abdomen. Stitching pains in abdomen and in the liver. Great pain in the region of the umbilicus, worse evening and night; worse from motion. Sore pains about the navel. The pains in abdomen come on or are worse when thinking of them. Obstructed flatus in the splenic flexure of the colon, causing pain in left hypochondrium. Stitching pains in liver, relieved by deep breathing.

Cramping pains in abdomen, worse at night with vomiting; worse from motion and from eating sugar. Chronic inflammation of the bowels. Extreme tenderness of the abdomen; chronic morning diarrhœa with cramping about the navel; tenesmus, renewed urging on lying down. Coffee brings on diarrhœa; stools watery; of mucus and blood; stools involuntary. The tenesmus during stool causes pain in head; constipation with difficult stool and the straining causes headache.

The renal region is painful and tender. Frequent urination; copious urine containing oxalate of lime; soreness of whole urinary tract; the urine causes soreness and burning of the urethra; when urinating there is pain in the glans penis; incontinence of urine in sleep; all the urinary symptoms are worse when thinking about them.

Tearing pains in the spermatic cords, worse from motion; marked tenderness in testes which become painful when walking. Strong sexual desire and erections when in bed; seminal emissions and sexual weakness; shooting pains along the spermatic cords.

Loss of voice with cardiac complaints; palpitation alternating with loss of voice; larynx sore, raw, with tickling and clutching; mucus forms in the larynx when talking; must constantly clear the larynx when talking; white mucus in the larynx; hawks up thick yellow and white mucus.

In complaints of the heart there is most difficult breathing. In feeble, nervous women there is paroxysmal breathing; violent rapid respiration with intervals of normal breathing; jerking inspiration and sudden, forced expiration in angina pectoris; dyspnœa with constriction in the larynx that is very painful; with wheezing and oppression of chest worse thinking of it.

Cardiac cough on slight exertion; choking feeling in larynx; tickling in larynx while walking in cold air.

Sharp, shooting pains in left lung, heart and left hypochondrium, with inability to breathe during perfect rest; soreness in chest; pain in middle of chest through to the back. Dullness in lower part of left lung.

Stitching tearing pains behind the sternum going to shoulders and arms; worse on left side, with blueness of nails and lips; cold sweat; paralysis of lower limbs; spasmodic respiration (compare *Latrodectus mactans*). Violent palpitation in rheumatic subjects, worse when thinking about it. Pulse irregular, intermittent, fast; cold sweat, blue nails, great weakness. It cures many cardiac complaints; endocarditis, pericarditis, valvular insufficiency, etc. *Fluttering heart.*

Pain under point of scapula, between shoulders, extending downward to small of back; stitches in chest, extending to scapula; violent aching pain in back and down the thighs, relieved by change of position. This symptom is an exception as the pains are generally worse from motion. Benumbing pains in the small of back better after stool. Numbness, pricking, causing a cold sensation with weakness in spine; weakness in loins and hips extending to lower limbs; pains shoot up back to head. Cold chills in lower part of back followed by evening fever, coming every day. Motion brings on many pains in spine with much drawing in muscles of back; paralysis from inflammation of spinal cord; limbs stiff; paroxysms of dyspnœa.

Numbness in shoulders to finger tips; sharp lancinating pains in arms; right wrist feels sprained; pain in right meta-carpus and fleshy part of right thumb with heat and numbness; hands almost helpless; *hands cold as if dead;* fingers and nails blue in heart complaints; pains in the points of flexed fingers. Twitching of muscles of shoulder, arm and fingers. The legs are stiff, numb and weak; lower limbs cold, blue and paralyzed. Violent pains in lower limbs. Burning in feet and hands. Rheumatism of joints.

Frightening dreams; wakens with palpitation, cold sweat and pain in limbs; sleepy during day but distressing sleep at night; feels better after passing flatus. Violent pains in stomach keep him awake.

Chilliness; shaking chill, cold body. Heat from slight exertion; flashes of heat then cold sweat; shaking chill in evening followed by internal heat and exetrnal sweat, hands cold. Cold sweat of face, hands and feet.

816

PETROLEUM

It is one of the abused remedies. It is used externally in rheumatism, bruises and all sorts of troubles, and the amelioration that comes is the result of establishing a disease on the surface, by counter-irritation, and not by homœopathic action. Crude Petroleum is extensively used in the oil regions on both man and beast as a "cure all".

It is a counter-irritant and, on the skin, produces irritation, eruptions and disturbances, like *Turpentine*. Among the early things that Petroleum does to a prover is that it puts him in a state of confusion of mind and dizziness; he is dazed so that he loses his way in the street. She has strange imaginations that there are people near her who are not present; that the atmosphere is full of strange forms; that her limbs are double; that another person is in the bed with her. Such things are found in the fevers. A woman after childbirth imagines there is another child in bed with her, and she wonders how she will take care of the two. These ideas are found in many diseases, have been often verified. In typhoids and low forms of sickness; in diarrhœas; when just awaking he is in confusion; in his dreams he had the idea of being two or more and the impression remains with him while he is in a semi-conscious state. He cannot reconcile the state, but when aroused to consciousness he is able to reason it away, and when semi-conscious again it returns. This annoys him day and night.

Skin symptoms. The surface symptoms are striking. The tendency is to throw out vesicles, herpetic vesicles which are isolated, and the tendency of the vesicles is to form thick yellow crusts, with considerable moisture. The vesicles break early. At times the vesicles do not form crusts, but break early and ulcerate underneath, and this changes into a phagedenic ulcer; this condition occurs about the fingers, scrotum, face and scalp. There is a special tendency to produce vesicular eruptions about the back of the neck. Papular, pustular, vesicular, dry, mealy eruptions, but most commonly moist; eruptions which extend deeply. it builds up eruptions on the site of old eruptions, with an increasing hardness in the base of the old eruption. When the crust dries down it indurates, and this induration takes place at the margin and builds up little rings about the margin. The induration cracks, bleeds, looks purple. Apply this to salt rheum, and eruptions about the hands. It is suitable when there are cracks about the ends of the fingers and on the backs of the hands. The skin is rough, ragged, exfoliates, cracks, bleeds; the tissues are hardened; this occurs sometimes about the palms of the hands and nails. This tissue ulcerates, and the ulcers eat and spread. All eruptions itch violently. He cannot rest until he scratches the skin off, when the part becomes moist, bloody, raw and inflamed. There is also itching, with no visible eruption. He scratches the skin until moisture oozes forth, and keeps on scratching until the skin bleeds and the part becomes *cold*. (This word makes me remark here that *coldness in spots* is quite a feature of this remedy. Coldness in spots; coldness in the stomach, in the abdomen, in the uterus; coldness in a spot between the scapulæ; coldness in the heart—sensation as if the heart were cold.) Various forms of eczema. Eczema of the scalp, especially of the occiput. Herpetic eruptions about the mouth (*Nat. m.*), about the genitals, lips, face, and the patches become crusty and ooze much.

The *mucous membrane,* or internal skin, has little patches of ulcers, with induration about the patch, and hence Petr. is useful in syphilitic ulcers. Ulcerous patches in the throat; aphthous patches in the mouth. There is inflammation of the mucous membranes everywhere, producing watery and finally thick yellow discharges. The nose is filled by tumefaction of the Schneiderian membrane. Old catarrhal complaints of the nose, crusts, thick yellow discharge, fœtid odor from the nose. The nose, posterior nares and pharynx become thickened and there is an accumulation of thick mucus, especially in the morning. The larynx is involved and there is loss of voice, and the trouble extends to the chest, causing a catarrhal condition with cough. He coughs especially at night, and there is emaciation of the body with pain and soreness of the chest. Dry, hacking cough, alternating with copious expectoration; emaciation about the chest. A striking feature of this drug is that the cough is worse at night, and the diarrhœa is worse during the day. Catarrh of the stomach and bowels. Catarrh of the rectum, much mucus with the stools. *Diarrhœa during the daytime, ameliorated at night,* while the patient is quiet and at rest. He cannot eat without pain, but he has a gnawing hunger which drives him to eat. (*Lach., Graph.*). There is an "all-gone," hungry feeling after stool, which drives him to eat. With the diarrhœa there is constant hunger, yet he cannot eat without pain; emaciation, skin eruptions, unhealthy ragged fingers which never look clean; he cannot wash them, as this causes them to chap.

Catarrh of the bladder and urethra; chronic catarrhal discharge; chronic gonorrhœa. Itching is common to the internal skin, and a striking feature in gonorrhœa is the itching in the posterior half of the urethra with the discharge. It almost drives him wild, keeps him awake at night. He rubs and manipulates the perinæum to relieve this itching. The gonorrhœal discharge is white or yellow. It is useful in that "last drop". Also in the early stages of gonorrhœa when the itching is troublesome.

Sore bruised feeling all over the body, especially in the joints. Rheumatic pain in the joints on motion; sore to touch; sensation as if bruised. It is analogous to *Arnica* in relation to bruises.

Petroleum is suitable in old stubborn *occipital headaches. Silicea* is the routine remedy for offensive foot sweat and periodic occipital headaches. Petroleum has also offensive foot sweat; offensive sweats all over, and especially so in the axilla, where it is so pungent that it can be observed on the patient entering the room. The pain often remains in the occiput, but when very severe it extends up over the top of the head to the eyes and forehead (*Silicea* has that condition). Petroleum is not so closely related to *Silicea* as it is to *Graphites* and *Carbo veg.*, which are carbonaceous substances; and all carbonaceous products affect the back of the head. "Pain from occiput over head to forehead and eyes, with transitory blindness; he gets stiff; loses consciousness." "Circumscribed pain in the occiput, aggravated on shaking the head." This remedy, unlike *Carbo veg.*, has oversensitiveness of the senses, hearing, touch and smell.

The Petroleum constitution produces a peculiar vertigo which comes on under regular circumstances, when on ship-board, or riding in a carriage, or on the cars. It suits occipital headache from riding on the cars, or from such motions, with nausea like seasickness. Seasickness is a trouble we cannot always meet, yet most people, when constitutionally treated, can be directed into a better state, so that they will not be troubled under ordinary conditions, such as riding on the cars or in a carriage. To a great extent the above condition is due to a lack of accommodation, a visual trouble; coming on, for example, from focusing the eyes on the waves as they retreat from the rear end of the ship, or on passing objects, the patient being relieved while in a dark state-room. Occipital headache, with the vertigo above mentioned, and an all-gone hungry feeling or pain in the stomach, driving him to eat, will be mitigated by Petroleum. The most common form of seasickness I have found to be the following: Awful deathly nausea, great pallor, cold body, profuse sweat and exhaustion, ameliorated by fanning, by the open air, by closing the eyes, by quiet and darkness, and aggravated by warmth. *Tabacum* is generally the remedy for such cases.

In Petroleum there is much disturbance of vision, but the catarrhal state of the eyes is striking. Vesicular formations, ulcerations, inflammation, redness and copious discharge; granular lids, thickening of the mucous membranes, cracks in the lids, fissures in the corners of the eyes with *great itching*. This itching is present in all congestions of the mucous membrane. *Eustachian tubes.* The mucous membrane is thickened, and deafness results. It is a catarrhal state, and is attended by great itching in the tube, which he cannot reach by any method; itching deep in the ear. He rubs the ear and tries to scratch it, but he cannot reach it. Itching in the pharynx; also in the external canal of the ear. Ear discharges.

Induration and inflammation of the glands of the body. In ear troubles the parotids enlarge; in troubles about the jaw the submaxillary and sublingual glands are involved; they become hard and tend to remain so. Face pale or yellow; sickly. "Nausea and qualmishness all day."

Stiffness in the back. Pain in the back on rising from a seat.

Heat and burning. Skin hot in places; with sensation of coldness in spots. Burning and itching of palms and soles; face and scalp burn. The itching and burning often go together; parts that burn itch much. Feet burn and have a sensation as if frozen. Chilblains which itch, burn and become purple. Parts frozen will, years after, itch, burn, sting and become red and hot. The patient can tell when it will thaw because of the itching in the chilblains. Petroleum cures the itching and burning in frozen parts, but not as prominently as *Agaricus*. *Agaricus* leads all other remedies, especially when the condition affects parts where the tissues are thin over the bones, as over the back of the toes.

Paretic conditions, especially left-sided. Weakness of muscles, weakness of the lower extremities, especially left-sided.

The eruptions on the surface and the state of induration are like *Graphites*, but the oozing in Petroleum is thin and watery, and in *Graphites* it is gluey, honey like, sticky, viscid. You have indurations and cracks of the fingers, and rhagades in both remedies, but the horn-like warty growths, lifting up the quick of the nails, you will find only in *Graphites*.

It is of wonderful use and competes with *Rhus* in eczema of the genitals of either male or female. Eruptions on the scrotum, penis, vulva. *Rhus* produces violent inflammation of the skin of the genitals in male and female; erysipelatous inflammation; nodules, vesicles and *large* blebs. Petroleum produces *small* vesicles which itch; sting and burn. Herpetic eruptions which tend to become erysipelatous. Petroleum and *Rhus* are the most common remedies for eruptions on the scrotum and genitals. "Herpetic itching, redness and moisture on scrotum; skin cracked, rough and bleeding; extending to perinæum and thighs." "Obstinate dry eruptions on genitals and perinæum." "Sweat and moisture of external genitals of both sexes."

Scurfy nipples; white, bran-like scurf; itching; always peeling off. If the woman is in run-down health, then the nipples inflame and become oversensitive to the touch of clothing.

Very sensitive to change of weather, like *Phos.* and *Rhod.;* aggravated before a thunder-storm. Often sensitive to air and cold. Lean, emaciated subjects; threatening consumption. Eruptions disappear of themselves or are suppressed. Hands and feet burn; wants the palms and soles out of bed. Do not be too sure of *Sulphur* because the soles burn, or too sure of *Silicea* because the feet sweat. Sweating of single parts. Eruptions in patches. Itching in patches. Coldness in parts. Complaints come in single parts. The most striking offensiveness is about the feet and in the axillæ. There are many strange sensations which are peculiar and striking. Study closely the skin symptoms and compare with *Graphites* and *Sulphur*.

PHOSPHORIC ACID

"Mental enfeeblement" is the thought that will come into the mind when considering what the Phosphoric acid patient says, does and looks. The mind seems tired. When questioned he answers slowly or does not speak, but only looks at the questioner. He is too tired to talk or even think. He says: "Don't talk to me; let me alone." This state is found in both acute and chronic diseases. He is so tired in mind, perfectly exhausted. In chronic diseases when brought on from long study; prolonged worry in business men; in feeble school girls, who become relaxed from very little effort. In acute diseases he, especially in typhoid fever, is averse to speaking or answering questions. He merely looks. Finally he rouses up and says: "Don't talk to me, I am so tired." He cannot think what he wishes to say, cannot frame his answers to questions. Another cause is sexual excesses in young men, or in those guilty of secret vice. Weakness; lack of reaction; state of stupor, with impotency; mental prostration, and as if the spine had given out.

In every case we find the *mental* symptoms are the first to develop. The remedy runs from the mental to the physical, from the brain to the muscles. This is so striking that it is contrasted with *Muriatic acid.* In the latter remedy the *muscular* prostration comes first, and the mind seems clear until long after the muscles are prostrated. In Phosphoric acid the muscles seem strong after the mind has given out. The patient seems vigorous physically. He says he is all right physically, can work, can exercise even violently; but the mind is tired, there is mental apathy, he cannot add up a column of figures, cannot read the newspaper and carry the trend of thought, cannot connect circumstances. He forgets the names of those in his family; a business man forgets the names of his clerks; he is in confusion. Yet he can exercise, can go out and walk; the weakness in the muscles will come later.

Phosphoric acid has also great physical weakness; so tired in the back; so tired in the muscles; so tired all over; a paralytic weakness. Later there is sexual impotence; aversion to coition; loss of sexual desire; no erections; penis becomes relaxed in the midst of an embrace and he cannot finish the act (*Nux.v*).

Ailments from business cares; prolonged grief; young women suffering from unrequited affection, or from the loss of a loved one. Some suffer more intensely than others; some seem more philosophical. "Ailments from care, grief, sorrow, chagrin, homesickness or disappointed love; particularly with drowsiness; night sweats towards morning; emaciation." The patient pines and emaciates, grows weaker and weaker, withered in the face; night sweats; cold sweat down the back; cold sweats on the arms and hands more than on the feet; cold extremities; feeble circulation, feeble heart; catches cold on the slightest provocation and it settles in the chest; dry, hacking cough; catarrhal conditions of the chest; tuberculosis; pallor with gradually increasing weakness and emaciation.

During this weakness there is vertigo. Vertigo while lying in bed; seems like floating while lying in bed. Limbs seem to be lifted up while the head does not seem to move; as if the limbs were floating.

Congestive headaches; in school girls from slight exertion of the mind and use of the eyes. Periosteal pains; bones ache as if scraped; ameliorated by motion; when lying the pain shifts to side lain on.

Most of the complaints are ameliorated from keeping warm, from absolute quiet, from being alone at peace. There is aggravation of the complaints from exertion, mental or physical, from being talked to. Morning headaches. He must lie down with the headaches. Headache aggravated from being talked to. He is sensitive to cold weather. He is sensitive to a warm room.

In the headache the pain often begins in the back of the head and spreads to the top of the head; feels as if a crushing weight were on the top of the head; worse from motion, talking and light. "Pressure as from a weight in head from above downward. These headaches are associated with mental weakness, brain-fag; so tired and exhausted. Vertigo with ringing in the ears and glassy eyes.

Its use in low fevers must be studied. The complaints come on slowly, slow decline, slowly increasing prostration. Such appearances as are found in advanced typhoid. It has the prostration, tympanitic abdomen, dry, brown tongue, sordes on the teeth, gradually approaching unconsciousness; little thirst increasing to intense thirst with craving for much water during perspiration; wants to be let alone; looks at the questioner with glassy eyes as if slowly comprehending the question; pupils contracted or dilated; eyes sunken; hippocratic countenance; continued fever; bleeding from the nose, lungs, bowels; hæmorrhage from any mucous membrane; sunken about the eyes; discolored lips, covered with sordes, becoming very black; prostration gradually increasing. From the beginning the mental state has been most marked, and finally comes the muscular weakness, which increases until the jaw drops and it seems that the patient must die of exhaustion. Such states of weakness may come on from hæmorrhages (*China* was the routine remedy among the older homœopaths). It checks the hæmorrhage and causes a rally, prevents the dropsy. There is a state like anæmia; pale lips and tongue; face, hands and feet waxy.

Pains and aches all over the body, ameliorated from motion and worse from cold. The pains seem deep-seated, often along the nerves, but especially along the long bones, as if the bones were scraped; as if a rough instrument were dragged over the bones. The pains are commonly worse at night. Severe bone pains.

The stomach refuses to do its work. The food remains in the stomach and sours. Sour vomiting. Old dyspeptics with brain-fag. Complaints from acid drinks, cold drinks and rich foods. Sinking sensation in the abdomen after a normal stool.

In most of the complaints of Phosphoric acid a marked feature is *milky* urine. Sometimes it is milky when passed; milky flakes in the urine. At times the male urethra seems to clog up and examination will show these little milk-like flakes. The urine becomes milky on standing, like flour, chalk or phosphate deposits stirred up in it.

In Phosphoric acid there is often an amelioration of complaints by their ending in a diarrhœa. Copious, thin, watery stool. From the quantity it would seem that the patient would be exhausted. Child with copious, watery stool in summer; so copious that the napkin seems of no use; the stool runs all over the mother's dress and on the floor forming great puddles; the stool is almost *odorless,* thin and watery, and the little one smiles as if nothing were the matter. The mother wonders where it all comes from, and yet the child seems well. The Phosphoric acid diarrhœa often ameliorates many of the symptoms and the patient feels better. Chronic diarrhœa, copious, thin and watery, whitish gray, and the patient feels comfortable, free and happy. If the diarrhœa slacks up the patient is worse and on come symptoms of tuberculosis, weakness prostration, brain-fag. Some patients say they are never comfortable unless they have diarrhœa. *Podophyllum* is the very opposite. Take the same child the stool is very copious and runs all over the floor, the mother wonders where it all comes from, but the stool is so *offensive,* a horrible stench, and the patient looks as if dying; mouth and nose drawn, countenance hippocratic almost unconscious. There is painless stool in both, but Phosphoric acid has not the great prostration. In Phosphoric acid the stool is whitish gray, like dirty white paint; in *Podophyllum* it is yellow. *Gratiola* has a similar state of prostration, but the fluid is green water; when seen it looks like light shining through a green glass; sometimes thicker, like green bile.

Abdomen much bloated, tympanitic; great soreness of the bowels as if in a typhoid state. "White or yellow, watery diarrhœa, chronic or acute, without pain or any marked debility or exhaustion." It is uncommon for the stool to be yellow when watery. It is yellow when it is mushy; when watery it is light colored, sometimes milky. When yellow it is like corn meal mush, pappy; as in the typhoid state, thin like thin mush. "Diarrhœa; not prostrating; after catching cold during heat of summer; water; chronic; violent, bilious or mucous of twenty months' standing; has the appearance of an old man; from acids in young persons who grow too rapidly; after eating, undigested greenish white; painless." When we have a diarrhœa from acids we sometimes find symptoms running to Phosphoric acid. In the diarrhœa from sour wine such as claret, from acids, vinegar, lemons, be sure to study *Antimonium crudum.* This is a very striking feature of that remedy. Useful in cholera.

Male sexual organs. Sexual weakness, prolonged exhaustion, impotency; masturbators; nightly pollutions with great exhaustion. "Prostatorrhœa; immediately after every erection discharge of prostatic fluid." Even when passing a soft stool the prostatic fluid is discharged.

Falling out of the hair is a striking feature; falling of the hair from the genitals, whiskers, eyebrows, head. It is closely related to *Natrum mur.* and *Selenium* in falling out of the hair. *Selenium* has falling out of the hair from the head, eyebrows and lashes, beard and genitals, from all over the body. *Natrum mur.* causes the hair to become very thin; during confinement the hair falls from the genitals.

Phosphoric acid produces a troublesome leucorrhœa; "yellow, mostly after menses, with itching; profuse, yellow; thin, acid mucus; with chlorosis." It suits the woman who has been nursing her child a long time, or nursing twins, and who gives much milk. She becomes tired and weakly. Loss of fluids, blood; prolonged nursing, and weakness from such causes.

The tendency of the Phosphoric acid patient at the end of the brain-fag and weakness is to run into *chest troubles.* If a diarrhœa comes on then the chest trouble is averted. Most awful results will ensue from the use of astringents, or any remedy that does not correspond to the patient, that will stop that diarrhœa. He goes into tuberculosis; difficult respiration; coughs and suffers in the chest, and the trouble culminates in structural changes in the lungs. The indications for Phosphoric acid are seldom found in the tissue changes, but they will be found in the *early* states of the patient, the nervous conditions, the milky urine and the diarrhœa, which have existed a long time. Chest complaints are acute; typhoid pneumonia; low forms of fever ending in chest troubles; not unlike *Phosphorus.* Prolonged pneumonia with the mental symptoms, lack of reaction, infiltration at the end of pneumonia. Hæmoptysis.

Prolonged fever ending in feeble heart, with palpitation and the mental symptoms. Palpitating during sexual excitement. Tendency to abscesses after a prolonged fever.

Limbs and joints become affected. Pain in the hip joint. Pains in the long bones between the joints, better by motion. Old gouty constitution. Tissues become weak. Red spots appear wherever the flesh is thin over the bones, and these spots become inflamed and form open ulcers. After fever, abscesses in the muscles, and state of molecular weakness about the ankles; over the tibia where the flesh is thin. Phosphoric acid has a special relation to the periosteum. Periostitis. Pains in the tibia at night. Bone feels as if scraped. Cold hands and hot feet. Ulcers on the legs with watery, offensive discharge.

Boils, abscesses, pustules and other moist eruptions. Suppurating eruptions; tissues become weak.

Nervous state; marked indifference; weak and trembling; fainting; great nervous exhaustion; hysterical affections. Creeping, tingling and crawling all over the body, especially where there is hair, as if in the roots of the hair; formication; especially in those debilitated from sexual excesses. "Formication over whole body." Sore spots in the spine; lame back. Backache.

"Itching between the fingers or in the bend of joints or on hands." Herpes; eczema, erysipelas. Large purple spots form on the skin, and extravasation of blood from the capillary veins; ecchymoses. Ulcers on the skin; carbuncles; warts; chilblains; wens; corns with stinging and burning, and parts become black; feeble circulation in the skin. Skin withered, old and gray, and the patient emaciates.

PHOSPHORUS

The complaints of Phosphorus are most likely to arise in the feeble constitutions, such as have been born sick, grown up slender, and grown too rapidly. Its complaints are found in such as are emaciated, and in those who are rapidly emaciating; in children who are going into marasmus, and in persons who have in them the foundation of consumption fairly well laid. Delicate, waxy, anæmic and emaciated subjects. In persons who are vehement, irascible. This expresses the person's disposition somewhat as well as his internal constitutional state. Internally he is in a turmoil. Subject to violent pulsations, complaints from electric changes in the atmosphere; violent palpitations and orgasms. In chlorotic girls who have grown too rapidly and have suddenly taken on weakness, pallor, green sickness, with menstrual difficulties. Ebullitions and congestions. Hæmorrhagic constitutions. Small wounds bleed much; the prick of the needle will bubble forth much bright red blood. Hæmorrhage from small wounds, from the nose, from the lungs, from the stomach, from the bladder and from the uterus. Bleeding from ulcerations. False granulations that bleed. Purpura hæmorrhagica. Black and blue spots. Blood settles beneath the conjunctiva, or beneath the skin anywhere. Bloody saliva; evidences of disorganized blood, or that the blood seems to become fluid. Small bruises take on broad blue spots. Blows much blood out of the nose. Petechiæ all over the body, such as are found in typhoid fever, low forms of continued fever with hæmorrhages. Fungous growths. Fatty degeneration is a marked feature of Phosphorus, and can be found in the liver, heart or kidneys. General dropsical condition. Bloating of the hands and feet, especially dropsical conditions after scarlet fever. The mucous membranes are all pale, such as is found after bleeding or in low forms of disease. A marked state of anæmia and relaxed condition of the muscles. Muscles flabby.

Fatty degeneration of the muscles. The genitals hang down. In the woman, relaxation of the pelvic organs, prolapsus and other displacements. Stiffness is a marked feature of Phosphorus. Stiffness on beginning to move. Limbs stiff like a foundered horse, especially in the morning. Rheumatic stiffness in all the limbs. Phosphorus has tearing, drawing pains in the limbs. Drawing, tearing pains in affected parts. Phosphorus complaints are worse in cold weather. The patient himself, generally considered, is sensitive to cold. All his complaints are worse from cold and cold applications, and better from heat and warm applications, except the complaints of the head and stomach, which are ameliorated from cold as will hereafter be described. Phosphorus has been very useful in weak, relaxed conditions of the joints following sprains, when the symptoms agree. Necrosis is another feature of Phosphorus, especially of the lower jaw, but may be useful in necrosis of any of the bones. Exostoses of the skull with tearing pains. Tearing, boring pains, especially at night. Phosphorus has cured polypi of the nose and ears. Scrofulous and glandular swellings. Glands enlarge, especially after contusions like *Bellis.* Glandular affections of weak, pale, sickly individuals, such as suffer from diarrhœa, such as suffer from exhaustive conditions, abscesses, fistulous openings, with hectic fever. Abscesses with copious discharge of yellow pus,. Malignant growths are greatly restrained by the use of Phosphorus, when the symptoms agree. Burning pains are observed everywhere. Burning in the brain, burning in the skin. Burning in the stomach in the chest, and in various parts.

The Phosphorus patient is very sensitive to all external impressions; slight odors, noises, touch. Slight causes lead to exhaustion of either body or mind. Trembling throughout the body from slight causes, using the hands, from slight exertion, from debility, from coughing. Weakness prevails in a marked degree, finally becoming paralysis or paralytic weakness such as occurs in most forms of typhoid fever, with sliding down in bed, trembling and jerking of the muscles. Paralysis with formication and tearing in the limbs. Paralysis that comes with apoplexy. Jerking and twitching of the muscles such as has been found in paralysis. Spasms of the paralyzed parts. Tearing, drawing, burning pains throughout the body. The Phosphorus patient wants to be rubbed. He is generally better after sleep. Always wants to rest. Always tired. The Phosphorus patient undergoes great excitement. Tremulousness. Wild thoughts. Excitability, keeping him awake at night. Violent imaginations. Excitability even to ecstacy and clairvoyance. The mind may be overactive or may be extremely passive with loss of meomry. Irritability of mind and body and great prostration of mind after slight mental effort, and of the body after slight physical exertion. Anxiety, gloomy forebodings. Fear that something will happen. Anxious at twilight. Anxious when alone. Apprehensiveness. Apprehensive during thunder-storms, which bring on many complaints;

palpitation, diarrhœa and trembling. Trembling of the whole body. Attacks of indigestion from fear. Fear in the evening, fear of death. Fear of strange old faces looking at him from the corner. Full of strange, insane imaginations. On the borderland of insanity. Inability to sustain a mental effort. Fear of apoplexy. Reflecting brings on headache and difficult breathing associated with apprehensiveness or sinking at the pit of the stomach. His fear seems to begin at the pit of the stomach. Apathy or indifference; indifferent to his friends and surroundings. Indifferent to his children. Answers no questions, takes no notice of his family and things about him, answers slowly, thinks sluggishly, seems dazed or in a stupor. Everything looks dark, he is weary of life, gloomy and says nothing. Dejected; a most marked case of hypochondriasis. Weeping, sad, hysterical; will uncover the body and expose his person. Violent, loquacious; delirium. Delirium of low forms of fever, or delirium of mania a potu. Maniacal attacks come on during sleep with fury and extreme violence, so that no one dares approach him, and this progresses to imbecility, silliness, weak brain, idiocy. Brain-fag from mental overwork and constant strain of eyes. Vertigo is a very common symptom throughout all of the complaints of Phosphorus. Staggering while walking as if intoxicated. Vertigo when in the open air; vertigo after eating; vertigo in the evening. Heaviness and confusion in the head and things go round; great weakness of the head. All of these mental symptoms are worse from mental exertion; aggravated from noise. All symptoms are worse in the dark; worse when alone; sometimes worse from music; worse from excitement; worse from playing the piano.

The headaches of Phosphorus are congestive and throbbing. The blood mounts to the head. The headaches are ameliorated from cold and worse from heat, worse from motion, and better from rest, worse lying down. The patient is often compelled to sit upright, with great pressure upon the head and cold applications. The face is flushed and hot; burning in the brain. The warm room, warm surroundings, warm food, putting the hands into warm water will increase the headache. The complaints of the head like the complaints of the stomach are worse from heat, warm applications and from warm food, and better from cold things; while the complaints of the body are better from warmth and worse from cold. The headaches are most violent and are often attended with hunger or preceded by hunger; headaches with vomiting, red face, and scanty urine; uræmic headaches; violent neuralgic pains darting, tearing, shooting through the head; pressing pains in the head. Periodical headaches, headaches brought on from mental exertion. Great heat in the head and stiffness in the muscles of the face and jaws. This is sometimes attended with coldness in the back of the head. Shocks through the brain. The headaches are worse from noise, from light; apoplectic congestion of the head. It has cured acute hydrocephalus and hydrocephaloid symptoms.

Chronic inflammation of the meninges of the brain; softening of the brain; imbecility; insanity. Violent head pains; atrophy of the brain; medulla oblongata. The scalp is covered with dandruff; the hair falls out in patches, leaving bald places here and there. Great heat in the scalp; tension in the scalp and face and forehead as if bound by a bandage. Scaly eruptions on the bald places of the head; exostoses on the skull. The complaints of the head are brought on from becoming overheated. Sensation as if the hair were pulled; great soreness of the scalp; must let the hair hang down during headaches.

The eye symptoms are very numerous; burning, redness, congestion, enlargement of the blood-vessels. Objects look red and often blue in the field of vision, or objects sometimes look green and gray as is observed in incipient cataract. Colors, also, appear black before the eyes. Vision is vague; the eyes give out while reading; sees better in the morning. in the twilight. The eye symptoms, like Phosphorus in general, have amelioration after rest. Momentary blindness like fainting; seems to suddenly become blind; paralysis of the optic nerve; blindness after electric shocks, or after a stroke of lightning. It has cured glaucoma. It has cured inflammation of the retina in Bright's disease. It has cured opacity of the vitreous humor. It has cured paralytic weakness of the various muscles of the eyes. It has cured paralysis of the third pair of nerves where there is falling of the lids; sub-acute inflammation of the eyes. Burning, redness, and smarting ameliorated from cold applications. The eyelids twitch and tremble; swelling of the eyelids; dropsical swelling of the eyelids; great darkness around the eyes; great circles around the eyes. It is a very useful remedy in malignant growths involving the eye, restraining very much the progress of the disease. The eye symptoms like the head and mind symptoms are such as often come on in brain workers; working under a bright light causing much determination of blood to the head in which the eyes as well as other parts suffer.

Phosphorus has a peculiar deafness. One of the most striking features of Phosphorus is inability to understand the articulations of the human voice. Hearing is difficult. He sometimes feels as if there were something over the ears; as if the ears were covered, obstructing the waves of sound. Violent itching in the ears; congestion of the external ear; itching, tearing, throbbing, burning pains within the ear. It has cured polypi in the ears.

The nose symptoms are also very numerous; inveterate nasal catarrh. He takes cold in the nose, but the most common seat of the Phosphorus. cold is in the chest, and most of his difficulties begin in the chest, but Phosphorus cures nasal catarrh and coryza. There is painful dryness in the nose; constant sneezing and running from the nose of bloody water. Frequent alternations of fluent and stopped-up conditions of the nose; coryza with sore throat; stoppage of the nostrils; much sneezing and stopping of the nose alternating with dryness of the nose in scarlet fever; nostrils filled with green mucus; a copious nasal discharge of greenish-yellow, bloodstreaked mucus, worse in the morning; bad odor from the nose; frequent blowing of blood from the nose; copious hæmorrhage from the nose of bright red blood; swelling of the nose, redness and shining; very sensitive to touch; necrosis of the bones of the nose. It has cured polypi of the nose, especially bleeding polypi. Fan-like motion of the nose, like *Lycopodium*.

The Phosphorus patient presents a sickly face, earthy, sunken and pale, such as we find in consumption and those about to go into consumption, and those suffering from deep-seated constitutional conditions; haggard, anæmic. The color is changeable; swollen, œdematous face; puffed under the eyes; lips and eyelids swollen. Again, red spots upon the cheeks, which appear in hectic fever; the hectic blush. Tension of the skin and of the face; tearing, shooting pains all through the face and about the eyes, from the temples and vertex down to the zygoma. Jerking, tearing pains in the teeth. The pains of the teeth are often ameliorated by warmth, while those of the head are ameliorated by cold. The pains of the teeth are worse when talking and eating, and worse after eating. It has violent neuralgias of the face involving the jaw and temples, with hot, bloated face, worse from talking and from eating. It has caries of the lower jaw, with great heat, burning and fistulous openings Neuralgia of the face and teeth; has to be wrapped up at night; worse in windy weather. The countenance is sickly, sunken, declining, as if a serious sickness was coming.

The lips are parched, dry and bleeding. The lips become black, brown and cracked as in low forms of fever, and with necrosis of the lower jaw. Inflammation of the parotid gland, especially when it suppurates or there are fistulous openings. Rapid decay of the teeth. The gums bleed and settle away from the teeth.

Phosphorus is very useful for the bright red hæmorrhage after the extraction of teeth. The tongue is swollen and speech is difficult. It is difficult to articulate. The taste in the mouth is bitter or sour, especially sour after taking milk; sometimes salty or sweetish; bitter after eating. Taste of hydrogen sulphide in the morning. The tongue is coated like fur; sometimes chalky white, sometimes yellow; dry, cracked and bleeding; sordes on the teeth. Crusts form upon the mucous membranes of the mouth, gums, lips and tongue. The tongue is swollen and the papillæ are engorged.

Dryness of the mouth and throat; sore, excoriated mucous membranes of the mouth and throat. The mouth may be covered with thrush, as in nursing sore mouth; bloody erosions of the mouth; nursing sore mouth. Much watery saliva and bloody saliva flows from the mouth. The saliva is copious, tasting sweetish, saltish or foul. The mucous membranes of the throat are like those of the mouth. Great dryness, roughness, rawness. excoriation, bleeding, and inflammation of the tonsils; inflammation of the throat; sensation of cotton in the throat; sensation of velvet in the throat. The tonsils are much swollen. Intense pain in the throat and burning in the throat that extends into the œsophagus. Inability to swallow any nourishment because of paralysis of the œsophagus or acute inflammation of the mucous membranes of the throat and œsophagus; constriction of the œsophagus. In Phosphorus there is violent hunger and very soon after eating the hunger returns again. Must eat during the chill. Must get up in the night to eat. Feels faint and is driven to eat. Ravenous hunger during headache; he knows that the headache is coming on because of his violent hunger; in periodical headaches. The hunger is often spasmodic, because at times there is aversion to food. Again, he wants to eat and as soon as the food is offered he does not want it. Thirst is one of the most constant features of Phosphorus. In acute and chronic complaints there is violent thirst; thirst for ice-cold drinks. Wants something refreshing; is ameliorated momentarily by drinking cold things, but the thirst appears as soon as the water gets warm in the stomach. Vomiting comes on as soon as the water becomes warm in the stomach, but there are many conditions where the ice-cold water agrees. Unquenchable thirst. When the water is vomited there is always unquenchable thirst. He wants cold food as well as cold drinks; refreshing, spicy things, juicy things; desire for wines and sour things. Phosphorus often cures the violent longing in inebriates for alcohol. It simply resembles the congestion of the mucous membrane of the stomach. Aversion to sweets, to meat, to boiled milk, to salt fish, to beer, to puddings, to tea and coffee.

Many of the complaints of Phosphorus are ameliorated by eating. The nervous symptoms of Phosphorus drive the patient to eat and he feels better for a little while, and then he must eat again or the nervous symptoms will come on. Often he can sleep better after eating and cannot go to sleep until he eats something.

The stomach symptoms are numerous—pains, nausea, vomiting, burning. The stomach symptoms are ameliorated by cold things and aggravated by warm things. The nausea and vomiting are brought on by putting the hands into warm water, from being in a warm room, from warm things and from taking warm things into the stomach. The nausea of pregnancy is cured when the woman cannot put the hands into warm water without bringing on vomiting. Another marked feature of Phosphorus is eructations of food. The food is eructated by mouthfuls until the stomach is emptied of the last meal. Constant nausea except when something cold is in the stomach. As soon as water becomes warm in the stomach it comes up. This very much resembles the vomiting and nausea of *Chloroform,* and Phosphorus is a great friend to the surgeon because he can nearly always antidote the stomach affections of *Chloroform* by Phosphorus. Vomiting of blood and violent vomiting of sour fluids; vomiting of bile and mucus; vomiting of black substances, coffee-ground substances. Awful sinking, gone feeling in the stomach. This sometimes comes at 11 o'clock like *Sulphur.* Pressing pains, burning pains, tearing pains in the stomach; pain in the stomach after eating; sensitiveness in the pit of the stomach; inflammation of the stomach. It has been a very useful remedy in cancer of the stomach, with coffee-ground vomiting and burning; coldness, as if freezing, in the pit of the stomach; paroxysms of knife-like pains in the stomach. The pains in the stomach are ameliorated by ice-cold things for a moment; spasmodic contractions of the stomach; hæmorrhage from the stomach; vomiting of great quantities of clotted blood; long-standing dyspepsia; much flatulence; regurgitation of food; distended stomach and abdomen; ulceration of the stomach.

The liver furnishes us many symptoms of Phosphorus. Congestion of the liver, fulness, pain, hardness, fatty degeneration of the liver, hyperæmia of the liver. Phosphorus is one of our most useful liver remedies; hard, large liver. With the stomach and liver symptoms there is commonly jaundice.

Very sensitive abdomen; painful to touch, rolling and rumbling. Sensation of emptiness in the abdomen; sunken feeling in the abdomen. The abdomen feels as if relaxed; hanging down sensation and sensation of great weight in the abdomen. Tympanitic abdomen such as occurs in typhoid fever. A marked feature in Phosphorus is the peculiar gurgling which begins in the stomach and gurgles along down through the intestines, attended with involuntary stool. This occurs in typhoid fever. The gurgling that occurs in *Arsenicum* is down the œsophagus. Flatulence; colic; rending, tearing, cutting pains throughout the abdomen; stitching pains in the abdomen; violent neuralgic pains in the abdomen; inflammation of the bowels, of the peritoneum; appendicitis. Yellow, brown spots on the abdomen; petechiæ over the abdomen during typhoid fever. Phosphorus is rich in symptoms of the rectum and stool; involuntary discharges from the bowels; copious emission of fluids, fœtid, gushing stools; horribly offensive, yellow, watery stools. The patient lies as if dying, the stools passing involuntarily; stools of white mucus stools of slime intermingled with little specks like tallow; involuntary oozings from the constantly wide open anus. Hæmorrhage from the bowels in typhoids in low forms of disease; bloody discharges like meat washings, involuntary on every motion. Burning in the rectum during stool. Protrusion of the rectum protrusion of hæmorrhoidal tumors. Sharp, stitching pains from the coccyx up the spine to the base of the brain drawing the neck backward, and this symptom occurs during stool. It has occurred during involuntary stool. After stool painful cramps in the rectum; burning in the anus; violent tenesmus sinking feeling in the abdomen; obliged to lie down; exhaustion and fainting

The copious diarrhœa is like the profuse flow of water from a hydrant. It is useful in cholera times and in cholera morbus. It is a useful medicine for chronic diarrhœa with soft, thin stools. It has been a very useful remedy in cholera infantum. It has also cured dysentery with bloody mucus, scanty stools with violent tenesmus. It also cures inveterate constipation. The stool is hard, long, and slender, described in the books as like that of a dog. Alternating diarrhœa and constipation in old people. Spasms of the rectum. Paralysis of the bowels so that it is impossible to strain at stool. Hœmorrhage from the bowels. It has cured polypi of the rectum; inflammation of the rectum. It has many times cured bleeding, protruding hæmorrhoids; hæmorrhoids that burn. It has cured fissures of the anus. Among many of these bowel symptoms the anus feels as if wide open.

Phosphorus is a useful remedy in diseases of the kidneys, especially diabetes, with sugar in the urine when there is great thirst for ice-cold things and ice-cold water. Gradual emaciation; gradual weakness; considerable heat of the head; coldness of the extremities, and sugar in the urine. Phosphorus will cure fatty degeneration of the kidneys. Renal calculi. No desire to pass urine though the bladder is full. There is a paralytic weakness which resembles the paralytic weakness throughout all the muscles of the body. He is unable to strain to pass the urine because such straining increases pain in the region of the bladder. Profuse, pale, watery urine; frequent and scanty or completely suppressed urine. Turbid, whitish urine; curdled like milk. Albuminous urine. Involuntary urination during sleep. Tearing in the urethra; twitching and burning in the urethra. Periodical sick headaches sometimes are preceded by scanty urine and sometimes by a copious watery flow of urine.

The male sexual organs furnish many symptoms of Phosphorus. Violent sexual desire driving him frantic. Erections frequent and painful day and night. Seminal emissions at night even without lascivious dreams. Sexual debility from the inordinate use of table salt. Impotence after excessive excitement and secret vice, preceded by over-excitement of the sexual organs. Frequent discharges day and night of thin, slimy, colorless fluid from the urethra. Sexual abuse with spinal disease. Discharges of prostatic fluid during a hard stool. Chronic urethral discharges due to hypertrophy of the prostate gland; gleety discharge. Swelling and soreness of the testes and cord; inflammation of the testes and cord. It has cured hydrocele following gonorrhœa.

In the woman it is equally useful. Phosphorus has cured many cases of sterility supposed to depend upon violent sexual excitement. Violent sexual excitement with aversion to coition. Violent pain in the ovaries extending down the inner side of the thighs during menstruation caused by inflammation of the ovaries. Inflammation of the uterus during menstruation and during pregnancy or during pyæmia. Copious hæmorrhages from uterus, bright red, clotted blood after confinement, during menstruation or during the climacteric period. Frequent and protuse hæmorrhages from the uterus caused from cancerous affections. The menstrual period is too early, flow bright red, lasting too long; is copious; during the menstrual period ice-cold feet and hands; nausea; pain in the back as if broken; blue rings around eyes; loss of flesh; much fearfulness. It has also menstrual suppression in consumptives with cough, bleeding from the nose, and spitting of blood. Violent sexual excitement driving to secret vice. Copious yellow leucorrhœa with great weakness; leucorrhœa instead of menses; white, watery leucorrhœa, acrid, excoriating; milky leucorrhœa copious when walking. The leucorrhœa is so excoriating that blisters form upon the genitals. Burning and smarting in the vagina. Stitching pains upward from the vagina into the pelvis. While there is violent sexual excitement during coition there is lack of sensation in the vagina, as if it were numb. Condylomata appear like fig-warts and excrescences about the genitals and in the vagina. Bleeding warts. Erectile tumors on the external genitals. Dropsical swelling of the labia. Cauliflower excrescences with much bleeding. Painful, hard, large nodosities in the female mammary glands. Fibroid tumors of the breast. Fibroid tumors of the uterus with copious hæmorrhages.

During pregnancy and lactation violent sexual desire; vomiting of pregnancy. Much prostration, sinking, and trembling, puerperal convulsions; pain in the back, as if it would break. Increased secretion of milk out of season. Inflammation of the mammary glands with much heat, weight, and suppuration. Erysipelas of the breasts or of the genitals.

Inflammation of the larynx with hoarseness in the morning; husky voice; great sensitiveness of the larynx to touch and cold air; pain and burning in the larynx on talking; weakness in the vocal cords; violent tickling of the larynx while talking; constriction and spasms of the larynx; constant irritation to cough in the larynx; tuberculous condition of the larynx; bleeding; loss of voice; cannot speak a word on account of pain in the larynx; sensation of velvet in the larynx; rawness and smarting in the larynx. Phosphorus has cured many cases of croup, membranous croup, when all the symptoms were present. Every change of weather, from becoming overheated, and cold, settle in the larynx, producing loss of voice and hoarseness, especially in public speakers and singers. Hoarseness and loss of voice; great dryness in the larynx and all of the air passages. Hard, dry, rasping cough that shakes the whole body from irritation in the larynx. The irritation travels down the air passages, affecting the trachea, along with difficult respiration; asthmatic breathing; clutching in the larynx; suffocation; dyspnœa; spasms and constrictions of the chest. Violent, stridulous inspiration in the evening or falling asleep; fear of suffocation; labored breathing. Paralysis of the lungs; fulness in the chest after eating, much irritation in the larynx; difficult breathing; scraping of mucus from the larynx after eating.

In the chest, Phosphorus produces oppression; anxiety, weakness and constriction going along with its chest complaints. Heaviness as if a great weight were lying upon the chest. With the cough, bronchitis, pneumonia and cardiac symptoms there is always more or less constriction of the chest as if bound, or as if bandaged, or as if tied tight with a string. Tightness felt over the sternum, and with all complaints great weakness of the chest; pressure as of a weight over the middle of the sternum; feeling of a rush of blood to the chest with or without violent pulsations. Sensation of heat in the chest mounting to the head; flushes of heat in the chest extending upward. Stitching pain in the chest; spasmodic pains in the chest; violent stitching pains in the left side of the chest better by lying on the right side. These are pains likely to occur in pleurisy or in pleurisy with pneumonia. Complaints of chest, worse in cold air. Rawness in the trachea extending into the lungs; burning in the chest; acute pain in the lower part of the lungs; violent pain in the chest with coughing. The patient is compelled to hold the chest with the hand. Inflammation of the lungs with anxiety, oppression, and expectoration of bright red blood. The Phosphorus patient suffers from copious hæmorrhages from the lungs in phthisical conditions, in inflammation, inflammation of the bronchial tubes with intense fever and violent shaking cough; the body trembles with the cough; tearing pains in the sternum with the cough; suffocation and constriction of the chest. Pain in the larynx. The expectoration may be bloodstreaked or rust-colored as it is in pneumonia. It may be purulent. In the later stages it becomes thick, yellow, sweetish. Phosphorus is a useful remedy in old bronchial catarrhs, in complaints that date from pneumonia or from bronchitis. Every cold settles in the chest. The lungs seem to be weak. Again, in hepatization during pneumonia with hard, dry, hacking cough; in hepatization of the lungs during pneumonia Phosphorus, *Sulphur* and *Lycopodium* are the most frequently indicated medicines. Phosphorus is often the remedy to follow *Arsenic* when *Arsenic* has been suited to the restlessness, prostration, and anxiety that comes to a place where because of hepatization it is capable of accomplishing no more toward the cure of a case. If, then, the patient has thirst for ice-cold water, constriction of the chest, dry, hacking cough, paralytic weakness of the lungs, and expectoration of blood or frothy mucus Phosphorus is the best remedy. In pneumonia, there may be burning in the chest, burning in the head, hot cheeks, and fever; gesticulation and delirium; violent thirst for ice-cold water; fan-like motion of the nose; difficult breathing; catchy inspiration; lying on the back with the head thrown far back; short, dry cough. The carotids pulsate. Rawness in the chest; bruised feeling in the chest; pains are cutting, burning or sharp and tearing in the lungs when coughing. Suffocation, or inspiration almost impossible, especially at the beginning of hepatization when the face becomes livid and the features pointed with cold sweat and quick, hard pulse. Frothy expectoration in low forms of pneumonia known as typhoid pneumonia. Threatened paralysis of the lungs. Again, Phosphorus is a useful remedy when tuberculosis is about to make its appearance, in persons who are narrow-chested, slender, and of feeble vitality. All colds settle in the chest. After each cold, much rattling, hard cough that shakes the whole body, in persons who are feeble, pale, sickly, and disposed to hæmorrhages. Cough comes on in cold air. Emaciation; emaciation of the chest and neck. Along with these conditions comes hectic fever in the last stages of phthisis; intense fever, red face, and night sweats; fever coming on in the afternoon and lasting until after midnight. A powder of Phosphorus very high will reduce this fever and make the patient comfortable until death. In all incurable cases after the fever has been reduced, Phosphorus should not be given, as it will intensify the fever and do just what it was given to avoid. It is not uncommon for a crisis to follow the administration of Phosphorus. Prolonged sweat and diarrhœa, these should never be interfered with as they will soon stop of their own accord and the patient will be left in a state of quietude. Phosphorus is a dangerous medicine to give very high in same cases of phthisis, in the last stages of phthisis. In this case they should have received Phosphorus when they were yet curable. In these cases Phosphorus 30th may sometimes be used with safety and it will act as a test in doubtful cases to see whether reaction can be brought about. In such cases where reaction can be brought about the administration later of a still higher potency may be found useful, but in the beginning with Phosphorus in phthisical cases far advanced it is better not to go higher than the 30th or 200th. Phosphorus very low will act as a poison in really Phosphorus cases and the only safety some patients have had who have received. Phosphorus so very low was due to the fact that the Phosphorus was not similar enough to either kill or cure.

Phosphorus has violent palpitation; worse from motion, and from lying on the left side especially in the evening; worse at night on waking, with orgasms of blood in the chest, accompanied by much suffocation. Tightness in the chest and palpitation over the body; pressure in the region of the heart. Phosphorus has cured endocarditis. Phosphorus has cured enlargement of the heart and dilatation and also fatty degeneration. With fatty degeneration where there is much veinous stagnation, puffiness of the face, particularly under the eyelids. Phosphorus is often the remedy. In all of these cardiac affections thirst for very cold water will always be present. Internal heat; he wants something cold to cool his insides. Violent orgasms of blood in the chest from every excitement, from worry, and from anticipation. Phosphorus has many neuralgic pains upon the outer chest and yellow brown spots. 'There are many symptoms in the back; stiffness in the back and in the back of the neck, between the shoulders, and in the small of the back. Stiffness on rising from a seat. Sensation of intense heat in the back running up the back. The patient complains of a hot spine. Soreness in places up and down the spine; soreness to touch between the shoulders; pulsations in various places in the back and in the whole spine. The coccyx is sensitive to pressure; pain in the coccyx as if ulcerated, preventing motion. Pain in the back during menstruation and during confinement as if the back would break. Spinal affections and inflammations. Weakness of the limbs after mental exertion, prolonged physical exertion; being overheated, sunstroke and sexual excesses; paralytic weakness. Myelitis; softening of the spine; progressive spinal paralysis. Phosphorus has been a useful remedy in locomotor ataxia, palliating many of the symptoms; the pains; restoring the reflexes. Phosphorus is often suitable and restrains the progress in multiple sclerosis where there is much weakness and trembling of the extremities. Phosphorus has cured caries of the vertebræ in scrofulous children. Phosphorus is a broad remedy in various diseases of the spine.

In the limbs we have paralytic weakness extending to both arms and legs, with trembling and numbness; paralysis of one or of both lower extremities or of the upper extremities with trembling and numbness. The hands and arms become very cold. The limbs emaciate and the veins become distended; the arms burn; periodical constriction of the fingers; numbness increasing to complete insensibility of the fingers; finger tips feel numb and insensible. Great restlessness in the lower limbs; weariness in the lower limbs; weakness in the lower limbs, especially observed on walking, unsteady and trembling gait; paralysis of the lower limbs. Acute inflammation of the joints of the knees and hip joint. Burning, tearing., pains in the limbs from exposure to cold. Rheumatism of the joints and muscles; stiffness of the joints on becoming cold. All complaints of the limbs are ameliorated by heat, while complaints of the head and stomach are ameliorated by cold. The complaints of the chest are ameliorated by heat. The lower limbs are covered with fœtid sweat. The lower limbs are gangrenous. Inflammation of the periosteum of the tibia. Ulcers upon the lower limbs; feet icy-cold. The Phosphorus patient wants to lie down; exhausted; he is unable to walk; staggers when walking from weakness and from vertigo. A gradual progressing weakness creeps over him; weakness; trembling; faintness. Jerking and twitching of the muscles; spasms of the paralyzed parts. Epilepsy; convulsions; neuralgic pains of the various parts of the body and of the limbs especially, ameliorated by heat. It has cured multiple neuritis.

Restless sleep; starts in sleep; feels in the morning as if he has not slept enough, yet most of the complaints and aches are ameliorated by sleep, especially the head symptoms; walks in his sleep. He sleeps on the right side. Lying on the left side causes anxiety and pain in the heart and palpitation. Late falling to sleep in the evening; lies awake thinking about the affairs of the day and borrownig trouble. Phosphorus is a usual remedy in low forms of typhoid fever on the symptoms previously mentioned.

There are many eruptions in Phosphorus. The eruptions are dry and scaly; dry furfuraceous herpes; blood blisters; purple spots; yellow spots on the chest and abdomen; formication and itching in the paralyzed parts; numbness of the skin; irregular brown spots upon the body; psoriasis of the knees, legs, elbows, and eyebrows; hives and blood boils; phlegmonous inflammation. Chronic suppurating openings with hectic fever; fistulous openings; ulcers bleed on appearance of the menses; deep eating ulcers; indolent ulcers; malignant ulcers. Very useful in cancerous ulcers that bleed and take on fungous appearance, and in low forms of scarlet fever where the rash is very dusky or disappears and suppuration begins in various places about the neck or upon the extremities or upon the ends of the fingers and there is violent thirst for cold water, purple appearance in the throat, and dry, hacking, shaking cough.

PHYTOLACCA

This is a very imperfectly proved remedy, and it is only possible to present fragments of it. The mental symptoms have not been brought out, but the remedy has some striking features.

You will notice the resembalnce of this drug to *Mercury,* and it is an antidote to *Mercury.* In those lingering mercurial bone pains, where the patient has been salivated; the pains come on at night from the warmth of the bed; the body aches; a chronic, sore, bruised state; soreness of the periosteum where the flesh is thin, over the tibia; joints; soreness of the muscles; drawing and cramping; drawing in the muscles of the back; backache, worse at night; worse from the warmth of the bed. The patient suffers from these symptoms in cold, damp weather, as in *Mercury.* Tendency to ulceration, hence its usefulness in syphilis; old, chronic, syphilitic ulcers; the patient has been salivated; had *Mercury* rubbed in; he became saturated with it, but it no longer helps. Ulcers in the throat; on the skin; on mucous membranes anywhere.

Spasmodic conditions; drawing in the muscles; this may extend to violent spasms; opitsthotonos; sometimes the cervical region is affected And the head is drawn back; jerking and twitching of the muscles.

Phytolacca is a *glandular* remedy. The glands become inflamed and hard. It produces sore throats, with inflammation of the glands of the neck, particularly the submaxillary and parotid. Inflammation of the throat with the accumulation of thick, tenacious mucus; swelling of the tonsils. Low grade inflammation like erysipelas.

The symptoms are aggravation at night, on cold days, in a cold room, and from the heat of the bed; so that there is a controversy between heat and cold.

It seems that the remedy centers in the *mammary glands.* Soreness and lumps in the breasts from each cold, damp spell; becomes chilled and a sore breast results; sore breast in connection with the menses; a nursing woman is exposed to the cold, the breast inflames and the milk becomes stringy; coagulated milk. This comes out in the proving, but poke root has been extensively used by cattle raisers when the cow's milk became thick and there were lumps in the bag, and when the condition was brought on from the cow standing out in the rain.

Almost any excitement centers in the mammary gland; fear or an accident; lumps form, pains, heat, swelling, tumefaction; even violent inflammation and suppuration. No other remedy in the Materia Medica centers, so in the mammary gland. *Mercury* is similar; when the patient takes cold the glands become sore. If every tribulation makes the glands sore in a nursing woman, give her Phytolacca. When a mother says she has no milk, or that the milk is scanty, thick, unhealthy; dries up soon; Phytolacca becomes then a constitutional remedy if there are no contraindicating symptoms. A bloody watery discharge which continued for five years after weaning the infant was cured by Phyto. The breast is so sore that, when she nurses the child, she almost goes into spasms, with the pain extending down the back and limbs all over the body.

Diphtheria. in certain epidemics; great tumefaction of the throat; swelling of the glands of the neck, parotid and submaxillary; aching in the bones; foetor from the mouth, with heavily coated tongue; great aching in the back; nose bleed; soreness of the muscles. Analogous to *Mercurius;* they are closely related in diphtheria. At times in diphtheria we can only obtain the foetor, loaded tongue, exudation, swollen glands and stiff neck. This looks like *Mercurius* or one of the *Mercuries.* The *Protoiodide* is *right sided,* and stays there or may go to the left side. The *Biniodide* goes from *left* to *right.* The *Merc. cyanide* has a thick, green membranous cast, extending from the nose to the throat. In Phytolacca we have many features of *Mercury.*

It has cured syphilitic nodes on the skull and shin bones.

Many eruptions. "Squamous eruptions; pityriasis, psoriasis." "Ringworm." "Barber's itch." "Rash on body; measles; scarlet eruption all over the body." It is not surprising that it cures scarlatina, as it has this scarlet rash, the sore throat and glandular involvement.

It has the ability to delay the formation of malignant growths, especially in the breast; glandular tumors that become hard and scirrhous. Until this remedy was known there was but one remedy for the old cicatrices in the mammary gland. Women who were confined years before, had abscesses of the breast which were poulticed and lanced had a cicatrix left, and now in the present confinement they have trouble; inflammation in the old cicatrices; ulceration which eats off the lacteal glands or turns the ducts aside and twists them; high inflammation; throbbing and pain; milk bloody. *Graphites* was the old routine remedy, but Phytolacca is a better remedy and suits the general concomitants oftener. The symptoms usually found in an inflamed breast after confinement are: Aching in the back and bone pains; fever and shivering. Phytolacca has these and falls into the very nature of the case. *Graphites* has it only in a limited way. If there is high fever; congestion to the head; throbbing carotids; much redness, and the redness radiates from the nipple, *Belladonna* is the remedy. When the entire gland is as heavy as a stone, and hard, and the patient is sensitive to motion and touch, *Bryonia*. *Mercury* when the general symptoms agree. *Hepar* and *Silicea* after suppuration is inevitable, especially when the only comfort is obtained from heat. *Hepar* when there is extreme pain and soreness, irritability and this relief from heat; it limits the extent of the suppuration and opens the part without pain.

The most distressing, lingering, inveterate, old catarrhs with destruction of the bones of the nose. "Total obstruction of the nose; when riding must breathe through the mouth." "Coryza and cough, with redness of eyes and lachrymation; photophobia; feeling of sand in the eyes, with soreness and burning." "Syphilitic ozæna, with bloody, sanious discharge and disease of bone." "Noli me tangere and cancerous affections of nose."

It is somewhat like *Graphites*, in that it seeks out fissures in which to establish inflammation, induration and eruptions. Where the circulation is feeble it has the tendency to establish induration.

"Face sunken, pale, hippocratic; blue around eyes; yellowish complexion; looking blue and suffering." "Pains in bones of head and face at night." "Swelling around left ear and side of face like erysipelas; thence over scalp; very painful." "Lips everted and firm. Tetanus." "Ulcers on lips." "Parotid and submaxillary glands swollen." "Tongue thickly coated on back; coated yellow and dry." This is found in all acute complaints and is like *Mercury*. Phytolacca holds a reputation among the Eclectics, and in their results we see a shadow of its homœopathic action. In Cincinnati they used three drops in a tumbler of water and gave it for ulcers in the mouth. It was a standard remedy with them and they made some homœopathic cures. "Ulcerated sore mouth." Syphilitic ulcers find a curative remedy in Phytolacca, when the symptoms agree.

There are several pages in the *Guiding Symptoms* showing homœopathic cures of the throat; diphtheria; sore throat; inflamed glands; aching bones worse at night; violent cases, With difficult swallowing, pains in the tonsils; enlarged tonsils; tendency to slough. Syphilitic and mercurial sore throats. The sore throats are often aggravated from warm drinks; he wants cool things;

and there is an aggravation at night. Here is a summary: "Diphtheria; sick and dizzy when trying to sit up; frontal headache; pains shooting from throat into ears, especially on trying to swallow; face flushed; tongue much coated, protruded, thickly coated at back, fiery red at tip; breath fœtid; putrid; vomiting; difficulty of swallowing; tonsils swollen, covered with membrane, first upon left; three or four patches; tonsils, uvula and back part of throat covered with ash-colored exudation. Pain in the root of the tongue on putting out."

Old gout and rheumatism of the limbs; in acute rheumatism which is prolonged, worse at night, worse from the warmth of the bed, worse from warm applications. Gouty rheumatism; syphilitic cases; pains as if in the bones. "Sharp cutting pains in hip, drawing; legs drawn up; cannot touch floor." "Syphilitic or gonorrhœal sciatica, etc." "Ulcers and nodes on the legs."

A certain class of physicians used to call *Podophyllum* "vegetable *Mercury*". Phytolacca ought to be called "vegetable *Mercury*" because it is so full of symptoms analogous to *Mercury*.

PICRIC ACID

The weakness of body and mind is the first impression wrought upon the mind of the reader who goes carefully over this proving. It is progressive, passing from weariness to paralysis. The evidences of softening of brain and cord are strong. He soon becomes sensitive to heat and desires the cool air which ameliorates his head and bodily condition. Cold air and cold bathing are grateful to him. He is sensitive to wet weather. Numbness of many parts, trembling, lassitude, heaviness, must lie down, worse from least exertion are marked features. Loss of sleep, mental worry, mental labor, are the exciting causes of symptoms. Extreme indifference.

It is a typical brain-fag remedy with indifference and lack of will-power, aversion to talk, think, or perform any mental exertion. He is quickly prostrated from the least mental work, and it brings on many complaints, such as soreness and lameness, diarrhœa, burning along the spine, general weakness and heaviness of limbs and back. He loses all interest in things; becomes irritable from any mental exertion. In young school children we have a common use for this very valuable but neglected remedy. When the child begins to learn the alphabet, headaches come, and return with every repeated effort, often with dilated pupils. After every examination at school come these violent headaches. A young man at school with the following symptoms was cured promptly: Student's headache, vertigo when remaining standing, heaviness in the head, epistaxis, dilated pupils, congestion of conjunctiva, inability to bear artificial light, loss of appetite, bitter taste in mouth, vomiting, jaundice.

Vertigo from mental exertion, lameness from stooping, walking, ascending, from raising the head from the pillow, cannot sit up, soon nausea comes from it. It is often associated with the head pains. For headaches of students, teachers, professional men, and overworked business men, it is a most useful remedy. For headaches with great nervous weakness from grief and depressing emotions, it has been often overlooked. It has violent pain in vertex, forehead and occiput, extending down the spine with much heat. Congestive headaches. The head must be cool, it is worse from warm room, and wrapping up the head or body, and better from rest of mind and body.

The headaches often begin and increase with the day, and are better by sleep at night. The patient is wholly incapacitated in the daytime, but comfortable from rest and sleep during the night. Extreme prostration often comes with these headaches. Extreme sexual excitement often comes with the headache as with many of its "complaints," but it is not an essential concomitant.

The eye symptoms are due to loss of tone in the eye muscles of such as are suffering from brain-fag. Looking, reading fine print and exertion of vision will bring on the headache and eye symptoms (*Onosmodium*). Sensation of sand in the eyes, smarting, acrid tears, sparks, fog before the eyes, near sighted, dim vision, objects confused, pupils dilated, severe pain over eyes. Thick mucus in eyes. The symptoms from the eye are worse from artificial light.

Small boils and pustules in external auditory canal.

Eructations, abortive, sour. Nausea in the morning worse on rising and moving about.

There is evidence of liver trouble, and the patient is jaundiced.

Rumbling in the abdomen, diarrhœa from mental exertion. Yellow, watery or thin fæcal, oily stool; smarting after stool; stool like yellow cornmeal gruel. Great weakness after stool, in debilitated persons.

Urine contains sugar and albumen. Urine of high specific gravity. Urine heavy with urates, uric acid, phosphates, and poor in sulphates. Dribbling after urination. Weakness of the bladder. Great waste of phosphates.

In the proving it turns the normal sexual sphere into lust, and salacity with violent erections, especially during the night. It has many times cured these symptoms even when of long standing. Pain in occiput and spine, heaviness of limbs and sexual excitement. Where great restlessness of feet is present the *Zincum picricum* acts better. It cures impotency and spermatorrhœa when the mind is unable to control the lustful state.

Burning heat in the spine from mental or physical exertion. Weakness of the spine and heaviness of the limbs, especially the lower limbs. The back is so tired that he cannot sit up erect, he must slide down in the chair or lie down. He is relieved while lying. It has been very useful in myelitis, with the weak limbs and a sensation as if body and limbs were bandaged or constricted;

PLATINUM 841

also with anæsthesia of legs and as if he had on elastic stockings. In locomotor ataxia where there are tormenting erections and emissions as soon as he falls asleep. Many cases of spinal weakness have been cured by this remedy.

Weakness of the lower limbs with trembling, numbness and constriction. Formication and prickling as from needles. Marked coldness of the feet. Physical exertion greatly intensifies all these symptoms; after long rest he is ameliorated.

Tired after least exertion in limbs and whole body; *excessive lassitude.* Great muscular weakness. Sleepiness in day-time and sleepless at night, especially after mental labor.

PLATINUM

The Platinum proving represents the woman's mind perverted. It is especially suited to hysterical women such as have undergone fright, prolonged excitement, or from disappointment, shock, or prolonged hæmorrhages. She becomes arrogant and haughty. One of the most striking characteristics of this drug is pride and over-estimate of one's self. She imagines that she is of a high born family and that her friends and relatives are of lowly origin and looks down upon them. Her acquaintances are inferior to herself. A strange thing about this remedy is that this imagination extends to the body. She imagines that her body is large and that the bodies of other people are smaller in comparison with her own. She is in a contemptuous mood, anxious and serious over matters that are not serious, irritable about trifling things, is moody and sulky over slight vexations, anxious, weeping. Palpitation, trembling in all limbs during every little excitement, fears death and loathes life. Fear is a very prominent feature in this remedy. Fears that something will happen, fears that her absent husband will never return to her, though he comes back regularly. Restless disposition, excitable, walking, moving about, and weeping.

The mental symptoms alternate with the physical symptoms. Strange illusions of fancy. Imagines that she does not belong to this race and becomes insane over religious matters, sits in the corner and broods and says nothing. Takes on insanity; becomes a sexual pervert, utters unchaste speech and trembles. Spasms will come on from vexation or anger. Whistles, sings, and dances. Talks constantly about fanciful things. She may go into melancholy or into mania. Any disturbance of her pride will bring on her symptoms. Sexual excitement will bring on her symptoms. The usual mental symptoms are intermingled with trembling of the limbs, sexual excitement, and numbness of various parts of the body and limbs. Compressing sensations, pressing pains, pressure of the limbs as if bandaged or constricted, tension of the skin of the limbs as if bandaged. These characteristic features prevail throughout the various regions of the body and modify many particulars. Sensation of numbness of the scalp with pressing pain in the head, boring, compression of the head. Tension of the scalp, cramplike constrictions of the scalp gradually increasing to violence, cramp like pains gradually increasing to violence. Squeezing sensation in the head. These pains may he in the temple, in the top of the head, or in the forehead. Again, there is crawling, creeping, numbness of the scalp. Sudden shocks in the head. There is no symptom in the head more persistent than numbness of the scalp, it prevails throughout all sensations and pains. All headaches gradually increase until they are severe. Violent neuralgia in the head with sensitiveness in hysterical persons. Sometimes numbness in the head is described as if the brain were numb. Headaches come on from chagrin, from fear, from vexation, from hæmorrhages, and from sexual excitement.

Sparks before the eyes, spasms of the lids, and objects appear smaller than they really are. Sensation of coldness in the eyes, spasms, spasmodic trembling and twitching of the muscles of the eyes. Cramping pain in the ears, coldness in the ears, numbness of the external ears. The numbness of the ears extends to the face, nose and scalp. Platinum is a hæmorrhagic remedy. Bleeding from various parts of the body and mucous membranes. The hæmorrhages wherever observed are black clots with fluid. On examining the symptoms of the nose hæmorrhage is observed. Black, coagulated blood from the nose. Oversensitive to smell Violent crampy pains at the root of the nose with redness of the face.

Sensation of coldness of the face, numbness of the face, cramping, pressing pains in the face. Neuralgia of the face. Coldness, crawling, numbness of the face. Numbness of the malar bone. Tearing boring pain in the face.

Pulsating and digging through the lower jaw, especially the right side, together with numbness and coldness. The pains come gradually and go gradually. Sensation as if the tongue were scalded, crawling in the tongue. Loss of appetite on account of the depressed mood or at other times a ravenous appetite; hasty eating, eats everything around her. Much flatulence, fermentation in the stomach. Jerking of the muscles of the stomach and abdomen. Sensation as if the whole abdomen were tightly constricted or bandaged. Tension of the skin of the abdomen. Violent, cramping pains in the abdomen, drawing pains in the navel as if by a string, which causes a sensation of retraction of the abdomen. Pressing, bearing down pains in the abdomen. These pains are much like *Plumbum* and Platinum has been used as an antidote to *Plumbum*. Pressing, drawing pains from incarcerated flatus. The torpor of the intestinal canal is much like that which is found in *Plumbum*. Inveterate constipation, much flatus.

The stool is half digested and papescent or hard as if burnt, or may be scanty and very difficult, or may be glutinous and adherent to the anus like soft clay. Frequent urging to stool and inability to strain at stool, inveterate constipation and unsuccessful urging to stool. Pain in the abdomen after lead poisoning and colic after lead poisoning. Constipation in travellers. Prolonged efforts to pass a stool. Aching pains, burning pains and protrusion of hæmorrhoids during stool. Burning in the rectum during stool. Itching, tickling, and tenesmus of the anus, especially in the evening. Extreme sexual erethism is found in both male and female. In the male there is great sexual erethism driving to secret vice. It has cured epilepsy arising from onanism. Sexual erethism is one of the most prominent features of Platinum in women. Unbearable sexual excitement and voluptuous crawling in the genitals. Such extreme sensitiveness of the external genitals that it is impossible for the woman to wear a napkin during menstruation. Such extreme sensitiveness of the vagina that it is impossible for the physician to make an examination with the index finger. It is not an inflammation but a hyperæsthesia. Increased sexual excitement in young girls, in hysterical girls. Violent sexual desire in married women with itching, tingling, and voluptuous sensations. Pain in the ovarian region, especially the left. It has cured sterility of long standing, especially sterility that is supposed to come from excessive sexual excitement. Burning, stitching pains in the ovaries. Inflammation of the ovaries coming with hæmorrhage of the uterus, and during the menstrual period. It has cured ovarian tumors and cystic tumors. Inflammation of the uterus, bearing down, as in prolapsus. Prolapsed uterus and dragging in the pelvis. Polypus of the uterus and uterine hæmorrhages. Copious menstrual flow. The flow is dark, even black, and clotted with much fluid blood. These nervous women constantly feel as if the menstrual flow was going to appear. The menstrual flow comes too early, is too profuse, and then generally of short duration. The hæmorrhage is somewhat like the menstrual flow in old women. The menstrual periods sometimes return every fourteen days or the menstrual flow may be entirely absent. The vulva and vagina are extremely sensitive during coition, sometimes preventing the act. The woman suffers from albuminous leucorrhœa mostly in the daytime without much sensation. There are many complaints of pregnancy, threatened abortion, exhausting hæmorrhages, discharges of black clotted blood. During labor the contractions are interrupted by sensitiveness of the vagina and internal parts. It is impossible for the obstetrician to make the usual examination. Cramping in the limbs during parturition or profuse hæmorrhage; hysterical convulsions, puerperal convulsions. After every mental exertion palpitatoin, trembling, numbness, quivering, and excitement in the limbs. Tremulous restlessness in the legs with numbness. Cold feet. Pains in the great toe as if bandaged. This sensation prevails throughout. The limbs feel as if bandaged about the thigh or leg. The nerves are in a great state of excitement most of the time. The patient is prostrated. Paralytic weakness, which is worse during rest. Numbness, stiffness and coldness. Painful tremulousness all over the body, with throbbing in the blood vessels. Numbness of the scalp, of the feet, of the hands, of the limbs. Shifting, neuralgic pains. Spasmodic affections of hysterical women. Spasms from sexual erethism. Coldness, crawling, and numbness of the skin, especially during fever.

PLUMBUM METALLICUM

This drug illustrates a doctrine of Hahnemann—the doctrine of attenuation. When you think of the insolubility of lead, and then think of it as spread on the wall of a room, and then remember how many become sick from sleeping in a newly painted room, you will then wonder how much lead it took to make them sick. Many patients cannot sleep in a newly painted room—they come down with lead colic or the acute affections of lead. Many people are sensitive to lead. This sensitivity is more marked than is observed in painters, who may use it for years with impunity, but all at once become susceptible to it. You wonder how much he gets, given off in the air. It is too attenuated to be examined by the microscope and yet enough to make him sick. We have no measure by which to find out how much he gets. We make use of such susceptibility, the lead palsy of lead workers, the lead colic in painters—these things add to the proper proving and give a well-rounded image of Plumbum

If we study the whole symptomatology of Plumbum, we will be struck with the general paralytic state in this remedy. The activities of the body, the functions of the organs, are slowed down in pace. The nerves do not convey their messages with the usual activity. The muscles are slow in action sluggish. There is first paresis and finally paralysis, of parts first and finally of the whole. The mind is impaired, slow. Perception is slow. He memorizes with difficulty. Comprehension is difficult. He cannot recall words to express himself. The operations of the mind are slow. When in conversation with such a patient you will wonder what he is thinking about while making up his mind to answer. There is sluggishness also in the skin. You may prick him and a second later he says, "Oh," showing the slowness in feeling. You would expect him to feel the prick instantly. When you begin to conclude that he does not feel at all, his limb will jerk. Anæsthesia of the skin. There is a state of hyperæsthesia in the acute affections, but the chronic affection are characterized by loss of sensation. Numbness of fingers and toes, soles and palms, and this extends to the skin, towards the spine.

The trophic functions are slow in that they do not keep up with the waste, and so we see emaciation until the patient becomes almost a skeleton. The skin is wrinkled, puckered, shrivelled, and drawn over the bones. The emaciation is sometimes local. When local it is generally associated with a painful part; the painful part withers. Pains down the sciatic nerve; burning, shooting; as if the bone were being pulled out of place; as if being scraped and the limb emaciates. Pain down the arm, in the shoulder; violent pains in the brachial plexus and the arm withers. Neuralgia of one side of the face and that side withers. Paralysis of single muscles and these muscles wither There is paralysis of both extensors and flexors, but especially extensors. The paralysis begins in the extensors, so that we have wrist drop. He cannot raise or lift anything with the hand. Extension is difficult. This occurs in piano players; they cannot lift their fingers sufficiently rapid to keep up the pace, while flexion is all right. *Curare* is another remedy which corresponds to this state in piano players; a paralysis from overexertion of the extensor muscles. When the mucles become fatigued from playing fixed exercises, scales, etc., for hours at a time, when the player has to do the same thing over and over again, *Rhus* comes in, but it is an acute remedy and only holds for a short time. It is especially a *Rhus* condition when certain muscles become overused and the patient takes cold and a weakness sets in; after a cold bath or plunge the muscles take on paresis; getting wet when tired brings on the *Rhus* state. For the chronic state which follows, Plumbum and sometimes *Curare* will be indicated.

Paresis of the intestines; constipation; cannot strain at stool. The patient can use the abdominal muscles, but the rectum is in a state of paresis and he cannot expel the fæces.

The bladder is also paretic; cannot expel the urine, the muscles do not co-operate to void the urine and there is retention. Plumbum has both retention and suppression of urine.

The paralyses are found in the chronic state. In the acute we have the fever, the colic, the sudden constipation; tearing pains in the intestines; indigestion with vomiting. Everything eaten turns sour.

Violent vomiting of everything eaten. Chronic gastric catarrh with vomiting albuminous mucus and sweetish substance. Vomiting of stercoraceous matter, blackish blood and green fluid. Sour eructations.

The remedy is slow and insidious; it works continuously; it does not leave the economy but holds on and establishes a miasm of its own. It, therefore, suits slow and insidious chronic cases, with no tendency to recovery. Progressive muscular atrophy; progressive paralysis. Chronic constipation; chronic retention of urine; chronic giving way of the mind.

Aside from the slowness of the mind, which is a general, the remedy is full of melancholia, sadness, feeling as if something terrible would happen; that she has sinned away the day of grace; that she has committed the unpardonable sin. The body and mind are weak. "Deep melancholy with timidity and restlessness." In the mental state, while he is slow to think, yet in this slow thinking he does a great amount of thinking; he makes an effort to think. His thoughts trouble him all night and prevent sleep. Insomnia; sleepless from the continual effort to think. The mind will not operate, yet the patient is full of imaginations and emotions. Inability to comprehend and to remember. Now this progresses from periods of insomnia to periods of coma and this coma is associated with suppression of urine. Uræmic coma. Uræmia. Perhaps it will fix it in your mind if I tell you something clinical about it. Some years ago a physician came to me in regard to his wife. She had been unconscious for two days and had passed no urine for days and the catheter showed there was none in the bladder. She had quite an array of symptoms, but they were common symptoms. She had had the slowness for days before, and complained of a sensation of a continual pulling at the navel, as if a string were drawing it back to the spinal column, and then the coma came on. In the middle of the night this doctor came to me in great distress. He said she was pale as death and breathing slow. A single powder of Plumbum high was given, and she passed urine in a few hours, roused up and lever had such an attack again.

Violent spasmodic palpitation of the heart, worse lying on the left side, with marked anxiety in the cardiac region. Hypertrophy and dilatation of the heart. Stitching pain in the heart.

Hysterical diathesis; hysterical contractures; cramping of the fingers; hysterical motions; convulsions of parts, hands, feet, whole body; an apparent delirium; cardiac pains; numbness in parts—all hysterical phenomena.

Plumbum produces an inclination to deceive, to cheat. The *Acetate of lead produced* in a woman, who took a little of it for suicide, a confirmed hysterical state. She would be in a hysterical condition for hours when any one was looking at her. When she thought no one was near she would get up, walk about, look in the glass to see how handsome she was, but when she heard a foot on the steps she would lie on the bed and appear to be unconscious. She would hear much pricking and you could scarcely tell she was breathing. Plumbum establishes a hysterical state in the economy; an inclination to deceive, to feign sickness; to exaggerate one's ills; and it goes to the root of the evil providing the symptoms agree.

Changeable; continually changing from one thing to another, from one group of imaginations to another, from one group of emotions to another. The whole remedy is intensely emotional. While the intellect is slowed down, yet most of the symptoms are emotional.

Plumbum cures kidney affections with albumen and sugar in the urine. The urine is dark, scanty, and of high specific gravity. Retention of urine from lack of sensation that the bladder is full.

Apoplexy. Stupor, when *Opium* is sufficiently similar to remove the cerebral congestion which always surrounds the apoplectic clot, Plumbum may follow. Plumbum, *Phosphorus* and *Alumina* are three sheet anchors. They conform to the symptoms often when the first state has been like *Opium*. The paralysis of muscles, the paralytic weakness of one side of the body, or single parts of the body, show its relation to such cases.

There is another feature of the upper part of the body, of the head and mind, which is not clear in the books and which is worthy of your attention. The mental symptoms, the emotional symptoms, and the head symptoms are greatly exaggerated by any exertion, especially exertion in the open air. While walking in the open air the patient becomes hot in the head, pale in the face, and cold in the extremities; hands and feet cold as ice, as if dead; and if he continues the exertion the face becomes fairly cadaveric. Persons cannot exercise and continue it without cold extremities. An irritable brain; pain in the base of the brain, back of the neck, in the nerve centers. Cold extremities from exertion; yet can do considerable mental exertion without becoming cold. It is from physical exertion like walking in the open air. Paroxysmal pain in the limbs, evening and night; better by pressure and worse from motion. Lightning-like pains. Jerking and trembling of all the limbs.

The Plumbum patient is cold and emaciated, needs much clothing even in warm weather, not about the head, but over the body. Extremities cold, blue, numb, and emaciated. Sweat on the extremities, and on the feet it is stinking. Feet and toes withered like a washerwoman's hands. Toes blistered; blisters between the toes, smarting. Ulcerations. Molecular death and even gangrene of the skin of the fingers and toes. Calluses about the feet, corns and bunions.

With the chronic affection of the head there is contraction of the muscles of the back and neck; drawing and twitching indicating meningeal troubles; spasmodic jerking. "Swelling of the submaxillary and sublingual glands." Convulsions often like tetanus, with lockjaw. "Distinct blue line along the margins of the gums." "Gums pale, swollen, show a lead-colored line; blue, purple, or brown; painful with hard tubercles." "Tongue dry, brown, cracked; coated yellow or green; dry, red, glazed in chronic gastritis." Breath fœtid, dryness of mouth, ulceration, aphthæ. "Sensation of a plug in the throat; globus hystericus." "Paralysis of throat and inability to swallow," a paralysis of the œsophagus.

The stomach has no ability to digest food. Assimilation is also destroyed. Pains in the abdomen, tearing, like colic, doubling the patient up. Constant sensation of pulling at the navel as by a string; as if the abdomen were drawn in. At times the abdomen does become concave, as if the abdomen and back were too close together.

Constipation is a common and well known feature. The constipation, colic, and abdominal symptoms are commonly associated. "Constipated stools, hard, lumpy like sheep's dung; with urging and terrible pain from constriction or spasms of anus; knotty fæces in form of balls." No matter how much straining he cannot expel the stool. "Constriction of intestines; navel and anus violently retracted." "Excessive pain in abdomen radiating from thence to all parts of the body." "Severe colic; contracted abdomen; bends backward, motor nerves most affected." Rumbling and flatulence. Impaction of fæces. Vaginismus in keeping with the spasmodic action.

"Inclination to take strange attitudes and positions in bed." Anæmia, chlorosis, emaciation, muscular atrophy. wandering pains, dropsical swellings, yellow skin, jaundice."

Burning in ulcers is in keeping with the remedy everywhere.

PODOPHYLLUM

This remedy is seldom used except in acute affections, but it is a long acting and deep acting drug; it produces a powerful impression on the economy; it relates to the deep-seated miasms.

It affects profoundly the abdominal viscera. It shows its symptoms largely on the abdominal organs, the pelvic organs, and the liver. The abdomen seems to be the earliest seat of attack. It produces such an impression upon the stomach and intestinal canal that the healthy action is impaired, digestion and assimilation cease. Everything taken into the stomach becomes sour. The glands of the stomach are as if paralyzed; there is no digestion; this goes on until we have vomiting and diarrhœa. During this there is a wonderful disturbance in the abdomen; rumbling; gurgling as if animals were floundering about; clinically, as if fish were turning and tossing in a pond, as we have seen them before a storm. Rumbling and rolling. This is attended with severe, cramping pains doubling her up. Abdomen is sensitive; so sore she cannot endure pressure. The soreness extends to the stomach, intestines and finally to the liver. The whole abdominal viscera are sore, sensitive to pressure. After this comes a gurgling, watery stool, pouring out of the anus. A tremendous outpouring so that the patient wonders where all the fluid comes from, and soon it comes on again. Copious, enormous, and very frequent. This soreness, cramping, and rumbling precedes the stool, but sometimes it continues during the stool. Commonly the patient is relieved by the stool. There is much flatus and spluttering, but not so marked as in *Aloe*. The colic often comes and goes without stool. Painless stools, in which compare *China* which has stool coming on at night and after eating. Putrid or not, and of inky color. Podophyllum is rarely indicated when the discharge is not offensive. After a while the abdomen again becomes tumultuous, and this is again relieved by a stool. This process is repeated over and over. It seems as if the blood vessels would empty themselves into the abdominal cavity, and then into the outer world. Not unlike cholera and cholera morbus, and these two are the common manifestations of disease for which this remedy is used in routine practice. The cholera morbus coming on in the latter part of the night, especially about 3, 4, or 5 o'clock. resembles Podophyllum. Tumultuous action of the bowels with rumbling, pain, and soreness, and the prostration is so marked that if not relieved in a day or two, it seems he must die. Rice-water stools, jelley-like on standing.

With this tumultuous action, she has an indescribable sensation; an all-gone feeling, a deathly sick feeling, described by some as an emptiness, as if fasting, yet averse to food. An awful, hungry, empty weakness, as if the whole intestines would drop out. No wonder they think so, because this remedy produces an astonishing amount of relaxation. Described by some as a sensation of dragging down. The uterine ligaments become relaxed and there is prolapsus. The rectum protrudes for inches. The sensation of dragging down as if all the parts would be pushed out into the world is a common feature. It seems to begin with the liver, as if all the parts were let down. Weakness attended with soreness.

Dragging down in the region of the ovary and the ovary is congested. The uterus is extremely sore and is enlarged; sore to touch so that light clothing aggravates. Sensitiveness of the abdomen in diarrhœa and vomiting; in cholera morbus; in women when menstruating. Indicated if there is a copious diarrhœa during the menstrual period, and great soreness in the uterus. Much pain in the ovaries, in one or both, extending down the crural region, down the front of the thigh. Pain in the ovaries, especially the right; pain in the ovaries during the menstrual period, griping pain in the bowels during the menstrual period. Great soreness of the abdomen before and during the menstrual period. (*Apis, Cimicifuga, Vespa, Lachesis,* but these are not so likely to have diarrhœa and, if so, it is not as copious.)

Alternating condition is a feature of this remedy. If a Podophyllum patient takes cold, has any mental excitement, overexerts himself, eats boiled food, cabbage, fruits, and overloads his stomach with rich food he has a diarrhœa, and following this a constipation lasting for weeks, no stool except in lumps; difficult, scanty stool and as soon as he disorders his stomach again comes a diarrhœa. This alternating diarrhœa and constipation is a Podophyllum state rather than a chronic diarrhœa, which is a continued state found in many remedies. The diarrhœa is periodic, alternating with constipation.

Another alternating feature is the headache. Chronic headache, periodic headache, sick headache, congestive in character, as if all the blood were in the head, as if the head would burst, and the pains most violent in the back of the head, bursting, and then on comes a diarrhœa which relieves the head. Sometimes when the diarrhœa slacks up too suddenly, a headache is the result. It is a common feature after giving a high potency of Podophyllum in a diarrhœa, that a headache comes on after the diarrhœa is stopped. It means that the medicine has acted suddenly and the headache will pass away soon.

Headache alternating with liver disturbances. The patient lies on the side or abdomen. Rending pains towards the duodenum. You will wonder if it is not gall-stone colic. Periodic, violent headaches; alternating diarrhœa and constipation; he strokes the region of the liver from behind forward and in this way gets relief, yet the liver is so sore that he can hardly bear the pressure. Liver sensitive to touch. Soreness about the liver; pain through to the back; dull aching pain, finally jaundice; becomes extremely yellow. Uneasiness and distress about two or three hours after eating, with jaundice; horrible nausea; aversion to food; empty all-gone feeling in the bowels. Vomiting, greenish, profuse, watery, vomits everything; vomiting of milk (*Calc., Æth.*—the latter sometimes retains water); hunger after vomiting; deathly, overpowering nausea and prostration. Prolapse of rectum and anus during vomiting. (*Mur. ac.*) A condition commonly called duodenal catarrh; a chronic state; rouses into a Podophyllum diarrhœa every once in a while.

Mental symptoms troublesome. A torpid liver is often associated with a torpid fluctuating state of the mind; also a slow, sluggish pulse; palpitation. Great depression of spirits, melancholia, sadness, dejection; everything goes wrong; the clouds are very dark, there is no light; thinks he may die or that he is going to become ill; that his disease will become chronic; that he has organic disease of the heart and liver; that he has sinned away his day of grace, and other such delusions. Mind easily fatigued; fidgety and restless; cannot sit still, whole body fidgety.

In this mental state with jaundice, all-gone sensation, aversion to food, even the thought or smell of food; stuffed feeling and distension in the region of the liver. The tongue is covered with thick slime; pasty, yellow coating as if mustard were spread upon it; imprint of the teeth upon the tongue; breath foul. For such a condition the ancients gave *Calomel.*

Gall-stone colic; enlargement of the liver; gastric weakness; unable to digest; duodenal catarrh; catarrh of intestines with copious diarrhœa. If you notice the Podophyllum discharge in the commode, you will see a great amount of water, on the bottom a sediment like cornmeal gruel; as if cornmeal had been stirred in. If you see it early it is yellow, muddy, or yellow-green, profuse, offensive, cadaverous; the odor penetrates the whole house; stool gushes away like water from a bung-hole; gurgling and much flatus. With the stool there is very commonly a prolapse of the rectum; a gush of watery stool and a prolapse of the rectum; a soft stool with great straining and a prolapse of the rectum.

Prolapsus of the uterus; prominent are *Murex, Sepia, Natrum mur. Sepia* is better sitting or lying; worse walking. Aversion to coition; hot flushes; constipation with sense of lump in the rectum, or better by stool. *Murex* has the following: The only relief is to press on the vulva; not better lying down; she then has pains in the back and hips compelling her to walk, yet this aggravates. Strong sexual desire. Pain in right ovary, which crosses entire body to left breast. Pain shooting up in the uterus.

The word bile is a striking feature in Podophyllum. You must connect the vomiting and the stool with this color. The patient declares he is "bilious;" his "liver is out of order;" bitter taste in the mouth; spitting up bile and the color is yellow; in diarrhœa it is a green substance.

In children subject to copious diarrhœa, with prolapsus of the anus—no other symptom—Podophyllum often cures.

A feature of infancy is the following: Child may not have diarrhœa, may even be constipated, but it lies in bed and rolls the head in sleep. *Bell.* and *Apis* roll head. *Apis* lies on back with the head on its side. Chewing motion of the jaws; sometimes a sucking; a grinding of the teeth in those who are old and have teeth; rolling the head from side to side; if you lift the eyelids you will find a strabismus. Provers felt as if the eyes were drawn inward. It has cured such a strabismus in congestion of the brain following a suddenly suppressed diarrhœa.

A child who should have a colored stool has instead a white one like chalk (*Calc. c.*). In adults, a bileless, white stool.

The body is offensive; offensive sweat; compare *Sepia, Merc., Aloe, Sulph., Murex, Nux.*

PSORINUM

Psorinurn is closely allied to *Sulphur.* The patient dreads to he washed. The skin over the body, especially of the face, looks filthy, though it has been well washed. A dingy, dirty, foul look, as if covered with dirt. Skin rough and uneven, cracks easily, bleeding fissures; it becomes rough and scaly. He cannot wash it clean. The skin of the hands is rough, chaps easily, becomes thick and scaly, easily cracks, breaks out in little scaly eruptions; looks unwashed; he always appears to have dirty hands. Many of the complaints of the skin are worse from bathing and from the warmth of the bed. The skin itches when warm; itches when wearing woolens. Itching when warm in bed; he scratches until the part becomes raw, and then it becomes scabby. When healing takes place there is itching and then he has to scratch. Legs and arms raw and scabby from scratching. Violent itching from the warmth of the bed, even without any eruption. The skin is unhealthy, looks dirty, dingy; studded with capillary blood vessels and enlarged veins. This is the state before the eruption appears. Scabs form from scratching and then comes the eruption. Papules, pimples, crusts, boils, vesicles, and eruptions ooze a watery moisture. When the eruption has gone on for some time the crusty formation and vesicles mingle; the skin becomes thickened and indurated, and new crops come out under the old crusts; rawness, itching, tingling, crawling, bleeding.

Eczema of the scalp and face; the crusts cover the scalp; the hair falls out; the oozing lifts up the crusts and exposes new vesicles; it looks like raw beef, and it tingles so that the child cannot keep its fingers off it; worse at night, worse from the warmth of the bed, worse from warm applications, anything that would keep the air away from it; ameliorated by cool air and worse from covering. This is the opposite of the general Psorinum state, which is aggravated from the open air. He has an aversion to the open air.

The eruption goes on, spreads, and the true skin becomes elevated, thickened, indurated, with an increased vascularity and redness. The oozing is offensive like carrion or decomposed meat; nauseating odor from the oozing fluid.

Offensiveness runs through Psorinum in such a characteristic way that it is worth while mentioning it here; foetid odors, foetid breath; discharges and oozings from the skin smelling like carrion; stool so offensive that the odor permeates the whole house, in diarrhœa, summer complaint, cholera infantum; perspiration foetid; leucorrhœa abominably offensive; eructations taste as if he had eaten hard boiled eggs and they had spoiled, and they smell so to others; stool, flatus, and eructations smell like spoiled eggs; offensive to sight and smell is the subject who needs this medicine.

The skin grows increasingly thick and bleeds, and the eruption spreads to other parts. Eruptions on the lips, on the genitals; very offensive; soreness and rawness about the anus; the vulva ulcerates and is very offensive; ulcers on the legs; on the tibiæ; on the backs of the hands; on the dorsum of the foot; behind the ears and upon the ears; over the scalp; over the cheek bones; on the wings of the nose and on the nose and eyelids. Greasy skin. The eruption is accompanied by redness of the mucous membranes of the nose, mouth, lips and eyes. Eyelids thickened and turned out, like ectropion; granulation and induration of mucous membranes, so that they become like gristle; redness and ulceration. Ulceration of the cornea; lachrymation; turning out of the lids with loss of the eyelashes. He looks frightful with his red eyes, eruption on the face, red skin oozing a thick yellow discharge. In the early stages the oozing is a whitish thin or whitish thick moisture. In old eruptions ulceration takes place beneath the crusts and there is a thick, yellow, purulent discharge. Yellow green discharge from the eyes and nose. Horribly offensive discharge from the nose; gluey discharge from the nose; offensive like *Merc., Sil., Calc. p., Hep.* Accumulation of foetid pus in the eyes.

Coryza with thick, yellow discharge. Always taking cold. In the coryza the nose dries up part of the time and runs part of the time; he must use the handkerchief continually; must blow the nose all the time. In the early stages of the coryza he blows it all the time, but there is no discharge or relief. This state is so marked that some think of it as a continuous hay fever, which runs all the year and ripens up in the Fall. It is closely related to hay fever; stuffing up of the nose in the Fall; catarrhal state of the eyes and nose. Hay fever is one of the most difficult conditions to fit a remedy to. It belongs to a low constitution which must be built up before the hay fever will cease. It is an expression of psora which comes once a year, and the psoric miasm must be changed. In a few years most subjects can be changed, but not in one season, so do not be disappointed. In catarrhal states, hay fever often dates back to low fever improperly treated.

The Psorinum patient himself is one of debility. He wants to go home after a short walk. He is worse in the open air. He cannot breathe in the open air; cannot breathe while he is standing up; *wants to go home and lie down so that he can breathe.* Asthma or cardiac dyspnœa, when the patient wants to go home and lie down so that he can breathe. Usually this condition is relieved by sitting up and from the open air. Not so with Psorinum, he wants a warm place and to lie down and to be let alone.

Psorinum is slowed down in all of its functions; a state of paretic weakness. He does not rally after a fever; his digestion is slow; the stool is normal, yet it requires a great effort to expel it; the bladder is full of urine, yet it passes slowly and he feels that some remains; he can never finish stool or urination; he has to go back several times. Although the stool is soft and perfectly normal it cannot be expelled at one sitting.

A psoric patient comes down with typhoid; the typhoid has been arrested or has run its course and it is time for convalescence. The fever has subsided, but the patient has no appetite; he does not convalesce; he wants to lie down and does not desire to be moved; he is worse when sitting up, lies upon his back; he has troublesome breathing and lies with *his arms abducted from his side,* thrown across the bed; this relieves his breathing and allows the chest to operate properly; so tired and so weak; one dose of Psorinum will cause a reaction, stop his sweat, increase his appetite, cause better breathing.

The Psorinum complex of symptoms is one in which remedies cause improvement but a short time and then the symptoms change and another remedy must be selected. It is a state of feeble reaction.

The mental symptoms present some strong features. Sadness, hopelessness; he sees no light breaking through the clouds above his head;

all is dark about him. He thinks his business is going to be a failure; that he is going to the poor house; that he has sinned away his day of grace. It is a fixed idea during the day and he dreams about it at night, Overwhelming sadness; dejection; he takes no joy in his family; feels that these things are not for him. His business is prosperous, yet he feels as if he were going to the poor house. No joy or realization of benefit. Extremely irritable, wants to be alone. Does not want to be washed. Full of anxiety, even of suicide. Despair of recovery if sick.

Though there is no eruption at night he is driven to despair by the continual itching. If he throws the covers off then he becomes chilly; if he covers up then there is itching. Sensitive to cold yet the skin is worse from heat. Tingling, itching, formication, crawling like ants running over the surface, as of insects in the skin.

Especially suited to broken down individuals, who have vertigo as soon as they go into the open air; become dizzy and want to go home and lie down; afraid they will lose their breath.

Old chronic periodic *headaches with hunger,* and often the hunger lasts during the whole headaches; *must get up at night to get something to eat.* The headache is sometimes improved by eating. If he goes without a meal he has a headache. Violent rush of blood to the head, hot face, hair wet with the perspiration, hunger. Every one, two, or three weeks a recurrent headache. Every time the air blows on his head it slacks up the catarrh and a headache comes on. Either coryza or headache from catching cold. Headache is violent, throbbing, pecking as of little hammers, red face, hot head —congestive; at times sweat. Hungry headache in such as have a dry cough in winter. Dry, teasing, racking cough with no expectoration. If the cough ceases he has a periodic headache. So complaints alternate. Headache goes and cough appears or eruption in winter alternating with headache.

Scalp cold; wears fur cap in summer; worse uncovering the head (*Sil.*), worse from getting the hair cut (*Bell., Glon., Sep.*). *Hepar* is also worse from cold.

Salt rheum, psoriasis in winter. Dry, cold weather, cold wet weather; washing in cold water; dish washing, aggravate the salt rheum.

"Hair dry, lusterless, tangles easily, glues together; must comb it continually."

Chronic offensive otorrhœa; thick, purulent, offensive, yellow discharge from the ears; smells like stinking meat; continuous discharge; eruptions about and behind ears. Discharge resulting from scarlet fever; abscess in middle ear; otitis media; rupture of drum; prolonged discharge from such an abscess; fœtid discharge. "Otorrhœa with headache; thin, ichorous and horribly offensive like spoiled meat; very offensive, purulent; brown offensive from left ear, for almost four years." Otorrhœa associated with watery, offensive diarrhœa. Scurfs in ears, and humid scurfy behind cars.

Teeth. Rigg's disease; the teeth become loose; the gums settle away, spongy, bleed easily, humid, blue, the teeth fall out. Ulcers about the tongue and mouth; ulcers as found in infancy; aphthæ, thrush; ulcerated sore mouth, sore throat, chronic ulcers of throat. Chronic thickening and elongation of the uvula. Enlargement of tonsils, parotids and submaxillary glands; they become hard and tender to touch; swelling from taking cold. Glands of the neck sore.

Chronic abdominal affections with disturbances. of stool. He will strain to pass a soft stool (*Nux mos., Alumina*). Chronic diarrhœa; horribly offensive; frequent stool day and night (unlike *Sulphur,* the remedy it most resembles). He must go several times to pass a normal stool.

Chronic vomiting; ulcer of the stomach, distension of stomach are commonly associated. Always sour belching, sour stomach. Vomiting of blood and bloody stools. This is not strange, because Psorinum has a tendency to hæmorrhages, especially from the uterus. All sorts of menstrual disorders, especially a prolonged menstruation. When a woman has passed through an abortion and the placenta has come away, but every few days a little gush of fresh, bright red blood and clots, or going days and weeks with a little oozing of bright red blood; every time she gets on her feet there is a new start of the flow; no tendency to permanent recovery. Two remedies 'that fit this state are *Sulphur* and Psorinum. A marked state of relaxation, sub-involution. The uterus does not go back to its normal size and there is this tendency to bleed; a state of inertia.

"Soft stool, passed with difficulty," do not forget this. Obstinate constipation. Hæmorrhage from the rectum. Cholera infantum; often in the early days the stool is horribly offensive, slimy, undigested; there is vomiting and prolonged weakness and the whole child has an offensive odor; child dirty; nose sunken in (*Ant. t.*), sunken countenance. Psorinum causes reaction and cures, or brings the child into such a condition that a simple remedy completes the cure. It is not the sourness of *Hepar*; in spite of washing, the child smells so sour; like sour milk; the diaper, urine, and fæces and perspiration are sour. This is a strong general feature of *Hepar.* The stool smells like spoiled eggs, so also the eructations and flatus. The offensiveness of the stool is horrible, but not so permeating as *Bapt.,* which is thick and clay-like, while the Psorinum stool is watery, brown, gushing and may be bloody. Chronic diarrhœa, early morning, urgent. Hot flatus, burning the anus; smells of spoiled eggs, *Arn.* and *Staph.* Involuntary stool at night (*China* has a black, profuse, watery stool at night and after meals). In Psorinum we find the haste of *Sulphur,* the flatulence of *Olean.* and *Aloe,* and difficulty of expelling a soft stool like *Alumina, China* and *Nux mosch.*

There is prostration in some Psorinum cases; prostration of the genitals. It is nor such an unusual thing in the female to have aversion to sexual intercourse, but man is not often subject to the complaints that cause aversion to coition. Yet we have in man as well as in the woman actual aversion or a state of no enjoyment. He can perform the act and he has no difficulty in obtaining an erection, so it is not impotence, but there is no enjoyment. Impotence comes later. "Absence of erections; parts flabby, torpid." "Aversion to coition; impotence; want of emission during coitus." "Prostatic fluid discharged before urinating.

Old gleet, painless discharge; the "last drop;" relaxed and cold genitals; a drop of white or yellow pus after a well selected remedy. (*Sepia, Sulphur, Alumina,* Psorinum.) Psorinum is indicated above all others if there is an unusually offensive state of the genitals. *Thuja,* if the odor is of a nauseating, sweet character; warts exposed by rolling back the foreskin; sweet odor in spite of washing.

Psorinum cures many heart complaints. Palpitation from the least exertion, better lying. Stitching pain better lying. Cardiac murmurs of either side. Mitral regurgitant murmur. Pericarditis of rheumatic origin. Heart symptoms with general weakness, dusky face, dazed look. Weak, irregular and rapid pulse.

But mark the modalities. Aggravation in the open air, aggravation when sitting up, aggravation when sitting at the writing table; wants to lie down wants to rest the chest and breathing apparatus by lying down. Asthmatic dyspnœa ameliorated by lying down, and worse the nearer the arms are brought to the body. Such symptoms are found in very few remedies and in none so marked as in Psorinum.

Febrile state. Intermittents, bilious fever, fever from a cold. The patient is so hot that the hand under the covers feels as though in a steam bath and the sensation of heat causes one to draw it back. It is not the dry heat of *Belladonna,* yet it is as intense. It is a steam. He is covered with a boiling sweat in fevers. Head and body hot and hot air or steam beneath the covers (*Opium* has this, but it is in a violent congestion to the head, an apoplectic condition.) In intermittents he is taken on the street with difficult breathing He wants to go home; he is weak and exhausted, crawls up stairs on the hands and knees. The chill is not marked, but the heat is intense and the sweat copious. He is almost in a stupor, befogged, bewildered, cannot answer questions; face red, puffed, mottled. "Sweat profuse, cold, clammy from least exertion." This is another form which comes on in the weak, broken down state. After typhoids, he sweats if he turns in bed, after the least exertion and the sweat is cold. Profuse night sweats. Night sweats of phthisis; when there is that tremendous heat under the covers, a copious hot sweat; mental state as if dazed.

Marasmus; shrivelling of the skin; dirty skin; cannot wash it clean. Offensive discharge from the bowels; great emaciation; increased growth of hair on the face; a fuzz (*Natr. m.,* Psor., *Sulph, Calc.*); horribly offensive in spite of washing; ravenous appetite yet grows thin. Fœtid odors would lead one to think of Psorinum.

PULSATILLA

It is said to be a very good medicine *for women,* for blondes, especially for *tearful blondes.* It is one of the polychrests and one of the medicines most frequently used, as well as often abused.

The Pulsatilla *patient* is an interesting one, found in any household where there are plenty of young girls. She is tearful, plethoric, and generally has little credit for being sick from her appearances; yet she is most nervous, fidgety, changeable, easily led and easily persuaded. While she is *mild, gentle* and *tearful,* yet she is remarkably irritable, not in the sense of pugnacity, but easily irritated, extremely touchy, always feels slighted or fears she will be slighted; sensible to every social influence. Melancholia, sadness, weeping, despair, religious despair, fanatical; full of notions and whims; imaginative; extremely excitable. She imagines the company of the opposite sex a dangerous thing to cultivate, and that it is dangerous to do certain things well established in society as good for the human race. These imaginations belong to eating as well as thinking. They imagine that milk is not good to drink, so they will not take it. They imagine that certain articles of diet are not good for the human race. Aversion to marriage is a strong symptom. A man takes it into his head that it is an evil thing to have sexual intercourse with his wife and abstains from it. Religious freaks; an especial tendency to dwell on religious notions; fixed ideas concerning the Scripture; he misuses and misapplies the Scriptures to his own detriment; dwells on sanctification until he becomes fanatical and insane; thinks he is in a wonderfully sanctimonious state of mind, or that he has sinned away his day of grace. This goes on until he becomes insane on other subjects, and then the tendency is to sit day after day in a taciturn way. He will not answer questions unless hard pressed, when all he will say is "Yes" or "No," or he will merely shake his head. Puerperal insanity in a woman who was mild, gentle and tearful, later sad and taciturn, and then she sits in her chair all day answering nothing or merely nodding her head for "Yes" or "No".

Many of the complaints are associated with weakness of the stomach and indigestion, or with menstrual disorders. Women who abort; various irregularities of the menstrual flow; false conception. The mental symptoms are often associated with the ovarian and uterine difficulties.

With such a mental state the general state of the body is *worse in a warm room* and *relieved by motion.* Tearful, sad and despondent, ameliorated walking in the open air, especially when it is crisp, cool, fresh and bright. Suffocation and an increase of the pains, and even chilliness in a warm room; a nervous chilliness when the patient perspires from the heat of a room. The inflammatory symptoms, neuralgias and rheumatisms are relieved by a cold, by eating and drinking cold things, by cold applications, or cold hands. Cold drinks relieve, even though the patient is *not thirsty.* Cold foods are digested while hot foods make the body warm from which symptoms are worse. Ice cold water feels good going down the œsophagus, and is retained in the stomach, though there is no thirst.

Many symptoms worse after eating. It is often only a lump in the stomach, but the mental and nervous symptoms also are worse after eating. The stomach symptoms are worse in the morning, the mental symptoms worse in the evening. *Aggravation from fats and rich foods.* Complaints brought on by eating fat, pork, greasy things, cakes, pastries and rich things. The Pulsatilla stomach is slow to digest. Hours after eating there is a sense of fulness in the stomach, a lump in the stomach, ameliorated by *slow walking in the open air.* The patient is commonly relieved from *slow motion in the open air,* becomes frantic when trying to keep still, worse during rest, ameliorated by doing something, generally slow, moderate motion. This relief from motion and aggravation from rest, relief in the open air, and aggravation in a warm room give us a good summary of this beautiful remedy.

In Pulsatilla patients the skin feels feverish and hot, while the temperature of the body is normal. There is aggravation from much clothing; she wants to wear a thin dress even in moderately cold weather. Does not need to dress warmly. Much clothing and covering aggravate. Often he cannot wear flannels or woolen clothing because they irritate the skin, causing itching and eruptions like *Sulphur,* and this is not surprising, as Pulsatilla and *Sulphur* are antidotes. There is no remedy like Pulsatilla to antidote *Sulphur* when it has been used every Spring to "cleanse the blood". Some people use *Sulphur* until the skin becomes red, hot, easily irritated, and aggravated by clothing. Pulsatilla is the antidote. Old cases of psoriasis; little flat, brownish patches about the size of the thumb nail, which itch tremendously, in old *Sulphur* patients are cured by Pulsatilla. A general feature of the skin is itching and burning, but a more marked Pulsatilla state is a *Lachesis* appearance of the skin. It is mottled erysipelatous; spotted, purplish in spots; veins engorged; capillaries tumid; a vasomotor paralysis of the capillaries or veins producing a mottled appearance. Pulsatilla has an unusually *venous* constitution. The veins are engorged, in a state of stasis, hence there is over-heat of the skin. This unusual fulness redness and purple aspect of the face is a false plethora. It often goes on to a puffiness and swelling, and especially at the menstrual periods. Considerable bloating of the face and eyes, bloating of the abdomen; feet puffed so that she cannot wear shoes, feet red and swollen at the menstrual period, ameliorated by the menstrual flow. Many women are late and are preparing for a week or ten days; face purple, red, puffed and bloated; abdomen distended; dyspnœa; and all this is relieved by the menstrual flow. She feels these symptoms perhaps one or two weeks, and is relieved by slow motion in the open air. Cannot breathe in a warm room; wants the windows open; chokes and suffocates in a warm lied at night. This increases until the menstrual flow starts. The stomach is so full and distended that she cannot eat. No appetite or desire for food.

With the engorgement of veins *ulcers* surrounded by varicose veins are common in this remedy. Ulcers bleed black blood which coagulates early; little black clots; bleeding is not copious; clots easily, dark, tarry, offensive. Ulcers bleed and ooze, discharge a bloody watery fluid or there is a very thick yellow or green flow.

This brings us to the *catarrhal state.* Wherever there is mucous membrane there is catarrh. The mucous membrane is covered with purple spots, dry spots; tumid, puffed, looks erysipelatous. Wherever there is inflammation of the mucous membrane it looks purple; a venous congestion. *Thick, green, yellow catarrhal discharges* are most characteristic. The catarrhal discharges are *bland* with the exception of that from the vagina, which is excoriating, causing rawness of the parts. From the eyes, ears, nose and chest there are thick, yellow, green, *bland* discharges, but there is thick yellow green *excoriating* leucorrhœa. Remember, however, that Pulsatilla has a bland leucorrhœa, in keeping with the general state. Discharges are often offensive, sometimes bloody, watery, but even then mingled with yellow green purulent fluid.

The Pulsatilla patient suffers from *vertigo* from affections of the eyes, ameliorated by wearing well-adjusted glasses; attended by nausea which is worse lying down, worse from motion, worse from the motion of the eyes, and ameliorated in a cold room, and by riding in a carriage in the cold air. As soon as she enters a room that is warm she has nausea, even to vomiting. Vertigo with vomiting after eating.

Pulsatilla has violent *headaches.* Headaches in school girls who are about to menstruate. Headache accompanying menstruation. Headache associated with suppressed menses, with menstrual disorders; not caused *from* them, but associated with them. Pains through the temples and sides of the head are common Pulsatilla headaches. Headaches before, during and after menstruation; but more commonly before, when there is a general state of congestion, stasis, and tumefaction of the veins, and amelioration of the headache when the menses set in if the flow is normal. It is common to have the head and nervous symptoms through the menses, because the flow is so scanty, often little more than a leucorrhœa, and for a single day a little clot of dark blood. *One-sided headaches* and *one-sided complaints* are peculiar to Pulsatilla. Perspiration on one side of head and face; fever on one side of the body; one side cool and normal and the other side hot. I remember a case of puerperal fever with sweat on one side of the body and dry heat on the other and confusion of other symptoms. Pulsatilla was given and the patient recovered.

The Pulsatilla headache is a throbbing congestive headache; much heat in the head, ameliorated by the application of cold, by external pressure, and sometimes by slow motion, aggravated by lying and sitting quiet, ameliorated by walking slowly in the air; becomes worse towards evening and gradually increases through the evening and night, worse from the motion of the eyes and from stooping. The pains are often constricting, throbbing and congestive. Periodic sick headaches, with vomiting of sour food. Headache when he overeats. Though he likes ice-cream, he has headache and congestion of the stomach after eating ice-cream.

Eyes. Catarrhal symptoms. Pustules about the lids and over the ball; on the cornea. Inflammatory features. Thick, yellow-green pus. Granular lids. Continued formation of little pustules. Isolated granules on lids, grow out here and there in hunches as large as pin leads. Eyelids inflamed and bleed easily. Every time he catches cold it settles in the eyes and nose. Eyes red, inflamed and discharge. In infants catarrhal diseases of the eyes of a gionorrhœal character; ophthalmia neonatorum. In early days the infant often needs the same constitutional remedy as the mother. Yellow green discharge from the eyes; eyes are ameliorated by washing in warm water, or tepid water; even cold water feels good to the eyes. The *Sulphur* patient is made worse by bathing; the eyes smart, burn and become increasingly red after washing in water. Pulsatilla causes a tendency to the formation of *styes;* recurrent styes; always having styes. Pustules, papules and little nodosites on the lids.

Prior to menstruation, in young girls especially, things get black before the eyes, like a gauze or a veil. Nervous manifestations, twitchings, spell of blindness and fainting. In the early stages of paralysis of the optic nerve Pulsatilla is a great remedy. The patient is always rubbing the eyes; whether or not there is mucus in the eyes it matters not; but it is a sensation of gauze before the eyes, ameliorated by rubbing. Pulsatilla has cured incipient cataract, *Itching of the eyes*, in keeping with the skin symptoms. Itching in the ears, nose, tickling in the throat, in the larynx.

In the *ears* we have the same catarrhal condition. Thick, yellow, offensive, purulent, bland discharge; very fœtid, sometimes bloody. Pulsatilla is commonly indicated in earache of children; when the child is a gentle, fat, plump, vascular red-faced child always pitifully crying. If it is a case of earache in a nondescript child Pulsatilla will also prove to be a temporary remedy, so closely is it related to pain in the ear. Pains in the ears in the evening or in the night, ameliorated by walking slowly about the room. In *Chamomilla* you have a snapping and snarling child, never pleased, scolds the nurse and mother; ameliorated by walking about. The irritability decides for *Chamomilla*. You can detect a pitiful cry from a snarling mad cry. Both are ameliorated by motion, by being carried. Both want this and that and are never satisfied; they want amusement. But the Pulsatilla child when not amused has a pitiful cry and the *Chamomilla* child a snarling cry. You will want to caress the one and spank the other.

Ear troubles with a ruptured drum and no healing; otitis media. Abscess in the middle ear; inflammation of the middle ear; copious thick bloody discharge, then yellow-green. The case goes on night and day until rupture takes place. I have found this condition as an endemic, in which *Merc., Hep.,* and Puls. were the most frequently indicated remedies. Ear troubles following eruptive diseases. Offensive catarrhal discharge dating back to scarlet fever or measles; badly treated and drugged patients. Inflammation and swelling of the external ear; erysipelatous purple conditions. Scabs on the tragus.

The patient is subject to repeated attacks of coryza, with sneezing and stuffing up of the nose; a febrile state; sometimes with chills, fever and sweat. Pains in the face through the nose. In the evening considerable watery discharge with sneezing; in the morning stuffing up of the nose with thick yellow-green discharge. Pulsatilla is suitable to chronic catarrhs, with thick yellow-green discharge which is bland; stuffing up of the nose; copious discharge; patient has a bad smell in the nose; smells various offensive things, sometimes like manure, but more commonly described as the offensiveness of a stinking catarrh. Large bloody, thick, yellow crusts accumulate in the nose, harden down and are blown out in the morning, accompanied by thick yellow pus. In old lingering cases, *loss of smell and taste.* The mucous membrane is in a state of thickening and suppuration, with the formation of crusts and ulcers. Fulness high in the nose; stuffing up and fulness in the posterior nares. Hawks up thick yellow mucus in masses, with crusts in the morning, very often offensive to others. Many Pulsatilla patients in this catarrhal state get relief from this horrible stench by blowing out great crusts. Thick clinkers of dried-up pus or dried mucus and pus accumulate for several days and this terrible catarrhal smell comes on; but as soon as he blows out these clinkers the odor goes away and he has relief until they form again in a few days. The patient *himself* feels better in the open air, and worse in a warm room. *He* breathes better in the open air; feels stuffy in a warm room. But there are times when his *nose* stuffs up more in a warm room, where he sneezes more in a warm room.

The loss of smell is present in chronic and acute catarrhs. Much stuffing up of the nose occurring in the evening; he blows the nose easily and cleans

it out during the day, but it stuffs up in the evening and he cannot clear it
out. Remember that the mental symptoms are worse in the evening. He gets
up in the morning with a stuffed up nose, but can clean it out; his mouth is
foul, tongue coated, rancid taste, requires much brushing of his teeth and
washing out of his mouth before he can take his breakfast. So you see the
mouth and stomach symptoms are worse in the morning, the mental symptoms
are worse in the evening and there is also a stuffing up of the nose in the
evening. Compare this with the cough. There is a *dry evening cough* in
Pulsatilla and a *loose morning cough.* Copious expectoration in the morning,
but a dry, tight, constricted feeling in the chest in the evening. Stuffed up in
the evening, making breathing difficult. To repeat, then, Pulsatilla is one of
our sheet anchors in old catarrhs with loss of smell, thick yellow discharge,
and amelioration in the open air; in the nervous, timid, yielding, with stuffing
up of the nose at night and copious flow in the morning.

With the catarrhs and acute colds there is often bleeding of the nose,
blowing blood from the nose; the crusts cling tight, and when blown out
they are torn loose, and this causes bleeding; but the nose bleeds easily,
subject to expistaxis. Nose-bleed during the menstrual period; nose-bleed
before the menstrual period; nose-bleed with suppressed menses; bleeding
dark, thick, clotted, almost black, venous blood. Especially do we find
catarrhal subjects in woman who have late, scanty, light colored menses;
scarcely more than a leucorrhœa; if bloody, then only a little black stain or
clot. Chlorotic patients who have their menses once every two or three months;
chlorotic girls who are irregular, and are subject to these catarrhal states.

Pulsatilla is very useful in hay fever. The management of hay fever requires
considerable study because you have to deal with the troublesome imaginations
of the patient, he will refuse to let you study him; he wants the hay fever
treated; he doesn't want the hæmorrhoids, the thick skin on the soles of the
feet, the pains in the sacrum, the diarrhœa which alternates with constipation,
talked about or inquired into; these are always better when the hay fever is
present. Sometimes he will tell you that he is always well except when he has
hay fever. He may feel well, but it is impossible for him to be well; he has always
had these complaints and he does not want you to bother with them. The hay
fever will hardly ever reveal the indications for a remedy for the patient.

Another individual has epilepsy, and if you expect to find in the fit the
remedy that cures the patient you will be mistaken. When an acute mimicking
manifestation of disease follows several times the same beaten track the details
are hard to find. He does not know much about his hay fever. If you suggest
several things he has them all. In nearly all these acute expressions you do
not find in the exaggerated attack the symptoms that will lead you to the
remedy. You will find these symptoms by getting the state of the patient

before he was taken with hay fever. These primitive symptoms are of more importance. Sometimes it is important to know what region was affected before the nose was affected. At times you will find spinal symptoms; great soreness in the back relieved by lying on something hard. Few remedies have that. They do not tell you that at first but continue to dwell on the hay fever. In many nervous women the attack comes on with sneezing and watery discharge and then a copious, thick, yellowish-green discharge. These are the natural symptoms of hay fever, but in the "back" symptoms you see something.

In Pulsatilla the menstrual symptoms and the prolapsus come in. When the hay fever comes on, all the other symptoms are better, she feels nothing except the hay fever, however, all the symptoms interweave with each other. The *Natrum mur.* symptoms will be worse in the morning and until toward noon, while in Pulsatilla they are worse in the evening, the nose filling up with thick, yellowish-green, ropy mucus, and when the nose has been cleared, a dry, burning, smarting feeling remains; if the room is warm at night, she cannot sleep. *Natrum mur.* is a little like that in the smarting and inability to sleep at night in a warm room. In *Natrum mur.*, too, the discharge may continue day and night. We have an acute class in which Pulsatilla is sometimes indicated—copious watery discharge which ends in sneezing. In the beginning we will think of *Carbo veg., Arsenic, Allium cepa, Euphrasia.*

With *Carbo veg.* there is a watery discharge and the irritation extends into the chest, with hoarseness and rawness. In *Allium cepa* we have one group of symptoms that points to this remedy. Excoriating discharge from the nose and bland discharge from the eyes; in the larynx, sensation as if books were there, and sometimes this extends below the larynx; this always means *Allium cepa;* it is also worse in a warm room like Puls. The *Euphrasia* looks like *Cepa*, only the discharge from the eyes is copious, watery and burning—the lachrymation burns the eyes and excoriates the cheeks; discharge from nose is bland like Pulsatilla; sometimes this goes into the chest, then it is no longer *Euphrasia.*

Iodine is worse in a warm room; thick discharge from nose which burns and excoriates and is yellowish-green; but there is one thing that differentiates it from all the others—the patient immediately begins to emaciate when the complaint comes on and is very hungry.

Kali hydr. with the thick yellowish discharge, worse in a warm room, there is a great amount of rawness and burning in the nose; external nose very sore to pressure; sensitiveness in the root of the nose; whole face aches and patient is extremely restless; wants to walk in the open air which does not fatigue him.

Iodide of Arsenic; anxiety, restlessness and weakness; frequent sneezing and copious watery nasal discharge that burns the lip. Burning, watery discharge from the eyes like *Arsenic. Arsenic* wants to be very warm; wants hot water applied to the eyes; the only relief is from sniffing hot water up the nose. The *Iodide of Arsenic* is worse in a warm room, and, for days after sneezing, the discharge thickens and becomes gluey, looking like *thick yellow honey,* this excoriates; much pain through the root of the nose and eyes; often rawness in the chest with dyspnœa. The remedies having the dyspnœa are *Arsenic, Iodide of Arsenic, Iodine, Kali hydr.,* and *Sahadilla;* these are the ones I have found most frequently indicated in the asthmatic forms of hay fever. If the complaint has been developed after being overheated about that time, you will find that *Silica,* Puls. and *Carbo veg.* must be carefully compared. There is another class of remedies having the stuffing up of the nose not relieved by the discharge. There is a constant desire to blow the nose, yet he gets no relief. This makes me think at once of *Lach., Kali bi., Psor., Naja* and *Sticta.*

Psorinum has the copious, watery, bland discharge from the nose, it may be excoriating, it has both. The stuffing up of the nose generally takes place in the open air; he is relieved in a warm, close room and by lying down; has some dyspnœa which is relieved by stretching the arms at right angles with the body. Hay fever is a psoric sickness. *Psorinum* given in a single dose will so develop the symptoms that the case will be more clear. The attack is not the best thing to prescribe for. If it is too violent, a short acting remedy may be selected that will mitigate it.

Nux vomica has a free, easy breathing in the open air, but when he goes into the warm room his nose stuffs up, which also occurs at night, though the water drips on the pillow yet he stuffs up like Puls., *Bry.,* and the *Iodine* preparations, *Iodide of Arsenic* and *Cyclamen.* Do not understand me to have given remedies for hay fever, we cannot lay down remedies for diseases. The whole constitution must be most carefully examined.

The face is sickly, often mottled, purple, intermixed with yellow and unhealthy colors; venous puffing; sensation of fulness; often a red face, like that of health, and the patient gets no sympathy; face often flushes; flushes of heat to the face; at times a sunken look; dark rings about the eyes; sallow, green, chlorotic. Subject to erysipelas; erysipelatous blotches on the face, spreading to the scalp, with stinging and burning; skin of face very sensitive to touch at such times.

Mumps and inflammation of parotid glands. If a woman suffering with mumps takes a decided cold the breasts swell, and there is an inflammation of the mammary gland. Girls take cold, the swelling of the parotid subsides too soon, and the corresponding mammary gland swells; sometimes both swell; or it may begin in one and go to the other. In men it is the testicle. Pulsatilla is one of the most important remedies in this form of metastasis; it breaks up complaints that flit about. Pulsatilla is the common remedy for enormously swollen testicles from mumps in a boy. *Carbo vegetabilis* is another remedy, but then you have a *Carbo veg.* patient. *Abrotanum* is also useful in wandering around symptoms. Pulsatilla has *wandering pains;* rheumatism goes from joint to joint, jumps around here and there; neuralgic pains fly from place to place; inflammations go from gland to gland. But here is the distinguishing feature—Pulsatilla *sticks to its own text;* it keeps jumping around, but it does not change to a new class of disease. *Abrotanum* has this metastasis, but it changes the whole diagnosis; that is, the allopath says, "This is a new disease today." The patient has a violent diarrhœa today, and an ignoramus suppresses it; an inflammatory rheumatism comes on, and he calls it a new disease. The suppression of a diarrhœa or a hæmorrhage, or the removal of piles, causes an out-cropping somewhere else. A child has a summer complaint suppressed and there follow symptoms referring to the brain, kidneys, liver, or a marasmus with emaciation from below upwards. Such things are in the nature of *Abrotanum.*

Stomach. Hours after eating the patient eructates mouthfuls of sour, rancid, bitter fluid; liquids roll up from the stomach; always belching up rancid food. Some patients cannot digest butter; cannot use olive oil on their food. All sorts of bad tastes in the mouth. Several hours after eating has not finished digesting food in the stomach. Sour vomiting and eructations. Digestion is slow, and the patient goes to the next meal hungry; eating does nor satisfy; assimilation is bad. Always bilious. Mouth is slimy and the taste is bad. All these symptoms are worse in the morning. "Accumulation of saliva and much mucus in the mouth." "Flow of sweetish or tenacious saliva." "Constant spitting of frothy, cotton-like mucus."

A striking feature of the Pulsatilla patient is that he never wants water. Dryness of the mouth, but *seldom thirsty.* Even in many of the fevers he is thirstless, but there is at times an exception to this—in high fevers there may be some thirst. "Thirstlessness, with moist or dry tongue." "Desire for sour, refreshing things." Often desires things he cannot digest; lemonade, herring, cheese, pungent things, highly-seasoned things, juicy things. "Aversion to meat, butter, fat food, pork, bread, milk, smoking." "Scraping sensation in stomach and œsophagus like heartburn." Many pains in the stomach when empty or when full. But the bloating, the gas and the sour stomach are most striking. Gastric catarrh. Craves ice cream; craves pastries, yet they will not digest, and make him worse. Craves things which make him sick. This is not uncommon. The whisky drinker craves his liquor, yet knows it will kill him. So in Pulsatilla with regard to pastries. Craves batter cakes, with maple syrup, yet knows they will be vomited. Craves *highly spiced* sausage, yet averse to pork alone.

Pulsatillla produces and cures jaundice. "Jaundice in consequence of chronic susceptibility to hepatitis and derangement of secretion of bile with looseness of bowels; duodenal catarrh; disordered digestion; feverishness and thirstlessness; after quinine."

Many troubles seem to manifest themselves in the abdomen by bloating, distension of the abdomen, flatulence, colicky pains, rumbling, fermentation of food, and from disorders of menstruation or diarrhœa. Great sensitiveness, tumefaction, tenderness; whole abdomen, stomach and pelvic organs sensitive to touch. Bloating after eating, especially after fats and rich foods. Fulness of the veins; general venous stasis. It, brings about especially a tumid fulness of the abdomen, such a stuffed feeling that she cannot breathe. In a woman about to menstruate, there is bloating of the abdomen, stuffed feeling, has to throw off her clothes, cannot wear stays, wants to get into a loose dress or to go to bed—so extremely puffed is she. Associated with this abdominal tumefaction the face and lips become bloated and puffed, the eyes red, and the feet puffed so that she cannot wear her shoes. There is also a sensation of dragging down, a sense of great weakness, commonly related to the menstrual disturbances or uterine disorders. The dragging down is recognized as prolapsus uteri. It is felt in the whole abdomen and is described as a funneling sensation, as if the parts would push out into the world, a dragging down. Oversensitiveness of the abdomen; especially in the lower part of the abdomen. She cannot stand on her feet or walk around much, because of the weight and dragging down. Labor-like pains in the uterus and back as if the menses would come on. It is not uncommon for the Pulsatilla patient to feel through the whole month as if she were about to menstruate.

The abdominal and bowel symptoms are associated. Cutting, flitting changing pains. Pains urging to stool. Griping, in the bowels associated with dysentery or diarrhœa; loose watery or green stools. A striking feature of the bowel symptoms is a loose, watery, green stool, *continually changing*; yellow, faecal, slimy. In summer complaints, when Pulsatilla is the indicated remedy, there will be hardly two stools alike; continually changing. This is characteristic of Pulsatilla in general; the pains wander; complaints change by metastases; the patient is scarcely ever twice alike. Diarrhœa alternating with constipation. Menstrual flow stops and starts, intermits and changes. In the Pulsatilla patient you never know what you will find next. Dysentery; dysenteric stools; scanty, slimy, bloody, green, watery stool with a little spurt; next stool might be diarrhœic, with quite a copious discharge; thus you have diarrhœa and dysentery together.

Troublesome chronic constipation; stool large, hard and difficult to expel. It has (like *Nux*) frequent urging to stool without any stool, or frequent urging with only a scanty stool; goes many times before can pass a stool, *Nux* and Pulsatilla. Frequent unsuccessful urging in a chronic case is looked on as a keynote to *Nux,* but many remedies have it. Pulsatilla is one. The diarrhœa and bowel symptoms of Pulsatilla are worse in the evening and during the night; that is, the stools are worse at night. The stomach, throat and mouth symptoms are worse in the morning. The mental symptoms are worse in the evening. The bowel and stool symptoms are aggravated by keeping perfectly still, and ameliorated by gentle motion. There is much restlessness in Pulsatilla. Amelioration from motion in the cool open air. Feels stuffed up in a close room, and wants the windows open. "Dysenteric stools of clear yellow, red or green slime; pain in the back, straining." "Stools of deep green mucus; pain in the abdomen; no thirst." You will remember the word *green* in Pulsatilla, as it relates extensively to the catarrhal discharges.

Most troublesome constipation with hæmorrhoids; violent pains in the hæmorrhoids, worse lying down, ameliorated from gentle motion, worse from the warmth of the bed, better moving about in the open air. She becomes so nervous in a room while at rest that the pains seem intensified and she must move about. "Hæmorrhoids; painful, protruding, blind, with itching and stitches in anus." The aggravation from lying down in extremely painful hæmorrhoids is contrasted with *Ammonium carb.* which has violently painful haemorrhoids relieved by lying flat on the back. In violently painful haemorrhoids, with intense burning, think of *Arsenicum* and *Kali carbonicum.* In those with sticking, tearing pains study *Æsculus.* Looking over a number of years I have been forced to use in these cases a remedy not yet fully proven. In painful hæmorrhoids, in a broken down constitution, where the whole disease seems to culminate in the hæmorrhoids; bleeding, protruding; a mere touch almost causes a convulsion; it causes her to scream out at the top of her voice; it is so painful that she feels that death would be a relief; she lies in bed holding the nates far apart with her hands; after every stool she has three or four hours of extreme suffering. In these cases look up the *Pæony.* The hæmorrhoids it cures look like the flowers of the plant, they are so inflamed, so red and bleeding; oozing; tender to touch; patient is so worn out with the pain. It has many times relieved the pain and cured these enormous hæmorrhoidal tumors. I have cured them after they had been operated on, and all sorts of violence done them, without relief. Do not go to this drug if you can find a remedy that covers *all the patient.* Many patients will not confess any other symptoms, and some of these will suffer so much from the hæmorrhoids alone that you will really need this remedy.

Urine frequent, scanty, with urging; Wonderful tenesmus; extremely painful, bloody, burning, smarting urine; there is scarcely a drop collects in the bladder but it must be expelled. She cannot *lie on the back without having a desire to urinate.* She may go all night without urinating if she does not lie on the back, but the minute she turns on her back she is wakened by the desire to urinate and she feels that if she does not hurry she will pass it involuntarily. Involuntary urination when coughing and sneezing, or from a sudden shock or surprise, or from sudden joy, or from laughing, or from the noise of the slam of a door or a pistol shot. Pulsatilla has dribbling of urine, dribbles on the slightest provocation. She must keep her mind continually on it, or she will lose her urine. As soon as she goes to sleep it flows away. Little, mild, gentle, florid, plethoric, warm-blooded girls, who kick the covers off at night and have nocturnal enuresis. Yellow, sallow, sickly girls who lose their urine in their first sleep call for *Sepia*. Losing the urine in the first sleep is looked upon as a strong symptom, but you can figure it out, and hence it is *not so*. All those cases that have to make an effort to hold the urine during the day lose it in their first sleep; for then the mind is taken off it, and as soon as the mind is taken off it the urine dribbles. *Causticum* and *Sepia* are remedies looked upon as curing involuntary urination during the first sleep, but I have cured it with many other remedies. A man past middle age flooded the bed at night as soon as he went to sleep. The medicines which have this are limited and he had received them all. I found I must figure it out on another basis. I ascertained that when moving about at his work he had no difficulty in holding the urine, but when he sat down he had to make an effort to control it. At the time this condition developed he had been in Atlantic City and had bathed much in the ocean. Here were the aggravation and amelioration of *Rhus,* and *Rhus* cured him. Few would think of *Bryonia* in urinary trouble. When he moves the urine dribbles, when he walks it flows. He is relieved only by keeping quiet. *Bryonia* is aggravated by motion; *Rhus* is relieved by motion.

Pulsatilla has relief from motion. A few remedies have relief from slow motion and of these Pulsatilla and *Ferrum* are the most striking. A few remedies are relieved by hurried motion; want to move fast. Such are *Bromine* and *Arsenicum.* The *Arsenic* child cannot be carried fast enough. The Pulsatilla baby is content with moderate motion. Any motion that *heats up* the Pulsatilla patient aggravates all the complaints. A wood sawyer working hard said his cough was relieved by moving about, but when he became heated up from sawing he had to sit down and rest on account of the violent spasmodic cough that would come on.

Pulsatilla has complaints from exposure to rain; getting feet wet. Urinary troubles worse when getting chilled (*Dulcamara*). Pulsatilla establishes a chronic, inveterate catarrh of the bladder. Copious mucous discharge, bloody discharge, especially after taking cold. Thick, ropy, purulent, green, offensive discharge.

Sexual desire unusually strong. "Long lasting morning erections." "Sexual excesses resulting in headache, backache; limbs heavy." "Burning and aching of the testicles, with or without swelling." Orchitis; inflammation and swelling of the testicles from suppressed gonorrhœa, from mumps, from catching cold, from sitting on damp ground, or on a cold stone when perspiring. Gonorrhœa suppressed by injections. "Cold" settles in the Testicles. Pulsatilla is the most frequently indicated remedy in gonorrhœa. in which the discharge is thick yellow or thick yellow and green, in those who are sensitive to heat, ameliorated walking in the open air. But also in persons with no other symptoms, and the gonorrhœal discharge is thick yellow or green; no symptoms contra-indicating it. Troublesome lingering discharges; an old glees rouses into a thick yellow discharge, when he takes cold or after coition. Frequent tenesmus; chordee; urging to urinate; burning urination and yellow discharge. Tumefaction about the penis. Foreskin dropsical. (*Nitric ac., Fluor. ac., Cann. sat.*) Pulsatilla is useful in cases of suppressed gonorrhœa, with complaints following. Inflammation of the prostate. In old sinners with enlarged prostate, hard, flat, packed farees, must always use a catheter; especially when the trouble has been brought on by sexual abuses, sexual excesses, vices. Pain in the testicles; tearing in the swollen testicles. Pain along the cord like cutting of knives; lacerating, tearing.

Exaggerated sexual desire; nymphomania; wild, beside herself with sexual thoughts; uncontrollable sexual desire. Inflammation of ovaries and uterus. Suppression of menses from getting feet wet. Menses too late, scanty. Face pale, yellow, sallow, or green like a chlorotic patient. It overcomes the tendency to miscarriage, false conception, moles, etc., and stops the growth of fibroids, other symptoms agreeing. In pregnancy and during confinement many symptoms call for Pulsatilla. Most often called for when the patient is not irritable and the pains are very feeble, lasting for several days, and doing nothing; irregular, flitting, changeable pains, now up the back, now down the limbs; a prolonged first stage or prolonged preparatory symptoms. *Chamomilla* is more suitable if the woman is extremely irritable. But in a mild, gentle, mental state, when the pains are irregular, the os dilated and the contractions have let up, the pains too short, Pulsatilla will terminate that labor in a short time. The next pain after the dose will be a good one. You very often see in these cases that the outside parts are relaxed and the conditions are such that everything ought to go on well, but there is inaction. For weak pains Pulsatilla stands high.

Violent menstrual colic, causing her to bend double; soreness in the region of the uterus and ovaries; distended abdomen; throws the covers off; wants the windows open; tearful; weeps without a cause. Suppression of the menstrual flow from getting feet wet. Flow slow in being established and then scarcely more than a leucorrhœa. Menstruation that has been painful since puberty in plethoric girls. I have seen Pulsatilla cure a great many girls of sixteen to eighteen years old. The mother comes to me saying her daughter has suffered since her first menses; she went in swimming, or got her feet wet, and has suffered since. The doctor says the parts are undeveloped and she must be operated on. Pulsatilla has established a normal flow in a few months. Now I will give you a contrast in another remdey. Scrawny girls who are sensitive to cold, have also taken a bath at the time the first menses should appear, or have got the feet wet, and the flow is partially suppressed, or has come on with an inflammation; a state of undevelopment is established, a stenosis; horrible menstrual colic; bearing down pains, as if everything would escape into the world, doubling the patient up; ameliorated by heat and aggravated by cold. *Calc. phos.* is the remedy. "In girls of mild disposition, when puberty is unduly delayed, or menstrual function is defectively or irregularly performed; they are pale and languid, complaint of headache, chilliness and lassitude." To develop these young girls Pulsatilla is a great remedy. Most troublesome cases of prolapsus. It competes with *Sepia, Belladonna. Natrum mur., Nux vomica* and *Secale;* all of these are remedies with great relaxation, bearing down; some have cured even procidentia. Pulsatilla cures many cases of gonorrhœa in females. I think it is most commonly indicated. A striking feature is, when the menstrual flow is present there is milk in the breasts. In girls at puberty—milk in the breasts; a premature establishment of milk. In non-pregnant women, milk in the breasts. (*Cyclamen* and *Mercurius.*)

The chest, respiratory organs, and cough furnish some most troublesome symptoms. Bronchitis; pneumonia. Dry, teasing cough and dyspnœa; wants the windows open, aggravated lying down. Cough, gagging and choking. Copious expectoration in the morning, of thick yellow-green mucus. Dry, teasing cough at night, worse lying down. Chronic loose cough after measles. Whooping cough.

In the larynx we have many symptoms; constriction; tickling causing cough. Dry, teasing cough, worse lying and in a warm room. Cough worse at night,

Bronchitis with loose morning and dry evening cough.

Dyspnœa; oppression from walking fast or becoming overheated after eating; stopping up nose; after emotions. Spasmodic contraction of larynx. Tightness of chest; dyspnœa when lying on left side; suffocation in the evening and during the night. Asthma of children from suppressed rash or in women from suppressed menses. Loud rattling in the chest when lying. Chronic loose cough after measles. Expectoration of copious, thick, yellow-green, or bloody mucus; salty; offensive. Chronic catarrh of chest. Sensation of fulness in the chest in the evening with pulsation preventing sleep. Palpitation from lying on the left side. Soreness in the walls of the chest. Pain in the chest sometimes relieved by lying on the opposite side; dryness and rawness in the chest. Wandering tearing pains in the chest; cutting pains in pleurisy; violent heat in the chest. Hæmorrhage of the lungs, dark blood. Dry cough in the evening, loose in the morning. Hæmorrhage with suppressed menses or instead of the menses. Pulsatilla is very useful in catarrhal phthisis in chlorotic girls.

In curvature of the spine Puls. is of great value. Pain in the back, lumbar and sacral regions; wandering pains; spinal irritation after sexual excesses. Rheumatic pains in the spine and limbs, worse during rest and better from slow motion. Pain in small of back as if sprained; sensation of cold water poured down back.

All the limbs are painful; drawing, tearing pains in the limbs, better from motion and after motion; worse from a warm room and better from cold applications. Swelling of the veins in the arms and hands. Varicose veins of the limbs like *Fl. ac.* Rheumatism of joints; pain in joints as if dislocated. Sciatica worse in the evening and better from slowly moving about. Drawing and tension of muscles in lower limbs in the evening in bed. Tearing, jerking pains in the limbs, changing place. Burning in the veins. Purple swelling with violent itching of the feet as if they had been frozen. Feet burn, and he must put them out of bed. Soles burn and are bruised when walking. Marked restlessness and twitching of the limbs and feet; numbness of the limb lain on; wandering pains in all the limbs.

Sleeps on the back with hands over head. Cannot sleep on the left side as it increases the palpitation and suffocation. Confused, frightful, anxious dreams. Late falling asleep; sleeplessness on account of flushes of heat. Pulsatilla cures intermittent fever, coming on from disordered stomach. Chill morning and evening daily. The chill begins in the hands and feet; pains in the limbs during the chill; one-sided coldness with numb feeling; fever one-sided. Thirst before the chill and seldom during the heat; heat with distended veins; sweat profuse all over or only on one side of the body. Vomiting of mucus during the chill.

PYROGEN

The potencies prepared from Heath's 3d of decomposed beef have been used by the author for many years against all forms of septic fever and sequelae, when the symptoms agree. Violent chill intermingled with heat and sweat, or dry heat with marked aching in the limbs; restlessness, > by motion and heat. The sore bruised condition is as marked as in *Arnica* and *Baptisia;* the aching in the bones like *Eupatorium,* the restlessness, > by motion and heat like *Rhus.* Pains all aggravated sitting. Complaints come on from becoming cold, and from cold damp weather.

These features are found in hectic fevers in the last stages of phthisis, as well as septic fevers. It aborts puerperal fever in a few hours when clearly indicated. In cases of typhoid where there is the confusion like that found in *Baptisia* and the heat is too intense for that remedy, Pyrogen should always be considered. When the temperature reaches 106° and there is great soreness and aching this remedy will make great changes in a single day; but if the pains are > by motion and heat it will abort the fever.

When the pulse is extremely high, and the temperature not correspondingly high this remedy will be useful. On the other hand, when the pulse and temperature are out of rhythm either way this remedy should be considered if the case is of septic origin. Great pain when the flow from an open abscess becomes scanty. *Violent burning in an abscess* (*Ars., Anthr., Tarent. C.*).

Offensiveness prevails extensively; even putrid and cadaveric odors of body, breath, sweat and discharges. Fevers from sewer gas poisoning; erysipelas from infection and surgical fevers. It cures many chronic complaints that date back to septic conditions. She has not been well since a puerperal fever many years ago, is a good reason for thinking of Pyrogen.

A young man of good inheritance suffered from blood poison and made a poor recovery, and for several years was affected with abscesses in various parts. He was pale and sickly, rheumatic and stiff; at this time there was an abscess of the calf slowly forming. He took Pyrogen and made a rapid and complete recovery. This time the abscess did not open. He has remained in good health now ten years.

It has cured Bright's disease that could be traced to septic origin. It is a most useful remedy when there is threatening heart failure in septic and zymotic fevers. Septic hæmorrhage, when the blood is dark. It will often save life in the most dangerous and rapid septic fevers.

Loquacity; can think and talk faster than ever before, especially during fever.

Irritable. Delirium and confusion of mind about his body and limbs (*Bapt.*).

Sensation as though he covered the whole bed.

Knew her head was on the pillow, but did not know where the rest of the body was.

Feels when lying on one side she is one person, and another when turning on the other side.

Sensation as though crowded with arms and legs.

These symptoms are much like *Baptisia,* but if the temperature runs very high *Baptisia* will not meet the condition so well as Pyrogen.

Violent congestion of the head *with pressing pain* and pulsation, > by pressure Copious sweat on the head. Pain in occiput on coughing; in the morning on walking.

The eyeballs are sore to touch, on turning them outwards or upwards. Septic bleeding from nose. Fan-like motion of alæ, nasi (*Lyc.*)

Face pale, sunken, and covered with cold sweat. Cheeks red and burning hot.

The mouth is foul, and the taste putrid. The tongue is coated, and brown. Brown streak down the center. Sordes on the teeth. Putrid odor from mouth.

Vomiting; of bile, blood; of putrid masses. Vomits water when it becomes warm in the stomach. Stercoraceous vomiting. Coffee ground vomiting. Thirst for cold drinks during chill and heat.

Distension and great sensitiveness of abdomen. Inflammation of peritoneum, intestines and uterus, of septic origin. Rumbling in bowels. Pain on deep breathing. Cutting, colicky pain. Pain in right side going through to the back < on every motion, talking and breathing; > by lying on right side; groaning with every breath.

Copious, liquid, putrid stools. Involuntary stool. Profuse, watery, painless stool. Stool carrion-like. The difficult constipated stool also like carrion in odor. Constipation with hard dry, black, putrid stools; small black balls like olives. Putrid bloody stools. Soft narrow stools with great straining. Hæmorrhage from bowels.

Urine scanty or suppressed. Red deposit, hard to wash off. Albuminous urine containing casts. Putrid urine. Frequent calls to urinate as the fever comes on. Intolerable tenesmus of the bladder; spasmodic contractions, involving rectum, ovaries, and broad ligaments (case cured by Yingling). Involuntary urine and stool in septic fevers.

Uterine hœmorrhage. *Putrid, scanty lochia. Suppressed lochia. Violent chill; puerperal fever.* Menses lasting one day, then bloody leucorrhœa. *Septic fever following abortion.* Prolapsus of uterus.

Wheezing when expiring. Weak and husky voice, and hoarseness. Cough with large masses of mucus from larynx, < by motion, and in warm room. Cough causes burning in larynx and bronchi. Putrid, thick, purulent expectoration. Cough < by lying, > by sitting up. Bloody or rusty expectoration. Cough, with copious, offensive night sweats. It is a great palliative in the last weeks of consumption. Abscesses in lung.

Heart failure in septic fevers, < by least motion. Every pulsation felt in distant parts. Anxiety and sinking sensation in region of heart. Distinct consciousness of the heart. Aching at the bifurcation of the trachea. Oppression of chest and heart. Fulness in region of heart. Feels as if the heart were pumping cold water (Yingling). Palpitation. Loud heart beats. Sensation of purring of the heart. *Rapid, irregular, fluttering pulse.*

Pulsation in the neck. Weak feeling in the back. Stitching in back on coughing.

Pain in all the limbs with great restlessness. Aching in bones all over the body. Soreness of the muscles and the bed feels hard, > by motion. Cold extremities. Numbness of extremities. Hands and arms numb. Hands cold and clammy. Pain in the thighs during chill and fever. Pain in the knees and legs during chill and fever, ameliorated from walking, and from heat. Aching in legs while sitting, > by walking. Aching above knee as if bone were broken, > by stretching of limbs and motion. Feet and legs dropsical. Numbness of feet.

Skin pale, cold, of ashy hue. Obstinate varicose offensive ulcers of old people. It has cured many old fever sores with putrid, thin, bloody discharges. Carrion-like perspiration. Putrid odors of the body. Must be covered in all stages. Chill ameliorated by warm bed. The chill is quotidian; it comes in the evening, generally at 7 P.M. The periodicity is regular. Cold sweat on the body. Hot sweat with high temperature. The sleep is full of frightful dreams. Persistent thoughts prevent sleep. Suffocation in sleep. Cries out in sleep from oppression of chest.

RANUNCULUS BULBOSUS

This buttercup gives off an acrid ethereal vapor very poisonous to such as are sensitive to it, and has been many times mistaken for *Rhus* poisoning. This common field buttercup is not used as often as it is indicated, and it must be that it is not as well known as many other remedies. It is a rheumatic remedy of great usefulness when the chest muscles are involved. Pain in the spinal nerves, pleura and costal muscles always with extreme soreness. It is as sensitive to motion as *Bryonia,* and to the cold, damp weather as *Dulcamara.* It has sudden weakness even to fainting, and it has cured epilepsy. It is extremely excitable, and resembles the much broken state of sensitive invalids; hence it has complaints from fright and vexation. Its complaints are worse in the evening and after any change in the weather, especially from warm to cold. The evening aggravations are quite marked; the headache, ear pain, the nasal symptoms, the fever, soreness in the short ribs, dyspnœa, oppression of chest and heart, tightness of chest, increased pulsation, trembling, chilliness, are all worse in the evening. He is extremely sensitive to cold and cold, open air. Cold air brings on headaches, rheumatism, neuralgia of chest, spine and ovaries, vertigo. Sudden exposure while overheated will bring on febrile symptoms, pleurisy or pneumonia. After exposure to cold air, his chest muscles are sore as if bruised. Draft of cold air causes sore pains in many parts. He is extremely sensitive to rainy and stormy weather. He is sore and bruised in many parts. *Stitching pains* in liver, ears, chest, abdomen, shoulder and other joints, spine, lumbar region to abdomen, between the shoulders in the back, stitching, burning pains radiating from the dorsal spine. *Burning pains* in cardiac orifice of stomach; in pit of stomach, neck of bladder, in cornea; in eruptions; in ulcers. *Pressing pain* in forehead; vertex; eyes; temples; root of nose; pit of stomach; shoulder; across the lower part of chest; middle of chest. It has creeping, crawling, tingling. Inflammation of the pleura with. dropsy of adhesion. With pleural effusion it is a very useful remedy when there is extreme soreness along the ribs, especially the lower ribs. It has cured lupus and epithelioma. Jaundiced.

It has great depression of spirits and desire to die. Fear of ghosts and very irritable, even quarrelsome. Confusion of mind.

Vertigo when going into the cold air. Sensation of enlargement of the head.

Cerebral hyperæmia with heat of the face. Headache with change of temperature, pressing headache in forehead and vertex worse when changing temperature, either to cold or warm room. Violent pains over right eye, worse lying, and better when walking and standing. All other pains worse from motion. This is a notable exception.

Pressure and burning in the eyes. Great pains in the eye, especially the right. Soreness and burning in *right lower lid.* Burning and soreness in outer canthus of the right eye. Bluish-black herpetic vesicles over the eye. It has cured hemiopia during pregnancy.

Stitching pains in the ears, especially the right, worse in the evening.

It has cured hay fever with burning in eyes and itching of the soft palate (like *Wyethia*), worse in the evening, pressing in the root of the nose. The skin of the nose is red and much inflamed.

It has caused vesicular eruption on the face with great burning. It has caused epithelioma of the face. Prickling of the face, nose and chin. Twitching of the lips.

Burning and soreness and redness in the throat, smarting and itching of the soft palate.

There is much thirst in the afternoon. It has cured many times the weak and tottering condition of patients suffering from prolonged use of stimulants, such as whisky and brandy. It is a great remedy for delirium tremens when he is besotted, has hiccoughs and is more or less convulsive. Epileptiform convulsions from alcoholic liquors. The hiccough is violent and convulsive. Frequent eructations.

Burning in the stomach and especially in the region of the cardiac orifice. Stomach is very sensitive to touch. Paroxysms of neuralgia of the stomach.

Sore bruised feeling in the short ribs, stitching pains in the liver, jaundiced. Soreness in liver on deep pressure; symptoms worse in the evening.

In the abdomen there is much flatulence, colic, burning and great soreness on pressure. Stitching pain in right side of abdomen under the ribs. The pains are much worse from motion, breathing and walking. Many stitching pains in abdomen. It has a watery diarrhœa and dysentery. It has herpes zoster with violent pains.

Excoriating leucorrhœa and sharp pains in the ovaries every cold change in the weather, from motion, and in the evening.

Heavy, short breathing with oppression of chest in the evening. Sighing breathing. Pressure and constriction of the chest. Pressing pains in the walls of the chest. Violent stitching pains in the chest walls. Stitching pains in region of fifth and sixth ribs. Painful soreness on touch or pressure on the floating ribs. Rheumatic pains in the chest. Chronic costal rheumatism. Soreness describing the attachments of the diaphragm. Inflammation of the diaphragm and pleura. Hydrothorax pains in chest from adhesions of the pleura. Sensitive as if inner parts were adhered. Pain worse from motion, in cold air, from becoming cold, on inspiration. Sensation of a cold wet cloth on going into cold air. Stitching pains every change of the weather from warm to cold. Sore spots here and there on the ribs. Pain in the region of heart from motion and inspiration and lying on left side. Rheumatic swelling of pectoral muscles with extreme soreness to touch. Pleurodynia with most violent cutting pains from inspiration, pressure, turning the body and cold air. Pulse full, hard and rapid in the evening and slow in the morning.

Sore spots in the spine. Pain along the inner margin of the left scapula. Stitching pains in the spine between the scapulæ. Pains in lower and inner margin of scapulæ in shoemakers, needle workers and writers from sitting bent. One scapula often becomes adhered to the back and it is immovable, and later burning pain comes on. Weak spine and great lassitude. Vesicular eruptions form upon the back and chest with blue contents, with severe pain.

Rheumatic pains, paroxysmal in character in the upper limbs. Stitching pains along the nerves in arms and hands. Tearing pains in forearm and hand. The pains are worse from cold, and worse from motion. Bluish vesicles in the palms and fingers. Seed warts on the thumb.

Great weakness in lower limbs in forenoon. Stitching burning from the spine along the sciatic nerve in cold, wet weather and in stormy weather, worse from motion and in cold air. Drawing pain in the thighs. Rheumatic pain in knees, stinging and soreness in foot and toes. Corns very painful, sore to touch, sting and burn. He suffers from complaints like chilblains.

He is late falling asleep. Sleepless from difficult breathing, from heat, and orgasms of blood.

Dark blue vesicles upon the skin. Horny scurf forms after the vesicles have opened. It has been used for vesicular eruptions; for burns; for herpes zoster; for pemphigus; for eczema. Flat burning, stinging, ulcers. Horn-like excrescences.

RHODODENDRON

This is a very useful remedy in gouty patients who suffer from rheumatic pains, sometimes wandering from joint to joint, aggravated during rest, aggravated before and during storms, aggravated in cold, wet weather and ameliorated from warm wrapping. These pains may be in the head or the limbs. it is a great palliative in old people who have suffered long from gout. Rheumatic swelling of joints. Pain in the aponeuroses at night, during rest. He can always fortell a thunderstorm. There are tearing, shooting pains. Sore bruised pains. Stiffness of joints, neck and back. Extremely sensitive to cold weather, and aggravated from becoming cold. Paralytic weakness during rest, yet he is weak from exertion. Continued motion is his only relief. Painfully sensitive to windy cold weather. Chorea before a storm. General amelioration from motion, even when the painful part is aggravated from moving the affected part.

Fear of thunder in nervous persons (*Phos.*), forgetful. While talking he forgets what he was talking about. Leaves out words in writing. Aversion to his business. Easily affected by wine.

Violent rheumatic headaches in morning in bed, ameliorated by moving about, by wrapping up the head; aggravated from drinking wine, aggravated in cold wet weather. Headaches come on before a storm. Pain in temples and forehead. The head feels sore as if bruised. External heat ameliorates the head pains.

Pain in the eyes before a storm, ameliorated by heat and motion. Weakness of the internal recti muscles with stitching pains before a storm.

Violent pains in ear, sometimes tearing, aggravated before a storm. Ameliorated by heat. Roaring, ringing and buzzing in the ears.

Neuralgia of the face in gouty subjects, aggravated from motion, aggravated from cold wind; ameliorated by applied heat. The patient is generally aggravated during rest; comes in stormy weather. Pains ameliorated by eating and warmth. Pain in the teeth before a storm. Pain in teeth with earache, ameliorated by heat; aggravated at night, from cold drinks.

Feels full after little food (*Lyc.*). Empty eructations. Green bitter vomiting after drinking cold water. Sinking at the stomach. Pressure in the stomach after eating.

Pains as from flatulence high up in sides of abdomen. Stitching in spleen from walking fast. Rumbling in abdomen and fulness after eating.

Much straining to pass a soft stool. Undigested, thin, brownish stool. Diarrhœa after eating, after fruit; from cold, wet weather, before a thunderstorm. Dysentery before a thunderstorm. Pulsating anus, drawing in anus extending o genitals.

Drawing pain in bladder with frequent urging to urinate.

Orchitis with much swelling in rheumatic patients from taking cold, from itting on a cold stone, from suppressed gonorrhœa; the right most affected. Drawing pain in spermatic cord, during rest, ameliorated by motion and heat. t has cured hydrocele in boys. Much itching of the scrotum.

Menses frequent and profuse. Serous cysts in the vagina.

Rheumatic stitching pains in chest in stormy weather during rest. Constriction of chest. Pain in heart.

Rheumatic pains and stiffness in neck and back. Pain in dorsal region extending to arms in cold, wet weather, aggravated during rest. Tearing pains in neck and back driving out of bed.

Rheumatic tearing pains in all the limbs in stormy weather, aggravated before a storm and during rest, aggravated at night; mostly in forearms and legs. Wandering pains in the limbs and joints. Pain in bone and periosteum. Pains drive him out of bed. Paralytic pains in limbs. Cannot sleep unless legs are crossed. Sleepless after midnight. Pain in the shoulder joint so severe that the arm cannot he moved—but the patient and the pain are ameliorated by walking about.

RHUS TOXICODENDRON

The complaints of this remedy come on from cold damp weather, from being exposed to cold damp air when perspiring. The patient is sensitive to cold air and all his complaints are made worse from cold and all are better from warmth. In a general way, the aching pains, the bruised feelings over the body, restlessness throughout the limbs, and amelioration from motion are features that prevail throughout all conditions of Rhus. While he is better from motion and better from walking, if he continues to walk he become exhausted. Any continued exertion of the body or mind exhausts the Rhus patient. He suffers from rheumatic conditions with pains in the bones lameness in the muscles, lameness in the tendons, ligaments, and joints from suppression of sweat, from becoming chilled. These occur with or without fever. Rhus is suitable in old chronic rheumatic conditions. He is stiff, lame and bruised on first beginning to move. This passes off on becoming warmed up, but soon he becomes weak and must rest. Then comes the restlessness and aching and uneasiness which drive him to move and which again make him better, but soon he becomes weak and these continue, so that he is never perfectly at ease and never finds rest. Inflammation of the glands and of the mucous membranes; inflammation of the muscles. Cellulitis of the pelvis, of the neck, about the glands with much swelling. Inflammation of the skin that becomes erysipelatous; purple; pitting upon pressure with large blisters that fill with serum, sometimes bloody. It has abscesses and carbuncles and vesicular eruptions. Inflammation of glands that are hot and very painful. They are hot and end in suppuration. Abscesses of the axillary glands and of the parotids. Scrofulous inflammation of the glands of the neck and low jaw. Inflammation of the periosteum and of the bones. Scrofulous and rickety affections. The prominent projections of bones become sore to touch, especially the cheek bones. Its complaints are more or less periodical. It has cured many cases of intermittent fever, is often suitable in remittent fever, and is a most useful remedy in continued fevers and in a low form of typhoid fever. The pains that run through Rhus are aching, tearing, and bruised pains often attended with numbness and paralytic weakness of the limbs. It has paralysis of the limbs with loss of sensation. In infantile paralysis Rhus is a very common remedy. The nurse-girls at the present time often bring on in the child this paralytic condition and spinal paralysis. The nurses take the infants to the park, take them out of their carriage and put them down upon the cold damp ground and in a few days the child comes down with infantile paralysis. Rhus will cure these cases because the symptoms take the Rhus type. Hemiplegia, especially of the right side. Twitching of the limbs and muscles. It has cured chorea brought on from taking a cold bath.

Most of the mental symptoms of Rhus are such as prevail during low forms of fever, especially in typhoid. There is then incoherent talking; answers questions hastily. There is anxiety, apprehensions, and fear. Intense fear at night. The complaints of Rhus often come on in the night. The mental symptoms are worse at night. The delirium is worse at night. The fears and anxiety are worse at night. The chronic mental symptoms of Rhus are despondency, mental prostration, inability to sustain a mental effort, disgust for life and thoughts of suicide. He wants to drown himself yet he has fear of death. He desires to die yet he has not the courage to commit suicide. In many instances he is filled with suicidal thoughts; sadness and weeping yet he knows not why. Irritability and anxiety as if he had met with some misfortune, restlessness, anxiousness and nervous in the extreme in acute and chronic complaints. Colds settle throughout the body and limbs. He is full of dizziness as if intoxicated; staggers when walking.

The headaches are commonly such as occur in fevers, in rheumatism, and in inflammation of the bladder. The brain feels loose or there is an undulating feeling in the head. Pain in the head as if the brain were torn. Stupefying headache with buzzing in the ears. Stitching pains in the head; feeling as if the parts were screwed together; feeling as if the brain were pressed. The muscles of the head are sore. The periosteum of the cranium is sore to touch. The pain in the back of the head is ameliorated by holding the head backwards. Tingling in the scalp. Rush of blood to the head. Humming in the ears. Fornication in the scalp. Pulsating headaches. Meningitis with high fever. Great restlessness with these Rhus symptoms. Cerebro-spinal meningitis with the anxiety and restlessness. Aching in the bones; amelioration from motion. Eruptions upon the scalp; very sensitive to touch. The scalp is very sensitive on the side lain on. Tearing, drawing pains in the periosteum of the head; pressure in the bones of the skull as if screwed together. From every exposure to cold, damp weather, or from suppressing the sweat upon the head comes pain in the head; rheumatic headaches. Headaches are worse from wetting the hair. Vesicular eruptions upon the scalp; erysipelas of the scalp with large blisters; eruptions upon the scalp that suppurate. It is a very useful remedy in the treatment of eczema of the scalp in infants; herpetic eruptions upon the scalp.

Inflammation of the eyes in rheumatic subjects from exposure to cold, damp weather, from suppressing the perspiration, with restlessness and fever. Pustules upon the cornea; photophobia; suppuration of the eves. Inflammation of the iris of a rheumatic character. There is much swelling and the eyes are closed from swelling. Very acute conjunctivitis; chemosis; eyes red and aggravated in the morning; scrofulous inflammation of the eyes from becoming cold. The lids are red; œdematous. The pains in the eyes are worse from moving the eyeballs, especially the bruised pain. Paralysis of the muscles of the eyeball the result of rheumatism and exposure to the cold, or from getting the feet wet. Red eyes and lachrymation; erysipelas of the lids; paralysis of the upper lids. The lids are agglutinated in the morning with a copious, purulent, mucous discharge. The Rhus patient is subject to styes on the lower lids; neuralgia in the eyes.

Neuralgia in the ears; erysipelatous inflammation of the external cars with visicles; inflammation of the parotid gland. Hæmorrhage from the nose; violent coryza. The nose is stopped up from every cold; great soreness in the nostrils; discharge from the nose of thick, yellow mucus; green, offensive mucus. Much swelling of the nose from erysipelas. The tip of the nose is red and sensitive. The nose is puffed and œdematous. Eruptions upon the nose and in the corners of the nose; eczema of the nose and much swelling.

Erysipelas of the face with burning, large blisters, and rapidly extending inflammation which becomes very purple and pits upon pressure. The erysipelas of the face often extends from left to right across the face. There is much burning, itching, and tingling, delirium, and high fever, and the mental state referred to above. Eczema of the face; chronic suppurating eruptions of the face. Stiffness of the jaws; rheumatic condition of the jaws and of the joints. The corners of the mouth ulcerate; fever blisters; lips dry and parched and covered with reddish-brown crusts in typhoid fever; lips bleed. We have many symptoms of the mouth especially in connection with typhoid fever. The tongue is sore, raw, and bleeding; burning of all the tissues in the mouth; red tongue. The taste is putrid and metallic. The teeth are covered with blood; fever in the gums with blood; blisters upon the tongue and the whole mouth appears to be raw and sometimes bleeding. The mouth is dry and an accumulation of saliva and sometimes bloody saliva in the mouth, which runs from the mouth during sleep.

In Rhus the thirst is often violent, but there is difficulty in swallowing solids from constriction of the throat; painful swallowing; inflammation of the throat; cellulitis of the throat internal and external with painful inflammation of the throat. Enlargement of the neck; swelling of the glands of the neck. The neck is stiff; sometimes erysipelatous inflammation of the parotids; neck greatly swollen. Rhus has cured diphtheria with these symptoms. Rhus is especially suitable for inflammation of the œsophagus. When it is acute from swallowing corrosive substances, because of the extensive cellulitis that such substances cause it makes the case like Rhus.

This remedy is very freaky. For instance, hunger, without appetite; hungry sensation or sensation of emptiness in the stomach without desire for food. Dryness of the mouth and throat with great thirst; unquenchable thirst for cold drinks especially at night with great dryness of the mouth. Yet the cold drinks bring on chilliness, bring on the cough.

Pain in the stomach and nausea. His desires are also strange. Desires oysters, cold milk, and sweets. Aversion to meat. Rhus has nausea and vomiting; bilious vomiting and nausea from drinking cold water; nausea after eating, with sudden vomiting; inordinate appetite with inclination to vomit; worse at night and after eating.

Pulsation in the pit of the stomach; gnawing pain in the stomach; fulness and heaviness in the stomach as from a load; pressure in the pit of the stomach as from a great weight; pain in the stomach and nausea, especially after cold things; pain in the stomach after ice cream; nausea after eating ice cream.

In the liver there is swelling and tenderness on pressure, so that he cannot lie on the right lobe of the liver. The soreness is increased on beginning to move; shooting pains in the region of the liver.

In the abdomen we have many of the complaints of Rhus. Distended abdomen during typhoid fever; extreme soreness of the tissues of the abdomen to touch; cannot bear any pressure; sensitive to clothing. Colic; pains and violent colic compelling him to lie on the back and draw up the limbs. Inflammation of any of the tissues of the abdomen; peritonitis; enteritis; typhlitis.

During these violent inflammatory conditions of the bowels, typhoid symptoms are likely to be present with involuntary stools. Inflammation and swelling of the glands of the abdomen and groin. With typhoid conditions there is diarrhœa, copious, watery, bloody stools or mushy stools; involuntary stools; frothy stools. Diarrhœa during typhoid fever; the diarrhœa is worse during the night and better during the day time; involuntary stools with great exhaustion. It has cured cholera infantum of a low type and it is often useful in dysentery with bloody, mucous stools. Violent tenesmus; violent tearing, pinching pains in the abdomen; involuntary stools; dysenteric stools; dysenteric discharges that drive him out of bed in the morning sometimes as early as 4 o'clock. Hæmorrhage of black blood from the bowels. Shooting pains in the rectum. It has cured hæmorrhoids when there is great soreness and when they are internal or protruding; protruding after stool with pressing in the rectum.

Urging to urinate with tenesmus and pain in the region of the prostate gland causing urging to stool, ameliorated by moving about. There are more or less tearing pains in the region of the kidneys. Albuminous urine; bloody urine; urine hot; muddy; white sediment, becoming turbid on standing; bloody drops of urine dribble away. Violent tenesmus of the bladder with dribbling of blood; retention of urine; urine is voided slowly from paralytic weakness of the bladder. There is sometimes complete paralysis of the bladder with involuntary urination at night in bed. Frequent urging to urinate day and night; weakness of the bladder in girls and women with frequent desire to urinate, especially in the women dribbling of the urine in cold air and on becoming very cold.

In the male sexual organs we have inflammation erysipelatous in character. Eczema of the genitals. The scrotum becomes thick and hard with intolerable itching; œdematous swelling of the genitals; erysipelas of the genitals; humid eruptions upon the genitals. In the female we have the same symptoms, especially erysipelatous swelling of the genitals; and some eruptions. The woman has prolapsus of the uterus from straining or lifting; weakness of all the pelvic muscles; labor-like pains in the abdomen from straining. Copious menstrual flow; clotted blood with labor-like pains. The menstrual period comes too soon, is too profuse, and lasts too long. The flow is acrid, causing excoriation of the parts. Every over-exertion brings on menorrhagia. Membranous tissue in the menstrual flow; suppressing of the menstrual flow from becoming wet, from getting the feet wet, or becoming chilled. Similar complaints come on in pregnancy from overstraining and a tendency to abortion. The after-pains are very torturesome. The woman suffers from cellulitis such as occurs in milk-leg. Typhoid symptoms come on and inflammation of the mammary glands. The milk vanishes.

In the larynx many of the colds locate producing hoarseness, rawness, and roughness. Soreness in the chest; muscular exhaustion of the larynx from loud and much exercise of the voice. Hoarseness on first beginning to sing, which wears off on singing a few notes or wears off after talking a little while; burning and rawness in the larynx. Rhus is suitable in many cases of influenza, such as begin in the nose and extend into the larynx with hoarseness and with Rhus symptoms. Respiration is hurried; oppression of the chest; very difficult and hard breathing, especially in pneumonia and bronchitis and in colds that settle in the chest. Rhus gets out of breath on exertion. The cough of Rhus is very tormenting; teasing cough; paroxysms of almost any kind; tormenting, dry, teasing cough before and during chill. He knows *that the chill is coming because of the dry, teasing cough;* cough with taste of blood in the mouth; dry, hoarse, racking, rheumatic cough, cough from rheumatic fever.

Inflammation of the lungs; inflammation of the pleura with stitching pains, much fever, progressing toward the typhoid state with aching in the bones; restlessness; general amelioration from motion; intense fever, marked thirst, great prostration; typhoid symptoms. The pneumonia is of a low type; pneumonia such as would denominate typhoid. Rhus has expectoration of blood from the lungs and from the mucous membranes of the air passages; hæmorrhage from the chest from overexertion; hæmorrhage from blowing wind instruments; hæmorrhage from the chest from violent mental excitement.

The heart is weak, tremulous with palpitation; violent palpitation when sitting still; pulsations move the whole body; anxious palpitation in the morning on waking; palpitation from exercise. It seems as if exertion had strained the muscles of the heart; hypertrophy of the heart from violent exercise; hypertrophy that comes on in athletes, in runners; organic diseases of the heart with sticking pains. *Numbness and lameness of the left arm with heart disease.*

In the back, we have stiffness and lameness. This is most noticeable on beginning to move, but wears off on moving about. Pains in the shoulder with stiffness; pains between the shoulders on swallowing food; rheumatic symptoms; painful tension between the shoulder blades. The small of the back aches while sitting. Painful stiffness on rising from a seat; pain in the hack as if bruised, sore and lame all over the back. The pain in the back is ameliorated by lying on something hard or from exercise. There are violent pains in the back, especially in the lumbar region, as if the back were broken. It is a remedy for lumbago brought on from getting wet, from overlifting, from taking cold, and from suppressing the sweat. He is ameliorated from motion and from moving about; worse on beginning to move. This remedy has many spinal symptoms with paralytic weakness either of the lower limbs or of one part of the body. Stiffness and lameness in the sacrum aggravated on resting after exercise. It might now be predicted that symptoms are to be found in the limbs from what has been said in general. There are stitching pains, pressing pains, all sorts of rheumatic lameness, and these pains are ameliorated from motion and are worse from keeping still. They are brought on from cold air and from suppressing the sweat, and as these pains grow worse they become tearing down the limbs, drawing pains. Paralytic pains, benumbing pains, and these are relieved from motion; numbness throughout the limbs; numbness and aching in the arms from heart disease; numbness in the joints; jerking, tearing pains in the joints. Paralysis of the arms; erysipelas with much swelling in the limbs; swelling of the hands and arms. When grasping anything a tingling and pricking is felt in the hands and fingers; crawling and numbness in the finger tips and fingers; swelling of the fingers; eruptions upon the hands and fingers. In the lower limbs, we find similar pains and similar modalities; pain in the hip when lying upon it; tearing, drawing pains in the lower limbs; sciatica with tearing, drawing pains in the lower limbs, worse during rest and ameliorated from motion, brought on from becoming chilled, from cold damp weather, from exposure, and from suppressing the sweat. In sprains such as occur in the ankles and in fact any of the joints, after *Arnica* has removed the first and most painful symptoms, Rhus becomes useful for weakness of tendons and muscular fibers such as always follows sprains. It is a routine remedy for this weakness in joints following sprains. The pains rush in streaks down the limbs; restlessness in the lower limbs at night, but amelioration from motion; must keep the limbs in constant motion; paralysis of the lower limbs; great weariness and heaviness of the lower extremities; weakness of the lower limbs on going up stairs; swelling of the joints of the lower limbs; stiffness of the knees and feet. Paroxysmal pains in the legs from getting wet, especially when sweating; complaints from living in damp houses; rheumatism in the lower limbs from living in damp houses. Ulcers on the legs. Intolerable itching of the legs at night in bed; eruptions upon the feet and legs; fœtid sweat of the feet in persons of rheumatic tendency. Eczema of the lower limbs. Rhus is a useful remedy in fevers. In typhoid sufficient has been said. It is a very useful remedy in scarlet fever with coarse rash. When the rash has been suppressed, with inflammation of the glands and much sore throat. During fever there is often violent urticaria which passes off during the sweat; night sweat with much itching eruption; fevers from suppressed foot sweat; rheumatic fevers; fevers worse at night; fevers that come with cold sores on the lips, remittent fevers and intermittent fevers take on the typhoid type and run through their course as symptomatic typhoid fever. Intolerable itching of the skin; tingling in the skin; eruptions burn and itch violently; much moisture with eruptions upon the skin. Large blisters form upon the skin either with or without erysipelas. The incessant itching is sometimes relieved by "scalding" the parts, as it is called by some who are poisoned with Rhus. by "scalding" with water as hot as it is possible to bathe the parts in Rhus. has cured shingles and the tendency to herpetic eruptions. It has made a grand record with humid eczema such as have raw surfaces; excoriated; oozing much. It is very commonly the remedy for hives that come on from getting wet or hives that come on during rheumatism or during chills and fever; hives that are worse in the cold air.

RUMEX CRISPUS

Rumex, the yellow dock, is a neglected remedy, and one that has been only partially proved. The mental symptoms have not been brought out but the catarrhal symptoms have been well expressed by provers.

There is a state of sadness; low spirited; aversion to work; irritable; mental excitability. This includes about all the mental state we know of this remedy as the provings were made with the lower potencies and tincture. The yellow dock has been used in domestic practice, as a blood medicine, to cure eruptions and boils. When used in this way it is a mild substance and hence the provings are somewhat in this form.

The catarrhal tendency is very striking. The nose, eyes, chest and trachea, the whole respiratory tract, gives forth a copious flow, copious mucous discharge. I have seen it so copious from the nose that it seemed as one continuous flow; so copious from the trachea and bronchial tubes that the patient continually hawked up, by the mouthful, thin frothy, white mucus, so that in a little while as much as half a pint of thin mucus, as thin as water, would be in the cuspidor. It also has marked dryness of the larynx and trachea with hard, dry, spasmodic cough.

At times it has taken the form of grippe, with a copious mucous discharge; thin, watery, frothy expectoration by the mouthful. This is only the first stage. Following this the discharge becomes thick, yellow, tough or thick, white and tenacious; so ropy and stringy and rough that in spite of blowing the nose and coughing he fails to get it up. Completely exhausted from his efforts to expectorate the tough, stringy, tenacious even gluey mucus. This catarrhal state is commonly accompanied by a morning diarrhœa, and these constitute the leading features.

"Catarrhal headache with great irritation of the larynx and trachea, clavicular pain and soreness behind sternum." Catarrhal headaches are headaches that come on during spells of dryness, alternating with a copious flux. Extreme rawness in the larynx and trachea; burning and smarting; unable to endure pressure on the throat pit. *Tickling in the throat pit causing cough.* Must sit without motion; cannot breathe deeply, hurriedly or irregularly because the burning is so much increased by any change in breathing. If he steps into the open air a paroxysmal cough takes his breath away; or if he passes from the open air into a warm room the same paroxysmal cough comes on. The paroxysm is so violent that in the morning, when he has a loose stool, he will pass it involuntarily with the cough. The urine also passes away with the cough. The headache returns when the discharges slack up.

A striking feature is pain under the clavicle; a sense of rawness under the clavicle; as if the parts inside were raw; as if the air came directly under the clavicle, producing rawness and burning. Rawness and burning from the inhalation of air.

"Nose obstructed; dry sensation even in posterior nares." Many times the coryza starts out by a marked dryness in the posterior nares, so that is constantly hawking; the irritation is so great that he cannot let it alone. There is a sensation of thickening in the nasopharynx, and he produces a peculiar noise in trying to get rid of it. "Sudden sharp tingling sensation in Schneiderian membrane." This is intense; tingling, sometimes described as an itching extending from the end of the nose to the pharynx; sometimes forces sneezing, blowing the nose and this peculiar noise, and sometimes a hawking to get the mucus when it is a little lower in the pharynx; hemming to get rid of it when in the larynx. The inflammation passes to the smallest bronchi, producing a capillary bronchitis and finally a pneumonia.

It suits acute and chronic catarrhal states. In old phthisical cases; every time he takes a cold, he is so sensitive to cold air and change of air that he sleeps with the bed clothes over this mouth. Every breath of air causes a spasmodic cough. The early expectoration is thin mucus, and then it becomes thicker and tenacious, and he cannot expectorate it; he hears the rattle; after many efforts which exhaust him he expectorates a little with hardly any relief. This is a great remedy to do patch work with in phthisis. Soreness, rawness and burning, especially down the trachea and under the sternum.

Violent sneezing, with fluent coryza, worse in the evening and at night. Many symptoms are worse in the evening. "Coryza. fluent, with sneezing with headache, worse evening and night." Some symptoms are worse in the early morning. Certain kinds of cough are worse at 11 P.M. *Lachesis* and Rumex furnish a puzzle in this cough and each has to be understood. In *Lachesis* young children cough in their early sleep, but if kept awake they will not cough. Therefore in *Lachesis* the 11 P.M. cough is an aggravation from sleep. In Rumex the cough will come on at 11 o'clock whether the child is asleep or not. "Accumulation of mucus in posterior nares." "Yellow mucous discharge through posterior nares." "Epistaxis, violent sneezing and painful irritation of, nostrils." "Influenza with violent catarrh, followed by bronchitis." "Scraping in the throat;" whenever this catarrhal state goes into the larynx and trachea, there is this continual scraping in the throat. Hoarse; cannot speak because the vocal cords are covered with tough mucus. Chronic cases have often been cured. *Phosphorus* has this hoarseness, but especially aphonia relieved by hemming up a little mucus from the vocal cords. The *Causticum* hoarseness is due to a weakness of the vocal cords. *Phosphorus* has an inflammatory state and the continual accumulation of mucus impedes speech. Rumex has the accumulation of tough, gelatinous, gluey mucus, and he continually scrapes the larynx.

"Sensation of a lump in the throat, not relieved by hawking or swallowing, it descends on deglutition, but immediately returns; this is also a strong feature in *Lachesis*. "Aching in the pharynx, with collection of tough mucus in the fauces." "Catarrhal affections of throat and fauces." This remedy shows the various stages of severe colds, but is especially indicated in constitutions that are constantly taking cold; worse from change of the weather; always shivering about the fire; want much clothing, want even the head covered up.

Many complaints are worse in the evening, from a bath, from becoming cold, from inhaling cold air. Rheumatic complaints are common and are aggravated by cold. Every cold seems to affect the joints. This is a marked feature of *Calcarea phos.;* every change to cold is felt in the joints; from bathing and getting chilled afterwards.

"Tight, suffocative, heavy ache in epigastrium, through to back; clothes seem too tight; weak feeling in epigastrium, all aggravated when talking; frequently takes a long breath." "Shooting from pit of stomach to chest; sharp pain in left chest; slight nausea; dull aching in forehead." "Aching and shooting in pit of stomach and above it on each side of sternum." The stomach will not digest food, or only the simplest food; the mucous membrane of the stomach is affected by this remedy like other mucous membranes. Various pains in the stomach; aching, shooting pains in the pit of the stomach. "Aching pain in the pit of stomach gradually becoming very severe; sharp stitching pains in stomach extending into chest, and below a sensation of pressure like a lump in pit of stomach, sometimes rising up under sternum, greatly aggravated from motion and somewhat from taking a long breath; generally aggravated after eating, ameliorated by lying perfectly quiet." It is strange how the stomach symptoms are aggravated by talking. The stomach feels sore, aggravated by talking, walking, inhaling cold air; wants warm things. Very flatulent; full of flatulent pains; pains relieved (*Carbo veg.*) by belching and passing flatus. Stomach and abdominal pains aggravated by talking, irregular breathing; must sit in a chair and breathe with perfect regularity. Irregular breathing will cause cough or Suffocation.

In the morning hurried to stool like *Sulphur.* "Stools, painless, offensive, profuse; brown or black, thin or watery; preceded by pain in abdomen; before stool sudden urging, driving him out of bed in morning." "Morning diarrhœa with cough from tickling in throat pit." It is common for phthisical cases to have a morning diarrhœa, and many of them look like *Sulphur.* When the morning diarrhœa is gushing, Rumex will palliate; it will allay the extreme sensibility of the lungs, will ward off the sensitiveness of cold and will patch him up. Rumex is not so deep as *Sulphur,* but it is an antipsoric. It is limited, however, to the early stages; will carry a chronic case so far, but it will require to be followed by another antipsoric. *Calcarea* follows it well.

Rumex is as sensitive to cold, to baths and chilly surroundings as *Rhus*. but it is aggravated by motion. *Bryonia* may be confused with it in this aggravation from motion and from talking, but *Bryonia* is not so sensitive to cold air, is often relieved from cold air and worse in a warm room; the complaints subside if the room becomes cool. In Rumex the nerves are sensitive to the open air; a nervous sensitiveness to open air as marked as *Nux*.

"Brown, watery diarrhœa, chiefly in morning, having stools from 5 to 9 A.M." "Serious attack of diarrhœa in an old man of seventy, after failure of *Sulphur.*" The *Sulphur* patient with a cough, especially in phthisis, commonly wants cool air, cooling things; though the stomach symptoms, are sometimes ameliorated from hot drinks, yet he wants cool, refreshing air.

"Aphonia after exposure to cold." "Tenacious mucus in throat or larynx, constant desire to hawk." *"Tickling in throat pit causing cough."* He fights off the cough as long as he can because of the burning and rawness. In the most violent coryza there is a lack of the febrile symptoms of *Bryonia, Rhus* and *Aconite.* It has not the constitutional symptoms, the aching of the limbs, the general soreness, the high fever and thirst. The condition seems to have localized itself.

"Hoarse, barking cough, in attacks every night at 11 P.M. and at 2 and 5 A.M. (children)." "Cough, with pain behind midsternum." "The most violent cough occurs a few moments after lying down, and at night, in some cases, complete aphonia."

"In women, every tit of coughing produces the passage of a few drops of urine."

Rumex is one of the most valuable palliatives in advanced phthisis; it will often carry a cast through another winter. With Rumex, *Pulsatilla, Senega, Arsenic* and *Nux vamica* you can patch up the last years of a phthisical patient. I would caution you also about the diarrhœa that occurs in most cases of phthisis. You will see *Acetic acid* recommended for the diarrhœa in phthisis. You had better let such conditions alone, unless they are very marked. If the diarrhœa is very exhausting use some simple medicine, like this one, to slack it up. But the phthisical patient is better off with a little diarrhœa, a loose morning stool. It is the same with night sweats; if he does not have them he will have something more violent. The allopath stops the diarrhœa and night sweats, and then has to feed *Morphine* to his patient because of the consequent sufferings. The more you undertake to relieve these outward conditions, these vents, the more harm you will do the patient, and if you go on you will have to abandon your Homœopathy and give *Morphine,* which is really a crime.

You will remove the sore, bruised, aching all over the body of a consumptive by *Arnica,* and it will suit the cough and gagging and retching, and make him sleep. Later *Pyrogen* may be needed for the aching in the bones and distressing cough. You patch him up year after year; sometimes *Arsenic* is the remedy, and it has to be more frequently repeated; sometimes it is *Lycopodium, Pulsatilla, Pyrogen* or *Arnica.* These medicines help him along and they have often to be changed, but finally the break down occurs, and these medicines are no longer suitable. An awful dyspnœa gradually creeps on the patient; there is craving for air; the breathing space is becoming diminished. Dropsy comes on in the extremities. The heart gives out; there is emaciation; the hippocratic countenance is seen; there is cold sweat, blue face sinking. Even now we can palliate with *Tarantula Cubensis.* Sometimes it has to be repeated. It will relieve for days and give an euthanasia, not a stupefaction as produced by *Morphia,* benumbing his senses, but an actual comforting.

RUTA GRAVEOLENS

Ruta is another remedy often overlooked. It is sometimes overlooked and *Rhus* or *Argentum nitricum* given, or other remedies not fully related to the case are given because Ruta is not well known. Many of its symptoms are difficult to classify in the Repertory. A knowledge of its *nature* must be obtained. It falls under a class of complaints that resemble *Rhus,* in that it is sensitive to cold, aggravated from cold, damp weather; aggravated from becoming cold, and the complaints are often brought on from straining the part; overstraining or overexertion of parts, but principally confined to parts that are of a tendinous character; aponeurotic fibers; white fibrous tissue; the flexor tendons especially; flexor tendons that are overstrained by exertion. *Rhus* has something like this, but nothing like what is found in Ruta. Ruta often suits in various surgical conditions; periosteal troubles from injury. Periosteal trouble where the flesh is thin over the bone; over the tibia. Bruises go away slowly and leave a hardened spot; thickening of periosteum; a knotty, nodular condition, it remains sore; slow repair. A lump in the periosteum that has existed for months or years; sensitive and sore and nodular; as a result of a blow with a stick or a hammer, or from humping the shin bone. In farmers, woodmen, mechanics, from holding a hammer or iron instrument, hard nodules form in the palm from clasping the hand over an iron instrument in projecting it forward, as from using a crowbar; a hardened mass of tissue in the tendons, like a bursa. Tendency to the formation of deposits in the periosteum, in bone, in tendons, about joints. The especial location is in the wrist; bursa and nodules form in this part. Overstraining of tendons and in the place where it is likely to give out a nodule will form in the tendon; lumps, bunches,, little tumors in the tendon. Gradually increasing contraction of flexors, so that the hands become permanently flexed; the foot becomes flexed so that the sole becomes increasingly concave, and the toes are drawn under from overstraining and violence to the flexors.

Overstraining of the muscles of the eye. These muscles are largely tendinous. Continual use until it becomes an overuse. Eyestrain followed by headache, and the effects are also on the globe of the eye, and coating of the eye, so that the overstrained eye is red. Pain in the eye, above and through the eye when he attempts to use the vision, that is, aggravation from the exertion of vision. From looking at fine print, fine sewing. This overexertion of vision brings about redness, pain and inability to concentrate vision on one point. Headache follows. Here *Argentum nitricum* resembles Ruta. *Arg. nit.* and *Natrum mur.* are the two remedies most frequently used, but *Onosmodium* is a very frequently indicated remedy for headaches from eyestrain. But they can be easily differentiated. Ruta is aggravated from cold, wants everything warm. *Arg. nit.* is aggravated from heat, wants to be in a cool place. The patient must he considered.

There is general exhaustion in Ruta. The legs give out on rising from a chair, the patient totters and makes several efforts on rising from a seat. Routinists give *Phosphorus* and *Conium* for this. Ruta and *Phosphorus* both have violent, unquenchable thirst for ice-cold water. *Compare Phos.* and *Con.* because of the weakness through the hips and thighs.

The remedy has not been proved sufficiently to bring out the mental symptoms. They are only common and belong to many other remedies. "Inclination to contradict and quarrel." "Dissatisfied with himself and others." "Anxious and low-spirited, with mental dejection." These symptoms are only common; they can be grouped in one of two classes. The patient can be irritable, or the opposite—good-natured. This remedy is classified among the irritable. "Despondent," that is, the opposite of happy—another of two classes. "Melancholy disposition toward evening." The only thing here is that it is aggravated toward evening. When things are brought out, so that they belong to one of two classes, they are important only in a mild degree.

Many of the complaints are worse lying down, especially the pains that are sharp, stinging, tearing in the nerves. Ruta is a painful medicine, but is slow in producing symptoms, hence its pains are of a chronic nature. Old neuralgias, stinging, tearing, burning pains especially in the lower extremities, about the eyes; faceaches. It has all the pains, described by all the adjectives that apply to pain, but it is worse lying down and worse from cold. Rending, tearing pains in the sciatic nerves. The severest forms of sciatica; pains commence in the back and go down the hips and thighs; tearing pains; comfortable during the day, but aggravated as soon as he lies down at night. *Gnaphalium* is a great sciatic remedy, and it also has this aggravation from lying down.

"Eyes feel hot like balls of fire." To use Ruta for a pure inflammation when the eyes feel hot would be a failure. *Euphrasia, Belladonna* and *Aconite* are used in simple inflammations from a cold, and the antipsorics when the case is chronic. But if a woman strains her eyes from long *sewing on fine work,* and the balls feel like fire, she needs Ruta. *Aconite* if, after exposure to cold winds, there is inflammation with lachrymation, and the eyes look like raw beef.

"Eyes burn, ache, feel strained; sight blurred; aggravated from using them in the evening." A part of the general aggravation in the evening. When, in copying, the manuscript is placed here, and the copy at a different distance, this necessitates a constant change of vision in looking from one to the other, and especially if the copying is done in a poor light, a headache will come on, which Ruta will cure. After overusing the eyes in this way, if the patient rides in a cold wind, a paralytic weakness results, and this is a further indication for Ruta. Lachrymation from exposure to the wind or riding in the cold. Paralysis of certain muscles of the eye, even strabismus; all sorts of disturbances of accommodation. "Loss of power over internal rectus." "Asthenopia; irritability of every tissue of eye from overwork or from *using eyes on fine work;* heat and aching in and over eyes; eyes feel like balls of fire at night; blurring of vision; letters seem to run together, lachrymation, etc."* Amblyopia, dependent upon overexertion of eyes, or anomalies of refraction; from writing by artificial light; *fine needlework,* etc.; in a weaver, could with difficulty distinguish one thread from another, and could not read at all; mistiness of sight, with complete obscuration at a distance.

Constipation is a striking feature, with prolapsus of the rectum at stool. "Frequent unsuccessful urging with prolapsus ani." "Protrusion of rectum after confinement." Pain in rectum when sitting. Great soreness in rectum as from ulceration. It is a useful remedy in piles and stricture of the rectum.

Back symptoms. It is a decided rheumatic remedy. All those remedies which are susceptible to cold, aggravated by cold, wet, stormy weather, are described as rheumatic remedies. Rheumatic symptoms of the back. "Pains as if bruised in lumbar vertebræ." "Pain in back or coccyx as from a fall or blow, or as if bruised." "Hamstrings feel shortened and weak; knees give way going up or down stairs." "Pain and lameness in the ankles after a sprain or dislocation." "Lameness after sprains, especially of the wrists and ankles." Immediately after a sprain, for the inflammatory state, you will most likely need to give *Arnica,* and *Rhus* will probably follow. But when nodules occur in the, tendons as a result of the strain Ruta is called for. Ruta is a great remedy for a mere sprain; it has all the soreness and weakness of tendons, *Arnica, Rhus* and *Calcarea* are often necessary in a routine way when there is absence of all symptoms, except the strain alone.

Paralytic weakness in the lower extremities after a sprain of the back.

Under the aggravation in the evening is melancholy disposition, burning in the eyes, green halo around the light; sight blurred; eyes ache; pain below right scapula.

Extreme restlessness like *Rhus*. So restless he can't keep still; a nervous restlessness.

"Bruised feeling all over as from a fall or blow, worse in the limbs and joints." "Bruises and other mechanical injuries of bones and periosteum; sprains; periostitis; erysipelas."

Ruta is related to and is an antidote to *Mercury.*

Eruptions on the skin with itching, which changes place after scratching like *Mezereum*. Compare *Phos*. in the thirst for cold water and the weakness of the lower extremities. In the rheumatism distinguish *Phytolacca*. Compare *Rhus, Sepia, Silicea* and *Sulphur*. Ruta is an antipsoric, but not so deep as *Silicea* and Sulphur.

SABADILLA

The Sabadilla patient is a shivering patient, sensitive to the cold air, a cold room, cold food. He wants to be well wrapped up; wants hot drinks to warm up his stomach. He is subject to catarrhal conditions, and in these he wants hot air. The catarrhal conditions of the throat require hot drinks and food. Warm things are grateful to him. It is difficult to swallow cold things; they increase the pain and difficulty in swallowing.

We often study remedies by contrast. This remedy travels from *left* to *right,* and at once a good prescriber connects it with *Lachesis*. The soreness, pain and inflammatory conditions of the throat commence on the left side and spread to the right in both Sabadilla and *Lachesis*. But warm things aggravate the pain in *Lachesis;* they cause a spasmodic condition, with a sensation of choking, and therefore he wants cold things, which relieve they are swallowed more easily and ameliorate the pain in the throat. Sabadilla on the other hand is relieved by heat, either outside or inside.

Catarrhal condition of the nose, with constant sneezing; sensation of great rawness in the nose: burning; stuffing up of the nose. Discharge at first of thin mucus and later thick mucus. It has all the appearance of a coryza. The coryza is ameliorated from inhaling hot air. He sits before an open grate or register, with the head close to it, inhaling the hot air. Especially useful when the catarrhal state of the nose is prolonged; a prolonged coryza, which does not yield to ordinary remedies; a lingering coryza, and the discharge i exaggerated by the odor of flowers. Even thinking of the odor of flower makes him sneeze and increases the flow from the nose. So, thinking of various things aggravates his complaints.

Many hay fever patients are sensitive to the odor of flowers, to the odor of the hay field, to dying vegetable matter; so oversensitive to the odor of fruit are some that apples have to be removed from the house. inhalation of odors that are beautiful, as that of the lavender, some hay fever patients cannot tolerate; such things may bring on an attack out of the season. Now Sabadilla is of this sort. Oversensitive to surroundings, to odors; these increase the catarrhal state of the throat and posterior nares. Sneezing and a flow of mucus from the nose; goes on even to ulceration. Periodical attacks; a rose cold in June; in autumn about August 20 as a hay fever. Hay fever is often an easy thing to palliate with short acting remedies; they will cut short an attack in a few days. But the cure requires years, and the patient must be treated in the interim and according to his symptoms. When the hay fever symptoms are present he has no others; one group is manifested at one time, and another group at another time. But the patient is sick and all the symptoms must be gathered together and the case treated accordingly.

Many of the annoyances of this individual seem to be imaginary. His mind is filled with strange things. Imaginations concerning persons or himself are strange. Imagines the body is withering, that the limbs are crooked, that the chin is elongated, and larger on one side than the other. She feels that this is so and believes it even in spite of her vision. It is a sensation which she believes, a delusion, an insanity. "Erroneous impressions as to the state of his body." "Imagines himself sick; imagines parts shrunken; that she is pregnant when she is merely swollen from flatus; that she has some horrible throat disease that will end fatally." The imaginations are groundless; nothing is visible, and the suffering is greater than if there was something to be seen. These patients often get no sympathy; they should really have a remedy. *Thuja* has erroneous impressions as to the state of the body; thinks she is made of glass; the idea is not that of transparency, but rather of brittleness, fears that she would break in pieces. There are but a few remedies which have fixed ideas; these ideas may be concerning politics, religion, clothing, things of the family and life. I once had an insane patient who would get out of the street car if anyone entered who wore a certain color, because she had a fixed idea that this was of evil import to her. The *Pulsatilla* mental state in a man is that a woman would be a detriment to his soul; it is a delusion, a fixed idea. *Iodine* is full of fixed ideas. *Anacardium* has a fixed idea that a devil is sitting on one shoulder talking into his ear, while an angel sits on the other shoulder talking into the other ear, and he halts between the two and says nothing.

"Delirium during intermittents." "Mental exertion aggravates the head ache and produces sleep." A sleepiness comes on from thinking, meditating, reading. While meditating in a chair he falls asleep like *Nux moschata* and *Phosphoric acid.*

Dizziness; vertigo. He wakens up at night with vertigo. Vertigo in the open air; under all sorts of circumstances. Full of headaches. Headaches on one side of the head. The meditation which drives him to sleep brings on headache. Headache in school girls. Feeble children, who have to be taken from school because of headache, come home with strange imaginations concerning school and themselves. Headache stupefying and associated with coryza; in the frontal sinuses, above the eyes. Fulness, bursting, stupefying aggravated by jarring, sneezing, walking. Stupefying headache with coryza. Often gets up with it in the morning, increases during the forenoon. Head covered with a cold sweat. Many of the symptoms are closely related to *Veratrum,* especially in the cold sweat on the forehead with complaints.

Hay fever when there is spasmodic sneezing, fluent coryza; nostrils stuffed up; inspirations through nose labored; snoring; itching in the nose; profuse bleeding from the nose; bright red blood comes from the posterior nares and is expectorated; very sensitive to the smell of garlic; coryza with severe frontal pains and redness of eyelids; violent sneezing; copious watery discharge from the nose.

A peculiar kind of itching coming on in some hay fevers is an itching in the roof of the mouth, on the soft palate, and for relief the patient must draw the tongue back and forth over the soft palate, with this coryza, sneezing, etc. *Wyethia* will cut the attack short.

When the itching extends to the larynx and trachea, with great irritability and sensitive to cold: *Nux vomica.*

When the discharge burns a red streak over the upper lip and about the wings of the nose, with sneezing and profuse, watery nasal discharge: *Arsenicum.*

Copious acrid lachrymation, and copious bland flow from the nose with sneezing: *Euphrasia.*

Copious, bland, watery discharge from the eyes and copious, acrid, watery discharge from the nose: *Allium cepa.*

But these are not the constitutional remedies; they do not cure, but only palliate during the severe attacks. These symptoms are the outcome of the psoric constitution, and this constitution must be treated by antipsorics. Sometimes the hay fever is so severe that it seems to be the only manifestation of psora in the patient, but if it is restrained or stopped up by bad treatment he is not well during the whole year. If let alone he has good health during the rest of the year. Many a time the hay fever goes through the whole winter and only by constitutional upbuilding can it be mitigated. But with constitutional treatment each yearly attack is lighter, and at the end of treatment he is able to live in his own climate unaffected. He must not go to the mountains to mitigate it. If to any place, he should go where the affection would be worse, so that all its manifestations would be apparent. The hay fever will only be cured if the *patient* is curable, but if not, if his constitution is so broken down that *he* is incurable, his hay fever will not be cured.

The most striking place of attack is the mucous membrane of the nose, throat, trachea and larynx. Violent acute inflammation of the mucous membrane of these parts.

Great thirst for hot drinks. The appetite is singular; it is commonly seen in pregnant women. She says she is never hungry; never wants anything to eat, and often there is an aversion to food; but when, from a matter of reason, she concludes to eat, and she takes a mouthful, it tastes good, it recalls the appetite, and she makes a good meal. At other times not only a loss of appetite, but a disgust and loathing of food. "Disgust for all food, for meat, for sour things, for coffee, for garlic." "Morbid hunger or loathing for food."

A routine remedy in pin worms, seat worms, all sorts of worms; stomach and tape worms. A careful prescriber never thinks of prescribing for worms. He takes all the symptoms of the patient, and these guide him to the remedy. I remember one time in a lady's house seeing a dog drag his hinder parts over the carpet as if to scratch the anus. She said: "Doctor, can't you give the dog a remedy?" I put a dose of Sabadilla in its mouth. Some time afterwards she asked me: "Doctor, what did you give the dog that medicine for?" I inquired why she asked. "Why," she said, "in a few days it passed an awful lot of worms." Sabadilla and *Sinapis nigra* are well adapted to cases in which pin worms are present. Often a remedy restores the patient to order in general and then all his particular parts are set in order.

Female sexual organs. "Nymphomania from ascarides." "Cutting pains, as from knives, in ovary." "Menses too late, with painful bearing down a few days previous; decreased, flow by fits and starts, sometimes stronger, sometimes weaker; blood bright red."

Hysterical patients; a patient with a strangely unbalanced mind, accompanied by various nervous manifestations. "Twitchings, convulsive tremblings, or catalepsy from worms." It is true that worms will not prosper in a perfectly healthy stomach, intestine or rectum. They can only thrive in the unhealthy. Many a time I have had a patient bring me a tape-worm in a bottle after I had put them on an antipsoric, even when I did not suspect its existence. Turn the economy into order and the parasites go. The same applies to germs. They only exist as a result of disease. They have never been known to exist without the disease having first existed. If you ignore the worm, but select the remedy on the totality of the symptoms, the patient will be restored to health, and, so far as the worm is concerned, go without a symptom. The

worm becomes smaller. shrivels and finally departs. It is rarely the case for
the worm to disappear inside of six weeks after the remedy. If, on the other
hand, you eject the worm by violent means, the patient may go for years with
troublesome symptoms, and you do not know why you fail to cure him.

Prescribe for the patient first. No results of disease should be removed
until proper constitutional treatment has been resorted to, and be sure that it
is proper.

SABINA

The use of this remedy is generally confined to symptoms of the kidneys,
bladder, uterus, rectum and anus; inflammatory and hæmorrhagic symptoms
principally of these parts. Sabina establishes a turmoil in the circulatory
system, with violent pulsations all over the body. The patient is disturbed by
heat, is worse in a warm room or from too much clothing. Wants the windows
open and to be in the open air (*Puls.*). This turmoil in the circulatory system
is such as might be expected in a hæmorrhagic remedy. Tendency to bleed
from all the mucous membranes, especially of the kidney, bladder and uterus.
It has a decided effect in diminishing knots, enlargements, or varices in veins.
The principal action is on the lower bowel, about the anus. Hæmorrhoidal
tumors which bleed copiously. Constipation with bleeding hæmorrhoids. A
sense of fulness in these parts. A sense of fulness in all the veins of the
body, a sense of distension, fulness, puffiness, bloating, with pulsations all
over, associated with repeated hæmorrhages from the mucous membranes.
Great burning and throbbing in the region of the kidneys. Severe suffering,
attended with inflammatory symptoms; bloody urine; inflammation of the
bladder with continuous urging to urinate, with the general aggravation from
heat and the throbbing all over.

Inflammation of the urethra, with a gonorrhœal discharge, or a catarrhal
discharge in the male. The most important sphere is menstrual symptoms, and
its relation to uterine hæmorrhage. In the menstrual symptoms the woman
suffers from bearing down, labor-like pains. Most distressing in dysmenorrhœa.
The menses last too long and are too copious, and at times in some subjects
the flow does not stop before the next period begins. Too frequent and
prolonged copious menses. A striking feature in this drug, as in a few other
remedies, is that the flow is liquid, bright red, intermingled with clots. It suits
many cases in which the flow slackens up and remains away for a while and
then labor-pains come on, and an enormous, partially decomposed dot is passed
and this is followed by a bright red flow. This occurs over and over again. Such
a state comes on after abortion, after labor and in dysmenorrhœa. Accompanying

the labor-like pains is a violent pain in the sacrum which shoots through to the front; pains extending from the sacrum to the uterus of pubes. Another striking feature is itching, shooting, knife-like pains, causing the patient to scream out, *shooting up* the vagina to the uterus, or up as far as the umbilicus. These two features, shooting pains from the back to the front and from below upwards, with hæmorrhages, are striking corroborations.

Belladonna and Sabina are the two most important remedies in abortion at three months. *Bell.* has the same bearing down pains which expel a clot followed by a copious, bright red flow. But the *Bell.* state is not like that of Sabina. In *Bell.* it is a hyperæsthesia, oversensitiveness to touch and jar; the patient will not allow the nurse to jar the bed, and the bright red flow is hot, so much so that it is noticeable; in parts over which the flow passes are so sensitive that the blood feels intensely hot to her. This is in keeping with the oversensitiveness of *Bell.,* to touch, light, motion, jar. If the physician jars the bed a scowl will immediately come over the patient's face. Bell. has many pains, not only shooting up but in every direction, irregular pains and hearing down pains. They come and go like lightning, appear suddenly and disappear suddenly, shooting in every direction. If these symptoms are present you will never need *Ergot* for its physiological effects. It has often been argued that in these cases of hæmorrhage you "won't have time to get the symptoms". The expert physician will often see all these symptoms in the twinkling of an eye. The actions of the patient, a word dropped by the nurse, and what he has observed himself, will have shown him the remedy.

As a medicine to prevent abortion it is one of the first to consider, because the symptoms we know are such as come during abortion, and it is most useful after the membranes have ruptured, or the ovum passed, or when the placenta is about to be expelled. It establishes the normal activities of the uterus so that it will expel whatever is left behind of these membranes. The curetting is never necessary with the homœopathic remedy. It suggests that there is something defective about the woman's organs.

"Inflammation of the ovaries or uterus after abortion or premature labor." Violent pains through ovaries and uterus. Aching in the sacrum as if broken, as if the hones would separate. Most violent tearing, rending, burning pains, with throbbing in the sacrum, with burning and throbbing all over the body, especially throbbing in parts, whether it be the uterus; or bladder. "Copious hæmorrhages, accompanied by uterine colic." Contractive labor-like pains extending from back to pubes and great urging to urinate. The uterine colic described is labor-like, drawing up like colic, but also bearing down as if to expel the clot. Metrorrhagia, resulting from false plethora; clotted and fluid blood; pain extending from sacrum or lumbar region to pubes; with severe bearing down, extending from lower part of hack around abdomen and down thighs; blood bright red, thin, liquid; labor-like pains in lumbar and uterine region, discharge of large clots of blood, bright red, coming in gushes, particularly profuse on motion, etc. This describes the symptoms from abortion or menstruation. "Menses too profuse, too early, last too long, partly fluid, partly clotted and offensive; flow in paroxysms; with colic and labor-like pains; pains from sacrum to pubes."

At another time, during the climacteric period, a woman is run down by overwork and much child bearing; she has repeated uterine hæmorrhages of this character, bright red intermingled with clots; pain from sacrum to pubes; she becomes exhausted and anæmic, but after a while she again builds up, her face becomes plump and she becomes plethoric, only to be broken by another hæmorrhage. Uterine hæmorrhage in fibroids.

Chronic catarrh of vagina with granulations, copious leucorrhœa. Bloody leucorrhœa. Old, prolonged, psoric cases. This medicine especially suits gonorrhœa in women. It has all the wart-like excrescences found in *Thuja*, and found in sycosis. The *Thuja* wart is a little sensitive wart, appears to be covered with a thin film, and bleeds from the slightest touch. Sabina cures warty excrescences about the anus, cauliflower excrescences, gonorrhœal warts about the vulva and about the male genitals.

In the uterine hæmorrhages compare it with *Ipecacuanha,* which has a gush of bright red blood fully as copious as Sabina, but at the beginning of that gush, before it has kept on long enough to produce exhaustion, the fact becomes pale, there is nausea and a feeling of faintness, syncope, all out of proportion to the amount of blood lost. *Millefolium* produces a gushing flow, but it has a continuous dribbling day after day, a continuous flow of bright red blood. *Secale* looks like Sabina, and when it is indicated it should never be given in large quantities. It has the expulsive, bearing down, labor-like pains, with the expulsion of large clots and copious flow, but the flow is dark and offensive and after a short time it becomes thin and watery, leaving a brown stain difficult to wash out; at times tarry, copious and continuous, as if the uterus had no ability to contract. If you observe the cases in which during labor or abortion crude *Ergot* had been used, you will notice that the patient has feeble uterine contractions as a resultant condition, and this will be seen during the menses or in the next labor. The symptoms of *Ergot* last for years; it is another psora. Large doses may kill the fœtus and cause abortion, but she will continue to bleed; the uterus will not contract when she most needs contractions. It produces a paralytic condition, and this is the state we prescribe *Secale* for. We seldom prescribe it for its primary effect, but rather for the state of sub-involution, when the uterus retains the secundines. There is a continuous oozing of dark and offensive flow. The picture is more complete if we find that no matter how cool the room is she does not want heat, but wants to be uncovered, and she is a lean, shrivelled, scrawny, hungry patient with dusky skin; she never takes on fat; is not robust: It produces varicoses of the skin and the skin about the toes becomes dusky, and over the shin bones are dark spots, and she wants to lie with the extremities uncovered. Such patients lose flesh and become shrivelled.

In old, troublesome, lingering hæmorrhages, starting up fresh on the slightest provocation, Sabina will stop the gush, the acute stage, but it does not hold, the hæmorrhage recurs, and then an antipsoric is needed. *Sulphur* is very commnoly the remedy, but *Psorinum,* though not laid down in the books for hæmorrhages, after *Sulphur,* has exhausted itself, will often follow for this oozing and frequent recurrence.

Phosphorus is somewhat like Sabina. It has a copious bright red flow, which may or may not contain clots. The striking features are outside the flow. There is pinched countenance, extremely dry tongue and mouth; violent, unquenchable thirst, craving ice-cold water. The hæmorrhage is bright red, in a gush or continuous oozing.

In this way we must study well the hæmorrhagic remedies. The physician must he acquainted with the emergency remedies, such as belong to the violent diarrhœas, cholera, violent sufferings and hæmorrhages. He must have them at his finger ends, and he must be able to compare instantaneously. Blood must be stopped.

Atony of the uterus is a striking feature of Sabina. The uterus will not contract on itself until it has something to contract on, like a clot or mole. Hæmorrhages from other parts as well. But other remedies have taken its. place in these regions because the individualizing symptoms have nor been brought out.

Much rheumatism and gout; gouty nodosities in the joints; they burn so and are so hot that the patient is compelled to put the hands or feet out of bed. Gouty cases, especially when the constitutional state changes; an alternation; when the gout is present there will be no hæmorrhages, and when there are hæmorrhages the gout will be relieved. An alternation of states. The gouty condition of the veins is often a hæmorrhagic state.

SANGUINARIA

Blood root is an old domestic remedy. A great many eastern farmers' wives will not go into the winter without blood root in the house. In the cold winter days, when the coryzas come on, a "cold" in the head, throat and chest, then they get the blood root ready and make a tea of it. With them it is a routine remedy for "colds". They give it to combat all complaints, and there is no doubt but that even in this crude form it does break up "colds," because the provings show its relation to chest troubles and "colds" that go to the chest.

Periodic headaches, when the headache comes once in seven days; it begins in the morning on waking or wakes the patient up. It begins in the occiput and travels upward and settles over the right eye and in the right temple. It gets worse during the day and is aggravated by light, so that he is driven into a dark room and compelled to lie down. Vomiting comes on and the vomited matter is bile, slime, bitter substance and food, and then comes relief of the pain. The headaches are relieved from passing flatus up or down. If the patient suffers when he goes to bed with hot palms and soles, so that he must put them out of bed, this an additional striking feature.

Take an individual who has missed his chronic headache, by some means, for a considerable time, but since then he has become increasingly sensitive to cold, and "colds" settle in the nose, throat and broncial tube, and these parts feel as if on fire, with rawness and burning; the expectoration is thick, tenacious mucus; disturbance of the belly, with much belching, and the belching is especially noticed after a violent attack of coughing.

It is not a very long acting remedy. When a periodic sick headache is interrupted by Sanguinaria, if a deeper drug, an antipsoric, is not given, the headache will return or something worse will come on, as Sanguinaria does not go deep into the nature of the case. I remember a case in which the patient missed his Sanguinaria headache and an epithelioma developed, which was cured by *Phosphorus*. I am convinced that if *Phosphorus* had been given at the end of the attack the cancer would not have developed, as *Phosphorus* was his constitutional remedy. If a chronic sick headache is interrupted the patient will tend to phthisis. Chest troubles come on and grow worse and worse. Its ability to palliate phthisis is very well known.

A patient much debilitated with bronchial catarrh; susceptible to cold, to every change in the weather, from change to damp weather, to every draft, to change of clothing; always taking new "cold". There is burning in the chest behind the sternum; thick, tough, ropy expectoration; spasmodic cough, and every cough ends in belching; eructations of gas; empty eructations. If to the burning in the chest, the severe pains in the larynx and trachea when talking, and cough ending in belching, you add heat in the palms and soles, Sanguinaria will patch him up and mitigate the trouble. Many such cases get *Sulphur,* but to their destruction. There is a class of remedies that suits these phthisical patients better than *Sulphur, Silicea* and *Graphites*; remedies such as *Pulsatilla,* Sanguinaria, *Senecio gracilis* and *Coccus cacti,* which palliate, mitigate his sufferings, and may even build him up so that he could take a medium potency of a deep remedy. But the deeper remedies ought to be avoided if the vital force is low, if the body is too much damaged to be repaired. Hahnemann warned against the use of *Phosphorus* in such cases of deficient vitality. Sanguinaria is a surface remedy; it does excellent palliation.

Catarrhal conditions of nose and throat, especially those due to colds and to poisonous plants; also rose colds. The Sanguinaria patient has "rose colds" in June. Sensitive to flowers and odors; subjects with hay fever. Hay fever patients with burning in the nose, in the throat, as if dry; as if the mucous membrane would crack open. Dryness and burning in the larynx, with hoarseness; dryness and burning throughout the chest, with asthma; associated with burning of the palms and soles. Examination shows the palms to be dry, wrinkled and hot to the touch; so, also, the soles, where the skin is thickened and indurated. Corns that burn; the toes burn and the patient puts the feet out of bed for relief.

When the headache is present it seems to he a general congestive headache; although beginning in the morning, coming up the back and extending to the right eye, the whole head is hot and aches.

Sulphur, Silicea and Sanguinaria have periodic weekly headaches. *Arsenicum* has a headache every two weeks. Not that these remedies will not cure other headaches, for Sanguinaria has also a headache every three days. The majority of headaches coming every two weeks are cured by *Arsenicum* or greatly mitigated in broken down constitutions. The attempt to cure a chronic sick headache should be made before the senile decline.

"Pulsations in the head with bitter vomiting; aggravated by motion." The headache is generally aggravated by motion, but not so strikingly as in *Bryonia.* When the Sanguinaria headache increases towards the afternoon or night, it becomes so severe he must go to bed; and the head becomes sore, and then a step or jar is extremely painful. A severe headache is likely to be disturbed by light, noise, motion, etc.

"Headache as if forehead would burst with chill, and burning in stomach?" "Headache over right eye." This is a characteristic. feature. "Periodic sick headache; begins in the morning, increases during the day, lasts till evening; head feels as if it must burst, or as if eyes would be pushed out; throbbing, lancinating pains through brain, worse on the right side, especially in the forehead and vertex:, followed by chills, nausea, vomiting of food or bile; must lie down or remain quiet; ameliorated by sleep." Some of these things are not found in every case, but they all go to make up a Sanguinaria headache.

All sorts of neuralgic pains; cutting, tearing, lacerating pains; as if the muscles were torn, or put on a stretch. Tearing pains anywhere, neuralgic or rheumatic. Pains about the scalp, but more particularly about the shoulder and neck; stiff neck; cannot turn over in bed; cannot raise the arm, though he can swing it back and forth. Pain streaks up the neck; pain in the deltoid. It prefers the right side, but also cures the left side. Rheumatic pains in the right shoulder so that he cannot raise the arm and all the muscles of the neck and back of the neck become involved; stiff neck. If the pain comes on in the day it increases as the day advances to night. Complaints are worse at night in Sanguinaria.

A patient comes to you after exposure to cold; he cannot raise the arm; it hangs by his side; pain worse at night in bed, worse turning over (as he uses the shoulder muscle to turn over). It is probably in the deltoid, but you need not speculate on the tissues involved.

It competes with *Ferrum*. All red-faced, highly-flushed people, who cannot raise the arm and have pain which is worse in the daytime, not night, and ameliorated by slow motion need *Ferrum*. Sanguinaria is not relieved by motion; it is aggravated by such motion as calls the arm into use. *Ferrum* has relief from slow motion, aggravated from rapid motion and the pain comes in the daytime. While *Ferrum* has a uniformly red, plethoric face, Sanguinaria has a pale face. In the chest complaints Sangunaria has a circumscribed red spot over the malar bones, such as seen in hectic patients

Headache from stomach disturbances, overeating, rich food, drinking wine. Almost as useful as *Nux* in old drinkers. Those who disorder their stomachs and weaken their digestion by beer drinking; they cannot eat; vomiting of even a teaspoonful of water. No food or drink stays on the stomach. Headaches associated with such troubles. Vomiting and diarrhœa with complaints.

Catarrhal affections are prominent. Chronic catarrh of the throat; apparent thickening of the mucous membranes of the throat. Nose and pharynx fill with mucus. He hawks it out; there is a dry burning sensation, but the burning is most marked every time he takes a fresh cold.

Acridity of discharges is another feature. Acrid mucus forms in the nose, causing burning in the throat. Acrid, hot fluids eructated from the stomach, excoriating the throat and mouth. The diarrhœa is accompanied by an acrid watery stool; especially in infants; the nates become raw and red. This burning extends all through the bowels; burning in the abdomen and stomach in old gastric troubles; vomiting of even a teaspoonful of water with burning; old gastric irritation; dyspepsia; all sorts of disorders of the stomach.

Tongue red and burns as if in contact with something hot. Burning in pharynx and œsophagus, burning in roof of mouth. Tonsillitis with burning. "Heat in throat, ameliorated by inspiring cold air; throat so dry it seems as if it would crack." This burning excoriated feeling applies to all the mucous membranes affected.

Patient suddenly taken to bed with a chill; burning in the chest; symptoms of pneumonia; rusty expectoration; violent cough; every cough felt as a concussion at the bifurcation of the trachea; as if a knife were in the parts; as if torn as under; and after the cough copious, loud, empty eructations. No other remedy has this.

"Nausea with burning at the stomach, with much spitting." Nausea not relieved by vomiting. Keeps on vomiting and retching. Burns as if on fire. *Arsenic* is often given by mistake, because of the great burning.

"Vomiting of bitter water; of sour, acrid fluids; of ingesta; of worms; preceded by anxiety; with headache and burning in stomach; head relieved afterwards; with prostration." Such symptoms occur in headache, disordered stomach, sour stomach. The sour stomach is manifested by sour eructations or sour vomiting. A patient often speaks of "a sour stomach," and you must find out whether he means sour eructations or sour vomiting. He says he "spits up" sour food.

With the headache and many complaints Sanguinaria has a faintness; like a hunger, yet not for food. A sinking, faint, "all gone," empty feeling. It is like *Phosphorus with* its "hungry headache". *Psorinum* leads all others in "hungry headaches," but *Psorinum* wants to eat and cannot get enough. Sanguinaria has a hunger, but it is not for food; aversion at the thought and smell of food. *Psorinum* can eat a wolf meal, and so can *Phosphorus*. It is a false hunger with the headache in Sanguinaria. "Burning in stomach; with headache and chill."

Belching up of acrid fluids in asthma; hay asthma. Sanguinaria palliates asthma associated with stomach disorders. Do not forget *Nux* in asthma from stomach troubles.

Liver complaints; pains and aches and sense of fulness. Bilious trouble described in general terms. It seems as if the liver makes an enormous quantity of bile, but there is a gastro-duodenal catarrh, so that the bile is regurgitated into the stomach instead of going down, and it is eructated as bitter, green, yellow fluid; vitiated bile. This is a peculiar thing. If you watch a chronic Sanguinaria patient you will notice that the stomach will be disordered for a week; spitting up bile; much flatulence; sour hot eructations; then all at once this will disappear, and a diarrhœa, which fairly floods him, comes on suddenly; a bilious, liquid, gushing stool. *Natrum sulph.,* Sanguinaria, *Pulsatilla* and *Lycopodium* cure this alternation of diarrhœa and constipation.

"Os uteri ulcerated; fœtid, corrosive leucorrhœa." "Distension of abdomen in the evening and flatulent discharges by vagina from os uteri, which was constantly open; at same time a pain passing in rays from nape of neck to head."

"Chronic dryness in throat, sensation of swelling in the larynx and expectoration of thick mucus when associated with dryness, rawness, burning and smarting." "Whooping cough; constricted, spasmodic action across throat beneath jaws; cough worse at night with diarrhœa." Cough worse at night with diarrhœa is the feature this remedy is prescribed for. "Severe cough occurring after whooping cough, when patient takes cold, which partakes of the spasmodic nature of whooping cough." An adult takes cold and has a spasmodic cough, like whooping cough. He says it is a stomach cough, because there is a gagging with it. In all there is burning and diarrhœa:

"Distressing, dry, spasmodic, exhaustive coughs, especially in children, worse towards night, lying down, going into a cold room to sleep; feeling of rawness and burning in bronchi." The trachea seems so sore; and it is sore; a bolus of food passing down the œsophagus can he plainly felt; he can outline the part where the food passes.

SARSAPARILLA

Sarsaparilla is suitable in low forms of chronic disease, especially in complex states resulting from mixed miasms; especially in cases of sycosis and syphilis; cases made complex by *Mercury,* sycosis, syphilis, and psora. Weakness stamps itself on the whole economy, as in *Merc., Lach.* and other remedies. The tissues become flabby, refuse to heal when injured, ulcerate from slight causes. After an injury an open sore remains and is indolent or becomes phagedenic and spreads like *Ars., Lach* and *Merc. cor.* Weakness over the whole body; a paralytic feeling. In the mental sphere it manifests itself in a dazed state, he is unable to comprehend, the mind is slow, it is a weakness bordering on imbecility, which in the end it may reach. Weakness of the mind and the tissues.

All the organs are slowed down, weak, sluggish, become congested. Weakness and dilatation of the veins, tendency to form varices in the limbs, varicose ulcers, hæmorrhoids, varicose veins of the face and body. The face is often red and discolored in patches. When the circulation is feeble the parts turn blue, over the shin bones; on the backs of the feet, toes; blue spots like approaching senile gangrene. Useful in old age when black and blue spots appear on the backs of the hands and elsewhere.

Moist, itching, scurfy, and scabby eruptions. The skin of the backs and the palms of the hands becomes thick and indurated with a bran-like scurf resembling psoriasis, intermingling with blue spots.

This remedy has many features as to cold and heat. The use of heat internally aggravates all complaints, but there is an external coldness relieved by heat; taking warm food and drink aggravates; wants cold food, but heat applied externally is grateful.

Secale also produces great weakness of tissue, with venous stasis, ulceration and gangrene. But the two remedies, though similar in appearance, differ in regard to heat and cold.

The stomach is in a most miserable condition. Flatulence, continuous nausea, eructations and vomiting of sour food. Always complaining of fermentation and uneasiness of the stomach as if he had overeaten or as if the food had spoiled; digestion is slow and feeble.

Organs become tumid and congested. The throat, tongue, and mouth look as if about to ulcerate; purple spots look as if they would break down, but remain intact for weeks and months.

Œdema of tissues, of the lower extremities, pitting on pressure; dropsical conditions; Bright's disease.

Suitable in old syphilitics whose complaints have been suppressed by *Mercury;* mind and body in a state of prostration; paralytic weakness of the lower extremities, no endurance; the heart palpitates on exertion; suffocation on the least exertion; always tired; ulcers here and there on the body; the skin is flabby and full of distress at night. *Bone-pains worse at night.* Sars. antidotes the *Merc.* and establishes reaction.

Marasmus of children from hereditary syphilis; emaciation about the neck; dry, purple, copper-like eruptions; no assimilation.

The child is always passing sand in its diaper, yellowish, or whitish like chalk; the child screams when it is about to urinate, because it remembers how painful the passing of urine is. Sometimes at the close of urination it gives forth an unearthly yell. This symptom is found in old broken down constitutions, a clutch in the bladder just as it shuts down causes him to cry out; pain at the end of urination.

Old debauches, enfeebled by wine and women, with weak heart, lungs, brain, and bladder, emaciated and shrivelled. Prematurely old, a man of forty looks to be eighty, feet swollen, totters about on a staff. *Nux* will palliate in early periods of breakdown, but the time comes when he is weak in body and mind and must have such remedies as Sars., *Lach., Secale, etc.*

Children emaciated; face looks like old people; big belly; dry, flabby skin; mushy passages.

Eruptions appear in the Spring. All the venous remedies are braced up by Winter and go down in the Spring, as *Lach., Secale* and *Hamam.*

Catarrh of the bladder and kidneys. Involuntary urination of children at night in bed, in feeble children. There is a spasmodic condition of the sphincter when sitting to urinate, which makes the act impossible in that position, but *when he stands up the urine flows freely.* This is especially important when the symptom occurs in women, because they have great difficulty in urinating while standing. Copious urine at night; he floods the bed, but during the day he can pass it only when standing.

It is fifteen years since I reported the following case and the man has remained well ever since: "A man, at 52, addicted to whiskey for years, had a copious flow of blood from the bowels some four months ago; the exertion of walking a few blocks causes suffocation; after the loss of blood, feet began to swell, both limbs to middle of thigh very œdematous, has had two or three nondescript chills; a few months ago, sudden paralytic weakness of left arm and leg, passed off in three hours, leaving a numbness in left hand and a tearing pain in left side of face and head; no appetite; bloody discharge with stools; feels as if in a dream all the time; loss of memory; face covered with varicose veins and very red; general venous stasis; feeling on the top of the head as if struck with a hammer; must pass urine several times in a night; urine thick and cloudy after standing; but clear when first passed; has had much worry from financial troubles; cannot pass urine when sitting at stool, but flows freely when he is standing, albumen in the urine." When Sars. can take such a man, 52 years old, and restore him to health it is worth considering.

"Jerking sensation along the male urethra." "Each time she makes water, air passes out of the urethra with a gurgling noise." This symptom is common in catarrh of the bladder; it is caused by fermentation of the mucus and consequent formation of gas. "Frequent ineffectual urging to urinate with diminished secretion."

This medicine has many times dissolved a stone in the bladder; it so changes the character of the urine that it is no longer possible for the stone to build up, and it grows smaller by the continual dissolving off from the surface. I have seen the high colored, bloody, and mucous urine cleared up after the administration of Sars., but on standing, the sand would appear. When the urine again becomes cloudy, it is time for another dose. The urine holds in solution, that is, actually dissolves the substance of the stone.

Some years ago there was an old man upon whom a surgeon was expected to operate. They had sounded his bladder and said that he had a stone, but he came to the conclusion that he would not permit the operation. In spite of their warnings he sent for me and I took charge of his case. His symptoms called for Sars. The enormous amount of sand he passed in the next year was wonderful. It mitigated the catarrh and kept the bladder comfortable. At the end of a year, after a night of great suffering, he passed a stone—the size of a pea. He passed several small stones after that and then returned to health.

A young man passed so much crusty deposit that I ordered him to use one commode and let it settle, pouring off the urine. At the end of a month there was a layer a sixteenth of an inch thick. This patient under Sars. had no stone. The sand continued to pass, but was held in solution and deposited only on cooling. In the course of time it disappeared. He was of a gouty nature and this was relieved.

Sars. has gouty nodes with extreme soreness. After the remedy has been given, there is a deposit of sand in the urine, which shows the good action of the remedy and should not be stopped.

"Obstinate constipation with violent urging to urinate; urging to stool with contraction of the intestines; excessive pressure from above downward, as if the bowels were pressing out; during stool, violent tearing, cutting in the rectum. Stool small, with much bearing down."

"Old, dry, sycotic warts remaining after *Mercurial* treatment for gouty pains."

SECALE CORNUTUM

The best provers of Secale, those who are most susceptible to its action, are scrawny people, and they are the ones who will most likely need it as their curative remedy. Of course, it is not necessarily contra-indicated in fat people. Certain constitutions are mentioned in connection with a remedy as being suited to it, but it must not be inferred that no action will result in others when the symptoms agree. Scrawny people are especially related to Secale.

Emaciated, withered, wrinkled, unhealthy appearance of the skin; purplish, bluish skin, general or in spots; purplish spots on withered skin, especially where the circulation is feeble as on the back of the hands and feet and on the tibia. These parts become numb, tingle and wither. The extremities prickle, burn, and tingle; creeping and crawling, as of insects under the skin, as if between the skin and the flesh; numb, dead, wooden sensation in the fingers and especially in the toes. The toes become black, gangrenous. A senile withering, such as is found in feeble old people; the blood-vessels close up; no blood goes to the toes and they become numb and black, devoid of sensation. Hence, Secale improves the circulation of the aged and postpones senile gangrene.

Burning is a feature of this remedy; the skin burns; the extremities burn, sensation of burning when the parts feel cold to the touch and really are cold, a sensation of heat with coldness. Burning, especially of internal parts. Dryness with burning; burning in the stomach and bowels; dryness and burning in the mouth and throat, the nose and air passages; burning in the lungs.

This remedy produces ulceration even to sloughing. Old ulcers take on a strange, withered appearance; dryness with no granulations; a shiny, blackish aspect and all at once blackish granulations shoot out, indolent, and finally forming a black sphacelus which slowly separates; the part is dry: there is no discharge except now and then a little bleeding of black blood.

Oozing of black, liquid blood, oozing when there is no inflammation; nosebleed of dark, venous, offensive, fluid blood, bleeding from the throat, lungs, bladder, and rectum, of dark blood; urine like ink. Prolonged uterine hæmorrhage so that one menstrual nisus runs into another; withered subjects; considerable flow on the first day, fluid, and blackish; this goes on for a couple of weeks and then a dark, watery flow comes on which lasts until the next period. Then comes the thick, black fluid, horribly offensive flow again. Such a state is found in the woman who has taken ergot to produce abortion, or in sensitive women who have been dosed with it to facilitate delivery. Of course, if the woman is not sensitive you will not get the lingering provings.

Some women are so insane that though they die they will get rid of their offspring. On all hands women say, "I have had no health since I aborted." The worst state of health is produced by ergot; it establishes a miasm as deep as psora itself. The desire to destroy the offspring is an engraftment on psora and by ergot she rakes on a miasm as dangerous as sycosis or syphilis.

I have patients who took ergot to cause abortion, and I can do nothing more than palliate them. They have Secale symptoms, sequellæ, and their psoric symptoms are suppressed, held down, just as syphilis holds down psoric manifestations; only by covering the Secale miasm and getting at the psora can we help the patient. They have placed themselves beyond the help of the physician and the ergot will shorten their lives many years unless they are fortunate enough to have careful prescribing continuously while they live.

The general constitutional state is aggravated from heat; there are only a few exceptions to this. Wants cold though the limbs are cold as ice, wants to be uncovered, wants the windows open; a patient with hæmorrhages wants the covers off though the room is cold. A patient with ulcers wants to be uncovered; in inflammaotry condition of the stomach and bowels, wants the abdomen uncovered.

At times there is a lingering state of heat of the skin and the patient wants to be covered up; there are also sharp, stinging neuralgic pains, which burn like fire and cut like a knife and are relieved by the "application of heat; headache worse in cold air. But the general state is *ameliorated from uncovering, in a cold room, and from cold air blowing on the patient.*

Violent inflammation of any part of the body; gangrenous pneumonia; gastritis; peritonitis; inflammation of the uterus and ovaries. In inflammatory conditions it competes with *Ars.* The symptoms are so nearly alike in both that it is difficult to differentiate; both have violently distended abdomen; tympanites; burning like coals of fire; violent thirst; extreme sensitiveness and tenderness to touch, so that motion or jar is unbearable; vomiting of blood; expulsion of blood-clots; horrible, offensive, bloody discharge from the bowels; but they are different in the generals. *Ars.* wants to be covered up, to be kept warm, to have hot applications, either wet or dry, while Secale wants to be uncovered, wants the cold air.

Convulsions of single parts or of the whole muscular system; opisthotonos; cramps in the calves, thighs, soles of the feet, and hands; hysterical contractures, a hysterical diathesis. Convulsions begin in the face, Active manias with great excitement; exposes her body and tears at the genitals; Puts her finger in the vagina and scratches until the lips bleed; all idea of modesty lost.

The spasms, nervous, and mental symptoms are worse while she is flowing, so that a puerperal convulsion comes on in the midst of a hæmorrhage.

From the hæmorrhagic tendency and the ability to destroy the red blood corpuscle, there is anæmia. The face looks like dried beef, wrinkled, shrivelled, scrawny, as if it had not been washed; as if grey dirt had dried on the skin, and this especially on the extremities, a dirty, grey appearance.

Catarrhal affections of all mucous membranes; they are dry and bleed; blood oozes from the catarrhal surfaces, liquid, black, and offensive, coagulating slowly or not at all. "Nosebleed, blood dark, runs continually, with great prostration, small thread-like pulse; in old people or drunkards; of young women; from debility."

Those poisoned by ergot become victims of opacity of the lens as in senile debility; cataract of old persons.

The withered scrawny person with tendency to ulcerations, unhealthy skin and *aggravation from heat,* is striking in both acute and chronic states.

Chronic diarrhœa, exhaustive, watery discharges, cholera. It is related to *Camphor.* Scrawny people take cholera, skin cold and blue; better from cold. Violent and continued thirst.

Diarrhœa and hæmorrhages are likely to come together; diarrhœa of bloody water of dark liquid blood.

Large doses produce such contractures of the uterus that its contents are expelled and an exhausting hæmorrhage follows; expulsion of large clots and in the early stages mixed with some red blood, but the most striking feature is liquid, black discharge.

"Asiatic cholera with collapse, sunken, distorted face, particularly the mouth, crawling sensation as of ants."

Paretic condition; paralysis of lower extremities; of one side; of one arm or one leg; paralysis of the upper extremities with tingling, numbness, and prickling. Numbness and burning down the whole length of the spine; general emaciation or only of diseased part.

Eruptions, abscesses, boils, carbuncles; green pus discharged; a green, purplish appearance; boils small with green contents, mature and heal slowly.

Establishes sterility; so weak is the uterus that it can never hold the fœtus, hence the value in sterility and repeated abortions.

Dwindling of the mammæ. Absence of milk after confinement.

"Thin, scrawny children with shrivelled skin, spasmodic twitchings, sudden cries, feverishness."

Purpura Hæmorrhagica. Paralysis of the extremities. Spinal irritation. Cachectic females with rough skin, pustules tending to gangrene.

SELENIUM

Marked mental and physical weakness following prolonged fevers, after sexual excesses, from secret vice, from exposure to the heat of the sun in summer. Great fatigue from which he seems unable to recuperate from rest. Slight exertion brings great fatigue and weakness and especially in hot weather. Sudden weakness in hot weather. Great weakness in the back, almost paralytic after typhoid fever or other temporary diseases. Extremely sensitive to a draft of air, cool, warm or damp. Marked general emaciation, also special emaciation of face, thighs and hands. The diseased limb withers. The hair falls out all over the body, head, eyebrows, whiskers and genitals. All his nervous symptoms are aggravated after coition. Pulsation in all the limbs and in the abdomen after eating. *Extreme sadness.* Some complaints are worse from wine, tea and lemonade. It is of great value in drunkards. Irresistible desire for alcoholic stimulants. Symptoms worse after sleep, especially on a hot day. Irritable after emissions. He is indifferent to his surroundings, and his mind is dull and in confusion. He is very forgetful during his waking hours, but in sleep he dreams what he has forgotten. Makes mistakes in syllables and mispronounces words. Stammering speech. Often fails to understand what he hears or reads. He has become unfit for his business. He is excitable and talkative in the evening. Mental exertion is exhaustive and he dreads company. His mind dwells on lascivious thoughts, yet he is sometimes impotent. All the mental symptoms are worse after coition.

Vertigo on rising from bed or seat, on moving about, with nausea, vomiting and faintness, worse aster breakfast and dinner.

Headaches from strong odors, after wine, tea, lemonade and alcoholic stimulants, violent stinging over left eye when walking in the heat of the sun. Increased flow of urine in headaches. Headaches in old drunkards.

The hair falls out from the whole head, leaving the scalp smooth and hairless; also the hair falls from the eyebrows and face, giving a strange appearance. In syphilitics it often checks the falling of the hair. It has cured eczema, tingling and itching of the scalp. The scalp feels as though tightly drawn over the bones of the skull.

Itching vesicles on the edges of the eyelids and spasmodic twitching of left eyeball.

The ear is stopped and ear wax becomes hard, from which he has hardness of hearing.

Dark clotted blood from nose. Nose full of thick, yellow, jelly-like mucus. Itching of nose and he bores into his nose with the fingers. Chronic obstruction of nose. Coryza followed by watery diarrhœa.

The face is sickly, looking greasy and shiny. Great emaciation of the face. Twitching of the muscles of the face.

Toothache from drinkng tea.

Aversion to food much salted. White tongue and he does not relish his breakfast. *Irresistible longing for strong drink.* After eating pulsation all over the body, especially in the abdomen. Symptoms are worse from sugar, salt food, tea and lemonade.

Soreness in liver from pressure and inspiration, with rash over the right. hypochondrium. Searehing pain in right hypochondrium, worse on deep breathing. The liver is enlarged. Stitching pains in liver from motion and pressure.

Constipation with inactivity of the rectum. *Most difficult stool, even impaction. Stool large, hard and very dry,* requires mechanical aid. Soft pasty stool. Watery diarrhœa.

Involuntary urination while walking, after urination and after stool. Twinge of pain outward along the urethra with a sensation as though drops were pouring out. Sensation as if biting drop was forcing itself out. The urine is dark, scanty, red in evening. Sediment coarse, red and sandy. It has caused inflammation of the prostate gland. In chronic gonorrhœa it is a very useful remedy.

Extreme weakness of the male genitalia. Though the desire is strong there are no erections, or the act of coition is unsatisfactory and incomplete. Frequent emissions and constant flow of prostatic fluid. Erections in the morning without sexual desire, but on attempting coition the penis becomes relaxed. Itching and formication of genitalia.

Menses copious and dark. Pulsating in the abdomen during pregnancy. worse after eating.

The weakness and failure of the voice is in keeping with the general weakness. Hoarseness on beginning to use the voice. Hoarseness from weakness after over-use of the voice for a long time. Much clear, starchy mucus scraped from the larynx. Must frequently clear the larynx. It is a very useful remedy in tubercular laryngitis; glands of neck large and hard.

Dry, hacking cough in the morning, weak feeling in the chest. Expectoration of lumps of bloody mucus. Difficult breathing from any exertion and from mucus in the chest and air passages. Pain in right side of chest under lowest ribs extending to kidneys which are tender to pressure.

Weak back and spine as if he would be paralyzed after typhoid fever, and other lingering diseases. Stiffening neck on turning head; lameness in back in the morning.

It has cured syphilitic psoriasis of the palms. Itching palms. Hands withered. Tearing pains in hands at night.

Emaciation of the legs. Great weakness of lower limbs. Itching of the ankle in the evening, blisters on the toes. Flat ulcers on the legs and about the ankles. Cramps in calves and soles.

He is sleepless until midnight. Sleeps in short naps. Awakens early and *always at same hour.* Symptoms worse after sleep.

Chill alternates with heat. Burning heat in spots. Sweat, profuse on chest, armpits and genitals staining yellow. Sweat from least exertion.

Moist itching spots here and there on the skin and tingling after eruptions have been treated locally. Flat ulcers. Itching about finger joints and between fingers.

It is said to be incompatible with *China.* It is much like *Sulphur* in general action, and *Phos. acid* in its action upon the nervous system and genitals. The chest symptoms and expectoration are like *Argentum met., Stannum.* Its constipation is much like *Alumen* and *Alumina.* It should be carefully compared with these remedies.

SENECIO AUREUS

In some parts of the country where it grows it is called *Golden Ragwort,* in others *Huckleroot.* It is an old domestic remedy and one only proved in a fragmentary way. Many of these medicines that have become household remedies should be properly proved. Only in this way can their power and influence be known, *i.e.,* they can be used properly only when indicated by the symptoms they can produce.

Senecio is to be studied in relation to young girls with menstrual irregularities. Those who have *suppression* of the menstrual flow from getting wet, from getting the feet wet; those who have *menorrhagia,* a copious menstrual flow which continues until they are anæmic; and those also who suffer from *dysmenorrhœa,* the pains being most violent. In this remedy, with these general features, the young girl gradually tends toward catarrhal phthisis. The menstrual flow is suppressed sometimes many months, she begins to look pale, has a dry, hacking cough, with bleeding from the lungs instead of the menstrual flow, a vicarious spitting of blood. There is a catarrhal state throughout the chest. They are pallid and weakly girls. They tell you they have lost their menstrual flow, and have a chronic cough, are sensitive to every draft of air, are always taking cold and finally expectorate profusely. The phthisis may go on as catarrh of the chest for years, but at last a miliary tuberculosis sets in and takes the patient off with what is known as acute consumption. Especially is this condition associated with disorder of the menstrual flow and a general catarrhal state. "Phthisis, with obstructed menstruation." When the symptoms agree in this kind of a case Senecio is a most useful medicine for establishing the menstrual flow. You will know that it is acting well by the fact that the cough gradually diminishes. Of course a great many medicines will be suited to such general states, but this one has an unusually marked and special relation to these cases. In certain regions Senecio has been used as a domestic medicine, an old woman's remedy for, bringing on the menstrual flow.

You will be struck on reading over this remedy with the *tendency to hæmorrhage* from all the mucous membranes of the body. There is coryza with nose-bleed; spitting of blood from the throat and chest; hæmorrhage from the lungs; a catarrhal condition of all the mucous membranes with a, tendency to hæmorrhage; congestion and inflammation of the kidneys with hæmorrhage. You know how commonly these cases end in dropsy. These waxy, anæmic, chlorotic girls, who have lost their menstrual flow, become dropsical after slow hæmorrhage from the uterus, kidneys and bladder. "Dropsy from anæmia." It is a medicine of the highest order for hæmorrhages in catarrhal conditions.

It has also in its proving many distressing symptoms of the *urinary organs.* Painful urination. Uncomfortable heat in the neck of the bladder. Renal colic, the pains being so great that they produce nausea. Renal dropsy. Intense pain over right kidney, etc. The whole urinary tract is painful and subject to bleeding. But bleeding especially in the absence of the menstrual flow is the feature of this remedy. Wherever there is an inflammatory spot or catarrhal condition of the mucous membrane it will bleed in case the menstrual flow does not appear. We have other medicines having the symptoms of vicarious hæmorrhage, such as *Hamamelis, Phosphorus* and *Bryonia,* but Senecio has this condition strikingly and is one of the newer remedies for such condition.

"Dysmenorrhœa with urinary symptoms; cutting in sacral and hypogastric regions." "Hacking cough at night." "Amenorrhœa from a cold; nervous irritability; lassitude; dropsy." "Menstrual irregularities in consumptive patients." "Mucous rattling with suppressed cough."

Leucorrhœa especially in chlorotic girls. It is a marked remedy in chlorosis, in the anæmic state with a green hue, called "green sickness" by the laity.

SENEGA

Senega is an old lung tonic, and I suspect it has been an ingredient in most of the lung medicines for the last one hundred years. It has been only partially proved, and needs further proving to bring out its particulars. When a medicine has been *fully proved,* it can be said of it that its symptoms are so well known that they can be examined as an image, *i.e.,* the drug has affected *all* portions of man in such a manner as to stamp itself upon all of his natural actions and functions in a way peculiar to itself. This remedy has done some wonderful things, and these results in many instances can be only attributed to mere guesswork. This is about all that can be said in favour of careless and loose prescribing.

Senega is more especially a chest medicine. It is full of chest symptoms, and its relation to the air passages makes it worthy of consideration, although many of the individualizing symptoms have not yet been brought out. From its most striking action on the mucous membrane of the air passages, its chief use has been in chest complaints, asthmatic complaints, in various forms of dyspnœa, cardiac and asthmatic.

There are violent pains in the chest, especially like those of pleurisy. It has also symptoms like pneumonia; one of its most useful spheres is in pleuro-pneumonia. The pleuro-pneumonia of cattle has almost found its specific in Senega. The finding of specifics is more likely to be true of animals than of human beings, as a remedy that is only partially indicated may cure an animal, but it requires much finer discrimination among remedies in dealing with human beings. A violent attack of pleurisy associated with pneumonia, too deep and too vicious for *Bryonia,* often finds its remedy in Senega. Senega is a sort of cross between *Bryonia* and *Rhus tox.* The violent symptoms are those of *Bryonia,* yet it is worse from rest, unlike *Bryonia.* The symptoms of Senega are not so much like *Rhus tox.,* but it has an amelioration like that of *Rhus tox.,* better from motion, the pains being worse when at rest. The chest pains, rheumatic pains and inflammatory pains are worse during rest, but the cough is made worse from motion and the asthmatic troubles are made worse from the slightest motion. The Senega patient cannot walk uphill; he cannot walk against the wind, because it brings on chest symptoms and dyspnœa.

The rattling in the chest is as marked as in *Antimonium tartaricum; the* tenacious mucus is as copious, as gluey and stringy as in *Kali bichromicum,* so much is this the case that he can get it only part way up, and with a spasmodic effort he swallows it, like *Spongia* and *Causticum.* Senega is a remedy of deep action, as well as an acute remedy. It is filled with sharp and acute sufferings, sufferings that come on with rapidity, from taking cold, or from a cold that involves the whole chest.

There are some eye symptoms in the text that are worthy of attention. "Paralysis of the muscles of the eyes." "Iritis and specks upon the cornea." "Paresis of the superior oblique." "Aching over the orbits." "Eyes pain as if pressed out." "Blepharitis." It has cured opacity of the vitreous humor.

Of the larynx the text says, "Aphonia from severe cold or excessive use of the voice." "Constant tickling and burning in the larynx, leaving the patient nut a moment's rest and preventing him from lying down; fear of suffocation." When Senega is indicated there is a dryness in the mouth and throat, and the cough is incessant; there is a constant metallic coppery taste in the mouth and throat, as if he were coughing up pulverized copper. A very little of this medicine in proving will produce such a dryness and metallic taste in the mouth, and such a tickling at the root of the tongue, the pharynx and larynx, and it will finally end in a copious, thick, gluey discharge. "Grippe, with stitches in right eye when coughing." "Laryngeal phthisis." "Copious accumulation of tough mucus in air-tubes, which causes the greatest, often ineffectual, efforts at coughing and hawking for its expulsion." This thick, tough mucus will lead most routine prescribers to give such medicines as *Kali bichromicum, Lachesis* and *Mercurius corrosvuns,* entirely overlooking the usefulness of Senega.

It is a remedy of very wide range in complaints of the chest, larynx and trachea, in the severe "colds" that settle in these parts, especially when associated with tenacious mucus, so tenacious that he cannot cough it up; it seems at times that he will strangle; he will cough and vomit in the effort to expel the mucus, but it seems to disappear and he does not know where it goes.

"Sensation as if the chest were too narrow." "Most violent suffocation with asthma." "Short breathing and oppression of chest when going up stairs." "Dyspnœa especially during rest."

"Dry cough with aphonia; worse in cold air and from walking," is like *Phosphorus* and *Rumex.* Those two remedies cause a cough, which commences when he first goes into the air. Senega has another feature like *Phosphorus*, in that the cough is so violent that it makes him shake from head to foot; it brings on a tremulous feeling all over the body. He coughs from inhaling cold air; the cough is violent and the expectoration most difficult. In old, chronic catarrh of the chest, for the earlier stages of which *Bryonia* was the most similar remedy, with this thick, tough, ropy mucus, Senega is most suitable, and even when the patient is in the last stages of consumption. The symptoms become most troublesome, the gagging and coughing and effort to expectorate because of the thick, ropy mucus, are very distressing. He breaks out in a cold swear, especially on the upper part of the body. The chest is full of coarse rales from the tough mucus which he cannot expectorate. We think in such a case of remedies like *Antimonium tartaricum, Pyrogen, Kali bichromicum, etc.,* but this remedy is just as suitable, especially when there is a great amount of dryness in the throat and larynx, dryness in the throat during sleep and observed on waking, and inability to expectorate the tough ropy mucus. "Shaking cough," *i.e.,* the cough is so violent that it shakes the whole frame. The concussion from the cough causes discharge of urine involuntarily, and causes violent pains in the head and over the eyes. Senega is called for especially in those cases where the pleura has been involved at one stage or the other. The pains are increased and it seems as if the chest would be torn on coughing. "Walls of the chest sensitive or painful when touched." *"Profuse secretion of mucus in lungs of old people."* Senega is one of the leading remedies for the tough mucus and coarse rales in old people without any other symptoms. It very often clears the throat and helps to patch up an old man when he is breaking down. "Great rattling of mucus in chest and flying pains in chest."

It has sometimes cured pleuro-pneumonia when there was the extreme exhaustion of *Phosphorus* and *Arsenicum.* In such cases Senega has caused reaction; it has such weakness. Especially is it suited in the advanced cases of phthisis, when those symptoms that I have mentioned are present. It acts as a palliative. It does excellent patch work without serious aggravations, as it relates more especially to superficial conditions. It is not as deep acting as *Sulphur* and *Silicea.* We give such remedies only when we have a reasonable assurance that we can cure, when the patient is yet curable. But when we have given up all hope, then we pay more attention to the most painful parts; we pay more attention to the local symptoms, to the group which causes the most suffering and attempt to do patch work. If the sufferings in the chest and the exhaustion become most severe it is true that *Arsenicum* will patch him up a little and make him feel more like life, and he will go on to the end with more comfort. If the pains in the chest are most severe such medicines as Senega or *Bryonia* will help him; if he is sore and feels as if bruised and he must move from side to side *Arnica* will relieve; but these are not the remedies to go deep into the life and eradicate a deep-seated disease like phthisis. Yet with these one may take a consumptive patient in comfort to the very grave, by simply patching him up and prescribing for his immediate sufferings. Homœopathic remedies give these incurable sufferers much greater comfort than sprays and anodynes

The pains of the chest are worse during rest and on inspiring. Stitching pains in the chest when lying on the right side. Great soreness in the walls of the chest. Pain under right scapula when coughing. The chest pains are better while walking in the open air.

SEPIA

Sepia is suited to tall, slim women with narrow pelvis and lax fibers and muscles; such a woman is not well built as a woman. A woman who has the hips of a well-built man is not built for child bearing, she cannot perform the functions of a woman without becoming relaxed in the pelvic organs and tissues. Such a build is a Sepia build, very tall, slim, narrow, straight from the shoulders all the way down.

One of the strongest features of the Sepia patient is found in the mind, the state of the affections. To a great extent, the remedy seems to abolish the ability to feel natural love, to be affectionate. To illustrate it in the language of the mother: "I know I ought to love my children and my husband, I used to love them, but now I have no feeling on the subject." The love does not go forth into affection, there is a lack of realization, a lack of ability to register such affections; the love does not manifest itself. Upon reflection it will be seen that the love itself cannot be so changed, but the affections can be as they are the expression of the love. It is a striking feature of this remedy that the affections are stilled; all things seem strange; she does not realize; she may even be estranged and turned aside from those she loves. This is on the border land of insanity; it is quite a different state of affairs from that when a woman abused by her husband knows in her rational mind that she does not love him.

This state is brought out in a woman during confinement, after uterine and other hæmorrhages, after prolonged indigestion; high living with disturbance in the circulation, pallor, enfeeblement of body and mind. It is seldom manifested in a man, but it is a striking feature in the woman. It often comes on when nursing a child, from nursing an over-vigorous child or twins who require much lacteal fluid and drag her down. It may be brought out in a woman who has an over-vigorous husband. Excessive sexual excitement and over-indulgence brings on coldness and she becomes a cold woman.

She who has been excitable, nervous, and fidgety becomes the opposite, cold, takes on a stoical state of mind. Yet Sepia has all the excitability of any medicine, aggravated by noises, excitement, company, extreme irritability of tissue and mind; an excitable suicidal patient; melancholy, sirs and says nothing; taciturn; answers questions in monosyllables when pressed to answer. An absence of all joy, inability to realize that things are real; all things seem strange; no affection for the delightful things of life; no joy; life has nothing in it for her. She is worse in company yet dreads to be alone; and when she is in company she is spiteful, in the midst of her dullness of mind she is spiteful; she vents her spite on those she loves best. The Sepia woman permits no opposition to her opinions. The best impression of her is lost if controversy arises.

The next most general state is a peculiar sallowness which you will need to see to fix in your mind. Sepia has jaundice, yet this peculiar sallowness is a waxy, anæmic appearance, mottled with yellow, a yellow, sallow tint across the nose and the cheeks described as a yellow saddle across the nose and down the sides of the face. It is also common for the whole face to be covered with enormous freckles, great brown patches as in pregnancy, brown spots on the cheeks, brown warts, warts that have been red or pink become pigmented; liver spots on the face, chest, and abdomen. The skin of the face is sallow and doughy, looks as if the muscles were flabby; you will seldom see Sepia indicated in the face that shows sharp lines of intellect; a person who has been thinking a long time has the lines and sharp angles of a thinking person, of one who possesses will and intellect. The Sepia subject is one who is rather stupid and dull, thinks slowly and is forgetful; the mind is anything but active and we see it in the face. In many instances, however, the Sepia patient is a quick patient, but the dullness of intellect is the most striking feature and it reflects itself upon the face. The face is generally puffed, often smooth and rounded and marked by an absence of intellectual lines and angles.

This patient is anæmic, pale lips and ears, pale, sallow face, fingers and hands become shrivelled, sallow, waxy, bloodless. Sepia establishes a progressing emaciation of the body and the skin becomes wrinkled; the person looks prematurely old; wrinkles intermingled with sallow spots on the face in one who is 35 years of age, making him look as if he were fifty. A child looks like a shrivelled dried up old person.

With all complaints there is constipation. The bowels lose their ability to expel their contents and the patient is always constipated; constipation during pregnancy; slow, difficult stool; stool like sheep dung. Always has a feeling of a lump in the rectum, never able to empty the bowels; though he goes to stool there is always a sensation of a lump remaining in the rectum When the stool passes into the lower bowel, it is not expelled until there is an accumulation, which presses the stool out.

Another feature present in most Sepia patients is a gnawing hunger, seldom satisfied; even though he eats plentifully he feels a gnawing, empty, hungry feeling in the stomach, not relieved by eating or relieved only for a moment. This is striking especially when associated with the constipation and the peculiar state of the affections.

When these symptoms are associated with prolapsus, Sepia will certainly cure, no matter how bad the prolapsus has been or what kind of displacement there is. It is the result of the state of relaxation of all the internal parts as if they were let down, wants a bandage to hold the parts up or wants to place the hand or napkin on the parts; a funneling sensation, better sitting down *and crossing the limbs.*

When these symptoms group themselves together, the gnawing hunger, the constipation, the dragging down, and the mental condition, it is Sepia and Sepia only. One is not sufficient but it is the combination.

Sepia has a marked catarrhal tendency, tendency to milky discharges from mucous membranes. Long after digestion has ceased and the stomach is empty comes nausea and sometimes vomiting. It is a catarrhal state of the stomach and when it persists with the milky vomiting, Sepia is very valuable. This is not an uncommon feature in the vomiting of pregnancy. Vomits up food and after emptying the stomach of its contents, vomits or eructates a milky fluid; morning vomiting, first of food, then a milky substance. Do not confound this with vomiting of milk. Some medicines vomit milk alone and Sepia does this also.

Whitish, milky discharges from the posterior nares, from the vagina, excoriating, milky leucorrhœa, which at times takes on the appearance of curds, thick, cheesy, and horribly offensive; it has also thick, green and yellow discharges; it has dry crusty formations on mucous membranes.

Prolonged inveterate catarrh of the nose, thick, green, and yellow crusts are blown from the nose and sometimes are hawked from the posterior nares, thick, leathery formations. Loss of taste and smell. The smell of cooking food, meat and broth causes nausea. Catarrh of the chest with thick, tenacious, yellow expectoration, accompanied with a violent cough, retching, gagging, violent prolonged retching, vomiting; dry cough and yet there is rattling. Whooping cough; asthmatic cough with retching and loss of urine. The cough is a violent one. Cough during first sleep (*Lach.,* in irritable children *Cham.*). Tuberculosis. Quick consumption after a suppressed gonorrhœa; if given soon enough it will check. Spasmodic dry cough in the evening until midnight; holds the chest during the cough (*Bry., Natr.sulph.,Phos.*).

Eruptions of the skin. Tendency to produce herpetic eruptions about the genitals, lips and mouth; ringworm upon the face and body. It has cured zona, and herpetic eruptions of the labia and foreskin. Vesicular eruptions in the axilla, upon the tips of the elbows; eruptions that pile up in great crusts on the elbows; thick crusts form upon the joints; eruptions between the fingers; moist eruptions that pour out a watery fluid, or thick, yellow, purulent fluid.

Sepia produces the induration that belongs to some forms of eruption like epithelioma; indurations will form on the lips and crack and bleed. The scaly eruption that looks like epithelioma is especially Sepia. When the scales come off a yellow, green, ichorous base remains, and as soon as one crust peels off, another forms; finally if torn off prematurely, it bleeds. Sepia has cured epithelioma of the lips, wings of the nose, and eyelids. It has cured old indurations caused by the use of a clay pipe, where it continues to form, and beneath it is seen this thick, yellow, purulent exudation. It is indicated in lumps and lupoid formation on the skin, where there is infiltration; sometimes healing from the centre to form a ring; this is a typical Sepia condition. The hardness and purple color are what are peculiarly Sepia. Sepia stands on a par with *Lach.* for this purple aspect.

Sepia has a hysterical diathesis. Breaks out in spells of weeping, is sad one minute, gentle, yielding, and in another she is disagreeable, excitable, obstinate. You do not know what she is going to do next. She says and does strange things, makes errors, no dependence can be placed on her; no mental endurance; no affection for her family; whole mind weak and disordered, not when there is fever, but it is a chronic manifestation of psora or sycosis. Fear of ghosts; that something unusual will happen; atmosphere full of figures, not seen, but she knows that they are there, departed friends or other forms and very often in accordance with religious belief. Never happy unless annoying some one; relating her grievances; sarcastic; insulting; fear of insanity, poverty. "Fears to starve, is peevish and feels mortified, easily frightened and full of forebodings." "Passionate, irritable; the greatest irritability from slight causes, very easily offended. Vexed and disposed to scold."

The headaches are nervous, bilious, periodic, violent, involving the whole head; congestive. Generally better lying down, keeping perfectly quiet; worse from ordinary motion, but relieved by violent motion, like most Sepia symptoms in general; she can walk off her sufferings. Stasis of the brain, slowness of thought, mind will not work and mental labor aggravates the headache. A good substantial sleep relieves it, but if she is awakened after sleeping a short time, the headache is worse. The same is seen in regard to motion; moving the eyes, head, or body, moving about in a warm room aggravates the pain, but a good, long walk in the open air until she becomes heated up, relieves. It is a sluggish state of the body which requires exercise, and violent exercise to keep it in a state of comfort. The Sepia symptoms are worse in the open air unless combined with continued motion, better from exercise in the open air and worse in the house. The headache is worse from stooping, motion, coughing, going up stairs, jarring, light, turning the head, lying on the back and from thinking, but continued, hard exercise relieves, as does a tight bandage, and the application of heat, though worse in a warm room.

There are Sepia headaches that particularly affect the occiput, worse in the morning; great pain through the eyes and temples; relieved by sweat, worse on beginning to move; throbbing felt on stooping, worse on going up stairs.

The *Phos.* headache is relieved by sleep, but continued, rapid motion aggravates. Cannot endure it. Sepia is suited to the old fashioned bilious headaches. It is better from vomiting; the pain gradually increases, loathing of food; then nausea, vomiting and the patient falls asleep and wakens without the headache. *Sang.* resembles it, is better vomiting; better in a dark room; the direction is different, however.

Neuralgia of the head; periodic sick-headaches in gouty people; violent, congestive headaches in young women sensitive to noise, women of extremely delicate fiber, especially those with dark eyes, dark skin, and who become sallow from sickness. Jaundice often sets in with the headaches; at the close of the headache vomiting, and in a few days jaundice, which passes away but returns again with the next headache. Headache every morning with nausea; the smell of food repulsive.

Sepia takes on a stupid state of mind as mentioned above; will not work; will not answer questions; as if intoxicated, benumbed; eyes and face swollen, sclerotics yellow and jaundice. This sometimes ends in violent vomiting spells. Craves spicy, pungent, bitter things like beer—in old drunkards with headache;

threatening apoplexy. "Apoplexy in men addicted to drinking and· sexual excesses, with a disposition to gout and hæmorrhoids, etc." "Threatening apoplexy in a dissipated, middle-aged man, who is subject to arthritic and hæmorrhoidal complaints; they have usually passed through several light attacks of apoplexy and are frequently visited with prodromic symptoms."

Under external head we have eruptions and falling out of the hair; yellow crusts; oozing of pus and other fluids; vesicles; eczema of infants.

Eyes; catarrhal symptoms with vesicles and pustules; granular lids; ulcers and psoric manifestations; various infiltrative conditions of the eyes and about the eyes; pustules on the margins of the lids, pustules on the globe of the eye, seems as if looking through a gauze; tarsal tumors, agglutination of lids, styes, etc.

The ears discharge thick, yellow pus; offensive.

The nose is a favorite locality; loss of smell; yellow or green thick crusts fill the nose and cannot be blown out; inveterate discharge of thick yellow pus. "Large offensive-smelling plugs from the nose, often so large that they have to be drawn back into the mouth and expectorated, causing vomiting. Dry coryza especially of left nostril. Blowing of large lumps of yellow or green mucus or yellow-green crusts with blood from the nose." This is descriptive of the worst forms of catarrh; very few will let it run on thus far, they apply local treatment and heal the nose up, and, the process at once going to the chest, phthisis pituitosa comes on.

The gums settle away from the teeth. Toothache and neuralgia from taking cold.

Sensation of a lump in the throat (like *Lach.*), but the latter is better from swallowing. (The same in worm troubles indicates *Cina.*). Uneasiness of the collar and corsets like *Lach.* Worse in the first sleep like *Lach.*

Sepia brings out many things in connection with the appetites, thirst, eating, drinking and stomach, etc. The Sepia patient is generally conscious of a spoiled stomach, sour and bitter eructations of food, of mucus and bile, sour and bitter vomiting of food and mucus; all-gone, hungry, empty feeling in the stomach sometimes not relieved by eating. At times a gnawing pain, a sinking, a gnawing hunger which is not always relieved by eating. Almost constant nausea, especially in the morning, nausea and eructations and vomiting of milky fluid; when the stomach is empty, vomiting, spitting up. eructations of milky fluid. Aversion to food, to the smell of food cooking, like *Colch.* and *Ars.* The patient gets up in the morning with an all gone feeling, distress and fulness in the stomach followed by belching and uprisings of mucus, and milky fluids; vomiting of pregnancy; vomiting of milky water in the morning; this is a characteristic of Sepia.

Acrid, burning eructations; heartburn; rancid eructations, excoriating the throat; pyrosis which is another form of eructation; acrid, sour fluids burning all the way up, causing contraction, tingling, smarting.

Nausea violent; deathly sinking accompanied with an awful anxiety in the stomach.

Phos. has more of the typical hunger which is relieved by eating. The *Ignatia* patient is always sighing; cannot get rid of "that feeling".

Oleander has an all-gone empty feeling as if he would die; food does not relieve, is not digested, but passes undigested the next day.

Lyc. has an all-gone feeling sometimes not better by eating, felt as markedly before as after eating, and after eating there comes a throbbing.

Kali carb. has it also, without the amelioration from taking food; it is even intensified by eating, which is followed by a sensation of fulness and throbbing.

In severe liver and heart affections the stomach is not able to keep up assimillation; palpitation, great weakness, liver congested, white stool. *Digitalis* comes in here with its deathly sinking not better by eating. In Sepia this symptom is associated with the loss of affections, the lump in the rectum, with the constipation, etc.

"Pain in the stomach after the simplest food. Stitches and burning in the stomach. Pain in the stomach worse by vomiting." This is peculiar, for vomiting usually relieves the distress. The Sepia stomach becomes like a leather bag, fill it up and the food comes up just as eaten or at times sour or mixed with bile.

Inflammation of the liver, enlargement with jaundice, pain, fulness, distension, distress in the region of the liver.

Abdomen distended with flatus, rumbling and distension. These disturbances are often chronic as in pot-bellied mothers; abdomen covered with brown spots.

Sepia has removed tape-worm.

Chronic diarrhœa, stools jelly-like, lumpy; alternating diarrhœa and constipation; a great amount of mucus with the stools, whether constipated or diarrhœic; hard stool covered with a great quantity of jelly-like mucus. Goes for days without a stool and then sits and strains until a copious sweat breaks out and yet no stool, but after assistance with the finger and prolonged strain a little stool is passed, followed by a cupful of jelly-like mucus, yellow or yellow-white and very offensive.

The acute diarrhœa and dysenteries with jelly-like stools are more in keeping with *Kali bi.* and *Colch.* This is chronic diarrhœa or in constipation with stool covered with or followed by jelly-like mucus is Sepia.

Do not confound with *Graph.,* which has an enormous stool with much straining and sweating, and coated with and mixed with a substance looking like the cooked white of egg, as if covered with albumen.

In Sepia there is much offensiveness; the odor of the stool is unusual loose stools horribly offensive, fœtid; the sweat is fœtid, the urine is fœtid. "The stool has a putrid, sourish, fœtid smell, expelled suddenly and the whole of it at once." Sepia is given in a routine way for constipation, when there are few symptoms. There is always a sense of fulness in the rectum after stool; ineffectual straining and sweating in the effort because the patient is weak and exhausted. Sepia has the ineffectual urging like *Nux*. She may go for days with no urging and then the effort is as if she were in labor. Prolapse of the rectum. Weight as of a ball in the anus not relieved by stool. Soreness of the anus. Expulsion of ascarides. Oozing moisture from the rectum, soreness between the buttocks.

Hæmorrhoids soon form when the rectum is so packed with fæces, and they give additional trouble.

There is much urinary trouble; involuntary urination as soon as the child goes to sleep at night. Sepia is compelled to keep the mind on the neck of the bladder or she will lose the urine; urine is lost when coughing, sneezing, laughing, the slam of a door, a shock, or when the mind is diverted. Frequent, constant urging to urinate with milky urine that burns like fire and after standing a while a milky, greyish deposit will form which is hard to wash off the vessel. Bloody urine, scanty and suppressed, great pain in the kidneys and bladder with great bearing down; sudden desire with tenesmus as if the uterus would come out. Sudden desire to urinate with cutting like knives and chill all over the body, if unable to pass it, as a lady in company. I remember a pitiable case. A saleswoman was obliged to go to the closet every few minutes; a violent pain like a knife cutting came with the desire to urinate, and if the urine was not passed this pain would hold right on. She was compelled to keep her mind on the urine or she would lose it. She was tall, slim, with sallow face, distressed look, worn and tired. Sepia cured her and she was never troubled again.

The Sepia patient aborts at the third month. All sorts of ulcerative conditions, displacements, dragging down and relaxations. Retained placenta. Subinvolution, all the pelvic organs are tired and weak. Metrorrhagia during the climacteric or during pregnancy, especially at the fifth and seventh months.

Both male and female have aversion to the opposite sex. In the female there is a state as if she had indulged to excess, when this is not the case. No endurance, tired after coition, sleepless nights, sleep full of dreams, jerking of muscles, twitching, leucorrhœa, congestion of the pelvis. A woman who has been normal in her relations with her husband brings forth a child, and then the thought of sexual relations causes nausea and irritability.

The menstrual symptoms are of all sorts, no particular derangement characterizes Sepia. At one time it was thought that scanty menstruation was the more striking feature, but this is not necessarily so; from provings and clinical observations, it has cured profuse as well as scanty flow.

Most violent dysmenorrhœa in girls of delicate fiber, sallow girls.

Sepia comes in when the woman ought to menstruate when the child ceases to nurse; sometimes the child dies and menses ought to be established but do not appear, and the mother runs down, pines away; Sepia will establish the flow.

Calc. is the opposite; the menses come on while the child is nursing. Thick greenish acrid or milky leucorrhœa. Leucorrhœa in little girls.

In the male, old sycotic discharge that has resisted injection. Profuse yellow, or milky discharge from the urethra, or the "last drop," painless. Gonorrhœa after the acute symptoms have subsided. Urine loaded with urates, stains everything red and often excoriates, very fœtid, associated with prostatitis. "Gleet; no pain; discharge only during the night, a drop or so staining the linen yellowish; yellowish discharge, no burning on urinating; painless; of a year and a half's standing; orifice of urethra stuck together in the morning, particularly when the sexual organs are debilitated by long continuance of disease or through frequent seminal emissions."

Warts on the genitals; Sepia is useful when these organs have been overused and take on such an appearance. Impotence in the male, loss of sexual feeling in the female.

The close relation between this remedy and *Murex* is worth considering. The muscular relaxation, dragging down in the abdomen and pelvis, aggravated from exertion and walking, ameliorated by sitting with the limbs crossed and ameliorated by pressure on the genitalia would be like both remedies but add to this copious menstrual flow and violent sexual desire and *Murex* must be considered and Sepia eliminated. Both have extreme empty feeling in the stomach. Sepia has diminished sexual desire and often aversion. *Murex* has great soreness and congestion of the uterus, and she is constantly reminded of the uterus. *Murex* has acute pain in right side of uterus which crosses the body diagonally upward to left side of chest, or left breast. It cures violent dysmenorrhœa. It has been useful in cancer of the uterus. Watery; greenish, thick, bloody leucorrhœa, causing itching.

One of Sepia's most general characteristics is the amelioration from violent exercise; worse on beginning to move but better by getting warmed up. This condition is closely related to the back symptoms. There is a great amount of soreness in the back, the spine aches all the way down. Pressure on the spine reveals sore places, spinal irritation. Aching in the back mostly from the loins to the coccyx, often coming on from sitting, and ameliorated from violent exercise. A peculiar feature is amelioration from hard pressure. The patient commonly puts a book low down on the chair and presses the back against it. Sepia does not seem to get the amelioration from lying upon the back as *Natrum mur.* does. Stooping aggravates the backache. "Backache worse from kneeling."

Under symptoms of the lower extremities we find great numbness of the feet. "Coldness of the legs and feet especially in the evening in bed; when the feet get warm the hands get cold; icy coldness of the feet; profuse sweat of the feet or sweat of unbearable odor causing soreness between the toes. Swelling of the limbs better while walking."

The sleep is full of dreams and distress; cannot sleep upon the left side because of palpitation of the heart. Palpitation in sleep, with pulsations and trembling all over the body, pulsations to the finger tips.

In old cases of suppressed malaria, Sepia brings back the chill, but its most useful sphere is after a bad selection of the remedy and the case becomes confused. Where a remedy has been selected for only a part of the case and changed it a little but the patient gets no better. It will be seen that the fever, chili, and sweat are just as erratic as can be. *Natrum mur.* is one of the greatest malarial remedies, but it is full of order like *China,* Sepia is full of disorder. In a case confused by remedies think of *Calc., Ars., Sulph.,* Sepia and *Ipecac.* Never give *China* or *Natrum mur* for irregular symptoms and stages.

Sepia is complementary to *Natrum mur.* Aside from the stupid condition of the mind it has an excitable condition of the general nervous system that is often marked in *Natrum mur.,* as, for instance, being disturbed by a noise, the slam of a door, etc. It produces jerking of the muscles in sleep; constantly wakes from imaginary noises, thinks someone has called her; the least disturbance about the house wakens her.

Worse before and during menses; during pregnancy; after eating; during first sleep; change of weather; during a thunderstorm; overwhelming fear.

SILICA

The action of Silica is slow. In the proving, it takes a long time to develop the symptoms. It is, therefore, suited to complaints that develop slowly. At certain times of the year and under certain circumstances peculiar symptoms will come out. They may stay with the prover the balance of his life. Such are the long-acting, deep-acting remedies; they are capable of going so thoroughly into the vital order that hereditary disturbances are routed out. The Silica patient is chilly; his symptoms are developed in cold, damp weather, though often better in cold, dry weather; symptoms come out after a bath.

The mental state is peculiar. The patient lacks stamina. What Silica is to the talk of grain in the field, it is to the human mind. Take the glossy, stiff, outer covering of a stalk of grain and examine it, and you will realize with what firmness it supports the head of grain until it ripens; there is a gradual deposit of Silica in it to give it stamina. So it is with the mind; when the mind needs Silica it is in a state of weakness, embarrassment, dread, a state of yielding. If you should listen to the description of this state by a prominent clergyman or a lawyer, or a man in the habit of appearing in public with self-confidence, firmness and fulness of thought and speech, he would tell you he had come to a state where he dreads to appear in public, he feels his own selfhood so that he cannot enter into his subject, he dreads it, he fears that he will fail, his mind will not work, he is worn out by prolonged efforts at mental work. But he will say that when he forces himself into the harness he can go on with ease, his usual self-command returns to him and he does well; he does his work with promptness, fulness, and accuracy. The peculiar Silica state is found in the dread of failure. If he has any unusual mental task to perform, he fears he will make a failure of it, yet he does it well. This is the early state; of course there comes a time when he cannot perform the work with accuracy and still he may need Silica.

Another case is illustrated in a young man who has studied for years and is now nearing the end of his course. He dreads the final examinations but he goes through them all right, then a fatigue comes upon him and for years he is unable to enter his profession. He has this dread of undertaking anything.

Irritable and irascible when aroused; when let alone he is timid, retiring, wants to shirk everything; mild, gentle, tearful women. The Silica child is cross and cries when spoken to. It is the natural complement and chronic of *Puls.* because of its great similarity; it is a deeper, more profound remedy. Religious melancholy, sadness, irritability, despondency. *Lyc.* is stupid, the dread of undertaking anything is from a general knowledge of inability. In Silica it is imaginary.

Silica is not suitable for the irritability and nervous exhaustion coming on from business brain-fag, but more for such brain-fag as belongs to professional men, students, lawyers, clergymen. A lawyer says, "I have never been myself since that John Doe case." He went through a prolonged effort and sleepless nights followed. Silica restores the brain.

The remedy produces inflammation about any fibrinous nidus and suppurates it out. It acts upon constitutions that are sluggish and inflame; fibrous deposits about old imbedded missiles. Stow nutrition; if the indivi dual receives a slight injury it suppurates and the cicatrix indurates, is hard and nodular. Along the track of a knife-cut, is a fibrinous deposit due to inferior and slow nutrition. An old ulcer heals with induration. Where cicatrical tissue forms, it is indurated, shiny, glassy. If Silica is given in such cases, it will throw out abscesses in these cicatrices and open them out. It will open up old ulcers and heal them with a normal cicatrix.

In ordinary people if a splinter lodges in the tissues, a suppuration will slough it out, but in these feeble constitutions a plastic deposit takes place about it and it remains. This is not the highest state of order. Suppuration takes place about a bullet and pushes it out, that is the best state that can be asked for.

Silica, therefore, hastens the formation of abscesses and boils. It suppurates out old wens and indurated tumors. It has cured recurrent fibroids and old indurated tumors.

If there is a deposit of tubercle in the lungs, Silica establishes an inflammation and throws it out, and if the whole lung be tubercular a general suppurative pneumonia will be the result; hence, the danger of giving such remedies and the danger of repeating them in advanced stage of phthisis. Not only Silica but many other remedies have the power to suppurate out deposits, the result of poor nutrition.

Warty growths on the skin, moist eruptions, pimples, pustules, abscesses. Suppurating cavities. It establishes healing in old fistulous openings with indurated margins. Catarrhal suppurations; copious muco-purulent discharge from the eyes, nose, ears, chest, vagina, etc.

Complaints from the suppression of discharges; suppressed sweat. These suppressions produce a state in the economy that threatens what little order is left. An offensive foot-sweat ceases after getting the feet wet, and is followed by chills and violent complaints. Silica cures long lasting foot-sweat when the symptoms agree, or complaints that have lasted since the suppression of a foot-sweat. Thick, yellow catarrhal discharges. They say, "I have had this discharge so many years," and when you investigate, you find that there has been some shock, a cold, that suppressed the foot-sweat and it has not appeared since. Silica will bring back that sweat, cause the catarrhal discharge to cease and in time cure the foot-sweat. Catarrhal discharges from the nose and other places, indurations, tumors, chronic gastritis, brain-fag, all dating back to the suppression of foot-sweat or otorrhœa, or to the healing up of a fistula.

Chronic sick-headache attended with nausea and even vomiting. Headache commencing in the back of the head in the morning or towards noon going to the forehead, worse towards night, from noise; better from heat; supra-orbital neuralgias; better from pressure and heat and attended with profuse head-sweat. Cold, clammy, offensive sweat on the forehead. When a Silica patient exerts himself he sweats on the face, the lower part of the body is dr~ or nearly so. It requires great exertion to produce general sweat. A striking feature is the sweat about the upper parts of the body and the head. Headache once a week (*Gels., Lyc., Sang., Sulph.*). Headache up through the back of the neck and especially to the right side of the head. Resembles *Sang.* Weight in the occiput as if it would be drawn back, with a rush of blood to the head, like *Carbo veg.* and *Sepia.* Headache worse from cold air. *Psor.* wears a fur cup even in summer. *Magn. mur.* is better from wrapping up the head but still wants to be in the air. *Rhus* sweats on the body; the head is dry. *Puls.* sweats on one side of the head.

Vertigo to fainting; with nausea; vertigo creeping up the spine into the head.

It is especially necessary for the Silica patient to avoid the cold air, must have the head well wrapped up, especially the part that is painful, and this part perspires copiously.

'Headache worse from mental exertion, excessive study, noise, motion, even jarring from foot-steps, light, stooping, pressing at stool, talking, cold air, touch."

Moist, scaly eruption on the scalp, eczema capitis.

Silica is suited to the phagedenic ulcers of syphilis, eating and spreading ulcers on the scalp. Inflammatory conditions between the scalp and skull, tumors forming, filled with a grumous fluid; as in infancy; it will remove blood tumors. Cephalatoma neonatorum, enchondroses. Silica is especially of use in the treatment of affections of the cartilages, growths about the joints, about the fingers and toes.

The complaints of Silica are associated with hardened glands, but especially about the neck, the cervical, salivary, and particularly the parotid glands; large, hard parotids. The parotids enlarge from every cold and get hard. (*Bar. carb., Catc., Sulph.*)

Puls. suits the acute inflammation of the parotid, but Silica is indicated in the more chronic forms due to psora, "scrofulous glands".

Many inflammations and conditions of the eyes. Ulcers on the cornea; pustules on the lids, falling of the lashes, suppuration of the margins of the lids with burning, stinging and redness. Intense photophobia in all eye complaints. Scrofulous cases with sore eyes; the most inveterate and chronic cases; suppuration; thin, watery, copious discharge, or bloody, thick and yellow like pus, with ulceration. Syphilitic iritis. "Perforating or sloughing ulcer on the cornea. Spots and cicatrices on the cornea. Fungus hæmatodes. Eyes inflamed from traumatic causes; foreign particles have lodged in the eyes; abscesses; boils around the eyes and lids; tarsal rumors, styes, Affections appearing in the angles of the eyes; fistula lachrymalis; stricture of lachrymal duct." This is a general survey of the eye affections in Silica.

There is no deeper remedy than Silica in eradicating the tubercular tendency, when the symptoms agree; most tubercular cases are worse from cold, wet weather; better in cold dry weather.

The most inveterate cases of catarrh of the ear; old offensive, thick, yellow otorrhœa; following scarlet fever; all sorts of abnormalities in hearing, ever to deafness. Roaring in the ears associated with many diseases and hardness of hearing; hissing, roaring like steam; like a train of cars, many times from mechanical cause and other times from a condition of the nerves. It is commonly the beginning of a dry catarrh of the middle ear; the remedy is especially useful when, in catarrh of the middle ear and Eustachian tube, the deafness goes on for some time and the hearing returns with a snap, due to the escape of the accumulation of fluids somewhere and described by the patient as a snap or report. Sudden reports in the ear like a cannon, distant noises with return of hearing. "Otorrhœa, offensive, watery, curdy, with soreness of inner nose and crusts on upper lip, after abuse of *Mercury,* with caries." Caries of bone in any part of the body, but especially of the small bones of the ear, nose and mastoid process. "Scabs behind the ears." Rupture of the drum of the ear. Catarrhal conditions of the internal ear and Eustachian tube, with "feeling of sudden stoppage in the ear, better by gaping or swallowing."

Especially with ear troubles, there will be associated indurated parotid glands.

Accumulation of hard crusts in the nose, loss of taste and smell; epistaxis, thickening of the mucous membrane; most vicious catarrh with discharge of bone from the nose. Horrible, fœtid ozæna, old syphilitic cases where the nasal bones are destroyed and the nose becomes a flabby bag, is sunken in or ulcerated away, leaving an opening. Silica may cure and an artificial nose be made afterwards.

Hepar competes with Silica in syphilitic nasal catarrhs where the parts are phagedenic; *Hepar, Merc. cor.* and *Ars.,* are the principal antisyphilitics when there is phagedenic ulceration of the nose. Babies suffer from bloody nasal discharge. This is often *Calc. sul.*

The aspect of the Silica face is silky, anæmic, waxy, tired. Pustular and vesicular eruptions spread over the face, the wings of the nose crack, the lips easily fissure; crusts form on the margin between the mucous membrane and the skin; eruptions and crusts, indurations form under the crusts, they peel off and there is no healing. These indurations are the same kind of inferior tissue that is found under lupus and epithelioma, a low tissue formation, a low state of eczema that favors infiltration. The small blood-vessels that lead to them become thicker and thicker until they become gristly. There is a tendency to make the soft tissues harder and the hard tissues harder.

In childhood the bones become softer and even necrose or there is an inflammation of the periosteum and a consequent necrosis. Caries of the shaft of the long bones, the head of the bones and the cartilaginous portions; abscesses in cartilages, enchondromata. Bones break down and form fistulous openings. Necrosis of the jaw, the joints, the hip-joint, the tibia, necrosis of the spine, of the vertebræ, so that there is curvature of the spine, lateral especially. The homœopathic physicians may treat these affections of the bones with the help of accessory contrivances or supports.

The Silica patient has rough lips, they crack and peel; rhagades. Scaly appearances at the margins of the lips, fissures in the corners of the mouth that indurate. There is often a line of fissure about the margin of the crust. Little crusts like epirhelioma form upon the wings of the nose and when picked off leave a raw surface with no tendency to heal. Crusty formations upon the ears.

The teeth break down, lose their enamel surface; the dentine is made up largely of the silicate of lime and the surface of the tooth becomes rough, loses its shiny appearance and caries sets in. This often takes place at the margin of the gum; ulcers form on the tip of the fangs. The teeth suffer when it is cold or damp; toothache in wet weather, and the teeth are yellow, decay rapidly, and the gums settle away from them. All the neuralgias and toothaches are better in a warm room and from hot drinks. Abscesses about the gums and face, better by warmth. Severe pain in the jaw, rending, tearing at night, better from heat; these pains often end in abscesses about the teeth. Sometimes relieved by pressure unless the part is extremely sore from inflammation.

The tongue takes on inflammation of gouty character; inflammation with threatening abscess, it fills the whole mouth; rending, tearing pains, worse at night and better from heat.

In the throat and neck we have inflammation and swelling of all the glands, external and internal, all at once or singly. Quinsy with great pain in the tonsils, one or both; threatening suppuration. Inflammation of the parotid, sublingual and much less frequently the submaxillary and cervical glands; painful, tumid and hard, with pain in the neck, shoulders and head, even in acute inflammations. But then we have the opposite state of affairs. In an old chronic case broken down with suffering the symptoms are worse after a bath, he wants warmth, dreads the cold, is always shivering. But when in the neck there is an acute inflammation the very opposite is present; he suffers from flushes of heat, an irregular, flushing fever, cold extremities while the upper part of the body is hot, sweat about the head and neck, sensation of heat and suffocation in a warm room. This will be present in quinsy and abscesses of the glands of the neck, if acute. Silica here shows its relation to *Puls.* The latter in its chronic manifestations is overburdened with heat, but in an acute trouble is chilly. They are reversed as to their acute and chronic states. *Puls.* in the beginning is chilly and sweating.

Silica is full of throat symptoms but is seldom indicated in acute forms because its pace is too slow; it comes on after there has been a series of colds, such colds as are ameliorated a number of times by *Bell.* or other acute remedies, but still continue to settle in the tonsils and in the glands of the neck. Silica breaks up the tendency. There is a catarrhal state in the throat that is roused up by every cold into an increased flux, with hoarseness, settling back into the chronic state again; chronic catarrhs of the pharynx. It competes with *Natrum mur.* in inveterate sore throat.

Silica disturbs the stomach, causes hiccough, nausea and vomiting; disturbs the liver. All these symptoms are connected and are hard to separate. Decided aversion to warm foods desires cold things, wants his tea moderately cold, he is willing to have his food cold, dislikes warm food. Sometimes there is a decided aversion to meat, but if he does take it, he prefers cold, sliced meat. He likes ice cream, ice water, and feels comfortable when it is in the stomach; it is sometimes impossible for him to drink hot fluids, they cause sweat about the face and head and cause hot flushes (*Bar. c.*).

Silica is disturbed by the extremes of heat and cold, easily affected in changes even of a few degrees; he has complaints from being overheated; he gets overheated easily, sweats easily from a slight change in the temperature and comes down with a cold.

Case: A physician waiting on an obstetrical case, had a little difficulty in the last stage and he became overheated; putting on his overcoat and hat he went out on the porch to cool off and was taken down with asthma. Violent cough, copious expectoration with gagging and vomiting which lasted him for months. The acute remedies he had taken only palliated, but a dose of Silica cured him almost as quickly as he was taken down; he could not tolerate a warm room; the acute complaints of Silica are often worse in a warm room and from heat.

Silica has an aggravation from milk. Many times the infant is unable to take any kind of milk and, hence, the physician is driven to prescribe all the foods in the market if he does not know the right remedy. *Natrum carb.* and Silica are both useful when the mother's milk causes diarrhœa and vomiting. The routinist is likely to give such medicines as *Æthusa,* entirely forgetting Silica. The latter, as well as *Natrum carb.,* has sour vomiting and sour curds in the stool. "Aversion to the mother's milk and vomiting." "Diarrhœa from milk." Put these two together.

Although the patient has an aversion to hot things and desires to eat cold things, yet in chest complaints cold water, ice cream and cold things in general, increase the cough to gagging, and then the retching is dreadful; violent, retching, gagging cough. Retching from an endeavor to expectorate is usually controlled by *Carbo veg.,* but Silica has it.

"Water brash, with chilliness, with brown tongue; nausea and vomiting of what is drunk, worse in the morning; water tastes bad; vomits after drinking."

The Silica stomach is weak, in a do-nothing state; old dyspeptics that have been vomiting a long time, especially those who have an aversion to hot food, who cannot take milk, are averse to meat, where the mental and bodily symptoms agree.

Silica was one of the greatest remedies for the chronic diarrhœa in the soldiers of our Civil War. It cured a fair percentage of those sick from sleeping on damp ground, eating all sorts of food until the stomach and bowels were prostrated, from long marehes, from going into the South from the cold North, from becoming overheated. It is like *Sulphur* in these symptoms.

Silica has some pain in the stomach and bowels, but there is more soreness to pressure; colic and flatulence and tenderness to pressure; a chronic soreness in the stomach and if it goes on too long, a tubercular state comes on. Abdominal pain relieved by heat; distension of the bowels with flatulence and rumbling. Enlarged abdomen in children and adults (*Bar. c.*); tightness across the abdomen. Disturbed by the pressure of the clothes and worse after eating; the decided feature is the amelioration from heat.

Constipation from inability of the rectum to expel the fæces. It is seldom that the stool lies in the rectum without urging like *Alumina;* there is much urging to stool but inability to expel. The stool may be in small balls or large and soft or large and hard, but there is much straining and sweating about the head and great suffering while straining; the rectum becomes impacted, he strains until he is weak and exhausted, *the stool slips back;* and he gives up in despair. The only way he can relieve himself is by some mechanical method. Great straining at stool belongs to many remedies, but especially to *Alumina, Alumen, China, Natr. mur., Nux vom., Nux mosch.,* and Silica.

Silica has removed tape-worm, when the symptoms agree (*Calc., Sul.*).

It has also cured fistulous openings. Patients who have a tendency to phthisis are subject to abscesses about the region of the rectum, that break inside or out and form complete or incomplete openings. These seem to take the place of what would otherwise come, and if healed by operation or other external means, the tendency is to end in chest trouble, either in form of a fixed catarrh or tubercular infiltrations. Silica is one of the remedies that turns the constitution into order and in one to five years the opening ceases to be necessary and it will heal. Surgeons heal it up at once, and for a time the patient is comfortable, but in a few years he breaks down.

Caust., Berb., Calc. c., Calc. phos., Graph., Sulph., etc., are suitable in such cases. Silica here follows *Thuja* well.

Suppurative conditions in the urinary tract, catarrh of the mucous membranes; old inveterate catarrh of the bladder with pus and blood in the urine; copious, stringy deposits in the urine. Prostatitis, suppuration, thick, fœtid pus from the urethra. Gonorrhœa, pus, or pus-like discharge from the urethra, slight, shreddy discharge, bloody, pufulent discharge. It is sometimes thick, or is curdy; this is from any mucous membrane.

Abscesses along the penis, in the perineum, prostate gland, testes.

Chronic inflammation and induration of the testes with much pain; testes feel as if squeezed, sensitive, painful. Hydrocele in boys or adults.

In the male, impotence, weakness of the genitals after coition, easily exhausted, lacks power; exhausted if he has coition with anything like ordinary frequency; it takes him a week or ten days to rest up (*Agar.*). Much sweating of the genitals with exhaustion, tired out in the spine, weak back.

Involuntary discharge of urine at night; enuresis in little boys and girls.

In women a prostrated condition of the sexual functions. Serous cysts in the vagina, fistulous openings and abscesses about the vulva, which heal with hard nodules or do not heal at all; little oozing fistulæ, offensive, cheesy discharge. They heal in little nodules and then break out again in the same nidus. Women who are subject to these abscesses.

Bloody discharge between the periods. In Silica there is very easy flow of blood from the uterus; a hæmorrhagic flow comes on before the menses from excitement, and especially when nursing; when the child is put to the breast a flow of blood starts. Notice the distinction between *Calc.* and Silica. *Calc.* has a tendency to flow during lactation, but not when the child is put to the breast.

Silica cures hydrosalpinx and pyosalpinx, with copious, watery discharge from the uterus. Sometimes a woman has a lump on one or the other side of the uterus, which steadily increases and all at once there is a flooding of watery, bloody, purulent fluid and the lump disappears, soon to fill up again and empty in the same way in a gushing flow. Such are the manifestations of hydrosalpinx and pyosalpinx.

Entire absence of the menses for months; amenorrhœa.

Serous cysts in the vagina as large as a pea or an orange, projecting from the vagina or projecting upwards and flattened out in conformation with it. Many little cysts like hickory-nuts grouped together. *Rhod.* and Silica have cured these even when there is a paucity of other symptoms.

"Leucorrhœa, profuse, acrid, corroding, milky, preceded by cutting around the navel, causing biting pain, especially after acrid food; during urination; in gushes; with cancer of the uterus. Hard lumps in the mammæ."

Threatened abscesses of the breasts. If the remedy is given in time, it will abort the entire trouble. Where the remedy has come too late and suppuration is inevitable, Silica comes in for its share. There may be throbbing, tenderness, and weight, yet the remedy controls the pain, hastens the conclusion, and the opening comes naturally, discharges little and closes at once. As sure as an anodyne is given, a hot poultice applied, you will fail with your remedies. There is too much blood in the part, and the application of a poultice increases the trouble; it causes an increased determination of blood to the part, and if suppuration takes place it causes more breaking down of tissue. Instead of a thimbleful of pus you will have cupfuls for days and half of the gland is destroyed.

Women who are so weak they tend to abort, or no conception takes place. It would seem if the organs were tired out and unable to perform their functions.

The infant has all sorts of troubles. It grows up sickly; cannot tolerate its mother's milk or indeed any kind of food; vomiting and diarrhœa. A healthy child will digest even unwholesome milk.

The Silica cough is a dangerous one; the remedy suits the early stage of phthisis, when the lung is not extensively involved; it suits a cough of catarrhal character when the symptoms agree. If there is a small abscess in the lung with no tendency to heal, it brings about repair, causes contraction of its walls. Inveterate cases of catarrh of the chest with asthmatic wheezing, overexertion. After violent exertion and overheating, gets in a draft, or takes cold from a bath, becomes chilled. Humid asthma, coarse rattling, the chest seems filled with mucus, seems as if he would suffocate. Especially the asthma of old sycotics, or in children of sycotic parents. It competes with *Natr. sul.* in such cases. The patient is pale, waxy, anæmic, with great prostration and thirst.

Asthmatic attacks from suppressed gonorrhœa, with liability to develop complaints from over-exertion and over-heating, as in most sycotics.

Dry, teasing cough with hoarseness, threatening tuberculosis of the larynx, peculiar cracked voice from thickening of the laryngeal mucous membrane or tubercular involvement; soreness of the chest threatening miliary tuberculosis, with aggravation from cold and amelioration from warm drinks. Pulmonary affections in stone-cutters. The fine dust causes chronic irritation. Silica establishes a suppuration and throws off these particles of stone.

Expectoration profuse, fœtid, green, purulent; only during the day; viscid, milky, acrid mucus, at times pale, frothy blood.

Chronic tendency for colds to settle in the chest and bring on asthmatic symptoms. Chronic bronchitis; inflammation of the lungs with suppuration. Silica especially suits the later stages of pneumonia and the old, chronic complaints following pneumonia. Slow recovery after pneumonia (*Lyc., Sulph., Phos.,* Sil., *Calc.*). Flushes, rattling in the chest. Flushes in the face during the day (*Sulph., Sep., Lach.*), rattling like *Ant. tart.,* flushes like *Sulph.* and *Lyc.*

Phthisis; thick, yellow, green, fœtid sputa, more pronounced coldness than *Calc* and head sweat, pains in the lungs, sore lungs, stitches.

In the extremities we have inflammation of the periosteum. Corns (*Ant. cr., Graph.*). Ingrowing toe-nails. Rheumatism of the soles of the feet. Cannot walk (*Ant. cr., Med., Ruta,* Sil.).

Begins to sweat as soon as he falls asleep (*Puls., Con.*).

Epilepsy; aura in the solar plexus creeping into the chest and stomach. Complementary to *Calc, Puls.,* and *Thuja.*

SPIGELIA ANTHELMINTICA

Spigelia is especially known by its pains. It is indicated in persons who are debilitated from taking cold and who have become rheumatic, run down, victims of pain. Hardly a nerve in the body escapes; shooting, burning, tearing, neuralgic pains; they are most marked about the eyes and jaws, neck, face, teeth, shoulders, burning like hot needles through the face and neck in any direction, stitching, tearing, worse from motion, from doing anything, even thinking, mental exertion, worse from eating. Pains in the neck and shoulders are better from heat; those about the eyes are better from cold.

Shooting, tearing pains in the extremities like hot wires. Sometimes the pains are worse from lying down, but most commonly better from keeping still; worse from light, eating, motion, jarring; so sore in the painful region that any gentle exercise like going up or down stairs, or riding in a carriage that jars, makes the pain unbearable.

The Spigelia patient is sensitive to cold, to atmospheric changes, he is a rheumatic patient, but the nerves are attacked by neuralgia.

Violent pains about the eyes. Routine practice limits the use of the remedy to this region. Worse from hard pressure though sometimes better from it, if gentle and prolonged, firm pressure, but any movement of the pressing hand aggravates. The part is turgesced and inflamed. Eyes red and engorged.

Neuralgic affections of the muscles of the chest. Many of the Spigelia pains in the chest are attributed to the heart, but there is intercostal neuralgia; tearing pains shooting into the shoulders and neck, especially the left side and down the arm. Pains shooting hither and thither.

Irregularity of the heart. Painful complaints associated with valvular troubles, especially growing out of rheumatism. Pericarditis and endocarditis of rheumatic character. Thrusting pains in the chest like a knife, in the eye like a knife.

This remedy needs further proving, its mental symptoms are scarcely known. "Weak memory; disinclination to work; restless and anxious, solicitude about the future; gloomy, suicidal mood; afraid of pointed things, pins, etc.; easily irritated or offended." This is all that is thought worthy of admission into the Guiding Symptoms, showing that the mental state has not been well brought out.

Many complaints are manifested in the morning; tired in the morning and full of tearing pains.

Old anæmic subjects where there has been a transfer of the complaints to the nerves; broken down, pallid, nervous, with neuralgia, palpitation, irregular pulse. Vertigo on rising; gets up with violent pains and dizziness. So nervous that she must "fly," full of excitement, cannot keep still, cannot keep control of herself.

Pulsating and stitching in the head; sometimes better lying with the head high; worse from stooping, motion, and from noise. Sometimes better from washing in cold water when the pain is about the eyes and head, but worse after washing; better while the cold water is applied. With these headaches and neuralgias there is stiff neck and shoulders, an apparent stiffness in that he cannot move on account of pain. He sits in a chair as if transfixed, is aggravated from noise, light, from seeing things move in the room, which he must follow with his eyes. "Fine burning, tearing pains in the brain." It seems to be in the brain, but is more likely in the nerves of the scalp. "Violent pain in the left parietal bone on motion or walking or making a misstep; toward evening—violent pressure and pressing outward in the forehead, worse from stooping, worse from pressure with the hand; tensive tearing pain in the forehead, especially beneath the frontal eminence, extending towards orbitis." Notice the intensity of the pains. Burrowing, tearing pain in the occiput, in the left side of the vertex and forehead, worse from motion, from loud noise, and when he speaks loudly or even on opening the mouth slightly; better when lying down. Pressive pain in the right side of the forehead, involving the right eye, in the morning in bed, but still more after rising; pain deeply seated, unaffected by pressure, very acute on motion, on suddenly turning the head, the brain seemed to be loose; worse from every jar, step, or straining at stool. When moving the muscles of the face, there is a sensation as if the head would burst. Sensation as if a band were about the head. Neuralgic pain settles in and above the left eye, or below it, from cold in damp, rainy weather; hyperæsthesia of the filaments of the fifth pair.

On the pain first beginning, there is not so much hyperæsthesia, but as it goes on this increases and the eye becomes congested. I have seen the pains so severe that they produced perfect prostration, cold sweat, vomiting.

The *Hepar* patient is so sensitive to pain that he becomes unconscious; faints with the pain.

Cham. feels pain with such intensity that he gives way to violent frenzy, irritability, and outbursts of anger.

The Spigelia patient suffers intensely and the pain leaves its mark, the part becomes red and inflamed and sensitive. The head pains are worse from warmth; better temporarily from cold, the pains in other regions are the reverse.

The *Phos.* head and stomach symptoms are better from cold; the chest and body are better from warmth. In *Ars.* the head is often better by washing in cold water, while the patient himself is sensitive to the cold and wants warmth in the rest of his complaints.

Spigelia is full of visual symptoms; visual symptoms bring on complaints; at times he can do nothing but look straight ahead, for he has vertigo even when there is no pain, from looking downwards, everything goes round in a whirl. Such a state is common to many people when they look down from a height, but Spigelia has it from looking down along his nose, so he sits and looks straight ahead.

Esophoria; exophoria; disturbances in accommodation; all sorts of tiny spasmodic conditions; it is most difficult to fit glasses; no settled focus, no fixed vision. Spigelia has from a mere neuralgic state what *Ruta* has from eye strain. Latent errors of vision.

Eyes that are always changing need a remedy. Stabbing pains in and around the eye, often radiating in every direction from one point. Eye-ball sensitive to touch. Eyes worse when thinking about them. Worse at night. Intolerable, pressing pain, worse on turning the eye, dizzy on attempting to move the eyes, must turn the whole head to see. Pain radiates to the frontal sinuses and head. Sensation as if the eye were too large for its orbit.

I remember a patient who had been travelling about from oculist to oculist, who had many visual troubles and no glasses would suit. She had one sharp, stinging pain over the left eye day and night and she could only sleep when worn out. *Lac fel.* cured. Constant, fine, stinging pain over left eye was brought out by the provers of cat's milk.

This medicine has cured a pterygium, probably a false pterygium, that came from violent neuralgia, prolonged and lasting for months.

Stitching pains in the chest, worse from the least movement, breathing, sensation of tearing in the chest; trembling feeling in the chest when moving the arms or from any movement. Can lie only on the right side with the head high. Rheumatic troubles especially in the left side of the chest. Feeling as if the heart were compressed with a hand. Purring feeling over the region of the heart, wave-like motion not synchronous with the pulse. Waving palpitation not synchronous with the pulse. Trembling of the carotids. Acute pericarditis with anxiety and weight in the præcordium. These troubles following a rheumatic attack, at its close or many months after the fever has subsided. Spigelia is seldom indicated in rheumatism of the heart in phlegmatic persons who do not feel intensely.

When a rheumatic affection attacks the venous side of the heart, and there is a sense of stuffiness, of fulness through the whole body, limbs swollen, but do not pit on pressure, face mottled, it is a serious case and may end in Bright's disease and death.

SPONGIA TOSTA

The mental symptoms of Spongia show that it is a heart remedy. When a remedy produces the anxiety, fear, and dyspnœa found in Spongia, it will most likely turn out to be a cardiac remedy, unless these conditions are connected with irritation and inflammatory diseases of the brain. In this drug we find without any cerebral symptoms, marked anxiety, fear of death, and suffocation, associated with palpitation and uneasiness in the region of the heart. It is especially related to cases where there is pain and a sense of stuffiness and fulness in the cardiac region, in the chest, with dyspnœa, anxiety, fear of death, fear of the future, fear that something dreadful is going to happen. Wakens at night in great fear and it is some time before he can rationalize his surroundings (*Æsc., Lyc., Samb., Lach., Phos.,* and *Carbo veg.*).

Spongia is closely related to *Aconite,* which also excites the heart, brings on anxiety, fear, and restlessness, fear of death, predicts the hour of death, but this is associated with a marked febrile excitement. Spongia has febrile excitement in a minimum degree. It is much deeper in its action than *Aconite.* Its cardiac diseases tend to develop slowly, with actual tissue changes, enlargement of the heart, it takes on a steady growth and the valves become changed, do not fit, hence, there are blowing and whizzing sounds, regurgitation with the mental symptoms. The two are similar in croup, but Spongia is deeper, slower in onset, taking several days for its development. *Aconite* from exposure to a dry cold wind takes a cold today and, of course, comes down with croup to-night in the first sleep. Before midnight has a dry spasmodic cough; hoarse cough; Spongia has taken a cold yesterday or the day before. First there is roughness and dryness of the mucous membranes, sneezing. Both remedies have croup before midnight with dry, hoarse, harking cough, sawing respiration and dry air passages. They are so similar that when *Aconite* only partially controls the condition and it returns the next night, or lasts on beyond midnight, Spongia becomes its natural follower. Spongia comes in because it was probably the remedy in the beginning. Cases that grow worse each succeeding night, hoarse barking and crowing before midnight, though it also has a croup after midnight. It is a deep-acting remedy though its complaints sometimes come on suddenly.

Hepar is worse at night and in the morning. And when *Aconite has* apparently controlled, but the croup returns the next morning, *Hepar* comes in. Or if it comes on again the next evening with rattling *Hepar* will also be suitable. Dry, with no rattling is Spongia. If the child wants to be covered or says that it is chilly, *Hepar.* If it says the room is too warm and kicks the covers off, it needs *Calc. sul.*

The Spongia patient is worse from a warm room, from heat. Wants to be cool like *Iodine,* but is better from warm drinks, like *Ars., Nux, Lyc.*

The tendency to affect the glands is striking. As a matter of fact all the glands are affected; they gradually and become increasingly hard. Glands that have undergone inflammation and are increased in size become hard, or they take on hypertrophy. Hypertrophy of the heart (*Kalmia, Sepia, Naja*). Spongia has cured endocarditis, cardiac croup and many other inflammatory diseases of the heart resulting from rheumatism. Hypertrophy of the thyroid, goitre, when the heart is affected and the eyes protruding. Cervical glands enlarged; inveterate cases of enlarged testes; orchitis from a suppressed gonorrhœa, a cold or other causes; gradually increasing hardness.

The whole respiratory apparatus is acted upon; cardiac dyspnœa and the most severe forms of asthma: Dryness of the air passages with whistling and wheezing, seldom rattling, must sit up and bend forward; at times after great dyspnœa, white, tough mucus forms in the air passages, difficult to expectorate; it comes up and often has to be swallowed (*Arn., Caust., Lach., Kali c., Kali s., Nux mos., Sep., Staph.*).

Dyspnœa worse lying down. The modality is common to its other complaints; violent, basilar headache forces him to sit up in bed and keep still. Holding the head in the upright position relieves the dull pressure in the occiput.

There are many headaches. In the occiput, in the forehead, congestive headaches, but most of them are associated with goitre, cardiac affections and asthma; they are due, probably, to sluggish circulation in the brain.

Face distressed in croup; anxious; livid; pale and bloated; blue, pale with sunken eyes; red with anxious expression; alternating red and pale; cold sweat. These symptoms are the natural effects of difficult breathing and are, therefore, not essential in the selection of a remedy. As primary symptoms, they would probably indicate *Ars.,* but when due to cardiac difficulties, they are unimportant.

"Sore throat worse after eating sweet things. Thyroid gland swollen even with the chin; at night, suffocating spells, barking cough, with stinging in the throat and soreness in the abdomen" Enlargement of the tonsils. Difficult swallowing.

Spongia is the remedy when dyspnœa and cough are relieved by warm food; may be better from warm drinks.

Laryngeal troubles with great hoarseness, in individuals tending towards phthisis, with tubercular heredity, cachectic aspect, weak lungs, but no deposit of tubercle. But all at once hoarseness sets in. There is a tendency for the larynx to become involved in phthisical patients that need Spongia. This patient takes an acute cold and it settles in the larynx with hoarseness. Look out for that patient, for there is a tendency for tubercles to deposit where there is inflammation, and the infiltration instead of being fibrinous may become tubercular. Tendency for the larynx to be first involved in phthisical patients.

In Spongia do not look for the exudative, but the infiltrative form of croup..

Hoarseness with loss of voice, great dryness of the larynx from a cold; coryza, sneezing, the whole chest rings, is as dry as a horn; voice hissing, croupy, nose dry. There is very little accumulation of mucus, but at a late date ulceration begins and then there may be a copious expectoration of mucus. In proportion to the extent of rattling, this remedy is decreasingly indicated. *Hepar* has the coarse rattling with much mucus.

At times an adult takes cold and rawness of the larynx and trachea is the result. On going to bed she is taken with a spasmodic constriction of the larynx. Laryngismus stridulus is commonly found in women. *Ign., Gels., Lauroc.* and Spongia. *Ign.* and *Gels.* will cure eight out of ten cases.

The larynx is sensitive to touch in croup, etc., like *Phos.*

Dry, spasmodic cough, troublesome cough; cold things taken into the stomach aggravate. (*Veratr.* is better from cold water, but the cough is worse.) If the room becomes too warm, there is a dry, tickling, teasing, croupy spasmodic cough.

In cardiac and asthmatic troubles it resembles *Lach.,* in the rousing up from sleep in suffocation; after the sleep the dyspnœa is worse.

The *Phos.* dyspnœa is often increased after sleeping, with suffocation. *Lach.* has it in a marked degree; in phthisis when the patient is about to die, there is sweat on going to sleep; dyspnœa on going to sleep and on waking. *Lach.* palliates and must be repeated.

Cardiac affections accompanied with thick, green or yellow expectoration like pus and dyspnœa on falling to sleep so that he must keep awake as long as he can, fear of sleep in advanced chest troubles. *Grindelia robusta* will palliate such a case and if the condition is only catarrhal and not tuberculous, it will cure.

Study especially the cardiac symptoms. "The symptoms of circulation are worse; from mental lassitude, from coughing, from lying on the right side, before menses, after lying down, sitting bent forward, from smoking, from going up stairs. Awakens in fright and feels as if suffocating. Falling asleep early at night, suffocation awakens." I have mentioned these symptoms, but read them for emphasis.

Ebullitions, distended veins; dropsy in cavities of the body. Especially suits young persons of tubercular parents, who remain weak, are pallid and do not thrive. Tubercular diathesis.

Itching but no eruption. Seems always ready for an eruption to appear. Has only simplest herpetic eruptions. Itching all over and no visible eruption.

In acute endocarditis, the principal remedies are Spongia, *Abrot., Sepia,* and *Kalmia.* Naja in valvular diseases.

SQUILLA

Squilla was given in the olden times by the old school in all lung, bronchial, and kidney affections; pneumonia, asthma, scanty urine and dropsical affections.

Cough: Has a loose morning cough and a dry evening cough (*Alum., Carbo veg., Phos, ac., Sep., Stram., Puls.,* Squilla) *Puls.* and Squil., being strong here, but Squil. has a hard cough; coughs, gags, sneezes; urine escapes and quite frequently fæces; the patient coughs until he is covered with sweat; he gags and coughs and finally succeeds in raising two or three little lumps of white, tenacious mucus; it is a spasmodic cough caused by mucus in the trachea or a tickling, creeping sensation in the chest.

The loose morning cough is worse than the dry evening cough. Patient chilly; cannot have the least draft; wants plenty of clothing and is very sensitive to cold; not so in *Puls.* Urine is generally copious, watery, colorless.

About 11 A.M. to 12 or 1 P.M. there is the most dyspnœa from filling up of the chest with mucus; this same feeling returns during the hour, but it is from cardiac weakness. Copious, colorless urine is one of its important symptoms and resembles *Ign.,* but Squil. is not a hysterical patient like *Ign.* Quite similar to *Can. Ind.* or *Gels,* in brain affections, but Squil. has not many brain affections nor many febrile symptoms. *Phos.* has inflammation of the brain and when the dangerous turn comes this increase of urine is a bad sign. *Puls.* tearful, then copious urine. Squil. copious, colorless urine in diabetes; when this seems to disappear and chest symptoms appear, these troubles disappear and kidney troubles appear, these would disappear and dropsy comes up; when the urine would get copious again these dropsical symptoms would disappear and Squil. acts a long time.

There is a copious, colorless flow from the nose, more especially in the morning; the cough is similar to *Tart. emet.*

Squil. in its internal nature is quite like *Thuja* in regard to its spurting urine and its spasmodic cough; with the escape of urine there is more or less of escape of fæces of a dark brown or black fluid in frothy bubbles, very offensive, painless, involuntary.

Respiration difficult with stitches in the chest when breathing and coughing. Great dyspnœa, the child cannot drink; seizes the cup eagerly, but can drink only in sips; frequently obliged to take a deep breath which provokes a cough; shortness of breath on every exertion. Pains in the chest aggravated in the morning. Dull rheumatic pains aggravated when exercising; ameliorated while at rest. Evening dry cough with sweetish expectoration. Great heat in the body. Follows well after *Bry.* Absolute lack of sweat is a characteristic.

Dry cough at 11 P.M.. worse from cold water and cold air (*Rumex*). *Bell.* has cough at 11 P.M. worse from uncovering, red face, congestion in head. *Lach.* soon after going to sleep, which may be 11 P.M.

Nasal discharge acrid, corroding, worse in the morning; violent sneezing. Stool dark brown or black.

Seldom much cough during day. Pneumonia: Stitches when inhaling, jerking pains; always right side; catarrh of the chest and threatened pneumonia after hæmorrhage from the lungs. Soreness in the chest, worse from motion. *Bry.* will often palliate and the case will go into Squilla.

STANNUM METALLICUM

Stannum is especially suited to persons who have long been growing feeble. This is so striking that it may be said that some deep-seated constitutional state must be present. There is a history of increasing weakness, cachexia, catarrhal conditions, and neuralgia dating back over years. There is sensitiveness to pain and an increasing aversion to doing anything, aversion to business in a man, and in a woman, to going about her housework; always tired, all work becomes irksome.

The countenance becomes increasingly sallow, even to a waxy, cachectic aspect. One who has been growing weaker and develops neuralgia of the face, eyes, stomach, and intestines; not the shooting, tearing pains often described, but a pain beginning gradually, increasing steadily and then disminishing gradually. The pain sometimes begins with sunrise, increases until noon and gradually diminishes, and ceases with sunset. On the other hand, it may begin at any time, as often at 10 A.M.. and increasing for ten or twenty minutes, then gradually decrease until gone. A few other remedies have these sun headaches. *Kalmia* has a similar headache, not so regularly increasing and diminishing, but especially worse at noon. *Cactus* has a sun headache. *Natrum mur* has never been known to cause it, but has cured it, especially when beginning at 10 A.M. and worse from 2 to 3 P.M. *Sang.* has headache coming and going with the sun.

The phthisical tendency of Stannum is closely allied to the neuralgias. If these patients settle down into a neuralgic constitution, the deposit of tubercles is postponed, but most of them then seek palliation with the inevitable result of hastening the end. If the Stannum neuralgia is suppressed, we will see phthisis making its appearance, particularly phthisis pituitosa. Nature seems to be able to throw off effects through mucous discharges. If

the neuralgia is not permitted to have sway the patient becomes oversensitive
to cold, takes cold easily. When let alone every cold settled in the nerves and
every draft caused neuralgias about the eyes, sensitive to every change in
the wea er, the hydrogenoid constitution of Grauvogl. But when palliated in
any way by *Quinine* and inappropriate homœopathic remedies that have the
tendency to catch cold in the chest like *Phos.,* he after a while does not get
over his cold, but there is a continuous catarrh of the chest, and later he will
die of miliary tuberculosis Stannum is useful in warding off phthisis, and is a
wonderful palliative in that disease.

The pain has been likened to the pulling of a string, gradually increasing
and gradually letting up.

The *Puls.* pain is somewhat similar in its first half; it gradually becomes
intense, but suddenly lets up with a snap; comes gradually and stops suddenly.

Remember what is said about the *Bell. pain.* It comes suddenly and reaches
its intensity at once, where it may remain for hours, but ceases suddenly.

The Stannum pain is at times so severe that there is a throbbing pulsating intermingled with it, and the mind seems stunned.

"Headache every morning, over one or the other eye, mostly the left,
gradually extending over the whole forehead and increasing and decreasing
gradually, often with vomiting." "Violent, glowing, beating pain." It is
sometimes attended with burning. "Felt as if the head would burst with inward
blows. Neuralgia of the left eye gradually increasing from 10 A.M. to noon,
then gradually decreasing, with lachrymation during pain. Intermittent supra-
orbital neuralgia from 10 A.M. to 3 or 4 P.M., gradually increasing and attaining
its acme, and then again gradually decreasing, after the abuse of quinine."
This is when the body is weak, with sallow countenance and tendency to
phthisis, full of pain, and the earlier history shows that instead of taking cold
in the chest or nose, as others take cold, every cold settles in the nerves.
Finally he begins to take cold in the chest, with dyspnœa, violent, racking
cough, gagging, retching, vomiting, and the most intense sufferings. Copious,
thick, yellow-green, bloody expectoration, which tastes sweetish (*Phos.*).
Retching when coughing is marked; thick, white, yellow or green tenacious
mucus. Cannot walk, cannot do anything without cough. Always tired; it is an
effort to work. Wakens in the morning with the chest filled with mucus, and
coughs and expectorates, and yet some remains; he gags, retches and vomits,
and it strings out of the mouth *tasting sweetish,* sometimes salty or sour.

This great weakness is manifested in the voice; hoarseness, loss of voice;
the vocal cords will not respond; a paralytic weakness. Talking makes him
feel weak, especially in the chest. "Hoarseness, weakness, emptiness in the
chest on beginning to sing, so that she was constantly obliged to stop and
take a deep breath; at times a few expulsive coughs removed the hoarseness

for a few minutes. Rawness in the larynx." Rawness in the trachea and smarting all the way down when coughing. Irritation to cough, as from mucus in the trachea; or breathing, with cough either loose or dry, felt more while sitting bent over than when walking. "Accumulation of great quantities of mucus in the trachea, easily thrown off by coughing. Oppressed breathing from ascending, from the slightest movement, when lying down, in the evening, from coughing." "Cough in fatiguing paroxysms; epigastric region painful as if beaten; violent, shattering, deep, short, from time to time, as from weakened chest, with a hoarse, weak sound. Cough caused by talking, singing, laughing, lying on the side and from drinking anything warm." "Sputa like white of egg; yellow, green pus; sweetish, putrid, sour or saltish during day. Chest so weak that he cannot talk; empty feeling in the chest." This remedy is frequently indicated in cases where the routinist would prescribe *Bry.*, etc., in low potencies to loosen the cough. Stannum is not dangerous in phthisis, and will palliate the case if it is incurable. It will not rouse up the whole economy like *Silica,* but there may be an aggravation of the nervous symptoms; if there is anything to build on it will cause the patient to rally. If it brings back his old neuralgic pains, and you know he has not a long time to live, and seems to suffer much, *Puls.* is the natural antidote.

When a loose, easy cough is turned into one that is violent, dry and racking under Stannum, and seems to be inclined to be prolonged, *Puls.* will restore the loose cough. This is not a good action of the remedy; in incurable cases you can get the best results by not going too high.

Another feature is seen in women. If you ever meet with a case who has suffered with violent neuralgia and she says since the obliteration of these pains she has had a copious, thick, yellow, green leucorrhœa, think of Stannum. There is great weakness, which seems to proceed from the chest. The leucorrhœa has saved her from consumption.

Menses too early and too profuse; bearing down in the uterine region; prolapsus uteri and vaginæ.

Paralytic symptoms; writers' cramp; women cannot let go of the broom (*bros.* cures most cases).

"Constipation; stools hard, dry, knotty, or insufficient and green." Inactive rectum, *i.e.,* a paralytic state; even though there is much urging there is inability to pass the stool, which at times is soft. Colic better from pressure, lying on the stomach (*Coloc., Cupr.*); worse from motion; better from bending double.

"Very much exhausted from talking or reading aloud. Great lassitude from walking; weariness of the whole body, especially when ascending stairs; great sense of weakness in larynx and chest, thence all over the body; trembling worse from slow exercise."

STAPHISAGRIA

The mental symptoms are very important, and the impressions made. upon the mind and thence upon the body guide to Staphisagria as a remedy Excitable, easily aroused to anger, but seldom irascible, that is, easily disturbed and excited, but seldom manifests it. Suitable in cases where complaints come from pent up wrath, suppressed anger, suppressed feelings. The person becomes speechless from suppressed indignation; anger with indignation. Complaints brought on by these causes; irritable bladder with frequent urging to urinate, lasting many days after suppressed wrath, after insults. "Great indignation about things done by others or by himself; grieves about consequences."

A gentleman comes in contact with one beneath his station and an altercation takes place, an argument which ends in insult, and the gentleman turns his hack on the other. He goes home and suffers; he does not speak it out, but controls it and then suffers from it. He has sleepless nights and many days of fatigue, brain-fag; for days and weeks he cannot add nor subtract, makes mistakes in writing and speaking, has irritability of the bladder, colic, etc. Loss of memory with a sense of weight between the eyes; it is difficult to say whether this is a feeling in the head or an effort to describe a dulness of mind. Feels as if a ball of wood were in the forehead, or as if the whole cerebrum were made of wood; it feels numb. It is difficult to state whether it is a condition of the mind or head. Accompanying this sensation of a lump in the forehead is a feeling as if the whole back of the head were hollow; the patient may describe it as a feeling of numbness or a lack of sensation.

"Indifferent, low-spirited, dulness of mind after onanism." Staph. cures these conditions when they are the result of sexual excitement, masturbation, excesses in venery, allowing the mind to dwell too much on venereal subjects. Thinking on sexual relations. These patients are irritable, easily fatigued, most excitable, and when they have to control their emotions.; they suffer intensely. One who is in health can easily put aside a controversy, knowing that he has done what is right, but a Staph. patient when he has to control himself goes all to pieces, trembles from head to foot, loses his voice, his ability to work, cannot sleep and a headache follows.

Many a time a man has come into my office with blue lips, trembling hands, pains about the heart and all over, and he thinks he is going to die. He tells a story of an altercation and pent up wrath, and Staph. stops his trembling and quiets him. Without it he would have sleepless nights, brain-fag, prostration and headache. This state belongs especially to those who have indulged in sexual excesses.

Now, the next step. The senses are in this same irritable state, so that the tips of the fingers are sensitive, the ears are sensitive to noise, the tongue is sensitive to tastes and the nose to odors; so sensitive that everything is painfully sensated. Every little inflamed spot will have in its center sensitive points, little nerve spots; ulcers when touched cause the patient to go all to pieces and a convulsion threatens.

Hæmorrhoidal tumors are so sensitive that they cannot be touched. Little aerve tumors form in the skin, little polypoid growths the size of a wheat grain and denuded of epithelium, covered with moisture, red, inflamed, blue, and a mere touch will throw the patient into convulsions and suffering for days and nights. A hyper-sensitive nerve growth will come out on the hand or on the back. Sometimes it turns black. Again, a little wart will come out, especially about the genitals and anus, little caruncular growths about the urethra and vagina, so sensitive that if nipped between the fingers the patient will go into spasms, especially if a woman.

Staph. suits all three of the miasms.

These nervous stares run all through the complaints. Look for a case of Staph. where the whole mind and nervous system are in a fret.

The Staph. headache is a numb, dull pain in the occiput and forehead, especially in these nervous constitutions. "Sensation as of a round ball in the forehead, sitting firmly there even when shaking the head." Headaches from vexation and indignation.

Crusty, squamous eruptions on the scalp. "Painful sensitiveness of the scalp, skin peels off, with itching and smarting, worse in the evening and from getting warm." The scales are lifted up by a watery exudate and the denuded surface is extremely sensitive to touch.

New growths about the lids and balls of the eyes, extremely painful to the touch. Meibomian tumors (*Con., Thuja*), in irritable children (*Kreos.*).

Another feature in Staph. is its action on the glands; scrofulous glands: glands of the neck enlarge; enlarged and indurated ovaries and testes stitching, tearing pains in the glands everywhere. Hardness and chronic induration.

Stitching, tearing pains along the course of the nerves; in the heart, and as in such a nervous patient the mind is likely to he on the heart, the stitching pains in the intercostals are supposed to be in the heart. Stitching pains directly through the chest to the back.

Swelling of the tonsils after the abuse of *Mercury*. Chronic tonsillitis, Tonsils are not large but hard from previous attacks of acute tonsillitis; strumous diathesis; cross and irritable. "Pains come on after eating."

The Staph. patient has much difficulty in the bowels. Subject to chronic diarrhœa and to constipation. Colic, twitching, tearing pains in the abdomen. Diarrhœa from cold water, from eating, from indignation, anger, with flatulence of a terribly offensive odor like spoiled eggs. "Chronic diarrhœa or dysentery of weakly, sickly children after anger; after being punished, after emotions." (*Coloc.* and *Cham.*)

Staph. and *Coloc.* resemble each other. In both, eating and drinking cause griping and stool, both have colic as if stones were squeezing; Staph. in the intestines, head and testes; *Coloc.* in the intestines and ovaries; both are worse from anger. *Caust,.Coloc.* and Staph. follow each other like *Sulph, Calc.* and *Lyc.*

It often happens that nervous women soon after marriage are attacked with frequent and painful urging to urinate which becomes extremely troublesome and may last many days. Staph. is very comforting to the young wife. Great teasing and tearing all night long; bloody urine; involuntary discharge of urine, acrid and corroding, with burning, worse from motion. Profuse discharge of pale urine with burning and urging. Burning during and after urination.

Staph. has cured enlarged prostate with frequent urging to urinate, especially in old men; continued teasing with dribbling. "Frequent urging to urinate, with scanty discharge in thin stream or discharge of urine in drops;" may be followed by a sensation as if the bladder were not fully emptied.

The most distressing symptom of the male genitals is excitability, but there is also impotence, great weakness of the sexual organs; the sexual desire is greatly increased but there is impotence. Useful in the results of secret vice, long practiced. "Seminal emissions followed by great chagrin and mortification, prostration, dyspnœa. Effects of onanism or sexual excesses; loss of memory, hypochondriasis, taciturnity, face sunken, abashed look, nocturnal emissions, backache, weak legs, relaxed organs, deficiency of vital heat and tendency to take cold, deep sunken, red, and lusterless eyes, hair falls out; loss of prostatic fluid and impairment of sexual desire; dull and contusive pains in the testicles, voluptuous itching of the scrotum, atrophy of the testicles." Think of the extremely nervous patient.

Dry, sensitive warts about the genitals, from sycosis or from the abuse of *Mercury,* which causes a tendency to warty growths. Moist, red offensive warts belong to *Thuja.*

The testes dwindle as well as become inflamed and swollen; genitals waste away.

Sensation as if there were worms crawling over him. Crawling, etc., in the female external genitals, *Coff., Plat.,Petrol., Apis, Tarant. Hisp.,* the latter has: While outer parts feel as if insects were biting and crawling, better from heat or cold.

In the female there is violent sexual excitement, nymphomania with extreme mental and physical impressions; mind has been dwelling too much on sexual subjects. "Very sharp, shooting pains in the ovary, which is exquisitely sore to touch; pains extend along crural regions and thighs.

Menses irregular, late and profuse, sometimes wanting; first of pale blood, then dark and clotted. Scorbutic diathesis, vegetations of the vagina; stinging, itching of the vulva."

Stitching in the region of the heart; trembling of the body with nervous excitement is an excellent indication for Staph.

Effects from loss of blood, shock, from surgical operations, injuries from sharp instruments, incised wounds. Stinging, etc., in surgical wounds, cuts; colic after lithotomy, urging to stool, qualmishness, worse from drinking.

Tetter on the hands, itches and burns in the evening after scratching; numbness in the tips of the fingers; arthritic nodosities on the fingers. I remember a patient suffering from gouty nodosities; he had lived a life of peculiar continence, dwelling on his vices, broken down in body. Staph. brought out an eruption on his legs as high up as the knees that looked like a pair of trousers. One continuous coat of crusts which lasted a year before it dwindled, but he was greatly improved in his body and his enlarged joints gradually improved. The eruption was yellow, crusty, tough, leathery, and, when lifted up by the moisture beneath, it had to be cut off like a bandage; he was practically crippled; new crops came out on the parts clipped off. It was with difficulty that he walked, for the crusts cut him.

Bone troubles, exostoses, inflammation of the periosteum.

Acute articular rheumatism of fast or debilitated men, with shifting pains. Mercurial bone diseases, ulcers, caries, injuries caused by sharp, cutting instruments. Nightly bone pains.

Asaf., Merc., Sil.

STRAMONIUM

When considering Stram. the idea of violence comes into mind. One cannot look upon a patient who needs Stram., or who has been poisoned with it, without wondering at the tremendous turmoil, the great upheaval taking place in mind and body. Full of excitement, rage, everything is tumultuous, violent; the face looks wild, anxious, fearful; the eyes are fixed on a certain object; face flushed, hot raging fever with hot head and cold extremities, violent delirium. In his anxiety he often turns away from the light, wants it dark, is aggravated especially if the light is bright. High fever with delirium; the heat is so intense that it may be mistaken for *Bell.,* but it is usually a continued fever, only at times remittent, while the intense fever of *Bell.* is remittent always.

Stram. is like an earthquake in its violence. The mind is in an uproar; cursing, tearing the clothes, violent speech, frenzy, erotomania, exposing of the person. These symptoms are found in continued fevers, insanity, cerebral congestion. It is useful in violent typhoids.

It is useful in mania that has existed for some time; attacks of mania coming on in paroxysms, appearing with more or less suddenness, so that a single attack would look like *Bell.*, but the history differentiates. *Bell.* would hardly be more than a palliative in the first attack, and the second exhibition of it would do nothing.

When the delirium is not on, the patient has the appearance of great suffering, forehead wrinkled, face pallid, sickly, haggard. In head-pains this anxious look, indicative of intense suffering from meningeal involvement.

"Delirium bland, murmuring; violent, foolish, joyful, loquacious, incoherent chattering with open eyes; vivid; merry with spasmodic laughter: furious, raving, wild; attempts to stab and bite; with queerest notions; with sexual excitement; fear as if a dog were attacking him."

Strange ideas about the formation of his body, that it is ill-shapen, elongated, deformed; strange feelings concerning his physical state. All sorts of illusions and hallucinations. One must distinguish between these states. An illusion is an apperance in the vision or mind which the patient knows is not true. A hallucination is a state that appears to be true. A delusion is a more advanced state, when the patient thinks it is true and cannot he reasoned out of it. Fear and great anxiety on hearing running water.

He sees animals, ghosts, angels, departed spirits, devils, and knows they are not real, but later he is confident of it. He has these hallucinations especially in the dark. At times he has an aversion to a bright light which is painful, and again he must sit and look into an open fire, but this may cause cough and other symptoms.

"Sings amorous songs and utters obscene speech. Crazy with distress, jumps out of bed, acts as if the bed were being drawn from under him. Screams until he is hoarse or loses his voice. Screeches and screams day and night with fever, with forms of mania. Hasty, hurries with all his might if he wants to go to another place." Violent laughter with sardonic expression on his face.

"Child awakens terrified, knows no one, screams with fright, clings to those near."

Hyosc. has wild, maniacal delirium, but with very little fever. In Stram. there is considerable fever. In *Bell.* the fever is in the afternoon and evening, 9 P.M. to 3 A.M., and then a remission.

Violent convulsions involving every muscle of the body, opisthotonos, violent distortions, contraction of the limbs, biting of the tongue and bleeding from the passages. During spasms, covered with cold sweat; sometimes almost as cold as ice; cold sweat in mania; this feature is equalled only by *Camphor.*

Hysterical convulsions of long standing, associated with spinal trouble; worse from fright. Convulsions in nervous, excitable people brought on by fright.

Puerperal convulsions and insanity. It has the septic nature. Those cases going on for a while as melancholic, low spirited; she believes she has sinned away her day of grace, yet she has lived an upright life; sad; imagines strange things, does strange things, until finally violent delirium comes on; she screams aloud; exhorts people to repent; face red, and eyes flashing; exhorts and prays in incoherent speech. In such cases Stram. should be compared with *Veratr.*

In cerebral congestions, the delirium subsides into unconsciousness; the patient has the appearance of profound intoxication; pupils dilated or contracted (in *Bell.* they are dilated). Marked stupor, stertorous breathing, lower jaw dropped. So in typhoid and the low forms of fever, fœtor, oozing of blood from the mouth and other passages. Throat and month dry; tongue dry, swollen, so that it fills the mouth, pointed, red like a piece of meat, bleeding from the mouth, sordes on the teeth, lips dry and cracked; at times violent thirst yet dread of water. Diarrhœa copious, involuntary; abdomen tympanitic, involuntary urination.

Basilar meningitis from suppressed ear-discharge. The Old School have no remedy for such cases. Forehead wrinkled, eyes glassy, staring, dilated pupils and scarcely any fever; awful pain through the base of the skull and there is a history of necrosis about the ear.

Violent headache from walking in the sun, and from the hear of the sun. Aggravated all day and at night the patient must sit up because of increased pain on lying down; he is worse from every motion or jar;. eyes fixed and glassy, face flushed, but later it is pale, eyes fixed on a corner of the room, motionless; delirium, says strange things. Pain in the occiput.

High grade inflammation which it carries to the finish. Pus forms abscesses with excruciating pain (*Hepar, Merc., Sil., Sulph.*). Violent catarrhal inflammations, vicious, septic states. Chronic abscesses, carbuncles, boils, abscesses in the joints, the left hip-joint is a special locality. You will often be able to abort a case of hip-disease, and even when pus is present or fistulous openings have formed it is very useful. Fulness, suppuration, and pain in the cartilages.

Stram. stands alone among the deep acting remedies, in its violence of mental symptoms.

Stram. cures eye troubles and irritation of the brain from overstudy; in students who are obliged to do much night work to keep up with day lectures. The patient seems almost blind; there is much pain in the eyes in dim light, relieved in intense light. The mental symptoms, cough, headache, etc., are worse from light.

"Dryness of throat and fauces, not benefited by any sort of drink,
Swallowing difficult and impeded with stinging pain in the throat, with
pain in the submaxillary glands with convulsions; particularly fluids from
constriction of throat." Choking on attempting to swallow water. It has done
some good work in hydrophobia. (*Hyosc., Bel., Canth., Hydroph.*)

In old cases of suppuration of the lungs where the cough is worse from
looking into the light, Strain. is often a great palliative and causes no
aggravation.

Retention of urine, cannot pass it if he ceases to strain; old men who have
lost power over the bladder, stream flows slowly, cannot make haste.

Cardiac affections with great constriction of the chest, mental irritability,
delusions as to personal identity, inability to sleep in the dark, great anxiety
when on a train going through a tunnel, pulse irregular, heart feeble.

Sleep full of dreams and turmoil.

SULPHUR

Sulphur is such a full remedy that it is somewhat difficult to tell where to
begin. It seems to contain a likeness of all the sicknesses of man, and a
beginner on reading over the proving of Sulphur might naturally think that he
would need no other remedy, as the image of all sickness seems to be contained
in it. Yet you will find it will not cure all the sicknesses of man, and it is not
well to use it indiscriminately any more than you would any other remedy. It
seems that the less a physician knows of the Materia Medica the oftener he
gives Sulphur, and yet it is very frequently given, even by good prescribers
so that the line between physicians' ignorance and knowledge cannot be
drawn from the frequency with which Sulphur is prescribed by them.

The Sulphur *patient* is a lean, lank; hungry, dyspeptic fellow with stoop
shoulders, yet many times it must be given to fat, rotund, well-fed people.
The angular, lean, stoop-shouldered patient, however. is the typical one, and
especially when he has become so from long periods of indigestion, bad
assimilation and feeble nutrition. The Sulphur state is sometimes brought
about by being long housed up and adapting the diet to the stomach. Persons
who lead sedentary lives, confined to their rooms in study, in meditation, in
philosophical inquiry, and who take no exercise, soon find out that they must
eat only the simplest foods, foods not sufficient to nourish the body, and
they end up by going into a philosophical mania.

There is another class of patients in whom we see a Sulphur appearance
in the face; dirty, shrivelled, red-faced people. The skin seems to be easily
affected by the atmosphere. He becomes red in the face from riding in the air,

both in very cold and in damp weather. He has a delicate, thin skin, blushing on the slightest occasion, *always red and dirty looking,* no matter how much he washes it. If it be a child, the mother may wash the face often, but it always looks as if it had been perfunctorily washed.

Hering called the Sulphur patient *"the ragged philosopher".* The Sulphur scholar, the inventor, works day and night in threadbare clothes and battered hat; he has long, uncut hair and a dirty face; his study is uncleanly, it is untidy; hooks and leaves of books are piled up indiscriminately; there is no order. It seems that Sulphur produces this state of disorder, a state of untidiness, a state of uncleanliness, a state of "don't care how things go," and a state of selfishness. He becomes a *false philosopher,* and the more he goes on in this state the more he is disappointed because the world does not consider him the greatest man on earth. Old inventors work and work, and fail. The complaints that arise in this kind of case, even the acute complaints, will run to Sulphur. You take such a patient and you will notice that he has on a shirt that he has worn many weeks; if he has not a wife to attend to him, he would wear his shirt until it fell off from him.

Cleanliness is not a great idea with the Sulphur patient; he thinks it is not necessary. *He is dirty;* he does not see the necessity of putting on a clean collar and cuffs and a clean shirt; it does not worry him. Sulphur is seldom indicated in cleanly people, but it is commonly indicated in those who are not disturbed by uncleanliness. When attending the public clinic I have many times noticed that after Sulphur an individual begins to take notice of himself and puts on a clean shirt, whereas his earlier appearances were in the one same old shirt. And it is astonishing how the Sulphur patients, especially the little ones, can get their clothing dirty so fast. Children have the most astonishing tendency to be filthy. Mothers tell you of the filthy things that little ones will do if they be Sulphur patients. The child is subject to 'catarrhal discharges from the nose, the eyes and from other parts, and he often eats the discharge from the nose. Now, that is peculiar, because offensive odors are the things that the Sulphur patient loathes. He is *oversensitive to filthy odors,* bur filthy substances themselves he will eat and swallow. He becomes nauseated even from the odor of his own body and of his own breath. The odor of the stool is so offensive that it will follow him around all day. He thinks he can smell it. Because of his sensitiveness to odors he is more cleanly about his bowels than anything else. It is an exaggerated sense of smell. He is always imagining and hunting for offensive odors. He has commonly such a strong imagination that he smells the things which he has only in memory.

The Sulphur patient has *filthiness* throughout. He is the victim of *filthy odors.* He has a filthy breath, he has an intensely fœtid stool; he has filthy-smelling genitals, which can be smelled in the room in spite of his clothing, and he himself smells them. The discharges are always more or less fœtid, having strong, offensive Odors. In spite of constant washing the axillæ give out a pungent odor, and at times the whole body gives off an odor like that coming from the axillæ.

The *discharges* of Sulphur from every part of the body, besides being offensive, are *excoriating*. The Sulphur patient is afflicted with *catarrhs of all mucous membranes,* and the catarrhal discharges everywhere excoriate him. Often with the coryza the discharge excoriates the lips and the nose. At times the fluid that remains in the nose smarts like fire, and when it comes in contact with the child's lip it burns, so acrid is it; almost-like the condition under *Sulphuric acid,* so red will be the parts that are touched by it. There is copious leucorrhœa that excoriates the genitals. The thin fæces cause burning and rawness around the anus. In women if a drop of urine remains about the genitals it will burn; very often it is not sufficient to wipe it away, it must be washed away to relieve the smarting. In children we find excoriation about the anus and between the buttocks; the whole length of the fissure is red, raw and inflamed from the stool. From this tendency a keynote has been constructed, and not a bad one either, "all the fluids burn the parts over which they pass," which is the same as saying that the fluids are acrid and cause smarting. This is true everywhere in Sulphur.

The Sulphur patient has all sorts of *eruptions*. There are vesicular, pustular, furuncular, scaly eruptions, all attended *with much itching,* and some of them with discharge and suppuration. The skin, even without any eruption, itches much, itches from the warmth of the bed and from wearing woolen clothing. Many times the Sulphur patient cannot wear anything except silk or cotton. The warmth of the room will drive him to despair if he cannot get at the itching part to scratch it. After scratching there is burning with relief of the itching. After scratching or after getting into the warmth of the bed great white welts come out all over the body, with much itching, and these he keeps on scratching until the skin becomes raw, or until it burns, and then comes a relief of the itching. This process goes on continuously; dreadful itching at night in bed, and in the morning when he wakes up he starts in again and the eruptions itch and ooze. Crops of boils and little boil-like eruptions come out and this makes it useful in impetigo.

This remedy is useful in *suppurations*. It establishes all sorts of suppurating cavities, small abscesses and large abscesses; abscesses beneath the skin, in the cellular tissues and in internal organs. The suppurative tendency is very marked in Sulphur. The glands become inflamed and the inflammation goes on to suppuration.

Wherever there is a Sulphur complaint you will find *burning*. Every part burns; burning where there is congestion; burning of the skin or a sensation of heat in the skin; burning here and there in spots; burning in the glands, in the stomach, in the lungs; burning in the bowels, in the rectum; burning and smarting in the hæmorrhoids; burning when passing urine, or a sensation of heat in the bladder. There is heat here and there, but when the patient describes something especially typical of Sulphur she says: "Burning of the soles of the feet, in the palms of the hands, and on the top of the head." Burning of the soles of the feet will very often be noticed after the patient becomes warm in bed. The Sulphur patient has so much heat and burning of the soles at night in bed that he puts the feet out from beneath the clothes, sleeps with the feet outside the covering. The soles and palms of the Sulphur patient when examined present a thick skin which burns on becoming *warm* in bed.

Many *complaints* come on *from becoming warm in bed.* The Sulphur patient cannot stand heat and cannot stand cold, though there is a strong craving for the open air. He wants an even temperature; he is disturbed if the temperature changes much. So far as his breathing is concerned, when he has much distress he wants the doors and windows open. The body, however, he is frequently forced to have covered, but if he is warmly clad he is bothered with the itching and burning of the skin.

As to *time aggravations, nightly complaints* are a feature. Headaches begin after evening meal and increase into the night; he cannot get to sleep because of the pain. There is nightly aching and nightly thirst; nightly distress and symptoms of the skin coming on after becoming warm in bed. "Intermittent periodic neuralgia, worse every 24 hours, generally at 12 A.M. or 12 P.M." *Midday* is another time of aggravation of the Sulphur complaints. It has chills at noon, fevers increase at noon, increase of the mental symptoms at noon, headache worse at noon. *Complaints* that come *once a week,* a seven-day aggravation, is another peculiar condition of Sulphur.

It is a common feature for a Sulphur patient to have a peculiar kind of diarrhœa which has been long known as "a Sulphur diarrhœa" though many other remedies have a similar condition, viz.: *diarrhœa coming on early in the morning.* The Sulphur diarrhœa belongs to the time between midnight and morning, but more commonly the time that he begins to think about rising. The *diarrhœa drives him out of bed.* It is generally thin, watery; there is not much gushing, and it is not very copious, sometimes quite scanty, sometimes yellow fæcal. After this morning stool he has, in many cases, no further trouble till next morning. There are many people who go on year after year with this urging to stool driving out of bed in the morning. The patient suffers from pain, griping, uneasiness, and burning soreness through the bowels. The stool burns while it is passing, and all parts that it comes in contact with are made sore and raw, and there is much chafing.

The Sulphur patient is very *thirsty.* He is always drinking water. He wants much water.

He also speaks of a *hungry feeling,* a desire for food, but when he comes to the table he loathes the food, turns away from it, does not want it. He eats almost nothing, takes only the simplest and lightest things. There is a craving for stimulants, for alcohol, and an aversion to milk and meat; these latter make him sick and he loathes them. One of the old men invented out of these things the keynote "drinks much and eats little". This is true under Sulphur, but many other remedies have the same thing. As to the use of keynotes I would impress on you that it is well to gather together all the symptoms with their associations. It will not do to place much dependence on one little symptom, or even on two or three little symptoms. The symptoms of the whole case must be considered and then, if the keynotes and characteristics and everything else cause the remedy to be well rounded out and full, and to look like the whole patient, only then is it suitable.

There is *emptiness occurring at 11 o'clock in the forenoon.* If there is any time in the whole twenty-four hours that he feels hungry it is at 11 o'clock. It seems as though he cannot wait for his dinner. There is this also about the Sulphur patient: he is very hungry about his customary meal-times and, if the meal is delayed, he becomes weak and nauseated. Those that are accustomed to eat at about 12 o'clock will have that all-gone hungry feeling at 11 A.M. Those accustomed to eat about 1 or 1.30 will have it about 12 o'clock. The all-gone sensation is about one hour before the accustomed time of eating with many people.

In a sort of condensed way a strong Sulphur group is this: an all-gone hungry feeling in the stomach at 11 A.M., burning of the soles and heat in the top of the head. These three things have been looked upon as a *sine qua non* of Sulphur, but they are scarcely the beginning of Sulphur.

There is an *unhealthy condition of the skin* in Sulphur aside from the eruptions. The skin will not heal. Small wounds continue to suppurate; abscesses formed under the skin become little discharging cavities with fistulous openings, and these leak and discharge for a long time.

Sulphur produces an *infiltration* in inflamed parts, so that they become indurated and these indurations last for years. When the inflammation is in a vital organ, like the lungs, this infiltration cannot always be endured; it leaves infiltrations after pneumonia called hepatization. Sulphur produces this same tendency in inflamed parts throughout the body and hence its great use in hepatization.

Sulphur is a very useful remedy *when the patient does not react* after a prolonged disease, because of a condition in the economy, a psoric condition. When a patient is drawing near the end of an acute disease he becomes weak and prostrated. The inflammatory state ends in suppuration and infiltrations; the patient is in a state of weakness, much fatigued, and prostrated, and has night sweats. He does not convalesce after a typhoid or other acute disease. There is slow repair and a slow, tired economy, and order is not restored after the acute disease. Sulphur often becomes very useful in such conditions. Old drunkards become debilitated and have violent craving for alcohol; they cannot let liquor alone. They crave strong and pungent things, want nothing to eat, but want cold water and alcoholic drinks. They go on drinking till greatly exhausted and then their complaints come on. Sulphur will for a while take away this craving for drink and build him up.

The *tissues* seem to *take on weakness,* so that very little pressure causes soreness, sometimes inflammation and suppuration. Bed sores come on easily in a Sulphur patient, as there is feeble circulation. *Induration from pressure* is also a strong feature. Sulphur has corns from pressure, callosities from pressure. These affections come easily. If a shoe presses anywhere on the skin a great corn or bunion develops. Where the teeth come in contact with the tongue and other parts of the buccal cavity nodules form and these little nodules in course of time commence to ulcerate. It is a slow process with burning and stinging. They may go into cancerous affections. They may be postponed for a long time and afterwards take on a state of malignancy. Cancer is an outgrowth of a state in the body, and that state may come on from a succession of states. It is not one continuous condition, but the malignant state may follow the benign. Sulphur removes these states when the symptoms agree.

We notice a marked evidence of disturbance of the veins under Sulphur. It is a *venous remedy,* has much vein trouble. The veins seem to be relaxed and there is sluggish circulation. There is a flushed appearance of the face here and there from slight irritation, from the weather, from irritation of the clothing. Tumefaction of the face. Sulphur has varicose veins; most marked of these are hæmorrhoidal veins, which are enlarged and burn and sting. Varices of the extremities. The veins even ulcerate, rupture and bleed. When going out of a cold into a warm atmosphere the patient suffers from enlarged veins, from puffiness of the hands and feet, from a sense of fulness throughout the body.

The Sulphur patient emaciates, and a peculiar feature is the *emaciation of the limbs with distended abdomen.* The abdomen is tumid, with rumbling, burning and soreness, and with the distended abdomen there is emaciation of all other parts. The muscles of the neck, back, thorax and limbs wither, and the muscles of the abdomen are also wasted, but there is much distension of the abdomen itself. This condition of affairs is found in marasmus. You will find a similar state under *Calcarea;* and, in women needing *Calcarea,* you will notice great enlargement, distension and hardness of the abdomen with shrivelling of all other parts of the body.

Under Sulphur there are *flashes of heat* to the face and head, like those which women have at the climacteric period. The flash of heat in Sulphur begins somewhere in the heart region, generally said to be in the chest, and it feels as if, inside the body, a glow of heat is rising to the face. The face is red, hot and flushed, and finally the heat ends in sweat. Flashes of heat with sweat and red face; the head is in a glow. Sometimes the patient will describe a feeling as if hot steam were inside the body and gradually rising up, and then she breaks out in a sweat. At times you will see a woman having little shiverings followed by flashes of heat and red splotches in the face, and then she fans vigorously; cannot fan fast enough, and she wants the doors and windows open. Such is Sulphur as well as *Lachesis* and many others. When the flashes begin in the chest, about the heart, it is more like Sulphur, but when in the back or in the stomach it is more like *Phosphorus.*

Among other general aggravations we have an *aggravation from standing in* Sulphur. All complaints are made worse by standing for a length of time. Standing is the most difficult position for a Sulphur patient, and there is an aggravation of the confusion of mind, dizziness, the stomach and abdominal symptoms, and a sense of enlargement and fulness of the veins and dragging down in the pelvis in women, from standing. The patient must sit down or keep moving, if on her feet. She can walk fairly well, but is worse when standing quiet.

An *aggravation after sleep* fits into many of the complaints of Sulphur, but especially those of the mind and sensorium. Most of the complaints of Sulphur are also *worse after eating.*

The Sulphur patient is *aggravated from bathing.* He dreads a bath. He does not bathe himself and from his state in general he belongs to "the great unwashed". He cannot take a bath without catching "cold".

Children's complaints. Dirty-faced, dirty-skinned little urchins, who are subject to nightly attacks of delirium, who suffer much from pains in the head, who had brain troubles, who are threatened with hydrocephalus, who had meningitis, need Sulphur. Sulphur will clear up the constitutional state when remedies have failed to reach the whole case because they are not deep enough. If the infant does not develop properly, if the bones do not grow, and there is slow closing of the fontanelles, *Calcarea carbonica may* be the remedy and Sulphur is next in importance for such slow growth.

You would not suppose that the Sulphur patient is so *nervous* as he is, but he is full of excitement, is easily startled by noise, wakens from sleep in a start as if he had heard a cannon report or seen a "spook". The Sulphur patient is the victim of much trouble in his sleep. He is very sleepy in the fore part of the night, at times sleeping till 3 A.M., but from that time on he has restless sleep, or does not sleep at all. He dreads daylight, wants to go to sleep again, and when he does sleep he can hardly be aroused, and wants to sleep late in the morning. That is the time he gets his best rest and his soundest sleep. He is much disturbed by dreadful dreams and nightmare.

When the symptoms agree, Sulphur will be found a curative medicine in erysipelas. For erysipelas as a name we have no remedy, but when the patient has erysipelas and his symptoms conform to those of Sulphur, you can cure him with Sulphur. If you hear that distinction in mind you will be able to see what Homœopathy means; it treats the patient and not the name that the sickness goes by.

The Sulphur patient is annoyed throughout his economy with *surgings of blood* here and there—surging, with fulness of the head, which we have heretofore described as flashes of heat. It has marked febrile conditions and can be used in acute diseases. It is one of the natural complements of *Aconite,* and when *Aconite* is suitable to the acute exacerbations and removes them, very often Sulphur corresponds to the constitutional state of the patient.

Sulphur is suitable in the most troublesome *"scrofulous" complaints* in broken-down constitutions and defective assimilation. It has deep-seated, ragged ulcers on the lower extremities, indolent ulcers, ulcers that will not granulate. They burn, and the little moisture that oozes out burns the parts round about It is indicated often in varicose ulcers that bleed easily and burn much.

In old cases of *gout,* Sulphur is a useful remedy. It is a deep-acting remedy, and in most instances it will keep the gout upon the extremities, as its tendency is outward from centre to circumference. Like *Lycopodium* and *Calcarea,* when suitably administered in old gouty conditions, not where there is much organic change present, it will keep the rheumatic state in the joints and extremities.

Sulphur, like *Silicea,* is a *dangerous medicine* to give *where there is structural disease* in organs that are vital, especially in the lungs. Sulphur will often heal old fistulous pipes and turn old abscesses into a normal state, so that healthy pus will follow, when it is indicated by the symptoms. It will open abscesses that are very slow, doing nothing, it will reduce inflamed glands that are indurated and about to suppurate, when the symptoms agree. But it is a dangerous medicine to administer in advanced cases of phthisis, and, if given, it should not be prescribed in the highest potencies. If there are symptoms that are very painful, and you think that Sulphur must be administered, go to the 30th or 200th potency. Do not undertake to stop with Sulphur the morning diarrhœa that commonly comes with phthisis. Do not undertake to stop the night sweats that come in the advanced stages, even if Sulphur seems to be indicated by the symptoms; the fact is, it is not indicated. A remedy that is dangerous in any case ought not to be considered as indicated, even though the symptoms are similar.

In old cases of *syphilis,* when the psoric state is uppermost, Sulphur may be needed. Sulphur is rarely indicated when the syphilitic symptoms are uppermost, but when these have been suppressed by *Mercury* and the disease is merely held in abeyance, Sulphur will antidote the *Mercury* and allow the symptoms to develop and the original condition to come back in order to be seen. The great mischief done by allopaths is due to the fact that they want to cover up everything that is in the economy; they act as if ashamed of everything in the human race; whereas Homœopathy endeavors to reveal everything in the human race and to antidote those drugs that cover up, and to free those diseases that are held down. It is true that many patients will not have Homœopathy because they do not want their syphilitic eruption brought to view; they do not want the evidences of their indiscretion brought to light; but Homœopathy endeavors to do that. Conditions that are in the economy will come out under proper homœopathic treatment. Sulphur brings complaints to the surface, so that they can be seen. It is a *general broad antidote.* It is a medicine often called for in the *suppression of eruptions* from cold and from drugs, and even from Sulphur. It is a great medicine to develop these things which have been covered up, hence you will see Sulphur in all the lists of remedies useful for suppressed eruptions or for anything suppressed by drugs. Even when acute eruptions have been suppressed Sulphur becomes a valuable remedy. In suppressed gonorrhœa Sulphur is often the remedy to start up the discharge and re-establish the conditions that have been caused to disappear. Symptoms that have been suppressed must return or a cure is not possible.

Sulphur has been the remedy from the beginning of its history, from the time of Hahnemann, and on his recommendation, to be thought of *when there is a paucity of symptoms to prescribe on,* a latent condition of the symptoms due to psora. In this stare it has been administered with so much benefit that the routine prescriber has learned the fact. When apparently (superficially) well-indicated remedies fail to hold a patient, and symptoms cannot be found for a better remedy, it is true that Sulphur takes a deep hold of the economy and remedies act better after it. This is well established from experience. You will find at times when you have given a remedy which seems well indicated, that it does not hold the case, and then you give the next best indicated remedy, and then the next, with the same result. You will begin to wonder why this is, but you will see that, although the case does not call clearly for Sulphur, yet on its administration it so closely conforms to the underlying condition (and psora is so often the underlying condition) that it makes the remedies act better. This is an observation that has been confirmed since the time of Hahnemann by all the old men. Such things are only necessary when there is a paucity of symptoms, where after much study it is necessary to resort to what seem the best measures, measures justifiable to a certain extent, based upon observation and upon a knowledge of the conditions underlying the constitution of the whole race. We know that underlying these cases with few symptoms there is a latent condition, and that it is either psora, syphilis or sycosis. If it were known to he syphilis we would select the head of the class of remedies looking like syphilis. If known to be sycosis, we would select the head of the class of remedies looking like sycosis. Sulphur stands at the head of the list of remedies looking like the underlying psora; and so, if the underlying constitution is known to be psoric, and it is a masked case, Sulphur will open up the latent cause, and, even if it does not act on, a positively curative basis, it is true that a better representation of the symptoms comes up. And as Sulphur is to psora, so is *Mercurius* to syphilis, and *Thuja* to sycosis.

In the coal regions of Pennsylvania, those who work in the mines and those living in the vicinity of the mines often need Sulphur. We know that the coal is not made up of Sulphur; there is a good deal in it besides; but those who handle the coal often need Sulphur. Persons who are always grinding kaolin and the various products that are used in the manufacture of china, and the workers among stone, especially require *Calcarea* and *Silicea,* but those who work in the coal mines often need Sulphur. The patients look like Sulphur patients; they have the aspect. and even when their symptoms are localized and call for other remedies, you will get no good action from these remedies until you give them a dose of Sulphur, after which they go on improving. Some believe this is due to the fact that there is so much Sulphur in the coal. We may theorize about these things as much as we have a mind to, but we do not want to fall into the habit of antidoting the lower patencies with the high. Only use that method as a *dernier ressort.* When *there are no symptoms* to indicate the remedy, then it is time for us to experiment, and then it is justifiable only when it is carried on by a man of the right sort, because such a man keeps within the limit. He knows how to give his remedy. Such a man is guided by the symptoms in each case so far as symptoms speak out.

In inflammatory conditions a purplish appearance of the inflamed parts, a venous engorgement, is seen under Sulphur. *Measles,* when they come out with that purplish color, very often require Sulphur. Sulphur is a great remedy in measles. The routinist can do pretty well in this disease with *Pulsatilla* and Sulphur, occasionally requiring *Aconite* and *Euphrasia.* Especially will Sulphur modify the case when the skin is dusky and the measles do not come out. This *purplish color may* be seen anywhere, in the erysipelas, in the sore throat, often on the forearms, legs and face.

The dreadful *effects of vaccination are* often cured by Sulphur. In this it competes with *Thuja* and *Malandrinum.*

In the *mental state,* which gives out the real man, shows forth the real interior nature, we see that Sulphur vitiates his affections, driving him to a most marked state of selfishness. He has no thought of anybody's wishes or desires but his own. Everything that he contemplates is for the benefit of himself. This selfishness runs through the Sulphur patient. There is absence of gratitude.

Philosophical mania is also a prominent feature. Monomania over the study of strange and abstract things, occult things; things that are beyond knowledge; studying different things without any basis to figure upon; dwelling upon strange and peculiar things. Sulphur has cured this consecutive tracing one thing to another as to first cause. It has cured a patient who did nothing but meditate as to what caused this and that and the other thing, finally tracing things back to Divine Providence, and then asking "Who made God?" She would sit in a corner counting pins and wonder, pondering over the insolvable question of "Who made God?" One woman could never see any handiwork of man without asking who made it. She could never be contented until she found out the man who made it, and then she wanted to know who his father was; she would sit down and wonder who he was, whether he was an Irishman, and so on. That is a feature of Sulphur. It is that kind of reasoning without any hope of discovery, without any possible answer. It is not that kind of philosophy which has a basis and which can be followed up, reasoning in a series, reasoning on things that are true, but a fanatical kind of philosophy that has no basis, wearing oneself out. Sulphur has an aversion to follow up things in an orderly fashion, an aversion to real work, an aversion to systematic work. The Sulphur patient is a sort of *inventive genius.* When he gets an idea in his mind he is unable to get rid of it. He follows it and follows it until finally accidentally he drops into something, and many times that is how things are invented. Such is a Sulphur patient. He is often ignorant but imagines himself to be a great man; he despises education and despises literary men and their accomplishments, and he wonders why it is everyone cannot see that he is above education.

Again, this patient takes on *religious melancholy,* not meditating upon the rational religion, but on foolish ideas about himself. He prays constantly and uninterruptedly, is always in his room, moaning with despair. He thinks he has sinned away his day of grace.

A patient needing Sulphur is often in a state of *dulness and confusion of mind,* with inability to collect the thoughts and ideas; lack of concentration. He will sit and meditate on no one thing continuously, making no effort to concentrate his mind upon anything. He wakes up in the morning with dulness of mind and fulness in the head and vertigo. Vertigo in the open air. In the open air comes on coryza with this fulness in the head and dulness, so that there is a confusion of the mind.

In the books there *is* an expression that has been extensively used. "Foolish happiness and pride; thinks himself in possession of beautiful things;

even rags seem beautiful." Such a state has been present in lunatics and in persons who were not lunatics in any other way except on that one idea.

The Sulphur patient has an *aversion to business.* He will sit around and do nothing, and let his wife take in washing and "work her finger-nails off" taking care of him; he thinks that is all she is good for. A state of refinement seems to have gone out of the Sulphur patient. Sulphur is the very opposite of all things fastidious. *Arsenicum* is the typical fastidious patient, and these two remedies are the extremes of each other. *Arsenicum* wants his clothing neat and clean, wants everything hung up well upon the pegs, wants all the pictures hung up properly upon the wall, wants everything neat and nice; and hence the *Arsenicum* patient has been called "the gold-headed-cane patient," because of his neatness, fastidiousness and cleanliness. The very opposite of all that is the Sulphur patient.

"Indisposed to everything, work, pleasure, talking or motion; indolence of mind and body." "Satiety of life; longing for indolence of mind and body." "Satiety of life; longing for death." "Too lazy to rouse himself up, and too unhappy to live." "Dread of being washed (in children)." Yes, they will cry lustily if they have to be washed. The Sulphur patient dreads water and takes cold from bathing.

As to its *relationship,* Sulphur should not be given immediately before *Lycopodium.* It belongs to a rotating group, Sulphur, *Calcarea, Lycopodium.* First Sulphur, then *Calcarea* and then *Lycopodium,* and then Sulphur again, as it follows *Lycopodium* well. Sulphur and *Arsenicum are* also related. You will very often treat a case with Sulphur for a while and then need to give *Arsenicum* for some time, and then back to Sulphur. Sulphur follows most of the acute remedies well.

The Sulphur patient is troubled with much *dizziness.* When he goes into the open air or when he stands any length of time, he becomes dizzy. On rising in the morning his head feels stupid, and on getting on his feet he is dizzy. He feels stupid and tired, and not rested by his sleep, and "things go round". It takes some time to establish an equilibrium. He is slow in gathering himself together after sleep. Here we see the aggravation from sleep and from standing.

The *head* furnishes many symptoms. The Sulphur patient is subject to periodical sick headaches; congestive headaches, a sensation of great congestion with stupefaction, attended with nausea and vomiting. Sick headache once a week or every two weeks, the characteristic seven-day aggravation. Most headaches coming on Sunday in working men are cured by Sulphur. You can figure this out. Sunday is the only day he does not work, and he sleeps late in the morning and gets up with a headache that involves the whole head, with dulness and congestion. Being busy and active prevents the headache during the week. Others have periodical headaches every seven to ten days, with nausea and vomiting of bile. Again he may have a headache lasting two or three days; a congestive headache. Headache with nausea and no vomiting or headache with vomiting of bile. The headache is aggravated by stooping, generally ameliorated in a warm room and by the application of warmth; aggravated from light, hence the desire to close the eyes and to go into a dark room; aggravated by jarring, and after eating. The whole head is sensitive and the eyes are red, and there is often lachrymation, with nausea and vomiting. Headaches at times in those who suffer constantly from great heat in the vertex; the top of the head is hot and burns and he wants cold cloths applied to the top of the head. These headaches associated with heat are often ameliorated by cold, but otherwise the head is ameliorated in a warm room. The head feels stupid and sometimes he cannot think. Every motion aggravates and he is worse after eating and drinking, worse from taking cold drinks into the stomach and better from hot drinks. When the headaches are present the face is engorged; bright red face. Headaches in persons who have a red face, a dirty face or sallow, a venous stasis of the face; the eyes are engorged and the skin is engorged; the face is puffed and venous in appearance. Sulphur is useful in, persons who get up in the morning with headache, dizziness and red face; in persons who say they know they are going to have the headache some time during the day because the face feels very full and is red in the morning, and the eyes are red. Before the headache comes on there is a flickering before ,the eyes, a flickering of color. Scintillations, stars, saw teeth, zig-zags are forewarnings of a headache. Some Sulphur headaches that have known present a peculiar appearance before the eyes; a rhomboidal figure, obliquely placed, with saw teeth on the upper side and the body filled with spots. Sometimes this figure is seen toward one side of the object looked at, sometimes on the other side, but it is seen equally distinct with both eyes at the same time. These saw teeth are flashes of light, and the base of the figure grows increasingly darker until you get all the colors of the rainbow. Whenever he disorders his stomach he has this peculiar vision. Sometimes it comes in the morning after eating and sometimes at noon after eating. It comes also when he is hungry in the evening and delays his eating. These zig-zags come very often with that hungry all-gone feeling in the stomach. We have the same state of affairs, similar apperance of zig-zags and flickerings in both *Natrum muriaticum* and *Psorinum* before the headache. They are warning of headaches. These zig-zags, flickerings, sparks, stars and irregular shapes appear before the eyes periodically, and may last an hour or so. In the head there is much throbbing. Morning headaches and headaches coming on at noon. Headaches also, as mentioned before, that begin after the evening meal and increase into the night, hindering sleep.

Upon the *external head* the itching is indescribable; constant itching, itching when warm in bed. It is worse from the warmth of the bed and yet it is also worse from cold. Itching eruptions; scaly, moist and dry eruptions; vesicles, pimples, pustules and boils; eruptions in general upon the scalp. Much dandruff in the hair, and loss of hair. There is slow closing of the fontanelles. "Humid, offensive eruption on top of the head, filled with pus, drying up into honey-like scabs. Tinea capitis." "Humid offensive eruption with thick pus, yellow crusts, bleeding and burning." Hair dry, falling off, etc.

It has many symptoms, such as in olden times would be called scro-fulous but which we recognize as psoric. There is a tendency for every "cold" to settle in the eyes. Discharge of mucus and pus from the eyes. Ulceration and thickening of the eyelids, lids rolled outwards or inwards, loss of eyelashes; red and disturbed condition. Now, if we would say "complaints of the eyes in a Sulphur patient," it would cover all kinds of eye troubles. Sulphur has extensive eye symptoms. Eye symptoms with eruptions on the face and scalp, with itching of the skin, especially when warm in bed. Catarrhal eye symptoms that are made worse from washing. When not only the eyes are aggravated by bathing, but the patient himself is aggravated from bathing and he dreads to bathe, and he has itching which is made worse from the warmth of the bed, and is subject to chronic sick headaches and has heat on top of the head, with such concomitants his eye symptoms, no matter what, will be cured by Sulphur. Sulphur has cured cataract and iritis, inflammatory conditions and opacities, and all sorts of "hallucinations of sight" (coming with headaches). "Flickering before the eyes" (as described) "small dark specks; dark points and spots; black flies seem to float not far from the eyes; gas or lamp light seems to be surrounded with a halo," etc. There are so many of these peculiar images before the eyes, but all have the Sulphur constitution. "Burning heat in the eyes, painful smarting." Every "cold" settles in the eyes, i.e., the eye symptoms, when present, are increased and, when he has no eye symptoms, these are brought on from every "cold".

The *ears* are subject to catarrh. You have learned in the generals, that the catarrhal state is a very strong feature of Sulphur. No mucous membrane of the body escapes, all have catarrhal discharges, copious, sometimes purulent, sometimes bloody. The eyes and ears are no exception. The catarrhal state goes on in a patient until deafness follows. Thickening of the mucous membrane and of the drum. All sorts of strange noises in the ear until the hearing is lost. After structural changes have taken place and deafness comes on even if there is no cure for the deafness, you may cure the patient. When a patient wants to know if he can be cured of his deafness you can never tell him. Many of the troubles are in the middle ear, and as you cannot examine it, you do not know how much structural change has taken place. You can only say that if the *patient* can be sufficiently cured then it can be ascertained. If the structural changes are not very great they will disappear after the patient is cured. If the internal parts are destroyed, if there is a dry, atrophic catarrh of the middle ear, you can hardly expect to restore that middle ear. It has been destroyed; the parts that are necessary for sensation no longer register sensation. because they have become atrophied. You can only talk to the patient about the prospects of curing *him.* Do not entertain in your mind the idea of curing an organ. Keep that idea out of your mind as much as possible, and, when people want you to locate the 'disease in organs, keep quiet, because only the *patient* is sick. Think as much as possible about the sick patient and as little as possible about the name or the pathological conditions of organs. So, when patients say, "Doctor, can you cure my hearing?" answer them: "First, *you* must be cured. The first and most important thing is to cure *you. "* Cure the patient and then it will be seen afterwards what can be done for the ear, for the hearing. That keeps your mind in proper form, keeps you in right relation to the patient. If you were all the time talking of the ear, the patient would worry your life out about his ear. "When are you going to do something for my ear? When am I going to hear?" Start out with the understanding that the whole patient is to be treated. *Remember the patient first,* and let him understand that. The idea of a patient going to a specialist for diseases of the ears should be discouraged unless a homœopathist is at hand. It is a disease of the whole body that is to be treated. There is no such trouble as an ear trouble considered apart from the constitutional state of the patient himself. Sulphur has "frequent stoppages of the ears, especially when eating or blowing one's nose." "Sounds in ears." Inflammation of various kinds. Discharges from the ears in a Sulphur patient. You see I have avoided saying that Sulphur is a remedy for the ears. Many times you will cure patients of these "local diseases" if you select remedies for the patients, when the local symptoms would never have led you to the remedy. You would never have thought of Sulphur for the ear alone, or for the prolapsus of the uterus, yet the patient needs Sulphur, and, having given it, you are astonished to see how the organs are turned into order after the constitution of the patient has been made orderly. Now and then pails that are located here and there in the body are prescribed at by the physician, and failure follows. He hunts a remedy through and through to find some particular kind of pain that resembles the pain which the patient has. You should treat the patient and not bother about trifling pains. Leave it out if you want to, but get a remedy for the patient. If that pain is in the remedy well and good, but if not do not bother about it. Do not bother about the little symptoms. You may even leave out a most prominent *keynote* in treating the *patient.* Sometimes that particular pain is the only symptom the patient wants cured, but if it is an old symptom, it will he the last thing to go away. Under such circumstances the patient will bother your life out wanting to know when that pain is going to be cured, but if you have knowledge of the matter you will not expect to relieve that pain the first time; if you do relieve it you know that you have made a mistake, for the *later* symptoms should all go away *first. It* is sometimes necessary, in order to hold a patient, to say, "That symptom must not be cured first, but these little symptoms that you do not care much about will go away first." You will hold that patient for life simply because you have told the truth, simply because you have exhibited to her that you *know.* Such business is honestly acquired business.

The catarrhal affections of the *nose* are extremely troublesome in Sulphur. "Smell before the nose as of an old catarrh," and so troublesome is the Sulphur nose, so troublesome is this catarrhal state that with odors he is made sick. He thinks he smells his own catarrh, and thinks others also smell it. The smell of this old catarrh, or of filthy things, keeps him nauseated. He is subject to coryzas; constant sneezing, stoppage of the nose. Under coryza we read "fluent like water trickling from the nose." All the nasal discharges are acrid and burning.

This is a state in Sulphur. Every time he takes "cold," it brings on a coryza. He cannot take a bath, he cannot become overheated, he cannot get into a cold place and cannot overexert himself without getting this "cold in the nose". Changes of the weather establish a new attack. I have observed in numbers of those old people who are in the habit of taking large quantities of Sulphur in the spring for boils, and as a spring cleanser, that for the rest of the year they suffer from coryza and the various complaints of Sulphur. If you can hunt out some of these old Sulphur takers, you will have a very good picture of Sulphur, interesting for the homœopathic physician to look upon. He is also subject to nose-bleed, dry ulcers and scabs in the nose.

I have quite sufficiently described the general aspect of the *face* in Sulphur, but we must especially remember the venous stasis, the dirty appearance, the red spots, the sickly look, the appearance of false plethora. It is a face that changes from pale to red, a pallid face that becomes easily disturbed, flushed from excitement, flushed in a warm room, flushed from slight stimulation, especially flushed in the morning. Eruptions upon the face

Periodical neuralgias of the most violent character, especially on the right side of the face. Long and tedious right-sided neuralgias. Persistent neuralgias in those that live in a malarial climate, when the short-acting remedies given for the neuralgia, such as *Belladonna* and *Nux vomica,* have only for a short time mitigated the suffering. If upon studying the whole case you find he turns out to be a Sulphur patient, Sulphur will permanently cure the neuralgia.

Sulphur cures erysipelatous inflammation of the face. In Sulphur the erysipelas commences on the right side of the face and about the right car, and there is considerable swelling of the right ear, and it spreads slowly, moves with sluggishness and is unusually purple. The whole patient is an offensive, filthy patient; in spite of washing, his skin looks wrinkled, shrivelled and like dried beef. Sulphur is not so suitable, in the cases that come on with rapidity and great violence, with vesicles and enormous blebs, but it suits those cases in which at first there is the appearance of a mottled dusky red spot on the face, and a little distance from it another spot and then another, and these, as it were, all run together, and after a week or so it develops into a sluggish erysipelatous state, and the veins seem to be distended, and he is passing into a state toward unconsciousness. You will be astonished to see what Sulphur will do in such a case, which comes slowly as if there were a lack of vitality to develop it, a slow, sluggish. erysipelatous inflammation. Whereas, if it be *Arsenicum, Apis* or *Rhus tox.,* it spreads with rapidity. *Arsenicum* and *Apis* burn like fire and *Rhus* has blisters upon the erysipelatous patches.

The whole face in Sulphur is covered at times with patches of moist, scaly, itching, eczematous eruptions. Crusta lactea that involves the scalp and the ears, with moisture, thick yellow crusts, piling up, with much itching, which is worse when warm in bed. The child sleeps without covers. If there is itching in parts that are covered, when the parts become warm the itching increases. These eruptions are associated with eye diseases, catarrhal affections of the eyes and nose.

The Sulphur patient has thick incrustations upon the lips, scabby lips, chapped lips, cracks about the lips and corners of the mouth. The saliva oozes out of the mouth making red streaks. Eruptions with itching and burning about the lower part of the, face. Herpetic eruptions about the mouth. All of these burn and become excoriated from the fluids of the mouth. Round about the under jaw there is swelling of the glands. Swelling and suppuration of the sub-maxillary glands; swelling of the parotids. The glands of the neck are enlarged.

In the Sulphur constitution the teeth become loose; the gums settle away from the teeth and bleed and burn. The teeth decay. There is a general unhealthy condition of the *mouth* and tongue. Foul taste and foul tongue. Ulceration of the mouth and burning in the ulcers. In the aphthæ there is burning, stinging. White patches in the mouth. Sulphur is a very useful remedy in sore mouth of nursing infants, and such as occurs in the mother during lactation. It has also deep-seated phagedenic ulcers that eat around the inner surface of the cheek. Peculiar little nodules form upon the tongue and upon the sides of the mouth where the unhealthy teeth press. When these nodules come along the edge of the tongue they are so painful that he cannot talk and cannot swallow. He must live on substances that he can take without having to move the tongue. Sometimes they involve the whole tongue, and have been called cancerous affections even when benign.

Sulphur is a wonderful medicine for chronic sore throat when the symptoms agree. The old Sulphur patient suffers from a general catarrhal state, as has been said, and the throat symptoms are of that sort. There is a catarrhal state which goes on even to ulceration. The tonsil is enlarged, and of a purplish aspect lasting for weeks and months, a general sore and painfully sensitive condition of the throat; but it has also an acute sore throat. It is especially useful in inflammation of the tonsil with suppuration, when the aspect is purplish, venous, and not a bright red inflammation. The *purplish,* dusky color is especially a Sulphur color. There is often burning in the throat, stitching, rawness, smarting, inflammation and difficult swallowing. It has cured diphtheria.

I have sufficiently covered appetite, desires and aversions under the generals. The Sulphur patients are commonly dyspeptics, patients who can digest almost nothing. They must live on the simplest forms of food in order to have any comfort at all; cannot digest anything like ordinary diet. The *stomach* is sensitive to touch with the all-gone hungry feeling before mealtimes. The Sulphur patient cannot go long without eating; he becomes faint and weak. Great heaviness in the stomach after eating but little, after eating meat, or after eating foods that require a healthy stomach to digest. Then he becomes the victim of pain. He will describe the pains in his stomach as burning pains and great soreness; he has a mobrid feeling in the stomach; smarting and rawness in the stomach. He will describe this sensation as "Pain in the stomach after eating. Sensation of weight in the stomach after eating," etc. The Sulphur stomach is a weak stomach, is slow in digesting. There is acid and bilious. vomiting, as a result of the disordered stomach. Sour taste in the mouth from the welling up of acids from the stomach.

The *liver* is a very troublesome organ. There is enlargement and induration, with much painfulness, pressure and distress. With congestion of the liver, the stomach also takes on its usual symptoms, or, if present already, they are aggravated. The patient becomes jaundiced, with sensation of engorgement or fulness of the liver, dull aching in the liver. He is subject to gall-stones; tearing pains in the region of the gall duct, coming periodically, attended with much increase of his sallowness. The Sulphur liver patient is the victim of chronic sallowness, which increases and decreases. When this patient takes "cold" it settles in the liver; every "cold," every bath he takes, every change of weather, aggravates his liver symptoms, and when these are worse he has less of other troubles. It localizes itself in attacks of bilious vomiting, in attacks of "bilious headaches," as he calls them. At times the stool is black as tar, at others it is green and thick, and there are times when the stool is white. These stools alternate and change about with the engorgement of his liver, and then he is subject to gall-stones.

The Sulphur patient suffers from great distension of the *abdomen;* rolling in the abdomen; soreness in the abdomen. He cannot stand because the abdominal viscera hang down so; they seem to be falling. There is rawness, soreness, distension and burning, with diarrhœa, with chronic diarrhœa, and then this goes on to more serious trouble, towards tubercle in the abdomen. The mesenteric glands become infiltrated with tubercle. There is nightly itching with the eruptions upon the abdomen, the itching being worse when warm in bed. Shingles come our about the sides and seem inclined to encircle the body.

He is also a *flatulent* patient. There is much belching, much distension, much rumbling and passing of flatus. He has spells of colic without being flatulent; the wind is confined. Dreadful spells of colic, cutting, tearing pains relieved in no position; burning and smarting in the whole abdomen and soreness of the intestines. Catarrh of the whole intestinal tract. That which he vomits is acid and smarts the mouth, and that which he passes by the anus is acrid and makes the parts raw. The liquid stool burns while it is passing, and there is much burning when passing moist flatus. He is often called to stool, but while sitting at stool he passes only a little fluid or a little moisture with flatus, and that fluid burns like coals of fire, and the anus becomes raw.

The stool may be thin faces, yellow, watery, mucous, green, bloody, excoriating. The stool is *offensive;* often sickening, of a penetrating odor which permeates the room, and "the smell of the stool follows him around, as if he had soiled himself".

The diarrhœa comes on especially in the morning and it is commonly limited to the forenoon. It drives. him out of bed in the morning; as soon as he wakes up and moves in bed; he feels the urging to stool and must make great haste, or he will lose it; it is with difficulty that he can hold it until he reaches the commode. The morning is the typical time, but a diarrhœa that comes on any time after midnight, from midnight till noon, may be a Sulphur diarrhœa. Very seldom would you expect to cure with Sulphur a diarrhœa that is in the habit of coming on during the afternoon. Sulphur has some evening aggravations in diarrhœa, but these are exceptions; it is the morning diarrhœa that we look to Sulphur to cure.

Sulphur is a wonderful remedy in cholera and in those cases of diarrhœa that occur in cholera times, when the diarrhœa begins in the morning. It is also of great value in dysentery, when the stool is bloody mucus with constant straining. As in *Mercurius* he must sit long at stool because of a feeling as if he could not finish. Such is the typical *Mercurius* state—a slimy stool with the sensation as if he could not finish. Sulphur often cures this state after *Mercurius* fails. It is the natural follower of *Mercurius* when the latter has been misunderstood and given. In dysentery, when this tenesmus is of the most violent character, when the stool is pure blood, when it is attended also with much urging to urinate, *Mercurius corrosivus* gives the quickest relief. If the tenesmus is less violent, and there is not much straining to urinate, or it is altogether absent, *Mercurius solubilis* is the more natural remedy. These medicines run very close to Sulphur in dysentery, but are more commonly indicated than Sulphur. In Sulphur *patients* of course Sulphur will be the suitable remedy in dysentery.

He is subject to *hæmorrhoids,* external and internal; great bunches that are sore and raw, burning and tender, and that bleed and smart with the liquid stool.

The *urinary* symptoms, and those of the *bladder* and *male sexual organs,* combine to give a very important group in Sulphur. There is a catarrhal state of the bladder, constant urging to urinate and burning and smarting while urinating. The urine scalds the urethra while passing and the smarting is so great that it lasts a long time after urination. It is indicated in broken-down constitutions, in old inventors, in old philosophers who have been leading sedentary lives, who suffer from enlarged prostate, burning in the urethra during and after the flow of urine, and a urethral discharge not unlike gonorrhœa, but really a chronic catarrhal state. Mucus in the urine, sometimes pus. In old cases of gleet, in old broken-down patients, when the ordinary gonorrhœa remedies, and the remedies especially fitted to the discharge itself, only palliate; when the patient himself is a Sulphur patient. Such a patient has had a gonorrhœa and has been treated by remedies adapted to the new appearance, to the discharge itself, but a catarrhal stare of the urethra follows, with burning in the urethra, swelling of the meatus, a red, swollen, pouty condition of the meatus, and only a drop collects, just enough to soil the linen, and this keeps up week after week, and sometimes for years he will be cured of this discharge by allowing potentized Sulphur to act long enough.

Sulphur has cured patients with sugar in the urine, in the early stage of diabetes. Sulphur cures involuntary urination during sleep. It cures troubles brought on by taking "cold". Every "cold" in some patients settles in the bladder. This is like *Dulcamara,* and when *Dulcamara* will no longer hold, or when it has been suitable in earlier stages, Sulphur follows it well. Continuous smarting of urine and frequent urging; burning, stinging, smarting in the urethra for a long time after micturition.

On the *genitals* there are many eruptions. Itching of the genitals, worse from warmth of the bed; much sweat about the genitals; coldness of the genitals. In the male, impotency; the sexual desire is fairly strong, but he is unable to secure suitable erections; or there is discharge of semen before intromission, or too soon after intromission. There is an inflammatory condition around the glans and foreskin. Herpetic eruptions under the foreskin, itching and burning. This patient has much annoyance from itching eruptions on the genitals. The prepuce becomes narrow and cannot be drawn back; inflammatory phimosis; thickening or restriction of the prepuce. Inflammatory phimosis can be cured by remedies, if the phimosis depends upon some trouble that is in itself curable. Congenital phimosis cannot be cured by remedies. The genitals are extremely offensive both to the patient and to the examining physician. The patient is likely to be very uncleanly; he does not bathe himself, and the genitals accumulate their natural filth. Discharge of prostatic fluid when at stool.

Under *female sexual organs* we have sterility. We have irregularity in the menstrual flow, menstrual flow suppressed from the slightest disturbance. Hæmorrhage in connection with the menstrual flow; uterine hæmorrhage; prolonged uterine hæmorrhage.

In an *abortion* you may have selected *Belladonna,* which was suitable while the woman was aborting, and it may have overcome the present state; or you may have selected *Apis* or *Sabina,* which was suitable for the early state, and it either postpones or checks the hæmorrhage for the time or hurries the expulsion of the foetus; but the hæmorrhage starts in again and with its return we have prolonged tribulation. In many of these cases we can do nothing until we put the patient on Sulphur. If the symptoms are masked, Sulphur stands very high. When *Belladonna* has been given you will often have to follow it with Sulphur. *Sabina,* which has the most violent gushing hæmorrhage in abortions, very commonly needs to be followed by Sulphur. In such haemorrhagic affections, however, i.e., in a prolonged recurring hæmorrhage, a chronic condition, not in the first or most exciting time, not in the time of the earliest gushing, there are two very frequently indicated remedies, viz.: Sulphur and *Psornum.* The flow keeps coming back in spite of ordinary remedies, and in spite of remedies selected upon the group of symptoms related to the pelvis. In many instances we go to a hæmorrhage and the pelvic symptoms are prominent and all other symptoms clouded; there is a gushing flow, the blood is hot, etc., and there are only a few symptoms; but the next time you see the woman she is quiet enough to give other symptoms, and in the course of a few days more symptoms come out, as the haemorrhagic state is an outcome of the chronic condition. This is unlike measles. You do not have to look into the chronic state until the measles or scarlet fever or small-pox is finished; these are acute miasms. But the hæmorrhage is a part of her constitutional state; it is not a miasm; and hence when it is violent, calling for a remedy, probably the best adapted will be the short acting remedies, such as *Belladonna* or even *Aconite;* but then look into the constitutional state for it is likely some remedy will have to follow the *Aconite* or the *Belladonna,* and commonly it is Sulphur;

the acute remedy being suitable to the violent action and then followed by its complementary medicine.

Women needing Sulphur are full of *hot flashes,* such as they are likely to have at the climacteric period, and here it competes with *Lachesis* and Sepia. Sulphur and *Sepia* are suitable in the most violent cases of dysmenorrhœa in girls and even in those of advanced age. Most violent cases that have existed a long time, since the beginning of menstruation, in women who always needed Sulphur. If you select a remedy merely on the kind of pain, on the sensitiveness of the uterus, on the appearance of the flow, i.e., on the pelvic symptoms, you will make a failure. You must treat the *patient,* even if the pelvic symptoms do not fall under the generals; when the generals agree Sulphur will cure dysmenorrhœa even though you cannot fit it to the pelvic symptoms. The *generals* always precede and rule in every case.

Sulphur has violent burning in the vagina. Troublesome itching of the vulva. Great offensiveness from the genitals. Perspiration copious and fœtid coming from about the genitals, down the inside of the thighs and up over the abdomen. She is so offensive that the odors nauseate her, and this general state is true, it is not the imagination. Remember the over-sensitiveness to odors. Leucorrhœa copious, offensive, burning, sticky; it may be whitish or yellow; it is offensive, acrid, and causes itching about the parts and excoriation.

There is much *nausea during gestation,* or only during the early period of gestation. In those women needing Sulphur, it will stop the nausea, and they will go into labor easily, with few protracted pains; they will go through their labor with only the contractions, and these comparatively painless. The only pains in such cases will be those from the pressure of the child's head. Labor is painful we know, but it is comparatively easy when the woman is upon a suitable remedy. Sulphur is indicated then in women who have suffered from the most dreadful agony in confinement; prolonged labor. Troublesome after-pains. Suitable also in swelling of the mammary glands.

Then we have *septicaemic conditions,* with purulent lochia or suppression of the lochia. You may go to a case in which, on the third day, there has been a chill, the lochia has been suppressed, the woman has a high temperature and is covered from head to foot with sweat. As you put your hand under the covers you feel steam come up from the body so that you want to take your hand away; it is so hot. She is dazed and is sensitive over the whole abdomen. You know now the meaning of the suppression of the lochia; you have a *puerperal fever* on hand. *Study closely for* Sulphur instead of hunting around among *Aconite, Bryonia, Belladonna, Opium, etc.* With these you will make a total failure in most instances, but Sulphur fits into just such a state and has cured many cases of puerperal fever. If it is but a milk fever or mammary indisposition and the chill is only acute, then your short-acting remedies will do very well and even *Aconite* has been useful, but when it is a case of septicaemia Sulphur goes to the very root of it. When the feet burn, when there is a hungry feeling in the stomach, the night aggravation with sinking and exhaustion, and when throughout the body there is a sensation of steam rising or hot flashes, one after another, you must give Sulphur. Now, on the other hand, if in such a case, with the hot sweat and other general features, you have one rigor following another in rapid succession and no end to them, you cannot get out of that case without *Lycopodium,* which goes as deeply into the case as Sulphur. When there is a continuous intermingling of little chillinesses and little quiverings throughout the body and the pulse has lost its proper relationship to the temperature, *Pyrogen* must be administered. If there is a purplish appearance of the body, cold sweat all over, if there are remittent or intermittent chills, with thirst during the chill, and at no other time, and the face is red during the chill, you must give *Ferrum,* as no other remedy looks just like that. When one side of the body is hot and the other side is cold and you find the woman in a tearful state, trembling with fear, nervous excitement and restlessness, give *Pulsatilla,* which also has a septic state and is sufficient to overcome the septic condition.

Sulphur is suitable in surgical fever when it takes this form of flashes of heat and steaming sweat.

In these deep-seated septic states, somewhere from beginning to end, Sulphur will most likely be wanted. You may see in the earlier stages of that septic state a number of *Bryonia* symptoms, but *Bryonia* cannot take hold of that case. Remember that in a septic state you want to get ahead of it in the first twenty-four hours; you do not want to let it run on, and if *Bryonia* has only mitigated it in its beginning then it is too late for Sulphur. Go to Sulphur at once. Now, another thing, even if you have made a mistake in giving Sulphur and you find it does not take hold of the case, it always simplifies it, does good and never spoils it. It gives you a good basis to begin on. It goes to the bottom and simplifies the matter, and, if you have mental and nervous symptoms left still you have overcome that violent septic state which must be met at once, and the remaining symptoms in many instances are simple. Sulphur is a general remedy to begin with in those cases where the symptoms are not perfectly clear for another.

This remedy is full of *difficult breathing,* shortness of breath from very little exertion, copious sweat, so exhausted; asthmatic breathing and much rattling in the chest. Every time he gets "cold", it settles in the chest or in the nose. In both these instances the catarrhal state hangs on and holds a long time; it seems never to be finished, always remains as a catarrhal state. "Every cold he takes ends in asthma," calls for *Dulcamara,* but very often the fag end of that attack will remain and the physician has to give a deep-acting remedy. After *Dulcamara* has done all it can do Sulphur comes in as its complementary remedy. *Calcarea carb.* has a similar relationship to *Dulcamara..*

The *nose,* the *inner chest* and *lungs* furnish us localities for much trouble. The patient has had pneumonia and it has gone on to the period of infiltration; you have taken the case in this advanced stage after *Bryonia* has overcome the threatening features, and now when the patient should rally he does not rally; he perspires all over, is tired and has a strange and singular consciousness that "there is something wrong in there; a load in there;" difficult breathing; flashes of heat and yet not much fever; sometimes coldness alternating with flashes of heat. I have often heard them say, "There is a great load in there, doctor. I cannot get rid of it." Upon close examination you find there is hepatization and now comes the time for such remedies as *Phosphorus, Lycopodium* and Sulphur, and Sulphur leads them all. When *Bryonia* has been sufficient for the earlier symptoms. or when *Aconite* has cleared them up, there has been too much for these remedies to relieve, then hepatization comes on. If this is confined to only a small area it will keep up quite a chronic course, but Sulphur will clear it up. If, however, it is a double pneumonia, or the hepatization involves a considerable portion of the lung, and the remedy given has not been sufficient, and the case is advancing towards a fatal issue, it may be that all at once at one, two or three o'clock in the morning, he begins to sink, his nose becomes pinched, his lips are drawn, he takes on a hippocratic countenance, is covered with cold sweat, he is too feeble in every part of his body to move; he only moves his head a little in a restless' manner. Unless you are called at once and give him a dose of *Arsenicum* he will die. You give the *Arsenicum,* and you have done well, but *Arsenicum* has no ability to remove the results of inflammation. But though it cannot *cure* that hepatized lung it acts as a vital stimulant; it warms up the patient and makes him feel he is going to get better; hut, mark this, in twenty-four hours he will die unless you follow the *Arsenicum* with the proper remedy. You must not wait on your remedy too long in these cases. Just as soon as he rallies and the reaction is at its highest pitch, give him the antidote and natural follower, of *Arsenicum,* which is Sulphur, and in twenty-four hours the patient will say, "I am getting better." As sure as you exist today, it will do just that thing. There are times when you will see clearly that *Phosphorus* is the medicine to follow *Arsenicum* with. If such a patient, rallying under *Arsenicum,* goes into a fever, if a hot fever comes on with burning thirst and he cannot get enough ice-cold water, you must follow it with *Phosphorus,* and it will do in that case what Sulphur will do in the other. You will not see these cases in your own practice because you will not let your cases get into that state; if such cases have power enough to live when prescribed for properly in that state, they have power enough to let you break up the whole nature of the case in the beginning. But go back to that patient who had only a circumscribed hepatization and felt well enough to get up and go around. He has a lingering cough, and now six months or a year after the attack he says, "Doctor, I have never been right since I had an attack of chest trouble. The doctor called it pneumonia." He can tell you about the rusty sputum and the other little things that belong to pneumonia; that is all you need to know. He has had a chronic cough ever since that attack and now he has chilliness. There is fibrinous infiltration, not a tuberculous state, but the remains of hepatization that nature could not cure. If that is allowed to go on he will go into catarrhal phthisis, asthmatic conditions of chronic bronchitis and troubles of various sorts, and finally he will die from these. Sulphur will very often confirm to all of his symptoms; it especially has the ability to clear up the lungs that were not properly cleared up at the time of his illness.

Sulphur cures bronchitis. It cures asthmatic bronchitis when the symptoms agree. Sulphur has a most violent cough that racks the whole frame; it seems that the head will fly off; pain in the head when coughing; the head is jarred by the cough. Then he has expectoration of blood, bleeding from the lungs; in all of these cases threatening phthisis, when there is yet not too much deposit of tubercle, when there is only the beginning of tubercular deposit. The low, stricken-down constitution, the emaciated subjects that have inherited phthisis who have the all-gone hungry feeling in the stomach, heat on the top of the head and uneasiness from the warmth of the bed. These cases would be better if they had plenty of eruptions come out upon the body; but as a matter of fact the skin has no eruptions; there is no relief; it is all going on in his internals and he is gradually breaking down. Sulphur will in such instances rouse that patient out of his phthisical state and he will return to health, or, if he is too bad for that he may be kept for years from his troubles. Look out for it in the advanced state of phthisis. You have had sufficient said concerning its administration in such a condition. It increases the suppuration, and brings on little pneumonias wherever there is a tubercle; it tends to suppurate these out. Every cell that is incapable of carrying on its function will be sloughed out by Sulphur.

The striking thing in Sulphur as to the *back* is pain in the back on rising from a seat, compelling him to walk bent, and he can only straighten up slowly after moving. The pain is principally in the lumbo-sacral region. The *extremities* are covered with eruptions. Eruptions upon the back of the hands and between the fingers, and sometimes upon the palm; vesicular and scaly eruptions which itch; pustules, boils and little abscesses; irregular erysipelatous patches here and there upon the extremities; a dirty appearance of the skin. Itching of the skin from the warmth of the bed.

Enlargement of the joints. Rheumatic affections; great stiffness of the joints; tightness in the hollow of the knees; tightness of the tendons, of rheumatic and gouty character. Cramps in the legs and soles of the feet. Burning of the soles of the feet in bed; he puts them out of bed to cool them off. The soles cramp and burn and itch. At times you will find the soles are cold, and then again burning, and these states alternate with each other. Distress of the body with coldness of the limbs, but after going to bed they burn so much that he must put them out. The corns, which he is a victim of and suffers from almost constantly, burn and sting in the warmth of the bed.

The *skin* of a Sulphur patient ulcerates and suppurates easily; a splinter under the skin will cause it to ulcerate; wounds heal slowly and fester. Every little prick of a pin festers as in *Hepar.*

The *eruptions* of Sulphur are too numerous to mention. They are of all sorts, but there are a few characterizing features in all, such as the burning, stinging and itching and the aggravation from the warmth of the bed. The skin is rough and unhealthy. Upon the face are many "blackheads," acne, pimples and pustules. Sulphur is full of boils and abscesses in all parts of the body, squamous eruptions, vesicular eruptions, etc. They are all present in Sulphur and they burn and sting.

SULPHURIC ACID

The sensation of quivering all over the body and in the limbs without visible trembling is a very strong symptom of Sulphuric acid, and especially if it is associated with weakness that has been of long standing. The exhaustion, excitability and hurried feeling are constant factors. The hæmorrhagic disposition with many complaints. Black fluid blood from all the orifice, of the body. Small red spots enlarging rapidly to resemble purpura hæmorrhagica. Blue-black spots on the skin from slight injury. Blood-red spots on the skin like those on a brook trout sometimes after injuries. Chafing easily, followed by ulceration. Boils and bedsores. It has many of the complaints found in old people. The morning aggravation of symptoms is also a strong feature. Sensitive to cold and emaciation. The pains are bruised, burning, tearing, stitching, shooting and jerking. The pain comes on slowly and departs suddenly. The discharges are dark, thin blood or blood-streaked; or thin, yellow and bloody. The discharges are excoriating. General sweat after eating. The symptoms predominate on the right side. It is often indicated in sour-smelling babies like *Hepar,* and it is as sensitive to touch and nearly as sensitive to cold. When it has cured the sensitiveness to cold the patient often becomes worse and requires *Pulsatilla,* which is the complement and antidote.

Prostration of mind and body, with extreme sadness, weeps continuously. Nothing can be done to please him. Fretful and irritable over the slightest cause. He cannot eat and work fast enough. No one does anything to please him; in such a hurry if doing anything or going anywhere. All things must be done at once. Unwilling to answer. Irresolution.

Vertigo in close room. Better walking in the open air. Better lying. Sometimes compelling him to keep his bed.

Tension in the forehead with coryza.

The brain seems loose and seems to fall to side lain on, better sitting perfectly still, worse walking. The blood flows strongly to the head and the feet become cold. Electric shocks in forehead and temples in forenoon and again in evening. Sensation as though a plug were being driven into the skull by strong blows. The pains in the head come on slowly and cease suddenly. Violent headaches in debilitated people. Extreme soreness in the periosteum such as is found in syphilis. The hair falls out or turns gray. Ulceration of the scalp. Extremely sensitive eruptions. Lachrymation when reading. Chronic inflammation of the eye, with enlarged veins and ulceration. Sensation of foreign body in right outer canthus. Soreness in the eyes with coryza.

Severe ear pains that increase gradually and cease suddenly. Gradual loss of hearing. Bloody discharge from ear. Buzzing in the ear.

Slowly oozing, dark, thin blood from the nose in the evening. It cures acrid, bloody discharge from nose in feeble patients when the generals are covered by it. The coryza is dry or fluid with loss of smell and taste.

The face of the Sulphuric acid patient is a most sickly one. Pale, sickly and sometimes jaundiced. The expression of long suffering is marked. The deep lines of pain, depletion and emaciation. Tension of the face or a sensation as though white of egg had dried on it. Violent neuralgic pains of the face coming on gradually and ceasing suddenly, ameliorated by warmth and lying on the painful side. Small red spots or specks on the face gradually increasing in size. Inflammation of the submaxillary gland.

The teeth decay early. Violent neuralgia of the teeth, coming on slowly and ceasing suddenly. Worse from cold and better from heat, worse in the evening in bed. The teeth are on edge. Loss of taste during coryza. The sore mouth is one of its most important features. It is our most frequently indicated remedy for *nursing sore mouth*. The *aphthous mouth of infant or mother* with yellowish or whitish ulcers. Bloody saliva from mouth; vesicles in the mouth. Breath very offensive. Bleeding from the mucous surfaces of mouth and gums with or without purpura hæmorrhagica. Rapidly spreading ulcers in the mouth.

Inflammation of the throat that is aphthous or follicular. Denuded mucous membrane. Diphtheritic exudate *yellowish* or white with aphthous surroundings and bleeding from nose, gums or other parts. Diphtheria with

more than ordinary exhaustion and fœtor. The uvula is œdematous. The throat
is full of spreading ulcers. Painful sore throat with painful, difficult swallowing.
During the throat troubles fluids drunk run out of nose. Salivation, glands of
throat swollen and there is great swelling of the tonsils, soft palate and
throat in general. Dark fluid blood from throat and mouth.

He craves brandy and fruit. Loss of appetite and progressive weakness
are strong features. Aversion to the smell of coffee. He cannot drink cold
water, as it feels so cold in the stomach and makes him chilly. Violent,
spasmodic hiccough, such as occurs in drunkards. *Chronic heart burn. Sour
belching. Sour vomiting.* The teeth are always on edge from sour eructations.
Sour vomiting during pregnancy. Vomiting of drunkards in the morning.
(Compare *Arsenicum.*) Sour and very foul. Nausea and shivering. Coughing
and belching sour fluids. The stomach seems to *hang down as if relaxed.*
Vomiting after drinking cold water. Violent, spasmodic pains in the stomach.
The pains come gradually and cease suddenly. The sour vomiting is most
like *Robinia.*

She does not vomit food, but cannot eat, as it causes pain in stomach and
she vomits mucus.

After intermittent fever had existed some time the spleen enlarges, and is
painful on coughing and sore to touch. Stitching pains in spleen and liver. It
has many times overcome the poison of lead and lead colic. Sinking, weak
feeling in abdomen after stool. Weak feeling in abdomen, as though menses
would come on. Labor-like pains in abdomen, extending to hips and back.

Diarrhœa with great general weakness and sensation of trembling. With
weak, *sinking sensation in the abdomen after stool.* Chronic diarrhœa with
much suffering. Excoriating stools, burning in rectum during stool. Diarrhœa
brought on from the least indiscretion in eating, after fruit, especially if unripe,
after oysters. Stool watery orange yellow, stringy, mucous, mixed with blood,
greenish, black, undigested smelling like spoiled eggs. Hæmorrhoids very
sore, itching, painful during stool, in drunkards. In constipation the stool is
in small balls.

Pain in the bladder if the desire to pass urine is postponed. It has cured
diabetes. Scanty urine. Bloody urine. Cuticle in the urine.

The menses are too frequent and copious and the flow is dark and thin.
Many symptoms come before the menses. Nightmare before menses. Has
nightmare at the close of the menses. The vagina is prolapsed and
gangrenous. Leucorrhœa bloody, acrid, milky or albuminous, yellow. The
woman at the climacteric period has many symptoms peculiar to Sulphuric
acid. The flashes of heat, weakness, sensation of trembling, a nervous hurry
in all her actions and feelings, bleeding from uterus and other parts of blood
that does not coagulate, and constipation with small, hard balls like sheep's

dung are symptoms common to the critical period. It often causes the vomiting of pregnancy. Vomiting *preceded by cough.*

It has cured sterility when it was supposed to depend upon the copious and frequent menstrual flow. Violent itching of the vulva.

Pain and soreness in the larynx. Pain in the larynx on swallowing. Hoarseness with a dry feeling and sensation of roughness in the larynx.

Weak chest and great dyspnœa. Rapid movement of the wings of nose like *Lycopodium.* Rapid moving up and down of the larynx during the dyspnœa. Short of breath.

Except in the morning the cough is dry and hacking. Sometimes in two coughs. He coughs in the open air, either walking or riding, worse from cold drinks and from the odor of coffee. Cough followed by itching and vomiting. The irritation is felt in the chest. The expectoration is in the morning of dark, thin blood, or of thin, yellowish, blood-streaked mucus tasting sour.

Weakness in the chest with burning and stitching pain. Pressure on left side of chest. Profuse hæmorrhage from the lungs of dark fluid blood, after pneumonia, and during the climacteric period. Ulceration of lungs (compare *Kali carb.*). Oppression of the chest and suffocation unless he lets the legs hang down. It has been a very useful remedy in the first steps of phthisis with profuse sweat and great weakness, but where given in the last stage it has appeared to bring on hæmorrhage and increase of the inflammatory condition in the lungs. Stitching pains in the heart, palpitation. It has been useful in pleuritic exudation.

Great weakness in the spine, felt mostly when standing and sitting. Pain in the lumbar region. Soreness between shoulder blades when coughing. Stiffening of the back in the morning on rising. Large abscess on the right side of the neck.

Black and blue spots on the limbs. Stitching pain in the shoulder joint on lifting the arm. Stitches in finger joints. Chafing of thighs after rising. Marked weakness in knees and ankles. Swollen veins of feet. Chilblains of frostbitten parts. Twitching of fingers during sleep.

Late falling asleep and wakens too early. Nightmare before menses.

It has chilliness, flashes of heat with sweat. Copious sweat, mostly on upper part of body, from motion, sour, cold, after eating warm food. Morning sweats. Night sweats. Typhoid fever with great prostration. Bleeding from capillaries. Dark, thin blood.

Hæmorrhage of dark, thin blood from the bowels. Putrid forms of continued fever. Cadaveric countenance.

Echymoses, purpura hæmorrhagica. Old cicatrices turn red and become painful. Itching and prickling with eruptions. Pimples. Red itching blotches on the skin. Livid spots. Contusions, bedsores. Boils and abscesses. Nodular urticarias. It cures old indolent ulcers that bleed easily a dark blood. Sensitive painful spreading ulcers. Stinging burning pain in ulcers. It has cured putrid ulcers on legs. It is useful in ulcers of drunkards, in ulcers following a low form of fever. Thin yellow or bloody discharge.

SULPHUR IODATUM

This is a very profound and long-acting remedy affecting all parts of the body with aggravations morning, afternoon, *evening,* NIGHT, and after midnight. Desires open air, *which ameliorates* the most of his symptoms. There is an indescribable feeling throughout the body like a *general physical anxiety,* which compels him to hurry in all his work and when walking. Atrophy of glands, chronic jerking of muscles and a sensation of a band around parts. He takes cold on the slightest provocation, while he desires to be in a cool place, and in the cold air he takes cold from becoming cold. There is a convulsive tendency in the remedy; hysterical and epileptiform. The cavities become dropsical. Some symptoms are better after eating, and others are worse. Emaciation is marked and it should be of great service in marasmus of children, with increased appetite. Slight exertion brings on all the symptoms: Weankess and palpitation; faint and fainting spells, with palpitation; feels unusually weak when hungry, warm food brings on much distress; formication all over; full feeling in body and limbs; body feels distended, as if there were great vascular engorgement; hemorrhage from internal parts; *great heat of the body,* which is only a sensation; heaviness of body and limbs; INDURATION OF GLANDS hard, knotty lymphatic glands in the neck like ropes; induration of muscles. This feature points to its usefulness in carcinoma of glands. When used early it is often able to cure promptly. Inflammation of organs and glands. Injuries with extravasations. Lack of reaction and marked lassitude. The symptoms are worse while lying, but sometimes better after lying a long time. Worse lying on the back and worse in a warm bed. It is an antidote to the over-use of mercury. Though he is restless and desires to move, the motion increases his symptoms. From all mucous membranes there is an increased flow. There is numbness in single parts and in suffering parts. There is a marked surging of blood in the body with general pulsation and hot sensations. Pain in bones and glands. These bruised, burning, cutting, jerking, *pressing,* stitching and tearing pains; when heated he sweats much and cannot cool off without taking cold. Its complaints are such as are found in plethoric, full-blooded, vascular people. Any kind of hurry or running creates a flush and surging in the body with palpitation and weakness. Many symptoms are one-sided, especially the *right.* Sluggishness is a marked feature of the whole complex of symptoms; many symptoms are worse sitting and better standing. He is much worse in the heat of summer, and in the sun's heat. *Swelling of glands.*

Its symptoms are such as are often found in the advanced stages of syphilis, and it is especially useful in such as have been heavily charged with mercury. The symptoms are worse from touch and pressure. Throughout the body there is a feeling of tension. Trembling, internal and external. The muscles twitch and the limbs jerk. The symptoms are worse from walking. The symptoms are worse *from warmth; warm air, warm bed, warm room, warm wraps.* Marked weariness in the morning; from ascending stairs; after diarrhœa; during menses; from walking. He is worse in wet weather, and better in winter.

Anxiety driving him to keep on the go. Apathy. Aversion to company. When reading and thinking cannot control the mind. Lost confidence in his own ability. Confusion of mind in the morning and evening, and when he exerts the mind. Over-conscientious about small matters. Says he is becoming timid, even cowardly. There are times in the night when he is almost delirious. Illusions of fancy. Sees dead people. Despair, cannot see any brightness in life. Discontented and discouraged. Dullness of mind. Very excitable. The whole mental state is worse from mental exertion. Dread of exertion. Fear that some unknown trouble is coming to him; of insanity; of misfortune; of people. He finds himself doing things in a great hurry. Walks fast and in a hurry. Strongly inclined to hysterical conduct. Very impatient, cannot wait, but must keep on the go. At times indifferent to all surroundings. She becomes indolent and neglects her housework. She cannot compel herself to attend to her duties. Her mood is very changeable; irritable or mirthful. Mental prostration. Very restless, and forced to keep on the move although moving causes weakness and increases her bodily symptoms. *Marked sadness,* and dullness of the senses. Would like to sit, but too restless. Starting during sleep. Stupefaction of mind. Persistent thoughts torment her. Weeps much in the evening.

Vertigo in the morning on rising, while lying, during menses, rising from bed, rising from a seat, *stooping,* walking.

The following particulars will yield to this remedy whenever the general symptoms above mentioned strongly predominate.

The scalp feels cold to the patient. Congestion on coughing and during menses, eruptions on the scalp; crusts, eczema. Itching eruptions and itching without eruptions. Heat in the head and the hair falls out. The hair stands on end. The head feels heavy. Pain in the head in the morning on rising; in the forenoon; in the afternoon. Headache is better in the open air, by cold applications, by motion. Headache worse by binding up the hair, from fasting, from becoming heated, before and during menses, from heat of sun, from talking, from *warm room* and from warm wraps on the body. Pain in forehead, over eyes, in the evening, worse from motion. Pain in occiput in the afternoon. Pain in both sides of the head and again on only one side. Pain in temples and vertex. Pressing pains in forehead, over eyes; in occiput; *sides of head;* temples; vertex. Shooting pains in head; in the temples when stooping. Sore, bruised feeling in head; stitching pains in occiput; sides of head; temples; *vertex.* Tearing pain in temples. Perspiration on scalp; on forehead. *Pulsation in head;* in the temples. Tension in the forehead. Wrapping up head brings on headache.

Dullness of eyes, inflammation of conjunctiva. Catarrhal inflammation in psoric patients. The lids feel heavy. Inflammation of the iris in syphilitic subjects. Copious lachrymation in cold air. Pressing, sore, stitching pains. Protrusion of the eyes. Pupils dilated. Redness of eyes and lids. Staring eyes. Sunken eyes with swollen lids. Twitching of the lids. Jaundiced eyes. *Dim,* foggy vision, and there is *flickering* and sparks. Diplopia.

Discharge of pus from ear. The ears are hot. Inflammation of eustachian tubes. Buzzing, humming, ringing, and roaring noises in ears. Itching in ears. Aching, pressing, shooting, stitching and tearing pains. Stopped sensation. Hearing acute for noise. Hearing impaired.

It cures our most obstinate catarrhal conditions, with discharges, as follows: Bloody, *copious, excoriating, greenish,* hard, dry masses; purulent, *thick,* YELLOW Excoriation and itching in nose. Redness of the nose. Coryza fluent in the open air, coryza with cough, long continued. It is a very useful remedy in hay fever Burning in the nose on blowing it. Pressing pain in roof of nose, loss of smell, sneezing in the *evening.* The nose is swollen. There are small ulcers up in the nose.

Cold face. Discoloration; red, circumscribed redness, *sallow, yellow.* Drawn face. Eruptions, acne, boils, pimples, crusty eruptions on the nose. Dry and hot. The expression is haggard and *sickly.* The face is Hippocratic. Induration of the parotid and submaxillary glands. The face is sunken with pain. Burning heat of the face. Swollen glands. Swollen parotid and submaxillary glands. Twitching of the face.

Copious aphthæ. Bleeding gums. Tongue coated at base, red at points. Cracked tongue. The gums are detached from the teeth. The *tongue is dry.* It overcomes the bad effect of the mercury. Much mucus forms in the mouth. Offensive, even putrid, odor from the mouth. Burning tongue. Salivation. Stammering speech. *Swollen gums.* The taste is bad, *bitter,* putrid, sour. Ulcers in the mouth and on the gums. Toothache after eating. Tearing pain in teeth.

Choking, constriction of oesophagus. Dryness of throat. Gray exudation in the throat. Tough, viscid, yellow or white mucus in throat. Pain in throat on coughing; when swallowing. Burning in throat and oesophagus. Pressing pain in throat. Sore throat in the morning. Scraping n throat. Swallowing of liquids difficult. Swelling of throat and uvula. Ulce s in throat. It has cured goitre. It has cured indurated lymphatic glands in the neck where they were like knotted ropes. Sore lymphatic glands of neck. Swelling of the lymphatic glands of the neck.

Appetite INCREASED; RAVENOUS; *with diarrhœa;* with emaciation; with marasmus in children; without relish of food; appetite wanting. Aversion to food. Desires stimulants, acids, pickles and lemonade. The stomach is easily disordered. Marked distension from gas and sensation of emptiness. Eructations empty, sour, waterbrash. Eructations ameliorate. There is fulness, heartburn, heaviness after eating and hiccough. Chronic indigestion, nausea, at night after eating. Pain in stomach after eating relieved by eructations. Burning, cramping, cutting, gnawing, pressing, stitching pain in stomach. Tenderness of stomach. Pulsation in stomach. Retching from the cough. Sensation of tightness. Thirst in the evening; burning, extreme, unquenchable. Vomiting on coughing; with diarrhœa, after drinking; after eating; after milk. Vomiting bloody bile; food, sour, watery.

Atrophy of the liver. Suppurating bubos. Tympanitic, distension of abdomen. Enlarged abdomen. Enlarged liver, mesenteric glands, spleen, lymphatic glands of groin. Much flatulence. HARDNESS OF LIVER, *spleen* and glands of groin. Inflammation of spleen. It cures many complaints of the liver. Pain in abdomen after eating, before and during menses. Pain in *liver,* in hypogastrium, in inguinal region; in *spleen,* in region of umbilicus. Burning and cramping in umbilical region. Cutting during stool. Pressing in liver, in hypogastrium, in groin. Soreness and stitching pains in liver. Rumbling and pulsation in abdomen. Suppuration of inguinal glands. Swelling of *mesenteric glands and glands of groin.*

Constipation with no desire to go to stool for a long time, and great straining to pass a stool. The stool is incomplete and unsatisfactory. Constipation alternating with diarrhœa. The stool is hard, knotty and light colored. There is diarrhœa in the *morning* and evening, worse after eating. Diarrhœa in emaciated people and in aged people. The diarrhœa stools are variable; black, brown, frequent frothy, offensive, purulent, watery, white, yellow. There is also dysenteric stools of bloody mucus, frequent, purulent, scanty, with tenesmus. Hemorrhoids, heat and *itching of the anus* and much flatus passes. Burning in anus after stool.

Retention of urine. Frequent urging to urinate, worse during the night. The urine passes by dribbling, and there is involuntary dribbling. Frequent urination at night. Also in the morning. Prostate gland is enlarged. The urine is albuminous, cloudy, dark, red, copious, milky, offensive, with red sediment. The urine smells like raspberries. There is a cuticle on the urine, and it sometimes become scanty.

Erections incomplete, without sexual desire or wanting. Erections troublesome at night. It has cured hydrocele of small boys. Induration of the testes. Itching of the penis; in the urethra. Perspiration of the scrotum. Relaxed genitals. Seminal emissions. Swelling of the testes. It has cured tuberculosis of testes and spermatic cords.

It has cured predisposition to abort. In cancer of the uterus it greatly restrains the progress of the disease and palliates the sufferings where the patient is very vascular, is losing flesh, has a strong appetite and very sensitive to heat. Increased sexual desire. Inflammation of the uterus. COPIOUS LEUCORRHŒA, acrid, bloody, *burning,* thick and sometimes thin, *yellow,* before and after menses. Menses absent, *copious,* frequent, *irregular,* painful, or short duration, suppressed. Metrorrhagia. Hard pain in ovaries. Great tenderness of vulva and *ovaries.* Prolapsus of uterus.

Catarrh of larynx and trachea. Dryness, crawling and constriction in the larynx. Much hawking. Inflammation of the larynx. Irritation of larynx and trachea. Laryngismus. Much mucus in the larynx and trachea; dark, purulent. Pain,, soreness and stitching in the larynx. For laryngeal phthisis, is a most useful remedy; where the general symptoms are present. Roughness in the larynx. Tickling in the larynx and trachea in a warm room. *Hoarseness* in the morning. Voice rough, weak and lost.

Respiration is fast; *asthmatic, irregular, rattling,* short, *suffocative,* and wheezing; difficult at night, on ascending and from least exertion. Desire for deep breath.

It is a highly important cough remedy. Cough *morning* and evening, asthmatic, choking and very exhausting. It *is paroxysmal, spasmodic, rattling* and suffocative. Cough during fever. Dry cough in the morning. Hard cough during the early part of the night. It also has a less cough. Cough from talking and smoking. The cough is relieved in the open air, from becoming cold and from expectoration; worse lying down and better from sitting up. Short hacking cough. Irritation to cough in the larynx and trachea. Expectoration morning and evening; *bloody, copious,* difficult, *greenish,* mucous, *offensive, purulent,* sweetish, tough, *viscid, yellow.*

Feeling of anxiety in the chest. It is of great service in cancer of the mammae. It is a most valuable remedy in catarrh of the bronchial tubes, *constriction of chest* and heart, dropsy of the pleura, eruptions of the chest. Great heat of chest. Induration of the mammary glands. Inflammation of lungs and bronchial tubes. Inflammation of the pleura, especially where neglected. Itching of the skin. Where the milk becomes suppressed in the nursing woman. Oppression of the chest. Pain in chest on coughing; pain in sides of chest, worse on the right side. Pain in the region of the heart. Aching, burning and cutting. Cutting in the region of the heart. Pressing in sides of chest on coughing. Stitching in chest on coughing. *Palpitation* at night, *on exertion,* during menses, on motion. It is a very useful remedy in phthisical conditions of the lungs; in ulcerative conditions and cavities. Swelling of the axillary glands. Feeling of weakness in chest.

Itching of the lumbar region. Pain and soreness under scapulæ. Pain in lumbar region during menses. Pain in sacrum and coccyx. Stitching in the back; in the lumbar region. Weakness of spine.

Painful gouty nodosities of the fingers. Coldness in upper limbs; hands; legs; *feet at night*. Convulsive action of muscles in upper limbs. Old corns become painful. Cramps in thighs, *legs;* feet. Vesicles on the limbs. Heat of hands. Heaviness of the limbs; feet. Itching of upper limbs; lower limbs. Numbness of limbs; fingers; legs. Gouty and rheumatic pains in the joints and bones. The soles ache and burn when standing. Pain in upper limbs, worse on motion. Rheumatic pain in limbs. Pain in elbow. Pain in hip; thigh; *knee;* calf; foot. Drawing pains in lower limbs; thighs; knees. Pressing pains in upper limbs. Sore bruised pains in shoulder, upper arms and thighs. *Stitching in knees.* Tearing in upper limbs; elbows; knees; legs. Paralysis of lower limbs. Perspiration of hands, cold palms; *feet*. Pulsation in limbs. Stiffness of limbs; fingers. Dropsical swelling of limbs; hands; lower limbs; knees; legs; feet. Trembling of all the limbs. Twitching in thighs, weakness of limbs; knees.

Dreams amorous; anxious; of dead people; distressing; nightmare; vivid; sleep is restless. Sleepiness in the evening. Sleepiness during daytime and sleepless at night. Sleeplessness after midnight; waking too early.

Chill at night in bed, better after rising. Internal chill. Warm room does not relieve. Warm bed does not relieve. Shaking chill worse from motion. Quartan or tertian. Fever in the afternoon alternating with chill. External heat. FLASHES OF HEAT It is a very useful remedy in hectic fever. Internal heat with external chill. Fever without sweat. Chill followed by heat. Wants to be uncovered during heat. Perspiration morning and night in bed. Clammy, cold, exhausting sweat. *Sweat from slight exertion;* from motion. Profuse sweat during the night. The sweat smells sour.

Anæsthesia. The skin sometimes burns: again it is cold. The skin des- quamates. Discoloration; liver spots, red spots; yellow skin; yellow spots. The skin is dry. Eruptions; boils; blood boils; herpes; pimples; psoriasis; pustules; rash; scaly; urticaria. Where eruptions have been suppressed by ointments. Erysipelatous inflammation of the skin. The skin becomes excor- iated easily. Excrescenses form upon the skin. Formication. Freckles. Inactivity of the skin. Itching, burning and stitching. Burning in swollen skin. Burning in erysipelas. Pale, spongy, dropsical swelling of skin. Tension of skin. Ulcers: Bleeding; cancerous, *indolent;* indurated; sensitive; *spongy;* suppurating. The discharges from ulcers are bloody; copious, corrosive, thin, watery, yellow.

SYPHILINUM

Whenever the symptoms that are representative of the patient himself have been suppressed in any case of syphilis, and nothing remains but weakness and a few results of the storm that has long ago or recently passed, this nosode will cause reaction and restore order and sometimes do much curing, and the symptoms that must always be present, that represent the disordered state of the economy will appear to guide to a restoration of health. When a syphilitic patient has suffered from a course of typhoid he may be very slow in convalescing, but a single dose of Syphilinum high will cause him to eat and feel stronger and gain rapidly. How does the old school treatment of syphilis differ from barbarism? One might well ask. The strong drugging by *Mercurius* and iodides so debilitate that all who pass through are invalids and weak; even then they are not cured of syphilis—if they were cured we could not cause to come back the symptoms that have been removed. Syphilinum often does bring back the ulcers in the throat and the eruptions. When there are violent neuralgias of the head, in sides of head and over the eyes, great soreness in bones of legs and head, and the multitude of symptoms of nerve syphilis all nondescript, then it is that the patient will be made free from suffering, and given sleep, strength and appetite. But the ulcers and eruptions will come back in some cases, and it is all the better if they do. It is by no means limited to patients who have had syphilis. It can be used like any remedy against the symptoms of the provings, or such as are similar to symptoms common to the disease or against the symptoms like the numerous verified clinical symptoms. Many symptoms are worse at night in bed, many come on in the evening and last till morning. *From sundown to sunrise* marks the time of many violent pains and sufferings. Some are better from heat, and some are better from cold air and cold applications. There is great prostration in the morning on waking. It has cured many cases of epilepsy. Epileptic convulsions after menses. *Sleeplessness,* sometimes only one-half of the night, again the whole night. The blood feels hot flowing through the arteris during the night, Wandering pains here and there all over the body. Pain in the periosteum, nerves and joints. Pains sometimes increase gradually and decrease gradually. Sharp pains here and there. Complaints worse in the cold weather of winter and heat of summer. Extreme emaciation. Abscesses. Paralysis of limbs. Caries of bone. Curvature of spine. Gummata. *Dwarfish children.* Curvature of bones. Enlarged glands. Offensive odor of the body. Soreness to touch in many parts, especially bones. It has often been observed that in syphilized invalids remedies act but a few days and must be changed. This always calls for the nosode. When there is only great weakness and few symptoms it will act well. When there is ulceration of legs, throat, mouth or other parts with no repair. Fistulous openings, exostoses, fissures, tubercles and warts have been cured promptly. When it has been used against the primary manifestations of the disease and in the earlier phenomena it has generally resulted in failure. It is seldom the best remedy for syphilis *per se,* but for marked and suppressed syphilis it seems to restore a sort of order and bring better reaction. The author has many times observed that gummata in throat and anus will take on desctructive ulceration in old broken-down casts after *Sulphur* has been given, and that Syphilinum will restrain it and establish repair. *Sulphur* often produces prolonged aggravation when there are many tissue changes in advanced cases of syphilis. Such changes are most likely gummata. The effort of *Sulphur* is to remove the results of disease, which the patient cannot stand. It often causes suspicion of latent syphilis when such aggravations are very severe after *Sulphur* high. *Sulphur* low will not be followed by such results. After such prolonged aggravations Syphilinum should be considered Latent syphilis often exists where it is least expected. This nosode should be used only in high potencies.

Forgetful, Weak Minded. Laughing and weeping without cause. He cannot remember faces: names, dates, events, books or places. He cannot calculate. Despair of recovery. Melancholia. Fears he is going insane. *Imbecility.* Indifferent to his friends, and feels no delight in anything. Dreads the night and dreads the morning, as the weakness and soreness are worse on waking. He always says he is not himself and he cannot feel like himself. A middle-aged man who had suffered many years from latent syphilis abandoned his business and remained at home lamenting and sad. His wife supported the family by keeping boarders. After receiving a few doses of Syphilinum he took on new energy and became industrious and prosperous. Much vertigo. Aphasia. In some of these cases of brain syphilis *Sulphur* and *Causticum* have caused prolonged suffering and weakness. Syphilinum will act favourably.

Syphilitic invalids are often sufferers from violent neuralgic headaches. Violent pains in sides of head, forehead or temples. Pain from temple to temple, from ear to ear, one eye to occiput; supraorbital pains. Pain sometimes ameliorated by warmth. Bursting pains; fulness of head. Maddening pains all night, causing sleeplessness. Headache and delirium. Neuralgia of head beginning at 4 P.M., growing gradually worse until midnight and then gradually better, ceasing at daylight. Great soreness of the pericranium. Many pains are confined to a direct line and are called *linear headaches.* Violent crushing pains in occiput. Stupefying headaches in the forehead or occiput. Cutting pains in occiput. Headache through the temples, thence vertically, like an inverted letter T. Headaches involving the whole top of the head as if head would be crushed in. Violent pain in whole head with red face, enlarged veins of face, restlessness and sleepless nights. Aggravated nights. Tubercles all over the scalp. Exostoses in the cranium, very sore and painful. The hair is falling out.

Paralysis of the eye muscles is common. Strabismus. Diplopia. Amaurosis. Atrophy of the optic nerve. The retina is pale, gray and spotted. Myopia.

Iritis. Ptosis. Paralysis of the superior oblique. Chronic recurrent phlyctenular inflammation of the cornea. Conjunctivitis with ulceration. Ulceration of the cornea. Interstitial keratitis. Spots on the cornea. Left eye covered with fungus-like growth, pain intense, aggravated at night. Acute ophthalmia neonatorum when one of the parents has syphilis. Copious purulent discharge from eyes. Lids enormously swollen. Eyes cannot be opened because of swelling. Iritis with intense pain at night, and photophobia. Pain in eye from sundown to sunrise. Scalding tears.

Sharp pains in ear. Purulent watery discharge from ear. Caries of mostoid. Paralysis of auditory nerve. Calcareous deposit on tympanum.

This remedy has cured many cases of offensive green or yellow discharge from nose in children with specific history. Dryness of nose; obstructed at night. Frequent attacks of coryza. Always taking cold in nose. Syphilitic ozæna. Bones of nose destroyed by caries and nose depressed. The whole nose destroyed by ulceration. Epistaxis from ulcers. Hard plugs in nose.

Neuralgia of face. Paralysis of one side of face. Tubercles and copper-colored eruptions on face. It has palliated cancerous ulceration of face. Scabby eruption on face. It has cured rupia on the cheek. Papules and pustules. The lips are fissured and ulcerated. Ulcers on chin, lips, and wing of nose. Wing and side of nose eaten away by an ulcer. It has cured many cases of lupus of face.

The teeth are deformed, distorted, spotted; decay early; cup shaped in children. Violent pain in teeth. Crawling in the roots of the teeth, like a worm.

Mouth and tongue ulcerated. Breath fœtid. Tongue soft, spongy, easily indented in persons who have long taken *Mercury*. Paralysis of tongue, one-sided. Tongue red, excoriated, cracked and sore. Patches on tongue. Denuded patches. Red spots. Copious viscid saliva in mouth. Ulceration of soft palate. Caries of hard palate. Soft palate entirely destroyed. Bleeding from ulcers.

Throat studded with ulcers. Inflammation of throat and tonsils. Soft palate swollen and nodular. Post nasal catarrh and ulceration. Posterior nares plugged with crusts.

The appetite is perverted. Longing for strong drink. Thirst. Aversion to food, to meat. No desire to eat. All food disagrees. Flatulence. Heart-burn; nausea; vomiting. Ulceration of stomach.

The rectum is the seat of many symptoms and conditions. Ulceration, fissures, piles, nodules, gummata; copious bleeding; cutting, burning pains. Condylomata. Constipation. Paralysis of rectum; prolapsus of anus. Relaxed protruding rectum.

This nosode has cured nodular formations in testes, spermatic cord and scrotum. It has cured herpetic eruptions on prepuce and scrotum. Induration of testes and spermatic cord.

Nodular formations in vagina and labia. Ulceration of os uteri, Induration of cervix uteri. Copious yellow-green leucorrhœa. Leucorrhœa in little girls, of specific history, acrid water, leucorrhœa aggravated nights from warmth of bed. Pain in ovaries during the night. Itching in the vulva. Sharp pains in uterus. Cystic ovaries. Ovarian tumor. Cutting pain in ovary during coition at moment of orgasm. Uterine and ovarian complaints when there is a specific history

Ulceration of larynx and loss of voice. Aphonia before menses. Continuous sharp pain in larynx from evening to sunrise every night compelling him to walk the floor all night cured by Syphilinum very high, one dose.

Asthma in warm damp weather during night. Dyspnœa. Attacks of spasmodic bronchial asthma for twenty-five years; at night in bed or during a thunderstorm, preventing sleep for many nights. Dyspnœa from 1 to 4 A.M.

Cough at night. Dry rasping cough during the night. Rawness in chest. Thick purulent expectoration. Dry cough from lying on right side. Mucopurulent expectoration, grayish, greenish, greenish-yellow, tasteless. Clear white mucous expectoration. Rattling in the chest. Pain and pressure behind the sternum. Eruptions on the chest.

Rheumatic stiffness and lameness in back. Aching in whole spine. Pain in region of kidneys, aggravated after urinating. Pain in sacrum, aggravated while sitting. Caries of cervical and dorsal vertebræ. Enlarged glands of neck. It has cured indurated cervical glands. Pain in back, hip and thighs during the night. It has cured Hodgkin's disease.

Inflammation of joints. Rheumatism, muscles are caked in hard knots or lumps. Pain in limbs ameliorated by heat, aggravated from sunset to sunrise. Stiffness of all the joints. Rheumatic pains and swelling of joints of upper limbs. Rheumatism of deltoid, painful on raising the arm. Pains in arms on motion. Ulcers on back of hands. Nightly pain and swelling in legs. Pains in lower extremities, preventing sleep, aggravated from hot applications, ameliorated by pouring cold water on them. Weakness in knees and hips. Severe bone aches in legs at night in bed. Pain in back of feet and toes at night in bed. Pains often aggravated in warm bed at night. Pains drive him, out of bed at night. Tearing in hip and thigh, aggravated during night, ameliorated at day-break, ameliorated by walking, not affected by weather (improved by Syph.). Ulcers on the legs. Large crusts on the legs. Tubercles on the lower limbs. Tension of the tendons of the legs and soles. The extremes of cold and heat often bring out the symptoms of these old sufferers. Neuralgia of limbs gradually increasing, aggravated as the night goes on. Extreme sensitiveness of the tibia.

There are fevers, chilliness, but the night sweats and great weakness are striking.

The eruptions are numerous, but may be studied better by consulting the numerous works on syphilis, as this is not a study of the disease, but the nosode.

TARENTULA HISPANICA

The terrible poison should never be used except in attenuations. The nervous manifestations of this remedy are almost indescribable and too numerous to mention. Anxiety and restlessness are words that prevail through all the conditions in it. It is much like *Ars.* The anxiety is felt sometimes in the mind, sometimes in the whole body, sometimes in the limbs and in the stomach. Cardiac anxiety is a strong feature. A strong aversion to colours, such as green, red and black. Depraved imaginations prevail through all the proving Loss of all shame. Desire to run about, to dance and jump up and down. Great fantastic dancing. Sometimes music ameliorates all the symptoms and at other times it aggravates them. He becomes violently excited from music.

Emaciation is so marked that it may be said sometimes that the flesh falls off from him. Creeping and crawling in the skin all over the body. Paralysis of any part of the body, or of all the limbs. Trembling and jerking convulsions. It has an appearance very much like St. Vitus' Dance and hence has cured chorea when it was better from music. But it will also cure when worse from music. The extreme restlessness of the limbs is like *Ars.* and it is a deep acting medicine like *Ars.,* and it sometimes has cured where *Ars.* has failed, although it seemed well selected. Anxiety, restlessness, constant motion of the arms, legs, trunk and head. Restlessness of the limbs in the evening, in bed before going to sleep, like *Ars.* and *Lyc.* It is full of pains in the body and limbs; pains in the bones; pains in the arms and in the joints. Periodicity is so well marked that it has been a marked curative remedy in intermittent fevers with restlessness of limbs, with aching of the bones, with stitching pains, with the anxiety, especially when these come in the evening and the fever lasts all night. Chill in the evening followed by fever without sweat is a marked feature.

The patient himself is always sensitive to cold, so the pains in the limbs are worse in cold air and from becoming cold. Cold damp weather aggravates all his symptoms. Walking in the open air when not cold ameliorates most of his symptoms. Open air ameliorates, rubbing ameliorates. There is weakness of all the limbs. Violent pains in the bowels and in the bladder. Burning is a strong symptom in many parts, but especially in the rectum; in the palms and soles and in the uterus. It is one of our high grade remedies for hysterical women. He is inclined to walk in his sleep. Excessive hyperæsthesia; all the symptoms are worse from grief and excitement. When choreic symptoms are present he can run better than he can walk.

Impairment of memory. Great irritability. In the hysterical symptoms she is better from music. Her motions are ludicrous and she is even lascivious in her conduct. Great excitement from music; she sings until she falls with exhaustion. Fox-like cunning and destructiveness. Paroxysms of insanity with restlessness of the legs and threatening words. When questioned she does not answer. Frequently imagines that she has been insulted. Dementia with great sadness. Excitement with singing, dancing and weeping. She sees monsters, animals, faces, insects and ghosts. She sees strangers in the room. Tarentula patients feign all sorts of sickness, especially fainting. They not only imagine themselves sick, but they pretend to be sick when they are not. Aversion to red, green and black and all striking colors. She pulls her own hair and presses her hands upon her head. Constantly complaining and threatening; threatens her nurse and her attendants; she strikes her head with her hands; she strikes her body; strikes her attendants and her best friends. Violence is a strong feature of the remedy. Violence with anger. Tears his clothing. Consolation causes weeping.

The mental symptoms are better in the evening after eating. Many physical symptoms are worse in the evening, especially the febrile conditions.

A desire to lie down in the dark and not be talked to. She has many insane ideas, one is that she wants to hide because she imagines that she will be assaulted. Angered from contradiction.

Frequent attacks of dizziness, even so great that she falls to the ground. Dizziness comes on in the night; when descending stairs. Dizziness with rush of blood to the head and dizziness when fixing the eyes upon objects.

The head symptoms are also very numerous. Contortions and jerking of the head. Constantly rubs the head against something, sometimes it is the pillow when in bed. Throws the head from side to side, here and there. She has a sensation of hammers in the head. Burning heat in the head. Headache in the evening; in the morning on waking. Cannot open the eyes. Bending head forward aggravates. Pains are pressing and often wander around from place to place in the head; violent pain in the occiput and temples at the same time.

Eyes are staring, spasmodically wide open. Dim vision usually worse in the right eye. Severe pain in the right eye. Sensation of sand or splinters in the eyes. Itching in the eyes. Burning, worse in the right eye. Photophobia is marked. It will therefore be seen that the right eye is more affected. Many symptoms of the body are confined to the right side.

Discharge from the ears profuse. Violent pains in the ear. Stinging in the meatus. Dulness of hearing. Dull pains in the right ear. tearing pains in the right ear. Buzzing and whizzing and dizziness. Ringing as of bells in the ear on waking in the morning. The right ear is most affected.

It has many catarrhal symptoms in the nose. Dryness and burning; sneezing with the coryza and bleeding from the nose. The acute and chronic nasal symptoms are worse on the right side.

The face looks sickly and has the appearance of terror.

Tearing pains in the teeth. Pain in the angle of the inferior maxilla as if the teeth would fall out.

There is inflammation of the throat and tonsils, worse on the right side. Pain in the right tonsil extending to the ear. Shooting pain in the throat. Pain and constriction on swallowing. It has cured diphtheria. The throat is much swollen externally and there is high fever.

Aversion to food; aversion to meat especially, though craves raw food. Thirst for cold water. Has nausea and vomiting. Has bitter eructations. Has an empty all-gone feeling in the stomach, an anxious feeling in the stomach. Vomits all food taken. Burning pain in the stomach.

There is burning in the abdomen that extends down through the intestines. Burning in the rectum. Sharp pain in the spleen. The liver is painful to touch and is swollen. Pain in both sides of the abdomen. The abdomen is distended with flatus. Subject to much colic. Shooting pains in the abdomen, anus and vagina at the same time. Women who have been poisoned by the Tarentula were found to have fibroid tumors in the abdomen and uterus. Severe pains in the lower abdomen.

It has cured most terrible and alarming constipation after cathartics and injections failed to effect a movement. The symptoms that guide to it are the continual tossing, anxiety, restlessness, rolling from side to side and rubbing the head against the pillow. There is no desire for stool. With the stool there is much blood. In the rectum there is pain, smarting, tenesmus and in the abdomen colic. Most difficult stool. It also has diarrhœa with nausea and vomiting. Diarrhœa has been brought on after washing the hair attended with dark fœtid stool.

Many toxicological symptoms are found. Sugar in the urine and it has cured diabetes; diabetes with grief, anxiety, weakness and bruised pain all through the body. There is involuntary urination when coughing. Many pains in the kidneys. Most difficult urination and it has cured renal colic. In the pathogenesis the symptoms are much like cystitis and it has cured inflammation of the bladder. In keeping with these general symptoms there is spasmodic action of the bladder; spasmodic retention of urine; copious urine with emaciation and sugar. Pain in the urethra, drawing after urination. Copious sand in the urine, and the urine is fœtid.

There is uncontrollable sexual desire and he seems in a state of mind wherein he has no desire to control himself and his sexual passions; lasciviousness almost to insanity. Onanism followed by prostatic troubles. Seminal emissions; semen is bloody; pain in the genitals; testes relaxed and painful; pain in the groin; the penis is swollen; tumor in both testicles; pains in the spermatic cords and testes with swelling; drawing pains in the spermatic cords.

In the female also there is violent, uncontrollable sexual erethism. Menstrual flow too early and copious. Violent itching of the genitals extending far up into the vagina, worse at night. Pain and violent cramps in the uterus. Nymphomania has been cured by this remedy. Coition intensifies the desire and is followed by no relief. Extreme hyperæsthesia of the genitals. Fibroid tumors have been cured. Great relaxation of the muscles and displacement of the uterus. Strong bearing down feeling in the pelvis. Burning in the uterus; swelling and induration of the uterus. Violent cramps with burning in the uterus with nausea and vomiting. The uterus is extremely sensitive to pressure. Contracting pains of the uterus are labor-like and such as are often found in abrotion. Shooting pains in the genitals.

It has been a very useful remedy in complaints of the air passages. Constantly scraping of larynx and trachea to clear them of mucus. Loss of voice and hoarseness; loss of voice when talking. Dryness in the larynx and trachea. Burning from the throat down into the chest.

It is very rich in cough symptoms. Dry frequent cough, worse in the evening dry spasmodic cough with retching, with gagging on every effort to expectorate; cough with involuntary urination; cough with smarting in the larynx and bronchial tubes; night cough. Again dry cough in the morning. It has a loose cough with thick yellow expectoration in the morning.

It has great difficulty in breathing very much like that which is found in cardiac troubles, such a pressure upon the chest with panting respiration and suffocative catarrh. Oppression in the chest when raising the arms and when lying on the left side. Rheumatic pains. Many pains through and in the chest.

It has numerous heart symptoms. It has cured palpitation with mitral murmurs and sensation of trembling in the heart with irregular pulse; extreme anxiety in the heart; tumultuous bearing of the heart; sudden thumping in the heart as from fright but when not frightened. Constant want of air and desire for fresh air and sensation as if the heart turned over; a sensation as if the heart were squeezed or compressed. It has cured angina pectoris and it has many symptoms of the heart like angina pectoris.

Upon the back there are boils, abscesses and carbuncles, especially on the back of the neck and between the shoulder blades. Violent pain in the lumbar region. Violent pains under the scapulæ, worse from motion. Rheumatic pains in the whole back. Pain in the shoulder blades. Neck is stiff and painful on motion. It is a great remedy for soreness of the spinal column, or spinal irritation, pressure aggravates and touch aggravates.

The symptoms of the limbs are too numerous to mention; only a few can be spoken of. Weakness, numbness and restlessness are always present. Rheumatic pains are numerous. The pains of the limbs are so great that he, cannot stand the weight of the clothing. Heaviness and numbness of the upper limbs. Pain in the arm as if squeezed. Heart pains and many pains of the shoulders. Burning pains are very numerous; rheumatic tearing pains. Must move the hands constantly and pick the fingers from nervousness. There is numbness of the left upper extremity and right lower. Paralysis of the lower limbs with pain in the back on motion. Restlessness of the lower limbs with constant desire to cry. (*Ars.*) Fatigue and pain in the evening. In the lower limbs there is numbness which changes to a drawing in the muscles. Restlessness in the lower limbs with aching pain during the chill in intermittent fever. Hard pain in the hips during the night. Pain in the hips and coccyx in the evening while sitting; strong desire to jump. Pains in the nates beginning at 6 A.M. and lasting until evening. Pain in the thighs as if bandaged when walking; shooting pains in the thighs. He is moving the legs constantly; heaviness in the legs; bruised pains in the legs; shooting pains in the right tendo-Achilles; he must walk the floor in the evening, like *Ars.* It is much like *Ars.*, going from chair to chair and from bed to bed, walking the floor.

Sleeplessness before midnight is very marked.

Itching, biting and creeping all over the body, marked in the limbs. Itching and burning. It has cured a dry itching eczema of the extremities and other parts of the skin after *Ars.* and *Sulph*. have failed. It is a very deep acting, long acting remedy and a most useful remedy in skin affections.

THERIDION

Hysterical sensitivity with extreme aggravation from noise, motion and exertion marks this remedy as unique. The pains are aggravated from noise, and motion, and the nerves are in such a state of sensitivity that a painful thrill passes over the body in waves and nausea follows. Nausea from noise is strikingly strange. It cures the most stubborn cases of spinal irritation, when the symptoms agree. Chronic catarrh of the nose. Necrosis of bone. Quick consumption. Emaciation. Enlargement of glands. Constant hunger and thirst. It was a remedy with the old masters for scrofulous conditions. Great lassitude. Complaints are ameliorated by warmth, and during rest. Fainting from least exertion. Chilliness, trembling and anxiety. So restless that she must keep busy, though she accomplishes nothing. The bones are sore.

Sadness and mental depression. Hysterical conduct, hilarity. Aversion to work, and to his business. Joyousness and singing with headache.

Vertigo on *closing the eyes,* from motion, from stooping, on board a vessel, *from every noise,* with nausea, vomiting, and cold sweat. Awakens at 11 P.M. with vertigo and slow pulse. Vertigo with dim vision and pain in eyes. Vertigo and nausea from closing the eyes when kneeling in church. Vertigo like seasickness.

The headache is most violent, aggravated on motion, aggravated talking, aggravated from warm drinks, with nausea and vomiting. Sensitive to light and noise. Pain in forehead extending to occiput, aggravated from noise, motion, and cold air. Headache on beginning to move. Sensation as if vertex did not belong to her, as though she could lift it off. Pain deep in eyes. Complaints from sunstroke. Pressing pain in temples. Pulsating pain over left eye and across forehead. Cannot lie down with the headache. Itching of scalp, and nape in evening.

This remedy cures many nervous eye symptoms. Flickering, even when eyes are closed. Like a veil before the eyes. Double vision. Sensitive to light. Diplopia. Fluttering. Nausea, and cold hands. Pressing pain behind eyes. On closing eyes, nausea and vomiting.

The hearing is very acute. Every least noise penetrates the whole body, especially the teeth, aggravates vertigo and causes nausea. Rushing noises in ears like a waterfall. Pressure about the ears. Fulness behind the ears.

It has cured most obstinate catarrh of nose with offensive thick yellow or greenish yellow discharges. Pressing pain at root of nose. Dryness in nose. Paroxysms of violent sneezing.

The face is pale and sickly. Lockjaw in morning on waking. Foam, at mouth with chill. Teeth sensitive to cold water and shrill sounds. Toothache causes weeping. Burning in teeth. Salty taste in mouth. The tongue feels as if burnt. Mouth feels numb. Taste impaired.

Desires wine and sour drinks. Much thirst. Desires food, but does not know what.

Nausea with many complaints and from many causes. Nausea in the morning on rising, from noise, on closing the eyes, when looking too long at one object, on motion, from talking, from fast riding in a carriage, from riding on the cars or on a ship. Nausea with headache, with vertigo; nausea aggravated from warm drinks. In seasickness of nervous women, when they close the eyes to get rid of the motion of the vessel they become deathly sick. Tenderness of stomach.

This is a useful remedy in many liver conditions, with burning pain, aggravated from touch, motion and noise, and bilious vomiting.

Pain in groin in a man after coitus; on motion, and on drawing up the limb. Constipation, with difficult, soft stool. Contraction of anus. Enlarged prostate gland with sensation of a lump in perineum.

Must arise several times during the night to pass urine. Copious urine during the night.

Feeble erection and diminished desire. Seminal emissions during sleep in the afternoon.

Sore bruised pain in the ovarian region, aggravated by motion. Menses suppressed.

Sighing and short breath on ascending stairs.

Stitching in chest beneath left shoulder to throat. Quick consumption. Anxiety about heart.

Very sensitive spine, aggravated from motion, noise, a jar, stepping. Pain between scapulae. Spinal anæmia. Itching of back and nape.

Drawing in thigh with a cold sensation, ameliorated by warmth. Violent itching of calf. Swelling of feet. Heaviness of the limbs. Pains in bones as if broken.

Shaking chill. Sweats easily. Icy cold perspiration with fainting, vertigo and vomiting at night.

Violent itching of skin.

THUJA OCCIDENTALIS

The general appearance of the Thuja subject, if he has a characteristic picture, is that of a waxy, shiny face, it looks as if it had been smeared over with grease, and is often transparent, he is a sickly looking individual, looks as if entering upon some cachexia. This is often the case in the sycotic constitution and the cancerous cachexia, weakly, cachetic, yellowish, or often very pallid.

The skin manifests many symptoms. The perspiration is peculiar; it is sweetish in odor and smells like honey, sometimes like garlic, strong and pungent. A pungent odor emanates from the genitals, sweetish honey-like odor to the sweat from the genitalia, he smells his genitals. The odor is also like burnt horn, burnt feathers or burnt sponge. These peculiar strong odors are particularly present when there are fig-warts upon the genitals such as Thuja cures.

The skin looks unhealthy everywhere about the body and there is a copious sweat on first going to sleep, like *Arsenic*. If you had only the waxiness such as *Arsenic* and Thuja produce, you might prescribe *Arsenic*. *Arsenic* is often the acute and Thuja the chronic. You remember that *Arsenic* is usually a chronic remedy.

A peculiar asthmatic condition is found in sycosis and *Arsenic* appears to be indicated for the symptoms, but it only relieves, it does not control the predisposition, it acts like *Aconite* in acute diseases and only ameliorates for a moment. Asthmatic and many other sycotic conditions seem to call for *Arsenic*, but it will do nothing but palliate, the constitutionality is not reached by *Arsenic*, its fundamental symptoms are not similar. In syphilis and psora *Arsenic* acts a long time and eradicates the complaints, when similar to them, but it is not similar to sycosis. *Arsenic* does not go to the bottom of the trouble, but Thuja and *Natrum sulph.* will take up the work and cure. *Natrum sulph.* and Thuja bring back the primitive manifestation that has been suppressed for years.

The tendency of the Thuja patient is to throw out wart-like excrescences, which are soft and pulpy and very sensitive, they burn, itch and bleed easily when rubbed by the clothing. Horny excrescences that form on the hands and split open, form upon a pedicle and crack around the base. Cauliflower excrescences upon the cervix uteri, about the anus (like *Nitric acid),* about the labia majora and mucous membranes generally. Horny excrescences, more upon the skin. Warts of a brownish color, especially if upon the abdomen; great brown spots, like liver spots, form upon the abdomen.

Zona around the chest, herpetic eruptions everywhere, here and there. like Sepia, herpes labialis and preputialis. Zona is a herpetic formation, great vesicular patches come out upon the body called "shingles," here we should compare Thuja, *Rhus, Graph., Kali hydr.* and *Mezereum.*

This condition is attended with a great amount of suffering and neuralgic pains. In cases that are sycotic, Thuja is especially a grand remedy. You will have a class of cases where the warts have been caused to disappear by calomel, which makes them shrivel up and fall off, such is the old school treatment. Sometimes a patient comes to you with erratic symptoms and you may study for hours over these symptoms, and see very little order in them, you will realize that the leading features have been left out and that something is lacking. Some one has applied *Nitric acid,* calomel or something else, and driven these fig-warts away. These condylomata could not come without having some constitutional basis, these warts have a cause, and that cause seems to be less able to make the patient sick if he has the warts, he feels better when he has the warts. Strange to say, when these warts have been suppressed, we get symptoms of *Nitric acid,* Thuja, *Mercurius* and *Staphisagria.*

Thuja leads all medicines for symptoms coming from suppressed fig-warts.

Thuja is pre-eminently a strong medicine when you have a trace of animal poisoning in the history, as snake bite, small-pox and vaccination.

There are probably several varieties of urethral discharges, but there is one that is sycotic, and when that has been suppressed, it has produced a miasm with soreness in the bottom of the feet and in the knees and particularly through the back and loins and sciatic nerves, in the knees and ankle joints. Sometimes it affects the upper extremities, but particularly the lower. Most violent aggravation when keeping still, like *Rhus,* great aching that increases so long as he keeps still, he is very often compelled to keep the bed, and then he constantly moves and turns. An antisycotic must be selected. While this group of symptoms would be cured by *Rhus* when the case is not sycotic, when these symptoms come from suppressed gonorrhœa *Medorrhinum* or Thuja will cure.

Thuja enters into this particular sphere and takes hold of this particular case where sycosis is at the bottom.

Sometimes when the discharge has been suppressed, orchitis comes on and then *Pulsatilia* will be the remedy, and very seldom Thuja.

Thuja affects the left testicle with intense squeezing pain, but most generally you will find *Pulsatilla* the remedy.

As we continue to study Thuja, we see that it has a profound action upon the glands, stitching, tearing pains in the glands, the pains are as if the gland were being torn to pieces. That may be true of glands in general, but one particular gland, the ovary, is more affected than any other and especially the left. This is so true, that if you meet a violent pain in the left ovary, coming on at the time of menstruation and continuing during the flow and extending down the thighs, but may be in every direction, it increases as the flow comes on, stinging, tearing, burning, bursting pains, as if the parts were being torn out, makes her cry aloud, she goes into a hysterical state. This is a very strong Thuja group. It has the opposite of *Zinc.* and *Lachesis,* for ir these, relief comes with the flow.

Many women suffer from grumbling pains in the ovaries all the time, they have a sense of the organ, which they should not feel; pain from taking cold or in change of weather; the increase of the pain in the left ovary is the first sign; sometimes the pain is so severe that the right one suffers apparently from sympathy. Where the ovaries have been affected for some time there will be mental symptoms, a most violent irritability, jealousy, quarrelsomeness, ugliness. This irritability is likely to be shown towards indivduals about the house, toward the husband and the mother; she is yet able to control herself among strangers and the doctor may not be able to find out about it, because she has in her nature a disposition to cheat; she wants to be alone and takes upon herself fixed ideas, that she is pregnant, or that an animal is in her bowels, she feels the motion of a child's arm, thinks she is followed, or that someone is walking beside her, thinks that soul and body are separated.

Now, these are fixed ideas, and there is no use trying to reason them out of her. It seems to her that she is very delicate, that she is made of glass and that she will break. The idea is that she will break, and not that she is transparent. Associated with this condition, we have violent, intense, tearing headaches, tearing in the eye, ameliorated by heat. The eye-ball pains are better from heat and the rest are better in the cool open air.

Pain localized in small spots. A nail driven in the head, side of head and forehead, like *Ignatia* and *Anacardium*. These pains are intensified into tearing pains, and affect the eye-ball, making it so sore that it can hardly be touched; worse from heat and worse from lying down; worse in a warm room and better in the open air.

Rheumatic head symptoms are worse in damp air. They are worse from sour things and also from stimulating and exciting things.

Crude drugs do not impress the vital force so lastingly, but an individual who is thoroughly sensitive and properly sensitive, as sensitive as contagion, then if you undertake to prove by giving it night and morning, you will rivet upon him a life-long miasm.

If you have given a medicine, wait for the symptoms to come and go in the natural manner. To a great extent, this is the tendency with sycosis, the tendency is rather outward.

We see in the proving of a drug what we see in disease. When a gonorrhœa is contracted, it goes through the prodromal period and then comes the disease, which, if let alone, has in its nature a tendency to eradicate itself from the economy, and then the patients do not suffer from lasting conditions.

In the old school, they always suppress the discharge, and there are those in the new school who do little better.

The frequent repetition by which one is exposed, would not increase the gonorrhœa itself, because the susceptibility is satisfied.

The taking of more of the drug to prove it does not do so much harm, provided the one who is directing the proving realizes, when the symptoms begin to rise, and then stops the drug. Now if we go on with the proving by repeating the doses after the symptoms come on, we force the drug into the economy when he is already poisoned, and by this means we get a confusion in the symptoms, the drug disease engrafted upon that individual for life.

Many of the provings of Thuja give us that kind of confusion, so that we see only now and then symptoms cropping out that are striking; in fact, the great hulk of the Thuja provings has been wasted, because there is so much confusion in the great number of symptoms, while the earlier provings brought out many of the characteristics, the Vienna provings, to a great extent, confused the image of Thuja. So that, by clinical experience only, we have been able to draw out the finer features of Thuja. It requires more than a school boy to do that.

The new provings must be carried on in a different manner.

Thuja has some striking bowel symptoms; gushing, watery morning diarrhœa, like water coming out of a bunghole.

There is also a general catarrhal condition running through the body; catarrh of the nose, ears and chest. In the catarrh of the chest it produces an intense hacking cough, with expectoration in the morning of greenish mucus, sometimes a copious expectoration.

It is often suited to old cases of pneumonia, in such individuals as have suppressed gonorrhœa, fig-wart gonorrhœa.

The kidneys and urinary symptoms are also striking; congestion and inflammation of the kidneys, sharp pain in the kidneys; burning urine; inflammation of the bladder and urethra that is not gonorrhœal; pus from the bladder; paralysis of the bladder, must wait a long time for the urine to start; retention of urine, continuous urging to urinate, tearing in the urethra, feeling as if the urine were constantly running along the urethra, like *Kali bich.* and *Petros.*

In the urethral disease of sycotic character, Thuja leads all other remedies. In the non-sycotic variety, *Cannabis sativa* is sufficient, but those cases that have proved to be sycotic *Cann. sat.* left uncured, it ameliorated the burning during and after urination and the thick yellowish-green discharge. but some other remedy had always to follow, when they were shown to be sycotic. It is not so with Thuja, because it is capable of finishing the case.

In the most violent cases, with bloody urine, extreme salacity, great torment, bloody, watery discharge from the urethra and bladder, tic, rest day or night, *Cantharis* comes in, it is capable of finishing the case in a few days. Such a patient must be in excellent health, which is not generally the case. They are drinking men and smokers. Tobacco is one of the most troublesome things you will run across, many cases will not recover promptly if they are tobacco users and great smokers, wine drinkers or convivial men, they run around a good deal and are high livers and with such you have a slow case on hand

With the system so broken down from high living, you may not get a decided curative action until you have forced him to abandon his way of living. Put him on light diet, diminish his smoking, get rid entirely of the drinking, and put him on a perfectly bland living. This is the first thing. If he is a man of family we have to contend with great mental distress, and not less so if a woman. So it may well be said, that usually the sycotic miasm is a troublesome one to begin with and one that will bother the young physician.

You cannot substitute the right method for a wrong one, which will make him a cripple for life.

The suppression of the disease, as usually tried, cannot be thought of by the sincere and earnest homœopath.

If he wants it checked suddenly, let him go somewhere else, but warn him what will take place, and that he will have untold disease and suffering.

TUBERCULINUM BOVINUM

I want to take up the study of Tuberculinum. The preparation which I use is a little different from that which is generally found in the market. This preparation I procured through a Professor of Veterinary Surgery. In Pennsylvania there came a time when a handsome herd of cattle had to be slaughtered because of tuberculosis. Through the Veterinary Surgeon of the Pennsylvania University I secured some of the tubercular glands from these slaughtered cattle. I selected from these the most likely specimen. This was potentized by Boericke & Tafel as far as the 6th, and has since been prepared on the Skinner machine, the 30th, 200th, 1000th and the higher potencies. This preparation I have been using for fifteen years. Many of my friends have been using it, as they have procured it from me.

From observing the effects of this preparation I have been gathering these notes in my inter-leaved Hering's Guiding Symptoms, and they now guide me in the use of Tuberculinum. I do not use Tuberc. merely because it is a nosode, or with the idea that generally prevails of using nosodes; that is, a product of the disease for the disease, and the results of the disease. This I fear is too much the prevailing thought in using nosodes. In certain places it prevails and is taught that any thing relating to syphilis must be treated with *Syphilinum;* that anything relating to gonorrhœa must be treated with *Medorrhinum,* anything psoric must be treated with *Psorinum,* and anything that relates to tuberculosis must be treated with Tuberculinum. That will go out of use some day; it is mere isopathy, and it is an unsound doctrine. it is not the better idea of Homœopathy. It is not based upon sound principles. It belongs to a hysterical Homœopathy that prevails in this century. Yet much good has come out of it.

It is hoped that provings may be made so that we may be able to prescribe Tuberc. on the symptoms of Tuberc. just as we would use any drug. It is deep acting, constitutionally deep, because it is a product of disease from a very deep-seated constitutional condition, like *Silica* and *Sulphur.* It goes deep into the life; it is antipsoric; it is long acting, and it affects constitutions more deeply than most remedies; and when our deepest remedies act only a few weeks, and they have to be changed, this remedy comes in as one of the remedies—when the symptoms agree—and brings a better state of reaction, so that remedies hold longer. It may well be considered a species of *Psorinum.*

One of the most prominent uses of this remedy is in intermittent fever. Some of our most stubborn cases of intermittent fever will relapse and continue relapsing, even when such remedies as *Silica* and *Calcarea* and the deeper-acting remedies have been indicated, have acted well, have broken the fever, and in a few weeks, from exposure to cold, from sitting in a draft, from becoming fatigued, from mental exertion, from over-eating and from disordering the stomach this ague has returned. Any of these circumstances will bring back these stubborn cases of intermittent fever when Tuberc. is needed. When a patient is travelling toward phthisis and he is exposed and intermittent comes out. He is of a feeble constitution and his complaints have a tendency to relapse, and remedies well selected do not hold long, though they act well at first—they must soon be changed—changing symptoms.

It is not an indication for Tuberc. when the well selected remedy fails to act. Well selected is a relative expression and involves too much of human opinion. It may be thought to be well selected when it is not related to the case. When the well selected remedy has acted and the constitution shows a tendency to break down, and the well selected remedy does not hold, because of vital weakness and because of deep-seated tendencies; then it is that this remedy sometimes fits in. Such a case is often tuberculous in inclination, even though no evidence is present of a pathological character.

Burnett dropped an idea, that has been confirmed many times. Patients who have inherited phthisis, patients whose parents have died of phthisis are often of feeble vitality. They do not throw off their inherited tendencies. They are always tired. They take on sicknesses easily. They become anæmic; nervous; waxy or pale. These conditions are sometimes met, when the finer symptoms agree, although Burnett evidently used this medicine in a sort of routine way for this kind of constitution, which he called "Consumptiveness". Persons who had inherited phthisis, who were debilitated and anæmic.

It seems from looking over the record of many cures that this remedy has been given many times for just that state on a paucity of symptoms, and if the records can be believed it has many times balanced up to the constitution in that anæmic state, where the *inheritance has been phthisis*. It is not the best indication for Tuberc., but where the symptoms agree in addition to that inheritance, then you may have indications for the remedy.

If Tuberculinum bovinum be given in 10m., 50m. and cm. potencies, two doses of each potency at long intervals, all children and young people who have inherited tuberculosis may be immuned from their inheritance and their resiliency will be restored. It cures most cases of adenoids and tuberculous glands of the neck.

The notes that have guided me to its use I will attempt to explain. The mental symptoms that I have seen give way while the patient was under treatment, and the mental symptoms that I have seen crop out under the provings, and the mental symptoms that I have so often seen associated when the patient is poisoned by the tubercular toxines are such as belong to many complaints and are cured by Tuberc. hopelessness in many complaints.

Aversion to mental work. Anxiety evening, until midnight. Anxiety during fever. Loquacity during fever. Weary of life. Cosmopolitan. Tormenting, persistent thoughts during the night. Thoughts intrude and crowd upon each other during the night. These I will say are the common mental features, and have often yielded when the remedy has been prescribed. Anyone who has inherited phthisis, anyone who has been in a state of debility, who has had intermittent fever with continual relapses, and these mental symptoms are present, you may think of Tuberc. Loquacity during fever is a common feature in hectic fever when the patient is decidedly affected by the toxines of tuberculosis. A person gradually running down, never finding the right remedy, or relief only momentarily; has a constant desire to change, and travel, and go somewhere, and do something different, or to find a new doctor. The desire to travel, that cosmopolitan condition of the mind belongs so strongly to the one who needs Tuberc. It comes out so often in clinical experience, is found so often in the *Calcareas,* and especially in *Calc. phos.,* always wanting to go somewhere. Such is the condition of those about to go into insanity, about to go into some lingering disease. Persons on the borderland of insanity. It is true that phthisis and insanity are convertible conditions, the one falls into the other. Many cases that are treated and cured, and phthisis of the lungs has just been turned aside, finally become insane. Persons who have been cured of insanity go into phthisis and die, showing the deep-seated character of their nature. The intellectual symptoms and the lung symptoms are interchangeable.

Tuberculinum cures the most violent and the most chronic periodical sick headaches, periodical nervous headaches. Coming every week; every two weeks; and the irregular periodicity coming under certain conditions, in damp weather, after overwork, from mental excitement, from over-eating, disordered stomach—Tuberc. breaks up the tendency to this chronic periodical headache when the symptoms agree.

It has been observed in the hands of good prescribers that when chronic constitutional headaches have been broken up sometimes the patient has a tendency to lose flesh and become feeble. An entire transformation scene takes place; a cough sets in; the headache has been removed, but the patient is feeble. Whenever that takes place Tuberc. is a most useful remedy. A new manifestation comes; a new organ is affected.

Sore bruised feeling all over the body. Aching of the bones. Sore bruised condition of the eyeballs, sensitive to touch, and on turning the eye sideways. Persons who have long felt the weakness of tuberculosis, tubercular conditions, and are subject to cold sweat on the head. This was brought out in the provings of *Calcarea,* and those about to go into phthisis have many times been cured by *Calcarea.* The relationship between Tuberc. and *Calc.*

is very close. They are interchangeable; that is, the one may be indicated for a while, and then the other. They are both deep-acting remedies—also *Silica* is closely related to Tuberc., on the same plane of action, going deep into the life in a similar way; *Calcarea,* Tuberc. and *Silica,* and the *Silicates.*

In the Guiding Symptoms is a record, "Pain in the head, as if the head had a tight hoop of iron around it," an iron band.

Headache, with frequent sharp cutting pains. Headache, worse from motion. In the Guiding Symptoms, "A sullen, taciturn, irritable" condition of mind. "Screams in his sleep. Is very restless at night. Sister died of tubercular meningitis." That symptom was given by Burnett. It has cured hydrocephalus.

Many years ago Doctor Biegler cured a case of tubercular meningitis with Tuberc. In many instances it has cured tubercular meningitis and tubercular diseases of the brain in the early stages.

The face becomes red, even to purple, during the chill, and during the heat. Aversion to all foods. Such aversion to meat that it becomes impossible to eat it. Thirst during the chill and heat, for large quantities of cold water. It has cured tubercular meningitis with effusion, where the head was greatly enlarged. Craving for cold milk. Emptiness in the abdomen, with faint feeling. Anxiety in the abdomen and stomach, much like the *Sulphur* sensation described. An all-gone, hungry feeling, that drives him to eat. This has been cured by Tuberc. after *Sulphur* had failed.

All know what a marked feature emaciation is in persons who are going into phthisis. The emaciation often begins before there is any sign of phthisis, gradually losing flesh. A gradually growing weakness, a gradually increasing fatigue. This is a prominent place for Tuberc.—if the symptoms agree. Always let that stand out boldly, IF THE SYMPTOMS AGREE, and WHEN THE SYMPTOMS AGREE. Of course it will be said that Tuberc. has cured when there are few symptoms; this is granted, but should not be lauded as a clinical practice.

It is a common feature of tubercular affections of the brain and of the meninges to suffer from constipation. Stool large and hard; or, constipation alternating with diarrhœa. It is a well-known clinical fact. Constipation is a strong feature of Tuberc. "Constipation, stool large and hard; then diarrhœa. Itching of the anus. Sudden diarrhœa before breakfast, with nausea. Inguinal glands indurated and visible. Excessive sweat in chronic diarrhœa." That symptom was brought out by Burnett. It was merely a clinical symptom. Burnett dwells on this phase of it; "Tabes Mesenterica". "Swelling on left side, also on right; complains of a stitch in side after running; languid and indisposed to talk. Nervous and irritable. Talks in his sleep; grinds his teeth. Appetite poor. Hands blue. Indurated and palpable glands everywhere. A drum-belly. Spleen region bulging out." That was one of Burnett's clinical cases. That was cured by Burnett's *Ertelllinum*. In most instances, I am informed, he used the *Bacillinum* 200th.

It is a common feature of *Sulphur* to be driven out of bed in the morning by a diarrhœa. It is a very common feature in cases of phthisis, and patients going into phthisis. In advanced stage of phthisis, driven out of bed with a diarrhœa; or, diarrhœa worse in the morning than at any other time in the twenty-four hours. This is a common feature of phthisis that Tuberc. has cured, and it has been verified many times, although it is a clinical symptom.

General relaxation. Weakness and hanging down of the genitals. Relaxed scrotum.

Menses too early, too profuse, long lasting. *Amenorrhœa. Dysmenorrhœa.* Cough before, and during chill.

Suffocation; worse in a warm room. Tubercular deposits in apices of lungs (left).

The uterus sags down and is heavy. At the menstrual period, a relaxation, as if the inner parts would come out.

Dry hacking cough before the evening chill (*Rhus t.*), and the hacking cough lasts sometimes during the chill, and sometimes during the fever, but he knows the chill is coming by the cough. The patient has been cured perhaps a number of times by remedies. Intermittent fever has been cured a number of times by remedies well selected. The fever goes away promptly under the action of the remedy; but from slight exposure, as was mentioned, it comes back again. Now at the end of three, four or five weeks—often two or three— he says, "I know my old chills are coming back again, because of the cough I have." The previous remedies have not been successful. They are not deep enough acting, they are not long enough acting. When the homœopathic remedy is really and truly able to cure the diseased condition it will hold that case, so that when the symptoms come back again the same remedy will be indicated, and only a changed potency perhaps will be necessary. The same remedy is called for; but it is an indication for Tuberc. when at every coming back of the case it calls for a new remedy. *Calcarea* breaks up the case once, and the next time it comes back it calls for something else, and the next time for something else, and it keeps turning around. Perhaps a number of times it calls for the same remedies again. Changing about. That very changing and unsatisfied symptom image is a strong indication for this medicine.

Suffocation in a warm room. Can find easy breathing only when riding in the cold wind. When phthisical patients find no comfort except riding in the cold wind—which is a rare symptom, but has been noticed. This was a symptom, specially marked in the lamented Gregg, of Buffalo. He would ride out in the cold winds by the lake for hours. *Arg. nit,* many times relieved that, but it is a strong symptom of Tuberc. He finally died of tuberculosis.

Desire for deep breathing. Longs for the open air. Wants the doors and windows open. Sits in the room covered with a cold sweat, but wants the air, wants fresh air. When covered with cold sweat he cannot have the wind blowing on him because he takes cold, he is sensitive to it, but he wants the fresh air, he wants the open air. Especially when the tubercular deposits begin in the apex of the left lung, which is the indication that has been verified by quite a number of observers.

"Hard, dry cough. Hard, dry, shaking cough," were symptoms noticed by Boardman—regardless of phthisis. The expectoration is thick, yellow, often yellowish-green in catarrhal conditions. Hacking cough in young girls, where there is a suppression of the menstrual flow, of the first menses. They come on once or twice or three times, and the patient is yellow, is puny, is tired, has a hacking cough, and a suspicious chest. If the tubercular deposits have not gone too far, Tuberc. may arrest the progress of the disease. Tuberc. often gives immunity if taken before the tuberculosis begins in those who have inherited it. It immunes the constitution.

Another marked feature recorded by Burnett was ringworms. Burnett was of the opinion that ringworms commonly formed upon those who had inherited phthisis. He thought it was a sign of approaching phthisis, that it was a very common feature of those who have inherited phthisis; and he used the *Bacillinum* 200th. He used it somewhat as a routine remedy on every child with ringworm.

Patients who suffer from weakness in the evening. Rapid pulse in the evening. Every evening for years he has noticed the pulse has been rapid. Palpitation after the evening meal.

Jerking of the muscles on going to sleep, and during sleep. Rheumatic pain in the right elbow. Sore bruised condition of the bones and periosteum. Aching, drawing pains in the limbs during rest, better by walking. A strong feature of this remedy is that its pains and aches are better by motion. I have seen this aching distress in the limbs many times where *Rhus* has acted only temporarily or has failed; where *Rhus* seemed to be the remedy, but was not deep enough to hold its action. Where *Rhus* was superficially indicated—or the deep action of the disturbance, the deep inheritance—the tired constitution, the chronic nature of the case prevents the action of *Rhus,* and Tuberc. cures these cases. Especially in girls that are bookkeepers, and shop-keepers, who have inherited phthisical constitutions, who have aches and pains during damp weather, in rainy weather, during a storm, when the weather changes, when the weather becomes cold; then it is that Tuberc. cures after such remedies as *Rhus* have failed; these patients are better by motion, better by walking; worse during rest. While sitting the pains become so severe that he is driven to travel, driven to walk. Aching, drawing pains in limbs during rest, better walking. Coldness of left foot and leg, evening in bed. Stitching pains in limbs during rest. Wandering pains in limbs—in joints. Pains all over the body, but mostly in lower limbs. Aching, drawing, tearing, as if in bones, and nerves, during rest; better walking. Pains in bones of lower limbs. Stiffness on beginning to move. Sore bruised joints. Pains all ameliorated by heat. Drawing pains in thighs. Stiching pains in limbs. Restless. Stiffness of lower limbs, evening Physical exertion aggravates.

Complaints worse standing; must move. This is as marked in this remedy as in *Sulphur*.

Intermittent fever, with drawing in limbs during rest. Chill 7 P.M. Chilliness, evening; better in bed. Chill 5 P.M., with thirst. Cough before chill, during chill, and vomiting during fever. Wants to be covered during all stages Extreme heat, with chilliness. Relapsing intermittents.

Drawing in the limbs in the evening before the chill, and during the chill. He knows the chill is coming on because of the drawing in the limbs. Chill at 11 o'clock at night. Must be covered up during all stages, the chill, the fever and the sweat. The chilliness extends into the fever and into the sweat if there is any uncovering.

Aching in the bones of the head, with soreness of the periosteum and these are better by travelling about, like *Rhus*. Better by motion; worse keeping still.

Perspiration from mental exertion. Perspiration stains the linen yellow. Heat and perspiration during sleep. We know what a common feature it is in phthisis to have night sweats.

Formication in the skin. This remedy has cured tubercular eruptions of the skin. This remedy has cured red purplish eruptions that are nodular in character; the patient wants to sit all the time by the fire—itching in cold air, better by going to the fire, worse from scratching. Sensitive to every change of the weather, especially to cold, and to damp weather, and sometimes to warm damp weather, and to rainy weather. Always worse before a storm. Can feel every electric change in the weather. Becoming cold brings on all the symptoms, pains, aches, distresses and sufferings. A large list of symptoms of patients that have been cured in all their varying conditions may be found by looking up the Guiding Symptoms.

Periodicity, then, is a strong feature of this remedy, and sensitive to weather changes.

Fainting fits. Weakness after a short walk.

It has cured constitutional headaches, periodical headaches, that existed forty-five years. It cures even old people of these periodical complaints.

The pains will sometimes travel. Stitching, pinching, cramping, wandering; and always worse from cold, and from cold damp weather.

1008

VALERIAN

This remedy cures many nervous and hysterical phenomena in excitable women and children, and the complaints of the hypochondriac. Great nervous excitability, exaltation, hysterical contractures, trembling, palpitation, sense of levitation, paroxysmal respiration, stitching pains, tension in the limbs, jerking, twitching, globus hystericus. Sensation of something warm rising from the stomach, causing paroxysmal suffocation. All the nerves are in a fret. Oversensitiveness of all the senses; great nervous restlessness. All these general symptoms come on *during rest,* and are relieved by motion and moving about. Fainting easily. Slight exertion brings on symptoms. Complaints change about, and pains wander from place to place. It is a great remedy for the numerous nondescript nervous manifestations that come in spinal irritation when there is amelioration by motion and aggravation by much exertion. Exertion brings on headache in these cases. Stitching pains all over the body during rest.

The mental state is often ecstatic or hysterical. The mind undergoes rapid changes in disposition and ideas. The mental symptoms come on at night; sees images, animals and men. The mental state is one of extreme activity—tension, excitement, passes from one subject to another. Erroneous ideas; thinks she is some one else, moves to the edge of the bed to make room; imagines animals lying near her which she fears she may hurt. Fear in the evening in the dark. Symptoms aggravated in the dark. Great sadness and irritability. Morose, easily exasperated. Mental symptoms come on during rest, while sitting and lying, and go off on walking about.

Vertigo when stooping. Feels light as if floating in air.

Violent nervous headaches in evening during rest, ameliorated by motion. Stupefying pains in head. Stitching, tearing pain. Sensation of great coldness in head. Headache from exposure to the heat and light of the sun. Aggravated in the open air and from a draft. Pain in forehead and through the eyes. Tension and constriction of the scalp. Icy coldness in vertex.

Wild look in the eyes. Flashes of light before the eyes in the dark. Pressure in the eyes in the morning. Smarting in the eyes. Vision very sharp.

Hearing acute. Jerking pains. Hissing and ringing in ears.

Face red and hot in open air. Stitching in face and teeth. Sudden jerking pain in the face. Twitching in the muscles and drawing pain in face. Neuralgia of face, aggravated during rest.

Thickly coated tongue; rancid taste. Flat taste in mouth on waking. Sensation as if a thread were hanging down the throat with salivation and vomiting.

Voracious hunger with nausea. Symptoms aggravated when stomach is empty, ameliorated after breakfast. Complaints from fasting. Eructations, like spoiled eggs, morning. Eructation of rancid fluid. Nausea, faintness, body ice cold. Child vomits as soon as it nurses after mother has been angry. Child vomits curdled milk in lumps.

Distended abdomen. Cutting pain in abdomen. Colic. Cramps in hysterical women, in evening in bed and after dinner.

Watery diarrhœa with curds in infants. Greenish papescent stool and blood with cramp in abdomen and tenesmus, in children. Worms in the stool. Prolapsus of the anus when straining to pass urine.

Copious frequent urination in nervous women. Sediment of urine red and white.

Menses late and scanty.

Choking in throat pit on falling asleep; weakness as if suffocating. Inspirations grow less deep and more rapid until they cease; then she catches her breath by a sobbing effort, in spells. (Compare *Ignatia, Ox. ac.*) Paroxysmal respiration in hysterical and very nervous women. Globus hystericus.

Jerking stitching pain in chest. Oppression of the chest with lump in the throat. Stitching in right side of chest and liver. Stitching in heart with pulse quick, small and weak.

Pain in small of back during rest, ameliorated by walking. Rheumatic pains in scapulæ.

Rheumatic pains in all the limbs, aggravated during rest after previous exertion, ameliorated walking. Drawing, jerking of limbs, and twitching of muscles during rest. Heaviness in limbs, drawing, feels as though must move the limbs but cannot. Darting pains in arms and shoulders. Drawing in the muscles with stitching pains in arms. Hysterical contractures in hands and arms. Crampy darting, tearing, like an electrical shock, repeatedly through the humerus, intensely painful. Cramp in biceps when writing. Pain along the sciatic when standing, ameliorated walking. Tearing pain in thigh upward to hip. Tearing in calf when crossing limbs. Tearing in muscles of thighs during rest. Violent drawing, jerking pains in lower limbs during rest. Drawing in thighs, legs and tendo-Achillis when sitting, ameliorated walking. Pain in ankles after exertion, ascending stairs, ameliorated walking. Drawing in tarsal joints when sitting. Pains in heel during rest. Violent drawing, jerking pains in lower limbs and hip, aggravated standing. Hysterical cramps in lower limbs, calves and feet.

Sleepless before midnight. Cramps in hands and feet prevent sleep. Vivid dreams. Symptoms aggravated on walking.

VERATRUM ALBUM

You will be astonished at the wonderful coldness running through this remedy. Hardly a group of symptoms will arise without this accompanying coldness. Coldness of discharges, coldness of the body. You would also wonder at the remarkable prostration attending the various groups of symptoms, complete relaxation and exhaustion, coldness. Profuse sweat, vomiting and diarrhœa.

Profuse watery discharges. These conditions occur without apparent provocation. In cholera or cholera morbus, it seems that the fluids run out of the body. Lies in bed, relaxed prostrated, cold to the finger-tips, with corresponding blueness, fairly purple; lips cold and blue, countenance pinched and shrunken; great sensation of coldness as if the blood were ice-water; scalp cold; forehead covered with cold sweat; headache and exhaustion; coldness in spots over the body; extremities cold as death. Full of cramps; looks as if he would die. This state comes out during the menses, during colic with nausea, with mania and violent delirium, with headache, with violent inflammations.

Is it any wonder that Hahnemann predicted that Veratrum, *Camphor,* and *Cuprum* would become remedies in the cure of cholera he saw in their nature the ability to cure. He saw the similitude.

In cases of this sort which are characterized by superabundance of cramps, *Cuprum* is the simillimum. For those with coldness and blueness and scanty sweat, vomiting, and purging, *Camphor* is the remedy. These are called "dry cholera;" they sink down and die without exhaustive discharges. In proportion as there are coldness, blueness and scanty discharges, *Camphor* is indicated. In proportion as copiousness, blueness, and coldness are present, Veratrum is indicated. *Secale* has something of cholera in it. *Podo.* has exhaustive stools: *Ars.* anxious restlessness.

The mental symptoms are marked by violence and destructiveness; he wants to destroy, to tear something; he tears the clothes from the body. Always wants to be busy, to carry on his daily work. A cooper who was suffering from the Veratrum insanity would pile up chairs on top of one another. When asked what he was doing, he replied that he was piling up staves. When not occupied with this he was tearing his clothes, or praying for hours on his knees, and so loud that he could be heard blocks away.

Exalted state of religious frenzy, believes he is the risen Christ; screams and screeches until he is blue in the face; head cold as ice, cold sweat, reaches out and exhorts to repentance.

Exhorts to repent, preaches, howls, sings obscene songs, exposes the persons. Fear and the effects of fear; fear of death and of being damned; imagines the world is on fire.

"Mania with desire to cut and tear everything, especially the clothes, with lewdness and lascivous talk. Puerperal mania and convulsions, with violent cerebral congestion: bluish and bloated face; protruding eyes; wild shrieks, with disposition to bite and tear. Loquacity, he talks rapidly. She is inconsolable over a fancied misfortune; runs around the room howling and screaming or sits brooding, wailing and weeping." Alternate states of brooding, screaming, and screeching. A few such remedies would empty our insane asylums, especially of recent cases. Insanity is curable if there are no incurable results of disease.

Full of despair and hopelessness with approaching insanity. "Despair of his recovery, attempts suicide." Insane people are not hopeless, those approaching insanity are, but after they become insane, they think that everybody is crazy except themselves. Those bowed down by great grief and despair are likely to go into a state of violent mania. Veratrum carries them through the state of despair. "Melancholia, head hangs down, sits brooding in silence."

Young girls go on for years with menstrual difficulties, and preceding each menstrual nisus is a state of despair; never smiles, the world seems blue, everything is dark; these are preparing for a marked state of insanity. Veratrum is a remedy that would keep many women out of the insane asylum, especially those with uterine troubles. Girls at puberty suffer with dysmenorrhœa, hysterical mental states, diarrhœa, and vomiting. During the menses they become cold as death, lips blue, extremities cold and blue, dreadful pains, sensation of sinking, mania to kiss everybody, hysteria with coldness at the menstrual period, copious sweat, vomiting, and diarrhœa, etc.

Veratrum has troublesome headaches, neuralgic, of great violence, accompanied with coldness, vomiting of bile and blood, great exhaustion, profuse sweat. Vomiting and retching after the stomach is empty; spas-modic retching and cramping of the stomach; you can see the effort to empty the stomach and every little while a mouthful of bile comes up.

Violent rush of blood to the head, congestion of the head with coldness of the extremities. Head feels as if packed with ice, feels as if ice lay on the vertex and occiput (*Calc.*), tension in the head if the membranes were drawn tighter about the brain; compressive pains.

I remember a farmer who consulted me in the Summer. He had a strange sensation when he drank water, as if it ran down the outside and did not go down the œsophagus. It was so marked that he requested his friends to see if it did not run down the outside. Veratrum 2m, cured him. No remedy has produced that sensation, but I figured it out by analogy.

Violent thirst for cold water and for ice. "All fruits cause painful dis-tension of the stomach."

"Vomiting forcible and excessive. Nausea with weakness; is obliged to lie down; hysterical cramps in the stomach; cramps in the muscles of the abdomen like colic. Gastric catarrh, great weakness, cold, sudden sinking."

Full of rheumatic and neuralgic pains in the extremities; worse from the warmth of the bed; they drive him out of bed at night into the cold room and he must walk the floor for relief. You would naturally suppose that heat would be comforting; so it is at times to the abdomen and other parts when there is coldness, but it aggravates the pains (*Merc.*).

"Painful paralytic weakness in the limbs."

"Chill and heat alternating, now here, now there, on single parts. Internal sensation of chilliness running from head to toes coming on when drinking." Many of the complaints of Veratrum are aggravated when drinking.

Burning while in cold sweat. In the chronic mental troubles, the skin is dusky and dry with the exception of that on the forehead. But in acute complaints where physical symptoms predominate, as in dysmenorrhœa, acute insanity, etc., there is profuse sweat.

Gnawing hunger in spite of nausea and vomiting. Empty, all-gone feeling in the abdomen after stool.

VESPA VULGARIS

A young man in perfect health was stung by a large number of wasps. Frequent convulsions followed, involving all the muscles of the body, with loss of consciousness; the convulsions disappeared after three years, leaving him subject to attacks of unconsciousness when walking about. He often starts to go somewhere and finds himself several blocks beyond the place he started for.

The period of unconsciousness lasts several minutes. He does not fall nor does he drop things which he happens to hold in his hands.

If spoken to he does not answer nor seem to hear or notice anything; he looks into space. When he comes to himself, he has no memory of the moments that have passed; he is as bright as ever. He has no warning of the coming spell: A friend remarked that his eyes were glassy and blood-shot, and he looked as though he had no sense.

When standing upon the platform of a street car, he was noticed to grasp the iron railing and look wild; two men standing near him undertook to loosen his hands and put him in a seat, but they could not force him to let loose until he came to himself, and then he needed no aid. It was thought that he continued to grasp the railing about ten minutes, but time flies under excitement, and no one has, timed this period.

He becomes sick and faint near a warm stove or in a close room; often gets up and leaves a close warm room to prevent vomiting; craves cold washing of hands and face which makes him feel better. Anger or excitement will bring on a spell.

The usual antidotes have helped for a while, and then the symptoms have returned with about the same general features.

Mentally he is not strong, and the tendency is to grow weaker.

WYETHIA

When in the autumn our hay-fever patients report to us with violent symptoms of coryza, great depression of spirits, symptoms worse in the afternoon, easy sweat and languor, extreme dryness of the mucous membranes of nose, mouth and throat, with burning acrid copious flow of mucus, constant swallowing, itching of the soft palate, and compelled to scratch it with the tongue, Wyethia will cure for the season, and it has cured permanently in some cases.

ZINCUM METALLICUM

Zinc. has a full and substantial proving, including symptoms of every part of the body. It is an antipsoric, suitable in broken down constitutions, feeble constitutions; enfeeblement characterizes the whole proving.

The Zinc. patient is nervous and extremely sensitive, excitable, trembling, quivering, twitching of muscles, tearing pains along the course of the nerves, tingling, excited on the least provocation; over-sensitiveness in one part and lack of feeling in another. This extreme oversensitiveness is like *Nux;* which is inimical. The overworked and excitable persons belong to *Nux* and Zinc. *Nux* is sensitive to the higher potencies. Further, there is paralytic weakness, emaciation, prostration; full of brain and spinal symptoms.

All the functions are slow; eruptions appear slowly. The whole economy seems to be tired and feeble, so that when a girl approaches puberty, and it is time for the menses to be established, but the flow does not appear, she goes into a decline; she begins to manifest choreic symptoms, jerking and twitching, soreness in the back of the neck, burning of the whole spine, creeping and crawling of the extremities, hysterical manifestations of all sorts. Sensitive to every little noise, to people talking in the room, to crumpling of paper. "Talking or listening is distressing; much talking of other people, even of those of whom he is fond, affects his nerves and makes him morose."

Feeble children, feeble girls, mind feeble, memory poor. Tendency to be docile, but when aroused irascible. If the child comes down with scarlatina or measles. it goes into a stupor. The eruption does not come out. There is a tendency to convulsions, drawing in the extremities, suppression of urine, rolling of the head from one side to the other, and from stupor it goes into complete unconsciousness; inability to throw eruptions to the surface.

The stomach is slow in digesting; sour vomiting. The intestines are sluggish. The rectum becomes impacted. Difficult expulsion of urine; paralysis of the bladder and tedious constipation associated with spinal symptoms; urine slow in starting; can pass it only when sitting and in some cases only when sitting leaning back against the seat with hard pressure. Aching in the dorsal, lumbar, and sacral regions; better when walking and worse from rising from a seat. (In *Rhus,* the aching is in the sacral region, and better when walking and coming on while sitting. *Calc., Rhus., Phos , Sulph.* and *Sepia* have this in the highest degree. Zinc. occupies a lower grade in the aggravation when rising from a seat, as do *Petr.* and Ledum)

Numbness of the soles of the feet, with cutting pain and soreness in the heel when stepping; fulgurating pains, stitching, stabbing, and tearing; tabes dorsalis.

Limbs paralyzed; paresis and finally paralysis of one or both sides; jerking, trembling and prostration. Shocks and jerking during sleep.

Trophic centers in a state of anæmia; emaciation throughout the body; the skin looks withered; the face pallid, wrinkled, unhealthy, sickly. Always chilly; sensitive to the cold. Full of neuralgic pains; tearing pains in all parts of the body when exposed to a draft; tension and drawing in various places. Strange drawing about the eyes as if strabismus would come on; drawing in the muscles; neck drawn back; tension and drawing everywhere. When he comes to rest, the limbs want to draw up, hence, hysterical contractures; drawing the fingers all out of shape.

The mind is slow and the patient is weak and tired; weak memory; forgetful. "Repeats all questions before answering them." When an individual does this it is to make the mind comprehend. He must first realize what it means and then answers. Such a symptom is found in typhoid, when the patient does not convalesce; in *a* child after brain affections. Nervous prostration; waits a moment, looking blank, then the face lights up and he answers. If you look at the Zincum patient and do not address him, you would not realize that he was so weak, but put a question to him and he stares at you in perfect amazement, then says, "Oh," and answers.

Zinc. is not suitable in those who are naturally feeble-minded, when the child is in a state bordering upon idiocy. *Baryta carb.* feeds such a mind He rouses out of a semi-slumber and stares a moment without answering.

Stupor; aroused by every little noise, startles, twitches all over; but soon he goes beyond this, becoming less and less excitable, and finally passes into unconsciousness and cannot be aroused.

You will find some deep-seated brain troubles that will try your patience. Some cases go slowly and gradually into unconsciousness; rolling of the h⸗ d for days; eyes lusterless; body emaciated, involuntary discharges of fæces and urine in the bed; tongue dry and parched, so shrivelled that it looks like leather, lips also; face withered and each day looks older; paralysis of one hand or one foot, or it seems that the whole muscular system is paralyzed. Screaming out in pain although not so shrilly as in *Apis*. A dose of Zinc. will sometimes bring this patient back to life. In a few days after the remedy there will be a jerking and quivering in the parts that were motionless, or its action will be shown in a copious sweat, much vomiting; sudden arousing that is alarming, for it looks like a threatened sinking, but this is the beginning of reaction. Now, for days and nights while this little one is coming back to consciousness, the restoration of sensation in the parts is accompanied with the most tormenting formication, tingling, prickling, creeping, and crawling. The mother and the father and the neighbors will want something done for it, but if you antidote, the case will return to where it was before. This suffering is but the awakening to life. It will go on in this way for a week or two and then will begin to show signs of falling back; it needs another dose of Zinc., which will again be followed by a sweat, vomiting, etc. You will see this in spinal meningitis. The early stage will be that of congestion, and *Bell.* may palliate, but with the onset of the symptoms enumerated above, Zinc. is the only remedy that will cure. The *Bell.* case will have flushed face, hot head, rolling of the head, flashing eyes, throbbing carotids. The *Bry.* case will be docile, stupid, purple, sleepy; ameliorated by quiet. The *Helleborus* case will exhibit but little fever; cold extremities, tossing of the head, dilated pupils, unconsciousness, can hardly be aroused; rolling head from side to side, but when the reflexes are abolished, Zinc. comes in.

After the relief from *Gels.*, *Bell.*, or *Bry.* give Zinc. Rugged little fellows who hang on for weeks in this state, emaciating and unconscious.

You must take ,the mother aside and inform her what will happen if the child returns to consciousness. If you do not, you may be turned out of the house. A persons advanced in years cannot stand such an ordeal, but it is astonishing how the little ones can endure the prolonged congestion and inflammation. After scarlet fever and badly treated meningitis; tuber-cular meningitis. I have carried these severe forms of brain disease through on *Phosphorus,* which has a picture somewhat like that of Zincum. There is no record of any recovery from tubercular meningitis, but a homœopath can cure some of these cases, though it may take two or three months to go down and come up out of it, with two or three relapses.

Among the eye symptoms we have a peculiar thickening and opacity of the conjunctiva, which is infiltrated, leathery, has yellow spots on it and the corners are thickened like pterygium. Dunham made a remarkable cure of pterygium. The report of the case in the Guiding Symptoms is as follows: "Pterygiurn in right eye just encroaching on cornea; in left eye extending to the pupil from the inner canthus."

"Itching and stinging pain in inner angles of eyes with cloudiness of sight. Much burning of the eyes and lids in the morning and in the evening with feeling of dryness and pressure in them."

Zinc. has cured distressing thickening of the lids, ectropion and entropion; granular thickening of the lids. In a severe case of entropion where the lashes were playing up and down the ball with lachrymation, great inflammation and redness, Zinc. removed the whole trouble. Violent photophobia; it seems as if the light would blind him. Zinc. and *Euphr.* are closely related in eye troubles.

Strabismus after brain troubles. Ever since scarlet fever, he had strabismus. She has much trouble with the menses; dysmenorrhœa. But here is a striking symptom; no matter what the violent symptoms are, pain in the ovaries, in the uterus, hysterical excitement; as soon as the menstrual flow appears there is relief. Violent pains in the ovaries relieved by the flow. This is a great contrast to *Cimicifuga,* which has nervous excitement and hysteria during the flow, and the more copious it is, the more violent are the pains. The *Lach.* and Zinc. symptoms are worse before, and better with the flow, but in the former the pains all return when the flow slacks up again. *Cimicifuga* has at times an intermittent flow, then pain ceasing with each intermission, returning when the flow again appears.

The great nervousness of Zinc. is manifested in the feet. You will notice a child or a woman keeping one foot going all the time, cannot keep it still. Many medicines have nervous feet and many have relief of symptoms by motion of the feet. But this is marked in Zinc. A girl about twelve years of age had no congruity of symptoms and I could not find the remedy. The mother said the child mortified her by keeping one foot constantly going in church. On asking why she did this, she replied that if she stopped she would lose her urine. Zinc. cured the whole patient. In the text we find double-lined the two words, "Fidgety feet".

Zinc. has some striking heart symptoms. Consriction of the whole chest in weakly subjects.

ZINCUM PHOSPHORICUM

The times of aggravation of this remedy are *morning,* forenoon, AFTRENOON, EVENING, NIGHT.

He has a strong craving for warm, fresh air and is markedly sensitive to drafts; the open air ameliorates in general; marked general physical anxiety; many symptoms are worse from ascending. Hands and feet and other single parts go to sleep and become numb. Many symptoms come on from bathing. Some symptoms are worse after breakfast. It has been a very useful remedy in the treatment of chorea; lack of vital heat; sensitiveness to cold air. Symptoms come on from becoming cold and in cold, wet weather. There is constriction like a band around the body. There are convulsions: clonic; epileptiform; hysterical; internal; tonic. Some complaints are worse and some are better from eating. Complaints are worse after the least physical exertion. Frequent fainting spells. Several kinds of food seem to disagree; bread; milk; sweets; warm drinks; cold drinks ameliorate. Marked formication all over the body. There is marked *heaviness* in the body and limbs. Great sluggishness and *lack of reaction.* Violent JERKING in the body. Extreme LASSITUDE with desire to lie down yet lying in bed aggravates many symptoms. Worse before, DURING and *after* menstruation. Some symptoms are worse and some are better from motion. Most symptoms are worse on beginning to move; there is aversion to motion: NUMBNESS in many parts. Pains are very numerous; BITING; *boring;* bruised; burning external and INTERNAL; CUTTING; pressing external and INTERNAL; STITCHING; TEARING in MUSCLES and NERVES. Paralysis one-sided; of organs; painless. External and internal pulsation. Pulse: FAST; *intermittent; irregular; small;* weak. He desires to be rubbed and most symptoms are ameliorated by rubbing. Sensitiveness prevails throughout the whole proving especially to pain. Electric shocks are quite common. From looking at the proving as a whole it may well be said that the symptoms resemble the results of sexual excesses. The symptoms are quite often one-sided. The symptoms come on while SITTING, *standing* and during sleep. Throughout all the muscles a feeling of tension. Throughout the body and limbs extreme *trembling* and *twitching.* Uncovering aggravates. Walking ameliorates the restlessness and aggravates the weakness; ameliorates the pain in the back. There is marked weakness in the *morning* and evening; during menses; marked NERVOUS weakness; worse walking. A sensation of extreme weariness. The patient is very sensitive to wet weather, to *wind* and to *wine.*

Becomes angry from trifles and even violent and his symptoms become worse from anger. Anxiety in morning; afternoon; night; with fever during menses; on waking. Wants things which he does not need. Aversion to being alone. Concentration of mind is quite difficult; confusion of mind in morning; on waking; evening; after eating. Much annoyed by presentiment of death. Delirium: frightful; raving; rasping with fingers; picking at the bed clothes; violent. Delusions of fancy and even sees dead people; fire; images at night. DULLNESS OF MIND. EXCITEMENT. Attempts to escape. Mental exertion aggravates his symptoms. Exaltation of fancy. Constantly APPREHENSIVE; evening; night; of death; ghosts; of robbers; on waking. VERY FORGETFUL. His symptoms are worse from fright. He is heedless, impatient, impetuous, indifferent, extremely INDOLENT, and appears like one going into imbecility. It should become one of our. most useful remedies in insanity. Marked irresolution. Irritability in the morning; EVENING; with headache; during menses. Silly spasmodic laughter followed by loquacity. *Loathing of life.* Malicious ideas come frequently. *Memory very weak.* Hilarity in the evening. Moods are very changeable. Morose, obstinate and easily offended. MENTAL PROSTRATION and aversion to work. Restlessness in the morning; evening; night; anxious. SADNESS in the morning; afternoon; evening. Marked dullness of the senses. Sensitive to music and to NOISE. Sexual excess aggravates the mental symptoms, shrieking out in sleep. Inclination to sit in perfect silence; indisposed to speak. Speech at times is incoherent. Starting easily during sleep. Marked stupefaction with much vertigo. Thinks much about suicide. His thoughts wander and vanish. He talks in sleep. Unusual timidity. Unconsciousness from fainting. Much weeping; during menses. Vertigo in the morning in bed; forenoon; noon; night; during headache; after dinner; tendency to fall; with nausea; before menses; while sitting; while standing; while walking.

The forehead is cold. There is constriction of the forehead and even of the whole head. Heat in the head especially in the evening; forehead. Hyperæmia of the brain. Eruptions on the scalp. The hair falls out. The head feels heavy in the morning and in the evening; forehead; occiput. The scalp itches. Pain in the head: in the morning in bed; *afternoon; evening;* at night; BETTER IN THE OPEN AIR; worse on ascending steps; binding up the hair; better from cold applications; worse after eating; from becoming heated; with desire to lie down; lying sometimes aggravates and sometimes ameliorates; before and during menses; *from mental exertion;* NERVOUS AND SPINAL HEADACHES; worse from noises; paroxysmal; periodical every day; better from pressure; worse from the heat of the sun; from talking; while walking; warm room; WINE. Pain in the forehead in the morning; *above the eyes.* Pain in the *occiput; sides of the head; temples; vertex.* Burning pain in forehead. Sore bruised pain in the head. Burning pain in the forehead. Drawing pain in the forehead; occiput; temples. Pressing outward in the *forehead;* over the eyes; occiput; sides of head; temples; occiput; vertex. Stitching pains in the head on coughing; forehead; sides; temples; vertex. Stunning pains in the head. Tearing pains in the head; forehead; occiput; SIDES; *temples;* vertex. Perspiration of the whole head; *forehead.* Pulsation in the whole head; forehead. The brain is very sensitive especially during menses. Electric shocks in head.

Agglutination of the lids in the morning. It has cured cataract. Thick muco-purulent discharge from the canthi. The eyes are very dry and lustre-less. Heat and burning in the eyes. Inflammation of the lids. Itching of the lids and lachrymation in the open air. He lies with half open eyes. Pain in the eyes; biting; burning in the evening; *pressing;* shooting; *stitching;* tearing. Paralysis of the lids; *optic nerve.* Photophobia in sunlight. Pupils contracted and then dilated. Redness of the margin of the lids. Staring and sunken look. Œdematous lids: Before the eyes there are floating spots; green colors; a halo of colors around the light. The vision is dim. Exertion of vision brings on many symptoms. There is flickering before the eyes. *Vision becomes foggy.* Bloody or purulent discharge from the ear. Itching in the ears. Noises: evening; night; with vertigo; buzzing; fluttering; ringing; *roaring;* whizzing. PAIN IN THE EAR; behind the ear; burning; *stitching;* TEARING. Pulsation in the ear. There is swelling of the external ear and inside of the ears. Twitching of the ears. Hearing is impaired.

Catarrhal irritation of the nose with redness of the skin of the nose. Coryza worse in the evening; fluent alternating with dry. Discharge from the nose; bloody; *copious;* excoriating; purulent; thick; from posterior nares. A sensation of dryness in the nose. He blows blood from the nose. The nose feels obstructed. Itching inside the nose. Soreness inside the nose. Smell at first acute, later diminished. Frequent sneezing. The nose is red and swollen.

The lips are dry and cracked. Much discoloration of the face; bluish circles around the eyes; earthy or pale; sickly face. Eruptions on the nose; pimples on the face and forehead; vesicles. The expression is sickly and haggard. Much itching of the skin of the face. It has cured right-sided paralysis of the face. The face looks sunken and distressed. The lips are swollen. There is a twitching of the muscles of the face. Small ulcers of the lips and corners of the mouth.

The gums bleed and the tongue is cracked. The mouth is dry and the tongue is coated white. The gums are painful and sore and the tongue burns. The papillæ on the tongue are erect. Salivation with bloody saliva, scorbutic gums. The gums are much swollen. Taste, bad; bitter; insipid; metallic; saltish; sweetish. Small ulcers upon the gums. Vesicles upon the tongue. The teeth become loose. Pain in the teeth; masticating; from pressure; on going to sleep; burning; drawing; jerking; pulsating; sore; stitching; tearing.

Constriction and *dryness* in the throat; constriction of the œsophagus. Frequent hawking. Throat is much inflamed. Sensation of a lump in the throat. Constant formation of tenacious mucus in the throat. Constantly scraping the throat. Pain in the throat on swallowing; burning; pressing; rawness; soreness. Spasms of the œsophagus on swallowing. Difficult swallowing of solids or liquids. Swelling of the throat, tonsils, and uvula. Drawing and pressing in the sides of the throat externally.

Appetite is variable; capricious; diminished; increased, even ravenous; ravenous after eating; wanting at noon; wanting with thirst. Aversion to food; to cooked food; to meat; to sweets; to warm drinks; to wine.

Constrictive sensations in the stomach. Desires beer and cold drinks. A

SENSATION OF EMPTINESS IN THE STOMACH. Eructations; in the evening; ameliorated by; after eating; ineffectual; acrid; bitter; empty; tasting of the food eaten; sour after eating and after milk; waterbrash. Fulness after eating with heaviness. Hiccough after eating. Heaviness in the stomach. NAUSEA; in the morning; noon; after eating; during headache. Pain in the stomach: morning; evening; after eating; during menses; burning; cramping; cutting; gnawing; fuming; soreness; stitching. Sinking in the stomach with retching. Extreme thirst in the afternoon and evening. VOMITING: morning; after drinking; *after eating;* with headache; during pregnancy; *bile;* bitter; black; blood; brownish; food; green; mucus; sour; *watery;* yellow.

Sensation of coldness in the abdomen. Distension of the abdomen after eating. Enlarged liver. Obstructed flatulence. Fulness after eating. Heaviness in the abdomen; sensation of a weight in hypochondria. Sensation of movements in the abdomen with gurgling. Pain in the abdomen; in the morning; in the evening; as if diarrhœa would come on; after eating; before menses; during menses; paroxysmal; after stool; while walking; in hypochondria; in hypogastrium before menses; in the inguinal region; in the region of the umbilicus.

Cramping pain in the morning; in the sides of the abdomen; in the umbilical region. Cutting pain in the region of the umbilicus. Dragging Pain in the abdomen. Pressing in the hypogastrium and in the liver. Soreness in the hypochondria. Stitching pains in the abdomen; in the right hypochondrium; in the liver; in the sides of the abdomen. Tearing pains in the abdomen. A nervous feeling in the abdomen; tension in the abdomen with *rumbling.*

CONSTIPATION: alternating with diarrhœa; stool very *difficult*; rectum inactive; no desire for stool; unsatisfactory stool; ineffectual straining, the stool is dry; hard; large, light-colored. *Diarrhœa;* afternoon, evening; painless; involuntary; with brain affections. The stool is bloody; brown; copious; frequent; green; offensive; watery. Copious flatus which ameliorates symptoms; offensive. Formication and itching in the anus in the evening. Hæmorrhoids external; bleeding. Much moisture about the anus. Pain in the anus and rectum; during stool; burning, during and after stool; cutting; pressing; soreness; stitching; tearing, tenesmus after stool. Prolapsus of the anus. Inefficient urging to stool.

Pressing pain in the bladder. Paralytic weakness of the bladder. Retention of urine. Spasmodic contractions in the bladder. *Urging to urinate*; night; ineffecttual; sudden; must hasten or will lose the urine; sudden urging after urination. Urination dribbling; dysuria; feeble stream; frequent but worse at night; with interrupted stream. Urination involuntary but worse at night; during sleep; on coughing; after stool; weak bladder.

Pain in the kidneys; cutting in the ureters; stitching in the kidneys; suppression of urine. Emissions of prostatic fluid during difficult stool.

Hæmorrhage from the urethra. Burning in the urethra during urination. Cutting and stitching in the urethra. Urine; albuminous; bloody; burning; CLOUDY ON STANDING; dark; *copious;* SEDIMENT; cloudy; flocculent and sandy and red, sandy and white. It has cured where sugar was found in the urine. It has cured so-called nervous colorless watery urine.

Troublesome, painful, strong. even violent erections at night. Pain in the testes; drawing pain in the testes; stitching pains in the penis and glans. *Seminal emissions :* without dreams. Sexual passions increased and even violent. Swollen testes. In the female the sexual desire is also *increased.* Inflammation of the ovaries. *Leucorrhœa :* acrid; bloody; *after the menses; yellow;* white. Menses: absent; bright red; clotted; copious; frequent; late; scanty; protracted; suppressed. Pain in the vulva; in the ovaries; worse in the left; bearing down before the menses; soreness in the vulva. Prolapses of the uterus.

Constriction of the larynx. A sensation of dryness in the larynx. Accumulations of mucus in the larynx. Burning, rawness and soreness in the larynx and trachea. Tickling and scraping in the larynx. Hoarseness with coryza. Rough, weak voice. Respiration is accelerated, anxious and asthmatic, worse at night; spasmodic asthma; *difficult;* evening, night and after eating; *irregular; rattling;* short; suffocative. Cough: daytime; day and night; morning; afternoon; evening; night; asthmatic; from deep breathing; constant; after dinner; dry evening and night; exhausting; hacking; from irritation in the larynx and trachea; *a nervous cough;* paroxysmal; racking; during rest; short; worse sitting; better rising and moving about; spasmodic; *spinal cough;* tickling cough; violent. It has been a very useful remedy in whooping cough. Expectoration; daytime only; morning; bright; red blood; blood streaked; difficult; frothy; *greenish; mucus; tasting* putrid and sweetish; viscid; yellow.

An anxious feeling in the chest. Constriction as of a band; of the heart; in spinal affections. Pimples on the chest. *Oppression of the chest.* Pain in the chest; evening; during cough; on deep breathing; in the heart; aching in the chest; burning in the chest with rawness on coughing; cutting; *pressing;* soreness on coughing; soreness in mammæ. Stitching pains in the chest; on coughing; deep breathing; sides of chest; worse in the left side; in the heart *Palpitation :* she feels every beat of the heart; *anxious;* heart pounds like a hammer; on waking. When spinal affections change into phthisis. Spasms of the chest.

Sensation of great heat, even burning in the back. Itching and formication of the back. Convulsive motions of the muscles of the back even to opisthotonos. *Pain in the back* during chill; before menses; *on motion; rising from a seat;* WHILE SITTING; while standing; some pains are ameliorated walking; cervical region. Pain in the dorsal region; between the scapulæ; in the spine. Pain in the lumbar region; during menses; on motion; rising from a seat; while sitting; better walking. Pain in the sacrum. Pain in the coccyx, during menses. Violent pain in the spine while sitting, better walking. Aching in the lumbar region. Bruised pain in the back; cervical region. Burning pain in the back and spine; lumbar region. Drawing pain in the back; between the scapulæ in the lumbar region. Pressing pain in the back; lumbar region. The spine is very sore to touch; dorsal region; coccyx. It is a most useful remedy in spinal irritation. Stitching pains in the back; in scapulæ. Tearing pains in the hack; in the cervical region; in the scapulæ. Stiffness in the back; in the cervical region. Great *weakness* in the lumbar region.

Chilblains of the feet. A most useful remedy in chorea. Cold extremities; upper limbs; HANDS; finger tips; thighs in the morning; feet icy cold at night. Cramps in the lower limbs, calves and feet. Blueness of the hands. Dryness of the hands and fingers. Pimples and vescles on the extremities. Formication, especially of the feet. Heat of the palms and feet; burning soles. Heaviness of all the limbs. Itching of the skin of all the limbs. Jerking of the lower limbs; worse during sleep.

Numbness of all the limbs; Pain of all kinds in the limbs; rheumatic; upper limbs; shoulders; lower limbs; thighs and legs; in the heel. Pain down the sciatic nerve. Burning in the upper limbs; forearm; hands; lower limbs; thighs; feet; soles. Drawing in the limbs; upper limbs; upper arm; forearm; thighs, thighs in the evening ameliorated by motion, worse sitting, better walking; *knees;* legs. Sore bruised pain in the limbs; thighs; legs. Stitching pain in the limbs; upper limbs; shoulder; hands; lower limbs; hips; thighs. *Tearing pains in the limbs;* JOINTS; *upper limbs; shoulder; upper arms;* forearm; wrist; hand; fingers; *lower limbs;* hip; *thigh;* knee; leg; toes. Painless paralysis of the lower limbs. Perspiration of the hands; cold; lower limbs; FEET; offensive foot-sweat; suppressed foot-sweat. Restlessness of all the limbs, especially feet and legs. Stiffness of the lower limbs. Dropsical swelling of the feet. Tension in the hollow of the knee; in the legs; in the calf. Tension in the thigh; in the evening; worse sitting; better walking; better drawing up the limbs. Twitching of the upper limbs and thighs. Weakness of all the limbs but more especially of the lower limbs and legs.

Comatose sleep : Dreams, anxious, of falling; frightful, horrible; of misfortune; of great mental exertion; vivid. Late falling asleep. Sleepiness in the afternoon and after eating. Sleeplessness before midnight and after three (3) a.m.; sleepless after waking. He is unrefreshed in the morning after sleep. Wakes up too early; three (3) a.m.; frequent.

Chill; afternoon; evening; cold air; in bed; after eating; *external chill; shaking chill;* after sleep. Fever; evening; night; *alternating with chill* flushes of heat. Perspiration: at night; cold; profuse during sleep.

Diminished sensation in the skin. Sensation of biting after scratching.

Burning sensation in the skin after scratching. Objective coldness of the skin. The skin cracks easily. Red spots. Dryness with burning. Eruptions: boils; burning; herpetic; itching; moist; rash; scabby; worse after scratching; *smarting;* SUPPRESSED; suppurating; urticaria, worse after scratching; vesicular. FORMICATION all over the body. Itching; itching biting; itching burning; itching crawling; itching stinging; worse in a warm bed. Hyperæsthesia. Sticking pains in the skin. Ulcers; bleeding; burning; discharge bloody; *indolent;* itching; painless; smarting.

CHARACTERISTIC SYMPTOMS

Phosphorus—Patients in low fever want to be mesmerized, they are starving for vital energy. Sometimes Calcarea.

Lycopodium—Deep furrows in forehead and face with flapping nostrils in pneumonia or bronchitis.

Camphor—Vomiting and purging with cold, blue, dry skin.

Camphor—When the fever is present or when there are pains in the abdomen he covers up, but after these (both fever and pains) pass the skin becomes cold and he uncovers. Camphor only.

Stramonium—Eyes fixed upon dark side of the room away from the light; violent speech with wrinkled face.

Cuprum—Sudden blindness followed by convulsions.

Arnica—He goes into a rage when he sees the doctor, saying: "Go home, I am not sick, I did not send for you.' (Apis.)

Selenium—Shining face, impotency, prostatic dribbling.

Lycopodium—Old misers with wrinkled faces, when they get sick need Lycopodium.

Arscnicum—She cannot go to sleep because things in her room are out of place, and the room is not tidy.

Sulphur—Always theorizing—Apis, *Cannabis Ind.*

Kali Ars.—Copious, thin, brown, horribly offensive, acrid leucorrhœa.

Calcarea Ars.—Headache goes to the side not lain on.

Staphisagria—Headache with ball in forehead and hollowness in occiput.

(Copy these into your Materia Medica so as to have them when you can find them when needed.)

INDEX

A

Abies nigra. 808

Abrotanum 17, 32, 601, 670, 865, 941

Acetic acid 18, 888

Aconitum napellus 19, 52, 57, 59, 111, 136, 148, 164, 241, 271, 276, 279, 291, 300, 367, 372, 434, 543, 567, 572, 607, 671, 739, 769, 770, 888, 891, 938, 958, 960, 971, 972, 973, 974, 997

Actaea racemosa (Black Cohosh) 31, 634

Aesculus hippo. 35, 57, 69, 261, 397, 444, 867, 938

Aethusa cynapium 40, 850, 931

Agaricus musc. 42, 39, 131, 801, 819, 933

Agnus castus 48

Ailanthus gland. 49

Aletris farinosa 53

Allium cepa 54, 508, 806, 863, 894

Aloe 57, 45, 402, 621, 808, 848, 851, 85

Alumen 61, 66, 71, 73, 133, 138, 155, 336, 912, 932

Alumina 66, 61, 65, 66, 67, 68, 69, 133, 139, 245, 360, 466, 676, 728, 771, 798, 803, 847, 855, 856, 912, 932, 941

Alumina Phosphorica 78

Alumina Silicate 84

Ambra grisea 91, 186

Ammoniacum 111, 226, 227

Ammonium carb. 96, 101, 102, 358, 694, 867

Ammonium mur. 101

Anacardium orient. 103, 446, 481, 893, 999

Anagallis 481, 482

Ancistrodon contortrix 473

Anthracinum 477, 872

Antim. crud. 105, 111, 112, 113, 114, 358, 444, 704, 714, 823, 934

Antim. tart. 109, 65, 100, 135,. 305, 358, 606, 855, 914, 915, 934, 941

Apis mellif. 115, 43, 123, 124, 125, 126, 254, 280, 468, 473, 567, 620, 695, 701, 735, 736, 798, 812, 849, 851, 947, 967, 971, 1015

Apocynum cann. 123

Argentum met. 128, 75, 76, 104, 723, 726, 801, 889, 912

Argentum nit. 136, 45, 130,. 268, 546, 576, 741, 771, 798, 800, 804, 889, 890, 1005

Arnica mont. 142, 30, 156, 180, 298, 397, 478, 504, 588, 539, 590, 591, 695, 696, 722, 809, 817, 855, 871, 884, 889, 916, 939

Arsenicum alb. 148, 39, 44, 71, 101, 105, 107, 113, 125, 140, 144, 145, 166, 180, 209, 224, 244, 279, 285, 304, 305, 306, 310, 311, 319, 357, 358, 363, 367, 437, 444, 469, 477, 478, 505, 506, 507, 509, 510, 516, 562, 598, 599, 600, 605, 625, 633, 713, 716, 718, 728, 739, 752, 763, 633, 713, 716, 718, 728, 739, 752, 763, 800, 801, 830, 833, 863, 864, 867, 868, 872, 888, 889, 894, 901, 903, 904, 908, 916, 921, 925, 929, 936, 939, 962, 967, 974, 978, 990, 994, 996, 997, 1010

Arsenicum iod. 166, 863, 864

Arsenicum sulphuretum flavum 171

Arum triph. 178, 53, 224, 254, 284

Asarum europaeum 675

Atropine 638

Aurum arsenicum 187

Aurum iodatum 191

Aurum met. 194, 71, 104, 183, 185, 254, 319, 495, 516, 566, 567, 597, 670

[NOTE — Antique figures appearing against the particular medicine (remedies) denot
main remedies.]